COMPLETE GUIDE TO PRESCRIPTION & NON-PRESCRIPTION

DRUGS

By H. WINTER GRIFFITH, M.D.

Technical consultants:
John D. Palmer, M.D., Ph.D.
William N. Jones, B.S., M.S.

NEW!
Revised for 1988
NOW INCLUDES
over 5000 Brand Names
over 550 Generic Names

The Body Press

THE BODY PRESS
A division of Price Stern Sloan, Inc.
360 North La Cienega Boulevard
Los Angeles, California 90048

Library of Congress Cataloging-in-Publication Data

Griffith, H. Winter (Henry Winter), 1926-   )
  **Complete guide to prescription and non-prescription
drugs.**

  Includes index.
  1. Drugs—Popular works. 2. Drugs, Nonprescription—
Popular works. I. Title. II. Title: Complete guide
to prescription and non-prescription drugs. [DNLM:
1. Drugs—popular works. 2. Drugs, Non-Prescription—
popular works.   QV 55 G853c]
RM301.15.G75   1988   615'.1   87-25596
ISBN 0-89586-594-7
ISBN 0-89586-593-9 (pbk.)

©1983, 1985, 1987, 1988   HPBooks, Inc.
Printed in U.S.A.
Fifth Edition. 1st Printing

CONTENTS

ABOUT THE AUTHOR

H. Winter Griffith has authored several medical books, including the *Complete Guide to Symptoms, Illness & Surgery* and *Complete Guide to Sports Injuries,* both published by The Body Press. Others are *Instructions for Patients, Drug Information for Patients, Instructions for Dental Patients, Information and Instructions for Pediatric Patients* and *Pediatrics for Parents.* Dr. Griffith received his medical degree from Emory University in 1953. After 20 years in private practice, he established a basic medical-science program at Florida State University. He then became an associate professor of family and community medicine at the University of Arizona College of Medicine.

Technical Consultants

John D. Palmer, M.D., Ph.D.
   Associate professor of pharmacology, University of Arizona College of Medicine
   Associate professor of medicine (clinical pharmacology), University of Arizona
     College of Medicine

William N. Jones, Pharmacist, B.S., M.S.
   Clinical pharmacy coordinator, Veterans Administration Medical Center, Tucson,
     Arizona
   Adjunct assistant professor, Department of Pharmacy Practice, College of
     Pharmacy, University of Arizona

DRUGS AND YOU

My first day of pharmacology class in medical school started with a jolt. The professor began by writing on the blackboard, "Drugs are poisons."

I thought the statement was extreme. New drug discoveries promised to solve medical problems that had baffled men for centuries. The medical community was intrigued with new possibilities for drugs.

In the 30 years since then, many drug "miracles" have lived up to those early expectations. But the years have also shown the damage drugs can cause when they are misused or not fully understood.

As a family doctor and teacher, I have developed a healthy respect for what drugs can and can't do. I now appreciate my professor's warning.

A drug cannot "cure." It aids the body's natural defenses to promote recovery.

Likewise, a manufacturer or doctor cannot guarantee a drug will be useful for everyone. The complexity of the human body, individual responses in different people and in the same person under different circumstances, past and present health, age and sex influence how well a drug works.

All effective drugs produce desirable changes in the body, but a drug can also cause undesirable adverse reactions or side effects in some people.

Despite uncertainties, the drug discoveries of the last 40 years have given us tools to save lives and reduce discomfort.

Before you decide whether to take a drug, you or your doctor must ask, "Will the benefits outweigh the risks?"

The purpose of this book is to give you enough information about the most widely used drugs so you can make a wise decision. The information will alert you to potential or preventable problems. You can learn what to do if problems arise.

The information is derived from several expert sources. Every effort has been made to ensure accuracy and completeness. When information from different sources conflicts, I have used the majority's opinion, coupled with my clinical judgment and that of my technical consultants. Drug information changes with continuing observations by clinicians and users.

Information in this book applies to generic drugs in both the United States and Canada. Generic names do not vary in these countries, but brand names do.

BE SAFE! TELL YOUR DOCTOR

Some suggestions for wise drug use apply to all drugs. Always give the following information to your physician, dentist or other health-care professional. They must have complete information to prescribe drugs safely for you. This information includes your medical history, your medical plans and progress while under medication.

MEDICAL HISTORY

Tell the important facts of your medical history dealing with drugs. Include allergic or adverse reactions you have had to any medicine in the past. Name the allergic symptoms you have, such as hay fever, asthma, eye watering and itching, throat irritation and reactions to food. People who have allergies to common substances are more likely to develop drug allergies.

List all drugs you take. Don't forget vitamin and mineral supplements, skin, rectal or vaginal medicines, antacids, antihistamines, cold and cough remedies, aspirin and aspirin combinations, motion-sickness remedies, weight-loss aids, salt and sugar substitutes, caffeine, oral contraceptives, sleeping pills or "tonics."

FUTURE MEDICAL PLANS

Discuss plans for elective surgery, pregnancy and breast-feeding.

QUESTIONS

Don't hesitate to ask questions about a drug. Your doctor, nurse or pharmacist may be able to provide more information if they are familiar with you and your medical history.

YOUR ROLE

Learn the generic names and brand names of all your medicines. Write them down to help you remember. If a drug is a mixture, learn the names of its generic ingredients.

TAKING A DRUG

Never take medicine in the dark! Recheck the label before each use. You could be taking the *wrong* drug! Tell your doctor about any unexpected new symptoms you have while taking medicine. You may need to change medicines or have a dose adjustment.

STORAGE

Keep all medicines out of children's reach. Store drugs in a cool, dry place, such as a kitchen cabinet or bedroom. Avoid medicine cabinets in bathrooms. They get too moist and warm at times.

Keep medicine in its original container, tightly closed. Don't remove the label! If directions call for refrigeration, don't freeze.

DISCARDING

Don't save leftover medicine to use later. Discard it on the expiration date shown on the container. Dispose safely to protect children and pets.

REFILLS

All refills must be ordered by your doctor or dentist, either in the first prescription or later. Only the pharmacy that originally filled the prescription can refill it without checking with your doctor or previous pharmacy. If you go to a *new* pharmacy, you must have a new prescription, or the new pharmacist must call your doctor or original pharmacy to see if a refill is authorized. Pharmacies don't usually transfer prescriptions.

If you need a refill, call your pharmacist and order your refill by number and name.

Use one pharmacy for the whole family if you can. The pharmacist then has a record of all of your drugs and can communicate effectively with your doctor.

LEARN ABOUT DRUGS

Study the information in this book's charts regarding your medications. Read each chart completely. Because of space limitations, most information that fits more than one category appears only once.

Take care of yourself. You are the most important member of your health-care team.

GUIDE TO DRUG CHARTS

The drug information in this book is organized in condensed, easy-to-read charts. Each drug is described in a two-page format, as shown in the sample chart below and opposite. Charts are arranged alphabetically by drug generic names, and in a few instances, such as *ADRENOCORTICOIDS, TOPICAL*, by drug class name.

A *generic name* is the official chemical name for a drug. A *brand name* is a drug manufacturer's registered trademark for a generic drug. Brand names listed on the charts

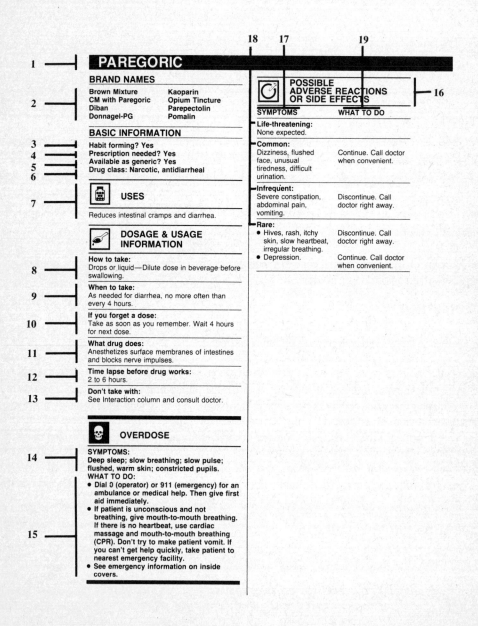

PAREGORIC

BRAND NAMES

Brown Mixture	Kaoparin
CM with Paregoric	Opium Tincture
Diban	Parepectolin
Donnagel-PG	Pomalin

BASIC INFORMATION

Habit forming? Yes
Prescription needed? Yes
Available as generic? Yes
Drug class: Narcotic, antidiarrheal

USES

Reduces intestinal cramps and diarrhea.

DOSAGE & USAGE INFORMATION

How to take:
Drops or liquid—Dilute dose in beverage before swallowing.

When to take:
As needed for diarrhea, no more often than every 4 hours.

If you forget a dose:
Take as soon as you remember. Wait 4 hours for next dose.

What drug does:
Anesthetizes surface membranes of intestines and blocks nerve impulses.

Time lapse before drug works:
2 to 6 hours.

Don't take with:
See Interaction column and consult doctor.

OVERDOSE

SYMPTOMS:
Deep sleep; slow breathing; slow pulse; flushed, warm skin; constricted pupils.
WHAT TO DO:
- Dial 0 (operator) or 911 (emergency) for an ambulance or medical help. Then give first aid immediately.
- If patient is unconscious and not breathing, give mouth-to-mouth breathing. If there is no heartbeat, use cardiac massage and mouth-to-mouth breathing (CPR). Don't try to make patient vomit. If you can't get help quickly, take patient to nearest emergency facility.
- See emergency information on inside covers.

POSSIBLE ADVERSE REACTIONS OR SIDE EFFECTS

SYMPTOMS	WHAT TO DO
Life-threatening: None expected.	
Common: Dizziness, flushed face, unusual tiredness, difficult urination.	Continue. Call doctor when convenient.
Infrequent: Severe constipation, abdominal pain, vomiting.	Discontinue. Call doctor right away.
Rare: • Hives, rash, itchy skin, slow heartbeat, irregular breathing.	Discontinue. Call doctor right away.
• Depression.	Continue. Call doctor when convenient.

include those from the United States and Canada. A generic drug may have one or many brand names.

To find information about a generic drug, look it up in the alphabetical charts. To learn about a brand name, check the index first, where brand names are followed by their generic ingredients and chart page numbers.

The chart design is the same for every drug. When you are familiar with the chart, you can quickly find information you want to know about a drug.

On the next few pages, each of the numbered chart sections below is explained. This information will guide you in reading and understanding the charts that begin on page 2.

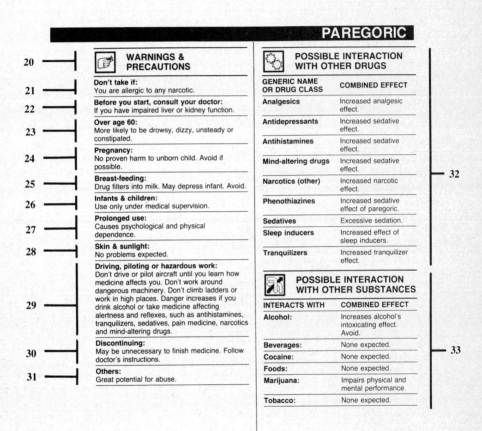

PAREGORIC

20 — 🖢 **WARNINGS & PRECAUTIONS**

21 — **Don't take if:**
You are allergic to any narcotic.

22 — **Before you start, consult your doctor:**
If you have impaired liver or kidney function.

23 — **Over age 60:**
More likely to be drowsy, dizzy, unsteady or constipated.

24 — **Pregnancy:**
No proven harm to unborn child. Avoid if possible.

25 — **Breast-feeding:**
Drug filters into milk. May depress infant. Avoid.

26 — **Infants & children:**
Use only under medical supervision.

27 — **Prolonged use:**
Causes psychological and physical dependence.

28 — **Skin & sunlight:**
No problems expected.

29 — **Driving, piloting or hazardous work:**
Don't drive or pilot aircraft until you learn how medicine affects you. Don't work around dangerous machinery. Don't climb ladders or work in high places. Danger increases if you drink alcohol or take medicine affecting alertness and reflexes, such as antihistamines, tranquilizers, sedatives, pain medicine, narcotics and mind-altering drugs.

30 — **Discontinuing:**
May be unnecessary to finish medicine. Follow doctor's instructions.

31 — **Others:**
Great potential for abuse.

⚙ **POSSIBLE INTERACTION WITH OTHER DRUGS**

GENERIC NAME OR DRUG CLASS	COMBINED EFFECT
Analgesics	Increased analgesic effect.
Antidepressants	Increased sedative effect.
Antihistamines	Increased sedative effect.
Mind-altering drugs	Increased sedative effect.
Narcotics (other)	Increased narcotic effect.
Phenothiazines	Increased sedative effect of paregoric.
Sedatives	Excessive sedation.
Sleep inducers	Increased effect of sleep inducers.
Tranquilizers	Increased tranquilizer effect.

— **32**

📇 **POSSIBLE INTERACTION WITH OTHER SUBSTANCES**

INTERACTS WITH	COMBINED EFFECT
Alcohol:	Increases alcohol's intoxicating effect. Avoid.
Beverages:	None expected.
Cocaine:	None expected.
Foods:	None expected.
Marijuana:	Impairs physical and mental performance.
Tobacco:	None expected.

— **33**

1—GENERIC NAME

Each drug chart is titled by generic name, or in a few instances, by the name of the drug class, such as *DIGITALIS PREPARATIONS*.

Sometimes a drug is known by more than one generic name. The chart is titled by the most common one. Less-common generic names appear in parentheses following the first. For example, vitamin C is also known as ascorbic acid. Its chart title is *VITAMIN C (ASCORBIC ACID)*. The index will include a reference for each name.

Your drug container may show a generic name, a brand name or both. If you have only a brand name, use the index to find the drug's generic name and chart.

If your drug container shows no name, ask your doctor or pharmacist for the name.

2—BRAND NAMES

A brand name is usually shorter and easier to remember than the generic name.

The brand names listed for each generic drug in this book may not include all brands available in the United States and Canada. The most-common ones are listed. New brands appear on the market, and brands are sometimes removed from the market. No list can reflect every change. In the few instances in which the drug chart is titled with a drug class name instead of a generic name, the generic and brand names all appear under the heading *BRAND AND GENERIC NAMES*. The *BRAND NAMES* are in lower case letters, and *GENERIC NAMES* are in capital letters.

Inclusion of a brand name does not imply recommendation or endorsement. Exclusion does not imply that a missing brand name is less effective or less safe than the ones listed. Some generic drugs have too many brand names to list on one chart. The most common brand names appear, or a complete list of common brand names for those drugs is on the page indicated on the chart.

Lists of brand names don't differentiate between prescription and non-prescription drugs. The active ingredients are the same.

If you buy a non-prescription drug, look for generic names of the active ingredients on the container. Common non-prescription drugs are described in this book under their generic components. They are also indexed by brand name.

Most drugs contain *inert,* or inactive, ingredients that are *fillers* or *solvents* for active ingredients. Manufacturers choose inert ingredients that preserve the drug without interfering with the action of the active ingredients.

Inert substances are listed on labels of non-prescription drugs. They do not appear on prescription drugs. Your pharmacist can tell you all active and inert ingredients in a prescription drug.

Occasionally, a tablet, capsule or liquid may contain small amounts of sodium, sugar or potassium. If you are on a diet that severely restricts any of these, ask your pharmacist or doctor to suggest another form.

BASIC INFORMATION

3—HABIT FORMING

A drug habit can be physical or psychological. A drug that produces physical dependence leads to addiction. It causes painful and sometimes dangerous effects when withdrawn.

Psychological dependence does not cause dangerous withdrawal effects. It may cause stress and unwanted behavior changes until the habit is broken.

4—PRESCRIPTION NEEDED?

"Yes" means a doctor must prescribe the drug for you. "No" means you can buy this drug without prescription. Sometimes low strengths of a drug are available without prescription, while high strengths require prescription.

The information about the generic drug applies whether it requires prescription or not. If the generic ingredients are the same, non-prescription drugs have the same dangers, warnings, precautions and interactions as prescribed drugs.

5—AVAILABLE AS GENERIC?

Some generic drugs have copyright restrictions that protect the manufacturer or distributor of that drug. These drugs may be purchased only by brand name.

In recent years, drug manufacturers have marketed more drugs under generic names. Drugs purchased by generic name sometimes are less expensive than brand names.

Some states allow pharmacists to fill prescriptions by brand names or generic names. This allows patients to buy the least-expensive form of a drug.

A doctor may specify a brand name because he or she trusts a known source more than an unknown manufacturer of generic drugs. You and your doctor should decide whether you should buy a medicine by generic or brand name.

Generic drugs manufactured in other countries are not subject to regulation by the U.S. Food and Drug Administration. Drugs manufactured in the United States are subject to regulation.

6—DRUG CLASS

Drugs that possess similar chemical structure and similar therapeutic effects are grouped into classes. Most drugs within a class produce similar benefits, side effects, adverse reactions and interactions with other drugs and substances. For example, there are 15 generic drugs in the narcotic drug class. All have similar effects on the body.

Some information on the charts applies to all drugs in a class. For example, a reference may be made to narcotics. The index lists the class—narcotics—and lists drugs in that class.

Drug classes are not standardized, so classes listed in other references may vary from the classes in this book.

7—USES

This section lists the disease or disorder for which a drug is prescribed.

Most uses listed are approved by the U.S. Food and Drug Administration. Some uses are listed if experiments and clinical trials indicate effectiveness and safety. Still, other uses are included that may not be officially sanctioned, but for which doctors commonly prescribe the drug.

The use for which your doctor prescribes the drug may not appear. You and your doctor should discuss the reason for any prescription medicine you take. You alone will probably decide whether to take a non-prescription drug. This section may help you make a decision.

DOSAGE & USAGE INFORMATION

8—HOW TO TAKE

Drugs are available in tablets, capsules, liquids, suppositories, injections, aerosol inhalers and topical forms such as drops, sprays, creams, ointments and lotions. This section gives general instructions for taking each form.

This information supplements drug-label information. If your doctor's instructions differ from the suggestions, follow your *doctor's* instructions.

Instructions are left out for how *much* to take. Dose amounts can't be generalized. They must be individualized for you by your doctor, or you must read the drug label.

9—WHEN TO TAKE

Dose schedules vary for medicines and for patients.

Drugs prescribed on a schedule should usually be taken at approximately the same times each day. Some *must* be taken at regular intervals to maintain a steady level of the drug in the body. If the schedule interferes with your sleep, consult with your doctor.

Instructions to take on an empty stomach mean the drug is absorbed best in your body this way. Many drugs must be taken with liquid or food because they irritate the stomach.

Instructions for other dose schedules are usually on the label. Variations in standard dose schedules may apply because some medicines interact with others if you take them at the same time.

10—IF YOU FORGET A DOSE

Suggestions in this section vary from drug to drug. Most tell you when to resume taking the medicine if you forget a scheduled dose.

Establish habits so you won't forget doses. Forgotten doses decrease a drug's therapeutic effect.

11—WHAT DRUG DOES

This is a simple description of the drug's action in the body. The wording is generalized and may not be a complete explanation of the complex chemical process that takes place.

12—TIME LAPSE BEFORE DRUG WORKS

The times given are approximations. Times vary a great deal from person to person, and from time to time in the same person. The figures give you some idea of when to expect improvement.

13—DON'T TAKE WITH

Some drugs create problems when taken in combination with other substances. Most problems are detailed in the Interaction column of each chart. This section mentions substances that don't appear in the Interaction column.

Occasionally, an interaction is singled out if the combination is particularly harmful.

OVERDOSE

14—SYMPTOMS

The symptoms listed are most likely to develop with accidental or purposeful overdose. An overdose patient may not show all symptoms listed. Sometimes symptoms are identical to ones listed as side effects. The difference is intensity and severity. You will have to judge. Consult a doctor or poison-control center if you have any doubt.

15—WHAT TO DO

If you suspect an overdose, whether symptoms are apparent or not, follow instructions in this section. Expanded instructions for emergency treatment for overdose are on the inside cover.

16—POSSIBLE ADVERSE REACTIONS OR SIDE EFFECTS

Adverse reactions or side effects are symptoms that may occur when you take a drug. They are effects on the body other than the desired therapeutic effect.

The term *side effect* implies expected and usually unavoidable effects of a drug. Side effects have nothing to do with the drug's intended use.

For example, the generic drug paregoric reduces intestinal cramps and vomiting. It also often causes a flushed face. The flushing is a side effect that is harmless and does not affect the drug's therapeutic potential.

The term *adverse reaction* is more significant. For example, paregoric can cause serious adverse allergic reaction in some people. This reaction can include hives, rash and severe itch.

Some adverse reactions can be prevented, which is one reason this information is included in the book. Most adverse reactions are minor and last only a short time. With many drugs, adverse reactions that might occur will frequently diminish in intensity as time passes.

The majority of drugs used properly for valid reasons offer benefits that outweigh potential hazards.

17—SYMPTOMS

Symptoms are grouped by various body systems. Symptoms that don't naturally apply to these body systems or which overlap systems are listed under "Others."

18—FREQUENCY

This is an estimation of how often symptoms occur in persons who take the drug. The four most common categories of frequency can be found under the **SYMPTOMS** heading and are as follows. **Life-threatening** means exactly what it says: Seek emergency treatment immediately. **Common** means these symptoms are expected and sometimes inevitable. **Infrequent** means the symptoms occur in approximately 1% to 10% of patients. **Rare** means symptoms occur in less than 1%.

19—WHAT TO DO

Carefully follow the instructions provided opposite the symptoms that apply to you.

20—WARNINGS AND PRECAUTIONS

Read these entries to determine special information that applies to you.

21—DON'T TAKE IF

This section lists circumstances that indicate the use of a drug may not be safe. On some drug labels and in formal medical literature, these circumstances are called *contraindications*.

22—BEFORE YOU START, CONSULT YOUR DOCTOR

This section lists conditions under which a drug should be used with caution.

23—OVER AGE 60

As a person ages, physical changes occur that require special consideration in drug use. Liver and kidney functions decrease, metabolism slows and the prostate gland enlarges in men.

Most drugs are metabolized or excreted at a rate dependent on kidney and liver functions. Small doses or longer intervals between doses may be necessary to prevent unhealthy concentration of a drug. Toxic effects and adverse reactions occur more frequently and cause more serious problems in this age group.

24—PREGNANCY

The best rule to follow during pregnancy is to avoid all drugs, including tobacco and alcohol. Any medicine—prescription or non-prescription—requires medical advice and supervision.

This section will alert you if there is evidence that a drug harms the unborn child. Lack of evidence does not guarantee a drug's safety. If safety is undetermined, and reasonable doubt exists, "No proven problems" is indicated.

25—BREAST-FEEDING

Many drugs filter into a mother's milk. Some drugs have dangerous or unwanted effects on the nursing infant. This section suggests ways to minimize harm to the child.

26—INFANTS & CHILDREN

Many drugs carry special warnings and precautions for children because of a child's size and immaturity. In medical terminology, *newborns* are babies up to 2 weeks old, *infants* are 2 weeks to 1 year, and *children* are 1 to 12 years.

27—PROLONGED USE

Most drugs produce no ill effects during short periods of treatment. However, relatively safe drugs taken for long periods may produce unwanted effects. These are listed. Drugs should be taken in the smallest dose and for the shortest time possible. Nevertheless, some diseases and conditions require an indefinite period of treatment. Your doctor may want to change drugs occasionally or alter your treatment regimen to minimize problems.

The words "functional dependence" sometimes appear in this section. This does not mean *physical* or *psychological addiction*. Sometimes a body function ceases to work naturally because it has been replaced or interfered with by the drug. The body then becomes dependent on the drug to continue the function.

28—SKIN & SUNLIGHT

Many drugs cause *photosensitivity,* which means increased skin sensitivity to ultraviolet rays from sunlight or artificial rays from a sunlamp. This section will alert you to this potential problem.

29—DRIVING, PILOTING OR HAZARDOUS WORK

Any drug that decreases alertness, muscular coordination or reflexes may make these activities hazardous. The effects may not appear in all people, or they may disappear after a short exposure to the drug. If this section contains a warning, use caution until you determine how a new drug affects you.

30—DISCONTINUING

Some patients stop taking a drug when symptoms begin to go away, although complete recovery may require longer treatment.

Other patients continue taking a drug when it is no longer needed. This section will tell you when you may safely discontinue a drug.

Some drugs cause symptoms days or weeks after discontinuing. This section warns you so the symptoms won't puzzle you if they occur.

31—OTHERS

Warnings and precautions appear here if they don't fit into the other categories. This section includes storage instructions, how to dispose of outdated drugs, weather influences on drug effect, changes in blood and urine tests, warnings to persons with chronic illness and other information.

32—POSSIBLE INTERACTION WITH OTHER DRUGS

Drugs interact in your body with other drugs, whether prescription or non-prescription. Interactions affect absorption, elimination or distribution of either drug. The chart lists interactions by generic name or drug class.

If a drug class appears, the generic drug interacts with any drug in that class. Drugs in each class that are included in the book are listed in the index.

Interactions are sometimes beneficial. You may not be able to determine from the chart which interactions are good and which are bad. Don't guess! Consult your doctor if you take drugs that interact. Some combinations are fatal!

Occasionally, drugs appear in the Interaction column that are not included in this book. These drugs are listed under Interactions for your safety.

Some drugs have too many interactions to list on one chart. The additional interactions appear on the page indicated at the bottom of the list.

33—POSSIBLE INTERACTION WITH OTHER SUBSTANCES

The substances listed here are repeated on every drug chart. All people eat food and drink beverages. Many adults consume alcohol. Many people use cocaine and smoke tobacco or marijuana. This section shows possible interactions between these substances and each drug.

DRUGS OF ABUSE

Each of the drug charts beginning on page 2 contains a section listing the interactions of alcohol, marijuana and cocaine with the therapeutic drug in the bloodstream. These three drugs are singled out because of their widespread use and abuse. The information is factual, not judgmental.

The long-term effects of alcohol and tobacco abuse are numerous. They have been well-publicized and information is provided here as a reminder of the inherent dangers of these drugs.

Drugs of potential abuse include those that are addictive and harmful. They usually produce a temporary, false sense of well-being. The long-term effects, however, are harmful and can be devastating to the body and psyche of the addict.

Refresh your memory frequently about the potential harm from prolonged use of *any* drugs or substances you take. Avoid unwise use of habit-forming drugs.

These are the most common drugs of abuse:

TOBACCO (NICOTINE)

What it does: Tobacco smoke contains noxious and cancer-producing ingredients. They include nicotine, carbon monoxide, ammonia, and a variety of harmful tars. Carcinogens in smoke probably come from the tars. Most are present in chewing tobacco and snuff as well as smoke from cigarettes, cigars, and pipes. Tobacco smoke interferes with the immune mechanisms of the body.

Short-term effects of average amount: Relaxation of mood if you are a steady smoker. Constriction of blood vessels.

Short terms effects of large amount inhaled: Headache, appetite loss, nausea.

Long term effects: Greatly enhanced chances of developing lung cancer. Impaired breathing and chronic lung disease (asthma, emphysema, bronchiectasis, lung abscess and others) much more likely. Heart and blood vessel disease more frequent and more severe when they happen. These include myocardial infarction (heart attack), coronary artery disease, heart beat irregularities, generalized atherosclerosis (hardening of the arteries making brain, heart, and kidney more vulnerable to disease), peripheral vascular disease such as intermittent claudication, Buerger's disease and others. Tobacco and nicotine lead to an increased incidence of abortion and significantly reduce the birth weight of children brought to term and delivered of women who smoke during pregnancy. Tobacco smoking causes higher frequency not only of lung cancer, but also increases the likelihood of developing cancer of the throat, larynx, mouth, esophagus, bladder, and pancreas.

Cigarette smoking has been linked to this many deaths per year in the U.S. alone:
    80,000 lung cancer
    22,000 other cancer
    15,000 chronic lung disease
    225,000 cardiovascular disease
    346,000 TOTAL

ALCOHOL

What it does:

- **Central Nervous System**

Depresses, does *not* stimulate, the action of all parts of the central nervous system, including the depression of normal mental activity and normal muscle function. Short term effects of an average amount: relaxation, breakdown of inhibitions, euphoria, decreased alertness. Short term effects of large amounts: nausea, stupor, hangover, unconsciousness, even death.

- **Gastrointestinal System**

Increases stomach acid, poisons liver function. Chronic alcoholism frequently leads to permanent damage to the liver.

- **Heart and Blood Vessels**

Decreased normal function, leading to heart diseases such as cardiomyopathy and disorders of the blood vessels and kidney such as high blood pressure. Bleeding from the esophagus and stomach frequently accompany chronic alcoholism.

- **Unborn Fetus (teratogenicity)**

Alcoholism in the mother carrying a fetus causes *fetal alcohol syndrome (FAS),* which includes the production of mental deficiency, facial abnormalities, slow growth and other major and minor malformations in the newborn.

Signs of Use:

Early signs: Prominent smell of alcohol on the breath, behavior changes (aggressive; passive; sexually uninhibited; poor judgment; outbursts of uncontrolled emotion, such as rage or tearfulness).

Intoxication signs: Unsteady gait, slurred speech, poor performance of any brain or muscle function, stupor or coma in *severe* alcoholic intoxication with slow, noisy breathing, cold and clammy skin, heartbeat faster than usual.

Long term effects:

Addiction: Compulsive use of alcohol. Persons addicted to alcohol have severe withdrawal symptoms when alcohol is unavailable. Even with successful treatment, addiction to alcohol (and other drugs that cause addiction) has a high tendency to relapse. (Memory of euphoric feelings plus family, social, emotional, psychological, and genetic factors probably are all important factors in producing the addiction.)

Liver disease: Usually cirrhosis; also, deleterious effects on the unborn child of an alcoholic mother.

Loss of sexual function: Impotence, erectile dysfunction, loss of libido.

Increased incidence of cancer: Mouth, pharynx, larynx, esophagus, liver, and lung.

Changes in blood: Makes it less likely for blood to clot efficiently.

Heart disease: Decreased normal function leading to possible damage and disease.

Stomach and intestinal problems: Increased production of stomach acid.

Interference with expected or normal actions of many medications: Detailed on every chart in this book, drugs such as sedatives, pain killers, narcotics, antihistamines, anti-convulsants, anticoagulants, and others.

MARIJUANA (CANNABIS, HASHISH)

What they do: Heighten perception, cause mood swings, relax mind and body.
Signs of use: Red eyes, lethargy, uncoordinated body movements.
Long-term effects: Decreased motivation. Possible brain, heart, lung and reproductive system damage.

AMPHETAMINES

What they do: Speed up physical and mental processes to cause a false sense of energy and excitement. The moods are temporary and unreal.
Signs of use: Dilated pupils, insomnia, trembling.
Long-term effects: Violent behavior, paranoia, possible death from overdose.

BARBITURATES

What they do: Produce drowsiness and lethargy.
Signs of use: Confused speech, lack of coordination and balance.
Long-term effects: Disrupts normal sleep pattern. Possible death from overdose, especially in combination with alcohol.

COCAINE

What it does: Stimulates the nervous system, heightens sensations and may produce hallucinations.

Signs of use: Trembling, intoxication, dilated pupils, constant sniffling.

Long-term effects: Ulceration of nasal passages where sniffed. Itching all over body, sometimes with open sores. Possible brain damage. Possible death from overdose.

OPIATES (CODEINE, HEROIN, METHADONE, MORPHINE, OPIUM)

What they do: Relieve pain, create temporary and false sense of well-being.

Signs of use: Constricted pupils, mood swings, slurred speech, sore eyes, lethargy, weight loss, sweating.

Long-term effects: Malnutrition, extreme susceptibility to infection, the need to increase drug amount to produce the same effects. Possible death from overdose.

PSYCHEDELIC DRUGS (LSD, MESCALINE)

What they do: Produce hallucinations, either pleasant or frightening.

Signs of use: Dilated pupils, sweating, trembling, fever, chills.

Long-term effects: Lack of motivation, unpredictable behavior, narcissism, recurrent hallucinations without drug use ("flashbacks"). Possible death from overdose.

VOLATILE SUBSTANCES (GLUE, SOLVENTS)

What they do: Produce hallucinations, temporary, false sense of well-being and possible unconsciousness.

Signs of use: Dilated pupils, flushed face, confusion.

Long-term effects: Permanent brain, liver, kidney damage. Possible death from overdose.

CHECKLIST FOR SAFER DRUG USE

- Tell your doctor about *any* drug you take (even aspirin, allergy pills, laxatives, vitamins, etc.) *before* you take *any* new drug.

- Learn all you can about drugs you may take *before* you take them. Information sources are your doctor, your nurse, your pharmacist, this book and other books in your public library.

- Don't take drugs prescribed for someone else—even if your symptoms are the same.

- Keep your prescription drugs to yourself. Your drugs may be harmful to someone else.

- Tell your doctor about any symptoms you believe are caused by a drug—prescription or non-prescription—that you take.

- Take only medicines that are *necessary*. Avoid taking non-prescription drugs while taking prescription drugs for a medical problem.

- Before your doctor prescribes for you, tell him about your previous experiences with any drug—beneficial results, adverse reactions or allergies.

- Take medicine in good light after you have identified it. If you wear glasses to read, put them on to check drug labels. It is easy to take the wrong drug at the wrong time.

- Don't keep any drugs that change mood, alertness or judgment—such as sedatives, narcotics or tranquilizers—by your bedside. These cause many accidental deaths by overdose. You may unknowingly repeat a dose when you are half asleep or confused.

- Know the names of your medicines. These include the generic name, the brand name and the generic names of all ingredients in a drug mixture. Your doctor, nurse or pharmacist can give you this information.

- Study the labels on all non-prescription drugs. If the information is incomplete or if you have questions, ask the pharmacist for more details.

- If you must deviate from your prescribed dose schedule, tell your doctor.

- Shake liquid medicines before taking.

- Store all medicines away from moisture and heat. Bathroom medicine cabinets are usually unsuitable.

- If a drug needs refrigeration, don't freeze.

- Obtain a standard measuring spoon from your pharmacy for liquid medicines. Kitchen teaspoons and tablespoons are not accurate enough.

- Follow diet instructions when you take medicines. Some work better on a full stomach, others on an empty stomach. Some drugs are more useful with special diets. For example, medicine for high blood pressure is more effective if accompanied by a sodium-restricted diet.

- Tell your doctor about any allergies you have. A previous allergy to a drug may make it dangerous to prescribe again. People with other allergies, such as eczema, hay fever, asthma, bronchitis and food allergies, are more likely to be allergic to drugs.

- Prior to surgery, tell your doctor, anesthesiologist or dentist about any drug you have taken in the past few weeks. Advise them of any cortisone drugs you have taken within two years.

- If you become pregnant while taking any medicine, including birth-control pills, tell your doctor immediately.

- Avoid *all* drugs while you are pregnant, if possible. If you must take drugs during pregnancy, record names, amounts, dates and reasons.

- If you see more than one doctor, tell each one about drugs others have prescribed.

- When you use non-prescription drugs, report it so the information is on your medical record.

- Store all drugs away from the reach of children.

- Note the expiration date on each drug label. Discard outdated ones safely.

- Pay attention to the information in the charts about safety while driving, piloting or working in dangerous places.

- Alcohol, cocaine, marijuana or other mood-altering drugs as well as tobacco—mixed with some drugs—can cause a life-threatening interaction, prevent your medicine from being effective or delay your return to health. Common sense dictates that you avoid them during illness.

DRUG CHARTS

ACEBUTOLOL

BRAND NAMES

Sectral

BASIC INFORMATION

Habit forming? No
Prescription needed? Yes
Available as generic? No
Drug class: Beta-adrenergic blocker

 USES

- Reduces frequency and severity of angina attacks.
- Stabilizes irregular heartbeat.
- Lowers blood pressure.
- Reduces frequency of migraine headaches. (Does not relieve headache pain.)

 DOSAGE & USAGE INFORMATION

How to take:
Tablet or capsule—Swallow with liquid. If you can't swallow whole, crumble tablet or open capsule and take with liquid or food.

When to take:
With meals or immediately after.

If you forget a dose:
Take as soon as you remember. Return to regular schedule, but allow 3 hours between doses.

What drug does:
- Blocks actions of sympathetic nervous system.
- Lowers heart's oxygen requirements.
- Slows nerve impulses through heart.
- Reduces blood-vessel contraction in several major organs and glands.

Time lapse before drug works:
1 to 4 hours.

Continued next column

 OVERDOSE

SYMPTOMS:
Weakness, slow or weak pulse, blood-pressure drop, fainting, convulsions, cold and sweaty skin.
WHAT TO DO:
- **Dial 0 (operator) or 911 (emergency) for an ambulance or medical help. Then give first aid immediately.**
- **See emergency information on inside covers.**

Don't take with:
Non-prescription drugs or drugs in interaction column without consulting doctor.

 POSSIBLE ADVERSE REACTIONS OR SIDE EFFECTS

SYMPTOMS	WHAT TO DO
Life-threatening:	
None expected.	
Common:	
• Drowsiness, numbness or tingling in fingers and toes, dizziness, diarrhea, nausea, fatigue, weakness.	Continue. Call doctor when convenient.
• Pulse slower than 50 beats per minute.	Discontinue. Call doctor right away.
• Cold hands and feet; dry mouth, skin or eyes.	Continue. Tell doctor at next visit.
Infrequent:	
• Hallucinations, nightmares, insomnia, headache, difficulty breathing.	Discontinue. Call doctor right away.
• Confusion, depression, reduced alertness.	Continue. Call doctor when convenient.
• Constipation.	Continue. Tell doctor at next visit.
Rare:	
• Sore throat, fever, rash.	Discontinue. Call doctor right away.
• Unexplained bleeding and bruising.	Continue. Call doctor when convenient.

 WARNINGS & PRECAUTIONS

Don't take if:
- You are allergic to any beta-adrenergic blocker.
- You have asthma.
- You have hay-fever symptoms.
- You have taken MAO inhibitors in past 2 weeks.

Before you start, consult your doctor:
- If you have heart disease or poor circulation to extremities.
- If you have hay fever, asthma, chronic bronchitis or emphysema.
- If you have overactive thyroid function.
- If you have impaired liver or kidney function.
- If you will have surgery within 2 months, including dental surgery, requiring general or spinal anesthesia.
- If you have diabetes or hypoglycemia.

Over age 60:
Adverse reactions and side effects may be more frequent and severe than in younger persons.

Pregnancy:
Risk to unborn child outweighs drug benefits. Don't use.

Breast-feeding:
Drug passes into milk. Avoid drug or discontinue nursing until you finish medicine. Consult doctor for advice on maintaining milk supply.

Infants & children:
Not recommended. Safety and dosage have not been established.

Prolonged use:
Weakens heart-muscle contractions.

Skin & sunlight:
No problems expected.

Driving, piloting or hazardous work:
Don't drive or pilot aircraft until you learn how medicine affects you. Don't work around dangerous machinery. Don't climb ladders or work in high places. Danger increases if you drink alcohol or take medicine affecting alertness and reflexes.

Discontinuing:
Don't discontinue without consulting doctor. Dose may require gradual reduction if you have taken drug for a long time. Doses of other drugs may also require adjustment.

Others:
May mask hypoglycemia.

POSSIBLE INTERACTION WITH OTHER DRUGS

GENERIC NAME OR DRUG CLASS	COMBINED EFFECT
Anesthetics used in surgery	Increased antihypertensive effect.
Antidiabetics	May make blood sugar more difficult to control.
Antihypertensives	Increased antihypertensive effect.
Anti-inflammatory drugs	Decreased antihypertensive effect.
Calcium-channel blockers	May worsen congestive heart failure.
Clonidine	Possible blood-pressure rise when clonidine is discontinued.
Digitalis preparations	Increased *or* decreased heart rate. Improves irregular heartbeat.

Diuretics	Increased antihypertensive effect.
Enalapril	Increased antihyperensive effect. Dosage of each may require adjustment.
Ketoprofen	Decreased antihypertensive effect of acebutolol.
Molindone	Increased tranquilizer effect.
MAO inhibitors	Possible excessive blood-pressure rise when MAO inhibitor is discontinued.
Pentoxifylline	Increased antihypertensive effect.
Reserpine	Possible excessively low blood pressure and slow heartbeat.
Suprofen	Decreased antihypertensive effect of acebutolol.
Sympathomimetics	Decreased effects of both drugs.
Timolol eyedrops	Possible increased acebutolol effect.
Xanthine bronchodilators	Decreased effects of both drugs.

POSSIBLE INTERACTION WITH OTHER SUBSTANCES

INTERACTS WITH	COMBINED EFFECT
Alcohol:	Excessive blood-pressure drop. Avoid.
Beverages:	None expected.
Cocaine:	Irregular heartbeat. Avoid.
Foods:	None expected.
Marijuana:	Daily use—Impaired circulation to hands and feet.
Tobacco:	Possible irregular heartbeat.

ACETAMINOPHEN

BRAND NAMES

See complete list of brand names in the *Brand Name Directory*, page 940.

BASIC INFORMATION

Habit forming? No
Prescription needed? No
Available as generic? Yes
Drug class: Analgesic, fever-reducer

 ## USES

Treatment of mild to moderate pain and fever. Acetaminophen does not relieve redness, stiffness or swelling of joints or tissue inflammation. Use aspirin or other drugs for inflammation.

 ## DOSAGE & USAGE INFORMATION

How to take:
- Tablet or capsule—Swallow with liquid.
- Effervescent granules—Dissolve granules in 4 oz. of cool water. Drink all the water.
- Suppositories—Remove wrapper and moisten suppository with water. Gently insert larger end into rectum. Push well into rectum with finger.

When to take:
As needed, no more often than every 3 hours.

If you forget a dose:
Take as soon as you remember. Wait 3 hours for next dose.

What drug does:
May affect hypothalamus—part of brain that helps regulate body heat and receives body's pain messages.

Time lapse before drug works:
15 to 30 minutes. May last 4 hours.

Continued next column

 ## OVERDOSE

SYMPTOMS:
Stomach upset, irritability, convulsions, coma.
WHAT TO DO:
- Call your doctor or poison-control center for advice if you suspect overdose, even if not sure. Symptoms may not appear until damage has occurred.
- See emergency information on inside covers.

Don't take with:
- Other drugs with acetaminophen. Too much acetaminophen can damage liver and kidneys.
- See Interaction column and consult doctor.

 ## POSSIBLE ADVERSE REACTIONS OR SIDE EFFECTS

SYMPTOMS	WHAT TO DO
Life-threatening: None expected.	
Common: Lightheadedness.	Continue. Call doctor when convenient.
Infrequent: Trembling.	Continue. Call doctor when convenient.
Rare:	
• Extreme fatigue; rash, itch, hives; sore throat and fever after taking regularly a few days; unexplained bleeding or bruising; blood in urine; painful or frequent urination; jaundice; anemia.	Discontinue. Call doctor right away.
• Decreased volume of urine output.	Continue. Call doctor when convenient.

WARNINGS & PRECAUTIONS

Don't take if:
- You are allergic to acetaminophen.
- Your symptoms don't improve after 2 days use. Call your doctor.

Before you start, consult your doctor:
If you have bronchial asthma, kidney disease or liver damage.

Over age 60:
Don't exceed recommended dose. You can't eliminate drug as efficiently as younger persons.

Pregnancy:
No proven harm to unborn child. Avoid if possible.

Breast-feeding:
No proven harm to nursing infant.

Infants & children:
Use only under medical supervision.

Prolonged use:
May affect blood system and cause anemia. Limit use to 5 days for children 12 and under, and 10 days for adults.

Skin & sunlight:
No problems expected.

Driving, piloting or hazardous work:
Avoid if you feel drowsy. Otherwise, no restrictions.

Discontinuing:
Discontinue in 2 days if symptoms don't improve.

Others:
No problems expected.

POSSIBLE INTERACTION WITH OTHER DRUGS

GENERIC NAME OR DRUG CLASS	COMBINED EFFECT
Anticoagulants (oral)	May increase anticoagulant effect. If combined frequently, prothrombin time should be monitored.
Phenobarbital	Quicker elimination of and decreased effect of acetaminophen.

POSSIBLE INTERACTION WITH OTHER SUBSTANCES

INTERACTS WITH	COMBINED EFFECT
Alcohol:	Drowsiness
Beverages:	None expected.
Cocaine:	None expected. However, cocaine may slow body's recovery. Avoid.
Foods:	None expected.
Marijuana:	Increased pain relief. However, marijuana may slow body's recovery. Avoid.
Tobacco:	None expected.

ACETAMINOPHEN & SALICYLATES

BRAND NAMES

See complete list of brand names in the *Brand Name Directory*, page 940.

BASIC INFORMATION

Habit forming? No
Prescription needed?
  High strength: Yes
  Low strength: No
Yes, for some combinations
Available as generic? Yes
Drug class: Analgesic, fever-reducer (acetaminophen and salicylates), non-steroidal anti-inflammatory (salicylates)

 ## USES

- Treatment of mild pain and fever.
- Salicylates are useful in the treatment of inflammatory conditions such as stiffness, swelling, joint pain of arthritis or rheumatism. For long term use for inflammatory problems, separate drugs instead of this combination may be safer and more effective.

 ## DOSAGE & USAGE INFORMATION

How to take:
- Tablet or capsule—swallow with liquid.
- Effervescent granules—dissolve granules in 4 oz. of cool water.

When to take:
As needed, no more often than every 3 hours or as prescribed by your doctor.

If you forget a dose:
Take as soon as you remember. Wait 3 hours for next dose.

What drug does:
- May affect hypothalamus, the part of the brain that helps regulate body heat and receives body's pain messages.

Continued next column

 ## OVERDOSE

SYMPTOMS:
Ringing in ears; nausea; vomiting; dizziness; fever; deep, rapid breathing; hallucinations; coma; unusual sweating; blood in urine.
WHAT TO DO:
- Dial 0 (operator) or 911 (emergency) for an ambulance or medical help. Then give first aid immediately.
- See emergency information on inside covers.

- May affect production of prostaglandins to reduce inflammation.

Time lapse before drug works:
15 to 30 minutes. May last 4 hours.

Don't take with:
- Other drugs with acetaminophen or aspirin or other salicylates. Too much can cause damage to liver, kidneys and peripheral nerves.
- Any laxative containing cellulose.
- If medicine you take has a buffering agent added, don't take with tetracyclines.

 ## POSSIBLE ADVERSE REACTIONS OR SIDE EFFECTS

SYMPTOMS	WHAT TO DO
Life-threatening:	
Wheezing and marked shortness of breath.	Seek emergency treatment immediately.
Common:	
• Jaundice, vomiting blood, black stools, cloudy urine, nausea and vomiting, discomfort on urinating, unexplained tiredness.	Discontinue. Call doctor right away.
• Indigestion or heartburn.	Continue. Call doctor when convenient.
Infrequent:	
Shortness of breath; wheezing (for medicines containing aspirin); urine volume decreased; feet swelling; black or tarry stools; pain on urinating; nausea and vomiting; skin rash, hives; sore throat, fever; easy bruising.	Discontinue. Call doctor right away.
Rare:	
• While taking medicine: Sudden decrease in urine volume.	Discontinue. Call doctor right away.
• After discontinuing medicine: Swelling of feet; rapid weight gain; bloating or puffiness; any urinary problems, such as painful, cloudy or bloody urine.	Check with doctor immediately.

WARNINGS & PRECAUTIONS

Don't take if:
- You are allergic to acetaminophen or any salicylates (see Glossary).
- Your symptoms don't improve after 3 days use.
- You take a buffered form and need to restrict sodium in your diet.
- You have a peptic ulcer.
- You have a bleeding disorder.

Before you start, consult your doctor:
- If you have ever had peptic ulcers.
- If you have had gout.
- If you have asthma or nasal polyps.
- If you have kidney disease or liver damage.

Over age 60:
Don't exceed recommended dose. More likely to be harmful to kidney and liver or cause hidden bleeding in stomach or intestines. Watch for black stools or decreased urine output.

Pregnancy:
Risk to unborn child outweighs drug benefits. Don't use.

Breast-feeding:
Drug passes into milk. Avoid drug or discontinue nursing until you finish medicine. Consult doctor on maintaining milk supply.

Infants & children:
Overdose frequent and severe. Keep bottles out of children's reach. Consult doctor before giving to persons under age 18 who have fever and discomfort of viral illness, especially chicken pox and influenza. Probably increases risk of Reye's syndrome (see Glossary).

Prolonged use:
High doses for severe inflammatory conditions taken for long periods may increase likelihood of kidney damage.

Skin & sunlight:
Aspirin combined with sunscreen may decrease sunburn.

Driving, piloting or hazardous work:
No problems expected unless you feel drowsy.

Discontinuing:
No problems expected.

Others:
- Children up to 12 years—Don't take more than 5 doses per day for more than 5 consecutive days.
- Adults—Don't take for more than 10 consecutive days.
- Urine test for sugar may be inaccurate.
- Don't take if container has a strong vinegar-like odor.

POSSIBLE INTERACTION WITH OTHER DRUGS

GENERIC NAME OR DRUG CLASS	COMBINED EFFECT
Allupurinol	Decreased allopurinol effect.
Antacids	Decreased acetaminophen and salicylates effect.
Anticoagulants	Increased anticoagulant effect. Abnormal bleeding.
Antidiabetics (oral)	Low blood sugar.
Anti-inflammatory drugs (non-steroid)	Risk of stomach bleeding and ulcers.
Aspirin and other salicylates	Likely toxicity.
Cortisone drugs	Increased cortisone effect. Risk of ulcers and stomach bleeding.
Furosemide	Possible salicylate toxicity.
Indomethacin	Risk of stomach bleeding and ulcers.
Methotrexate	Increased methotrexate effect.
Para-aminosalicylic acid (PAS)	Possible salicylate toxicity.
Phenobarbital	Decreased effect of acetaminophen and salicylates because of quicker elimination.

Continued page 961

POSSIBLE INTERACTION WITH OTHER SUBSTANCES

INTERACTS WITH	COMBINED EFFECT
Alcohol:	Increased chance of stomach irritation and bleeding.
Beverages:	None expected.
Cocaine:	None expected. However, cocaine may deter body's recovery. Avoid.
Foods:	None expected.
Marijuana:	Possible increased pain relief, but marijuana may deter body's recovery. Avoid.
Tobacco:	None expected.

ACETOHEXAMIDE

BRAND NAMES

Dimelor   Dymelor

BASIC INFORMATION

Habit forming? No
Prescription needed? Yes
Available as generic? No
Drug class: Antidiabetic (oral), sulfonurea

USES

Treatment for diabetes in adults who can't control blood sugar by diet, weight loss and exercise.

DOSAGE & USAGE INFORMATION

How to take:
Tablet—Swallow with liquid or food to lessen stomach irritation. If you can't swallow whole, crumble tablet and take with liquid or food.

When to take:
At the same times each day.

If you forget a dose:
Take as soon as you remember up to 2 hours late. If more than 2 hours, wait for next scheduled dose (don't double this dose).

What drug does:
Stimulates pancreas to produce more insulin. Insulin in blood forces cells to use sugar in blood.

Time lapse before drug works:
3 to 4 hours. May require 2 weeks for maximum benefit.

Don't take with:
See Interaction column and consult doctor.

OVERDOSE

SYMPTOMS:
Excessive hunger, nausea, anxiety, cool skin, cold sweats, drowsiness, rapid heartbeat, weakness, unconsciousness, coma.
WHAT TO DO:
- **Dial 0 (operator) or 911 (emergency) for an ambulance or medical help. Then give first aid immediately.**
- **See emergency information on inside covers.**

POSSIBLE ADVERSE REACTIONS OR SIDE EFFECTS

SYMPTOMS	WHAT TO DO
Life-threatening: Low blood sugar (hunger, anxiety, cold sweats, rapid pulse).	Seek emergency treatment immediately.
Common: • Dizziness.	Discontinue. Call doctor right away.
• Diarrhea, appetite loss, nausea, stomach pain, heartburn.	Continue. Call doctor when convenient.
Infrequent: Fatigue, itching or rash, ringing in ears.	Discontinue. Call doctor right away.
Rare: Sore throat, fever, unusual bleeding or bruising, jaundice.	Discontinue. Call doctor right away.

WARNINGS & PRECAUTIONS

Don't take if:
- You are allergic to any sulfonurea.
- You have impaired kidney or liver function.

Before you start, consult your doctor:
- If you have a severe infection.
- If you have thyroid disease.
- If you take insulin.
- If you have heart disease.

Over age 60:
Dose usually smaller than for younger adults. Avoid "low-blood-sugar" episodes because repeated ones can damage brain permanently.

Pregnancy:
No proven harm to unborn child. Avoid if possible.

Breast-feeding:
Drug filters into milk. May lower baby's blood sugar. Avoid.

Infants & children:
Don't give to infants or children.

Prolonged use:
None expected.

Skin & sunlight:
May cause rash or intensify sunburn in areas exposed to sun or sunlamp.

Driving, piloting or hazardous work:
No problems expected unless you develop hypoglycemia (low blood sugar). If so, avoid driving or hazardous activity.

Discontinuing:
Don't discontinue without consulting doctor. Dose may require gradual reduction if you have taken drug for a long time. Doses of other drugs may also require adjustment.

Others:
Don't exceed recommended dose. Hypoglycemia (low blood sugar) may occur, even with proper dose schedule. You must balance medicine, diet and exercise.

POSSIBLE INTERACTION WITH OTHER DRUGS

GENERIC NAME OR DRUG CLASS	COMBINED EFFECT
Anticoagulants (oral)	Unpredictable prothrombin times.
Anticonvulsants (hydantoin)	Decreased acetohexamide effect
Anti-inflammatory drugs (non-steroidal)	Increased acetohexamide effect.
Aspirin	Increased acetohexamide effect.
Beta-adrenergic blockers	Increased acetohexamide effect.May take blood sugar more difficult to control.
Chloramphenicol	Increased acetohexamide effect.
Clofibrate	Increased acetohexamide effect.
Contraceptives (oral)	Decreased acetohexamide effect.
Cortisone drugs	Decreased acetohexamide effect.
Diuretics (thiazide)	Decreased acetohexamide effect.
Epinephrine	Decreased acetohexamide effect.
Estrogens	Increased acetohexamide effect.
Guanethidine	Unpredictable acetohexamide effect.
Isoniazid	Decreased acetohexamide effect.

Labetolol	Increased antidiabetic effect, may mask hypoglycemia.
MAO inhibitors	Increased acetohexamide effect.
Oxyphenbutazone	Increased acetohexamide effect.
Phenylbutazone	Increased acetohexamide effect.
Phenyramidol	Increased acetohexamide effect.
Probenecid	Increased acetohexamide effect.
Pyrazinamide	Decreased acetohexamide effect.
Sulfa drugs	Increased acetohexamide effect.
Sulfaphenazole	Increased acetohexamide effect.
Thyroid hormones	Decreased acetohexamide effect.

POSSIBLE INTERACTION WITH OTHER SUBSTANCES

INTERACTS WITH	COMBINED EFFECT
Alcohol:	Disulfiram reaction (see Glossary). Avoid.
Beverages:	None expected.
Cocaine:	No proven problems.
Foods:	None expected.
Marijuana:	Decreased acetohexamide effect. Avoid.
Tobacco:	None expected.

BRAND NAMES

Lithostat

BASIC INFORMATION

Habit forming? No
Prescription needed? Yes
Available as generic? No
Drug class: Antibacterial, antiurolithic

 USES

- Treatment for chronic urinary-tract infections.
- Prevents formation of urinary-tract stones. Will not dissolve stones already present.

 DOSAGE & USAGE INFORMATION

How to take:
Tablet or capsule—Swallow with liquid. If you can't swallow whole, crumble tablet or open capsule and take with liquid or food.

When to take:
At the same time each day, according to instructions on prescription label.

If you forget a dose:
Take as soon as you remember up to 2 hours late. If more than 2 hours, wait for next scheduled dose (don't double this dose).

What drug does:
Stops enzyme action that makes urine too alkaline. Alkaline urine favors bacterial growth and stone formation and growth.

Time lapse before drug works:
1 to 3 weeks.

Don't take with:
Alcohol or iron. See Interaction column and consult doctor.

 OVERDOSE

SYMPTOMS:
Loss of appetite, tremor, nausea, vomiting.
WHAT TO DO:
Overdose unlikely to threaten life. If person takes much larger amount than prescribed, call doctor, poison-control center or hospital emergency room for instructions.

 POSSIBLE ADVERSE REACTIONS OR SIDE EFFECTS

SYMPTOMS	WHAT TO DO
Life-threatening: None expected.	
Common:	
• Appetite loss, nausea, vomiting.	Discontinue. Seek emergency treatment.
• Anxiety, depression, unusual tiredness.	Continue. Call doctor when convenient.
Infrequent:	
• Loss of coordination, slurred speech, severe headache, sudden change in vision, shortness of breath, clot or pain over a blood vessel, sudden chest pain, leg pain in calf (deep vein blood clot).	Discontinue. Seek emergency treatment.
• Rash on arms and face.	Discontinue. Call doctor right away.
Rare: Hair loss.	Continue. Call doctor when convenient.

WARNINGS & PRECAUTIONS

Don't take if:
You have severe chronic kidney disease.

Before you start, consult your doctor:
- If you are anemic.
- If you have or have had phlebitis or thrombophlebitis.

Over age 60:
Adverse reactions and side effects may be more frequent and severe than in younger persons.

Pregnancy:
Studies inconclusive on harm to unborn child. Animal studies show fetal abnormalities. Decide with your doctor whether drug benefits justify risk to unborn child.

Breast-feeding:
No proven problems. Avoid if possible.

Infants & children:
Not recommended. Safety and dosage have not been established.

Prolonged use:
No problems expected.

Skin & sunlight:
No problems expected.

Driving, piloting or hazardous work:
Don't drive or pilot aircraft until you learn how medicine affects you. Don't work around dangerous machinery. Don't climb ladders or work in high places. Danger increases if you drink alcohol or take medicine affecting alertness and reflexes, such as antihistamines, tranquilizers, sedatives, pain medicines, narcotics and mind-altering drugs.

Discontinuing:
Don't discontinue without consulting doctor. Dose may require gradual reduction if you have taken drug for a long time. Doses of other drugs may also require adjustment.

Others:
No problems expected.

POSSIBLE INTERACTION WITH OTHER DRUGS

GENERIC NAME OR DRUG CLASS	COMBINED EFFECT
Iron	Decreased effects of both drugs.

POSSIBLE INTERACTION WITH OTHER SUBSTANCES

INTERACTS WITH	COMBINED EFFECT
Alcohol:	Severe skin rash common in many patients within 30 to 45 minutes after drinking alcohol.
Beverages:	None expected.
Cocaine:	None expected.
Foods:	None expected.
Marijuana:	None expected.
Tobacco:	None expected.

ACETOPHENAZINE

BRAND NAMES

Tindal

BASIC INFORMATION

Habit forming? No
Prescription needed? Yes
Available as generic? Yes
Drug class: Tranquilizer, antiemetic
(phenothiazine)

 USES

- Stops nausea, vomiting.
- Reduces anxiety, agitation.

 DOSAGE & USAGE INFORMATION

How to take:

- Tablet or capsule—Swallow with liquid or food to lessen stomach irritation.
- Suppositories—Remove wrapper and moisten suppository with water. Gently insert into rectum, large end first.
- Drops or liquid—Dilute dose in beverage.

When to take:

- Nervous and mental disorders—Take at the same times each day.
- Nausea and vomiting—Take as needed, no more often than every 4 hours.

If you forget a dose:

- Nervous and mental disorders—Take up to 2 hours late. If more than 2 hours, wait for next scheduled dose (don't double this).
- Nausea and vomiting—Take as soon as you remember. Wait 4 hours for next dose.

What drug does:

- Suppresses brain's vomiting center.
- Suppresses brain centers that control abnormal emotions and behavior.

Continued next column

 OVERDOSE

SYMPTOMS:
Stupor, convulsions, coma.
WHAT TO DO:

- **Dial 0 (operator) or 911 (emergency) for an ambulance or medical help. Then give first aid immediately.**
- **See emergency information on inside covers.**

Time lapse before drug works:

- Nausea and vomiting—1 hour or less.
- Nervous and mental disorders—4-6 weeks.

Don't take with:

- Antacid or medicine for diarrhea.
- Non-prescription drug for cough, cold or allergy.
- See Interaction column and consult doctor.

 POSSIBLE ADVERSE REACTIONS OR SIDE EFFECTS

SYMPTOMS	WHAT TO DO
Life-threatening: None expected.	
Common:	
• Muscle spasms of face and neck, unsteady gait.	Discontinue. Seek emergency treatment.
• Restlessness, tremor, drowsiness.	Discontinue. Call doctor right away.
• Decreased sweating, dry mouth. stuffy nose, constipation.	Continue. Call doctor when convenient.
Infrequent:	
• Fainting.	Discontinue. Seek emergency treatment.
• Rash.	Discontinue. Call doctor right away.
• Difficult or painful urination, diminished sex drive, swollen breasts, menstrual irregularities.	Continue. Call doctor when convenient.
Rare: Change in vision, sore throat and fever, jaundice.	Discontinue. Call doctor right away.

12

WARNINGS & PRECAUTIONS

Don't take if:
- You are allergic to any phenothiazine.
- You have a blood or bone-marrow disease.

Before you start, consult your doctor:
- If you will have surgery within 2 months, including dental surgery, requiring general or spinal anesthesia.
- If you have asthma, emphysema or other lung disorder.
- If you take non-prescription ulcer medicine, asthma medicine or amphetamines.

Over age 60:
Adverse reactions and side effects may be more frequent and severe than in younger persons. More likely to develop involuntary movement of jaws, lips, tongue, chewing. Report this to your doctor immediately. Early treatment can help.

Pregnancy:
Risk to unborn child outweighs drug benefits. Don't use.

Breast-feeding:
Drug passes into milk. Avoid drug or discontinue nursing until you finish medicine. Consult doctor for advice on maintaining milk supply.

Infants & children:
Don't give to children younger than 2.

Prolonged use:
May lead to tardive dyskinesia (involuntary movement of jaws, lips, tongue, chewing).

Skin & sunlight:
May cause rash or intensify sunburn in areas exposed to sun or sunlamp. Skin may remain sensitive for 3 months after discontinuing.

Driving, piloting or hazardous work:
Don't drive or pilot aircraft until you learn how medicine affects you. Don't work around dangerous machinery. Don't climb ladders or work in high places. Danger increases if you drink alcohol or take medicine affecting alertness and reflexes.

Discontinuing:
- Nervous and mental disorders—Don't discontinue without doctor's advice until you complete prescribed dose, even though symptoms diminish or disappear.
- Nausea and vomiting—May be unnecessary to finish medicine. Follow doctor's instructions.

POSSIBLE INTERACTION WITH OTHER DRUGS

GENERIC NAME OR DRUG CLASS	COMBINED EFFECT
Anticholinergics	Increased anticholinergic effect.
Antidepressants (tricyclic)	Increased acetophenazine effect.
Antihistamines	Increased antihistamine effect. Possible oversedation.
Appetite suppressants	Decreased suppressant effect.
Dronabinol	Increased effects of both drugs. Avoid.
Levodopa	Decreased levodopa effect.
Mind-altering drugs	Increased effect of mind-altering drugs.
Molindone	Increased tranquilizer effect.
Narcotics	Increased narcotic effect.
Phenytoin	Increased phenytoin effect.
Quinidine	Impaired heart function. Dangerous mixture.
Sedatives	Increased sedative effect.
Tranquilizers (other)	Increased tranquilizer effect.

POSSIBLE INTERACTION WITH OTHER SUBSTANCES

INTERACTS WITH	COMBINED EFFECT
Alcohol:	Dangerous oversedation.
Beverages:	None expected.
Cocaine:	Decreased acetophenazine effect. Avoid.
Foods:	None expected.
Marijuana:	Drowsiness. May increase antinausea effect.
Tobacco:	None expected.

ACYCLOVIR (ORAL & TOPICAL)

BRAND NAMES

Zovirax   Zovirax Ointment

BASIC INFORMATION

Habit forming? No
Prescription needed? Yes
Available as generic? No
Drug class: Antiviral

 ## USES

- Treatment of severe herpes infections of genitals occurring for first time in special cases.
- Treatment of severe herpes infections on mucous membrane of mouth and lips in special cases.
- Used (although not yet approved by FDA) for shingles (herpes zoster) and chicken pox (varicella) in special cases.

 ## DOSAGE & USAGE INFORMATION

How to take:
- Tablet or capsule—Swallow with liquid.
- Ointment—Apply to skin and mucous membranes every 3 hours (6 times a day) for 7 days. Use rubber glove when applying. Apply 1/2-inch strip to each sore or blister. Wash before using.

When to use:
As directed on label.

If you forget a dose:
Take as soon as you remember up to 2 hours late. If more than 2 hours, wait for next scheduled dose (don't double this dose).

What drug does:
- Inhibits reproduction of virus in cells without killing normal cells.
- Does not cure. Herpes may recur.

Continued next column

 ## OVERDOSE

SYMPTOMS:
Hallucinations, seizures, kidney shutdown.
WHAT TO DO:
- Dial 0 (operator) or 911 (emergency) for an ambulance or medical help. Then give first aid immediately.
- See emergency information on inside covers.

Time lapse before drug works:
2 hours.

Don't take with:
See Interaction column and consult doctor.

 ## POSSIBLE ADVERSE REACTIONS OR SIDE EFFECTS

SYMPTOMS	WHAT TO DO
Life-threatening: None expected.	
Common: Rash, hives, itch, mild pain, burning or stinging of skin, lightheadedness, headache.	Continue. Call doctor when convenient.
Infrequent: Confusion, hallucinations, trembling.	Discontinue. Call doctor right away.
Rare: Abdominal pain, decreased appetite, nausea, vomiting, breathing difficulty, blood in urine, decreased urine volume.	Discontinue. Call doctor right away.

ACYCLOVIR (ORAL & TOPICAL)

WARNINGS & PRECAUTIONS

Don't take if:
You are allergic to acyclovir.

Before you start, consult your doctor:
- If pregnant or plan pregnancy.
- If breast-feeding.
- If you have kidney disease.
- If you have any nerve disorder.

Over age 60:
Adverse reactions and side effects may be more frequent and severe than in younger persons.

Pregnancy:
Risk to unborn child outweighs drug benefits. Don't use.

Breast-feeding:
Drug passes into milk. Avoid drug or discontinue nursing until you finish medicine. Consult doctor for advice on maintaining milk supply.

Infants & children:
Use only under special medical supervision by experienced clinician.

Prolonged use:
Don't use longer than prescribed time.

Skin & sunlight:
No problems expected.

Driving, piloting or hazardous work:
No problems expected.

Discontinuing:
May be unnecessary to finish medicine. Follow doctor's instructions.

Others:
- Women: Get Pap smear every 6 months because those with herpes infections are more likely to develop cancer of cervix. Avoid sexual activity until all blisters or sores heal. Don't get medicine in eyes.
- Protect from freezing.
- Check with doctor if no improvement in 1 week.

POSSIBLE INTERACTION WITH OTHER DRUGS

GENERIC NAME OR DRUG CLASS	COMBINED EFFECT
Interferon	Neurological abnormalities. Avoid.
Methotrexate	Neurological abnormalities. Avoid.
Other medications that can cause toxic effects on kidneys: Amikacin Amphotericin B Capreomycin Colistimethate Colistin Gentamycin Kanamycin Neomycin Netilmicin Polymixin B Probenecid Streptomycin Tobramycin Vancomycin	Increase kidney toxicity.

POSSIBLE INTERACTION WITH OTHER SUBSTANCES

INTERACTS WITH	COMBINED EFFECT
Alcohol:	Increased chance of brain and nervous system adverse reaction. Avoid.
Beverages:	No problems expected.
Cocaine:	Increased chance of brain and nervous system adverse reaction. Avoid.
Foods:	No problems expected.
Marijuana:	Increased chance of brain and nervous system adverse reaction. Avoid.
Tobacco:	No problems expected.

ADRENOCORTICOIDS (TOPICAL)

BRAND NAMES

Some of these brand names are available as oral medicine. Look under specific generic name for each brand. See complete list of brand names in the *Brand Name Directory*, page 941.

BASIC INFORMATION

Habit forming? No
Prescription needed? Yes
Available as generic? Yes
Drug class: Adrenocorticoid (topical)

 ## USES

Relieves redness, swelling, itching, skin discomfort of hemorrhoids, insect bites, poison ivy, oak, sumac, soaps, cosmetics and jewelry.

 ## DOSAGE & USAGE INFORMATION

How to use:
- Cream, lotion, ointment—Apply small amount and rub in gently.
- Topical aerosol—Follow directions on container. Don't breathe vapors.

When to use:
When needed or as directed. Don't use more often than directions allow.

If you forget an application:
Use as soon as you remember.

What drug does:
Reduces inflammation by affecting enzymes that produce inflammation.

Time lapse before drug works:
15 to 20 minutes.

Don't use with:
See Interaction column and consult doctor.

 ## OVERDOSE

SYMPTOMS:
None expected.
WHAT TO DO:
If person swallows or inhales drug, call doctor, poison-control center or hospital emergency room for instructions.

 ## POSSIBLE ADVERSE REACTIONS OR SIDE EFFECTS

SYMPTOMS	WHAT TO DO
Life-threatening: None expected.	
Common: None expected.	
Infrequent: Infection on skin with pain, redness, blisters, pus; skin irritation with burning, itching, blistering or peeling; acne-like skin eruptions.	Continue. Call doctor when convenient.
Rare: None expected.	

WARNINGS & PRECAUTIONS

Don't take if:
You are allergic to any topical adrenocorticoid (cortisone) preparation.

Before you start, consult your doctor:
- If you plan pregnancy within medication period.
- If you have diabetes.
- If you have infection at treatment site.
- If you have stomach ulcer.
- If you have tuberculosis.

Over age 60:
Adverse reactions and side effects may be more frequent and severe than in younger persons, especially thinning of the skin.

Pregnancy:
Risk to unborn child outweighs drug benefits. Don't use.

Breast-feeding:
No problems expected.

Infants & children:
- Use only under medical supervision. Too much for too long can be absorbed into bloodstream through skin and retard growth.
- For infants in diapers, avoid plastic pants or tight diapers.

Prolonged use:
- Increases chance of absorption into bloodstream to cause side effects of oral cortisone drugs.
- May thin skin where used.

Skin & sunlight:
No problems expected.

Driving, piloting or hazardous work:
No problems expected.

Discontinuing:
May be unnecessary to finish medicine. Follow doctor's instructions.

Others:
- Don't use a plastic dressing longer than 2 weeks.
- Aerosol spray—Store in cool place. Don't use near heat or open flame or while smoking. Don't puncture, break or burn container.

 POSSIBLE INTERACTION WITH OTHER DRUGS

GENERIC NAME OR DRUG CLASS	COMBINED EFFECT
Antibiotics (topical)	Decreased antibiotic effects.
Antifungals (topical)	Decreased antifungal effect.

 POSSIBLE INTERACTION WITH OTHER SUBSTANCES

INTERACTS WITH	COMBINED EFFECT
Alcohol:	None expected.
Beverages:	None expected.
Cocaine:	None expected.
Foods:	None expected.
Marijuana:	None expected.
Tobacco:	None expected.

ALBUTEROL

BRAND AND GENERIC NAMES

ALBUTEROL   Salbutamol
Proventil   Ventolin

BASIC INFORMATION

Habit forming? No
Prescription needed? Yes
Available as generic? Yes
Drug class: Bronchodilator,
           sympathomimetic

 USES

- Relieves wheezing and shortness of breath in bronchial asthma attacks, allergies, bronchitis, emphysema or other conditions that cause spasm of the bronchial tubes.
- Temporarily increases blood pressure.

 DOSAGE & USAGE INFORMATION

How to take:
- Oral liquid or tablet—Swallow with liquid or food to lessen stomach irritation.
- Inhaler—Follow instructions on package.

When to take:
When needed according to doctor's instructions. Don't take more than 2 doses 1 hour apart.

If you forget a dose:
Take when you remember. Wait 2 hours before next dose.

What drug does:
Relaxes smooth muscles to relieve constriction of bronchial tubes.

Continued next column

 OVERDOSE

SYMPTOMS:
Chest pain, irregular heartbeat, convulsions, coma.
WHAT TO DO:
- **Dial 0 (operator) or 911 (emergency) for an ambulance or medical help. Then give first aid immediately.**
- **If patient is unconscious and not breathing, give mouth-to-mouth breathing.**
- **If there is no heartbeat, use cardiac massage and mouth-to-mouth breathing (CPR). Don't try to make patient vomit. If you can't get help quickly, take patient to nearest emergency facility.**
- **See emergency information on inside covers.**

Time lapse before drug works:
5 to 30 minutes

Don't take with:
See Interaction column and consult doctor.

 POSSIBLE ADVERSE REACTIONS OR SIDE EFFECTS

SYMPTOMS	WHAT TO DO
Life-threatening:	
Severe chest pain, extremely rapid heart-beat (200/min or more).	Seek emergency treatment immediately.
Common:	
Dizziness, lightheadedness, headache, nausea or vomiting, large pupils, blurred vision.	Discontinue. Call doctor right away.
Infrequent:	
Difficult or painful urination, muscle cramps in legs, dry mouth.	Continue. Call doctor when convenient.
Rare:	
Light chest pain, hallucinations, mood changes.	Discontinue. Call doctor right away.

WARNINGS & PRECAUTIONS

Don't take if:
You are allergic to any sympathomimetic.

Before you start, consult your doctor:
- If you have irregular or rapid heartbeat, congestive heart failure, coronary-artery disease or high blood pressure.
- If you have diabetes.
- If you have overactive thyroid.

Over age 60:
Adverse reactions and side affects may be more frequent and severe than in younger persons.

Pregnancy:
Risk to unborn child outweights drug benefits. Don't use.

Breast-feeding:
Drug passes into milk. Avoid drug or discontinue nursing until you finish medicine. Consult doctor for advice on maintaining milk supply.

Infants & children:
Use only under medical supervision.

Prolonged use:
No problems expected.

Skin & sunlight:
No problems expected.

Driving, piloting or hazardous work:
Don't drive or pilot aircraft until you learn how medicine affects you. Don't work around dangerous machinery. Don't climb ladders or work in high places. Danger increases if you drink alcohol or take medicine affecting alertness and reflexes, such as antihistamines, tranquilizers, sedatives, pain medicine, narcotics and mind-altering drugs.

Discontinuing:
No problems expected.

Others:
- May change blood glucose laboratory determinations (increased).
- May increase serum lactic acid concentrations.

POSSIBLE INTERACTION WITH OTHER DRUGS

GENERIC NAME OR DRUG CLASS	COMBINED EFFECT
Antidepressant (tricyclic)	Increased effect of both drugs.
Beta-adrenergic blockers	Decreased albuterol effect and beta-adrenergic blocker effect.
Digitalis	Increased risk of heartbeat irregularity.
Hydralazine	Decreased hydralazine effect.
Levodopa	Increased risk of heartbeat irregularity.
Sympathomimetics (others)	Increased effects of both drugs, especially harmful side effects.

POSSIBLE INTERACTION WITH OTHER SUBSTANCES

INTERACTS WITH	COMBINED EFFECT
Alcohol:	Decreased albuterol effect.
Beverages:	None expected.
Cocaine:	Likely albuterol toxicity.
Foods:	None expected.
Marijuana:	Overstimulation. Avoid.
Tobacco:	No proven problems.

ALLOPURINOL

BRAND NAMES

Alloprin	Purinol
Aluline	Roucol
Apo-Allopurinol	Zurinol
Caplenal	Zyloprim
Lopurin	Zyloric
Novopurol	

BASIC INFORMATION

Habit forming? No
Prescription needed? Yes
Available as generic? Yes
Drug class: Antigout

 USES

- Treatment for chronic gout.
- Prevention of kidney stones caused by uric acid.

 DOSAGE & USAGE INFORMATION

How to take:
Tablet—Swallow with liquid or food to lessen stomach irritation.

When to take:
At the same times each day.

If you forget a dose:
- 1 dose per day—Take as soon as you remember up to 6 hours late. If more than 6 hours, wait for next scheduled dose (don't double this dose).
- More than 1 dose per day—Take as soon as you remember up to 3 hours late. If more than 3 hours, wait for next scheduled dose (don't double this dose).

What drug does:
Slows formation of uric acid by inhibiting enzyme (xanthine oxidase) activity.

Time lapse before drug works:
Reduces blood uric acid in 1 to 3 weeks. May require 6 months to prevent acute gout attacks.

Continued next column

 OVERDOSE

SYMPTOMS:
None expected.
WHAT TO DO:
Overdose unlikely to threaten life. If person takes much larger amount than prescribed, call doctor, poison-control center or hospital emergency room for instructions.

Don't take with:
See Interaction column and consult doctor.

 POSSIBLE ADVERSE REACTIONS OR SIDE EFFECTS

SYMPTOMS	WHAT TO DO
Life-threatening: None expected.	
Common: Rash, hives, itch.	Discontinue. Call doctor right away.
Infrequent: • Jaundice.	Discontinue. Call doctor right away.
• Drowsiness, diarrhea, stomach pain, nausea, vomiting.	Continue. Call doctor when convenient.
Rare: • Sore throat, fever, unusual bleeding or bruising.	Discontinue. Call doctor right away.
• Numbness, tingling, pain in hands or feet.	Continue. Call doctor when convenient.

 WARNINGS & PRECAUTIONS

Don't take if:
You are allergic to allopurinol.

Before you start, consult your doctor:
If you have had liver or kidney problems.

Over age 60:
Adverse reactions and side effects may be more frequent and severe than in younger persons.

Pregnancy:
Studies inconclusive on harm to unborn child. Animal studies show fetal abnormalities. Decide with your doctor whether drug benefits justify risk to unborn child.

Breast-feeding:
Drug passes into milk. Avoid drug or discontinue nursing.

Infants & children:
Not recommended.

Prolonged use:
No problems expected.

Skin & sunlight:
No problems expected.

Driving, piloting or hazardous work:
Avoid if you feel drowsy. Use may disqualify you for piloting aircraft.

Discontinuing:
Don't discontinue without doctor's advice until you complete prescribed dose, even though symptoms diminish or disappear.

Others:
Acute gout attacks may increase during first weeks of use. If so, consult doctor about additional medicine.

POSSIBLE INTERACTION WITH OTHER DRUGS

GENERIC NAME OR DRUG CLASS	COMBINED EFFECT
Ampicillin	Likely skin rash.
Anticoagulants (oral)	Increased anticoagulant effect.
Antidiabetics (oral)	Increased uric-acid elimination.
Azathioprine	Increased azathioprine effect.
Chlorthalidone	Decreased allopurinol effect.
Cyclophosphamide	Increased cyclophosphamide toxicity.
Diuretics (thiazide)	Decreased allopurinol effect.
Ethacrynic acid	Decreased allopurinol effect.
Furosemide	Decreased allopurinol effect.
Indapamide	Decreased allopurinol effect.
Iron supplements	Excessive accumulation of iron in tissues.
Mercaptopurine	Increased mercaptopurine effect.
Metolazone	Decreased allopurinol effect.
Probenecid	Increased allopurinol effect.

POSSIBLE INTERACTION WITH OTHER SUBSTANCES

INTERACTS WITH	COMBINED EFFECT
Alcohol:	None expected, but may impair management of gout.
Beverages: Caffeine drinks.	Decreased allopurinol effect.
Cocaine:	Decreased allopurinol effect. Avoid.
Foods:	None expected. Low-purine diet recommended (see Glossary).
Marijuana:	Occasional use—None expected. Daily use—Possible increase in uric-acid level.
Tobacco:	None expected.

ALPRAZOLAM

BRAND NAMES

Xanax

BASIC INFORMATION

Habit forming? Yes
Prescription needed? Yes
Available as generic? No
Drug class: Tranquilizer (benzodiazepine)

 USES

Treatment for nervousness or tension.

 DOSAGE & USAGE INFORMATION

How to take:
Tablet or capsule—Swallow with liquid. If you
can't swallow whole, crumble tablet or open
capsule and take with liquid or food.

When to take:
At the same time each day, according to
instructions on prescription label.

If you forget a dose:
Take as soon as you remember up to 2 hours
late. If more than 2 hours, wait for next
scheduled dose (don't double this dose).

What drug does:
Affects limbic system of brain—part that
controls emotions.

Time lapse before drug works:
2 hours. May take 6 weeks for full benefit.

Don't take with:
See Interaction column and consult doctor.

 OVERDOSE

SYMPTOMS:
Drowsiness, weakness, tremor, stupor,
coma.
WHAT TO DO:
- Dial 0 (operator) or 911 (emergency) for an
  ambulance or medical help. Then give first
  aid immediately.
- If patient is unconscious and not
  breathing, give mouth-to-mouth breathing.
  If there is no heartbeat, use cardiac
  massage and mouth-to-mouth breathing
  (CPR). Don't try to make patient vomit. If
  you can't get help quickly, take patient to
  nearest emergency facility.
- See emergency information on inside
  covers.

 POSSIBLE ADVERSE REACTIONS OR SIDE EFFECTS

SYMPTOMS	WHAT TO DO
Life-threatening: None expected.	
Common: Clumsiness, drowsiness, dizziness.	Continue. Call doctor when convenient.
Infrequent: • Hallucinations, confusion, depression, irritability, rash, itch, vision changes.	Discontinue. Call doctor right away.
• Constipation or diarrhea, nausea, vomiting, difficult or painful urination.	Continue. Call doctor when convenient.
Rare: • Slow heartbeat, breathing difficulty.	Discontinue. Seek emergency treatment.
• Mouth or throat ulcers, jaundice	Discontinue. Call doctor right away.

ALPRAZOLAM

WARNINGS & PRECAUTIONS

Don't take if:
- You are allergic to any benzodiazepine.
- You have myasthenia gravis.
- You are active or recovering alcoholic.
- Patient is younger than 6 months.

Before you start, consult your doctor:
- If you have liver, kidney or lung disease.
- If you have diabetes, epilepsy or porphyria.

Over age 60:
Adverse reactions and side effects may be more frequent and severe than in younger persons. You need smaller doses for shorter periods of time. May develop agitation, rage or "hangover" effect.

Pregnancy:
Risk to unborn child outweighs drug benefits. Don't use.

Breast-feeding:
Drug passes into milk. Avoid drug or discontinue nursing until you finish medicine. Consult doctor for advice on maintaining milk supply.

Infants & children:
Use only under medical supervision for children older than 6 months.

Prolonged use:
May impair liver function.

Skin & sunlight:
No problems expected.

Driving, piloting or hazardous work:
Don't drive or pilot aircraft until you learn how medicine affects you. Don't work around dangerous machinery. Don't climb ladders or work in high places. Danger increases if you drink alcohol or take medicine affecting alertness and reflexes.

Discontinuing:
Don't discontinue without consulting doctor. Dose may require gradual reduction if you have taken drug for a long time. Doses of other drugs may also require adjustment.

Others:
- Hot weather, heavy exercise and profuse sweat may reduce excretion and cause overdose.
- Blood sugar may rise in diabetics, requiring insulin adjustment.

POSSIBLE INTERACTION WITH OTHER DRUGS

GENERIC NAME OR DRUG CLASS	COMBINED EFFECT
Anticonvulsants	Change in seizure frequency or severity.
Antidepressants	Increased sedative effect of both drugs.
Antihistamines	Increased sedative effect of both drugs.
Antihypertensives	Excessively low blood pressure.
Cimetidine	Excess sedation.
Disulfiram	Increased alprazolam effect.
Dronabinol	Increased effects of both drugs. Avoid.
MAO inhibitors	Convulsions, deep sedation, rage.
Molindone	Increased tranquilizer effect.
Narcotics	Increased sedative effect of both drugs.
Sedatives	Increased sedative effect of both drugs.
Sleep inducers	Increased sedative effect of both drugs.
Tranquilizers	Increased sedative effect of both drugs.

POSSIBLE INTERACTION WITH OTHER SUBSTANCES

INTERACTS WITH	COMBINED EFFECT
Alcohol:	Heavy sedation. Avoid.
Beverages:	None expected.
Cocaine:	Decreased alprazolam effect.
Foods:	None expected.
Marijuana:	Heavy sedation. Avoid.
Tobacco:	Decreased alprazolam effect.

ALUMINUM, CALCIUM & MAGNESIUM ANTACIDS

BRAND NAMES

Camalox

BASIC INFORMATION

Habit forming? No
Prescription needed? No
Available as generic? No
Drug class: Antacids

USES

- Binds excess phosphate in intestine.
- Treatment for hyperacidity in upper gastrointestinal tract, including stomach and esophagus. Symptoms may be heartburn or acid indigestion. Diseases include peptic ulcer, gastritis, esophagitis, hiatal hernia.
- Constipation relief.

DOSAGE & USAGE INFORMATION

How to take:
- Tablet or capsule—Swallow with liquid.
- Chewable tablets or wafers—Chew well before swallowing.
- Liquid—Shake well and take undiluted.

When to take:
1 to 3 hours after meals unless directed otherwise by your doctor.

If you forget a dose:
Take as soon as you remember, but not simultaneously with any other medicine.

What drug does:
- Neutralizes some of the hydrochloric acid in the stomach.
- Reduces action of pepsin, a digestive enzyme.
- Stimulates muscles in lower bowel wall.

Continued next column

OVERDOSE

SYMPTOMS:
Dry mouth, diarrhea, shallow breathing, weakness, fatigue, stupor.
WHAT TO DO:
- **Dial 0 (operator) or 911 (emergency) for an ambulance or medical help. Then give first aid immediately.**
- **See emergency information on inside covers.**

Time lapse before drug works:
15 minutes.

Don't take with:
Other medicines at the same time. Decreases absorption of other drugs. Wait 2 hours between doses.

POSSIBLE ADVERSE REACTIONS OR SIDE EFFECTS

SYMPTOMS	WHAT TO DO
Life-threatening:	
Heartbeat irregularity in patient with heart disease.	Discontinue. Seek emergency treatment.
Common:	
• Constipation, headache, appetite loss, distended stomach.	Discontinue. Call doctor right away.
• Unpleasant taste in mouth, abdominal pain, laxative effect, belching.	Continue. Call doctor when convenient.
Infrequent:	
Bone pain, frequent urination, dizziness, urgent urination, muscle weakness or pain, nausea.	Discontinue. Call doctor right away.
Rare:	
Mood changes, vomiting, nervousness, swollen feet and ankles.	Discontinue. Call doctor right away.

WARNINGS & PRECAUTIONS

Don't take if:
- You are allergic to any antacid.
- You have a high blood-calcium level.

Before you start, consult your doctor:
- If you have kidney disease.
- If you have chronic constipation, colitis or diarrhea.
- If you have symptoms of appendicitis.
- If you have stomach or intestinal bleeding.
- If you have irregular heartbeat.

Over age 60:
Adverse reactions and side effects may be more frequent and severe than in younger persons. Diarrhea or constipation particularly likely.

Pregnancy:
Risk to unborn child outweighs drug benefits. Don't use.

Breast-feeding:
Drug passes into milk. Avoid drug or discontinue nursing until you finish medicine. Consult doctor for advice on maintaining milk supply.

Infants & children:
Use only under medical supervision.

Prolonged use:
- Decreased phosphate level in blood weakens bones.
- High blood level of calcium which disturbs electrolyte balance.
- Kidney stones, impaired kidney function.

Skin & sunlight:
No problems expected.

Driving, piloting or hazardous work:
No problems expected.

Discontinuing:
May be unnecessary to finish medicine. Follow doctor's instructions.

Others:
Don't take longer than 2 weeks unless under medical supervision.

POSSIBLE INTERACTION WITH OTHER DRUGS

GENERIC NAME OR DRUG CLASS	COMBINED EFFECT
Anticoagulants	Decreased anticoagulant effect.
Calcitonin	Decreased calcitonin effect.
Chlorpromazine	Decreased chlorpromazine effect.
Digitalis preparations	Decreased digitalis effect.
Diuretics	Increased calcium in blood.
Iron supplements	Decreased iron effect.
Isoniazid	Decreased isoniazid effect.
Levodopa	Increased levodopa effect.
Meperidine	Increased meperidine effect.
Nalidixic acid	Decreased effect of nalidixic acid
Oxyphenbutazone	Decreased oxyphenbutazone effect.

Para-aminosalicylic acid (PAS)	Decreased PAS effect.
Penicillins	Decreased penicillin effect.
Pentobarbital	Decreased pentobarbital effect.
Phenylbutazone	Decreased phenylbutazone effect.
Pseudoephedrine	Increased pseudoephedrine effect.
Quinidine	Increased quinidine effect.
Salicylates	Increased salicylate effect.
Sulfa drugs	Decreased sulfa effect.
Tetracyclines	Decreased tetracycline effect.
Vitamins A and C	Decreased vitamin effect.
Vitamin D	Too much calcium in blood.

POSSIBLE INTERACTION WITH OTHER SUBSTANCES

INTERACTS WITH	COMBINED EFFECT
Alcohol:	Decreased antacid effect.
Beverages:	No proven problems.
Cocaine:	No proven problems.
Foods:	Decreased antacid effect. Wait 1 hour after eating.
Marijuana:	No proven problems.
Tobacco:	Decreased antacid effect.

ALUMINUM HYDROXIDE

BRAND NAMES

See complete list of brand names in the
Brand Name Directory, page 941.

BASIC INFORMATION

Habit forming? No
Prescription needed? No
Available as generic? Yes
Drug class: Antacid, antidiarrheal

 USES

- Binds excess phosphate in intestine.
- Treatment for hyperacidity in upper gastrointestinal tract, including stomach and esophagus. Symptoms may be heartburn or acid indigestion. Diseases include peptic ulcer, gastritis, esophagitis, hiatal hernia.
- Treatment for diarrhea.

 DOSAGE & USAGE INFORMATION

How to take:
- Tablet or capsule—Swallow with liquid.
- Chewable tablets or wafers—Chew well before swallowing.
- Liquid—Shake well and take undiluted.

When to take:
1 to 3 hours after meals unless directed otherwise by your doctor.

If you forget a dose:
Take as soon as you remember, but not simultaneously with any other medicine.

What drug does:
- Neutralizes some of the hydrochloric acid in the stomach.
- Reduces action of pepsin, a digestive enzyme.

Time lapse before drug works:
15 minutes.

Continued next column

 OVERDOSE

SYMPTOMS:
Weakness, fatigue, dizziness.
WHAT TO DO:
Overdose unlikely to threaten life. If person takes much larger amount than prescribed, call doctor, poison-control center or hospital emergency room for instructions.

Don't take with:
Other medicines at the same time. Decreases absorption of other drugs. Wait 2 hours between doses.

 POSSIBLE ADVERSE REACTIONS OR SIDE EFFECTS

SYMPTOMS	WHAT TO DO
Life-threatening: None expected.	
Common: Constipation, appetite loss.	Continue. Call doctor when convenient.
Infrequent: • Lower abdominal pain and swelling, bone pain, muscle weakness, swollen wrists or ankles.	Discontinue. Call doctor right away.
• Mood changes, nausea, vomiting, weight loss.	Continue. Call doctor when convenient.
Rare: None expected.	

 WARNINGS & PRECAUTIONS

Don't take if:
You are allergic to any antacid.

Before you start, consult your doctor:
- If you have kidney disease.
- If you have chronic constipation, colitis or diarrhea.
- If you have symptoms of appendicitis.
- If you have have stomach or intestinal bleeding.

Over age 60:
Adverse reactions and side effects may be more frequent and severe than in younger persons. Diarrhea or constipation particularly likely.

Pregnancy:
Risk to unborn child outweighs drug benefits. Don't use.

Breast-feeding:
Drug passes into milk. Avoid drug or discontinue nursing until you finish medicine. Consult doctor for advice on maintaining milk supply.

Infants & children:
Use only under medical supervision.

Prolonged use:
Decreased phosphate level in blood weakens bones.

ALUMINUM HYDROXIDE

Skin & sunlight:
No problems expected.

Driving, piloting or hazardous work:
No problems expected.

Discontinuing:
May be unnecessary to finish medicine. Follow doctor's instructions.

Others:
Don't take longer than 2 weeks unless under medical supervision.

 ## POSSIBLE INTERACTION WITH OTHER DRUGS

GENERIC NAME OR DRUG CLASS	COMBINED EFFECT
Anticoagulants	Decreased anticoagulant effect.
Chlorpromazine	Decreased chlorpromazine effect.
Digitalis preparations	Decreased digitalis effect.
Iron supplements	Decreased iron effect.
Meperidine	Increased meperidine effect.
Nalidixic acid	Decreased effect of nalidixic acid.
Oxyphenbutazone	Decreased oxyphenbutazone effect.
Para-aminosalicylic acid (PAS)	Decreased PAS effect.
Penicillins	Decreased penicillin effect.
Pentobarbital	Decreased pentobarbital effect.
Phenylbutazone	Decreased phenylbutazone effect.
Pseudoephedrine	Increased pseudoephedrine effect.
Sulfa drugs	Decreased sulfa effect.
Tetracyclines	Decreased tetracycline effect.
Vitamins A and C	Decreased vitamin effect.

 ## POSSIBLE INTERACTION WITH OTHER SUBSTANCES

INTERACTS WITH	COMBINED EFFECT
Alcohol:	Decreased antacid effect.
Beverages:	No proven problems.
Cocaine:	No proven problems.
Foods:	Decreased antacid effect. Wait 1 hour after eating.
Marijuana:	No proven problems.
Tobacco:	Decreased antacid effect.

ALUMINUM & MAGNESIUM ANTACIDS

BRAND NAMES

See complete list of brand names in the *Brand Name Directory,* page 942.

BASIC INFORMATION

Habit forming? No
Prescription needed? No
Available as generic? Yes
Drug class: Antacids

 ## USES

- Binds excess phosphate in intestine.
- Treatment for hyperacidity in upper gastrointestinal tract, including stomach and esophagus. Symptoms may be heartburn or acid indigestion. Diseases include peptic ulcer, gastritis, esophagitis, hiatal hernia.
- Constipation relief.

 ## DOSAGE & USAGE INFORMATION

How to take:
- Tablet or capsule—Swallow with liquid.
- Chewable tablets or wafers—Chew well before swallowing.
- Liquid—Shake well and take undiluted.

When to take:
1 to 3 hours after meals unless directed otherwise by your doctor.

If you forget a dose:
Take as soon as you remember, but not simultaneously with any other medicine.

What drug does:
- Neutralizes some of the hydrochloric acid in the stomach.
- Reduces action of pepsin, a digestive enzyme.
- Stimulates muscles in lower bowel wall.

Time lapse before drug works:
15 minutes for acid relief.

Continued next column

 ## OVERDOSE

SYMPTOMS:
Weakness, fatigue, dizziness, dry mouth, diarrhea, shallow breathing, stupor.
WHAT TO DO:
- **Dial 0 (operator) or 911 (emergency) for an ambulance or medical help. Then give first aid immediately.**
- **See emergency information on inside covers.**

Don't take with:
Other medicines at the same time. Decreases absorption of other drugs. Wait 2 hours between doses.

 ## POSSIBLE ADVERSE REACTIONS OR SIDE EFFECTS

SYMPTOMS	WHAT TO DO
Life-threatening:	
Heartbeat irregularity in patient with heart disease.	Discontinue. Seek emergency treatment.
Common:	
• Constipation, headache, appetite loss, distended stomach.	Discontinue. Call doctor right away.
• Unpleasant taste in mouth, abdominal pain, laxative effect, belching.	Continue. Call doctor when convenient.
Infrequent:	
Bone pain, frequent or urgent urination, dizziness, muscle weakness or pain, nausea.	Discontinue. Call doctor right away.
Rare:	
Mood changes, vomiting, nervousness, swollen feet and ankles.	Discontinue. Call doctor right away.

 ## WARNINGS & PRECAUTIONS

Don't take if:
You are allergic to any antacid.

Before you start, consult your doctor:
If you have kidney disease, chronic constipation, colitis, diarrhea, symptoms of appendicitis, stomach or intestinal bleeding.

Over age 60:
Adverse reactions and side effects may be more frequent and severe than in younger persons. Diarrhea or constipation particularly likely.

Pregnancy:
Risk to unborn child outweighs drug benefits. Don't use.

Breast-feeding:
Drug passes into milk. Avoid drug or discontinue nursing until you finish medicine. Consult doctor for advice on maintaining milk supply.

Infants & children:
Use only under medical supervision.

ALUMINUM & MAGNESIUM ANTACIDS

Prolonged use:
Decreased phosphate level in blood weakens bones.

Skin & sunlight:
No problems expected.

Driving, piloting or hazardous work:
No problems expected.

Discontinuing:
May be unnecessary to finish medicine. Follow doctor's instructions.

Others:
Don't take longer than 2 weeks unless under medical supervision.

POSSIBLE INTERACTION WITH OTHER DRUGS

GENERIC NAME OR DRUG CLASS	COMBINED EFFECT
Anticoagulants (oral)	Decreased anticoagulant effect.
Chlorpromazine	Decreased chlorpromazine effect.
Digitalis preparations	Decreased digitalis effect.
Iron supplements	Decreased iron effect.
Isoniazid	Decreased isoniazid effect.
Levodopa	Increased levodopa effect.
Meperidine	Increased meperidine effect.
Nalidixic acid	Decreased effect of nalidixic acid.
Oxyphenbutazone	Decreased oxyphenbutazone effect.
Para-aminosalicylic acid (PAS)	Decreased PAS effect.
Penicillins	Decreased penicillin effect.
Pentobarbital	Decreased pentobarbital effect.
Phenylbutazone	Decreased phenylbutazone effect.
Pseudoephedrine	Increased pseudoephedrine effect.
Sulfa drugs	Decreased sulfa effect.
Tetracyclines	Decreased tetracycline effect.
Vitamin D	Too much calcium in blood.

POSSIBLE INTERACTION WITH OTHER SUBSTANCES

INTERACTS WITH	COMBINED EFFECT
Alcohol:	Decreased antacid effect.
Beverages:	No proven problems.
Cocaine:	No proven problems.
Foods:	Decreased antacid effect. Wait 1 hour after eating.
Marijuana:	No proven problems.
Tobacco:	Decreased antacid effect.

ALUMINUM, MAGNESIUM, MAGALDRATE & SIMETHICONE ANTACIDS

BRAND NAMES

See complete list of brand names in the *Brand Name Directory,* page 942.

BASIC INFORMATION

Habit forming? No
Prescription needed? No
Available as generic? No
Drug class: Antacid, antiflatulent

 ## USES

- Treatment for hyperacidity in upper gastrointestinal tract, including stomach and esophagus. Symptoms may be heartburn or acid indigestion. Diseases include peptic ulcer, gastritis, esophagitis, hiatal hernia.
- Relief of constipation or diarrhea (sometimes).
- Treatment for retention of abdominal gas.
- Used prior to x-ray of abdomen to reduce gas shadows.

 ## DOSAGE & USAGE INFORMATION

How to take:
- Tablet or capsule—Swallow with liquid.
- Liquid—Dissolve in water. Drink complete dose.
- Chewable tablets—Chew completely. Don't swallow whole.

When to take:
1 to 3 hours after meals unless directed otherwise by your doctor.

If you forget a dose:
Take as soon as you remember, but not simultaneously with any other medicine.

Continued next column

 ## OVERDOSE

SYMPTOMS:
Dry mouth, shallow breathing, diarrhea, weakness, fatigue, dizziness, stupor.
WHAT TO DO:
- Dial 0 (operator) or 911 (emergency) for an ambulance or medical help. Then give first aid immediately.
- See emergency information on inside covers.

What drug does:
- Neutralizes some of the hydrochloric acid in the stomach.
- Reduces action of pepsin, a digestive enzyme.
- Stimulates muscles in lower bowel wall.

Time lapse before drug works:
15 minutes.

Don't take with:
Other medicines at the same time. Decreases absorption of other drugs. Wait 2 hours between doses.

 ## POSSIBLE ADVERSE REACTIONS OR SIDE EFFECTS

SYMPTOMS	WHAT TO DO
Life-threatening:	
Heartbeat irregularity in patient with heart disease.	Discontinue. Seek emergency treatment.
Common:	
• Constipation, headache, appetite loss, distended stomach.	Discontinue. Call doctor right away.
• Unpleasant taste in mouth, abdominal pain, laxative effect, belching.	Continue. Call doctor when convenient.
Infrequent:	
Bone pain, frequent urination, dizziness, urgent urination, muscle weakness or pain, nausea.	Discontinue. Call doctor right away.
Rare:	
Mood changes, vomiting, nervousness, swollen feet and ankles.	Discontinue. Call doctor right away.

 ## WARNINGS & PRECAUTIONS

Don't take if:
You are allergic to any antacid or simethicone.

Before you start, consult your doctor:
If you have kidney disease, chronic constipation, colitis, diarrhea, symptoms of appendicitis, stomach or intestinal bleeding.

Over age 60:
Adverse reactions and side effects may be more frequent and severe than in younger persons. Diarrhea or constipation particularly likely.

ALUMINUM, MAGNESIUM, MAGALDRATE & SIMETHICONE ANTACIDS

Pregnancy:
Risk to unborn child outweighs drug benefits. Don't use.

Breast-feeding:
Drug passes into milk. Avoid drug or discontinue nursing until you finish medicine. Consult doctor for advice on maintaining milk supply.

Infants & children:
Use only under medical supervision.

Prolonged use:
Decreased phosphate level in blood weakens bones.

Skin & sunlight:
No problems expected.

Driving, piloting or hazardous work:
No problems expected.

Discontinuing:
May be unnecessary to finish medicine. Follow doctor's instructions.

Others:
Don't take longer than 2 weeks unless under medical supervision.

 POSSIBLE INTERACTION WITH OTHER DRUGS

GENERIC NAME OR DRUG CLASS	COMBINED EFFECT
Anticoagulants (oral)	Decreased anticoagulant effect.
Chlorpromazine	Decreased chlorpromazine effect.
Digitalis preparations	Decreased digitalis effect.
Iron supplements	Decreased iron effect.
Isoniazid	Decreased isoniazid effect.
Levodopa	Increased levodopa effect.
Meperidine	Increased meperidine effect.
Nalidixic acid	Decreased effect of nalidixic acid.
Oxyphenbutazone	Decreased oxyphenbutazone effect.
Para-aminosalicylic acid (PAS)	Decreased PAS effect.
Penicillins	Decreased penicillin effect.
Pentobarbital	Decreased pentobarbital effect.
Phenylbutazone	Decreased phenylbutazone effect.
Pseudoephedrine	Increased pseudoephedrine effect.
Sulfa drugs	Decreased sulfa effect.
Tetracyclines	Decreased tetracycline effect.
Vitamins A and C	Decreased vitamin effect.
Vitamin D	Too much calcium in blood.

 POSSIBLE INTERACTION WITH OTHER SUBSTANCES

INTERACTS WITH	COMBINED EFFECT
Alcohol:	Decreased antacid effect.
Beverages:	No proven problems.
Cocaine:	No proven problems.
Foods:	Decreased antacid effect. Wait 1 hour after eating.
Marijuana:	No proven problems.
Tobacco:	Decreased antacid effect.

ALUMINUM, MAGNESIUM & SODIUM BICARBONATE ANTACIDS

BRAND NAMES

Gas-Is-Gon   Triconsil

BASIC INFORMATION

Habit forming? No
Prescription needed? No
Available as generic? No
Drug class: Antacid, antiflatulent

 ## USES

- Binds excess phosphate in intestine.
- Treatment for hyperacidity in upper gastrointestinal tract, including stomach and esophagus. Symptoms may be heartburn or acid indigestion. Diseases include peptic ulcer, gastritis, esophagitis, hiatal hernia.
- Relief of constipation or diarrhea (sometimes).

 ## DOSAGE & USAGE INFORMATION

How to take:
- Liquid—Shake well and take undiluted.
- Powder—Dilute dose in beverage before swallowing.

When to take:
1 to 3 hours after meals unless directed otherwise by your doctor.

If you forget a dose:
Take as soon as you remember, but not simultaneously with any other medicine.

Continued next column

 ## OVERDOSE

SYMPTOMS:
Dry mouth, shallow breathing, diarrhea, weakness, fatigue, dizziness, stupor.
WHAT TO DO:
- Overdose unlikely to threaten life. Depending on severity of symptoms and amount taken, call doctor, poison-control center or hospital emergency room for instructions.
- Dial 0 (operator) or 911 (emergency) for an ambulance or medical help. Then give first aid immediately.
- See emergency information on inside covers.

What drug does:
- Neutralizes some of the hydrochloric acid in the stomach.
- Reduces action of pepsin, a digestive enzyme.
- Stimulates muscles in lower bowel wall.

Time lapse before drug works:
15 minutes.

Don't take with:
Other medicines at the same time. Decreases absorption of other drugs. Wait 2 hours between doses.

 ## POSSIBLE ADVERSE REACTIONS OR SIDE EFFECTS

SYMPTOMS	WHAT TO DO
Life-threatening:	
Heartbeat irregularity in patient with heart disease.	Discontinue. Seek emergency treatment.
Common:	
• Constipation, headache, appetite loss, distended stomach.	Discontinue. Call doctor right away.
• Unpleasant taste in mouth, abdominal pain, laxative effect, belching.	Continue. Call doctor when convenient.
Infrequent:	
Bone pain, frequent or urgent urination, dizziness, muscle weakness or pain, nausea, weight gain.	Discontinue. Call doctor right away.
Rare:	
Mood changes, vomiting, nervousness, swollen feet and ankles.	Discontinue. Call doctor right away.

WARNINGS & PRECAUTIONS

Don't take if:
You are allergic to any antacid.

Before you start, consult your doctor:
If you have kidney or liver disease, high blood pressure, congestive heart failure, chronic constipation, colitis, diarrhea, symptoms of appendicitis, stomach or intestinal bleeding.

Over age 60:
Adverse reactions and side effects may be more frequent and severe than in younger persons. Diarrhea or constipation particularly likely.

Pregnancy:
Risk to unborn child outweighs drug benefits. Don't use.

Breast-feeding:
Drug passes into milk. Avoid drug or discontinue nursing until you finish medicine. Consult doctor for advice on maintaining milk supply.

Infants & children:
Use only under medical supervision.

Prolonged use:
- Decreased phosphate level in blood weakens bones.
- Prolonged use with calcium supplements or milk leads to too much calcium in blood.

Skin & sunlight:
No problems expected.

Driving, piloting or hazardous work:
No problems expected.

Discontinuing:
May be unnecessary to finish medicine. Follow doctor's instructions.

Others:
Don't take longer than 2 weeks unless under medical supervision.

POSSIBLE INTERACTION WITH OTHER DRUGS

GENERIC NAME OR DRUG CLASS	COMBINED EFFECT
Anticoagulants (oral)	Decreased anticoagulant effect.
Chlorpromazine	Decreased chlorpromazine effect.
Digitalis preparations	Decreased digitalis effect.
Iron supplements	Decreased iron effect.
Isoniazid	Decreased isoniazid effect.
Levodopa	Increased levodopa effect.
Meperidine	Increased meperidine effect.
Nalidixic acid	Decreased effect of nalidixic acid.
Oxyphenbutazone	Decreased oxyphenbutazone effect.
Para-aminosalicylic acid (PAS)	Decreased PAS effect.
Penicillins	Decreased penicillin effect.
Pentobarbital	Decreased pentobarbital effect.
Phenylbutazone	Decreased phenylbutazone effect.
Pseudoephedrine	Increased pseudoephedrine effect.
Sulfa drugs	Decreased sulfa effect.
Tetracyclines	Decreased tetrcycline effect.
Vitamina A and C	Decreased vitamin effect.
Vitamin D	Too much calcium in blood.

POSSIBLE INTERACTION WITH OTHER SUBSTANCES

INTERACTS WITH	COMBINED EFFECT
Alcohol:	Decreased antacid effect.
Beverages:	No proven problems.
Cocaine:	No proven problems.
Foods:	Decreased antacid effect. Wait 1 hour after eating.
Marijuana:	Decreased antacid effect.
Tobacco:	No proven problems.

AMANTADINE

BRAND NAMES

Symmetrel

BASIC INFORMATION

Habit forming? No
Prescription needed? Yes
Available as generic? No
Drug class: Antiviral, antiparkinsonism

 ## USES

- Treatment for Type-A flu infections.
- Relief for symptoms of Parkinson's disease.

 ## DOSAGE & USAGE INFORMATION

How to take:
- Tablet or capsule—Swallow with liquid or food to lessen stomach irritation.
- Syrup—Dilute dose in beverage before swallowing.

When to take:
At the same times each day. For Type-A flu it is especially important to take regular doses as prescribed.

If you forget a dose:
Take as soon as you remember. Wait 4 hours for next dose. Return to schedule.

What drug does:
- Type-A flu—May block penetration of tissue cells by infectious material from virus cells.
- Parkinson's disease—Improves muscular condition and coordination.

Time lapse before drug works:
- Type-A flu—48 hours.
- Parkinson's disease—2 days to 2 weeks.

Don't take with:
- Alcohol
- See Interaction column and consult doctor.

 ## OVERDOSE

SYMPTOMS:
Heart-rhythm disturbances, blood-pressure drop, convulsions, toxic psychosis.
WHAT TO DO:
- Dial 0 (operator) or 911 (emergency) for an ambulance or medical help. Then give first aid immediately.
- See emergency information on inside covers.

 ## POSSIBLE ADVERSE REACTIONS OR SIDE EFFECTS

SYMPTOMS	WHAT TO DO
Life-threatening:	
None expected.	
Common:	
• Hallucinations, confusion, lightheadedness.	Continue. Call doctor when convenient.
• Dizziness, headache, purple blotches, appetite loss, nausea.	Continue. Tell doctor at next visit.
• Dry mouth.	No action necessary.
Infrequent:	
• Fainting, slurred speech.	Discontinue. Call doctor right away.
• Difficult or painful urination.	Continue. Call doctor when convenient.
Rare:	
• Rash, uncontrollable rolling of eyes, blurred vision, sore throat, fever.	Discontinue. Call doctor right away.
• Vomiting.	Continue. Call doctor when convenient.
• Constipation.	Continue. Tell doctor at next visit.

WARNINGS & PRECAUTIONS

Don't take if:
You are allergic to amantadine.

Before you start, consult your doctor:
- If you have had epilepsy or other seizures.
- If you have had heart disease or heart failure.
- If you have had liver or kidney disease.
- If you have had peptic ulcers.
- If you have had eczema or skin rashes.
- If you have had emotional or mental disorders or taken drugs for them.

Over age 60:
Adverse reactions and side effects may be more frequent and severe than in younger persons.

Pregnancy:
Studies inconclusive on harm to unborn child. Animal studies show fetal abnormalities. Decide with your doctor whether benefits justify risk to unborn child.

Breast-feeding:
Drug passes into milk. Avoid drug or discontinue nursing until you finish medicine. Consult doctor for advice on maintaining milk supply.

Infants & children:
Use only under medical supervision.

Prolonged use:
Skin splotches, feet swelling, rapid weight gain, shortness of breath. Consult doctor.

Skin & sunlight:
No problems expected.

Driving, piloting or hazardous work:
Don't drive or pilot aircraft until you learn how medicine affects you. Don't work around dangerous machinery. Don't climb ladders or work in high places. Danger increases if you drink alcohol or take medicine affecting alertness and reflexes.

Discontinuing:
- Parkinson's disease—Don't discontinue without doctor's advice until you complete prescribed dose, even though symptoms diminish or disappear.
- Type-A flu—Discontinue 48 hours after symptoms disappear.

Others:
- Parkinson's disease—May lose effectiveness in 3 to 6 months. Consult doctor.
- Amantadine may increase susceptibility to German measles.

POSSIBLE INTERACTION WITH OTHER DRUGS

GENERIC NAME OR DRUG CLASS	COMBINED EFFECT
Amphetamines	Increased amantadine effect. Possible excessive stimulation and agitation.
Anticholinergics	Increased benefit, but excessive anticholinergic dose produces mental confusion, hallucinations, delirium.
Appetite suppressants	Increased amantadine effect. Possible excessive stimulation and agitation.
Levodopa	Increased benefit of levodopa. Can cause agitation.
Sympathomimetics	Increased amantadine effect. Possible excessive stimulation and agitation.

POSSIBLE INTERACTION WITH OTHER SUBSTANCES

INTERACTS WITH	COMBINED EFFECT
Alcohol:	Increased alcohol effect. Possible fainting.
Beverages:	None expected.
Cocaine:	Dangerous overstimulation.
Foods:	None expected.
Marijuana:	None expected.
Tobacco:	None expected.

AMBENONIUM

BRAND NAMES

Mytelase

BASIC INFORMATION

Habit forming? No
Prescription needed? Yes
Available as generic? No
Drug class: Cholinergic (anticholinesterase)

 USES

- Treatment of myasthenia gravis.
- Treatment of urinary retention and abdominal distention.

 DOSAGE & USAGE INFORMATION

How to take:
Capsule—Swallow with liquid or food to lessen stomach irritation.

When to take:
As directed, usually 3 or 4 times a day.

If you forget a dose:
Take as soon as you remember up to 2 hours late. If more than 2 hours, wait for next scheduled dose (don't double this dose).

What drug does:
Inhibits the chemical activity of an enzyme (cholinesterase) so nerve impulses can cross the junction of nerves and muscles.

Time lapse before drug works:
3 hours.

Don't take with:
See Interaction column and consult doctor.

 OVERDOSE

SYMPTOMS:
Muscle weakness, cramps, twitching or clumsiness; severe diarrhea, nausea, vomiting, stomach cramps or pain; breathing difficulty; confusion, irritability, nervousness, restlessness, fear; unusually slow heartbeat; seizures.
WHAT TO DO:
- **Dial 0 (operator) or 911 (emergency) for an ambulance or medical help. Then give first aid immediately.**
- **See emergency information on inside covers.**

 POSSIBLE ADVERSE REACTIONS OR SIDE EFFECTS

SYMPTOMS	WHAT TO DO
Life-threatening:	
None expected.	
Common:	
• Mild diarrhea, nausea, vomiting, stomach cramps or pain.	Discontinue. Call doctor right away.
• Excess saliva, unusual sweating.	Continue. Call doctor when convenient.
Infrequent:	
• Confusion, irritability.	Discontinue. Seek emergency treatment.
• Constricted pupils, watery eyes, lung congestion, urgent or frequent urination.	Continue. Call doctor when convenient.
Rare:	
None expected.	

WARNINGS & PRECAUTIONS

Don't take if:
- You are allergic to any cholinergic or bromide.
- You take mecamylamine.

Before you start, consult your doctor:
- If you plan to become pregnant within medication period.
- If you have bronchial asthma.
- If you have heartbeat irregularities.
- If you have urinary obstruction or urinary-tract infection.

Over age 60:
Adverse reactions and side effects may be more frequent and severe than in younger persons.

Pregnancy:
No proven harm to unborn child. Avoid if possible. May increase uterus contractions close to delivery.

Breast-feeding:
No problems expected, but consult doctor.

Infants & children:
Not recommended.

Prolonged use:
Medication may lose effectiveness. Discontinuing for a few days may restore effect.

Skin & sunlight:
No problems expected.

Driving, piloting or hazardous work:
Don't drive or pilot aircraft until you learn how medicine affects you. Don't work around dangerous machinery. Don't climb ladders or work in high places. Danger increases if you drink alcohol or take medicine affecting alertness and reflexes, such as antihistamines, tranquilizers, sedatives, pain medicine, narcotics and mind-altering drugs.

Discontinuing:
Don't discontinue without doctor's advice until you complete prescribed dose, even though symptoms diminish or disappear.

Others:
No problems expected.

POSSIBLE INTERACTION WITH OTHER DRUGS

GENERIC NAME OR DRUG CLASS	COMBINED EFFECT
Anesthetics (local or general)	Decreased ambenonium effect.
Antiarrhythmics	Decreased ambenonium effect.
Antibiotics	Decreased ambenonium effect.
Anticholinergics	Decreased ambenonium effect. May mask severe side effects.
Cholinergics (other)	Reduced intestinal-tract function. Possible brain and nervous-system toxicity.
Mecamylamine	Decreased ambenonium effect.
Nitrates	Decreased ambenonium effect.
Quinidine	Decreased ambenonium effect.

POSSIBLE INTERACTION WITH OTHER SUBSTANCES

INTERACTS WITH	COMBINED EFFECT
Alcohol:	No proven problems with small doses.
Beverages:	None expected.
Cocaine:	Decreased ambenonium effect. Avoid.
Foods:	None expected.
Marijuana:	No proven problems.
Tobacco:	No proven problems.

AMILORIDE

BRAND NAMES

Midamor

BASIC INFORMATION

Habit forming? No
Prescription needed? Yes
Available as generic? Yes
Drug class: Diuretic

 ## USES

Treatment for high blood pressure and congestive heart failure. Decreases fluid retention and prevents potassium loss.

 ## DOSAGE & USAGE INFORMATION

How to take:
Tablet—Swallow with liquid.

When to take:
At the same time each day, preferably in the morning. May interfere with sleep if taken after 6 p.m.

If you forget a dose:
Take as soon as you remember up to 8 hours late. If more than 8 hours, wait for next scheduled dose (don't double this dose).

What drug does:
Blocks exchange of certain chemicals in the kidney so sodium is excreted. Conserves potassium.

Continued next column

 ## OVERDOSE

SYMPTOMS:
Rapid, irregular heartbeat; confusion; shortness of breath; nervousness; extreme weakness.
WHAT TO DO:
- **Dial 0 (operator) or 911 (emergency) for an ambulance or medical help. Then give first aid immediately.**
- **If patient is unconscious and not breathing, give mouth-to-mouth breathing. If there is no heartbeat, use cardiac massage and mouth-to-mouth breathing (CPR). Don't try to make patient vomit. If you can't get help quickly, take patient to nearest emergency facility.**
- **See emergency information on inside covers.**

Time lapse before drug works:
2 hours.

Don't take with:
See Interaction column and consult doctor.

 ## POSSIBLE ADVERSE REACTIONS OR SIDE EFFECTS

SYMPTOMS	WHAT TO DO
Life-threatening: None expected.	
Common: Headache, nausea, appetite loss, vomiting, diarrhea.	Continue. Call doctor when convenient.
Infrequent: • Cough, shortness of breath.	Discontinue. Call doctor right away.
• Dizziness, constipation, pain, bloating, muscle cramps.	Continue. Call doctor when convenient.
Rare: None expected.	

 ## WARNINGS & PRECAUTIONS

Don't take if:
- You are allergic to amiloride.
- Your serum potassium level is high.

Before you start, consult your doctor:
- If you plan to become pregnant within medication period.
- If you have diabetes.
- If you have heart disease.
- If you have kidney or liver disease.

Over age 60:
Adverse reactions and side effects may be more frequent and severe than in younger persons. More likely to exceed safe potassium blood levels.

Pregnancy:
No proven harm to unborn child. Avoid if possible.

Breast-feeding:
No problems expected, but consult doctor.

Infants & children:
Not recommended.

Prolonged use:
No problems expected.

Skin & sunlight:
No problems expected.

Driving, piloting or hazardous work:
Don't drive or pilot aircraft until you learn how medicine affects you. Don't work around dangerous machinery. Don't climb ladders or work in high places. Danger increases if you drink alcohol or take medicine affecting alertness and reflexes, such as antihistamines, tranquilizers, sedatives, pain medicine, narcotics and mind-altering drugs.

Discontinuing:
Don't discontinue without doctor's advice until you complete prescribed dose, even though symptoms diminish or disappear.

Others:
Periodic physical checkups and potassium-level tests recommended.

POSSIBLE INTERACTION WITH OTHER DRUGS

GENERIC NAME OR DRUG CLASS	COMBINED EFFECT
Acebutolol	Increased antihypertensive effect. Dosages may require adjustment.
Amiodarone	Increased risk of heartbeat irregularity due to low potassium.
Antihypertensives	Increased effect of both drugs.
Blood-bank blood	Increased potassium levels.
Calcium supplements	Increased calcium in blood.
Diuretics (other)	Increased effect of both drugs.
Enalapril	Possible excessive potassium in blood.
Labetolol	Increased antihypertensive effects.
Lithium	Possible lithium toxicity.
Nitrates	Excessive blood-pressure drop.
Oxprenolol	Increased antihypertensive effect. Dosages may require adjustment.
Pentoxifylline	Increased antihypertensive effect.
Potassium supplements	Increased potassium levels.
Sodium bicarbonate	Decreased potassium levels.

POSSIBLE INTERACTION WITH OTHER SUBSTANCES

INTERACTS WITH	COMBINED EFFECT
Alcohol:	Increased blood-pressure drop. Avoid.
Beverages: Low-salt milk.	Possible excess potassium levels. Low-salt milk has extra potassium.
Cocaine:	Blood-pressure rise. Avoid.
Foods: Salt substitutes.	Possible excess potassium levels.
Marijuana:	None expected.
Tobacco:	None expected.

AMILORIDE & HYDROCHLOROTHIAZIDE

BRAND NAMES

Moduretic

BASIC INFORMATION

Habit forming? No
Prescription needed? Yes
Available as generic? No
Drug class: Diuretic (thiazide),
antihypertensive

USES

- Controls, but doesn't cure, high blood pressure.
- Reduces fluid retention (edema), decreasing likelihood of congestive heart failure.

DOSAGE & USAGE INFORMATION

How to take:
Tablet or capsule—Swallow with liquid. If you can't swallow whole, crumble tablet or open capsule and take with liquid or food.

When to take:
At the same time each day, no later than 6 p.m.

If you forget a dose:
Take as soon as you remember up to 2 hours late. If more than 2 hours, wait for next scheduled dose (don't double this dose).

What drug does:
- Forces sodium and water excretion, conserves potassium, reducing body fluid.
- Relaxes muscle cells of small arteries.
- Reduced body fluid and relaxed arteries lower blood pressure.

Time lapse before drug works:
2-6 hours. May require several weeks to lower blood pressure.

Continued next column

OVERDOSE

SYMPTOMS:
Cramps, weakness, drowsiness, weak pulse, coma, rapid, irregular heartbeat.
WHAT TO DO:
- Dial 0 (operator) or 911 (emergency) for an ambulance or medical help. Then give first aid immediately.
- See emergency information on inside covers.

Don't take with:
- See Interaction column and consult doctor.
- Non-prescription drugs without consulting doctor.

POSSIBLE ADVERSE REACTIONS OR SIDE EFFECTS

SYMPTOMS	WHAT TO DO
Life-threatening: None expected.	
Common: • Increased thirst, irregular heartbeat, cramps in muscles, numbness and tingling in hands and feet, thready pulse, shortness of breath.	Discontinue. Call doctor right away.
• Tiredness, weakness, dry mouth, diarrhea, headache, appetite loss, nausea.	Continue. Call doctor when convenient.
Infrequent: Mood changes, constipation, decreased sex function, dizziness, lightheadedness.	Continue. Call doctor when convenient.
Rare: Jaundice; unusual bleeding or bruising; abdominal pain with nausea and vomiting; sore throat, fever, sores in mouth; hives, skin rash; joint pain.	Discontinue. Seek emergency treatment.

WARNINGS & PRECAUTIONS

Don't take if:
You are allergic to amiloride or any thiazide diuretic drug.

Before you start, consult your doctor:
- If you are allergic to any sulfa drug.
- If you have gout, diabetes, heart disease.
- If you have liver, pancreas or kidney disorder.

Over age 60:
Adverse reactions and side effects may be more frequent and severe than in younger persons, especially dizziness and excessive potassium loss.

Pregnancy:
Risk to unborn child outweighs drug benefits. Don't use.

Breast-feeding:
Drug passes into milk. Avoid drug or discontinue nursing until you finish medicine.

Infants & children:
Not recommended unless closely supervised.

Prolonged use:
You may need medicine to treat high blood pressure for the rest of your life.

Skin & sunlight:
May cause rash or intensify sunburn in areas exposed to sun or sunlamp. Avoid overexposure.

Driving, piloting or hazardous work:
Don't drive or pilot aircraft until you learn how medicine affects you. Don't work around dangerous machinery. Don't climb ladders or work in high places. Danger increases if you drink alcohol or take medicine affecting alertness and reflexes, such as antihistamines, tranquilizers, sedatives, pain medicine, narcotics and mind-altering drugs.

Discontinuing:
Don't discontinue without medical advice.

Others:
- Hot weather and fever may cause dehydration and drop in blood pressure. Dose may require temporary adjustment. Weigh daily and report any unexpected weight decreases to your doctor.
- May cause rise in uric acid, leading to gout.
- May cause blood-sugar rise in diabetics.
- Get periodic check-ups and potassium-level laboratory tests.

POSSIBLE INTERACTION WITH OTHER DRUGS

GENERIC NAME OR DRUG CLASS	COMBINED EFFECT
Acebutolol	Increased antihypertensive effect. Dosages of both drugs may require adjustments.
Allopurinol	Decreased allopurinol effect.
Antidepressants (tricyclic)	Dangerous drop in blood pressure. Avoid combination unless under medical supervision.
Antihypertensives (other)	Increased effect of both drugs.
Barbiturates	Increased hydrochlorothiazide effect.

Blood-bank blood	Increased potassium levels.
Cortisone drugs	Excessive potassium loss that causes dangerous heart rhythms.
Digitalis preparations	Excessive potassium loss that causes dangerous heart rhythms.
Diuretics (thiazide)	Increased diuretic effect.
Diuretics (other)	Increased effect of both drugs.
Indapamide	Increased diuretic effect.
Lithium	Possible lithium toxicity.
MAO inhibitors	Increased hydrochlorothiazide effect.
Nitrates	Excessive blood-pressure drop.
Oxprenolol	Increased antihypertensive effect. Dosages may require adjustment.
Probenecid	Decreased probenecid effect.
Sodium bicarbonate	Decreased potassium levels.

POSSIBLE INTERACTION WITH OTHER SUBSTANCES

INTERACTS WITH	COMBINED EFFECT
Alcohol:	Dangerous blood-pressure drop.
Beverages: Low-salt milk.	Possible excess potassium levels. Low-salt milk has extra potassium.
Cocaine:	None expected.
Foods: Salt substitutes.	Possible excess potassium levels.
Marijuana:	May increase blood pressure.
Tobacco:	None expected.

AMINOBENZOATE POTASSIUM

BRAND NAMES

KPAB
Potaba
Potassium
  Aminobenzoate

Potassium
Para-
  aminobenzoate

BASIC INFORMATION

Habit forming? No
Prescription needed? Yes
Available as generic? Yes
Drug class: Antifibrosis

USES

Reduces inflammation and relieves contractions in tissues lying under the skin that have become tight from such disorders as dermatomyositis, Peyronie's disease, scleroderma, pemphigus, morphea.

DOSAGE & USAGE INFORMATION

How to take:
- Tablets—Dissolve in liquid to prevent stomach upset.
- Capsules—Take with full glass of liquid.

When to take:
At the same times each day, according to instructions on prescription label. Usually taken with meals and at bedtime with a snack.

If you forget a dose:
Take as soon as you remember up to 2 hours late. If more than 2 hours, wait for next scheduled dose (don't double this dose).

What drug does:
May increase ability of diseased tissues to use oxygen.

Time lapse before drug works:
May require 3 to 10 months for improvement to begin.

Don't take with:
See Interaction column and consult doctor.

OVERDOSE

SYMPTOMS:
Nausea, vomiting.
WHAT TO DO:
Overdose unlikely to threaten life. If person takes much larger amount than prescribed, call doctor, poison-control center or hospital emergency room for instructions.

POSSIBLE ADVERSE REACTIONS OR SIDE EFFECTS

SYMPTOMS	WHAT TO DO
Life-threatening: None expected.	
Common: Appetite loss, nausea.	Continue. Call doctor when convenient.
Infrequent:	
• Low blood sugar (hunger, anxiety, cold sweats, rapid pulse).	Discontinue. Seek emergency treatment. (Note: Take sugar or honey on the way to emergency room.)
• Sore throat.	Discontinue. Call doctor right away.
Rare: None expected.	

WARNINGS & PRECAUTION

Don't take if:
You are allergic to aminobenzoate potassium or aminobenzoic acid (PABA).

Before you start, consult your doctor:
- If you have low blood sugar.
- If you have diabetes mellitus.
- If you have kidney disease.

Over age 60:
Adverse reactions and side effects may be more frequent and severe than in younger persons, particularly low blood sugar.

Pregnancy:
No proven problems.

Breast-feeding:
Drug passes into milk. Avoid drug or discontinue nursing.

Infants & children:
Not recommended. Safety and dosage have not been established.

Prolonged use:
No problems expected.

Skin & sunlight:
No problems expected.

Driving, piloting or hazardous work:
No problems expected.

Discontinuing:
No problems expected.

Others:
If you become acutely ill and cannot eat well for even a short while, tell your doctor. These circumstances can lead to low blood sugar, and dosage may need adjustment.

POSSIBLE INTERACTION WITH OTHER DRUGS

GENERIC NAME OR DRUG CLASS	COMBINED EFFECT
Sulfa drugs (sulfonamides)	Decreased sulfa effect.

POSSIBLE INTERACTION WITH OTHER SUBSTANCES

INTERACTS WITH	COMBINED EFFECT
Alcohol:	None expected.
Beverages:	None expected.
Cocaine:	None expected.
Foods:	None expected.
Marijuana:	None expected.
Tobacco:	None expected.

AMIODARONE

BRAND NAMES

Cordarone

BASIC INFORMATION

Habit forming? No
Prescription needed? Yes
Available as generic? No
Drug class: Antiarrhythmic

 USES

Prevents and treats life-threatening heartbeat irregularities involving both the large chambers of the heart (auricles and ventricles).

 DOSAGE & USAGE INFORMATION

How to take:
Tablets—Swallow whole with liquid or food to lessen stomach irritation. If you can't swallow whole, crumble tablet and take with liquid or food.

When to take:
According to prescription instructions.

If you forget a dose:
Skip this dose and resume regular schedule. Do not double the next dose. If you forget 2 doses or more, consult your doctor.

What drug does:
- Slows nerve impulses in the heart.
- Makes heart muscle fibers less responsive to abnormal electrical impulses arising in the electrical regulatory system of the heart.

Continued next column

 OVERDOSE

SYMPTOMS:
Irregular heartbeat, loss of consciousness, seizures.
WHAT TO DO:
- **Dial 0 (operator) or 911 (emergency) for an ambulance or medical help. Then give first aid immediately.**
- **If patient is unconscious and not breathing, give mouth-to-mouth breathing. If there is no heartbeat, use cardiac massage and mouth-to-mouth breathing (CPR). Don't try to make patient vomit. If you can't get help quickly, take patient to nearest emergency facility.**
- **See emergency information on inside covers.**

Time lapse before drug works:
2 to 3 days to 2 to 3 months.

Don't take with:
See Interaction column and consult doctor.

 POSSIBLE ADVERSE REACTIONS OR SIDE EFFECTS

SYMPTOMS	WHAT TO DO
Life-threatening:	
Shortness of breath, difficulty breathing, cough. (Not uncommon)	Discontinue. Seek emergency treatment.
Common:	
• Walking difficulty, fever, numbness or tingling in hands or feet, shakiness, weakness in arms and legs.	Discontinue. Call doctor right away.
• Constipation, headache, appetite loss, nausea, vomiting.	Continue. Call doctor when convenient.
Infrequent:	
• Skin color change to blue-gray, blurred vision, cold feeling, dry eyes, nervousness, scrotum swelling or pain, insomnia, swollen feet and ankles, fast or slow heartbeat, eyes hurt in light, weight gain or loss.	Discontinue. Call doctor right away.
• Bitter or metallic taste, diminished sex drive, dizziness, flushed face.	Continue. Call doctor when convenient.
Rare:	
Jaundice, skin rash.	Discontinue. Call doctor right away.

WARNINGS & PRECAUTIONS

Don't take if:
You are allergic to amiodarone.

Before you start, consult your doctor:
- If you have liver or kidney disease.
- If you have high blood pressure.
- If you have heart disease other than coronary artery disease.

Over age 60:
- Adverse reactions and side effects may be more frequent and severe than in younger persons. Ask about smaller doses.
- Pain in legs (while walking) considerably more likely.

Pregnancy:
Safety to unborn child unestablished. Avoid if possible.

Breast-feeding:
Drug passes into milk. Avoid drug or discontinue nursing until you finish medicine. Consult doctor for advice on maintaining milk supply.

Infants & children:
Use only under close medical supervision.

Prolonged use:
- Blue-gray discoloration of skin may appear.
- Don't discontinue without consulting doctor. Dose may require gradual reduction if you have taken drug for a long time. Doses of other drugs may also require adjustment.

Skin & sunlight:
May cause rash or intensify sunburn in areas exposed to sun or sunlamp. Avoid undue exposure.

Driving, piloting or hazardous work:
Avoid if you feel dizzy or lightheaded. Otherwise, no problems expected.

Discontinuing:
- Don't discontinue without consulting doctor. Dose may require gradual reduction if you have taken drug for a long time. Doses of other drugs may also require adjustment.
- Notify doctor if cough, fever, breathing difficulty or shortness of breath occur after discontinuing medicine.

Others:
Learn to check your own pulse. If it drops to lower than 50 or rises to higher than 100 beats per minute, don't take amiodarone until you consult your doctor.

POSSIBLE INTERACTION WITH OTHER DRUGS

GENERIC NAME OR DRUG CLASS	COMBINED EFFECT
Anticoagulants	Increased anticoagulant effect.
Antiarrhythmics (other)	Increased likelihood of heartbeat irregularity.
Beta-blockers (acebutolol, atenolol, labetolol, metaprolol, nadolol, oxprenol, pindolol, propranolol, sotalol, timolol)	Increased likelihood of slow heartbeat.
Digitalis	Increased digitalis effect.
Diltiazam	Increased likelihood of slow heartbeat.
Diuretics	Increased risk of heartbeat irregularity due to low potassium level.
Nifedipine	Increased likelihood of slow heartbeat.
Phenytoin	Increased effect of phenytoin.
Verapamil	Increased likelihood of slow heartbeat.

POSSIBLE INTERACTION WITH OTHER SUBSTANCES

INTERACTS WITH	COMBINED EFFECT
Alcohol:	Increased risk of heartbeat irregularity. Avoid.
Beverages:	None expected.
Cocaine:	Increased risk of heartbeat irregularity. Avoid.
Foods:	None expected.
Marijuana:	Possible irregular heartbeat. Avoid.
Tobacco:	Possible irregular heartbeat. Avoid.

AMOBARBITAL

BRAND NAMES

Amytal
Dexamyl
Isobec

Novamobarb
Tuinal

BASIC INFORMATION

Habit forming? Yes
Prescription needed? Yes
Available as generic? Yes
Drug class: Sedative, hypnotic (barbiturate)

USES

- Reduces anxiety or nervous tension (low dose).
- Relieves insomnia (higher bedtime dose).

DOSAGE & USAGE INFORMATION

How to take:
Tablet, capsule or liquid—Swallow with food or liquid to lessen stomach irritation. If you can't swallow whole, crumble tablet or open capsule and take with liquid or food.

When to take:
At the same times each day.

If you forget a dose:
Take as soon as you remember up to 2 hours late. If more than 2 hours, wait for next scheduled dose (don't double this dose).

What drug does:
May partially block nerve impulses at nerve-cell connections.

Continued next column

OVERDOSE

SYMPTOMS:
Deep sleep, weak pulse, coma.
WHAT TO DO:
- **Dial 0 (operator) or 911 (emergency) for an ambulance or medical help. Then give first aid immediately.**
- **If patient is unconscious and not breathing, give mouth-to-mouth breathing. If there is no heartbeat use cardiac massage and mouth-to-mouth breathing (CPR). Don't try to make patient vomit. If you can't help quickly, take patient to nearest emergency facility.**
- **See emergency information on inside covers.**

Time lapse before drug works:
60 minutes.

Don't take with:
- Non-prescription drugs without consulting doctor.
- See Interaction column and consult doctor.

POSSIBLE ADVERSE REACTIONS OR SIDE EFFECTS

SYMPTOMS	WHAT TO DO
Life-threatening: None expected.	
Common: Dizziness, drowsiness, "hangover" effect.	Continue. Call doctor when convenient.
Infrequent: • Rash or hives; swollen face, lips, eyelids; sore throat, fever.	Discontinue. Call doctor right away.
• Depression, confusion, slurred speech, nausea, vomiting, joint or muscle pain.	Continue. Call doctor when convenient.
Rare: • Agitation, slow heartbeat, breathing difficulty, jaundice.	Discontinue. Call doctor right away.
• Unexplained bleeding or bruising.	Continue. Call doctor when convenient.

WARNINGS & PRECAUTIONS

Don't take if:
- You are allergic to any barbiturate.
- You have porphyria.

Before you start, consult your doctor:
- If you have epilepsy.
- If you have kidney or liver damage.
- If you have asthma.
- If you have anemia.
- If you have chronic pain.
- If you will have surgery within 2 months, including dental surgery, requiring general or spinal anesthesia.

Over age 60:
Adverse reactions and side effects may be more frequent and severe than in younger persons. Use small doses.

Pregnancy:
Risk to unborn child outweighs drug benefits. Don't use.

Breast-feeding:
Drug passes into milk. Avoid drug or discontinue nursing until you finish medicine. Consult doctor for advice on maintaining milk supply.

Infants & children:
Use only under doctor's supervision.

Prolonged use:
- May cause addiction, anemia, chronic intoxication.
- May lower body temperature, making exposure to cold temperatures hazardous.

Skin & sunlight:
May cause rash or intensify sunburn in areas exposed to sun or sunlamp.

Driving, piloting or hazardous work:
Don't drive or pilot aircraft until you learn how medicine affects you. Don't work around dangerous machinery. Don't climb ladders or work in high places. Danger increases if you drink alcohol or take medicine affecting alertness and reflexes.

Discontinuing:
May be unnecessary to finish medicine. Follow doctor's instructions. If you develop withdrawal symptoms of hallucinations, agitation or sleeplessness after discontinuing, call doctor right away.

Others:
Great potential for abuse.

POSSIBLE INTERACTION WITH OTHER DRUGS

GENERIC NAME OR DRUG CLASS	COMBINED EFFECT
Anticoagulants (oral)	Decreased anticoagulant effect.
Anticonvulsants	Changed seizure patterns.
Antidepressants (tricyclics)	Decreased antidepressant effect. Possible dangerous oversedation.
Antidiabetics (oral)	Increased amobarbital effect.
Antihistamines	Dangerous sedation. Avoid.
Anti-inflammatory drugs (non-steroidal)	Decreased anti-inflammatory effect.
Aspirin	Decreased aspirin effect.
Beta-adrenergic blockers	Decreased effect of beta-adrenergic blocker.

Contraceptives (oral)	Decreased contraceptive effect.
Cortisone drugs	Decreased cortisone effect.
Digitoxin	Decreased digitoxin effect.
Doxycycline	Decreased doxycycline effect.
Dronabinol	Increased effects of both drugs. Avoid.
Griseofulvin	Decreased griseofulvin effect.
Indapamide	Increased indapamide effect.
MAO inhibitors	Increased amobarbital effect.
Mind-altering drugs	Dangerous sedation. Avoid.
Narcotics	Dangerous sedation. Avoid.
Pain relievers	Dangerous sedation. Avoid.
Sedatives	Dangerous sedation. Avoid.
Sleep inducers	Dangerous sedation. Avoid.
Tranquilizers	Dangerous sedation. Avoid.
Valproic acid	Increased amobarbital effect.

POSSIBLE INTERACTION WITH OTHER SUBSTANCES

INTERACTS WITH	COMBINED EFFECT
Alcohol:	Possible fatal oversedation. Avoid.
Beverages:	None expected.
Cocaine:	Decreased amobarbital effect.
Foods:	None expected.
Marijuana:	Excessive sedation. Avoid.
Tobacco:	None expected.

AMOXICILLIN

BRAND NAMES

Amoxil	Polymox
Augmentin	Robamox
Larotid	Sumox
Moxilean	Trimox
Novamoxin	Utimox
Penamox	Wymox

BASIC INFORMATION

Habit forming? No
Prescription needed? Yes
Available as generic? Yes
Drug class: Antibiotic (penicillin)

USES

Treatment of bacterial infections that are susceptible to amoxicillin.

DOSAGE & USAGE INFORMATION

How to take:
- Tablet or capsule—Swallow with liquid on an empty stomach 1 hour before or 2 hours after eating.
- Liquid—Take with cold beverage. Liquid form is perishable and effective for only 7 days at room temperature. Effective for 14 days if stored in refrigerator. Don't freeze.

When to take:
Follow instructions on prescription label or side of package. Doses should be evenly spaced. For example, 4 times a day means every 6 hours.

If you forget a dose:
Take as soon as you remember. Continue regular schedule.

What drug does:
Destroys susceptible bacteria. Does not kill viruses.

Continued next column

OVERDOSE

SYMPTOMS:
Severe diarrhea, nausea or vomiting.
WHAT TO DO:
Overdose unlikely to threaten life. If person takes much larger amount than prescribed, call doctor, poison-control center or hospital emergency room for instructions.

Time lapse before drug works:
May be several days before medicine affects infection.

Don't take with:
See Interaction column and consult doctor.

POSSIBLE ADVERSE REACTIONS OR SIDE EFFECTS

SYMPTOMS	WHAT TO DO
Life-threatening:	
Hives, rash, intense itching, faintness soon after a dose (anaphylaxis).	Seek emergency treatment immediately.
Common:	
Dark or discolored tongue.	Continue. Tell doctor at next visit.
Infrequent:	
Mild nausea, vomiting, diarrhea.	Continue. Call doctor when convenient.
Rare:	
Unexplained bleeding.	Discontinue. Call doctor right away.

WARNINGS & PRECAUTIONS

Don't take if:
You are allergic to amoxicillin, cephalosporin antibiotics, other penicillins or penicillamine. Life-threatening reaction may occur.

Before you start, consult your doctor:
If you are allergic to any substance or drug.

Over age 60:
You may have skin reactions, particularly around genitals and anus.

Pregnancy:
Studies inconclusive on harm to unborn child. Animal studies show fetal abnormalities. Decide with your doctor whether drug benefits justify risk to unborn child.

Breast-feeding:
Drug passes into milk. Child may become sensitive to penicillins and have allergic reactions to penicillin drugs. Avoid amoxicillin or discontinue nursing until you finish medicine. Consult doctor for advice on maintaining milk supply.

Infants & children:
No problems expected.

Prolonged use:
You may become more susceptible to infections caused by germs not responsive to amoxicillin.

Skin & sunlight:
No problems expected.

Driving, piloting or hazardous work:
Usually not dangerous. Most hazardous reactions likely to occur a few minutes after taking amoxicillin.

Discontinuing:
Don't discontinue without doctor's advice until you complete prescribed dose, even though symptoms diminish or disappear.

Others:
No problems expected.

POSSIBLE INTERACTION WITH OTHER DRUGS

GENERIC NAME OR DRUG CLASS	COMBINED EFFECT
Beta-adrenergic blockers	Increased chance of anaphylaxis (see emergency information on inside front cover).
Chloramphenicol	Decreased effect of both drugs.
Erythromycins	Decreased effect of both drugs.
Loperamide	Decreased amoxicillin effect.
Paromomycin	Decreased effect of both drugs.
Tetracyclines	Decreased effect of both drugs.
Troleandomycin	Decreased effect of both drugs.

POSSIBLE INTERACTION WITH OTHER SUBSTANCES

INTERACTS WITH	COMBINED EFFECT
Alcohol:	Occasional stomach irritation.
Beverages:	None expected.
Cocaine:	No proven problems.
Foods:	None expected.
Marijuana:	No proven problems.
Tobacco:	None expected.

AMPHETAMINE

BRAND NAMES

Amphaplex 10 & 20	Biphetamine
Benzedrine	Declobese
Bexedrine	Obetrol 10 & 20

BASIC INFORMATION

Habit forming? Yes
Prescription needed? Yes
Available as generic? Yes
Drug class: Central-nervous-system stimulant (amphetamine)

USES

- Prevents narcolepsy (attacks of uncontrollable sleepiness).
- Controls hyperactivity in children.

DOSAGE & USAGE INFORMATION

How to take:
- Tablet—Swallow with liquid.
- Extended-release capsules—Swallow each dose whole with liquid.

When to take:
- At the same times each day.
- Short-acting form—Don't take later than 6 hours before bedtime.
- Long-acting form—Take on awakening.

If you forget a dose:
- Short-acting form—Take up to 2 hours late. If more than 2 hours, wait for next dose (don't double this dose).
- Long-acting form—Take as soon as you remember. Wait 20 hours for next dose.

Continued next column

OVERDOSE

SYMPTOMS:
Rapid heartbeat, hyperactivity, high fever, hallucinations, suicidal or homicidal feelings, convulsions, coma.
WHAT TO DO:
- **Dial 0 (operator) or 911 (emergency) for an ambulance or medical help. Then give first aid immediately.**
- **See emergency information on inside covers.**

What drug does:
- Narcolepsy—Apparently affects brain centers to decrease fatigue or sleepiness and increase alertness and motor activity.
- Hyperactive children—Calms children, opposite to effect on narcoleptic adults.

Time lapse before drug works:
15 to 30 minutes.

Don't take with:
See Interaction column and consult doctor.

POSSIBLE ADVERSE REACTIONS OR SIDE EFFECTS

SYMPTOMS	WHAT TO DO
Life-threatening: None expected.	
Common:	
• Irritability, nervousness, insomnia.	Continue. Call doctor when convenient.
• Dry mouth.	Continue. Tell doctor at next visit.
Infrequent:	
• Dizziness; reduced alertness; blurred vision; fast, pounding heartbeat; unusual sweating.	Discontinue. Call doctor right away.
• Headache.	Continue. Call doctor when convenient.
• Diarrhea or constipation, appetite loss, stomach pain, nausea, vomiting, weight loss, diminished sex drive, impotence.	Continue. Tell doctor at next visit.
Rare:	
• Rash, hives; chest pain or irregular heartbeat; uncontrollable movements of head, neck, arms, legs.	Discontinue. Call doctor right away.
• Mood changes, swollen breasts.	Continue. Call doctor when convenient.

WARNINGS & PRECAUTIONS

Don't take if:
- You are allergic to any amphetamine.
- You will have surgery within 2 months, including dental surgery, requiring general or spinal anesthesia.

Before you start, consult your doctor:
- If you plan to become pregnant within medication period.
- If you have glaucoma.
- If you have heart or blood-vessel disease, or high blood pressure.
- If you have overactive thyroid, anxiety or tension.
- If you have a severe mental illness (especially children).

Over age 60:
Adverse reactions and side effects may be more frequent and severe than in younger persons.

Pregnancy:
Risk to unborn child outweighs drug benefits. Don't use.

Breast-feeding:
Drug passes into milk. Avoid drug or discontinue nursing.

Infants & children:
Not recommended for children under 12.

Prolonged use:
Habit forming.

Skin & sunlight:
No problems expected.

Driving, piloting or hazardous work:
Don't drive or pilot aircraft until you learn how medicine affects you. Don't work around dangerous machinery. Don't climb ladders or work in high places. Danger increases if you drink alcohol or take medicine affecting alertness and reflexes.

Discontinuing:
May be unnecessary to finish medicine. Follow doctor's instructions.

Others:
- This is a dangerous drug and must be closely supervised. Don't use for appetite control or depression. Potential for damage and abuse.
- During withdrawal phase, may cause prolonged sleep of several days.

POSSIBLE INTERACTION WITH OTHER DRUGS

GENERIC NAME OR DRUG CLASS	COMBINED EFFECT
Anesthesias (general)	Irregular heartbeat.
Antidepressants (tricyclic)	Decreased amphetamine effect.
Antihypertensives	Decreased antihypertensive effect.
Carbonic anhydrase inhibitors	Increased amphetamine effect.
Guanethidine	Decreased guanethidine effect.
Haloperidol	Decreased amphetamine effect.
MAO inhibitors	May severely increase blood pressure.
Phenothiazines	Decreased amphetamine effect.
Sodium bicarbonate	Increased amphetamine effect.

POSSIBLE INTERACTION WITH OTHER SUBSTANCES

INTERACTS WITH	COMBINED EFFECT
Alcohol:	Decreased amphetamine effect. Avoid.
Beverages: Caffeine drinks.	Overstimulation. Avoid.
Cocaine:	Dangerous stimulation of nervous system. Avoid.
Foods:	None expected.
Marijuana:	Frequent use—Severely impaired mental function.
Tobacco:	None expected.

AMPICILLIN

BRAND NAMES

Alpen	Penbritin
Amcill	Polycillin
Ampicin	Prinicipen
Ampilean	SK-Ampicillin
Novo-Ampicillin	Supen
Omnipen	Totacillin

BASIC INFORMATION

Habit forming? No
Prescription needed? Yes
Available as generic? Yes
Drug class: Antibiotic (penicillin)

USES

Treatment of bacterial infections that are susceptible to ampicillin.

DOSAGE & USAGE INFORMATION

How to take:
- Tablets or capsules—Swallow with liquid on an empty stomach 1 hour before or 2 hours after eating.
- Liquid—Take with cold beverage. Liquid form is perishable and effective for only 7 days at room temperature. Effective for 14 days if stored in refrigerator. Don't freeze.

When to take:
Follow instructions on prescription label or side of package. Doses should be evenly spaced. For example, 4 times a day means every 6 hours.

If you forget a dose:
Take as soon as you remember. Continue regular schedule.

What drug does:
Destroys susceptible bacteria. Does not kill viruses.

Time lapse before drug works:
May be several days before medicine affects infection.

Continued next column

OVERDOSE

SYMPTOMS:
Severe diarrhea, nausea or vomiting.
WHAT TO DO:
Overdose unlikely to threaten life. If person takes much larger amount than prescribed, call doctor, poison-control center or hospital emergency room for instructions.

Don't take with:
See Interaction column and consult doctor.

POSSIBLE ADVERSE REACTIONS OR SIDE EFFECTS

SYMPTOMS	WHAT TO DO
Life-threatening:	
Hives, rash, intense itching, faintness soon after a dose (anaphylaxis).	Seek emergency treatment immediately.
Common:	
Dark or discolored tongue.	Continue. Tell doctor at next visit.
Infrequent:	
Mild nausea, vomiting, diarrhea.	Continue. Call doctor when convenient.
Rare:	
Unexplained bleeding.	Discontinue. Call doctor right away.

WARNINGS & PRECAUTIONS

Don't take if:
You are allergic to ampicillin, cephalosporin antibiotics, other penicillins or penicillamine. Life-threatening reaction may occur.

Before you start, consult your doctor:
If you are allergic to any substance or drug.

Over age 60:
You may have skin reactions, particularly around genitals and anus.

Pregnancy:
Studies inconclusive on harm to unborn child. Animal studies show fetal abnormalities. Decide with your doctor whether drug benefits justify risk to unborn child.

Breast-feeding:
Drug passes into milk. Child may become sensitive to penicillins and have allergic reactions to penicillin drugs. Avoid ampicillin or discontinue nursing until you finish medicine. Consult doctor for advice on maintaining milk supply.

Infants & children:
No problems expected.

Prolonged use:
You may become more susceptible to infections caused by germs not responsive to ampicillin.

Skin & sunlight:
No problems expected.

Driving, piloting or hazardous work:
Usually not dangerous. Most hazardous reactions likely to occur a few minutes after taking ampicillin.

Discontinuing:
Don't discontinue without doctor's advice until you complete prescribed dose, even though symptoms diminish or disappear.

Others:
Urine sugar test for diabetes may show false positive result.

POSSIBLE INTERACTION WITH OTHER DRUGS

GENERIC NAME OR DRUG CLASS	COMBINED EFFECT
Beta-adrenergic blockers	Increased chance of anaphylaxis (see emergency information on inside front cover).
Chloramphenicol	Decreased effect of both drugs.
Erythromycins	Decreased effect of both drugs.
Loperamide	Decreased ampicillin effect.
Oral contraceptives	Occasionally impairs contraceptive efficiency.
Paromomycin	Decreased effect of both drugs.
Tetracyclines	Decreased effect of both drugs.
Troleandomycin	Decreased effect of both drugs.

POSSIBLE INTERACTION WITH OTHER SUBSTANCES

INTERACTS WITH	COMBINED EFFECT
Alcohol:	Occasional stomach irritation.
Beverages:	None expected.
Cocaine:	No proven problems.
Foods:	None expected.
Marijuana:	No proven problems.
Tobacco:	None expected.

ANDROGENS

BRAND AND GENERIC NAMES

See complete list of brand names in the *Brand Name Directory,* page 942.

BASIC INFORMATION

Habit forming? No
Available as generic? Yes
Prescription needed? Yes
Drug class: Androgens

 USES

- Corrects male hormone deficiency.
- Reduces "male menopause" symptoms (loss of sex drive, depression, anxiety).
- Decreases calcium loss of osteoporosis (softened bones).
- Blocks growth of breast-cancer cells in females.
- Corrects undescended testicles in male children.
- Reduces breast pain and fullness following childbirth.
- Augments treatment of aplastic anemia.
- Stimulates weight gain after illness, injury or for chronically underweight persons.
- Stimulates growth in treatment of dwarfism.

 DOSAGE & USAGE INFORMATION

How to take:
- Tablets—With food to lessen stomach irritation.
- Injection—Once or twice a month.

When to take:
At the same time each day.

If you forget a dose:
Take as soon as you remember up to 2 hours late. If more than 2 hours, wait for next scheduled dose (don't double this dose).

Continued next column

 OVERDOSE

SYMPTOMS:
None expected.
WHAT TO DO:
Overdose unlikely to threaten life. If person takes much larger amount than prescribed, call doctor, poison-control center or hospital emergency room for instructions.

What drug does:
- Stimulates cells that produce male sex characteristics.
- Replaces hormone deficiencies.
- Stimulates red-blood-cell production.
- Suppresses production of estrogen (female sex hormone).

Time lapse before drug works:
Varies with problems treated. May require 2 or 3 months of regular use for desired effects.

Don't take with:
See Interaction column and consult doctor.

 POSSIBLE ADVERSE REACTIONS OR SIDE EFFECTS

SYMPTOMS	WHAT TO DO
Life-threatening:	
Intense itching, weakness, loss of consciousness.	Seek emergency treatment immediately.
Common:	
• Acne or oily skin in females, deep voice, enlarged clitoris, frequent erections, swollen breasts in men.	Continue. Call doctor when convenient.
• Sore mouth, higher sex drive.	Continue. Tell doctor at next visit.
Infrequent:	
• Jaundice.	Discontinue. Seek emergency treatment.
• Depression or confusion, flushed face, rash or itch, nausea, vomiting, diarrhea, swollen feet or legs, vaginal bleeding.	Discontinue. Call doctor right away.
Rare:	
• Hives, black stool.	Discontinue. Seek emergency treatment.
• Sore throat, fever, abdominal pain.	Discontinue. Call doctor right away.

WARNINGS & PRECAUTIONS

Don't take if:
You are allergic to any male hormone.

Before you start, consult your doctor:
- If you might be pregnant.
- If you have cancer of prostate.
- If you have heart disease or arteriosclerosis.
- If you have kidney or liver disease.
- If you have breast cancer (males).
- If you have high blood pressure.
- If you have migraine attacks.
- If you have high level of blood calcium.
- If you have epilepsy.

Over age 60:
- May stimulate sexual activity.
- Can make high blood pressure or heart disease worse.
- Can enlarge prostate and cause urinary retention.

Pregnancy:
Risk to unborn child outweighs drug benefits. Don't use.

Breast-feeding:
Drug passes into milk. Avoid drug or discontinue nursing until you finish medicine. Consult doctor for advice on maintaining milk supply.

Infants & children:
Don't give to children younger than 2. Use with older children only under medical supervision.

Prolonged use:
- Reduces sperm count and volume of semen.
- Possible kidney stones.
- Unnatural hair growth and deep voice in women.

Skin & sunlight:
No problems expected.

Driving, piloting or hazardous work:
No problems expected.

Discontinuing:
No problems expected.

Others:
- May cause atrophy of testicles.
- Will not increase strength in athletes.

POSSIBLE INTERACTION WITH OTHER DRUGS

GENERIC NAME OR DRUG CLASS	COMBINED EFFECT
Anticoagulants	Increased anticoagulant effect.
Antidiabetics (oral)	Increased antidiabetic effect.
Chlorzoxazone	Decreased androgen effect.
Oxyphenbutazone	Decreased androgen effect.
Phenobarbital	Decreased androgen effect.
Phenylbutazone	Decreased androgen effect.

POSSIBLE INTERACTION WITH OTHER SUBSTANCES

INTERACTS WITH	COMBINED EFFECT
Alcohol:	None expected.
Beverages:	None expected.
Cocaine:	No proven problems.
Foods: Salt.	Excessive fluid retention (edema). Decrease salt intake while taking male hormones.
Marijuana:	Decreased blood levels of androgens.
Tobacco:	No proven problems.

ANESTHETICS (TOPICAL)

BRAND AND GENERIC NAMES

See complete list of brand names in the *Brand Name Directory,* page 942.

BASIC INFORMATION

Habit forming? No
Prescription needed?
  High strength: Yes
  Low strength: No
Available as generic? Yes
Drug class: Anesthetic (topical)

USES

- Relieves pain and itch of sunburn, insect bites, scratches and other minor skin irritations.
- Relieves discomfort and itch of hemorrhoids and other disorders of anus and rectum.

DOSAGE & USAGE INFORMATION

How to use:
- Suppositories—Remove wrapper and moisten suppository with water. Gently insert larger end into rectum. Push well into rectum with finger.
- All other forms—Use only enough to cover irritated area. Follow instructions on label.

When to use:
When needed for discomfort, no more often than every hour.

If you forget an application:
Use as needed.

What drug does:
Blocks pain impulses from skin to brain.

Time lapse before drug works:
3 to 15 minutes.

Don't take with:
See Interaction column and consult doctor.

OVERDOSE

SYMPTOMS:
If swallowed or inhaled—Dizziness, nervousness, trembling, seizures.
WHAT TO DO:
- **Dial 0 (operator) or 911 (emergency) for an ambulance or medical help. Then give first aid immediately.**
- **See emergency information on inside covers.**

POSSIBLE ADVERSE REACTIONS OR SIDE EFFECTS

SYMPTOMS	WHAT TO DO
Life-threatening: None expected.	
Common: None expected.	
Infrequent:	
• Nervousness; trembling; hives, rash, itch; inflammation or tenderness not present before application; slow heartbeat.	Discontinue. Call doctor right away.
• Dizziness, blurred vision, swollen feet.	Continue. Call doctor when convenient.
Rare:	
• Blood in urine.	Discontinue. Call doctor right away.
• Increased or painful urination.	Continue. Call doctor when convenient.

WARNINGS & PRECAUTIONS

Don't use if:
You are allergic to any topical anesthetic.

Before you start, consult your doctor:
- If you have skin infection at site of treatment.
- If you have had severe or extensive skin disorders such as eczema or psoriasis.
- If you have bleeding hemorrhoids.

Over age 60:
Adverse reactions and side effects may be more frequent and severe than in younger persons.

Pregnancy:
No proven harm to unborn child. Avoid if possible.

Breast-feeding:
No problems expected.

Infants & children:
Use caution. More likely to be absorbed through skin and cause adverse reactions.

Prolonged use:
Possible excess absorption. Don't use longer than 3 days for any one problem.

Skin & sunlight:
No problems expected.

Driving, piloting or hazardous work:
No problems expected.

Discontinuing:
May be unnecessary to finish medicine. Follow doctor's instructions.

Others:
No problems expected.

POSSIBLE INTERACTION WITH OTHER DRUGS

GENERIC NAME OR DRUG CLASS	COMBINED EFFECT
Sulfa drugs	Decreased effect of sulfa drugs for infection.

POSSIBLE INTERACTION WITH OTHER SUBSTANCES

INTERACTS WITH	COMBINED EFFECT
Alcohol:	None expected.
Beverages:	None expected.
Cocaine:	Possible nervous-system toxicity. Avoid.
Foods:	None expected.
Marijuana:	None expected.
Tobacco:	None expected.

ANTICOAGULANTS (ORAL)

BRAND AND GENERIC NAMES

ANISINDIONE	Melitoxin
Anthrombin-K	Miradon
Coumadin	Panwarfin
Danilone	PHENINDIONE
DICUMAROL	PHENPROCOUMON
Dufalone	WARFARIN
Hedulin	POTASSIUM
Liquamar	WARFARIN SODIUM
Marcumar	Warfilone
Marevan	Warnerin

BASIC INFORMATION

Habit forming? No
Prescription needed? Yes
Available as generic? Yes
Drug class: Anticoagulant

 ## USES

Reduces blood clots. Used for abnormal clotting inside blood vessels.

 ## DOSAGE & USAGE INFORMATION

How to take:
Tablet—Swallow with liquid. If you can't swallow whole, crumble tablet and take with liquid or food.

When to take:
At the same time each day.

If you forget a dose:
Take as soon as you remember up to 12 hours late. If more than 12 hours, wait for next scheduled dose (don't double this dose). Inform your doctor of any missed doses.

What drug does:
Blocks action of vitamin K necessary for blood clotting.

Time lapse before drug works:
36 to 48 hours.

Continued next column

 ## OVERDOSE

SYMPTOMS:
Bloody vomit and bloody or black stools, red urine.
WHAT TO DO:
- **Dial 0 (operator) or 911 (emergency) for an ambulance or medical help. Then give first aid immediately.**
- **See emergency information on inside covers.**

Don't take with:
See Interaction column and consult doctor.

 ## POSSIBLE ADVERSE REACTIONS OR SIDE EFFECTS

SYMPTOMS	WHAT TO DO
Life-threatening: None expected.	
Common: Bloating, gas.	Continue. Tell doctor at next visit.
Infrequent: • Black stools or bloody vomit, coughing up blood.	Discontinue. Seek emergency treatment.
• Rash, hives, itch, blurred vision, sore throat, easy bruising, bleeding, cloudy or red urine, back pain, jaundice, fever, chills, fatigue, weakness.	Discontinue. Call doctor right away.
• Diarrhea, cramps, nausea, vomiting, swollen feet or legs, hair loss.	Continue. Call doctor when convenient.
Rare: Dizziness, headache, mouth sores.	Discontinue. Call doctor right away.

 ## WARNINGS & PRECAUTIONS

Don't take if:
- You have been allergic to any oral anticoagulant.
- You have a bleeding disorder.
- You have an active peptic ulcer.
- You have ulcerative colitis.

Before you start, consult your doctor:
- If you take any other drugs, including non-prescription drugs.
- If you have high blood pressure.
- If you have heavy or prolonged menstrual periods.
- If you have diabetes.
- If you have a bladder catheter.
- If you have serious liver or kidney disease.
- If you will have surgery within 2 months, including dental surgery, requiring general or spinal anesthesia.

Over age 60:
Adverse reactions and side effects may be more frequent and severe than in younger persons.

Pregnancy:
Risk to unborn child outweighs drug benefits. Don't use.

Breast-feeding:
Drug filters into milk. May harm child. Avoid.

Infants & children:
Use only under doctor's supervision.

Prolonged use:
No problems expected.

Skin & sunlight:
No problems expected.

Driving, piloting or hazardous work:
- Avoid hazardous activities that could cause injury.
- Don't drive if you feel dizzy or have blurred vision.

Discontinuing:
Don't discontinue without consulting doctor. Dose may require gradual reduction if you have taken drug for a long time. Doses of other drugs may also require adjustment.

Others:
Carry identification to state you take anticoagulants.

POSSIBLE INTERACTION WITH OTHER DRUGS

GENERIC NAME OR DRUG CLASS	COMBINED EFFECT
Acetaminophen	Increased effect of anticoagulant.
Allopurinol	Increased effect of anticoagulant.
Amiodarone	Increased effect of anticoagulant.
Androgens	Increased effect of anticoagulant.
Antacids (large doses)	Decreased effect of anticoagulant.
Antibiotics	Increased effect of anticoagulant.
Anticonvulsants (hydantoin)	Increased effect of both drugs.
Antidepressants (tricyclic)	Increased effect of anticoagulant.
Antidiabetics (oral)	Increased effect of anticoagulant.
Antihistamines	Unpredictable increased or decreased effect of anticoagulant.
Aspirin	Possible spontaneous bleeding.
Barbiturates	Decreased effect of anticoagulant.
Benzodiazepines	Unpredictable increased or decreased anticoagulant effect.
Calcium supplements	Decreased anticoagulant effect.
Carbamazepine	Decreased effect of anticoagulant.
Ketoprofen	Increased risk of bleeding.
Suprofen	Increased risk of bleeding.

POSSIBLE INTERACTION WITH OTHER SUBSTANCES

INTERACTS WITH	COMBINED EFFECT
Alcohol:	Can increase or decrease effect of anticoagulant. Use with caution.
Beverages:	None expected.
Cocaine:	None expected.
Foods: High in vitamin K such as fish, liver, spinach, cabbage.	May decrease anticoagulant effect.
Marijuana:	None expected.
Tobacco:	None expected.

ANTICONVULSANTS (DIONE-TYPE)

BRAND AND GENERIC NAMES

PARAMETHADIONE   TRIMETHADIONE
Paradione   Tridione

BASIC INFORMATION

Habit forming? No
Prescription needed? Yes
Available as generic? No
Drug class: Anticonvulsant (Dione-type)

USES

Controls but does not cure petit mal seizures (absence seizures).

DOSAGE & USAGE INFORMATION

How to take:
Tablets, capsules or liquid: Take with food or milk to lessen stomach irritation.

When to take:
At the same time each day.

If you forget a dose:
Take as soon as you remember up to 2 hours late. If more than 2 hours, wait for next scheduled dose (don't double this dose).

What drug does:
Raises threshold of seizures in cerebral cortex. Does not alter seizure pattern.

Time lapse before drug works:
1 to 3 hours.

Don't take with:
See Interaction column and consult doctor.

OVERDOSE

SYMPTOMS:
Bleeding, coma.
WHAT TO DO:
- Dial 0 (operator) or 911 (emergency) for an ambulance or medical help. Then give first aid immediately.
- If patient is unconscious and not breathing, give mouth-to-mouth breathing. If there is no heartbeat, use cardiac massage and mouth-to-mouth breathing (CPR). Don't try to make patient vomit. If you can't get help quickly, take patient to nearest emergency facility.
- See emergency information on inside covers.

POSSIBLE ADVERSE REACTIONS OR SIDE EFFECTS

SYMPTOMS	WHAT TO DO
Life-threatening: None expected.	
Common: Dizziness, drowsiness, headache, rash.	Continue. Call doctor when convenient.
Infrequent: Itching, nausea, vomiting.	Continue. Call doctor when convenient.
Rare: • Changes in vision; sore throat with fever and mouth sores; bleeding gums; easy bleeding or bruising; smoky or bloody urine; jaundice; puffed hands, face, feet or legs; swollen lymph glands; unusual weakness and fatigue.	Discontinue. Call doctor right away.
• Sensitivity to light.	Continue. Call doctor when convenient.

ANTICONVULSANTS (DIONE-TYPE)

WARNINGS & PRECAUTIONS

Don't take if:
You are allergic to this drug or any anticonvulsant.

Before you start, consult your doctor:
- If you are pregnant or plan pregnancy.
- If you have blood disease.
- If you have liver or kidney disease.
- If you have disease of optic nerve or eye.
- If you will have surgery within 2 months, including dental surgery, requiring general or spinal anesthesia.

Over age 60:
Adverse reactions and side effects may be more frequent and severe than in younger persons.

Pregnancy:
Risk to unborn child outweighs drug benefits. Don't use.

Breast-feeding:
No problems proven. Avoid if possible. Consult doctor.

Infants & children:
Use only under close medical supervision of clinician experienced in convulsive disorders.

Prolonged use:
Have regular checkups, especially during early months of treatment.

Skin & sunlight:
Increased sensitivity to sunlight or sun lamp. Avoid overexposure.

Driving, piloting or hazardous work:
Don't drive or pilot aircraft until you learn how medicine affects you. Don't work around dangerous machinery. Don't climb ladders or work in high places. Danger increases if you drink alcohol or take medicine affecting alertness and reflexes, such as antihistamines, tranquilizers, sedatives, pain medicine, narcotics and mind-altering drugs. Be especially careful driving at night because medicine can affect vision.

Discontinuing:
Don't discontinue without consulting doctor. Dose may require gradual reduction if you have taken drug for a long time. Doses of other drugs may also require adjustment.

Others:
Arrange for eye exams every 6 months as well as blood counts and kidney-function studies.

POSSIBLE INTERACTION WITH OTHER DRUGS

GENERIC NAME OR DRUG CLASS	COMBINED EFFECT
Antidepressants (tricyclic)	Greater likelihood of seizures.
Antipsychotic medicines	Greater likelihood of seizures.
Anticonvulsants	Increased chance of blood toxicity.
Sedatives, sleeping pills, antihistamines, pain medicine, alchohol, tranquilizers, narcotics, mind-altering drugs.	Extreme drowsiness. Avoid.

POSSIBLE INTERACTION WITH OTHER SUBSTANCES

INTERACTS WITH	COMBINED EFFECT
Alcohol:	Increased chance of seizures and liver damage. Avoid.
Beverages: Caffeine drinks.	May decrease anticonvulsant effect.
Cocaine:	Increased chance of seizures. Avoid.
Foods:	No problems expected.
Marijuana:	Increased chance of seizures. Avoid.
Tobacco:	Decreased absorption of medicine leading to uneven control of disease.

ANTITHYROID MEDICINES

BRAND AND GENERIC NAMES

METHIMAZOLE   Tapazole
PROPYLTHIOURACIL   Thiamazole
Propyl-Thyracil

BASIC INFORMATION

Habit forming? No
Prescription needed? Yes
Available as generic? Yes
Drug class: Antihyperthyroid

USES

- Treatment of overactive thyroid (hyperthyroidism).
- Treatment of angina in patients who have overactive thyroid.

DOSAGE & USAGE INFORMATION

How to take:
Tablet or capsule—Swallow with liquid or food to lessen stomach irritation. If you can't swallow whole, crumble tablet or open capsule and take with liquid or food.

When to take:
At the same times each day.

If you forget a dose:
Take as soon as you remember up to 2 hours late. If more than 2 hours, wait for next scheduled dose (don't double this dose).

What drug does:
Prevents thyroid gland from producing excess thyroid hormone.

Time lapse before drug works:
10 to 20 days.

Don't take with:
- Anticoagulants
- See Interaction column and consult doctor.

OVERDOSE

SYMPTOMS:
Bleeding, spots on skin, jaundice (yellow eyes and skin), loss of consciousness.
WHAT TO DO:
Overdose unlikely to threaten life. If person takes much larger amount than prescribed, call doctor, poison-control center or hospital emergency room for instructions.

POSSIBLE ADVERSE REACTIONS OR SIDE EFFECTS

SYMPTOMS	WHAT TO DO
Life-threatening: None expected.	
Common: Skin rash, itching, dryness.	Discontinue. Call doctor right away.
Infrequent: Dizziness, taste loss, sore throat with chills and fever, abdominal pain, constipation, diarrhea.	Discontinue. Call doctor right away.
Rare: Headache; enlarged lymph glands; irregular or rapid heartbeat; unusual bruising or bleeding; backache; numbness or tingling in toes, fingers or face; joint pain; muscle aches; menstrual irregularities; jaundice; tired, weak, sleepy, listless; swollen eyes or feet.	Discontinue. Call doctor right away.

WARNINGS & PRECAUTIONS

Don't take if:
You are allergic to antithyroid medicines.

Before you start, consult your doctor:
- If you have liver disease.
- If you have blood disease.
- If you have an infection.
- If you take anticoagulants.

Over age 60:
Adverse reactions and side effects may be more frequent and severe than in younger persons.

Pregnancy:
Risk to unborn child outweighs drug benefits. Don't use.

Breast-feeding:
Drug filters into milk. May harm child. Avoid.

Infants & children:
Use only under special medical supervision by experienced clinician.

Prolonged use:
Adverse reactions and side effects more common.

Skin & sunlight:
No problems expected.

Driving, piloting or hazardous work:
Don't drive or pilot aircraft until you learn how medicine affects you. Don't work around dangerous machinery. Don't climb ladders or work in high places. Danger increases if you drink alcohol or take medicine affecting alertness and reflexes, such as antihistamines, tranquilizers, sedatives, pain medicine, narcotics and mind-altering drugs.

Discontinuing:
Don't discontinue without consulting doctor. Dose may require gradual reduction if you have taken drug for a long time. Doses of other drugs may also require adjustment.

Others:
No problems expected.

POSSIBLE INTERACTION WITH OTHER DRUGS

GENERIC NAME OR DRUG CLASS	COMBINED EFFECT
Anticoagulants	Increased effect of anticoagulants.
Antineoplastic drugs	Increased chance to suppress bone marrow.
Chloramphenicol	Increased chance to suppress bone marrow.

POSSIBLE INTERACTION WITH OTHER SUBSTANCES

INTERACTS WITH	COMBINED EFFECT
Alcohol:	Increased possibility of liver toxicity. Avoid.
Beverages:	No problems expected.
Cocaine:	Increased toxicity potential of medicines. Avoid.
Foods:	No problems expected.
Marijuana:	Increased rapid or irregular heartbeat. Avoid.
Tobacco:	Increased chance of rapid heartbeat. Avoid.

APPETITE SUPPRESSANTS

BRAND AND GENERIC NAMES

See complete list of brand names in the *Brand Name Directory,* page 943.

BASIC INFORMATION

Habit forming? Yes
Prescription needed? Yes
Available as generic? Yes
Drug class: Appetite suppressant

 ## USES

Suppresses appetite.

 ## DOSAGE & USAGE INFORMATION

How to take:
- Tablet or capsule—Swallow with liquid. You may chew or crush tablet.
- Extended-release tablets or capsules—Swallow each dose whole with liquid.

When to take:
- Long-acting forms—10 to 14 hours before bedtime.
- Short-acting forms—1 hour before meals. Last dose no later than 4 to 6 hours before bedtime.

If you forget a dose:
- Long-acting form—Take as soon as you remember up to 2 hours late. If more than 2 hours, wait for next scheduled dose (don't double this dose).
- Short-acting form—Wait for next scheduled dose. Don't double this dose.

What drug does:
Apparently stimulates brain's appetite-control center.

Continued next column

 ## OVERDOSE

SYMPTOMS:
Irritability, overactivity, trembling, insomnia, mood changes, rapid heartbeat, confusion, disorientation, hallucinations, convulsions, coma.
WHAT TO DO:
- Dial 0 (operator) or 911 (emergency) for an ambulance or medical help. Then give first aid immediately.
- See emergency information on inside covers.

Time lapse before drug works:
Begins in 1 hour. Short-acting form lasts 4 hours. Long-acting form lasts 14 hours.

Don't take with:
- Non-prescription drugs without consulting doctor.
- See Interaction column and consult doctor.

 ## POSSIBLE ADVERSE REACTIONS OR SIDE EFFECTS

SYMPTOMS	WHAT TO DO
Life-threatening: None expected.	
Common: Irritability, nervousness, insomnia, false sense of well-being.	Continue. Call doctor when convenient.
Infrequent: • Irregular or pounding heartbeat, urgent or difficult urination.	Discontinue. Call doctor right away.
• Blurred vision, unpleasant taste or dry mouth, constipation or diarrhea, nausea, vomiting, cramps, changes in sex drive, increased sweating.	Continue. Call doctor when convenient.
Rare: • Mood changes, rash or hives, breathing difficulty.	Discontinue. Call doctor right away.
• Hair loss.	Continue. Call doctor when convenient.

WARNINGS & PRECAUTIONS

Don't take if:
- You are allergic to any sympathomimetic or phenylpropanolamine.
- You have glaucoma.
- You have taken MAO inhibitors within 2 weeks.
- You plan to become pregnant within medication period.
- You have a history of drug abuse.
- You have irregular or rapid heartbeat.

Before you start, consult your doctor:
- If you have high blood pressure or heart disease.
- If you have an overactive thyroid, nervous tension or "anxiety."
- If you have epilepsy.
- If you will have surgery within 2 months, including dental surgery, requiring general or spinal anesthesia.

Over age 60:
Adverse reactions and side effects may be more frequent and severe than in younger persons.

Pregnancy:
Safety not established. Avoid.

Breast-feeding:
No proven problems. Consult doctor.

Infants & children:
Don't give to children younger than 12.

Prolonged use:
Loses effectiveness. Avoid.

Skin & sunlight:
No problems expected.

Driving, piloting or hazardous work:
Don't drive or pilot aircraft until you learn how medicine affects you. Don't work around dangerous machinery. Don't climb ladders or work in high places. Danger increases if you drink alcohol or take medicine affecting alertness and reflexes, such as antihistamines, tranquilizers, sedatives, pain medicine, narcotics and mind-altering drugs.

Discontinuing:
Don't discontinue without consulting doctor. Dose may require gradual reduction if you have taken drug for a long time. Doses of other drugs may also require adjustment.

Others:
Don't increase dose.

POSSIBLE INTERACTION WITH OTHER DRUGS

GENERIC NAME OR DRUG CLASS	COMBINED EFFECT
Appetite suppressants (other)	Dangerous overstimulation.
Caffeine	Increased stimulant effect of phentermine.
Guanethidine	Decreased guanethidine effect.
Hydralazine	Decreased hydralazine effect.
MAO inhibitors	Dangerous blood-pressure rise.
Methyldopa	Decreased methyldopa effect.
Molindone	Decreased suppressant effect.
Phenothiazines	Decreased appetite suppressant effect.
Rauwolfia alkaloids	Decreased effect of rauwolfia alkaloids.

POSSIBLE INTERACTION WITH OTHER SUBSTANCES

INTERACTS WITH	COMBINED EFFECT
Alcohol: Beer, chianti wines, vermouth.	Dangerous blood-pressure rise.
Beverages: • Caffeine drinks. • Drinks containing tyramine (see Glossary).	Excessive stimulation. Blood-pressure rise.
Cocaine:	Excessive stimulation.
Foods: Foods containing tyramine (see Glossary).	Blood-pressure rise.
Marijuana:	Frequent use—Irregular heartbeat.
Tobacco:	None expected.

ASPIRIN

BRAND NAMES

See complete list of brand names in the *Brand Name Directory*, page 943.

BASIC INFORMATION

Habit forming? No
Prescription needed? No
Available as generic? Yes
Drug class: Analgesic, anti-inflammatory (salicylate)

 ## USES

- Reduces pain, fever, inflammation.
- Relieves swelling, stiffness, joint pain of arthritis or rheumatism.

 ## DOSAGE & USAGE INFORMATION

How to take:
- Tablet or capsule—Swallow with liquid.
- Extended-release tablets or capsules—Swallow each dose whole.
- Suppositories—Remove wrapper and moisten suppository with water. Gently insert into rectum, large end first.

When to take:
Pain, fever, inflammation—As needed, no more often than every 4 hours.

If you forget a dose:
- Pain, fever—Take as soon as you remember. Wait 4 hours for next dose.
- Arthritis—Take as soon as you remember up to 2 hours late. Return to regular schedule.

What drug does:
- Affects hypothalamus, the part of the brain which regulates temperature by dilating small blood vessels in skin.

Continued next column

 ## OVERDOSE

SYMPTOMS:
Ringing in ears; nausea; vomiting; dizziness; fever; deep, rapid breathing; hallucinations; convulsions; coma.
WHAT TO DO:
- Dial 0 (operator) or 911 (emergency) for an ambulance or medical help. Then give first aid immediately.
- See emergency information on inside covers.

- Prevents clumping of platelets (small blood cells) so blood vessels remain open.
- Decreases prostaglandin effect.
- Suppresses body's pain messages.

Time lapse before drug works:
30 minutes for pain, fever, arthritis.

Don't take with:
- Tetracyclines. Space doses 1 hour apart.
- See Interaction column and consult doctor.

 ## POSSIBLE ADVERSE REACTIONS OR SIDE EFFECTS

SYMPTOMS	WHAT TO DO
Life-threatening:	
Black or bloody vomit, blood in urine. Hives, rash, intense itching, faintness soon after a dose (anaphylaxis).	Seek emergency treatment immediately.
Common:	
• Nausea, vomiting.	Discontinue. Seek emergency treatment.
• Heartburn, indigestion.	Continue. Call doctor when convenient.
• Ringing in ears.	Continue. Tell doctor at next visit.
Infrequent:	
None expected.	
Rare:	
• Black stools, unexplained fever.	Discontinue. Seek emergency treatment.
• Rash, hives, itch, diminished vision, shortness of breath, wheezing, jaundice.	Discontinue. Call doctor right away.
• Drowsiness.	Continue. Call doctor when convenient.

 ## WARNINGS & PRECAUTIONS

Don't take if:
- You need to restrict sodium in your diet. Buffered effervescent tablets and sodium salicylate are high in sodium.
- Aspirin has a strong vinegar-like odor, which means it has decomposed.
- You have a peptic ulcer of stomach or duodenum.
- You have a bleeding disorder.

Before you start, consult your doctor:
- If you have had stomach or duodenal ulcers.
- If you have had gout.
- If you have asthma or nasal polyps.

Over age 60:
More likely to cause hidden bleeding in stomach or intestines. Watch for dark stools.

Pregnancy:
Risk to unborn child outweighs drug benefits. Don't use.

Breast-feeding:
Drug passes into milk. Avoid drug or discontinue nursing until you finish medicine. Consult doctor for advice on maintaining milk supply.

Infants & children:
- Overdose frequent and severe. Keep bottles out of children's reach.
- Consult doctor before giving to persons under age 18 who have fever and discomfort of viral illness, especially chicken pox and influenza. Probably increases risk of Reye's syndrome.

Prolonged use:
Kidney damage. Periodic kidney-function test recommended.

Skin & sunlight:
Aspirin combined with sunscreen may decrease sunburn.

Driving, piloting or hazardous work:
No restrictions unless you feel drowsy.

Discontinuing:
For chronic illness—Don't discontinue without doctor's advice until you complete prescribed dose, even though symptoms diminish or disappear.

Others:
- Aspirin can complicate surgery, pregnancy, labor and delivery, and illness.
- For arthritis—Don't change dose without consulting doctor.
- Urine tests for blood sugar may be inaccurate.

 ## POSSIBLE INTERACTION WITH OTHER DRUGS

GENERIC NAME OR DRUG CLASS	COMBINED EFFECT
Acebutolol	Decreased antihypertensive effect of acebutolol.
Allopurinol	Decreased allopurinol effect.
Antacids	Decreased aspirin effect.
Anticoagulants	Increased anticoagulant effect. Abnormal bleeding.
Antidiabetics (oral)	Low blood sugar.
Anti-inflammatory drugs (non-steroid)	Risk of stomach bleeding and ulcers.

Aspirin (other)	Likely aspirin toxicity.
Cortisone drugs	Increased cortisone effect. Risk of ulcers and stomach bleeding.
Furosemide	Possible aspirin toxicity.
Gold compounds	Increased likelihood of kidney damage.
Indomethacin	Risk of stomach bleeding and ulcers.
Ketoprofen	Increased risk of stomach ulcer.
Methotrexate	Increased methotrexate effect.
Minoxidil	Decreased minoxidil effect.
Oxprenolol	Decreased antihypertensive effect of oxprenolol.
Para-aminosalicylic acid (PAS)	Possible aspirin toxicity.
Penicillins	Increased effect of both drugs.
Phenobarbital	Decreased aspirin effect.
Phenytoin	Increased phenytoin effect.
Probenecid	Decreased probenecid effect.
Propranolol	Decreased aspirin effect.
Rauwolfia alkaloids	Decreased aspirin effect.
Salicylates (other)	Likely aspirin toxicity.

Continued page 961

 ## POSSIBLE INTERACTION WITH OTHER SUBSTANCES

INTERACTS WITH	COMBINED EFFECT
Alcohol:	Possible stomach irritation and bleeding. Avoid.
Beverages:	None expected.
Cocaine:	None expected.
Foods:	None expected.
Marijuana:	Possible increased pain relief, but marijuana may slow body's recovery. Avoid.
Tobacco:	None expected.

ATENOLOL

BRAND NAMES

Tenormin

BASIC INFORMATION

Habit forming? No
Prescription needed? Yes
Available as generic? No
Drug class: Beta-adrenergic blocker

 USES

- Reduces angina attacks.
- Stabilizes irregular heartbeat.
- Lowers blood pressure.
- Reduces frequency of migraine headaches. (Does not relieve headache pain.)
- Other uses prescribed by your doctor.

 DOSAGE & USAGE INFORMATION

How to take:
Tablet or capsule—Swallow with liquid. If you can't swallow whole, crumble tablet or open capsule and take with liquid or food.

When to take:
With meals or immediately after.

If you forget a dose:
Take as soon as you remember. Return to regular schedule, but allow 3 hours between doses.

What drug does:
- Blocks certain actions of sympathetic nervous system.
- Lowers heart's oxygen requirements.
- Slows nerve impulses through heart.
- Reduces blood vessel contraction in heart, scalp and other body parts.

Time lapse before drug works:
1 to 4 hours.

Continued next column

 OVERDOSE

SYMPTOMS:
Weakness, slow or weak pulse, blood pressure drop, fainting, convulsions, cold and sweaty skin.
WHAT TO DO:
- **Dial 0 (operator) or 911 (emergency) for an ambulance or medical help. Then give first aid immediately.**
- **See emergency information on inside covers.**

Don't take with:
Non-prescription drugs or drugs in Interaction column without consulting doctor.

 POSSIBLE ADVERSE REACTIONS OR SIDE EFFECTS

SYMPTOMS	WHAT TO DO
Life-threatening:	
None expected.	
Common:	
• Pulse slower than 50 beats per minute.	Discontinue. Call doctor right away.
• Drowsiness, numbness or tingling in fingers or toes, dizziness, diarrhea, nausea, fatigue, weakness.	Continue. Call doctor when convenient.
• Cold hands or feet; dry mouth, eyes, skin.	Continue. Tell doctor at next visit.
Infrequent:	
• Hallucinations, nightmares, insomnia, headache, breathing difficulty, joint pain.	Discontinue. Call doctor right away.
• Confusion, depression, reduced alertness.	Continue. Call doctor when convenient.
• Constipation.	Continue. Tell doctor at next visit.
Rare:	
• Rash, sore throat, fever.	Discontinue. Call doctor right away.
• Unusual bleeding or bruising.	Continue. Call doctor when convenient.

 WARNINGS & PRECAUTIONS

Don't take if:
- You are allergic to any beta-adrenergic blocker.
- You have asthma.
- You have hay fever symptoms.
- You have taken MAO inhibitors in past 2 weeks.

Before you start, consult your doctor:
- If you have heart disease or poor circulation to the extremities.
- If you have hay fever, asthma, chronic bronchitis, emphysema.
- If you have overactive thyroid function.
- If you have impaired liver or kidney function.
- If you will have surgery within 2 months, including dental surgery, requiring general or spinal anesthesia.
- If you have diabetes or hypoglycemia.

Over age 60:
Adverse reactions and side effects may be more frequent and severe than in younger persons.

Pregnancy:
Risk to unborn child outweighs drug benefits. Don't use.

Breast-feeding:
Drug passes into milk. Avoid drug or discontinue nursing until you finish medicine. Consult doctor for advice on maintaining milk supply.

Infants & children:
Not recommended.

Prolonged use:
Weakens heart muscle contractions.

Skin & sunlight:
No problems expected.

Driving, piloting or hazardous work:
Don't drive or pilot aircraft until you learn how medicine affects you. Don't work around dangerous machinery. Don't climb ladders or work in high places. Danger increases if you drink alcohol or take medicine affecting alertness and reflexes.

Discontinuing:
Don't discontinue without consulting doctor. Dose may require gradual reduction if you have taken drug for a long time. Doses of other drugs may also require adjustment.

Others:
May mask hypoglycemia.

 POSSIBLE INTERACTION WITH OTHER DRUGS

GENERIC NAME OR DRUG CLASS	COMBINED EFFECT
Acebutolol	Increased antihypertensive effects of both drugs.
Albuterol	Decreased albuterol effect and Beta-adrenergic blocking effect.
Antidiabetics	Increased antidiabetic effect.
Antihistamines	Decreased antihistamine effect.
Antihypertensives	Increased effect of antihypertensive.
Anti-inflammatory drugs	Decreased effect of anti-inflammatory.
Barbiturates	Increased barbiturate effect. Oversedation.

Digitalis preparations	Increased or decreased heart rate. Improves irregular heartbeat.
Enalapril	Possible excessive potassium in blood.
Narcotics	Increased narcotic effect. Oversedation.
Nitrates	Possible excessive blood-pressure drop.
Pentoxifylline	Increased antihypertensive effect.
Phenytoin	Increased atenolol effect.
Quinidine	Slows heart excessively.
Reserpine	Increased reserpine effect. Excessive sedation and depression.
Tocainide	May worsen congestive heart failure.

 POSSIBLE INTERACTION WITH OTHER SUBSTANCES

INTERACTS WITH	COMBINED EFFECT
Alcohol:	Excessive blood pressure drop. Avoid.
Beverages:	None expected.
Cocaine:	Irregular heartbeat.
Foods:	None expected.
Marijuana:	Daily use—Impaired circulation to hands and feet.
Tobacco:	Possible irregular heartbeat.

ATROPINE

BRAND NAMES

See complete list of brand names in the *Brand Name Directory,* page 944.

BASIC INFORMATION

Habit forming? No
Prescription needed?
  Low strength: No
  High strength: Yes
Available as generic? Yes
Drug class: Antispasmodic, anticholinergic

USES

Reduces spasms of digestive system, bladder and urethra.

DOSAGE & USAGE INFORMATION

How to take:
Tablet—Swallow with liquid or food to lessen stomach irritation.

When to take:
30 minutes before meals (unless directed otherwise by doctor).

If you forget a dose:
Take as soon as you remember up to 2 hours late. If more than 2 hours, wait for next scheduled dose (don't double this dose).

What drug does:
Blocks nerve impulses at parasympathetic nerve endings, preventing muscle contractions and gland secretions of organs involved.

Time lapse before drug works:
15 to 30 minutes.

Don't take with:
See Interaction column and consult doctor.

OVERDOSE

SYMPTOMS:
Dilated pupils, rapid pulse and breathing, dizziness, fever, hallucinations, confusion, slurred speech, agitation, flushed face, convulsions, coma.
WHAT TO DO:
- **Dial 0 (operator) or 911 (emergency) for an ambulance or medical help. Then give first aid immediately.**
- **See emergency information on inside covers.**

POSSIBLE ADVERSE REACTIONS OR SIDE EFFECTS

SYMPTOMS	WHAT TO DO
Life-threatening:	
None expected.	
Common:	
• Confusion, delirium, rapid heartbeat.	Discontinue. Call doctor right away.
• Nausea, vomiting, decreased sweating,	Continue. Call doctor when convenient.
• Constipation.	Continue. Tell doctor at next visit.
• Dryness in ears, nose, throat.	No action necessary.
Infrequent:	
Headache, difficult or painful urination.	Continue. Call doctor when convenient.
Rare:	
Rash or hives, pain, blurred vision.	Discontinue. Call doctor right away.

WARNINGS & PRECAUTIONS

Don't take if:
- You are allergic to any anticholinergic.
- You have trouble with stomach bloating.
- You have difficulty emptying your bladder completely.
- You have narrow-angle glaucoma.
- You have severe ulcerative colitis.

Before you start, consult your doctor:
- If you have open-angle glaucoma.
- If you have angina.
- If you have chronic bronchitis or asthma.
- If you have liver disease.
- If you have hiatal hernia.
- If you have enlarged prostate.
- If you have myasthenia gravis.
- If you have peptic ulcer.
- If you will have surgery within 2 months, including dental surgery, requiring general or spinal anesthesia.

Over age 60:
Adverse reactions and side effects may be more frequent and severe than in younger persons.

Pregnancy:
Studies inconclusive on harm to unborn child. Animal studies show fetal abnormalities. Decide with your doctor whether drug benefits justify risk to unborn child.

Breast-feeding:
Drug passes into milk and decreases milk flow. Avoid drug or discontinue nursing until you finish medicine. Consult doctor for advice on maintaining milk supply.

Infants & children:
Use only under medical supervision.

Prolonged use:
Chronic constipation, possible fecal impaction. Consult doctor immediately.

Skin & sunlight:
No problems expected.

Driving, piloting or hazardous work:
Use disqualifies you for piloting aircraft. Otherwise, no problems expected.

Discontinuing:
May be unnecessary to finish medicine. Follow doctor's instructions.

Others:
No problems expected.

POSSIBLE INTERACTION WITH OTHER DRUGS

GENERIC NAME OR DRUG CLASS	COMBINED EFFECT
Amantadine	Increased atropine effect.
Anticholinergics (other)	Increased atropine effect.
Antidepressants (tricyclic)	Increased atropine effect. Increased sedation.
Antihistamines	Increased atropine effect.
Cortisone drugs	Increased internal-eye pressure.
Haloperidol	Increased internal-eye pressure.
MAO inhibitors	Increased atropine effect.
Meperidine	Increased atropine effect.
Methylphenidate	Increased atropine effect.
Molindone	Increased anticholinergic effect.
Nitrates	Increased internal-eye pressure.
Orphenadrine	Increased atropine effect.

Phenothiazines	Increased atropine effect.
Pilocarpine	Loss of pilocarpine effect in glaucoma treatment.
Potassium supplements	Possible intestinal ulcers with oral potassium tablets.
Vitamin C	Decreased atropine effect. Avoid large doses of vitamin C.

POSSIBLE INTERACTION WITH OTHER SUBSTANCES

INTERACTS WITH	COMBINED EFFECT
Alcohol:	None expected.
Beverages:	None expected.
Cocaine:	Excessively rapid heartbeat. Avoid.
Foods:	None expected.
Marijuana:	Drowsiness and dry mouth.
Tobacco:	None expected.

ATROPINE, HYOSCYAMINE, METHENAMINE, METHYLENE BLUE, PHENYLSALICYLATE & BENZOIC ACID

BRAND NAMES

Dolsed	Urinary Antiseptic
Hexalol	No. 2
Prosed	Urised
Trac Tabs	Urisep
U-Tract	Uritab
UAA	Urithol
Uramine	Uritin
Uridon Modified	Uroblue
Urimed	Uro-Ves

BASIC INFORMATION

Habit forming? No
Prescription needed? Yes
Available as generic? No
Drug class: Urinary tract analgesic,
　　　　　　antispasmodic, anti-infective

USES

A combination medicine to control infection,
spasms and pain caused by urinary tract
infections.

DOSAGE & USAGE INFORMATION

How to take:
Tablet—Swallow with liquid or food to lessen
stomach irritation.

When to take:
30 minutes before meals (unless directed
otherwise by doctor).

If you forget a dose:
Take as soon as you remember up to 2 hours
late. If more than 2 hours, wait for next
scheduled dose (don't double this dose).

Continued next column

OVERDOSE

SYMPTOMS:
**Dilated pupils, rapid pulse and breathing,
dizziness, fever, hallucinations, confusion,
slurred speech, agitation, flushed face,
convulsions, coma.**
WHAT TO DO:
● **Dial 0 (operator) or 911 (emergency) for an
ambulance or medical help. Then give first
aid immediately.**
● **See emergency information on inside
covers.**

What drug does:
Makes urine acid. Blocks nerve impulses at
parasympathetic nerve endings, preventing
muscle contractions and gland secretions of
organs involved. Methenamine destroys some
germs.

Time lapse before drug works:
15 to 30 minutes.

Don't take with:
See Interaction column and consult doctor.

POSSIBLE ADVERSE REACTIONS OR SIDE EFFECTS

SYMPTOMS	WHAT TO DO
Life-threatening:	
Heartbeat irregularity, shortness of breath or difficulty breathing.	Seek emergency treatment immediately.
Common:	
Dry mouth, throat.	Continue. Call doctor when convenient.
Infrequent:	
Flushed, red face; drowsiness; difficult urination; nausea and vomiting; abdominal pain; ringing or buzzing in ears; severe drowsiness; back pain.	Discontinue. Call doctor right away.
Rare:	
Blurred vision; pain in eyes; skin rash, hives.	Discontinue. Seek emergency treatment.

WARNINGS & PRECAUTIONS

Don't take if:
● You are allergic to any of the ingredients or
aspirin.
● Brain damage in child.
● You have glaucoma.

Before you start, consult your doctor:
● If you are on any special diet such as
low-sodium.
● If you have had a hiatal hernia, bronchitis,
asthma, liver disease, stomach or duodenal
ulcers.
● If you have asthma, nasal polyps, bleeding
disorder or enlarged prostate.
● If you will have any surgery within 2 months.

ATROPINE, HYOSCYAMINE, METHENAMINE, METHYLENE BLUE, PHENYLSALICYLATE & BENZOIC ACID

Over age 60:
- Adverse reactions and side effects may be more frequent and severe than in younger persons.
- More likely to cause hidden bleeding in stomach or intestines. Watch for dark stools.

Pregnancy:
Risk to unborn child outweighs benefits. Don't use.

Breast-feeding:
Drug passes into milk. Avoid or discontinue nursing until you finish medicine.

Infants & children:
Side effects more likely. Not recommended in children under 12.

Prolonged use:
May lead to constipation or kidney damage. Request lab studies to monitor effects of prolonged use.

Skin & sunlight:
No problems expected.

Driving, piloting or hazardous work:
May disqualify for piloting aircraft during time you take medicine.

Discontinuing:
May be unnecessary to finish medicine. Follow your symptoms and doctor's advice.

Others:
- Salicylates can complicate surgery, pregnancy, labor and delivery, and illness.
- Urine tests for blood sugar may be inaccurate.
- Drink cranberry juice or eat prunes or plums to help make urine more acid.

 ## POSSIBLE INTERACTION WITH OTHER DRUGS

GENERIC NAME OR DRUG CLASS	COMBINED EFFECT
Acebutolol	Decreased antihypertensive effect of acebutolol.
Allopurinol	Decreased allopurinol effect.
Amantadine	Increased atropine and belladonna effect.
Antacids	Decreased salicylate and methenamine effect.
Anticoagulants	Increased anticoagulant effect. Abnormal bleeding.

Anticholinergics (other)	Increased atropine and belladonna effect.
Antidepressants (other)	Increased hyoscyamine and belladonna effect. Increased sedation.
Antidiabetics (oral)	Low blood sugar.
Anti-inflammatory drugs (non-steroid)	Risk of stomach bleeding and ulcers.
Antihistamines	Increased atropine and hyoscyamine effect.
Aspirin	Likely salicylate toxicity.
Carbonic anhydrase inhibitors	Decreased methenamine effect.
Cortisone drugs	Increased internal-eye pressure, increased cortisone effect. Risk of ulcers and stomach bleeding.
Diuretics (thiazide)	Decreased urine acidity.
Furosemide	Possible salicylate toxicity.
Gold compounds	Increased likelihood of kidney damage.
Haloperidol	Increased internal-eye pressure.
Indomethacin	Risk of stomach bleeding and ulcers.
MAO inhibitors	Increased belladonna and atropine effect.

Continued page 961

 ## POSSIBLE INTERACTION WITH OTHER SUBSTANCES

INTERACTS WITH	COMBINED EFFECT
Alcohol:	Excessive sedation. Possible stomach irritation and bleeding. Avoid.
Beverages:	None expected.
Cocaine:	Excessively rapid heartbeat. Avoid.
Foods:	None expected.
Marijuana:	Drowsiness and dry mouth. May slow body's recovery.
Tobacco:	Dry mouth.

AZATADINE

BRAND NAMES

Optimine   Trinalin Repetabs

BASIC INFORMATION

Habit forming? No
Prescription needed? Yes
Available as generic? No
Drug class: Antihistamine

 USES

- Reduces allergic symptoms such as hay fever, hives, rash or itching.
- Induces sleep.

 DOSAGE & USAGE INFORMATION

How to take:
Tablet—Swallow with liquid or food to lessen stomach irritation.

When to take:
Varies with form. Follow label directions.

If you forget a dose:
Take as soon as you remember up to 2 hours late. If more than 2 hours, wait for next scheduled dose (don't double this dose).

What drug does:
Blocks action of histamine after an allergic response triggers histamine release in sensitive cells.

Time lapse before drug works:
30 minutes.

Don't take with:
See Interaction column and consult doctor.

 OVERDOSE

SYMPTOMS:
Convulsions, red face, hallucinations, coma.
WHAT TO DO:
- Dial 0 (operator) or 911 (emergency) for an ambulance or medical help. Then give first aid immediately.
- If patient is unconscious and not breathing, give mouth-to-mouth breathing. If there is no heartbeat, use cardiac massage and mouth-to-mouth breathing (CPR). Don't try to make patient vomit. If you can't get help quickly, take patient to nearest emergency facility.
- See emergency information on inside covers.

 POSSIBLE ADVERSE REACTIONS OR SIDE EFFECTS

SYMPTOMS	WHAT TO DO
Life-threatening: None expected.	
Common: Drowsiness; dizziness; dry mouth, nose, throat; nausea.	Continue. Tell doctor at next visit.
Infrequent:	
• Changes in vision.	Discontinue. Call doctor right away.
• Less tolerance for contact lenses, difficult urination.	Continue. Call doctor when convenient.
• Appetite loss.	Continue. Tell doctor at next visit.
Rare: Nightmares, agitation, irritability, sore throat, fever, rapid heartbeat, unusual bleeding or bruising, fatigue, weakness.	Discontinue. Call doctor right away.

WARNINGS & PRECAUTIONS

Don't take if:
You are allergic to any antihistamine.

Before you start, consult your doctor:
- If you have glaucoma.
- If you have enlarged prostate.
- If you have asthma.
- If you have kidney disease.
- If you have peptic ulcer.
- If you will have surgery within 2 months, including dental surgery, requiring general or spinal anesthesia.

Over age 60:
Don't exceed recommended dose. Adverse reactions and side effects may be more frequent and severe than in younger persons, especially urination difficulty, diminished alertness and other brain and nervous-system symptoms.

Pregnancy:
No proven harm to unborn child. Avoid if possible.

Breast-feeding:
Drug passes into milk. Avoid drug or discontinue nursing until you finish medicine. Consult doctor for advice on maintaining milk supply.

Infants & children:
Not recommended for premature or newborn infants. Otherwise, no problems expected.

Prolonged use:
Avoid. May damage bone-marrow and nerve cells.

Skin & sunlight:
May cause rash or intensify sunburn in areas exposed to sun or sunlamp.

Driving, piloting or hazardous work:
Don't drive or pilot aircraft until you learn how medicine affects you. Don't work around dangerous machinery. Don't climb ladders or work in high places. Danger increases if you drink alcohol or take medicine affecting alertness and reflexes, such as antihistamines, tranquilizers, sedatives, pain medicine, narcotics and mind-altering drugs.

Discontinuing:
No problems expected.

Others:
May mask symptoms of hearing damage from aspirin, other salicylates, cisplatin, paromomycin, vancomycin or anticonvulsants. Consult doctor if you use these.

POSSIBLE INTERACTION WITH OTHER DRUGS

GENERIC NAME OR DRUG CLASS	COMBINED EFFECT
Anticholinergics	Increased anticholinergic effect.
Antidepressants	Excess sedation. Avoid.
Antihistamines (other)	Excess sedation. Avoid.
Dronabinol	Increased effects of both drugs. Avoid.
Hypnotics	Excess sedation. Avoid.
MAO inhibitors	Increased azatadine effect.
Mind-altering drugs	Excess sedation. Avoid.
Molindone	Increased antihistamine effect.
Narcotics	Excess sedation. Avoid.
Sedatives	Excess sedation. Avoid.
Sleep inducers	Excess sedation. Avoid.
Tranquilizers	Excess sedation. Avoid.

POSSIBLE INTERACTION WITH OTHER SUBSTANCES

INTERACTS WITH	COMBINED EFFECT
Alcohol:	Excess sedation. Avoid.
Beverages: Caffeine drinks.	Less azatadine sedation.
Cocaine:	Decreased azatadine effect. Avoid.
Foods:	None expected.
Marijuana:	Excess sedation. Avoid.
Tobacco:	None expected.

AZT (AZIDOTHYMIDINE), Also Called ZIDOVUDINE

BRAND NAMES

Retrovir

BASIC INFORMATION

Habit forming? No
Prescription needed? Yes
Available as generic? No
Drug class: Antiviral

 USES

Treatment of selected adult patients with AIDS (autoimmune deficiency syndrome) and advanced ARC (AIDS Related Complex) who have a history of pneumonia caused by *Pneumocystis carinii.*

 DOSAGE & USAGE INFORMATION

How to take:
Tablet or capsule—Swallow with liquid.

When to take:
Every 4 hours around the clock unless instructed otherwise.

If you forget a dose:
Take as soon as you remember.

What drug does:
Inhibits reproduction of some viruses, including HIV virus (the virus that causes AIDS).

Time lapse before drug works:
May require several weeks of treatment for full effect.

Don't take with:
See Interaction column and consult doctor.

 OVERDOSE

SYMPTOMS:
No cases reported. However, if overdose occurs, follow instructions below.
WHAT TO DO:
- **Dial 0 (operator) or 911 (emergency) for an ambulance or medical help. Then give first aid immediately.**
- **See emergency information on inside covers.**

 POSSIBLE ADVERSE REACTIONS OR SIDE EFFECTS

SYMPTOMS	WHAT TO DO
Life-threatening: None expected.	
Common:	
• Anemia, low white-blood-cell count.	Discontinue. Call doctor right away.
• Severe headache, nausea, insomnia.	Continue. Call doctor when convenient.
Infrequent: Severe headache, sweating, fever, appetite loss, abdominal pain, vomiting, aching muscles, dizziness, numbness in hands and feet, shortness of breath, skin rash, strange taste.	Continue. Call doctor when convenient.
Rare: None expected.	

WARNINGS & PRECAUTIONS

Don't take if:
You are allergic to any component of this capsule.

Before you start, consult your doctor:
- If you know you have a low white-blood-cell count or severe anemia.
- If you have severe kidney or liver disease.

Over age 60:
Adverse reactions and side effects may be more frequent and severe than in younger persons. Ask doctor about smaller doses.

Pregnancy:
Effect unknown at present.

Breast-feeding:
Drug passes into milk. If possible, avoid drug or discontinue until you finish medicine. Consult your doctor for advice on maintaining milk supply.

Infants & children:
Not recommended.

Prolonged use:
Not recommended.

Skin & sunlight:
No problems expected.

Driving, piloting, or hazardous work:
Don't drive or pilot aircraft until you learn how medicine affects you. Don't work around dangerous machinery. Don't climb ladders or work in high places. Danger increases if you drink alcohol or take medicine affecting alertness and reflexes, such as antihistamines, tranquilizers, sedatives, pain medicine, narcotics and mind-altering drugs.

Discontinuing:
Don't discontinue without consulting your doctor. Dose may require gradual reduction if you have taken drug for a long time. Doses of other drugs may also require adjustment.

Others:
- Drug is still considered experimental so full safety and effectiveness are unknown.
- AZT does *not cure* HIV virus infections. Transfusions or dose modification may be necessary if toxicity develops.
- Have blood counts followed closely during treatment to detect anemia or lowered white-blood-cell count.
- AZT does not reduce risk of transmitting disease to others.

POSSIBLE INTERACTION WITH OTHER DRUGS

GENERIC NAME OR DRUG CLASS	COMBINED EFFECT
Acetaminophen	May increase toxic effects of AZT.
Acyclovir	Lethargy, convulsions.
Aspirin	May increase toxic effects of AZT.
Indomethacin	May increase toxic effects of AZT.
Probenecid	May increase toxic effects of AZT.

POSSIBLE INTERACTION WITH OTHER SUBSTANCES

INTERACTS WITH	COMBINED EFFECT
Alcohol:	Unknown. Best avoid.
Beverages:	None expected.
Cocaine:	Unknown. Best avoid.
Foods:	None expected.
Marijuana:	Unknown. Best avoid.
Tobacco:	None expected.

BACAMPICILLIN

BRAND NAMES

Spectrobid

BASIC INFORMATION

Habit forming? No
Prescription needed? Yes
Available as generic? No
Drug class: Antibiotic (penicillin)

 USES

Treatment of bacterial infections that are
susceptible to bacampicillin.

 DOSAGE & USAGE INFORMATION

How to take:
- Tablets or capsules—Swallow with liquid on
  an empty stomach 1 hour before meals or 2
  hours after eating.
- Liquid—Take with cold beverage. Liquid form
  is perishable and effective for only 7 days at
  room temperature. Effective for 14 days if
  stored in refrigerator. Don't freeze.

When to take:
Follow instructions on prescription label or side
of package. Doses should be evenly spaced.
For example, 4 times a day means every 6
hours.

If you forget a dose:
Take as soon as you remember. Continue
regular schedule.

What drug does:
Destroys susceptible bacteria. Does not kill
viruses.

Time lapse before drug works:
May be several days before medicine affects
infection.

Don't take with:
See Interaction column and consult doctor.

 OVERDOSE

SYMPTOMS:
Severe diarrhea, nausea or vomiting.
WHAT TO DO:
Overdose unlikely to threaten life. If person
takes much larger amount than prescribed,
call doctor, poison-control center or hospital
emergency room for specific instructions.

 POSSIBLE ADVERSE REACTIONS OR SIDE EFFECTS

SYMPTOMS	WHAT TO DO
Life-threatening:	
Hives, rash, intense itching, faintness soon after a dose (anaphylaxis).	Seek emergency treatment immediately.
Common:	
Dark or discolored tongue.	Continue. Tell doctor at next visit.
Infrequent:	
Mild nausea, vomiting, diarrhea.	Continue. Call doctor when convenient.
Rare:	
Unexplained bleeding.	Discontinue. Call doctor right away.

WARNINGS & PRECAUTIONS

Don't take if:
You are allergic to bacampicillin, cephalosporin antibiotics, other penicillins or penicillamine. Life-threatening reaction may occur.

Before you start, consult your doctor:
If you are allergic to any substance or drug.

Over age 60:
You may have skin reactions, particularly around genitals and anus.

Pregnancy:
Studies inconclusive on harm to unborn child. Animal studies show fetal abnormalities. Decide with your doctor whether drug benefits justify risk to unborn child.

Breast-feeding:
Drug passes into milk. Child may become sensitive to this and all penicillins. Avoid bacampicillin or discontinue nursing until you finish medicine. Consult doctor for advice on maintaining milk supply.

Infants & children:
No problems expected.

Prolonged use:
You may become more susceptible to infections caused by germs not responsive to bacampicillin.

Skin & sunlight:
No problems expected.

Driving, piloting, or hazardous work:
Usually not dangerous. Most hazardous reactions likely to occur a few minutes after taking bacampicillin.

Discontinuing:
Don't discontinue without doctor's advice until you complete prescribed dose, even though symptoms diminish or disappear.

Others:
Urine sugar test for diabetes may show false positive result.

POSSIBLE INTERACTION WITH OTHER DRUGS

GENERIC NAME OR DRUG CLASS	COMBINED EFFECT
Beta-adrenergic blockers	Increased chance of anaphylaxis (see emergency information on inside front cover).
Chloramphenicol	Decreased effect of both drugs.
Erythromycins	Decreased effect of both drugs.
Loperamide	Decreased bacampicillin effect.
Paromomycin	Decreased effect of both drugs.
Tetracyclines	Decreased effect of both drugs.
Troleandomycin	Decreased effect of both drugs.

POSSIBLE INTERACTION WITH OTHER SUBSTANCES

INTERACTS WITH	COMBINED EFFECT
Alcohol:	Occasional stomach irritation.
Beverages:	None expected.
Cocaine:	No proven problems.
Foods:	None expected.
Marijuana:	No proven problems.
Tobacco:	None expected.

BACLOFEN

BRAND NAMES

Lioresal

BASIC INFORMATION

Habit forming? No
Prescription needed? Yes
Available as generic? No
Drug class: Muscle relaxant (analgesic)

 USES

- Relieves spasms, cramps and spasticity of muscles caused by medical problems, including multiple sclerosis and spine injuries.
- Reduces number and severity of trigeminal neuralgia attacks.

 DOSAGE & USAGE INFORMATION

How to take:
Tablet or capsule—Swallow with liquid or food to lessen stomach irritation.

When to take:
3 or 4 times daily as directed.

If you forget a dose:
Take as soon as you remember up to 2 hours late. If more than 2 hours, wait for next scheduled dose (don't double this dose).

What drug does:
Blocks body's pain and reflex messages to brain.

Time lapse before drug works:
Variable. Few hours to weeks.

Continued next column

 OVERDOSE

SYMPTOMS:
Blurred vision, blindness, difficult breathing, muscle weakness, convulsive seizures.
WHAT TO DO:
- Dial 0 (operator) or 911 (emergency) for an ambulance or medical help. Then give first aid immediately.
- If patient is unconscious and not breathing, give mouth-to-mouth breathing. If there is no heartbeat, use cardiac massage and mouth-to-mouth breathing (CPR). Don't try to make patient vomit. If you can't get help quickly, take patient to nearest emergency facility.
- See emergency information on inside covers.

Don't take with:
See Interaction column and consult doctor.

 POSSIBLE ADVERSE REACTIONS OR SIDE EFFECTS

SYMPTOMS	WHAT TO DO
Life-threatening:	
None expected.	
Common:	
Dizziness, lightheadedness, confusion, drowsiness, nausea.	Continue. Call doctor when convenient.
Infrequent:	
• Rash with itching, numbness or tingling in hands or feet.	Discontinue. Call doctor right away.
• Headache, abdominal pain, diarrhea or constipation, appetite loss, muscle weakness, difficult or painful urination, male sex problems.	Continue. Call doctor when convenient.
Rare:	
• Fainting, hallucinations, depression, weakness, chest pain.	Discontinue. Call doctor right away.
• Ringing in ears, lowered blood pressure, pounding heartbeat.	Continue. Call doctor when convenient.

WARNINGS & PRECAUTIONS

Don't take if:
You are allergic to any muscle relaxant.

Before you start, consult your doctor:
- If you have Parkinson's disease.
- If you have cerebral palsy.
- If you have had a recent stroke.
- If you have had a recent head injury.
- If you have arthritis.
- If you have diabetes.
- If you have epilepsy.
- If you have psychosis.
- If you have kidney disease.
- If you will have surgery within 2 months, including dental surgery, requiring general or spinal anesthesia.

Over age 60:
Adverse reactions and side effects may be more frequent and severe than in younger persons.

Pregnancy:
Risk to unborn child outweighs drug benefits. Don't use.

Breast-feeding:
Avoid nursing or discontinue until you finish medicine.

Infants & children:
Not recommended.

Prolonged use:
Epileptic patients should be monitored with EEGs. Diabetics should more closely monitor blood sugar levels. Obtain periodic liver function tests.

Skin & sunlight:
No problems expected.

Driving, piloting or hazardous work:
Don't drive or pilot aircraft until you learn how medicine affects you. Don't work around dangerous machinery. Don't climb ladders or work in high places. Danger increases if you drink alcohol or take medicine affecting alertness and reflexes, such as antihistamines, tranquilizers, sedatives, pain medicine, narcotics and mind-altering drugs.

Discontinuing:
Don't discontinue without consulting doctor. Dose may require gradual reduction if you have taken drug for a long time. Doses of other drugs may also require adjustment.

Others:
No problems expected.

POSSIBLE INTERACTION WITH OTHER DRUGS

GENERIC NAME OR DRUG CLASS	COMBINED EFFECT
CNS depressants: antidepressants, antihistamines, muscle relaxants (other), narcotics, sedatives, sleeping pills, tranquilizers.	Increased sedation. Low blood pressure. Avoid.
General anesthetics	Increased sedation. Low blood pressure. Avoid.
Insulin and oral medications for diabetes	Need to adjust diabetes medicine dosage.

POSSIBLE INTERACTION WITH OTHER SUBSTANCES

INTERACTS WITH	COMBINED EFFECT
Alcohol:	Increased sedation. Low blood pressure. Avoid.
Beverages:	No problems expected.
Cocaine:	Increased spasticity. Avoid.
Foods:	No problems expected.
Marijuana:	Increased spasticity. Avoid.
Tobacco:	May interfere with absorption of medicine.

BECLOMETHASONE

BRAND NAMES

Beclovent Inhaler   Vancenase Inhaler
Beconase Inhaler   Vanceril Inhaler
Propaderm

BASIC INFORMATION

Habit forming? No
Prescription needed? Yes
Available as generic? No
Drug class: Cortisone drug (adrenal corticosteroid), antiasthmatic

 ## USES

Prevents attacks of bronchial asthma and allergic hay fever. Does not stop an active asthma attack.

 ## DOSAGE & USAGE INFORMATION

How to take:
Follow package instructions. Don't inhale more than twice per dose. Rinse mouth after use to prevent hoarseness, throat irritation and mouth infection.

When to take:
Regularly at the same times each day.

If you forget a dose:
Take as soon as you remember up to 2 hours late. If more than 2 hours, wait for next scheduled dose (don't double this dose).

What drug does:
Reduces inflammation in bronchial tubes.

Time lapse before drug works:
1 to 4 weeks.

Don't take with:
See Interaction column and consult doctor.

 ## OVERDOSE

SYMPTOMS:
Fluid retention, flushed face, nervousness, stomach irritation.
WHAT TO DO:
Overdose unlikely to threaten life. If person inhales much larger amount than prescribed, call doctor, poison-control center or hospital emergency room for instructions.

 ## POSSIBLE ADVERSE REACTIONS OR SIDE EFFECTS

SYMPTOMS	WHAT TO DO
Life-threatening: None expected.	
Common: Fungus infection with white patches in mouth, dryness, sore throat.	Continue. Call doctor when convenient.
Infrequent: • Rash.	Discontinue. Call doctor right away.
• Lung inflammation, spasm of bronchial tubes.	Continue. Call doctor when convenient.
Rare: None expected.	

BECLOMETHASONE

WARNINGS & PRECAUTIONS

Don't take if:
- You are allergic to beclomethasone.
- You have had tuberculosis.
- You are having an asthma attack.

Before you start, consult your doctor:
- If you take other cortisone drugs.
- If you have an infection.

Over age 60:
More likely to develop lung infections.

Pregnancy:
Risk to unborn child outweighs drug benefits. Don't use.

Breast-feeding:
Drug passes into milk. Avoid drug or discontinue nursing.

Infants & children:
Use only under medical supervision.

Prolonged use:
No problems expected.

Skin & sunlight:
No problems expected.

Driving, piloting or hazardous work:
No problems expected.

Discontinuing:
Don't discontinue without doctor's advice until you complete prescribed dose, even though symptoms diminish or disappear.

Others:
- Unrelated illness or injury may require cortisone drugs by mouth or injection. Notify your doctor.
- Consult doctor as soon as possible if your asthma returns while using beclamethasone as a preventive.
- Drug can reactivate tuberculosis.

POSSIBLE INTERACTION WITH OTHER DRUGS

GENERIC NAME OR DRUG CLASS	COMBINED EFFECT
Antiasthmatics (other)	Increased antiasthmatic effect.
Ephedrine	Increased beclomethasone effect.
Epinephrine	Increased beclomethasone effect.
Indapamide	Possible excessive potassium loss, causing dangerous heartbeat irregularity.
Isoetharine	Increased beclomethasone effect.
Isoproterenol	Increased beclomethasone effect.
Potassium supplements	Decreased potassium effect.
Terbutaline	Increased beclomethasone effect.
Theophylline	Increased beclomethasone effect.

POSSIBLE INTERACTION WITH OTHER SUBSTANCES

INTERACTS WITH	COMBINED EFFECT
Alcohol:	None expected.
Beverages:	None expected.
Cocaine:	None expected.
Foods:	None expected.
Marijuana:	Decreased beclomethasone effect.
Tobacco:	Decreased beclomethasone effect.

BELLADONNA

BRAND NAMES

See complete list of brand names in the *Brand Name Directory*, page 944.

BASIC INFORMATION

Habit forming? No
Prescription needed?
  Low strength: No
  High strength: Yes
Available as generic? Yes
Drug class: Antispasmodic, anticholinergic

USES

Reduces spasms of digestive system, bladder and urethra.

DOSAGE & USAGE INFORMATION

How to take:
- Tablet, elixir or capsule—Swallow with liquid or food to lessen stomach irritation.
- Drops—Dilute dose in beverage before swallowing.

When to take:
30 minutes before meals (unless directed otherwise by doctor).

If you forget a dose:
Take as soon as you remember up to 2 hours late. If more than 2 hours, wait for next scheduled dose (don't double this dose).

What drug does:
Blocks nerve impulses at parasympathetic nerve endings, preventing muscle contractions and gland secretions of organs involved.

Time lapse before drug works:
15 to 30 minutes.

Don't take with:
See Interaction column and consult doctor.

OVERDOSE

SYMPTOMS:
Dilated pupils, rapid pulse and breathing, dizziness, fever, hallucinations, confusion, slurred speech, agitation, flushed face, convulsions, coma.
WHAT TO DO:
- **Dial 0 (operator) or 911 (emergency) for an ambulance or medical help. Then give first aid immediately.**
- **See emergency information on inside covers.**

POSSIBLE ADVERSE REACTIONS OR SIDE EFFECTS

SYMPTOMS	WHAT TO DO
Life-threatening:	
None expected.	
Common:	
● Confusion, delirium, rapid heartbeat.	Discontinue. Call doctor right away.
● Nausea, vomiting, decreased sweating,	Continue. Call doctor when convenient.
● Constipation.	Continue. Tell doctor at next visit.
● Dryness in ears, nose, throat.	No action necessary.
Infrequent:	
Headache, difficult urination.	Continue. Call doctor when convenient.
Rare:	
Rash or hives, pain, blurred vision.	Discontinue. Call doctor right away.

WARNINGS & PRECAUTIONS

Don't take if:
- You are allergic to any anticholinergic.
- You have trouble with stomach bloating.
- You have difficulty emptying your bladder completely.
- You have narrow-angle glaucoma.
- You have severe ulcerative colitis.

Before you start, consult your doctor:
- If you have open-angle glaucoma.
- If you have angina.
- If you have chronic bronchitis or asthma.
- If you have hiatal hernia.
- If you have liver disease.
- If you have enlarged prostate.
- If you have myasthenia gravis.
- If you have peptic ulcer.
- If you will have surgery within 2 months, including dental surgery, requiring general or spinal anesthesia.

Over age 60:
Adverse reactions and side effects may be more frequent and severe than in younger persons.

Pregnancy:
Studies inconclusive on harm to unborn child. Animal studies show fetal abnormalities. Decide with your doctor whether drug benefits justify risk to unborn child.

Breast-feeding:
Drug passes into milk and decreases milk flow. Avoid drug or discontinue nursing until you finish medicine. Consult doctor for advice on maintaining milk supply.

Infants & children:
Use only under medical supervision.

Prolonged use:
Chronic constipation, possible fecal impaction.
Consult doctor immediately.

Skin & sunlight:
No problems expected.

Driving, piloting or hazardous work:
Use disqualifies you for piloting aircraft.
Otherwise, no problems expected.

Discontinuing:
May be unnecessary to finish medicine. Follow doctor's instructions.

Others:
No problems expected.

POSSIBLE INTERACTION WITH OTHER DRUGS

GENERIC NAME OR DRUG CLASS	COMBINED EFFECT
Amantadine	Increased belladonna effect.
Anticholinergics (other)	Increased belladonna effect.
Antidepressants (tricyclic)	Increased belladonna effect. Increased sedation.
Antihistamines	Increased belladonna effect.
Cortisone drugs	Increased internal-eye pressure.
Haloperidol	Increased internal-eye pressure.
MAO inhibitors	Increased belladonna effect.
Meperidine	Increased belladonna effect.
Methylphenidate	Increased belladonna effect.
Molindone	Increased anticholinergic effect.
Nitrates	Increased internal-eye pressure.
Orphenadrine	Increased belladonna effect.
Phenothiazines	Increased belladonna effect.

Pilocarpine	Loss of pilocarpine effect in glaucoma treatment.
Potassium supplements	Possible intestinal ulcers with oral potassium tablets.
Vitamin C	Decreased belladonna effect. Avoid large doses of vitamin C.

POSSIBLE INTERACTION WITH OTHER SUBSTANCES

INTERACTS WITH	COMBINED EFFECT
Alcohol:	None expected.
Beverages:	None expected.
Cocaine:	Excessively rapid heartbeat. Avoid.
Foods:	None expected.
Marijuana:	Drowsiness and dry mouth.
Tobacco:	None expected.

BELLADONNA ALKALOIDS & BARBITURATES

BRAND NAMES

See complete list of brand names in the *Brand Name Directory,* page 945.

BASIC INFORMATION

Habit forming? Yes
Prescription needed? Yes
Available as generic? Some yes, some no
Drug class: Antispasmodic, anticholinergic, sedative

 ## USES

- Reduces spasms of digestive system, bladder and urethra.
- Reduces anxiety or nervous tension (low dose).
- Relieves insomnia (higher bedtime dose).

 ## DOSAGE & USAGE INFORMATION

How to take:
- Tablet, liquid or capsule—Swallow with liquid or food to lessen stomach irritation. If you can't swallow whole, crumble tablet or open capsule and take with liquid or food.
- Extended-release tablets or capsules—Swallow each dose whole.
- Drops—Dilute dose in beverage before swallowing.

When to take:
At the same times each day.

If you forget a dose:
Take as soon as you remember up to 2 hours late. If more than 2 hours, wait for next scheduled dose (don't double this dose).

What drug does:
- May partially block nerve impulses at nerve-cell connections.

Continued next column

 ## OVERDOSE

SYMPTOMS:
Blurred vision, confusion, convulsions, irregular heartbeat, hallucinations, coma.
WHAT TO DO:
- **Dial 0 (operator) or 911 (emergency) for an ambulance or medical help. Then give first aid immediately.**
- **See emergency information on inside covers.**

- Blocks nerve impulses at parasympathetic nerve endings, preventing muscle contractions and gland secretions of organs involved.

Time lapse before drug works:
15 to 30 minutes.

Don't take with:
See Interaction column and consult doctor.

 ## POSSIBLE ADVERSE REACTIONS OR SIDE EFFECTS

SYMPTOMS	WHAT TO DO
Life-threatening:	
Unusual excitement, restlessness, fast heartbeat, breathing difficulty.	Seek emergency treatment immediately.
Common:	
• Dry mouth, throat, nose; drowsiness; constipation; dizziness; nausea; vomiting; "hangover" effect; depression; confusion.	Discontinue. Call doctor right away.
• Reduced sweating, slurred speech, agitation.	Continue. Call doctor when convenient.
Infrequent:	
Difficult urination; difficult swallowing; rash or hives; face, lip or eyelid swelling; joint or muscle pain.	Discontinue. Call doctor right away.
Rare:	
Jaundice; unusual bruising or bleeding; hives, skin rash; pain in eyes; blurred vision; sore throat, fever, mouth sores; unexplained bleeding or bruising.	Discontinue. Call doctor right away.

 ## WARNINGS & PRECAUTIONS

Don't take if:
- You are allergic to any barbiturate or any anticholinergic.
- You have porphyria, trouble with stomach bloating, difficulty emptying your bladder completely, narrow-angle glaucoma, severe ulcerative colitis.

Before you start, consult your doctor:
- If you have open-angle glaucoma, angina, chronic bronchitis or asthma, hiatal hernia, liver disease, enlarged prostate, myasthenia gravis, peptic ulcer, epilepsy, kidney or liver damage, anemia, chronic pain.
- If you will have surgery within 2 months, including dental surgery, requiring general or spinal anesthesia.

Over age 60:
Adverse reactions and side effects may be more frequent and severe than in younger persons. Ask your doctor about small doses.

Pregnancy:
Risk to unborn child outweighs drug benefits. Don't use.

Breast-feeding:
Drug passes into milk. Avoid drug or discontinue nursing until you finish medicine.

Infants & children:
Use only under doctor's supervision.

Prolonged use:
- May cause addiction, anemia, chronic intoxication.
- May lower body temperature, making exposure to cold temperatures hazardous.

Skin & sunlight:
May cause rash or intensify sunburn in areas exposed to sun or sunlamp.

Driving, piloting or hazardous work:
Don't drive or pilot aircraft until you learn how medicine affects you. Don't work around dangerous machinery. Don't climb ladders or work in high places. Danger increases if you drink alcohol or take medicine affecting alertness and reflexes.

Discontinuing:
May be unnecessary to finish medicine. Follow doctor's instructions. If you develop withdrawal symptoms of hallucinations, agitation or sleeplessness after discontinuing, call doctor right away.

Others:
Great potential for abuse.

POSSIBLE INTERACTION WITH OTHER DRUGS

GENERIC NAME OR DRUG CLASS	COMBINED EFFECT
Amantadine	Increased belladonna effect.
Anticoagulants (oral)	Decreased anticoagulant effect.
Anticholinergics (other)	Increased belladonna effect.

Anticonvulsants	Changed seizure patterns.
Antidepressants (tricyclics)	Possible dangerous oversedation. Avoid.
Antidiabetics (oral)	Increased barbiturate effect.
Antihistamines	Dangerous sedation. Avoid.
Anti-inflammatory drugs (non-steroidal)	Decreased anti-inflammatory effect.
Aspirin	Decreased aspirin effect.
Beta-adrenergic	Decreased effects of beta-adrenergic blocker.
Contraceptives (oral)	Decreased contraceptive effect.
Cortisone drugs	Increased internal-eye pressure. Decreased cortisone effect.
Digitoxin	Decreased digitoxin effect.
Doxycycline	Decreased doxycycline effect.
Dronabinol	Increased effects of both drugs. Avoid.
Griseofulvin	Decreased griseofulvin effect.
Haloperidol	Increased internal-eye pressure.
Indapamide	Increased indapamide effect.
MAO inhibitors	Increased belladonna and barbiturate effect.

Continued page 962

POSSIBLE INTERACTION WITH OTHER SUBSTANCES

INTERACTS WITH	COMBINED EFFECT
Alcohol:	Possible fatal oversedation. Avoid.
Beverages:	None expected.
Cocaine:	Excessively rapid heartbeat. Avoid.
Foods:	None expected.
Marijuana:	Drowsiness and dry mouth. Avoid.
Tobacco:	Decreased effectiveness of acid reduction in stomach.

BENDROFLUMETHIAZIDE

BRAND NAMES

Corzide   Rauzide
Naturetin

BASIC INFORMATION

Habit forming? No
Prescription needed? Yes
Available as generic? Yes
Drug class: Antihypertensive, diuretic
          (thiazide)

 ## USES

- Controls, but doesn't cure, high blood pressure.
- Reduces fluid retention (edema) caused by conditions such as heart disorders and liver disease.

 ## DOSAGE & USAGE INFORMATION

How to take:
Tablet or capsule—Swallow with liquid. If you can't swallow whole, crumble tablet or open capsule and take with liquid or food. Don't exceed dose.

When to take:
At the same time each day.

If you forget a dose:
Take as soon as you remember up to 2 hours late. If more than 2 hours, wait for next scheduled dose (don't double this dose).

What drug does:
- Forces sodium and water excretion, reducing body fluid.
- Relaxes muscle cells of small arteries.
- Reduced body fluid and relaxed arteries lower blood pressure.

Time lapse before drug works:
4 to 6 hours. May require several weeks to lower blood pressure.

Continued next column

 ## OVERDOSE

SYMPTOMS:
Cramps, weakness, drowsiness, weak pulse, coma.
WHAT TO DO:
- **Dial 0 (operator) or 911 (emergency) for an ambulance or medical help. Then give first aid immediately.**
- **See emergency information on inside covers.**

Don't take with:
- See Interaction column and consult doctor.
- Non-prescription drugs without consulting doctor.

 ## POSSIBLE ADVERSE REACTIONS OR SIDE EFFECTS

SYMPTOMS	WHAT TO DO
Life-threatening:	
None expected.	
Common:	
None expected.	
Infrequent:	
• Blurred vision, severe abdominal pain, nausea, vomiting, irregular heartbeat, weak pulse.	Discontinue. Call doctor right away.
• Dizziness, mood changes, headaches, weakness, tiredness, weight changes.	Continue. Call doctor when convenient.
• Dry mouth, thirst.	Continue. Tell doctor at next visit.
Rare:	
• Rash or hives.	Discontinue. Seek emergency treatment.
• Sore throat, fever, jaundice.	Discontinue. Call doctor right away.

WARNINGS & PRECAUTIONS

Don't take if:
You are allergic to any thiazide diuretic drug.

Before you start, consult your doctor:
- If you are allergic to any sulfa drug.
- If you have gout.
- If you have liver, pancreas or kidney disorder.

Over age 60:
Adverse reactions and side effects may be more frequent and severe than in younger persons, especially dizziness and excessive potassium loss.

Pregnancy:
Risk to unborn child outweighs drug benefits. Don't use.

Breast-feeding:
Drug passes into milk. Avoid this medicine or discontinue nursing.

Infants & children:
No problems expected.

Prolonged use:
You may need medicine to treat high blood pressure for the rest of your life.

Skin & sunlight:
May cause rash or intensify sunburn in areas exposed to sun or sunlamp.

Driving, piloting or hazardous work:
Don't drive or pilot aircraft until you learn how medicine affects you. Don't work around dangerous machinery. Don't climb ladders or work in high places. Danger increases if you drink alcohol or take medicine affecting alertness and reflexes, such as antihistamines, tranquilizers, sedatives, pain medicine, narcotics and mind-altering drugs.

Discontinuing:
Don't discontinue without medical advice.

Others:
- Hot weather and fever may cause dehydration and drop in blood pressure. Dose may require temporary adjustment. Weigh daily and report any unexpected weight decreases to your doctor.
- May cause rise in uric acid, leading to gout.
- May cause blood-sugar rise in diabetics.

POSSIBLE INTERACTION WITH OTHER DRUGS

GENERIC NAME OR DRUG CLASS	COMBINED EFFECT
Acebutolol	Increased antihypertensive effect. Dosages of both drugs may require adjustments.
Allopurinol	Decreased allopurinol effect.
Amiodarone	Increased risk of heartbeat irregularity due to low potassium.
Antidepressants (tricyclic)	Dangerous drop in blood pressure. Avoid combination unless under medical supervision.
Barbiturates	Increased bendroflumethiazide effect.
Calcium supplements	Decreased calcium in blood.
Cholestyramine	Decreased bendroflumethiazide effect.
Cortisone drugs	Excessive potassium loss that causes dangerous heart rhythms.

Digitalis preparations	Excessive potassium loss that causes dangerous heart rhythms.
Diuretics (thiazide)	Increased effect of other thiazide diuretics.
Indapamide	Increased diuretic effect.
Labetolol	Increased antihypertensive effects.
Lithium	Increased effect of lithium.
MAO inhibitors	Increased bendroflumethiazide effect.
Nitrates	Excessive blood-pressure drop.
Oxprenolol	Increased antihypertensive effect. Dosages of both drugs may require adjustments.
Potassium supplements	Decreased potassium effect.
Probenecid	Decreased probenecid effect.

POSSIBLE INTERACTION WITH OTHER SUBSTANCES

INTERACTS WITH	COMBINED EFFECT
Alcohol:	Dangerous blood-pressure drop.
Beverages:	None expected.
Cocaine:	None expected.
Foods: Licorice.	Excessive potassium loss that causes dangerous heart rhythms.
Marijuana:	May increase blood pressure.
Tobacco:	None expected.

BENZOYL PEROXIDE

BRAND NAMES

See complete list of brand names in the *Brand Name Directory,* page 945.

BASIC INFORMATION

Habit forming? No
Prescription needed? No
Available as generic? Yes
Drug class: Antiacne (topical)

 USES

- Treatment for acne.
- Decreases wrinkles in face.

 DOSAGE & USAGE INFORMATION

How to use:
Cream, gel, pads, sticks or lotion—Wash affected area with plain soap and water. Dry gently with towel. Rub medicine into affected areas. Keep away from eyes, nose, mouth.

When to use:
Apply 1 or more times daily. If you have a fair complexion, start with single application at bedtime.

If you forget an application:
Use as soon as you remember.

What drug does:
Slowly releases oxygen from skin, which controls some skin bacteria. Also causes peeling and drying, helping control blackheads and whiteheads.

Time lapse before drug works:
1 to 2 weeks.

Don't use with:
See Interaction column and consult doctor.

 OVERDOSE

SYMPTOMS:
None expected.
WHAT TO DO:
- **If person swallows drug, call doctor, poison-control center or hospital emergency room for instructions.**
- **See emergency information on inside covers.**

 POSSIBLE ADVERSE REACTIONS OR SIDE EFFECTS

SYMPTOMS	WHAT TO DO
Life-threatening:	
None expected.	
Common:	
None expected.	
Infrequent:	
• Rash, excessive dryness.	Discontinue. Call doctor right away.
• Painful skin irritation.	Continue. Call doctor when convenient.
Rare:	
None expected.	

WARNINGS & PRECAUTIONS

Don't take if:
You are allergic to benzoyl peroxide.

Before you start, consult your doctor:
- If you plan to become pregnant within medication period.
- If you take oral contraceptives.

Over age 60:
No problems expected.

Pregnancy:
No proven problems. Consult doctor.

Breast-feeding:
No proven problems. Consult doctor.

Infants & children:
Not recommended.

Prolonged use:
Permanent rash or scarring.

Skin & sunlight:
No problems expected.

Driving, piloting or hazardous work:
No problems expected.

Discontinuing:
- May be unnecessary to finish medicine. Discontinue when acne improves.
- If acne doesn't improve in 2 weeks, call doctor.

Others:
- Keep away from hair and clothing. May bleach.
- Store away from heat in cool, dry place.
- Avoid contact with eyes, lips, nose and sensitive areas of the neck.

POSSIBLE INTERACTION WITH OTHER DRUGS

GENERIC NAME OR DRUG CLASS	COMBINED EFFECT
Antiacne topical preparations (other)	Excessive skin irritation.
Skin-peeling agents (salicylic acid, sulfur, resorcinol, tretinoin)	Excessive skin irritation.

POSSIBLE INTERACTION WITH OTHER SUBSTANCES

INTERACTS WITH	COMBINED EFFECT
Alcohol:	None expected.
Beverages:	None expected.
Cocaine:	None expected.
Foods: Cinnamon, foods with benzoic acid.	Skin rash.
Marijuana:	None expected.
Tobacco:	None expected.

BENZTHIAZIDE

BRAND NAMES

Aquastat   Exna
Aquatag   Hydrex

BASIC INFORMATION

Habit forming? No
Prescription needed? Yes
Available as generic? Yes
Drug class: Antihypertensive, diuretic
      (thiazide)

 ## USES

- Controls, but doesn't cure, high blood pressure.
- Reduces fluid retention (edema) caused by conditions such as heart disorders and liver disease.

 ## DOSAGE & USAGE INFORMATION

How to take:
Tablet or capsule—Swallow with liquid. If you can't swallow whole, crumble tablet or open capsule and take with liquid or food. Don't exceed dose.

When to take:
At the same time each day.

If you forget a dose:
Take as soon as you remember up to 2 hours late. If more than 2 hours, wait for next scheduled dose (don't double this dose).

What drug does:
- Forces sodium and water excretion, reducing body fluid.
- Relaxes muscle cells of small arteries.
- Reduced body fluid and relaxed arteries lower blood pressure.

Time lapse before drug works:
4 to 6 hours. May require several weeks to lower blood pressure.

Continued next column

 ## OVERDOSE

SYMPTOMS:
Cramps, weakness, drowsiness, weak pulse, coma.
WHAT TO DO:
- **Dial 0 (operator) or 911 (emergency) for an ambulance or medical help. Then give first aid immediately.**
- **See emergency information on inside covers.**

Don't take with:
- See Interaction column and consult doctor.
- Non-prescription drugs without consulting doctor.

 ## POSSIBLE ADVERSE REACTIONS OR SIDE EFFECTS

SYMPTOMS	WHAT TO DO
Life-threatening:	
None expected.	
Common:	
None expected.	
Infrequent:	
• Blurred vision, severe abdominal pain, nausea, vomiting, irregular heartbeat, weak pulse.	Discontinue. Call doctor right away.
• Dizziness, mood changes, headaches, weakness, tiredness, weight changes.	Continue. Call doctor when convenient.
• Dry mouth, thirst.	Continue. Tell doctor at next visit.
Rare:	
• Rash or hives.	Discontinue. Seek emergency treatment.
• Sore throat, fever, jaundice.	Discontinue. Call doctor right away.

 ## WARNINGS & PRECAUTIONS

Don't take if:
You are allergic to any thiazide diuretic drug.

Before you start, consult your doctor:
- If you are allergic to any sulfa drug.
- If you have gout.
- If you have liver, pancreas or kidney disorder.

Over age 60:
Adverse reactions and side effects may be more frequent and severe than in younger persons, especially dizziness and excessive potassium loss.

Pregnancy:
Risk to unborn child outweighs drug benefits. Don't use.

Breast-feeding:
Drug passes into milk. Avoid drug or discontinue nursing.

Infants & children:
No problems expected.

Prolonged use:
You may need medicine to treat high blood pressure for the rest of your life.

Skin & sunlight:
May cause rash or intensify sunburn in areas exposed to sun or sunlamp.

Driving, piloting or hazardous work:
Don't drive or pilot aircraft until you learn how medicine affects you. Don't work around dangerous machinery. Don't climb ladders or work in high places. Danger increases if you drink alcohol or take medicine affecting alertness and reflexes, such as antihistamines, tranquilizers, sedatives, pain medicine, narcotics and mind-altering drugs.

Discontinuing:
Don't discontinue without medical advice.

Others:
- Hot weather and fever may cause dehydration and drop in blood pressure. Dose may require temporary adjustment. Weigh daily and report any unexpected weight decreases to your doctor.
- May cause rise in uric acid, leading to gout.
- May cause blood-sugar rise in diabetics.

POSSIBLE INTERACTION WITH OTHER DRUGS

GENERIC NAME OR DRUG CLASS	COMBINED EFFECT
Acebutolol	Increased antihypertensive effect. Dosages of both drugs may require adjustments.
Allopurinol	Decreased allopurinol effect.
Amiodarone	Increased risk of heartbeat irregularity due to low potassium.
Antidepressants (tricyclic)	Dangerous drop in blood pressure. Avoid combination unless under medical supervision.
Barbiturates	Increased benzthiazide effect.
Calcium supplements	Increased calcium in blood.
Cholestyramine	Decreased benzthiazide effect.
Cortisone drugs	Excessive potassium loss that causes dangerous heart rhythms.
Digitalis preparations	Excessive potassium loss that causes dangerous heart rhythms.

Diuretics (thiazide)	Increased effect of other thiazide diuretics.
Indapamide	Increased diuretic effect.
Labetolol	Increased antihypertensive effects.
Lithium	Increased effect of lithium.
MAO inhibitors	Increased benzthiazide effect.
Nitrates	Excessive blood-pressure drop.
Oxprenolol	Increased antihypertensive effect. Dosages of both drugs may require adjustments.
Potassium supplements	Decreased potassium effect.
Probenecid	Decreased probenecid effect.

POSSIBLE INTERACTION WITH OTHER SUBSTANCES

INTERACTS WITH	COMBINED EFFECT
Alcohol:	Dangerous blood-pressure drop.
Beverages:	None expected.
Cocaine:	None expected.
Foods: Licorice.	Excessive potassium loss that causes dangerous heart rhythms.
Marijuana:	May increase blood pressure.
Tobacco:	None expected.

BENZTROPINE

BRAND NAMES

Apo-Benztropine
Bensylate

Cogentin
PMS-Benztropine

BASIC INFORMATION

Habit forming? No
Prescription needed? Yes
Available as generic? Yes
Drug class: Antidyskinetic, antiparkinsonism

 USES

- Treatment of Parkinson's disease.
- Treatment of adverse effects of phenothiazines.

 DOSAGE & USAGE INFORMATION

How to take:
Tablets or capsules—Take with food to lessen stomach irritation.

When to take:
At the same times each day.

If you forget a dose:
Take as soon as you remember up to 2 hours late. If more than 2 hours, wait for next scheduled dose (don't double this dose).

What drug does:
- Balances chemical reactions necessary to send nerve impulses within base of brain.
- Improves muscle control and reduces stiffness.

Time lapse before drug works:
1 to 2 hours.

Continued next column

 OVERDOSE

SYMPTOMS:
Agitation, dilated pupils, hallucinations, dry mouth, rapid heartbeat, sleepiness.
WHAT TO DO:
- Dial 0 (operator) or 911 (emergency) for an ambulance or medical help. Then give first aid immediately.
- If patient is unconscious and not breathing, give mouth-to-mouth breathing. If there is no heartbeat, use cardiac massage and mouth-to-mouth breathing (CPR). Don't try to make patient vomit. If you can't get help quickly, take patient to nearest emergency facility.
- See emergency information on inside covers.

Don't take with:
- Non-prescription drugs for colds, cough or allergy.
- See Interaction column and consult doctor.

 POSSIBLE ADVERSE REACTIONS OR SIDE EFFECTS

SYMPTOMS	WHAT TO DO
Life-threatening: None expected.	
Common:	
• Blurred vision, light sensitivity, constipation, nausea, vomiting.	Continue. Call doctor when convenient.
• Difficult or painful urination.	Continue. Tell doctor at next visit.
Infrequent: None expected.	
Rare:	
• Rash, pain in eyes.	Discontinue. Call doctor right away.
• Confusion, dizziness, sore mouth or tongue, muscle cramps, numbness or weakness in hands or feet.	Continue. Call doctor when convenient.

WARNINGS & PRECAUTIONS

Don't take if:
You are allergic to any antidyskinetic.

Before you start, consult your doctor:
- If you have had glaucoma.
- If you have had high blood pressure or heart disease.
- If you have had impaired liver function.
- If you have had kidney disease or urination difficulty.

Over age 60:
More sensitive to drug. Aggravates symptoms of enlarged prostate. Causes impaired thinking, hallucinations, nightmares. Consult doctor about any of these.

Pregnancy:
Studies inconclusive on harm to unborn child. Animal studies show fetal abnormalities. Decide with your doctor whether drug benefits justify risk to unborn child.

Breast-feeding:
No problems expected.

Infants & children:
Not recommended for children 3 and younger. Use for older children only under doctor's supervision.

Prolonged use:
Possible glaucoma.

Skin & sunlight:
No problems expected.

Driving, piloting or hazardous work:
Don't drive or pilot aircraft until you learn how medicine affects you. Don't work around dangerous machinery. Don't climb ladders or work in high places. Danger increases if you drink alcohol or take medicine affecting alertness and reflexes, such as antihistamines, tranquilizers, sedatives, pain medicine, narcotics and mind-altering drugs.

Discontinuing:
Don't discontinue without consulting doctor. Dose may require gradual reduction if you have taken drug for a long time. Doses of other drugs may also require adjustment.

Others:
- Internal eye pressure should be measured regularly.
- Avoid becoming overheated.

 ## POSSIBLE INTERACTION WITH OTHER DRUGS

GENERIC NAME OR DRUG CLASS	COMBINED EFFECT
Amantadine	Increased amantadine effect.
Antidepressants (tricyclic)	Increased benztropine effect. May cause glaucoma.
Antihistamines	Increased benztropine effect.
Levodopa	Increased levodopa effect. Improved results in treating Parkinson's disease.
Meperidine	Increased benztropine effect.
MAO inhibitors	Increased benztropine effect.
Orphenadrine	Increased benztropine effect.
Phenothiazines	Behavior changes.
Primidone	Excessive sedation.
Procainamide	Increased procainamide effect.
Quinidine	Increased benztropine effect.
Tranquilizers	Excessive sedation.

 ## POSSIBLE INTERACTION WITH OTHER SUBSTANCES

INTERACTS WITH	COMBINED EFFECT
Alcohol:	None expected.
Beverages:	None expected.
Cocaine:	Decreased benztropine effect. Avoid.
Foods:	None expected.
Marijuana:	None expected.
Tobacco:	None expected.

BETA-ADRENERGIC BLOCKING AGENTS & THIAZIDE DIURETICS

BRAND AND GENERIC NAMES

ATENOLOL &
  CHLORTHALIDONE
Corzide
Inderide
Lopressor HCT
METOPROLOL &
  HYDROCHLORO-
  THIAZIDE
NADOLOL &
  BENDROFLUME-
  THIAZIDE

PINDOLOL &
  HYDROCHLORO-
  THIAZIDE
PROPRANOLOL &
  HYDROCHLORO-
  THIAZIDE
Tenoretic
Timolide
TIMOLOL & HYDRO-
  CHLOROTHIAZIDE
Viskazide

BASIC INFORMATION

Habit forming? No
Prescription needed? Yes
Available as generic? No
Drug class: Beta-adrenergic blocker, thiazide
        diuretic

 USES

- Controls, but doesn't cure, high blood pressure.
- Reduces fluid retention (edema).
- Reduces angina attacks.
- Stabilizes irregular heartbeat.
- Lowers blood pressure.
- Reduces frequency of migraine headaches. (Does not relieve headache pain.)
- Other uses prescribed by your doctor.

 DOSAGE & USAGE INFORMATION

How to take:
Tablet or capsule—Swallow with liquid. If you can't swallow whole, crumble tablet or open capsule and take with liquid or food.

Continued next column

 OVERDOSE

SYMPTOMS:
Irregular heartbeat (usually too slow), fainting, convulsions, coma.
WHAT TO DO:
- **Dial 0 (operator) or 911 (emergency) for an ambulance or medical help. Then give first aid immediately.**
- **See emergency information on inside covers.**

When to take:
At the same time each day.

If you forget a dose:
Take as soon as you remember up to 4 hours late. If more than 4 hours, wait for next scheduled dose (don't double this dose).

What drug does:
- Forces sodium and water excretion, reducing body fluid.
- Relaxes muscle cells of small arteries.
- Reduced body fluid and relaxed arteries lower blood pressure.
- Blocks some of the actions of sympathetic nervous system.
- Lowers heart's oxygen requirements.
- Slows nerve impulses through heart.
- Reduces blood vessel contraction in heart, scalp and other body parts.

Time lapse before drug works:
- 1 to 4 hours for beta-blocker effect.
- May require several weeks to lower blood pressure.

Don't take with:
Any other medicines, even OTC drugs such as cough/cold medicines, diet pills, nose drops, caffeine, without consulting your doctor.

 POSSIBLE ADVERSE REACTIONS OR SIDE EFFECTS

SYMPTOMS	WHAT TO DO
Life-threatening:	
Wheezing, chest pain, irregular heartbeat.	Seek emergency treatment immediately.
Common:	
• Dry mouth, weak pulse, vomiting, muscle cramps, increased thirst, mood changes.	Discontinue. Call doctor right away.
• Weakness, tiredness, dizziness, mental depression, diminished sex drive, constipation, nightmares, insomnia.	Continue. Call doctor when convenient.
Infrequent:	
Cold feet and hands, chest pain, breathing difficulty, anxiety, nervousness, headache, appetite loss, numbness and tingling in fingers and toes.	Discontinue. Call doctor right away.

BETA-ADRENERGIC BLOCKING AGENTS & THIAZIDE DIURETICS

Rare:

Hives, skin rash; joint pain; jaundice; fever, sore throat, mouth ulcers.

Discontinue. Call doctor right away.

WARNINGS & PRECAUTIONS

Don't take if:
- You are allergic to any beta-adrenergic blocker or any thiazide diuretic drug.
- You have asthma or hay fever symptoms.
- You have taken MAO inhibitors in past two weeks.

Before you start, consult your doctor:
- If you have heart disease or poor circulation to the extremities.
- If you have hay fever, asthma, chronic bronchitis, emphysema, overactive thyroid function, impaired liver or kidney function, gout, diabetes, hypoglycemia, liver, pancreas or kidney disorder.
- If you are allergic to any sulfa drug.
- If you will have surgery within 2 months, including dental surgery, requiring general or spinal anesthesia.

Over age 60:
Adverse reactions and side effects may be more frequent and severe than in younger persons, especially dizziness and excessive potassium loss.

Pregnancy:
Risk to unborn child outweighs drug benefits. Don't use.

Breast-feeding:
Drug passes into milk. Avoid drug or discontinue nursing until you finish medicine. Consult doctor for advice on maintaining milk supply.

Infants & children:
Not recommended.

Prolonged use:
- Weakens heart muscle contractions.
- You may need medicine to treat high blood pressure for the rest of your life.

Skin & sunlight:
May cause rash or intensify sunburn in areas exposed to sun or sunlamp.

Driving, piloting or hazardous work:
Don't drive or pilot aircraft until you learn how medicine affects you. Don't work around dangerous machinery. Don't climb ladders or work in high places. Danger increases if you drink alcohol or take medicine affecting alertness and reflexes, such as antihistamines, tranquilizers, sedatives, pain medicine, narcotics and mind-altering drugs.

Discontinuing:
Don't discontinue without consulting doctor. Dose may require gradual reduction if you have taken drug for a long time. Doses of other drugs may also require adjustment.

Others:
- May mask hypoglycemia.
- Hot weather and fever may cause dehydration and drop in blood pressure. Dose may require temporary adjustment. Weigh daily and report any unexpected weight decreases to your doctor.
- May cause rise in uric acid, leading to gout.
- May cause blood-sugar rise in diabetics.

POSSIBLE INTERACTION WITH OTHER DRUGS

GENERIC NAME OR DRUG CLASS	COMBINED EFFECT
Acebutolol	Increased antihypertensive effect of acebutolol. Dosage of both drugs may require adjustment.
Allopurinol	Decreased allopurinol effect.
Antidepressants (tricyclic)	Dangerous drop in blood pressure. Avoid combination unless under medical supervision.

Continued page 962

POSSIBLE INTERACTION WITH OTHER SUBSTANCES

INTERACTS WITH	COMBINED EFFECT
Alcohol:	Dangerous blood-pressure drop. Avoid.
Beverages:	None expected.
Cocaine:	Irregular heartbeat. Avoid.
Foods: Licorice.	Excessive potassium loss that causes dangerous heart rhythms.
Marijuana:	May increase blood pressure.
Tobacco:	May increase blood pressure and make heart work harder. Avoid.

BETAMETHASONE

BRAND NAMES

See complete list of brand names in the *Brand Name Directory*, page 945.

BASIC INFORMATION

Habit forming? No
Prescription needed? Yes
Available as generic? Yes
Drug class: Cortisone drug (adrenal corticosteroid)

 ## USES

- Reduces inflammation caused by many different medical problems.
- Treatment for some allergic diseases, blood disorders, kidney diseases, asthma and emphysema.
- Replaces corticosteroid deficiencies.

 ## DOSAGE & USAGE INFORMATION

How to take:
- Tablet or liquid—Swallow with liquid or food to lessen stomach irritation. If you can't swallow whole, crumble tablet and take with liquid or food.
- Inhaler—Follow label instructions.

When to take:
At the same times each day. Take once-a-day or once-every-other-day doses in mornings.

If you forget a dose:
- Several-doses-per-day prescription—Take as soon as you remember up to 2 hours late. If more than 2 hours, wait for next scheduled dose (don't double this dose).
- Once-a-day dose or less—Wait for next dose. Double this dose.

What drug does:
Decreases inflammatory responses.

Time lapse before drug works:
2 to 4 days.

Continued next column

 ## OVERDOSE

SYMPTOMS:
Headache, convulsions, heart failure.
WHAT TO DO:
- Dial 0 (operator) or 911 (emergency) for an ambulance or medical help. Then give first aid immediately.
- See emergency information on inside covers.

Don't take with:
See Interaction column and consult doctor.

 ## POSSIBLE ADVERSE REACTIONS OR SIDE EFFECTS

SYMPTOMS	WHAT TO DO
Life-threatening: None expected.	
Common: Acne, poor wound healing, thirst, indigestion, nausea, vomiting.	Continue. Call doctor when convenient.
Infrequent:	
• Bloody or black, tarry stool.	Discontinue. Seek emergency treatment.
• Blurred vision, halos around lights, sore throat, fever.	Discontinue. Call doctor right away.
• Mood changes, insomnia, restlessness, frequent urination, weight gain, round face, fatigue, weakness, TB recurrence, menstrual irregularities.	Continue. Call doctor when convenient.
Rare:	
• Irregular heartbeat.	Discontinue. Seek emergency treatment.
• Rash.	Discontinue. Call doctor right away.

 ## WARNINGS & PRECAUTIONS

Don't take if:
- You are allergic to any cortisone drug.
- You have tuberculosis or fungus infection.
- You have herpes infection of eyes, lips or genitals.

Before you start, consult your doctor:
- If you have had tuberculosis.
- If you have congestive heart failure.
- If you have diabetes.
- If you have peptic ulcer.
- If you have glaucoma.
- If you have underactive thyroid.
- If you have high blood pressure.
- If you have myasthenia gravis.
- If you have blood clots in legs or lungs.

Over age 60:
Adverse reactions and side effects may be more frequent and severe than in younger persons. Likely to aggravate edema, diabetes or ulcers. Likely to cause cataracts and osteoporosis (softening of the bones).

Pregnancy:
Risk to unborn child outweighs drug benefits. Don't use.

Breast-feeding:
Drug passes into milk. Avoid drug or discontinue nursing until you finish medicine. Consult doctor for advice on maintaining milk supply.

Infants & children:
Use only under medical supervision.

Prolonged use:
- Retards growth in children.
- Possible glaucoma, cataracts, diabetes, fragile bones and thin skin.
- Functional dependence.

Skin & sunlight:
No problems expected.

Driving, piloting or hazardous work:
No problems expected.

Discontinuing:
- Don't discontinue without doctor's advice until you complete prescribed dose, even though symptoms diminish or disappear.
- Drug affects your response to surgery, illness, injury or stress for up to 2 years after discontinuing. Inform doctor.

Others:
Avoid immunizations if possible.

 ## POSSIBLE INTERACTION WITH OTHER DRUGS

GENERIC NAME OR DRUG CLASS	COMBINED EFFECT
Amphoterecin B	Potassium depletion.
Anticholinergics	Possible glaucoma.
Anticoagulants (oral)	Decreased anticoagulant effect.
Anticonvulsants (hydantoin)	Decreased betamethasone effect.
Antidiabetics (oral)	Decreased antidiabetic effect.
Antihistamines	Decreased betamethasone effect.
Aspirin	Increased betamethasone effect.
Barbiturates	Decreased betamethasone effect. Oversedation.
Beta-adrenergic blockers	Decreased betamethasone effect.
Chloral hydrate	Decreased betamethasone effect.
Chlorthalidone	Potassium depletion.
Cholinergics	Decreased cholinergic effect.
Contraceptives (oral)	Increased betamethasone effect.
Digitalis preparations	Dangerous potassium depletion. Possible digitalis toxicity.
Diuretics (thiazide)	Potassium depletion.
Ephedrine	Decreased betamethasone effect.
Estrogens	Increased betamethasone effect.
Ethacrynic acid	Potassium depletion.
Furosemide	Potassium depletion.
Glutethimide	Decreased betamethasone effect.
Indapamide	Possible excessive potassium loss, causing dangerous heartbeat irregularity.
Indomethacin	Increased betamethasone effect.
Insulin	Decreased insulin effect.
Isoniazid	Decreased isoniazid effect.
Oxyphenbutazone	Possible ulcers.
Phenylbutazone	Possible ulcers.
Potassium supplements	Decreased potassium effect.
Rifampin	Decreased betamethasone effect.
Sympathomimetics	Possible glaucoma.

 ## POSSIBLE INTERACTION WITH OTHER SUBSTANCES

INTERACTS WITH	COMBINED EFFECT
Alcohol:	Risk of stomach ulcers.
Beverages:	No proven problems.
Cocaine:	Overstimulation. Avoid.
Foods:	No proven problems.
Marijuana:	Decreased immunity.
Tobacco:	Increased betamethasone effect. Possible toxicity.

BETHANECHOL

BRAND NAMES

Duvoid   Urecholine
Myotonachol

BASIC INFORMATION

Habit forming? No
Prescription needed? Yes
Available as generic? Yes
Drug class: Cholinergic

USES

Helps initiate urination following surgery, or for persons with urinary infections or enlarged prostate.

DOSAGE & USAGE INFORMATION

How to take:
Tablet or capsule—Swallow with liquid, 1 hour before or 2 hours after eating.

When to take:
At the same times each day.

If you forget a dose:
Take as soon as you remember up to 2 hours late. If more than 2 hours, wait for next scheduled dose (don't double this dose).

What drug does:
Affects chemical reactions in the body that strengthen bladder muscles.

Time lapse before drug works:
30 to 90 minutes.

Continued next column

OVERDOSE

SYMPTOMS:
Shortness of breath, wheezing or chest tightness, unconsciousness, coma.
WHAT TO DO:
- **Dial 0 (operator) or 911 (emergency) for an ambulance or medical help. Then give first aid immediately.**
- **If patient is unconscious and not breathing, give mouth-to-mouth breathing. If there is no heartbeat, use cardiac massage and mouth-to-mouth breathing (CPR). Don't try to make patient vomit. If you can't get help quickly, take patient to nearest emergency facility.**
- **See emergency information on inside covers.**

Don't take with:
See Interaction column and consult doctor.

POSSIBLE ADVERSE REACTIONS OR SIDE EFFECTS

SYMPTOMS	WHAT TO DO
Life-threatening: None expected.	
Common: None expected.	
Infrequent: Dizziness, headache, faintness, blurred or changed vision, diarrhea, nausea, vomiting, stomach discomfort, belching, excessive urge to urinate.	Continue. Call doctor when convenient.
Rare: Shortness of breath, wheezing, tightness in chest.	Discontinue. Call doctor right away.

WARNINGS & PRECAUTIONS

Don't take if:
You are allergic to any cholinergic.

Before you start, consult your doctor:
- If you plan to become pregnant within medication period.
- If you have asthma.
- If you have epilepsy.
- If you have heart or blood-vessel disease.
- If you have high or low blood pressure.
- If you have overactive thyroid.
- If you have intestinal blockage.
- If you have Parkinson's disease.
- If you have stomach problems (including ulcer).
- If you have had bladder or intestinal surgery within 1 month.

Over age 60:
Adverse reactions and side effects may be more frequent and severe than in younger persons.

Pregnancy:
Risk to unborn child outweighs drug benefits. Don't use.

Breast-feeding:
Drug filters into milk. May harm child. Avoid.

Infants & children:
Use only under medical supervision.

Prolonged use:
No problems expected.

Skin & sunlight:
No problems expected.

Driving, piloting or hazardous work:
Don't drive or pilot aircraft until you learn how medicine affects you. Don't work around dangerous machinery. Don't climb ladders or work in high places. Danger increases if you drink alcohol or take medicine affecting alertness and reflexes, such as antihistamines, tranquilizers, sedatives, pain medicine, narcotics and mind-altering drugs.

Discontinuing:
May be unnecessary to finish medicine. Follow doctor's instructions.

Others:
- Be cautious about standing up suddenly.
- Interferes with laboratory studies of liver and pancreas function.
- Side effects more likely with injections.

POSSIBLE INTERACTION WITH OTHER DRUGS

GENERIC NAME OR DRUG CLASS	COMBINED EFFECT
Cholinergics (other)	Increased effect of both drugs. Possible toxicity.
Nitrates	Decreased bethanechol effect.
Procainamide	Decreased bethanechol effect.
Quinidine	Decreased bethanechol effect.

POSSIBLE INTERACTION WITH OTHER SUBSTANCES

INTERACTS WITH	COMBINED EFFECT
Alcohol:	None expected.
Beverages:	None expected.
Cocaine:	None expected.
Foods:	None expected.
Marijuana:	None expected.
Tobacco:	None expected.

BIPERIDEN

BRAND NAMES

Akineton

BASIC INFORMATION

Habit forming? No
Prescription needed? Yes
Available as generic? No
Drug class: Antidyskinetic, antiparkinsonism

USES

- Treatment of Parkinson's disease.
- Treatment of adverse effects of phenothiazines.

DOSAGE & USAGE INFORMATION

How to take:
Tablets or capsules—Take with food to lessen stomach irritation.

When to take:
At the same times each day.

If you forget a dose:
Take as soon as you remember up to 2 hours late. If more than 2 hours, wait for next scheduled dose (don't double this dose).

What drug does:
- Balances chemical reactions necessary to send nerve impulses within base of brain.
- Improves muscle control and reduces stiffness.

Time lapse before drug works:
1 to 2 hours.

Continued next column

OVERDOSE

SYMPTOMS:
Agitation, dilated pupils, hallucinations, dry mouth, rapid heartbeat, sleepiness.
WHAT TO DO:
- **Dial 0 (operator) or 911 (emergency) for an ambulance or medical help. Then give first aid immediately.**
- **If patient is unconscious and not breathing, give mouth-to-mouth breathing. If there is no heartbeat, use cardiac massage and mouth-to-mouth breathing (CPR). Don't try to make patient vomit. If you can't get help quickly, take patient to nearest emergency facility.**
- **See emergency information on inside covers.**

Don't take with:
- Non-prescription drugs for colds, cough or allergy.
- See Interaction column and consult doctor.

POSSIBLE ADVERSE REACTIONS OR SIDE EFFECTS

SYMPTOMS	WHAT TO DO
Life-threatening: None expected.	
Common:	
• Blurred vision, light sensitivity, constipation, nausea, vomiting.	Continue. Call doctor when convenient.
• Difficult or painful urination.	Continue. Tell doctor at next visit.
Infrequent: None expected.	
Rare:	
• Rash, pain in eyes.	Discontinue. Call doctor right away.
• Confusion, dizziness, sore mouth or tongue, muscle cramps, numbness or weakness in hands or feet.	Continue. Call doctor when convenient.

WARNINGS & PRECAUTIONS

Don't take if:
You are allergic to any antidyskinetic.

Before you start, consult your doctor:
- If you have had glaucoma.
- If you have had high blood pressure or heart disease.
- If you have had impaired liver function.
- If you have had kidney disease or urination difficulty.

Over age 60:
More sensitive to drug. Aggravates symptoms of enlarged prostate. Causes impaired thinking, hallucinations, nightmares. Consult doctor about any of these.

Pregnancy:
Studies inconclusive on harm to unborn child. Animal studies show fetal abnormalities. Decide with your doctor whether drug benefits justify risk to unborn child.

Breast-feeding:
May inhibit milk secretion. Consult doctor.

Infants & children:
Not recommended for children 3 and younger. Use for older children only under doctor's supervision.

Prolonged use:
Possible glaucoma.

Skin & sunlight:
No problems expected.

Driving, piloting or hazardous work:
Don't drive or pilot aircraft until you learn how medicine affects you. Don't work around dangerous machinery. Don't climb ladders or work in high places. Danger increases if you drink alcohol or take medicine affecting alertness and reflexes, such as antihistamines, tranquilizers, sedatives, pain medicine, narcotics and mind-altering drugs.

Discontinuing:
Don't discontinue without consulting doctor. Dose may require gradual reduction if you have taken drug for a long time. Doses of other drugs may also require adjustment.

Others:
- Internal eye pressure should be measured regularly.
- Avoid becoming overheated.

POSSIBLE INTERACTION WITH OTHER DRUGS

GENERIC NAME OR DRUG CLASS	COMBINED EFFECT
Amantadine	Increased amantadine effect.
Antidepressants (tricyclic)	Increased biperiden effect. May cause glaucoma.
Antihistamines	Increased biperiden effect.
Levodopa	Increased levodopa effect. Improved results in treating Parkinson's disease.
Meperidine	Increased biperiden effect.
MAO inhibitors	Increased biperiden effect.
Orphenadrine	Increased biperiden effect.
Phenothiazines	Behavior changes.
Primidone	Excessive sedation.
Procainamide	Increased procainamide effect.
Quinidine	Increased biperiden effect.
Tranquilizers	Excessive sedation.

POSSIBLE INTERACTION WITH OTHER SUBSTANCES

INTERACTS WITH	COMBINED EFFECT
Alcohol:	None expected.
Beverages:	None expected.
Cocaine:	Decreased biperiden effect. Avoid.
Foods:	None expected.
Marijuana:	None expected.
Tobacco:	None expected.

BISACODYL

BRAND NAMES

Apo-Bisacodyl
Bisco-Lax
Cenalax
Clysodrast
Codylax
Dacodyl
Deficol

Dulcolax
Evac-Q-Kwik
Fleet Bisacodyl
Fleet Enema
Nulac
Theralax

BASIC INFORMATION

Habit forming? No
Prescription needed? No
Available as generic? Yes
Drug class: Laxative (stimulant)

 ## USES

Constipation relief.

 ## DOSAGE & USAGE INFORMATION

How to take:
- Tablet—Swallow with liquid.
- Suppository—Remove wrapper and moisten suppository with water. Gently insert larger end into rectum. Push well into rectum with finger.

When to take:
Usually at bedtime with a snack, unless directed otherwise.

If you forget a dose:
Take as soon as you remember.

What drug does:
Acts on smooth muscles of intestine wall to cause vigorous bowel movement.

Time lapse before drug works:
6 to 10 hours.

Don't take with:
- See Interaction column and consult doctor.
- Don't take within 2 hours of taking another medicine. Laxative interferes with medicine absorption.

 ## OVERDOSE

SYMPTOMS:
Vomiting, electrolyte depletion.
WHAT TO DO:
Overdose unlikely to threaten life. If person takes much larger amount than prescribed, call doctor, poison-control center or hospital emergency room for instructions.

 ## POSSIBLE ADVERSE REACTIONS OR SIDE EFFECTS

SYMPTOMS	WHAT TO DO
Life-threatening:	
None expected.	
Common:	
Rectal irritation.	Continue. Call doctor when convenient.
Infrequent:	
• Dangerous potassium loss.	Discontinue. Call doctor right away.
• Belching, cramps, nausea.	Continue. Call doctor when convenient.
Rare:	
• Irritability, confusion, headache, rash, breathing difficulty, irregular heartbeat, muscle cramps, unusual tiredness or weakness.	Discontinue. Call doctor right away.
• Burning on urination.	Continue. Call doctor when convenient.

WARNINGS & PRECAUTIONS

Don't take if:
- You have symptoms of appendicitis, inflamed bowel or intestinal blockage.
- You are allergic to a stimulant laxative.
- You have missed a bowel movement for only 1 or 2 days.

Before you start, consult your doctor:
- If you have a colostomy or ileostomy.
- If you have congestive heart disease.
- If you have diabetes.
- If you have high blood pressure.
- If you have a laxative habit.
- If you have rectal bleeding.
- If you take other laxatives.

Over age 60:
Adverse reactions and side effects may be more frequent and severe than in younger persons.

Pregnancy:
Risk to mother and unborn child outweighs drug benefits. Don't use.

Breast-feeding:
Drug passes into milk. Avoid drug or discontinue nursing until you finish medicine. Consult doctor for advice on maintaining milk supply.

Infants & children:
Use only under medical supervision.

Prolonged use:
Don't take for more than 1 week unless under doctor's supervision. May cause laxative dependence.

Skin & sunlight:
No problems expected.

Driving, piloting or hazardous work:
No problems expected.

Discontinuing:
May be unnecessary to finish medicine. Follow doctor's instructions.

Others:
Don't take to "flush out" your system or as a "tonic."

POSSIBLE INTERACTION WITH OTHER DRUGS

GENERIC NAME OR DRUG CLASS	COMBINED EFFECT
Antacids	Tablet coating may dissolve too rapidly, irritating stomach or bowel.
Antihypertensives	May cause dangerous low potassium level.
Cimetidine	Stomach or bowel irritation.
Diuretics	May cause dangerous low potassium level.
Ranitidine	Stomach or bowel irritation.

POSSIBLE INTERACTION WITH OTHER SUBSTANCES

INTERACTS WITH	COMBINED EFFECT
Alcohol:	None expected.
Beverages:	None expected.
Cocaine:	None expected.
Foods:	None expected.
Marijuana:	None expected.
Tobacco:	None expected.

BROMOCRIPTINE

BRAND NAMES

Parlodel

BASIC INFORMATION

Habit forming? No
Prescription needed? Yes
Available as generic? Yes
Drug class: Antiparkinsonism

 USES

- Controls Parkinson's disease symptoms such as rigidity, tremors and unsteady gait.
- Treats female infertility.
- Prevents lactation.

 DOSAGE & USAGE INFORMATION

How to take:
Tablet or capsule—Swallow with liquid or food to lessen stomach irritation. If you can't swallow whole, crumble tablet or open capsule and take with liquid or food.

When to take:
At the same times each day.

If you forget a dose:
Take as soon as you remember up to 2 hours late. If more than 2 hours, wait for next scheduled dose (don't double this dose).

What drug does:
Restores chemical balance necessary for normal nerve impulses.

Continued next column

 OVERDOSE

SYMPTOMS:
Muscle twitch, spastic eyelid closure, nausea, vomiting, diarrhea, irregular and rapid pulse, weakness, fainting, confusion, agitation, hallucination, coma.
WHAT TO DO:
- **Dial 0 (operator) or 911 (emergency) for an ambulance or medical help. Then give first aid immediately.**
- **If patient is unconscious and not breathing, give mouth-to-mouth breathing. If there is no heartbeat, use cardiac massage and mouth-to-mouth breathing (CPR). Don't try to make patient vomit. If you can't get help quickly, take patient to nearest emergency facility.**
- **See emergency information on inside covers.**

Time lapse before drug works:
2 to 3 weeks to improve; 6 weeks or longer for maximum benefit.

Don't take with:
See Interaction column and consult doctor.

 POSSIBLE ADVERSE REACTIONS OR SIDE EFFECTS

SYMPTOMS	WHAT TO DO
Life-threatening: None expected.	
Common:	
• Mood changes, uncontrollable body movements, diarrhea.	Continue. Call doctor when convenient.
• Dry mouth, body odor.	No action necessary.
Infrequent:	
• Fainting, severe dizziness, headache, insomnia, nightmares, rash, itch, nausea, vomiting, irregular heartbeat.	Discontinue. Call doctor right away.
• Flushed face, blurred vision, muscle twitching, discolored or dark urine, difficult urination.	Continue. Call doctor when convenient.
• Constipation, tiredness.	Continue. Tell doctor at next visit.
Rare:	
• High blood pressure.	Discontinue. Call doctor right away.
• Anemia, duodenal ucler.	Continue. Call doctor when convenient.

WARNINGS & PRECAUTIONS

Don't take if:
- You are allergic to bromocriptine.
- You have taken MAO inhibitors in past 2 weeks.
- You have glaucoma (narrow-angle type).

Before you start, consult your doctor:
- If you have diabetes or epilepsy.
- If you have had high blood pressure, heart or lung disease.
- If you have had liver or kidney disease.
- If you have a peptic ulcer.
- If you have malignant melanoma.
- If you will have surgery within 2 months, including dental surgery, requiring general or spinal anesthesia.

Over age 60:
Adverse reactions and side effects may be more frequent and severe than in younger persons.

Pregnancy:
Risk to unborn child outweighs drug benefits. Don't use.

Breast-feeding:
Drug filters into milk. May harm child. Avoid.

Infants & children:
Not recommended.

Prolonged use:
May lead to uncontrolled movements of head, face, mouth, tongue, arms or legs.

Skin & sunlight:
No problems expected.

Driving, piloting or hazardous work:
Don't drive or pilot aircraft until you learn how medicine affects you. Don't work around dangerous machinery. Don't climb ladders or work in high places. Danger increases if you drink alcohol or take medicine affecting alertness and reflexes, such as antihistamines, tranquilizers, sedatives, pain medicine, narcotics and mind-altering drugs.

Discontinuing:
Don't discontinue without doctor's advice until you complete prescribed dose, even though symptoms diminish or disappear.

Others:
Expect to start with small doses and increase gradually to lessen frequency and severity of adverse reactions.

POSSIBLE INTERACTION WITH OTHER DRUGS

GENERIC NAME OR DRUG CLASS	COMBINED EFFECT
Antiparkinsonism drugs (other)	Increased bromocriptine effect.
Haloperidol	Decreased bromocriptine effect.
MAO inhibitors	Dangerous rise in blood pressure.
Methyldopa	Decreased bromocriptine effect.
Papaverine	Decreased bromocriptine effect.
Phenothiazines	Decreased bromocriptine effect.
Pyridoxine (Vitamin B-6)	Decreased bromocriptine effect.
Rauwolfia alkaloids	Decreased bromocriptine effect.

POSSIBLE INTERACTION WITH OTHER SUBSTANCES

INTERACTS WITH	COMBINED EFFECT
Alcohol:	None expected.
Beverages:	None expected.
Cocaine:	Decreased bromocriptine effect. Avoid.
Foods:	None expected.
Marijuana:	Increased fatigue, lethargy, fainting. Avoid.
Tobacco:	Interferes with absorption. Avoid.

BROMODIPHENHYDRAMINE

BRAND NAMES

Ambenyl Expectorant   Ambodryl

BASIC INFORMATION

Habit forming? No
Prescription needed? Yes
Available as generic? No
Drug class: Antihistamine

 USES

- Reduces allergic symptoms such as hay fever, hives, rash or itching.
- Induces sleep.

 DOSAGE & USAGE INFORMATION

How to take:
Capsule or liquid—Swallow with liquid or food to lessen stomach irritation.

When to take:
Varies with form. Follow label directions.

If you forget a dose:
Take as soon as you remember up to 2 hours late. If more than 2 hours, wait for next scheduled dose (don't double this dose).

What drug does:
Blocks action of histamine after an allergic response triggers histamine release in sensitive cells.

Time lapse before drug works:
30 minutes.

Don't take with:
See Interaction column and consult doctor.

 OVERDOSE

SYMPTOMS:
Convulsions, red face, hallucinations, coma.
WHAT TO DO:
- Dial 0 (operator) or 911 (emergency) for an ambulance or medical help. Then give first aid immediately.
- If patient is unconscious and not breathing, give mouth-to-mouth breathing. If there is no heartbeat, use cardiac massage and mouth-to-mouth breathing (CPR). Don't try to make patient vomit. If you can't get help quickly, take patient to nearest emergency facility.
- See emergency information on inside covers.

 POSSIBLE ADVERSE REACTIONS OR SIDE EFFECTS

SYMPTOMS	WHAT TO DO
Life-threatening: None expected.	
Common: Drowsiness, dizziness, dry mouth or throat, nausea.	Continue. Tell doctor at next visit.
Infrequent:	
• Vision changes.	Discontinue. Call doctor right away.
• Less tolerance for contact lenses, difficult or painful urination.	Continue. Call doctor when convenient.
• Appetite loss.	Continue. Tell doctor at next visit.
Rare: Nightmares, agitation, irritability, sore throat, fever, rapid heartbeat, unusual bleeding or bruising, fatigue, weakness.	Discontinue. Call doctor right away.

WARNINGS & PRECAUTIONS

Don't take if:
You are allergic to any antihistamine.

Before you start, consult your doctor:
- If you have glaucoma.
- If you have enlarged prostate.
- If you have asthma.
- If you have kidney disease.
- If you have peptic ulcer.
- If you will have surgery within 2 months, including dental surgery, requiring general or spinal anesthesia.

Over age 60:
Don't exceed recommended dose. Adverse reactions and side effects may be more frequent and severe than in younger persons, especially urination difficulty, diminished alertness and other brain and nervous-system symptoms.

Pregnancy:
No proven harm to unborn child. Avoid if possible.

Breast-feeding:
Drug passes into milk. Avoid drug or discontinue nursing until you finish medicine. Consult doctor for advice on maintaining milk supply.

Infants & children:
Not recommended for premature or newborn infants. Otherwise, no problems expected.

Prolonged use:
Avoid. May damage bone-marrow and nerve cells.

Skin & sunlight:
May cause rash or intensify sunburn in areas exposed to sun or sunlamp.

Driving, piloting or hazardous work:
Don't drive or pilot aircraft until you learn how medicine affects you. Don't work around dangerous machinery. Don't climb ladders or work in high places. Danger increases if you drink alcohol or take medicine affecting alertness and reflexes, such as antihistamines, tranquilizers, sedatives, pain medicine, narcotics and mind-altering drugs.

Discontinuing:
No problems expected.

Others:
May mask symptoms of hearing damage from aspirin, other salicylates, cisplatin, paromomycin, vancomycin or anticonvulsants. Consult doctor if you use these.

POSSIBLE INTERACTION WITH OTHER DRUGS

GENERIC NAME OR DRUG CLASS	COMBINED EFFECT
Anticholinergics	Increased anticholinergic effect.
Antidepressants	Excess sedation. Avoid.
Antihistamines (other)	Excess sedation. Avoid.
Dronabinol	Increased effects of both drugs. Avoid.
Hypnotics	Excess sedation. Avoid.
MAO inhibitors	Increased bromodiphenhydramine effect.
Mind-altering drugs	Excess sedation. Avoid.
Narcotics	Excess sedation. Avoid.
Sedatives	Excess sedation. Avoid.
Sleep inducers	Excess sedation. Avoid.
Tranquilizers	Excess sedation. Avoid.

POSSIBLE INTERACTION WITH OTHER SUBSTANCES

INTERACTS WITH	COMBINED EFFECT
Alcohol:	Excess sedation. Avoid.
Beverages: Caffeine drinks.	Less bromodiphenhydramine sedation.
Cocaine:	Decreased bromodiphenhydramine effect. Avoid.
Foods:	None expected.
Marijuana:	Excess sedation. Avoid.
Tobacco:	None expected.

BROMPHENIRAMINE

BRAND NAMES

See complete list of brand names in the *Brand Name Directory,* page 945.

BASIC INFORMATION

Habit forming? No
Prescription needed? Yes
Available as generic? Yes
Drug class: Antihistamine

 USES

- Reduces allergic symptoms such as hay fever, hives, rash or itching.
- Induces sleep.

 DOSAGE & USAGE INFORMATION

How to take:
- Tablet, capsule or syrup—Swallow with liquid or food to lessen stomach irritation.
- Extended-release tablets or capsules—Swallow each dose whole.

When to take:
Varies with form. Follow label directions.

If you forget a dose:
Take as soon as you remember up to 2 hours late. If more than 2 hours, wait for next scheduled dose (don't double this dose).

What drug does:
Blocks action of histamine after an allergic response triggers histamine release in sensitive cells.

Time lapse before drug works:
30 minutes.

Don't take with:
See Interaction column and consult doctor.

 OVERDOSE

SYMPTOMS:
Convulsions, red face, hallucinations, coma.
WHAT TO DO:
- Dial 0 (operator) or 911 (emergency) for an ambulance or medical help. Then give first aid immediately.
- See emergency information on inside covers.

 POSSIBLE ADVERSE REACTIONS OR SIDE EFFECTS

SYMPTOMS	WHAT TO DO
Life-threatening: None expected.	
Common: Drowsiness; dizziness; dry mouth, nose or throat; nausea.	Continue. Tell doctor at next visit.
Infrequent: • Vision changes.	Discontinue. Call doctor right away.
• Less tolerance for contact lenses, difficult or painful urination.	Continue. Call doctor when convenient.
• Appetite loss.	Continue. Tell doctor at next visit.
Rare: Nightmares, agitation, irritability, sore throat, fever, rapid heartbeat, unusual bleeding or bruising, fatigue, weakness.	Discontinue. Call doctor right away.

WARNINGS & PRECAUTIONS

Don't take if:
You are allergic to any antihistamine.

Before you start, consult your doctor:
- If you have glaucoma.
- If you have enlarged prostate.
- If you have asthma.
- If you have kidney disease.
- If you have peptic ulcer.
- If you will have surgery within 2 months, including dental surgery, requiring general or spinal anesthesia.

Over age 60:
Don't exceed recommended dose. Adverse reactions and side effects may be more frequent and severe than in younger persons, especially urination difficulty, diminished alertness and other brain and nervous-system symptoms.

Pregnancy:
No proven harm to unborn child. Avoid if possible.

Breast-feeding:
Drug passes into milk. Avoid drug or discontinue nursing until you finish medicine. Consult doctor for advice on maintaining milk supply.

Infants & children:
Not recommended for premature or newborn infants. Otherwise, no problems expected.

Prolonged use:
Avoid. May damage bone marrow and nerve cells.

Skin & sunlight:
May cause rash or intensify sunburn in areas exposed to sun or sunlamp.

Driving, piloting or hazardous work:
Don't drive or pilot aircraft until you learn how medicine affects you. Don't work around dangerous machinery. Don't climb ladders or work in high places. Danger increases if you drink alcohol or take medicine affecting alertness and reflexes, such as antihistamines, tranquilizers, sedatives, pain medicine, narcotics and mind-altering drugs.

Discontinuing:
No problems expected.

Others:
May mask symptoms of hearing damage from aspirin, other salicylates, cisplatin, paromomycin, vancomycin or anticonvulsants. Consult doctor if you use these.

POSSIBLE INTERACTION WITH OTHER DRUGS

GENERIC NAME OR DRUG CLASS	COMBINED EFFECT
Anticholinergics	Increased anticholinergic effect.
Antidepressants	Excess sedation. Avoid.
Antihistamines (other)	Excess sedation. Avoid.
Dronabinol	Increased effects of both drugs. Avoid.
Hypnotics	Excess sedation. Avoid.
MAO inhibitors	Increased brompheniramine effect.
Mind-altering drugs	Excess sedation. Avoid.
Molindone	Increased antihistamine effect.
Narcotics	Excess sedation. Avoid.
Sedatives	Excess sedation. Avoid.
Sleep inducers	Excess sedation. Avoid.
Tranquilizers	Excess sedation. Avoid.

POSSIBLE INTERACTION WITH OTHER SUBSTANCES

INTERACTS WITH	COMBINED EFFECT
Alcohol:	Excess sedation. Avoid.
Beverages: Caffeine drinks.	Less brompheniramine sedation.
Cocaine:	Decreased brompheniramine effect. Avoid.
Foods:	None expected.
Marijuana:	Excess sedation. Avoid.
Tobacco:	None expected.

BUCLIZINE

BRAND NAMES

Bucladin-S

BASIC INFORMATION

Habit forming? No
Prescription needed?
  U.S.: No
  Canada: Yes
Available as generic? No
Drug class: Antihistamine, antiemetic

 USES

Prevents motion sickness.

 DOSAGE & USAGE INFORMATION

How to take:
Tablet—Swallow with liquid or food to lessen stomach irritation. If you can't swallow whole, crumble tablet and chew or take with liquid or food.

When to take:
30 minutes to 1 hour before traveling.

If you forget a dose:
Take as soon as you remember. Wait 4 hours for next dose.

What drug does:
Reduces sensitivity of nerve endings in inner ear, blocking messages to brain's vomiting center.

Time lapse before drug works:
30 to 60 minutes.

Don't take with:
See Interaction column and consult doctor.

 OVERDOSE

SYMPTOMS:
Drowsiness, confusion, incoordination, stupor, coma, weak pulse, shallow breathing.
WHAT TO DO:
- Dial 0 (operator) or 911 (emergency) for an ambulance or medical help. Then give first aid immediately.
- See emergency information on inside covers.

 POSSIBLE ADVERSE REACTIONS OR SIDE EFFECTS

SYMPTOMS	WHAT TO DO
Life-threatening: None expected.	
Common: Drowsiness.	Continue. Tell doctor at next visit.
Infrequent:	
• Headache, diarrhea or constipation, fast heartbeat.	Continue. Call doctor when convenient.
• Dry mouth, nose, throat.	Continue. Tell doctor at next visit.
Rare:	
• Rash or hives.	Discontinue. Call doctor right away.
• Restlessness, excitement, insomnia, blurred vision, frequent urination, difficult urination.	Continue. Call doctor when convenient.
• Appetite loss, nausea.	Continue. Tell doctor at next visit.

WARNINGS & PRECAUTIONS

Don't take if:
- You are allergic to meclizine, buclizine or cyclizine.
- You have taken MAO inhibitors in the past 2 weeks.

Before you start, consult your doctor:
- If you have glaucoma.
- If you have prostate enlargement.
- If you have reacted badly to any antihistamine.

Over age 60:
Adverse reactions and side effects may be more frequent and severe than in younger persons, especially impaired urination from enlarged prostate gland.

Pregnancy:
Studies inconclusive on harm to unborn child. Animal studies show fetal abnormalities. Decide with your doctor whether drug benefits justify risk to unborn child.

Breast-feeding:
Drug passes into milk. Avoid drug or discontinue nursing until you finish medicine. Consult doctor for advice on maintaining milk supply.

Infants & children:
No problems expected.

Prolonged use:
No problems expected.

Skin & sunlight:
No problems expected.

Driving, piloting or hazardous work:
Don't fly aircraft. Don't drive until you learn how medicine affects you. Don't work around dangerous machinery. Don't climb ladders or work in high places. Danger increases if you drink alcohol or take medicine affecting alertness and reflexes, such as antihistamines, tranquilizers, sedatives, pain medicine, narcotics and mind-altering drugs.

Discontinuing:
No problems expected.

Others:
No problems expected.

POSSIBLE INTERACTION WITH OTHER DRUGS

GENERIC NAME OR DRUG CLASS	COMBINED EFFECT
Amphetamines	May decrease drowsiness caused by buclizine.
Anticholinergics	Increased effect of both drugs.
Antidepressants (tricyclic)	Increased effect of both drugs.
MAO inhibitors	Increased buclizine effect.
Narcotics	Increased effect of both drugs.
Pain relievers	Increased effect of both drugs.
Sedatives	Increased effect of both drugs.
Sleep inducers	Increased effect of both drugs.
Tranquilizers	Increased effect of both drugs.

POSSIBLE INTERACTION WITH OTHER SUBSTANCES

INTERACTS WITH	COMBINED EFFECT
Alcohol:	Increased sedation. Avoid.
Beverages: Caffeine drinks.	May decrease drowsiness.
Cocaine:	None expected.
Foods:	None expected.
Marijuana:	Increased drowsiness, dry mouth.
Tobacco:	None expected.

BUMETANIDE

BRAND NAMES

Bumex

BASIC INFORMATION

Habit forming? No
Prescription needed? Yes
Available as generic? No
Drug class: Diuretic

 USES

Decreases fluid retention.

 DOSAGE & USAGE INFORMATION

How to take:
Tablet or capsule—Swallow with liquid or food to lessen stomach irritation. If you can't swallow whole, crumble tablet or open capsule and take with liquid or food.

When to take:
● 1 dose a day—Take after breakfast.
● More than 1 dose a day—Take last dose no later than 6 p.m. unless otherwise directed.

If you forget a dose:
● 1 dose a day—Take as soon as you remember up to 12 hours late. If more than 12 hours, wait for next scheduled dose (don't double this dose).
● More than 1 dose a day—Take as soon as you remember up to 2 hours late. If more than 2 hours, wait for next scheduled dose (don't double this dose).

What drug does:
Increases elimination of sodium and water from body. Decreased body fluid reduces blood pressure.

Time lapse before drug works:
1 hour to increase water loss.

Continued next column

 OVERDOSE

SYMPTOMS:
Weakness, lethargy, dizziness, confusion, nausea, vomiting, leg-muscle cramps, thirst, stupor, deep sleep, weak and rapid pulse, cardiac arrest.
WHAT TO DO:
● **Dial 0 (operator) or 911 (emergency) for an ambulance or medical help. Then give first aid immediately.**
● **See emergency information on inside covers.**

Don't take with:
See Interaction column and consult doctor.

 POSSIBLE ADVERSE REACTIONS OR SIDE EFFECTS

SYMPTOMS	WHAT TO DO
Life-threatening: None expected.	
Common: Dizziness.	Continue. Call doctor when convenient.
Infrequent: Mood changes, appetite loss, diarrhea, irregular heartbeat, muscle cramps, fatigue, weakness.	Discontinue. Call doctor right away.
Rare: Rash or hives; yellow vision; ringing in ears; hearing loss; sore throat, fever; dry mouth; thirst; side or stomach pain; nausea; vomiting; unusual bleeding or bruising; joint pain; jaundice.	Discontinue. Call doctor right away.

 WARNINGS & PRECAUTIONS

Don't take if:
You are allergic to bumetanide.

Before you start, consult your doctor:
● If you have liver or kidney disease.
● If you have gout.
● If you have diabetes.
● If you have impaired hearing.
● If you will have surgery within 2 months, including dental surgery, requiring general or spinal anesthesia.

Over age 60:
Adverse reactions and side effects may be more frequent and severe than in younger persons.

Pregnancy:
Risk to unborn child outweighs drug benefits. Don't use.

Breast-feeding:
Drug filters into milk. May harm child. Avoid.

Infants & children:
Use only under medical supervision.

Prolonged use:
- Impaired balance of water, salt and potassium in blood and body tissues. Request periodic laboratory studies of electrolytes in blood.
- Possible diabetes.

Skin & sunlight:
May cause rash or intensify sunburn in areas exposed to sun or sunlamp.

Driving, piloting or hazardous work:
No problems expected.

Discontinuing:
Don't discontinue without doctor's advice until you complete prescribed dose, even though symptoms diminish or disappear.

Others:
Frequent laboratory studies to monitor potassium level in blood recommended. Eat foods rich in potassium or take potassium supplements. Consult doctor.

POSSIBLE INTERACTION WITH OTHER DRUGS

GENERIC NAME OR DRUG CLASS	COMBINED EFFECT
Acebutolol	Increased antihypertensive effect. Dosages may require adjustment.
Amiodarone	Increased risk of heartbeat irregularity due to low potassium.
Amitracin, gentamycin, kanamycin, streptomycin, tobramycin, cisplatin, ethacrynic acid, furosemide, mercaptopurine, polymixins.	Increased possibility of hearing loss.
Amitriptyline	Increased amitriptyline effect.
Antihypertensives	Increased blood-pressure drop.
Calcium supplements	Increased calcium in blood.
Cephalosporin antibiotics	Increased possibility of hearing loss.
Enalapril	Possible excessive potassium in blood.
Indapamide	Increased diuretic effect.
Indomethicin	Decreased effect of bumetanide.

Labetolol	Increased antihypertensive effects.
Lithium	Increased possibility of lithium toxicity.
Nitrates	Excessive blood-pressure drop.
Oxprenolol	Increased antihypertensive effect. Dosages may require adjustment.
Pentoxifylline	Increased antihypertensive effect.
Potassium supplements	Decreased potassium effect.
Probenecid	Decreased effect of bumetanide.

POSSIBLE INTERACTION WITH OTHER SUBSTANCES

INTERACTS WITH	COMBINED EFFECT
Alcohol:	Blood-pressure drop. Avoid.
Beverages: Caffeine.	Decreased bumetanide effect.
Cocaine:	Dangerous blood-pressure drop. Avoid.
Foods:	None expected.
Marijuana:	Increased thirst and urinary frequency, fainting.
Tobacco:	Decreased bumetanide effect.

BUSPIRONE

BRAND NAMES

BuSpar

BASIC INFORMATION

Habit forming? Unknown
Prescription needed? Yes
Available as generic? No
Drug class: Antianxiety (tranquilizer)

 USES

Treats anxiety disorders with nervousness or tension. Not intended for treatment of ordinary stress of daily living. Causes less sedation than some antianxiety drugs.

 DOSAGE & USAGE INFORMATION

How to take:
Tablets—Take with a glass of liquid.

When to take:
As directed. Usually 3 times daily. Food does not interfere with absorption.

If you forget a dose:
Take as soon as you remember, but skip this dose and don't double the next dose if it is almost time for the next dose.

What drug does:
Chemical family azaspirodecanedione; *not* a benzodiazepine. Probably has an effect on neurotransmitter systems.

Time lapse before drug works:
1 or 2 weeks before beneficial effects may be observed.

Don't take with:
Alcohol, other tranquilizers, antihistamines, muscle relaxants, sedatives or narcotics.

 OVERDOSE

SYMPTOMS:
Severe drowsiness or nausea, vomiting, small pupils, unconsciousness.
WHAT TO DO:
- **Dial 0 (operator) or 911 (emergency) for an ambulance or medical help. Then give first aid immediately.**
- **See emergency information on inside covers.**

 POSSIBLE ADVERSE REACTIONS OR SIDE EFFECTS

SYMPTOMS	WHAT TO DO
Life-threatening:	
Chest pain; pounding, fast heartbeat (rare).	Discontinue. Seek emergency treatment.
Common:	
Lightheadedness, headache, nausea, restlessness.	Discontinue. Call doctor right away.
Infrequent:	
Drowsiness, dry mouth, ringing in ears, nightmares or vivid dreams, unusual fatigue.	Continue. Call doctor when convenient.
Rare:	
Numbness or tingling in feet or hands; sore throat; fever; depression or confusion; uncontrollable movements of tongue, lips, arms and legs.	Discontinue. Call doctor right away.

WARNINGS & PRECAUTIONS

Don't take if:
If you are allergic to buspirone.

Before you start, consult your doctor:
- If you have ever been addicted to any substance.
- If you have chronic kidney or liver disease.
- If you are already taking *any* medicine.

Over age 60:
Adverse reactions and side effects may be more frequent and severe than in younger persons.

Pregnancy:
No problems expected, but better to avoid if possible.

Breast-feeding:
Buspirone passes into milk of lactating experimental animals. Avoid if possible.

Infants & children:
Use only under close medical supervision.

Prolonged use:
Not recommended for prolonged use. Adverse side effects more likely.

Skin & sunlight:
No problems expected.

Driving, piloting or hazardous work:
Don't drive or pilot aircraft until you learn how medicine affects you. Don't work around dangerous machinery. Don't climb ladders or work in high places. Danger increases if you drink alcohol or take medicine affecting alertness and reflexes, such as antihistamines, tranquilizers, sedatives, pain medicine, narcotics and mind-altering drugs.

Discontinuing:
No problems expected.

Others:
Before elective surgery requiring local or general anesthesia, tell your dentist, surgeon or anesthesiologist that you take buspirone.

 POSSIBLE INTERACTION WITH OTHER DRUGS

GENERIC NAME OR DRUG CLASS	COMBINED EFFECT
Antihistamines	Excessive sedation. Sedative effect of both drugs may be increased.
Barbiturates	Excessive sedation. Sedative effect of both drugs may be increased.
Muscle relaxants	Excessive sedation. Sedative effect of both drugs may be increased.
Narcotics	Excessive sedation. Sedative effect of both drugs may be increased.
Other tranquilizers	Excessive sedation. Sedative effect of both drugs may be increased.
Sedatives	Excessive sedation. Sedative effect of both drugs may be increased.

 POSSIBLE INTERACTION WITH OTHER SUBSTANCES

INTERACTS WITH	COMBINED EFFECT
Alcohol:	Excess sedation. Avoid.
Beverages: Caffeine-containing drinks.	Avoid. Decreased antianxiety effect of busiprone.
Cocaine:	Avoid. Decreased antianxiety effect of busiprone.
Foods:	None expected.
Marijuana:	Avoid. Decreased antianxiety effect of busiprone.
Tobacco:	Avoid. Decreased antianxiety effect of busiprone.

BUSULFAN

BRAND NAMES

Myleran

BASIC INFORMATION

Habit forming? No
Prescription needed? Yes
Available as generic? No
Drug class: Antineoplastic,
                immunosuppressant

 USES

- Treatment for some kinds of cancer.
- Suppresses immune response after transplant and in immune disorders.

 DOSAGE & USAGE INFORMATION

How to take:
Tablet or capsule—Swallow with liquid after light meal. Don't drink fluids with meals. Drink extra fluids between meals. Avoid sweet or fatty foods.

When to take:
At the same time each day.

If you forget a dose:
Take as soon as you remember. Don't ever double dose.

What drug does:
Inhibits abnormal cell reproduction. May suppress immune system.

Time lapse before drug works:
Up to 6 weeks for full effect.

Continued next column

 OVERDOSE

SYMPTOMS:
Bleeding, chills, fever, collapse, stupor, seizure.
WHAT TO DO:
- **Dial 0 (operator) or 911 (emergency) for an ambulance or medical help. Then give first aid immediately.**
- **If patient is unconscious and not breathing, give mouth-to-mouth breathing. If there is no heartbeat, use cardiac massage and mouth-to-mouth breathing (CPR). Don't try to make patient vomit. If you can't get help quickly, take patient to nearest emergency facility.**
- **See emergency information on inside covers.**

Don't take with:
See Interaction column and consult doctor.

 POSSIBLE ADVERSE REACTIONS OR SIDE EFFECTS

SYMPTOMS	WHAT TO DO
Life-threatening: None expected.	
Common:	
• Unusual bleeding or bruising, mouth sores with sore throat, chills and fever, black stools, lip sores, menstrual irregularities.	Discontinue. Call doctor right away.
• Hair loss, joint pain.	Continue. Call doctor when convenient.
• Nausea, vomiting, diarrhea (unavoidable), tiredness, weakness.	Continue. Tell doctor at next visit.
Infrequent:	
• Mental confusion, shortness of breath, may increase chance of developing leukemia.	Continue. Call doctor when convenient.
• Cough.	Continue. Tell doctor at next visit.
Rare: Jaundice.	Discontinue. Call doctor right away.

WARNINGS & PRECAUTIONS

Don't take if:
- You have had hypersensitivity to alkylating antineoplastic drugs.
- Your physician has not explained the serious nature of your medical problem and risks of taking this medicine.

Before you start, consult your doctor:
- If you have gout.
- If you have had kidney stones.
- If you have active infection.
- If you have impaired kidney or liver function.
- If you have taken other antineoplastic drugs or had radiation treatment in last 3 weeks.

Over age 60:
Adverse reactions and side effects may be more frequent and severe than in younger persons.

Pregnancy:
Consult doctor. Risk to child is significant.

Breast-feeding:
Drug passes into milk. Don't nurse.

Infants & children:
Use only under care of medical supervisors who are experienced in anticancer drugs.

Prolonged use:
Adverse reactions more likely the longer drug is required.

Skin & sunlight:
No problems expected.

Driving, piloting or hazardous work:
No problems expected.

Discontinuing:
Don't discontinue without doctor's advice until you complete prescribed dose, even though symptoms diminish or disappear. Some side effects may follow discontinuing. Report to doctor blurred vision, convulsions, confusion, persistent headache.

Others:
May cause sterility.

POSSIBLE INTERACTION WITH OTHER DRUGS

GENERIC NAME OR DRUG CLASS	COMBINED EFFECT
Antigout drugs	Decreased antigout effect.
Antineoplastic drugs (other)	Increased effect of all drugs (may be beneficial).
Chloramphenicol	Increased likelihood of toxic effects of both drugs.

POSSIBLE INTERACTION WITH OTHER SUBSTANCES

INTERACTS WITH	COMBINED EFFECT
Alcohol:	May increase chance of intestinal bleeding.
Beverages:	No problems expected.
Cocaine:	Increases chance of toxicity.
Foods:	Reduces irritation in stomach.
Marijuana:	No problems expected.
Tobacco:	Increases lung toxicity.

BUTABARBITAL

BRAND NAMES

See complete list of brand names in the *Brand Name Directory,* page 945.

BASIC INFORMATION

Habit forming? Yes
Prescription needed? Yes
Available as generic? Yes
Drug class: Sedative, hypnotic (barbiturate)

 ## USES

- Reduces anxiety or nervous tension (low dose).
- Relieves insomnia (higher bedtime dose).

 ## DOSAGE & USAGE INFORMATION

How to take:
Tablet, capsule or liquid—Swallow with food or liquid to lessen stomach irritation. If you can't swallow whole, crumble tablet or open capsule and take with liquid or food.

When to take:
At the same times each day.

If you forget a dose:
Take as soon as you remember up to 2 hours late. If more than 2 hours, wait for next scheduled dose (don't double this dose).

What drug does:
May partially block nerve impulses at nerve-cell connections.

Time lapse before drug works:
60 minutes.

Don't take with:
- Non-prescription drugs without consulting doctor.
- See Interaction column and consult doctor.

 ## OVERDOSE

SYMPTOMS:
Deep sleep, weak pulse, coma.
WHAT TO DO:
- Dial 0 (operator) or 911 (emergency) for an ambulance or medical help. Then give first aid immediately.
- See emergency information on inside covers.

 ## POSSIBLE ADVERSE REACTIONS OR SIDE EFFECTS

SYMPTOMS	WHAT TO DO
Life-threatening: None expected.	
Common: Dizziness, drowsiness, "hangover" effect.	Continue. Call doctor when convenient.
Infrequent:	
• Rash or hives; swollen lips, face or eyelids; sore throat, fever.	Discontinue. Call doctor right away.
• Depression, confusion, slurred speech, diarrhea, nausea, vomiting, joint or muscle pain.	Continue. Call doctor when convenient.
Rare:	
• Agitation, slow heartbeat, breathing difficulty, jaundice.	Discontinue. Call doctor right away.
• Unexplained bleeding or bruising.	Continue. Call doctor when convenient.

 ## WARNINGS & PRECAUTIONS

Don't take if:
- You are allergic to any barbiturate.
- You have porphyria.

Before you start, consult your doctor:
- If you have epilepsy.
- If you have kidney or liver damage.
- If you have asthma.
- If you have anemia.
- If you have chronic pain.
- If you will have surgery within 2 months, including dental surgery, requiring general or spinal anesthesia.

Over age 60:
Adverse reactions and side effects may be more frequent and severe than in younger persons. Use small doses.

Pregnancy:
Risk to unborn child outweighs drug benefits. Don't use.

Breast-feeding:
Drug passes into milk. Avoid drug or discontinue nursing until you finish medicine. Consult doctor for advice on maintaining milk supply.

Infants & children:
Use only under doctor's supervision.

Prolonged use:
- May cause addiction, anemia, chronic intoxication.
- May lower body temperature, making exposure to cold temperatures hazardous.

Skin & sunlight:
May cause rash or intensify sunburn in areas exposed to sun or sunlamp.

Driving, piloting or hazardous work:
Don't drive or pilot aircraft until you learn how medicine affects you. Don't work around dangerous machinery. Don't climb ladders or work in high places. Danger increases if you drink alcohol or take medicine affecting alertness and reflexes.

Discontinuing:
May be unnecessary to finish medicine. Follow doctor's instructions. If you develop withdrawal symptoms of hallucinations, agitation or sleeplessness after discontinuing, call doctor right away.

Others:
High potential for abuse.

POSSIBLE INTERACTION WITH OTHER DRUGS

GENERIC NAME OR DRUG CLASS	COMBINED EFFECT
Anticoagulants (oral)	Decreased anticoagulant effect.
Anticonvulsants	Changed seizure patterns.
Antidepressants (tricyclics)	Decreased antidepressant effect. Possible dangerous oversedation.
Antidiabetics (oral)	Increased butabarbital effect.
Antihistamines	Dangerous sedation. Avoid.
Anti-inflammatory drugs (non-steroidal)	Decreased anti-inflammatory effect.
Aspirin	Decreased aspirin effect.
Beta-adrenergic blockers	Decreased effect of beta-adrenergic blocker.
Contraceptives (oral)	Decreased contraceptive effect.
Cortisone drugs	Decreased cortisone effect.
Digitoxin	Decreased digitoxin effect.

Doxycycline	Decreased doxycycline effect.
Dronabinol	Increased effects of both drugs. Avoid.
Griseofulvin	Decreased griseofulvin effect.
Indapamide	Increased indapamide effect.
MAO inhibitors	Increased butabarbital effect.
Mind-altering drugs	Dangerous sedation. Avoid.
Molindone	Increased sedative effect.
Narcotics	Dangerous sedation. Avoid.
Pain relievers	Dangerous sedation. Avoid.
Sedatives	Dangerous sedation. Avoid.
Sleep inducers	Dangerous sedation. Avoid.
Tranquilizers	Dangerous sedation. Avoid.
Valproic acid	Increased butabarbital effect.

POSSIBLE INTERACTION WITH OTHER SUBSTANCES

INTERACTS WITH	COMBINED EFFECT
Alcohol:	Possible fatal oversedation. Avoid.
Beverages:	None expected.
Cocaine:	Decreased butabarbital effect.
Foods:	None expected.
Marijuana:	Excessive sedation. Avoid.
Tobacco:	None expected.

BUTALBITAL & ASPIRIN
(Also contains caffeine)

BRAND AND GENERIC NAMES

Buff-A-Comp
BUTALBITAL,
  ASPIRIN &
  CAFFEINE
Butal Compound
Fiorinal

Isollyl (Improved)
Lanorinal
Marnal
Protension
Tenstan

BASIC INFORMATION

Habit forming? Yes
Prescription needed? Yes
Available as generic? Yes
Drug class: Analgesic, anti-inflammatory,
    sedative

USES

- Reduces anxiety or nervous tension (low dose).
- Reduces pain, fever, inflammation.

DOSAGE & USAGE INFORMATION

How to take:
- Tablet, liquid or capsule—Swallow with liquid or food to lessen stomach irritation. If you can't swallow whole, crumble tablet or open capsule and take with liquid or food.
- Extended-release tablets or capsules—Swallow each dose whole.
- Suppositories—Remove wrapper and moisten suppository with water. Gently insert into rectum, large end first.

When to take:
At the same times each day. No more often than every 4 hours.

Continued next column

OVERDOSE

SYMPTOMS:
Deep sleep, weak pulse, ringing in ears, nausea, vomiting, dizziness, fever, deep and rapid breathing, hallucinations, convulsions, coma.
WHAT TO DO:
- **Dial 0 (operator) or 911 (emergency) for an ambulance or medical help. Then give first aid immediately.**
- **See emergency information on inside covers.**

If you forget a dose:
Take as soon as you remember up to 2 hours late. If more than 2 hours, wait for next scheduled dose (don't double this dose).

What drug does:
- May partially block nerve impulses at nerve-cell connections.
- Affects hypothalamus, the part of the brain which regulates temperature by dilating small blood vessels in skin.
- Prevents clumping of platelets (small blood cells) so blood vessels remain open.
- Decreases prostaglandin effect.
- Suppresses body's pain messages.

Time lapse before drug works:
30 minutes.

Don't take with:
- Non-prescription drugs without consulting doctor.
- See Interaction column and consult doctor.

POSSIBLE ADVERSE REACTIONS OR SIDE EFFECTS

SYMPTOMS	WHAT TO DO
Life-threatening:	
Hives, rash, intense itching, faintness soon after a dose (anaphylaxis); wheezing; tightness in chest; black or bloody vomit; black stools; shortness of breath.	Seek emergency treatment immediately.
Common:	
Dizziness, drowsiness, heartburn.	Continue. Call doctor when convenient.
Infrequent:	
Jaundice; vomiting blood; easy bruising; skin rash, hives; confusion; depression; sore throat, fever, mouth sores; hearing loss; slurred speech; decreased vision.	Discontinue. Call doctor right away.
Rare:	
• Diminished vision, blood in urine, unexplained fever.	Discontinue. Call doctor right away.
• Insomnia, nightmares, constipation, headache, nervousness, jaundice.	Continue. Call doctor when convenient.

BUTALBITAL & ASPIRIN
(Also contains caffeine)

WARNINGS & PRECAUTIONS

Don't take if:
- You are allergic to any barbiturate.
- You have a peptic ulcer of stomach or duodenum, bleeding disorder, porphyria.

Before you start, consult your doctor:
- If you have had stomach or duodenal ulcers.
- If you have asthma, nasal polyps, epilepsy, kidney or liver damage, anemia, chronic pain.
- If you will have surgery within 2 months, including dental surgery, requiring general or spinal anesthesia.

Over age 60:
- Adverse reactions and side effects may be more frequent and severe than in younger persons.
- More likely to cause hidden bleeding in stomach or intestines. Watch for dark stools.

Pregnancy:
Risk to unborn child outweighs drug benefits. Don't use.

Breast-feeding:
Drug passes into milk. Avoid drug or discontinue nursing until you finish medicine. Consult doctor for advice on maintaining milk supply.

Infants & children:
- Overdose frequent and severe. Keep bottles out of children's reach.
- Use only under doctor's supervision.

Prolonged use:
- Kidney damage. Periodic kidney-function test recommended.
- May cause addiction, anemia, chronic intoxication.
- May lower body temperature, making exposure to cold temperatures hazardous.

Skin & sunlight:
May cause rash or intensify sunburn in areas exposed to sun or sunlamp.

Driving, piloting or hazardous work:
Don't drive or pilot aircraft until you learn how medicine affects you. Don't work around dangerous machinery. Don't climb ladders or work in high places. Danger increases if you drink alcohol or take medicine affecting alertness and reflexes, such as antihistamines, tranquilizers, sedatives, pain medicine, narcotics and mind-altering drugs.

Discontinuing:
May be unnecessary to finish medicine. Follow doctor's instructions. If you develop withdrawal symptoms of hallucinations, agitation or sleeplessness after discontinuing, call doctor right away.

Others:
- Aspirin can complicate surgery, pregnancy, labor and delivery, and illness.
- For arthritis—Don't change dose without consulting doctor.
- Urine tests for blood sugar may be inaccurate.
- Great potential for abuse.

POSSIBLE INTERACTION WITH OTHER DRUGS

GENERIC NAME OR DRUG CLASS	COMBINED EFFECT
Acebutolol	Decreased antihypertensive effect of acebutolol.
Allopurinol	Decreased allopurinol effect.
Antacids	Decreased aspirin effect.
Anticoagulants (oral)	Increased anticoagulant effect. Abnormal bleeding.
Anticonvulsants	Changed seizure patterns.
Antidepressants	Decreased antidepressant effect. Possible dangerous oversedation.
Antidiabetics (oral)	Increased butalbital effect. Low blood sugar.
Antihistamines	Dangerous sedation. Avoid.

Continued page 963

POSSIBLE INTERACTION WITH OTHER SUBSTANCES

INTERACTS WITH	COMBINED EFFECT
Alcohol:	Possible stomach irritation and bleeding, possible fatal oversedation. Avoid.
Beverages:	None expected.
Cocaine:	Decreased butalbital effect.
Foods:	None expected.
Marijuana:	Possible increased pain relief, but marijuana may slow body's recovery. Avoid.
Tobacco:	None expected.

123

BUTALBITAL, ASPIRIN & CODEINE
(Also contains caffeine)

BRAND NAMES

Buff-A-Comp 3   Isollyl with Codeine
Fiorinal with Codeine

BASIC INFORMATION

Habit forming? Yes
Prescription needed? Yes
Available as generic? No
Drug class: Narcotic, analgesic

 ## USES

- Reduces anxiety or nervous tension (low dose).
- Reduces pain, fever, inflammation.

 ## DOSAGE & USAGE INFORMATION

How to take:
- Tablet, liquid or capsule—Swallow with liquid or food to lessen stomach irritation. If you can't swallow whole, crumble tablet or open capsule and take with liquid or food.
- Extended-release tablets or capsules—Swallow each dose whole.

When to take:
When needed. No more often than every 4 hours.

Continued next column

 ## OVERDOSE

SYMPTOMS:
Deep sleep, slow and weak pulse, ringing in ears, nausea, vomiting, dizziness, fever, deep and rapid breathing, hallucinations, convulsions, coma.
WHAT TO DO:
- Dial 0 (operator) or 911 (emergency) for an ambulance or medical help. Then give first aid immediately.
- If patient is unconscious and not breathing, give mouth-to-mouth breathing. If there is no heartbeat, use cardiac massage and mouth-to-mouth breathing (CPR). Don't try to make patient vomit. If you can't get help quickly, take patient to nearest emergency facility.
- See emergency information on inside covers.

If you forget a dose:
Take as soon as you remember. Wait 4 hours for next dose.

What drug does:
- May partially block nerve impulses at nerve-cell connections.
- Affects hypothalamus, the part of the brain which regulates temperature by dilating small blood vessels in skin.
- Prevents clumping of platelets (small blood cells) so blood vessels remain open.
- Decreases prostaglandin effect.
- Blocks pain messages to brain and spinal cord.
- Reduces sensitivity of brain's cough-control center.

Time lapse before drug works:
30 minutes.

Don't take with:
- Non-prescription drugs without consulting doctor.
- See Interaction column and consult doctor.

 ## POSSIBLE ADVERSE REACTIONS OR SIDE EFFECTS

SYMPTOMS	WHAT TO DO
Life-threatening:	
Wheezing, tightness in chest, pinpoint pupils.	Seek emergency treatment immediately.
Common:	
Dizziness, drowsiness, heartburn, flushed face, depression, false sense of well-being, increased urination.	Continue. Call doctor when convenient.
Infrequent:	
Jaundice; vomiting blood; easy bruising; skin rash, hives; confusion; depression; sore throat, fever, mouth sores; difficult urination; hearing loss; slurred speech; blood in urine; decreased vision.	Discontinue. Call doctor right away.
Rare:	
Insomnia, nightmares, constipation, headache, nervousness, flushed face, increased sweating, unusual tiredness.	Continue. Call doctor when convenient.

BUTALBITAL, ASPIRIN & CODEINE
(Also contains caffeine)

WARNINGS & PRECAUTIONS

Don't take if:
- You are allergic to any barbiturate or narcotic.
- You have a peptic ulcer of stomach or duodenum, bleeding disorder, porphyria.

Before you start, consult your doctor:
- If you have had stomach or duodenal ulcers.
- If you have asthma, epilepsy, kidney or liver damage, anemia, chronic pain, gout.
- If you will have surgery within 2 months, including dental surgery, requiring general or spinal anesthesia.

Over age 60:
- Adverse reactions and side effects may be more frequent and severe than in younger persons.
- More likely to cause hidden bleeding in stomach or intestines. Watch for dark stools.
- More likely to be drowsy, dizzy, unsteady or constipated. Use only if absolutely necessary.

Pregnancy:
Risk to unborn child outweighs drug benefits. Don't use.

Breast-feeding:
Drug passes into milk. Avoid drug or discontinue nursing until you finish medicine. Consult doctor for advice on maintaining milk supply.

Infants & children:
- Overdose frequent and severe. Keep bottles out of children's reach.
- Use only under doctor's supervision.
- Consult doctor before giving to persons under age 18 who have fever and discomfort of viral illness, especially chicken pox and influenza. Probably increases risk of Reye's syndrome.

Prolonged use:
- Kidney damage. Periodic kidney-function test recommended.
- May cause addiction, anemia, chronic intoxication.
- May lower body temperature, making exposure to cold temperatures hazardous.

Skin & sunlight:
May cause rash or intensify sunburn in areas exposed to sun or sunlamp.

Driving, piloting or hazardous work:
Don't drive or pilot aircraft until you learn how medicine affects you. Don't work around dangerous machinery. Don't climb ladders or work in high places. Danger increases if you drink alcohol or take medicine affecting alertness and reflexes, such as antihistamines, tranquilizers, sedatives, pain medicine, narcotics and mind-altering drugs.

Discontinuing:
May be unnecessary to finish medicine. Follow doctor's instructions. If you develop withdrawal symptoms of hallucinations, agitation or sleeplessness after discontinuing, call doctor right away.

Others:
- Aspirin can complicate surgery, pregnancy, labor and delivery, and illness.
- For arthritis—Don't change dose without consulting doctor.
- Urine tests for blood sugar may be inaccurate.
- Great potential for abuse.

POSSIBLE INTERACTION WITH OTHER DRUGS

GENERIC NAME OR DRUG CLASS	COMBINED EFFECT
Acebutolol	Decreased antihypertensive effect of acebutolol.
Allopurinol	Decreased allopurinol effect.
Analgesics (other)	Increased analgesic effect.
Antacids	Decreased aspirin effect.
Anticoagulants (oral)	Increased anticoagulant effect. Abnormal bleeding.
Anticonvulsants	Changed seizure patterns.

Continued page 963

POSSIBLE INTERACTION WITH OTHER SUBSTANCES

INTERACTS WITH	COMBINED EFFECT
Alcohol:	Possible stomach irritation and bleeding, possible fatal oversedation. Avoid.
Beverages:	None expected.
Cocaine:	Increased cocaine toxic effects. Avoid.
Foods:	None expected.
Marijuana:	Possible increased pain relief, but marijuana may slow body's recovery. Impairs physical and mental performance. Avoid.
Tobacco:	None expected.

BUTAPERAZINE

BRAND NAMES

Repoise

BASIC INFORMATION

Habit forming? No
Prescription needed? Yes
Available as generic? Yes
Drug class: Tranquilizer, antiemetic
(phenothiazine)

 USES

- Stops nausea, vomiting.
- Reduces anxiety, agitation.

 DOSAGE & USAGE INFORMATION

How to take:
- Tablet or capsule—Swallow with liquid or food to lessen stomach irritation.
- Suppositories—Remove wrapper and moisten suppository with water. Gently insert into rectum, large end first.
- Drops or liquid—Dilute dose in beverage.

When to take:
- Nervous and mental disorders—Take at the same times each day.
- Nausea and vomiting—Take as needed, no more often than every 4 hours.

If you forget a dose:
- Nervous and mental disorders—Take up to 2 hours late. If more than 2 hours, wait for next scheduled dose (don't double this).
- Nausea and vomiting—Take as soon as you remember. Wait 4 hours for next dose.

What drug does:
- Suppresses brain's vomiting center.
- Suppresses brain centers that control abnormal emotions and behavior.

Time lapse before drug works:
- Nausea and vomiting—1 hour or less.
- Nervous and mental disorders—4-6 weeks.

Continued next column

 OVERDOSE

SYMPTOMS:
Stupor, convulsions, coma.
WHAT TO DO:
- Dial 0 (operator) or 911 (emergency) for an ambulance or medical help. Then give first aid immediately.
- See emergency information on inside covers.

Don't take with:
- Antacid or medicine for diarrhea.
- Non-prescription drug for cough, cold or allergy.
- See Interaction column and consult doctor.

 POSSIBLE ADVERSE REACTIONS OR SIDE EFFECTS

SYMPTOMS	WHAT TO DO
Life-threatening:	
None expected.	
Common:	
• Muscle spasms of face and neck, unsteady gait.	Discontinue. Seek emergency treatment.
• Restlessness, tremor, drowsiness.	Discontinue. Call doctor right away.
• Decreased sweating, dry mouth, stuffy nose, constipation.	Continue. Call doctor when convenient.
Infrequent:	
• Fainting.	Discontinue. Seek emergency treatment.
• Rash.	Discontinue. Call doctor right away.
• Difficult urination, diminished sex drive, swollen breasts, menstrual irregularities.	Continue. Call doctor when convenient.
Rare:	
Changes in vision, sore throat, fever, jaundice.	Discontinue. Call doctor right away.

WARNINGS & PRECAUTIONS

Don't take if:
- You are allergic to any phenothiazine.
- You have a blood or bone-marrow disease.

Before you start, consult your doctor:
- If you will have surgery within 2 months, including dental surgery, requiring general or spinal anesthesia.
- If you have asthma, emphysema or other lung disorder.
- If you take non-prescription ulcer medicine, asthma medicine or amphetamines.

Over age 60:
Adverse reactions and side effects may be more frequent and severe than in younger persons. More likely to develop involuntary movement of jaws, lips, tongue, chewing. Report this to your doctor immediately. Early treatment can help.

Pregnancy:
Risk to unborn child outweighs drug benefits. Don't use.

Breast-feeding:
Drug passes into milk. Avoid drug or discontinue nursing until you finish medicine. Consult doctor for advice on maintaining milk supply.

Infants & children:
Don't give to children younger than 2.

Prolonged use:
May lead to tardive dyskinesia (involuntary movement of jaws, lips, tongue, chewing).

Skin & sunlight: .
May cause rash or intensify sunburn in areas exposed to sun or sunlamp. Skin may remain sensitive for 3 months after discontinuing.

Driving, piloting or hazardous work:
Don't drive or pilot aircraft until you learn how medicine affects you. Don't work around dangerous machinery. Don't climb ladders or work in high places. Danger increases if you drink alcohol or take medicine affecting alertness and reflexes.

Discontinuing:
- Nervous and mental disorders—Don't discontinue without doctor's advice until you complete prescribed dose, even though symptoms diminish or disappear.
- Nausea and vomiting—May be unnecessary to finish medicine. Follow doctor's instructions.

Others:
No problems expected.

POSSIBLE INTERACTION WITH OTHER DRUGS

GENERIC NAME OR DRUG CLASS	COMBINED EFFECT
Anticholinergics	Increased anticholinergic effect
Antidepressants (tricyclic)	Increased butaperazine effect.
Antihistamines	Increased antihistam effect.
Appetite suppressants	Decreased suppressant effect.
Dronabinol	Increased effects of both drugs. Avoid.
Levodopa	Decreased levodopa effect.
Mind-altering drugs	Increased effect of mind-altering drugs.
Narcotics	Increased narcotic effect.
Phenytoin	Increased phenytoin effect.
Quinidine	Impaired heart functio Dangerous mixture.
Sedatives	Increased sedative effect.
Tranquilizers (other)	Increased tranquilizer effect.

POSSIBLE INTERACTION WITH OTHER SUBSTANCES

INTERACTS WITH	COMBINED EFFECT
Alcohol:	Dangerous oversedation.
Beverages:	None expected.
Cocaine:	Decreased butaperazine effect. Avoid.
Foods:	None expected.
Marijuana:	Drowsiness. May increase antinausea effect.
Tobacco:	None expected.

CAFFEINE

BRAND NAMES

See complete list of brand names in the *Brand Name Directory*, page 945.

BASIC INFORMATION

Habit forming? Yes
Prescription needed? No
Available as generic? Yes
Drug class: Stimulant (xanthine), vasoconstrictor

 ## USES

- Treatment for drowsiness and fatigue.
- Treatment for migraine and other vascular headaches in combination with ergot.

 ## DOSAGE & USAGE INFORMATION

How to take:
- Tablet—Swallow with liquid or food to lessen stomach irritation. If you can't swallow whole, crumble tablet or open capsule and take with liquid or food.
- Extended-release capsules—Swallow whole with liquid.

When to take:
At the same times each day.

If you forget a dose:
Take as soon as you remember up to 2 hours late. If more than 2 hours, wait for next scheduled dose (don't double this dose).

What drug does:
- Constricts blood-vessel walls.
- Stimulates central nervous system.

Time lapse before drug works:
30 minutes.

Continued next column

 ## OVERDOSE

SYMPTOMS:
Excitement, rapid heartbeat, hallucinations, convulsions, coma.
WHAT TO DO:
- **Dial 0 (operator) or 911 (emergency) for an ambulance or medical help. Then give first aid immediately.**
- **See emergency information on inside covers.**

Don't take with:
- Non-prescription drugs without consulting doctor.
- See Interaction column and consult doctor.

 ## POSSIBLE ADVERSE REACTIONS OR SIDE EFFECTS

SYMPTOMS	WHAT TO DO
Life-threatening:	
None expected.	
Common:	
• Rapid heartbeat, low blood sugar (hunger, anxiety, cold sweats, rapid pulse) with tremor, irritability.	Continue. Call doctor when convenient.
• Nervousness, insomnia.	Continue. Tell doctor at next visit.
• Increased urination.	No action necessary.
Infrequent:	
• Confusion, irritability.	Discontinue. Call doctor right away.
• Nausea, indigestion, burning feeling, in stomach.	Continue. Call doctor when convenient.
Rare:	
None expected.	

WARNINGS & PRECAUTIONS

Don't take if:
- You are allergic to any stimulant.
- You have heart disease.
- You have active peptic ulcer of stomach or duodenum.

Before you start, consult your doctor:
- If you have irregular heartbeat.
- If you have hypoglycemia (low blood sugar).
- If you have epilepsy.

Over age 60:
Adverse reactions and side effects may be more frequent and severe than in younger persons.

Pregnancy:
Risk to unborn child outweighs drug benefits. Don't use.

Breast-feeding:
Drug passes into milk. Avoid drug or discontinue nursing until you finish medicine. Consult doctor for advice on maintaining milk supply.

Infants & children:
Not recommended.

Prolonged use:
Stomach ulcers.

Skin & sunlight:
No problems expected.

Driving, piloting or hazardous work:
No problems expected.

Discontinuing:
Will cause withdrawal symptoms of headache, irritability, drowsiness. Discontinue gradually if you use caffeine for a month or more.

Others:
May produce or aggravate fibrocystic disease of the breast in women.

POSSIBLE INTERACTION WITH OTHER DRUGS

GENERIC NAME OR DRUG CLASS	COMBINED EFFECT
Contraceptives (oral)	Increased caffeine effect.
Isoniazid	Increased caffeine effect.
MAO inhibitors	Dangerous blood-pressure rise.
Sedatives	Decreased sedative effect.
Sleep inducers	Decreased sedative effect.
Sympathomimetics	Overstimulation.
Thyroid hormones	Increased thyroid effect.
Tranquilizers	Decreased tranquilizer effect.

POSSIBLE INTERACTION WITH OTHER SUBSTANCES

INTERACTS WITH	COMBINED EFFECT
Alcohol:	Decreased alcohol effect.
Beverages: Caffeine drinks.	Increased caffeine effect.
Cocaine:	Overstimulation. Avoid.
Foods:	No proven problems.
Marijuana:	Increased effect of both drugs. May lead to dangerous, rapid heartbeat. Avoid.
Tobacco:	Increased heartbeat. Avoid.

CALCIUM CARBONATE

BRAND NAMES

See complete list of brand names in the *Brand Name Directory,* page 946.

BASIC INFORMATION

Habit forming? No
Prescription needed? No
Available as generic? Yes
Drug class: Antacid

 ## USES

Treatment for hyperacidity in upper gastrointestinal tract, including stomach and esophagus. Symptoms may be heartburn or acid indigestion. Diseases include peptic ulcer, gastritis, esophagitis, hiatal hernia.

 ## DOSAGE & USAGE INFORMATION

How to take:
- Tablet—Swallow with liquid.
- Chewable tablets or wafers—Chew well before swallowing.

When to take:
1 to 3 hours after meals unless directed otherwise by your doctor.

If you forget a dose:
Take as soon as you remember.

What drug does:
- Neutralizes some of the hydrochloric acid in the stomach.
- Reduces action of pepsin, a digestive enzyme.

Time lapse before drug works:
15 minutes.

Don't take with:
Other medicines at the same time. Decreases absorption of other drugs.

 ## OVERDOSE

SYMPTOMS:
Weakness, fatigue, dizziness.
WHAT TO DO:
Overdose unlikely to threaten life. If person takes much larger amount than prescribed, call doctor, poison-control center or hospital emergency room for instructions.

 ## POSSIBLE ADVERSE REACTIONS OR SIDE EFFECTS

SYMPTOMS	WHAT TO DO
Life-threatening: None expected.	
Common: Constipation, appetite loss.	Continue. Call doctor when convenient.
Infrequent: • Lower abdominal pain and swelling, bone pain, muscle weakness, swollen wrists or ankles.	Discontinue. Call doctor right away.
• Mood changes, nausea, vomiting, weight loss.	Continue. Call doctor when convenient.
Rare: Difficult or painful urination, unusual tiredness or weakness.	Discontinue. Call doctor right away.

 ## WARNINGS & PRECAUTIONS

Don't take if:
- You are allergic to any antacid.
- You have a high blood-calcium level.

Before you start, consult your doctor:
- If you have kidney disease.
- If you have chronic constipation, colitis or diarrhea.
- If you have symptoms of appendicitis.
- If you have stomach or intestinal bleeding.
- If you have irregular heartbeat.

Over age 60:
Adverse reactions and side effects may be more frequent and severe than in younger persons. Diarrhea or constipation particularly likely.

Pregnancy:
Risk to unborn child outweighs drug benefits. Don't use.

Breast-feeding:
Drug passes into milk. Avoid drug or discontinue nursing until you finish medicine. Consult doctor for advice on maintaining milk supply.

Infants & children:
Use only under medical supervision.

Prolonged use:
- High blood level of calcium which disturbs electrolyte balance.
- Kidney stones, impaired kidney function.

Skin & sunlight:
No problems expected.

Driving, piloting or hazardous work:
No problems expected.

Discontinuing:
May be unnecessary to finish medicine. Follow doctor's instructions.

Others:
Don't take longer than 2 weeks unless under medical supervision.

POSSIBLE INTERACTION WITH OTHER DRUGS

GENERIC NAME OR DRUG CLASS	COMBINED EFFECT
Anticoagulants	Decreased anticoagulant effect.
Calcitonin	Decreased calcitonin effect.
Chlorpromazine	Decreased chlorpromazine effect.
Digitalis preparations	Decreased digitalis effect.
Diuretics	Increased calcium in blood.
Iron supplements	Decreased iron effect.
Meperidine	Increased meperidine effect.
Mexiletine	May slow elimination of mexiletine and cause need to adjust dosage.
Nalidixic acid	Decreased effect of nalidixic acid.
Oxyphenbutazone	Decreased oxyphenbutazone effect.
Para-aminosalicylic acid (PAS)	Decreased PAS effect.
Penicillins	Decreased penicillin effect.
Pentobarbital	Decreased pentobarbital effect.
Phenylbutazone	Decreased phenylbutazone effect.
Pseudoephedrine	Increased pseudoephedrine effect.
Quinidine	Increased quinidine effect.
Salicylates	Increased salicylate effect.
Sulfa drugs	Decreased sulfa effect.

Tetracyclines	Decreased tetracycline effect.
Vitamin A	Decreased vitamin effect.
Vitamin D (large doses)	Excessive absorption of vitamin D.

POSSIBLE INTERACTION WITH OTHER SUBSTANCES

INTERACTS WITH	COMBINED EFFECT
Alcohol:	Decreased antacid effect.
Beverages:	No proven problems.
Cocaine:	No proven problems.
Foods:	Decreased antacid effect if taken with food. Wait 1 hour after eating.
Marijuana:	No proven problems.
Tobacco:	Decreased antacid effect.

CALCIUM & MAGNESIUM ANTACIDS

BRAND AND GENERIC NAMES

Alkets
Bisodol
CALCIUM &
 MAGNESIUM
 CARBONATES
CALCIUM &
 MAGNESIUM
 CARBONATES &
 MAGNESIUM
 OXIDE

CALCIUM
 CARBONATE &
 MAGNESIA
Marblen
Ratio
Spastosed

BASIC INFORMATION

Habit forming? No
Prescription needed? No
Available as generic? Yes
Drug class: Antacid

USES

- Treatment for hyperacidity in upper gastrointestinal tract, including stomach and esophagus. Symptoms may be heartburn or acid indigestion. Diseases include peptic ulcer, gastritis, esophagitis, hiatal hernia.
- Constipation relief.

DOSAGE & USAGE INFORMATION

How to take:
- Tablet or capsule—Swallow with liquid.
- Chewable tablets or wafers—Chew well before swallowing.
- Liquid—Shake well and take undiluted.

Continued next column

OVERDOSE

SYMPTOMS:
Dry mouth, shallow breathing, diarrhea, weakness, fatigue, stupor.
WHAT TO DO:
- **Overdose unlikely to threaten life. Depending on severity of symptoms and amount taken, call doctor, poison-control center or hospital emergency room for instructions.**
- **Dial 0 (operator) or 911 (emergency) for an ambulance or medical help. Then give first aid immediately.**
- **See emergency information on inside covers.**

When to take:
1 to 3 hours after meals unless directed otherwise by your doctor.

If you forget a dose:
Take as soon as you remember, but not simultaneously with any other medicine.

What drug does:
- Neutralizes some of the hydrochloric acid in the stomach.
- Reduces action of pepsin, a digestive enzyme.
- Stimulates muscles in lower bowel wall.

Time lapse before drug works:
15 minutes for antacid effect.

Don't take with:
Other medicines at the same time. Decreases absorption of other drugs. Wait 2 hours between doses.

POSSIBLE ADVERSE REACTIONS OR SIDE EFFECTS

SYMPTOMS	WHAT TO DO
Life-threatening:	
Heartbeat irregularity in patient with heart disease.	Discontinue. Seek emergency treatment.
Common:	
• Constipation, headache, appetite loss, distended stomach.	Discontinue. Call doctor right away.
• Unpleasant taste in mouth, abdominal pain, laxative effect, belching.	Continue. Call doctor when convenient.
Infrequent:	
Bone pain, frequent urination, dizziness, urgent urination, muscle weakness or pain, nausea, weight gain.	Discontinue. Call doctor right away.
Rare:	
Mood changes, vomiting, nervousness, swollen feet and ankles.	Discontinue. Call doctor right away.

CALCIUM & MAGNESIUM ANTACIDS

WARNINGS & PRECAUTIONS

Don't take if:
- You are allergic to any antacid.
- You have a high blood-calcium level.

Before you start, consult your doctor:
If you have kidney disease, chronic constipation, colitis, diarrhea, symptoms of appendicitis, stomach or intestinal bleeding, irregular heartbeat.

Over age 60:
Adverse reactions and side effects may be more frequent and severe than in younger persons. Diarrhea or constipation particularly likely.

Pregnancy:
Risk to unborn child outweighs drug benefits. Don't use.

Breast-feeding:
Drug passes into milk. Avoid drug or discontinue nursing until you finish medicine. Consult doctor for advice on maintaining milk supply.

Infants & children:
Use only under medical supervision.

Prolonged use:
- High blood level of calcium which disturbs electrolyte balance.
- Kidney stones, impaired kidney function.

Skin & sunlight:
No problems expected.

Driving, piloting or hazardous work:
No problems expected.

Discontinuing:
May be unnecessary to finish medicine. Follow doctor's instructions.

Others:
Don't take longer than 2 weeks unless under medical supervision.

POSSIBLE INTERACTION WITH OTHER DRUGS

GENERIC NAME OR DRUG CLASS	COMBINED EFFECT
Anticoagulants (oral)	Decreased anticoagulant effect.
Calcitonin	Decreased calcitonin effect.
Chlorpromazine	Decreased chlorpromazine effect.
Digitalis preparations	Decreased digitalis effect.
Iron supplements	Decreased iron effect.
Isoniazid	Decreased isoniazid effect.
Levodopa	Increased levodopa effect.
Meperidine	Increased meperidine effect.
Nalidixic acid	Decreased nalidixic acid effect.
Oxyphenbutazone	Decreased oxyphenbutazone effect.
Para-aminosalicylic acid (PAS)	Decreased PAS effect.
Penicillins	Decreased penicillin effect.
Pentobarbital	Decreased pentobarbital effect.
Phenylbutazone	Decreased phenylbutazone effect.
Pseudoephedrine	Increased pseudoephedrine effect.
Quinidine	Increased quinidine effect.
Salicylates	Increased salicylate effect.
Sulfa drugs	Decreased sulfa effect.

POSSIBLE INTERACTION WITH OTHER SUBSTANCES

INTERACTS WITH	COMBINED EFFECT
Alcohol:	Decreased antacid effect.
Beverages:	No proven problems.
Cocaine:	No proven problems.
Foods:	Decreased antacid effect. Wait 1 hour after eating.
Marijuana:	Decreased antacid effect.
Tobacco:	Decreased antacid effect.

CALCIUM SUPPLEMENTS

BRAND NAMES

See complete list of brand names in the
Brand Name Directory, page 946.

BASIC INFORMATION

Habit forming? No
Prescription needed? For some
Available as generic? Yes
Drug class: Antihypocalcemic

USES

- Treats or prevents osteoporosis (thin, porous, easily fractured bones). Frequently prescribed with estrogen beginning at menopause.
- Helps heart, muscle and nervous system to work properly.

DOSAGE & USAGE INFORMATION

How to take:
- Take in addition to foods high in calcium (milk, yogurt, sardines, cheese, canned salmon, turnip greens, broccoli, shrimp, tofu).
- Swallow with liquid or food to lessen stomach irritation. If you can't swallow whole, crumble tablet and take with food or liquid.
- Syrup—Take before meals.

When to take:
As directed. Don't take within 2 hours of any other medicine you take by mouth.

If you forget a dose:
Use as soon as you remember.

What drug does:
Participates in metabolism of all activities essential for normal life and function of cells.

Time lapse before drug works:
15 to 30 minutes.

Continued next column

OVERDOSE

SYMPTOMS:
Confusion, irregular heartbeat, depression, bone pain, coma.
WHAT TO DO:
- **Dial 0 (operator) or 911 (emergency) for an ambulance or medical help. Then give first aid immediately.**
- **See emergency information on inside covers.**

Don't take with:
- Any other medicine until 2 hours have passed since taking calcium.
- See Interaction column and consult doctor.

POSSIBLE ADVERSE REACTIONS OR SIDE EFFECTS

SYMPTOMS	WHAT TO DO
Life-threatening:	
Irregular or very slow heart rate.	Discontinue. Seek emergency treatment.
Common:	
None expected.	
Infrequent:	
Constipation, diarrhea, drowsiness, headache, appetite loss, dry mouth, weakness.	Discontinue. Call doctor right away.
Rare:	
Frequent, painful or difficult urination; increased thirst; nausea, vomiting; rash; urine frequency increased and volume larger; confusion; high blood pressure; eyes sensitive to light.	Discontinue. Call doctor right away.

WARNINGS & PRECAUTIONS

Don't take if:
- You are allergic to calcium.
- You have a high blood-calcium level.

Before you start, consult your doctor:
If you have diarrhea, heart disease, kidney stones, kidney disease, sarcoidosis, malabsorption.

Over age 60:
No problems expected.

Pregnancy:
No problems expected, but ask your doctor.

Breast-feeding:
No problems expected.

Infants & children:
Use only under close medical supervision.

Prolonged use:
Side effects more likely.

Skin & sunlight:
No problems expected.

Driving, piloting or hazardous work:
No problems expected.

Discontinuing:
No problems expected.

Others:
- Exercise, along with vitamin D from sunshine and calcium, helps prevent osteoporosis.
- Don't use bone meal or dolomite as a source for calcium supplement (they may contain lead).

POSSIBLE INTERACTION WITH OTHER DRUGS

GENERIC NAME OR DRUG CLASS	COMBINED EFFECT
Anticoagulants	Decreased anticoagulant effect.
Calcitonin	Decreased calcitonin effect.
Chlorpromazine	Decreased chlorpromazine effect.
Digitalis preparations	Decreased digitalis effect.
Diuretics	Increased calcium in blood.
Estrogens and birth control pills	May increase absorption of calcium— frequently a desirable combined effect.
Iron supplements	Decreased iron effect.

Meperidine	Increased meperidine effect.
Mexiletine	May slow elimination of mexiletine and cause need to adjust dosage.
Nalidixic acid	Decreased effect of nalidixic acid.
Oxyphenbutazone	Decreased oxyphenbutazone effect.
Para-aminosalicylic acid (PAS)	Decreased PAS effect.
Penicillins	Decreased penicillin effect.
Pentobarbital	Decreased pentobarbital effect.
Phenylbutazone	Decreased phenylbutazone effect.
Pseudoephedrine	Increased pseudoephedrine effect.
Quinidine	Increased quinidine effect.
Salicylates	Increased salicylate effect.
Sulfa drugs	Decreased sulfa effect.
Tetracyclines	Decreased tetracycline effect.
Vitamins A and C	Decreased vitamin effect.

POSSIBLE INTERACTION WITH OTHER SUBSTANCES

INTERACTS WITH	COMBINED EFFECT
Alcohol:	Decreased absorption of calcium.
Beverages:	No problems expected.
Cocaine:	No proven problems.
Foods: Don't take within 1 or 2 hours of food.	Decreased absorption of calcium.
Marijuana:	Decreased absorption of calcium.
Tobacco:	Decreased absorption of calcium.

CAPTOPRIL

BRAND NAMES

Capoten

BASIC INFORMATION

Habit forming? No
Prescription needed? Yes
Available as generic? No
Drug class: Antihypertensive, A.C.E.
          inhibitor (See Glossary)

USES

Treatment for high blood pressure and congestive heart failure.

DOSAGE & USAGE INFORMATION

How to take:
Tablets—Swallow with liquid. Instructions to take on empty stomach mean 1 hour before or 2 hours after eating.

When to take:
At the same times each day, usually 3 times daily. Take first dose at bedtime and lie down immediately.

If you forget a dose:
Take as soon as you remember up to 2 hours late. If more than 2 hours, wait for next scheduled dose (don't double this dose).

What drug does:
• Reduces resistance in arteries.
• Strengthens heartbeat.

Time lapse before drug works:
60 to 90 minutes.

Don't take with:
See Interaction column and consult doctor.

OVERDOSE

SYMPTOMS:
Fever, chills, sore throat, fainting, convulsions, coma.
WHAT TO DO:
• Dial 0 (operator) or 911 (emergency) for an ambulance or medical help. Then give first aid immediately.
• See emergency information on inside covers.

POSSIBLE ADVERSE REACTIONS OR SIDE EFFECTS

SYMPTOMS	WHAT TO DO
Life-threatening: None expected.	
Common: Rash, loss of taste.	Discontinue. Call doctor right away.
Infrequent:	
• Swelling of mouth, face, hands or feet.	Discontinue. Seek emergency treatment.
• Dizziness, fainting, chest pain, fast or irregular heartbeat.	Discontinue. Call doctor right away.
Rare:	
• Sore throat, cloudy urine, fever, chills.	Discontinue. Call doctor right away.
• Nausea, vomiting, indigestion, abdominal pain.	Continue. Call doctor when convenient.

WARNINGS & PRECAUTIONS

Don't take if:
• You are allergic to captopril.
• You have any autoimmune disease, including AIDS or lupus.
• You are receiving blood from a blood bank.
• You take drugs for cancer.
• You will have surgery within 2 months, including dental surgery, requiring general or spinal anesthesia.

Before you start, consult your doctor:
• If you have had a stroke.
• If you have angina or heart or blood-vessel disease.
• If you have high level of potassium in blood.
• If you have kidney disease.
• If you are on severe salt-restricted diet.
• If you have lupus.

Over age 60:
Adverse reactions and side effects may be more frequent and severe than in younger persons.

Pregnancy:
Risk to unborn child outweighs drug benefits. Don't use.

Breast-feeding:
Drug passes into milk. Avoid drug or discontinue nursing.

Infants & children:
Not recommended.

Prolonged use:
May decrease white cells in blood or cause protein loss in urine. Request periodic laboratory blood counts and urine tests.

Skin & sunlight:
No problems expected.

Driving, piloting or hazardous work:
Avoid if you become dizzy or faint. Otherwise, no problems expected.

Discontinuing:
Don't discontinue without consulting doctor. Dose may require gradual reduction if you have taken drug for a long time. Doses of other drugs may also require adjustment.

Others:
- Stop taking diuretics or increase salt intake 1 week before starting captopril.
- Avoid exercising in hot weather.

 POSSIBLE INTERACTION WITH OTHER DRUGS

GENERIC NAME OR DRUG CLASS	COMBINED EFFECT
Acebutolol	Increased antihypertensive effect. Dosage of each may require adjustment.
Amiloride	Possible excessive potassium in blood.
Antihypertensives (other)	Possible excessive blood-pressure drop.
Enalapril	Possible excessive potassium in blood.
Chloramphenicol	Possible blood disorders.
Diuretics	Possible severe blood-pressure drop with first dose.
Nitrates	Possible excessive blood-pressure drop.
Oxprenolol	Increased antihypertensive effect. Dosage of each may require adjustment.
Pentoxifylline	Increased antihypertensive effect.
Potassium supplements	Excessive potassium in blood.
Spironolactone	Possible excessive potassium in blood.
Triamterene	Possible excessive potassium in blood.

 POSSIBLE INTERACTION WITH OTHER SUBSTANCES

INTERACTS WITH	COMBINED EFFECT
Alcohol:	Possible excessive blood-pressure drop.
Beverages: Low-salt milk.	Possible excessive potassium in blood.
Cocaine:	Increased dizziness and chest pain.
Foods: Salt substitutes.	Possible excessive potassium.
Marijuana:	Increased dizziness.
Tobacco:	May decrease captopril effect.

CAPTOPRIL & HYDROCHLOROTHIAZIDE

BRAND NAMES

Capozide

BASIC INFORMATION

Habit forming? No
Prescription needed? Yes
Available as generic? No
Drug class: Antihypertensive, diuretic (thiazide), A.C.E. inhibitor (See Glossary)

USES

- Treatment for high blood pressure and congestive heart failure.
- Reduces fluid retention.

DOSAGE & USAGE INFORMATION

How to take:
Tablets—Swallow with liquid. Instructions to take on empty stomach mean 1 hour before or 2 hours after eating.

When to take:
At the same times each day, usually 3 times daily. Take first dose at bedtime and lie down immediately.

If you forget a dose:
Take as soon as you remember up to 2 hours late. If more than 2 hours, wait for next scheduled dose (don't double this dose).

What drug does:
- Forces sodium and water excretion, reducing body fluid.
- Relaxes muscle cells of small arteries.
- Reduced body fluid and relaxed arteries lower blood pressure.
- Reduces resistance in arteries.
- Strengthens heartbeat.

Continued next column

OVERDOSE

SYMPTOMS:
Cramps, weakness, drowsiness, weak pulse, fever, chills, sore throat, fainting, convulsions, coma.
WHAT TO DO:
- **Dial 0 (operator) or 911 (emergency) for an ambulance or medical help. Then give first aid immediately.**
- **See emergency information on inside covers.**

Time lapse before drug works:
4 to 6 hours. May require several weeks to lower blood pressure.

Don't take with:
- Non-prescription drugs without consulting doctor.
- See Interaction column and consult doctor.

POSSIBLE ADVERSE REACTIONS OR SIDE EFFECTS

SYMPTOMS	WHAT TO DO
Life-threatening:	
Irregular heartbeat (fast or uneven).	Discontinue. Seek emergency treatment.
Common:	
• Dry mouth, thirst, tiredness, weakness, muscle cramps, vomiting, chest pain, skin rash.	Discontinue. Call doctor right away.
• Taste loss, dizziness.	Continue. Call doctor when convenient.
Infrequent:	
• Face, mouth, hands swell.	Discontinue. Call doctor right away.
• Nausea, diarrhea.	Continue. Call doctor when convenient.
Rare:	
None expected.	

WARNINGS & PRECAUTIONS

Don't take if:
- You are allergic to captopril, or any thiazide diuretic drug.
- You have any autoimmune disease, including AIDS or lupus.
- You are receiving blood from a blood bank.
- You take drugs for cancer.
- If you will have surgery within 2 months, including dental surgery, requiring general or spinal anesthesia.

Before you start, consult your doctor:
- If you have had a stroke.
- If you have angina, heart or blood-vessel disease, a high level of potassium in blood, lupus, gout, liver, pancreas or kidney disorder.
- If you are on severe salt-restricted diet.
- If you are allergic to any sulfa drug.

Over age 60:
Adverse reactions and side effects may be more frequent and severe than in younger persons, especially dizziness and excessive potassium loss.

Pregnancy:
Risk to unborn child outweighs drug benefits. Don't use.

Breast-feeding:
Drug passes into milk. Avoid drug or discontinue nursing until you finish medicine. Consult doctor for advice on maintaining milk supply.

Infants & children:
Not recommended.

Prolonged use:
May decrease white cells in blood or cause protein loss in urine. Request periodic laboratory blood counts and urine tests.

Skin & sunlight:
May cause rash or intensify sunburn in areas exposed to sun or sunlamp.

Driving, piloting or hazardous work:
Don't drive or pilot aircraft until you learn how medicine affects you. Don't work around dangerous machinery. Don't climb ladders or work in high places. Danger increases if you drink alcohol or take medicine affecting alertness and reflexes, such as antihistamines, tranquilizers, sedatives, pain medicine, narcotics and mind-altering drugs.

Discontinuing:
Don't discontinue without consulting doctor. Dose may require gradual reduction if you have taken drug for a long time. Doses of other drugs may also require adjustment.

Others:
- Hot weather and fever may cause dehydration and drop in blood pressure. Dose may require temporary adjustment. Weigh daily and report any unexpected weight decreases to your doctor.
- May cause rise in uric acid, leading to gout.
- May cause blood-sugar rise in diabetics.

POSSIBLE INTERACTION WITH OTHER DRUGS

GENERIC NAME OR DRUG CLASS	COMBINED EFFECT
Acebutolol	Increased antihypertensive effect. Dosages of both drugs may require adjustments.
Allopurinol	Decreased allopurinol effect.
Amiloride	Possible excessive potassium in blood.

Antidepressants (tricyclic)	Dangerous drop in blood pressure. Avoid combination unless under medical supervision.
Antihypertensives (other)	Possible excessive blood-pressure drop.
Barbiturates	Increased hydrochlorothiazide effect.
Chloramphenicol	Possible blood disorders.
Cholestyramine	Decreased hydrochlorothiazide effect.
Cortisone drugs	Excessive potassium loss that causes dangerous heart rhythms.
Digitalis preparations	Excessive potassium loss that causes dangerous heart rhythms.
Diuretics (thiazide)	Increased effect of other thiazide diuretics.
Indapamide	Increased diuretic effect.
Lithium	Increased effect of lithium.
MAO inhibitors	Increased hydrochlorothiazide effect.

Continued page 964

POSSIBLE INTERACTION WITH OTHER SUBSTANCES

INTERACTS WITH	COMBINED EFFECT
Alcohol:	Dangerous blood-pressure drop. Avoid.
Beverages: Low-salt milk.	Possible excessive potassium in blood.
Cocaine:	Increased dizziness, chest pain.
Foods: Salt substitutes.	Possible excessive potassium.
Marijuana:	Increased dizziness, may increase blood pressure.
Tobacco:	May decrease captopril effect.

CARBAMAZEPINE

BRAND NAMES

Apo-Carbamazepine   Tegretol
Mazepine

BASIC INFORMATION

Habit forming? No
Prescription needed? Yes
Available as generic? Yes
Drug class: Analgesic, anticonvulsant

 USES

- Decreased frequency, severity and duration of attacks of tic douloureaux (See Glossary).
- Prevents seizures.

 DOSAGE & USAGE INFORMATION

How to take:
Regular or chewable tablet—Swallow with liquid or food to lessen stomach irritation.

When to take:
At the same times each day.

If you forget a dose:
Take as soon as you remember up to 2 hours late. If more than 2 hours, wait for next scheduled dose (don't double this dose).

What drug does:
- Reduces transmission of pain messages at certain nerve terminals.
- Reduces excitability of nerve fibers in brain, thus inhibiting repetitive spread of nerve impulses.

Continued next column

 OVERDOSE

SYMPTOMS:
Involuntary movements, dilated pupils, flushed skin, stupor, coma.
WHAT TO DO:
- Dial 0 (operator) or 911 (emergency) for an ambulance or medical help. Then give first aid immediately.
- If patient is unconscious and not breathing, give mouth-to-mouth breathing. If there is no heartbeat, use cardiac massage and mouth-to-mouth breathing (CPR). Don't try to make patient vomit. If you can't get help quickly, take patient to nearest emergency facility.
- See emergency information on inside covers.

Time lapse before drug works:
- Tic douloureaux—24 to 72 hours.
- Seizures—1 to 2 weeks.

Don't take with:
See Interaction column and consult doctor.

 POSSIBLE ADVERSE REACTIONS OR SIDE EFFECTS

SYMPTOMS	WHAT TO DO
Life-threatening: None expected.	
Common: Blurred vision.	Continue. Call doctor when convenient.
Infrequent:	
• Confusion, slurred speech, fainting, depression, headache, hallucinations, hives, rash, mouth sores, sore throat, fever, unusual bleeding or bruising, unusual fatigue.	Discontinue. Call doctor right away.
• Diarrhea.	Continue. Call doctor when convenient.
Rare:	
• Back-and-forth eye movements; breathing difficulty; irregular, pounding or slow heartbeat; chest pain; uncontrollable body jerks; numbness, weakness or tingling in hands and feet; tender, bluish legs or feet; less urine; swollen lymph glands.	Discontinue. Call doctor right away.
• Frequent urination.	Continue. Call doctor when convenient.

WARNINGS & PRECAUTIONS

Don't take if:
- You are allergic to carbamazepine.
- You have had liver or bone-marrow disease.
- You have taken MAO inhibitors in the past 2 weeks.

Before you start, consult your doctor:
- If you have high blood pressure, thrombophlebitis or heart disease.
- If you have glaucoma.
- If you have emotional or mental problems.
- If you have liver or kidney disease.
- If you drink more than 2 alcoholic drinks per day.

Over age 60:
Adverse reactions and side effects may be more frequent and severe than in younger persons.

Pregnancy:
Studies inconclusive on harm to unborn child. Animal studies show fetal abnormalities. Decide with your doctor whether drug benefits justify risk to unborn child.

Breast-feeding:
Drug passes into milk. Avoid drug or discontinue nursing until you finish medicine. Consult doctor for advice on maintaining milk supply.

Infants & children:
Not recommended.

Prolonged use:
- Jaundice and liver damage.
- Hair loss.
- Ringing in ears.
- Lower sex drive.

Skin & sunlight:
May cause rash or intensify sunburn in areas exposed to sun or sunlamp.

Driving, piloting or hazardous work:
Don't drive or pilot aircraft until you learn how medicine affects you. Don't work around dangerous machinery. Don't climb ladders or work in high places. Danger increases if you drink alcohol or take medicine affecting alertness and reflexes.

Discontinuing:
Don't discontinue without doctor's advice until you complete prescribed dose, even though symptoms diminish or disappear.

Others:
Use only if less-hazardous drugs are not effective. Stay under medical supervision.

POSSIBLE INTERACTION WITH OTHER DRUGS

GENERIC NAME OR DRUG CLASS	COMBINED EFFECT
Anticoagulants (oral)	Decreased anticoagulant effect.
Anticonvulsants (hydantoin)	Decreased effect of both drugs.
Antidepressants (tricyclic)	Confusion. Possible psychosis.
Contraceptives (oral)	Reduced contraceptive protection. Use another birth-control method.
Digitalis preparations	Excess slowing of heart.
Doxycycline	Decreased doxycycline effect.
MAO inhibitors	Dangerous overstimulation. Avoid.
Tranquilizers (benzodiazepine)	Increased carbamazepine effect.

POSSIBLE INTERACTION WITH OTHER SUBSTANCES

INTERACTS WITH	COMBINED EFFECT
Alcohol:	Increased sedative effect of alcohol. Avoid.
Beverages:	None expected.
Cocaine:	Increased adverse effects of carbamazepine. Avoid.
Foods:	None expected.
Marijuana:	Increased adverse effects of carbamazepine. Avoid.
Tobacco:	None expected.

CARBENICILLIN

BRAND NAMES

Geocillin   Pyopen
Geopen

BASIC INFORMATION

Habit forming? No
Prescription needed? Yes
Available as generic? Yes
Drug class: Antibiotic (penicillin)

USES

Treatment of bacterial infections that are susceptible to carbenicillin.

DOSAGE & USAGE INFORMATION

How to take:
Tablets or capsules—Swallow with liquid on an empty stomach 1 hour before or 2 hours after eating.

When to take:
Follow instructions on prescription label or side of package. Doses should be evenly spaced. For example, 4 times a day means every 6 hours.

If you forget a dose:
Take as soon as you remember. Continue regular schedule.

What drug does:
Destroys susceptible bacteria. Does not kill viruses.

Time lapse before drug works:
May be several days before medicine affects infection.

Don't take with:
See Interaction column and consult doctor.

OVERDOSE

SYMPTOMS:
Severe diarrhea, nausea or vomiting.
WHAT TO DO:
Overdose unlikely to threaten life. If person takes much larger amount than prescribed, call doctor, poison-control center or hospital emergency room for instructions.

POSSIBLE ADVERSE REACTIONS OR SIDE EFFECTS

SYMPTOMS	WHAT TO DO
Life-threatening:	
Hives, rash, intense itching, faintness soon after a dose (anaphylaxis).	Seek emergency treatment immediately.
Common:	
Dark or discolored tongue.	Continue. Tell doctor at next visit.
Infrequent:	
Mild nausea, vomiting, diarrhea.	Continue. Call doctor when convenient.
Rare:	
Unexplained bleeding.	Discontinue. Call doctor right away.

WARNINGS & PRECAUTIONS

Don't take if:
You are allergic to carbenicillin, cephalosporin antibiotics, other penicillins or penicillamine. Life-threatening reaction may occur.

Before you start, consult your doctor:
If you are allergic to any substance or drug.

Over age 60:
You may have skin reactions, particularly around genitals and anus.

Pregnancy:
Studies inconclusive on harm to unborn child. Animal studies show fetal abnormalities. Decide with your doctor whether drug benefits justify risk to unborn child.

Breast-feeding:
Drug passes into milk. Child may become sensitive to penicillins and have allergic reactions to penicillin drugs. Avoid carbenicillin or discontinue nursing until you finish medicine. Consult doctor for advice on maintaining milk supply.

Infants & children:
No problems expected.

Prolonged use:
You may become more susceptible to infections caused by germs not responsive to carbenicillin.

Skin & sunlight:
No problems expected.

Driving, piloting or hazardous work:
Usually not dangerous. Most hazardous reactions likely to occur a few minutes after taking carbenicillin.

Discontinuing:
Don't discontinue without doctor's advice until you complete prescribed dose, even though symptoms diminish or disappear.

Others:
Injection forms may cause fluid retention (edema) with weakness and low potassium in the blood.

POSSIBLE INTERACTION WITH OTHER DRUGS

GENERIC NAME OR DRUG CLASS	COMBINED EFFECT
Beta-adrenergic blockers	Increased chance of anaphylaxis (see emergency information on inside front cover).
Chloramphenicol	Decreased effect of both drugs.
Erythromycins	Decreased effect of both drugs.
Loperamide	Decreased carbenicillin effect.
Paromomycin	Decreased effect of both drugs.
Tetracyclines	Decreased effect of both drugs.
Troleandomycin	Decreased effect of both drugs.

POSSIBLE INTERACTION WITH OTHER SUBSTANCES

INTERACTS WITH	COMBINED EFFECT
Alcohol:	Occasional stomach irritation.
Beverages:	None expected.
Cocaine:	No proven problems.
Foods:	Decreased effect of oral carbenicillin.
Marijuana:	No proven problems.
Tobacco:	None expected.

CARBIDOPA & LEVODOPA

BRAND NAMES

Dopar   Sinemet
Larodopa

BASIC INFORMATION

Habit forming? No
Prescription needed? Yes
Available as generic? Yes
Drug class: Antiparkinsonism

 USES

Controls Parkinson's disease symptoms such as rigidity, tremor and unsteady gait.

 DOSAGE & USAGE INFORMATION

How to take:
Tablet or capsule—Swallow with liquid or food to lessen stomach irritation. If you can't swallow whole, crumble tablet or open capsule and take with liquid or food.

When to take:
At the same times each day.

If you forget a dose:
Take as soon as you remember up to 2 hours late. If more than 2 hours, wait for next scheduled dose (don't double this dose).

What drug does:
Restores chemical balance necessary for normal nerve impulses.

Continued next column

 OVERDOSE

SYMPTOMS:
Muscle twitch, spastic eyelid closure, nausea, vomiting, diarrhea, irregular and rapid pulse, weakness, fainting, confusion, agitation, hallucination, coma.
WHAT TO DO:
- **Dial 0 (operator) or 911 (emergency) for an ambulance or medical help. Then give first aid immediately.**
- **If patient is unconscious and not breathing, give mouth-to-mouth breathing. If there is no heartbeat, use cardiac massage and mouth-to-mouth breathing (CPR). Don't try to make patient vomit. If you can't get help quickly, take patient to nearest emergency facility.**
- **See emergency information on inside covers.**

Time lapse before drug works:
2 to 3 weeks to improve; 6 weeks or longer for maximum benefit.

Don't take with:
See Interaction column and consult doctor.

 POSSIBLE ADVERSE REACTIONS OR SIDE EFFECTS

SYMPTOMS	WHAT TO DO
Life-threatening: None expected.	
Common:	
• Mood changes, uncontrollable body movements, diarrhea.	Continue. Call doctor when convenient.
• Dry mouth, body odor.	No action necessary.
Infrequent:	
• Fainting, severe dizziness, headache, insomnia, nightmares, rash, itch, nausea, vomiting, irregular heartbeat.	Discontinue. Call doctor right away.
• Flushed face, blurred vision, muscle twitching, discolored or dark urine, difficult urination.	Continue. Call doctor when convenient.
• Constipation, tiredness.	Continue. Tell doctor at next visit.
Rare:	
• High blood pressure.	Discontinue. Call doctor right away.
• Duodenal ulcer, anemia.	Continue. Call doctor when convenient.

WARNINGS & PRECAUTIONS

Don't take if:
- You are allergic to levodopa or carbidopa.
- You have taken MAO inhibitors in past 2 weeks.
- You have glaucoma (narrow-angle type).

Before you start, consult your doctor:
- You have diabetes or epilepsy.
- If you have had high blood pressure, heart or lung disease.
- If you have had liver or kidney disease.
- If you have a peptic ulcer.
- If you have malignant melanoma.
- If you will have surgery within 2 months, including dental surgery, requiring general or spinal anesthesia.

Over age 60:
Adverse reactions and side effects may be more frequent and severe than in younger persons.

Pregnancy:
Risk to unborn child outweighs drug benefits. Don't use.

Breast-feeding:
Drug filters into milk. May harm child. Avoid.

Infants & children:
Not recommended.

Prolonged use:
May lead to uncontrolled movements of head, face, mouth, tongue, arms or legs.

Skin & sunlight:
No problems expected.

Driving, piloting or hazardous work:
Don't drive or pilot aircraft until you learn how medicine affects you. Don't work around dangerous machinery. Don't climb ladders or work in high places. Danger increases if you drink alcohol or take medicine affecting alertness and reflexes, such as antihistamines, tranquilizers, sedatives, pain medicine, narcotics and mind-altering drugs.

Discontinuing:
Don't discontinue without doctor's advice until you complete prescribed dose, even though symptoms diminish or disappear.

Others:
Expect to start with small dose and increase gradually to lessen frequency and severity of adverse reactions.

POSSIBLE INTERACTION WITH OTHER DRUGS

GENERIC NAME OR DRUG CLASS	COMBINED EFFECT
Antiparkinsonism drugs (other)	Increased effect of carbidopa and levodopa.
Haloperidol	Decreased effect of carbidopa and levodopa.
MAO inhibitors	Dangerous rise in blood pressure.
Methyldopa	Decreased effect of carbidopa and levodopa.
Papaverine	Decreased effect of carbidopa and levodopa.
Phenothiazines	Decreased effect of carbidopa and levodopa.
Pyridoxine (Vitamin B-6)	Decreased effect carbidopa and levodopa.
Rauwolfia alkaloids	Decreased effect carbidopa and levodopa.

POSSIBLE INTERACTION WITH OTHER SUBSTANCES

INTERACTS WITH	COMBINED EFFECT
Alcohol:	None expected.
Beverages:	None expected.
Cocaine:	Decreased carbidopa and levodopa effect.
Foods:	None expected.
Marijuana:	Increased fatigue, lethargy, fainting.
Tobacco:	None expected.

CARBINOXAMINE

BRAND NAMES

Clistin   Clistin R-A

BASIC INFORMATION

Habit forming? No
Prescription needed? Yes
Available as generic? No
Drug class: Antihistamine

 ## USES

Reduces allergic symptoms such as hay fever, hives, rash or itching.

 ## DOSAGE & USAGE INFORMATION

How to take:
- Tablet—Swallow with liquid or food to lessen stomach irritation.
- Extended-release tablets—Swallow each dose whole. If you take regular tablets, you may chew or crush them.

When to take:
Varies with form. Follow label directions.

If you forget a dose:
Take as soon as you remember up to 2 hours late. If more than 2 hours, wait for next scheduled dose (don't double this dose).

What drug does:
Blocks action of histamine after an allergic response triggers histamine release in sensitive cells.

Time lapse before drug works:
30 minutes.

Continued next column

 ## OVERDOSE

SYMPTOMS:
Convulsions, red face, hallucinations, coma.
WHAT TO DO:
- Dial 0 (operator) or 911 (emergency) for an ambulance or medical help. Then give first aid immediately.
- If patient is unconscious and not breathing, give mouth-to-mouth breathing. If there is no heartbeat, use cardiac massage and mouth-to-mouth breathing (CPR). Don't try to make patient vomit. If you can't get help quickly, take patient to nearest emergency facility.
- See emergency information on inside covers.

Don't take with:
See Interaction column and consult doctor.

 ## POSSIBLE ADVERSE REACTIONS OR SIDE EFFECTS

SYMPTOMS	WHAT TO DO
Life-threatening: None expected.	
Common: Drowsiness; dizziness; nausea; dry mouth, nose, throat.	Continue. Tell doctor at next visit.
Infrequent: • Changes in vision.	Discontinue. Call doctor right away.
• Less tolerance for contact lenses, urination difficulty.	Continue. Call doctor when convenient.
• Appetite loss.	Continue. Tell doctor at next visit.
Rare: Nightmares, agitation, irritability, sore throat, fever, rapid heartbeat, unusual bleeding or bruising, fatigue, weakness.	Discontinue. Call doctor right away.

WARNINGS & PRECAUTIONS

Don't take if:
You are allergic to any antihistamine.

Before you start, consult your doctor:
- If you have glaucoma.
- If you have enlarged prostate.
- If you have asthma.
- If you have kidney disease.
- If you have peptic ulcer.
- If you will have surgery within 2 months, including dental surgery, requiring general or spinal anesthesia.

Over age 60:
Don't exceed recommended dose. Adverse reactions and side effects may be more frequent and severe than in younger persons, especially urination difficulty, diminished alertness and other brain and nervous-system symptoms.

Pregnancy:
No proven harm to unborn child. Avoid if possible.

Breast-feeding:
Drug passes into milk. Avoid drug or discontinue nursing until you finish medicine. Consult doctor for advice on maintaining milk supply.

Infants & children:
Not recommended for premature or newborn infants. Otherwise, no problems expected.

Prolonged use:
Avoid. May damage bone marrow and nerve cells.

Skin & sunlight:
May cause rash or intensify sunburn in areas exposed to sun or sunlamp.

Driving, piloting or hazardous work:
Don't drive or pilot aircraft until you learn how medicine affects you. Don't work around dangerous machinery. Don't climb ladders or work in high places. Danger increases if you drink alcohol or take medicine affecting alertness and reflexes, such as antihistamines, tranquilizers, sedatives, pain medicine, narcotics and mind-altering drugs.

Discontinuing:
No problems expected.

Others:
May mask symptoms of hearing damage from aspirin, other salicylates, cisplatin, paromomycin, vancomycin or anticonvulsants. Consult doctor if you use these.

POSSIBLE INTERACTION WITH OTHER DRUGS

GENERIC NAME OR DRUG CLASS	COMBINED EFFECT
Anticholinergics	Increased anticholinergic effect.
Antidepressants	Increased carbinoxamine effect. Excess sedation. Avoid.
Antihistamines (other)	Excess sedation. Avoid.
Dronabinol	Increased effects of both drugs. Avoid.
Hypnotics	Excess sedation. Avoid.
MAO inhibitors	Increased carbinoxamine effect.
Mind-altering drugs	Excess sedation. Avoid.
Molindone	Increased antihistamine effect.
Narcotics	Excess sedation. Avoid.
Sedatives	Excess sedation. Avoid.
Sleep inducers	Excess sedation. Avoid.
Tranquilizers	Excess sedation. Avoid.

POSSIBLE INTERACTION WITH OTHER SUBSTANCES

INTERACTS WITH	COMBINED EFFECT
Alcohol:	Excess sedation. Avoid.
Beverages: Caffeine drinks.	Less carbinoxamine sedation.
Cocaine:	Decreased carbinoxamine effect. Avoid.
Foods:	None expected.
Marijuana:	Excess sedation. Avoid.
Tobacco:	None expected.

CARBONIC ANHYDRASE INHIBITORS

BRAND AND GENERIC NAMES

Acetazolam
ACETAZOLAMIDE
Ak-Zol
Apo-Acetazolamide
Cetazol
Daranide
Dazamide

Diamox
Diamox Sequels
DICHLORPHENAMIDE
METHAZOLAMIDE
Neptazane
Oratrol

BASIC INFORMATION

Habit forming? No
Prescription needed? Yes
Available as generic? Yes
Drug class: Carbonic anhydrase inhibitor
(See Glossary)

 ## USES

- Treatment of glaucoma.
- Treatment of epileptic seizures.
- Treatment of body-fluid retention.
- Treatment for shortness of breath, insomnia and fatigue in high altitudes.

 ## DOSAGE & USAGE INFORMATION

How to take:
Tablets—Swallow whole with liquid or food to lessen stomach irritation.

When to take:
- 1 dose per day—At the same time each morning.
- More than 1 dose per day—Take last dose several hours before bedtime.

If you forget a dose:
Take as soon as you remember. Continue regular schedule.

Continued next column

 ## OVERDOSE

SYMPTOMS:
Drowsiness, confusion, excitement, nausea, vomiting, numbness in hands and feet, coma.
WHAT TO DO:
- Call your doctor or poison-control center for advice if you suspect overdose, even if not sure. Symptoms may not appear until damage has occurred.
- See emergency information on inside covers.

What drug does:
- Inhibits action of carbonic anhydrase, an enzyme. This lowers the internal eye pressure by decreasing fluid formation in the eye.
- Forces sodium and water excretion, reducing body fluid.

Time lapse before drug works:
2 hours.

Don't take with:
- Non-prescription drugs without consulting doctor.
- See Interaction column and consult doctor.

 ## POSSIBLE ADVERSE REACTIONS OR SIDE EFFECTS

SYMPTOMS	WHAT TO DO
Life-threatening: Convulsions.	Seek emergency treatment immediately.
Common: None expected.	
Infrequent: • Back pain.	Discontinue. Call doctor right away.
• Fatigue, weakness, tingling or burning in feet or hands.	Continue. Call doctor when convenient.
Rare: Headache; mood changes; nervousness; clumsiness; trembling; confusion; hives, itch, rash; sores; ringing in ears; hoarseness; dry mouth; thirst; sore throat; fever; appetite change; nausea; vomiting; black, tarry stool; breathing difficulty; irregular or weak heartbeat; easy bleeding or bruising; muscle cramps; painful or frequent urination; blood in urine.	Discontinue. Call doctor right away.

CARBONIC ANHYDRASE INHIBITORS

 ## WARNINGS & PRECAUTIONS

Don't take if:
- You are allergic to any carbonic anhydrase inhibitor.
- You have liver or kidney disease.
- You have Addison's disease (adrenal gland failure).
- You have diabetes.

Before you start, consult your doctor:
- If you have gout or lupus.
- If you are allergic to any sulfa drug.
- If you will have surgery within 2 months, including dental surgery, requiring general or spinal anesthesia.

Over age 60:
- Don't exceed recommended dose.
- If you take a digitalis preparation, eat foods high in potassium content or take a potassium supplement.

Pregnancy:
No proven harm to unborn child. Avoid if possible, especially first 3 months.

Breast-feeding:
Avoid drug or don't nurse your infant.

Infants & children:
Not recommended for children younger than 12.

Prolonged use:
May cause kidney stones, vision change, loss of taste and smell, jaundice or weight loss.

Skin & sunlight:
No problems expected.

Driving, piloting or hazardous work:
Avoid if you feel drowsy or dizzy. Otherwise, no problems expected.

Discontinuing:
Don't discontinue without medical advice.

Others:
Medicine may increase sugar levels in blood and urine. Diabetics may need insulin adjustment.

 ## POSSIBLE INTERACTION WITH OTHER DRUGS

GENERIC NAME OR DRUG CLASS	COMBINED EFFECT
Amphetamines	Increased amphetamine effect.
Anticonvulsants	Increased loss of bone minerals.
Antidepressants (tricyclic)	Increased antidepressant effect.
Antidiabetics (oral)	Increased potassium loss.
Aspirin	Decreased aspirin effect.
Cortisone drugs	Increased potassium loss.
Digitalis preparations	Possible digitalis toxicity.
Diuretics	Increased potassium loss.
Lithium	Decreased lithium effect.
Methenamine	Decreased methenamine effect.
Mexiletene	May slow elimination of mexilitene and cause need to adjust dosage.
Quinidine	Increased quinidine effect.
Salicylates	Salicylate toxicity.
Sympathomimetics	Increased sympathomimetic effect.

 ## POSSIBLE INTERACTION WITH OTHER SUBSTANCES

INTERACTS WITH	COMBINED EFFECT
Alcohol:	None expected.
Beverages:	None expected.
Cocaine:	Avoid. Decreased carbonic anhydrase inhibitor effect.
Foods: Potassium-rich foods (see Glossary).	Eat these to decrease potassium loss.
Marijuana:	Avoid. Increased carbonic anhydrase inhibitor effect.
Tobacco:	May decrease absorption of carbonic anhydrase inhibitors.

CARISOPRODOL

BRAND NAMES

Rela   Soma Compound
Soma   Soprodol

BASIC INFORMATION

Habit forming? No
Prescription needed? Yes
Available as generic? Yes
Drug class: Muscle relaxant (skeletal)

 ## USES

Treatment for sprains, strains and muscle
spasms.

 ## DOSAGE & USAGE INFORMATION

How to take:
Tablet or capsule—Swallow with liquid.

When to take:
As needed, no more often than every 4 hours.

If you forget a dose:
Take as soon as you remember. Wait 4 hours
for next dose.

What drug does:
Blocks body's pain messages to brain. May also
sedate.

Time lapse before drug works:
60 minutes.

Don't take with:
See Interaction column and consult doctor.

 ## OVERDOSE

SYMPTOMS:
Nausea, vomiting, diarrhea, headache. May
progress to severe weakness, difficult
breathing, sensation of paralysis, coma.
WHAT TO DO:
- Dial 0 (operator) or 911 (emergency) for an
  ambulance or medical help. Then give first
  aid immediately.
- See emergency information on inside
  covers.

 ## POSSIBLE ADVERSE REACTIONS OR SIDE EFFECTS

SYMPTOMS	WHAT TO DO
Life-threatening: None expected.	
Common:	
• Drowsiness, fainting, dizziness.	Continue. Call doctor when convenient.
• Orange or red-purple urine.	No action necessary.
Infrequent: Agitation, constipation or diarrhea; nausea; cramps; vomiting; wheezing; shortness of breath.	Discontinue. Call doctor right away.
Rare:	
• Black, tarry or bloody stool.	Discontinue. Seek emergency treatment.
• Rash, hives, or itch; sore throat; fever; jaundice; tiredness; weakness.	Discontinue. Call doctor right away.

WARNINGS & PRECAUTIONS

Don't take if:
- You are allergic to any skeletal-muscle relaxant.
- You have porphyria.

Before you start, consult your doctor:
- If you have had liver or kidney disease.
- If you plan pregnancy within medication period.

Over age 60:
Adverse reactions and side effects may be more frequent and severe than in younger persons.

Pregnancy:
No proven harm to unborn child. Avoid if possible.

Breast-feeding:
Drug passes into milk. Avoid drug or discontinue nursing until you finish medicine. Consult doctor for advice on maintaining milk supply.

Infants & children:
Not recommended.

Prolonged use:
Periodic liver-function tests recommended if you use this drug for a long time.

Skin & sunlight:
No problems expected.

Driving, piloting or hazardous work:
Don't drive or pilot aircraft until you learn how medicine affects you. Don't work around dangerous machinery. Don't climb ladders or work in high places. Danger increases if you drink alcohol or take medicine affecting alertness and reflexes, such as antihistamines, tranquilizers, sedatives, pain medicine, narcotics and mind-altering drugs.

Discontinuing:
Don't discontinue without doctor's advice until you complete prescribed dose, even though symptoms diminish or disappear.

Others:
No problems expected.

POSSIBLE INTERACTION WITH OTHER DRUGS

GENERIC NAME OR DRUG CLASS	COMBINED EFFECT
Antidepressants	Increased sedation.
Antihistamines	Increased sedation.
Dronabinol	Increased effect of dronabinol on central nervous system. Avoid combination.
Mind-altering drugs	Increased sedation.
Muscle relaxants (others)	Increased sedation.
Narcotics	Increased sedation.
Sedatives	Increased sedation.
Sleep inducers	Increased sedation.
Testosterone	Decreased carisoprodol effect.
Tranquilizers	Increased sedation.

POSSIBLE INTERACTION WITH OTHER SUBSTANCES

INTERACTS WITH	COMBINED EFFECT
Alcohol:	Increased sedation.
Beverages:	None expected.
Cocaine:	Lack of coordination, increased sedation.
Foods:	None expected.
Marijuana:	Lack of coordination, drowsiness, fainting.
Tobacco:	None expected.

CARPHENAZINE

BRAND NAMES

Proketazine

BASIC INFORMATION

Habit forming? No
Prescription needed? Yes
Available as generic? Yes
Drug class: Tranquilizer, antiemetic
           (phenothiazine)

 USES

- Stops nausea, vomiting.
- Reduces anxiety, agitation.

 DOSAGE & USAGE INFORMATION

How to take:

- Tablet or capsule—Swallow with liquid or food to lessen stomach irritation.
- Suppositories—Remove wrapper and moisten suppository with water. Gently insert into rectum, large end first.
- Drops or liquid—Dilute dose in beverage.

When to take:

- Nervous and mental disorders—Take at the same times each day.
- Nausea and vomiting—Take as needed, no more often than every 4 hours.

If you forget a dose:

- Nervous and mental disorders—Take up to 2 hours late. If more than 2 hours, wait for next scheduled dose (don't double this dose).
- Nausea and vomiting—Take as soon as you remember. Wait 4 hours for next dose.

What drug does:

- Suppresses brain's vomiting center.
- Suppresses brain centers that control abnormal emotions and behavior.

Time lapse before drug works:

- Nausea and vomiting—1 hour or less.
- Nervous and mental disorders—4-6 weeks.

Continued next column

 OVERDOSE

SYMPTOMS:
Stupor, convulsions, coma.
WHAT TO DO:

- **Dial 0 (operator) or 911 (emergency) for an ambulance or medical help. Then give first aid immediately.**
- **See emergency information on inside covers.**

Don't take with:

- Antacid or medicine for diarrhea.
- Non-prescription drug for cough, cold or allergy.
- See Interaction column and consult doctor.

 POSSIBLE ADVERSE REACTIONS OR SIDE EFFECTS

SYMPTOMS	WHAT TO DO
Life-threatening:	
None expected.	
Common:	
• Muscle spasms of face and neck, unsteady gait.	Discontinue. Seek emergency treatment.
• Restlessness, tremor, drowsiness.	Discontinue. Call doctor right away.
• Decreased sweating, dry mouth, stuffy nose, constipation.	Continue. Call doctor when convenient.
Infrequent:	
• Fainting.	Discontinue. Seek emergency treatment.
• Rash.	Discontinue. Call doctor right away.
• Difficult urination, diminished sex drive, swollen breasts, menstrual irregularities.	Continue. Call doctor when convenient.
Rare:	
Changes in vision, sore throat, fever, jaundice.	Discontinue. Call doctor right away.

WARNINGS & PRECAUTIONS

Don't take if:
- You are allergic to any phenothiazine.
- You have a blood or bone-marrow disease.

Before you start, consult your doctor:
- If you will have surgery within 2 months, including dental surgery, requiring general or spinal anesthesia.
- If you have asthma, emphysema or other lung disorder.
- If you take non-prescription ulcer medicine, asthma medicine or amphetamines.

Over age 60:
Adverse reactions and side effects may be more frequent and severe than in younger persons. More likely to develop involuntary movement of jaws, lips, tongue, chewing. Report this to your doctor immediately. Early treatment can help.

Pregnancy:
Risk to unborn child outweighs drug benefits. Don't use.

Breast-feeding:
Drug passes into milk. Avoid drug or discontinue nursing until you finish medicine. Consult doctor for advice on maintaining milk supply.

Infants & children:
Don't give to children younger than 2.

Prolonged use:
May lead to tardive dyskinesia (involuntary movement of jaws, lips, tongue, chewing).

Skin & sunlight:
May cause rash or intensify sunburn in areas exposed to sun or sunlamp. Skin may remain sensitive for 3 months after discontinuing.

Driving, piloting or hazardous work:
Don't drive or pilot aircraft until you learn how medicine affects you. Don't work around dangerous machinery. Don't climb ladders or work in high places. Danger increases if you drink alcohol or take medicine affecting alertness and reflexes.

Discontinuing:
- Nervous and mental disorders—Don't discontinue without doctor's advice until you complete prescribed dose, even though symptoms diminish or disappear.
- Nausea and vomiting—May be unnecessary to finish medicine. Follow doctor's instructions.

Others:
No problems expected.

POSSIBLE INTERACTION WITH OTHER DRUGS

GENERIC NAME OR DRUG CLASS	COMBINED EFFECT
Anticholinergics	Increased anticholinergic effect.
Antidepressants (tricyclic)	Increased carphenazine effect.
Antihistamines	Increased antihistamine effect.
Appetite suppressants	Decreased suppressant effect.
Dronabinol	Increased effects of both drugs. Avoid.
Levodopa	Decreased levodopa effect.
Mind-altering drugs	Increased effect of mind-altering drugs.
Narcotics	Increased narcotic effect.
Phenytoin	Increased phenytoin effect.
Quinidine	Impaired heart function. Dangerous mixture.
Sedatives	Increased sedative effect.
Tranquilizers (other)	Increased tranquilizer effect.

POSSIBLE INTERACTION WITH OTHER SUBSTANCES

INTERACTS WITH	COMBINED EFFECT
Alcohol:	Dangerous oversedation.
Beverages:	None expected.
Cocaine:	Decreased carphenazine effect. Avoid.
Foods:	None expected.
Marijuana:	Drowsiness. May increase antinausea effect.
Tobacco:	None expected.

CASCARA

BRAND NAMES

Aromatic Cascara
  Fluidextract
Cascara Sagrada
Cas-Evac

Milk of
  Magnesia-Cascara
Peri-Colace

BASIC INFORMATION

Habit forming? No
Prescription needed? No
Available as generic? Yes
Drug class: Laxative (stimulant)

 USES

Constipation relief.

 DOSAGE & USAGE INFORMATION

How to take:
- Tablet—Swallow with liquid. If you can't swallow whole, chew or crumble tablet and take with liquid or food.
- Liquid—Drink 6 to 8 glasses of water each day, in addition to one taken with each dose.

When to take:
Usually at bedtime with a snack, unless directed otherwise.

If you forget a dose:
Take as soon as you remember.

What drug does:
Acts on smooth muscles of intestine wall to cause vigorous bowel movement.

Time lapse before drug works:
6 to 10 hours.

Don't take with:
- See Interaction column and consult doctor.
- Don't take within 2 hours of taking another medicine. Laxative interferes with medicine absorption.

 OVERDOSE

SYMPTOMS:
Vomiting, electrolyte depletion.
WHAT TO DO:
Overdose unlikely to threaten life. If person takes much larger amount than prescribed, call doctor, poison-control center or hospital emergency room for instructions.

 POSSIBLE ADVERSE REACTIONS OR SIDE EFFECTS

SYMPTOMS	WHAT TO DO
Life-threatening: None expected.	
Common: Rectal irritation.	Continue. Call doctor when convenient.
Infrequent:	
• Dangerous potassium loss.	Discontinue. Call doctor right away.
• Belching, cramps, nausea.	Continue. Call doctor when convenient.
Rare:	
• Irritability, confusion, headache, rash, breathing difficulty, irregular heartbeat, muscle cramps, unusual tiredness or weakness.	Discontinue. Call doctor right away.
• Burning on urination.	Continue. Call doctor when convenient.

WARNINGS & PRECAUTIONS

Don't take if:
- You have symptoms of appendicitis, inflamed bowel or intestinal blockage.
- You are allergic to a stimulant laxative.
- You have missed a bowel movement for only 1 or 2 days.

Before you start, consult your doctor:
- If you have a colostomy or ileostomy.
- If you have congestive heart disease.
- If you have diabetes.
- If you have high blood pressure.
- If you have a laxative habit.
- If you have rectal bleeding.
- If you take other laxatives.

Over age 60:
Adverse reactions and side effects may be more frequent and severe than in younger persons.

Pregnancy:
Risk to mother and unborn child outweighs drug benefits. Don't use.

Breast-feeding:
Drug passes into milk. Avoid drug or discontinue nursing until you finish medicine. Consult doctor for advice on maintaining milk supply.

Infants & children:
Use only under medical supervision.

Prolonged use:
Don't take for more than 1 week unless under a doctor's supervision. May cause laxative dependence.

Skin & sunlight:
No problems expected.

Driving, piloting or hazardous work:
No problems expected.

Discontinuing:
May be unnecessary to finish medicine. Follow doctor's instructions.

Others:
Don't take to "flush out" your system or as a "tonic."

POSSIBLE INTERACTION WITH OTHER DRUGS

GENERIC NAME OR DRUG CLASS	COMBINED EFFECT
Antihypertensives	May cause dangerous low potassium level.
Diuretics	May cause dangerous low potassium level.

POSSIBLE INTERACTION WITH OTHER SUBSTANCES

INTERACTS WITH	COMBINED EFFECT
Alcohol:	None expected.
Beverages:	None expected.
Cocaine:	None expected.
Foods:	None expected.
Marijuana:	None expected.
Tobacco:	None expected.

CASTOR OIL

BRAND NAMES

Alphamul	Kellogg's
Emulsoil	Neoloid
Fleet Prep Kit	Purge
Granulex	Stimuzyme Plus
Hydrisinol	Unisoil

BASIC INFORMATION

Habit forming? No
Prescription needed? No
Available as generic? Yes
Drug class: Laxative (stimulant)

 ## USES

Constipation relief.

 ## DOSAGE & USAGE INFORMATION

How to take:
Liquid—Drink 6 to 8 glasses of water each day, in addition to one taken with each dose.

When to take:
Usually at bedtime with a snack, unless directed otherwise.

If you forget a dose:
Take as soon as you remember.

What drug does:
Acts on smooth muscles of intestine wall to cause vigorous bowel movement.

Time lapse before drug works:
2 to 6 hours.

Don't take with:
● See Interaction column and consult doctor.
● Don't take within 2 hours of taking another medicine. Laxative interferes with medicine absorption.

 ## OVERDOSE

SYMPTOMS:
Vomiting, electrolyte depletion.
WHAT TO DO:
Overdose unlikely to threaten life. If person takes much larger amount than prescribed, call doctor, poison-control center or hospital emergency room for instructions.

 ## POSSIBLE ADVERSE REACTIONS OR SIDE EFFECTS

SYMPTOMS	WHAT TO DO
Life-threatening: None expected.	
Common: Rectal irritation.	Continue. Call doctor when convenient.
Infrequent:	
● Dangerous potassium loss.	Discontinue. Call doctor right away.
● Belching, cramps, nausea.	Continue. Call doctor when convenient.
Rare:	
● Irritability, confusion, headache, rash, breathing difficulty, irregular heartbeat, muscle cramps, unusual tiredness or weakness.	Discontinue. Call doctor right away.
● Burning on urination.	Continue. Call doctor when convenient.

WARNINGS & PRECAUTIONS

Don't take if:
- You have symptoms of appendicitis, inflamed bowel or intestinal blockage.
- You are allergic to a stimulant laxative.
- You have missed a bowel movement for only 1 or 2 days.

Before you start, consult your doctor:
- If you have a colostomy or ileostomy.
- If you have congestive heart disease.
- If you have diabetes.
- If you have high blood pressure.
- If you have a laxative habit.
- If you have rectal bleeding.
- If you take other laxatives.

Over age 60:
Adverse reactions and side effects may be more frequent and severe than in younger persons.

Pregnancy:
Risk to mother and unborn child outweighs drug benefits. Don't use.

Breast-feeding:
Drug passes into milk. Avoid drug or discontinue nursing until you finish medicine. Consult doctor for advice on maintaining milk supply.

Infants & children:
Use only under medical supervision.

Prolonged use:
Don't take for more than 1 week unless under doctor's supervision. May cause laxative dependence.

Skin & sunlight:
No problems expected.

Driving, piloting or hazardous work:
No problems expected.

Discontinuing:
May be unnecessary to finish medicine. Follow doctor's instructions.

Others:
Don't take to "flush out" your system or as a "tonic."

 ## POSSIBLE INTERACTION WITH OTHER DRUGS

GENERIC NAME OR DRUG CLASS	COMBINED EFFECT
Antihypertensives	May cause dangerous low potassium level.
Diuretics	May cause dangerous low potassium level.

 ## POSSIBLE INTERACTION WITH OTHER SUBSTANCES

INTERACTS WITH	COMBINED EFFECT
Alcohol:	None expected.
Beverages:	None expected.
Cocaine:	None expected.
Foods:	None expected.
Marijuana:	None expected.
Tobacco:	None expected.

CEFACLOR

BRAND NAMES

Ceclor

BASIC INFORMATION

Habit forming? No
Prescription needed? Yes
Available as generic? No
Drug class: Antibiotic (cephalosporin)

 ## USES

Treatment of bacterial infections. Will not cure viral infections such as cold and flu.

 ## DOSAGE & USAGE INFORMATION

How to take:
- Tablet or capsule—Swallow with liquid. If you can't swallow whole, crumble tablet or open capsule and take with liquid or food.
- Liquid—Use measuring spoon.

When to take:
At same times each day, 1 hour before or 2 hours after eating.

If you forget a dose:
Take as soon as you remember or double next dose. Return to regular schedule.

What drug does:
Kills susceptible bacteria.

Time lapse before drug works:
May require several days to affect infection.

Don't take with:
See Interaction column and consult doctor.

 ## OVERDOSE

SYMPTOMS:
Abdominal cramps, nausea, vomiting, severe diarrhea with mucus or blood in stool.
WHAT TO DO:
Overdose unlikely to threaten life. If person takes much larger amount than prescribed, call doctor, poison-control center or hospital emergency room for instructions.

 ## POSSIBLE ADVERSE REACTIONS OR SIDE EFFECTS

SYMPTOMS	WHAT TO DO
Life-threatening:	
Hives, rash, intense itching, faintness soon after a dose (anaphylaxis).	Seek emergency treatment immediately.
Common:	
Rash, redness, itching.	Discontinue. Call doctor right away.
Infrequent:	
Rectal itching.	Continue. Call doctor when convenient.
Rare:	
Mild nausea, vomiting, cramps, severe diarrhea with mucus or blood in stool, unusual weakness, tiredness, weight loss, fever.	Discontinue. Call doctor right away.

WARNINGS & PRECAUTIONS

Don't take if:
You are allergic to any cephalosporin antibiotic.

Before you start, consult your doctor:
- If you are allergic to any penicillin antibiotic.
- If you have a kidney disorder.
- If you have colitis or enteritis.

Over age 60:
Adverse reactions and side effects may be more frequent and severe than in younger persons. More likely to itch around rectum and genitals.

Pregnancy:
No proven harm to unborn child. Avoid if possible.

Breast-feeding:
Drug passes into milk. Avoid drug or discontinue nursing until you finish medicine. Consult doctor for advice on maintaining milk supply.

Infants & children:
No special warnings.

Prolonged use:
Kills beneficial bacteria that protect body against other germs. Unchecked germs may cause secondary infections.

Skin & sunlight:
No problems expected.

Driving, piloting or hazardous work:
No problems expected.

Discontinuing:
Don't discontinue without doctor's advice until you complete prescribed dose, even though symptoms diminish or disappear.

Others:
No problems expected.

 ## POSSIBLE INTERACTION WITH OTHER DRUGS

GENERIC NAME OR DRUG CLASS	COMBINED EFFECT
Anticoagulants	Increased anticoagulant effect.
Loperamide	Reduced cefaclor effect.
Probenecid	Increased cefaclor effect.

 ## POSSIBLE INTERACTION WITH OTHER SUBSTANCES

INTERACTS WITH	COMBINED EFFECT
Alcohol:	None expected.
Beverages:	None expected.
Cocaine:	None expected, but cocaine may slow body's recovery. Avoid.
Foods:	Slow absorption. Take with liquid 1 hour before or 2 hours after eating.
Marijuana:	None expected, but marijuana may slow body's recovery. Avoid.
Tobacco:	None expected.

CEFADROXIL

BRAND NAMES

Duricef   Ultracef

BASIC INFORMATION

Habit forming? No
Prescription needed? Yes
Available as generic? No
Drug class: Antibiotic (cephalosporin)

USES

Treatment of bacterial infections. Will not cure viral infections such as cold and flu.

DOSAGE & USAGE INFORMATION

How to take:
- Tablet or capsule—Swallow with liquid. If you can't swallow whole, crumble tablet or open capsule and take with liquid or food.
- Liquid—Use measuring spoon.

When to take:
At same times each day, 1 hour before or 2 hours after eating.

If you forget a dose:
Take as soon as you remember or double next dose. Return to regular schedule.

What drug does:
Kills susceptible bacteria.

Time lapse before drug works:
May require several days to affect infection.

Don't take with:
See Interaction column and consult doctor.

OVERDOSE

SYMPTOMS:
Abdominal cramps, nausea, vomiting, severe diarrhea with mucus or blood in stool.
WHAT TO DO:
Overdose unlikely to threaten life. If person takes much larger amount than prescribed, call doctor, poison-control center or hospital emergency room for instructions.

POSSIBLE ADVERSE REACTIONS OR SIDE EFFECTS

SYMPTOMS	WHAT TO DO
Life-threatening:	
Hives, rash, intense itching, faintness soon after a dose (anaphylaxis).	Seek emergency treatment immediately.
Common:	
Rash, redness, itching.	Discontinue. Call doctor right away.
Infrequent:	
Rectal itching.	Continue. Call doctor when convenient.
Rare:	
Mild nausea, vomiting, cramps, severe diarrhea with mucus or blood in stool, unusual weakness, tiredness, weight loss, fever.	Discontinue. Call doctor right away.

WARNINGS & PRECAUTIONS

Don't take if:
You are allergic to any cephalosporin antibiotic.

Before you start, consult your doctor:
- If you are allergic to any penicillin antibiotic.
- If you have a kidney disorder.
- If you have colitis or enteritis.

Over age 60:
Adverse reactions and side effects may be more frequent and severe than in younger persons. More likely to itch around rectum and genitals.

Pregnancy:
No proven harm to unborn child. Avoid if possible.

Breast-feeding:
Drug passes into milk. Avoid drug or discontinue nursing until you finish medicine. Consult doctor for advice on maintaining milk supply.

Infants & children:
No special warnings.

Prolonged use:
Kills beneficial bacteria that protect body against other germs. Unchecked germs may cause secondary infections.

Skin & sunlight:
No problems expected.

Driving, piloting or hazardous work:
No problems expected.

Discontinuing:
Don't discontinue without doctor's advice until you complete prescribed dose, even though symptoms diminish or disappear.

Others:
No problems expected.

POSSIBLE INTERACTION WITH OTHER DRUGS

GENERIC NAME OR DRUG CLASS	COMBINED EFFECT
Anticoagulants	Increased anticoagulant effect.
Loperamide	Reduced cefadroxil effect.
Probenecid	Increased cefadroxil effect.

POSSIBLE INTERACTION WITH OTHER SUBSTANCES

INTERACTS WITH	COMBINED EFFECT
Alcohol:	None expected.
Beverages:	None expected.
Cocaine:	None expected, but cocaine may slow body's recovery. Avoid.
Foods:	Slow absorption. Take with liquid 1 hour before or 2 hours after eating.
Marijuana:	None expected, but marijuana may slow body's recovery. Avoid.
Tobacco:	None expected.

CEPHALEXIN

BRAND NAMES

Ceporex   Novolexin
Keflex

BASIC INFORMATION

Habit forming? No
Prescription needed? Yes
Available as generic? No
Drug class: Antibiotic (cephalosporin)

 USES

Treatment of bacterial infections. Will not cure viral infections such as cold and flu.

 DOSAGE & USAGE INFORMATION

How to take:
- Tablet or capsule—Swallow with liquid. If you can't swallow whole, crumble tablet or open capsule and take with liquid or food.
- Liquid—Use measuring spoon.

When to take:
At same times each day, 1 hour before or 2 hours after eating.

If you forget a dose:
Take as soon as you remember or double next dose. Return to regular schedule.

What drug does:
Kills susceptible bacteria.

Time lapse before drug works:
May require several days to affect infection.

Don't take with:
See Interaction column and consult doctor.

 OVERDOSE

SYMPTOMS:
Abdominal cramps, nausea, vomiting, severe diarrhea with mucus or blood in stool.
WHAT TO DO:
Overdose unlikely to threaten life. If person takes much larger amount than prescribed, call doctor, poison-control center or hospital emergency room for instructions.

 POSSIBLE ADVERSE REACTIONS OR SIDE EFFECTS

SYMPTOMS	WHAT TO DO
Life-threatening:	
Hives, rash, intense itching, faintness soon after a dose (anaphylaxis).	Seek emergency treatment immediately.
Common:	
Rash, redness, itching.	Discontinue. Call doctor right away.
Infrequent:	
Rectal itching.	Continue. Call doctor when convenient.
Rare:	
Mild nausea, vomiting, cramps, severe diarrhea with mucus or blood in stool, unusual weakness, tiredness, weight loss, fever.	Discontinue. Call doctor right away.

WARNINGS & PRECAUTIONS

Don't take if:
You are allergic to any cephalosporin antibiotic.

Before you start, consult your doctor:
- If you are allergic to any penicillin antibiotic.
- If you have a kidney disorder.
- If you have colitis or enteritis.

Over age 60:
Adverse reactions and side effects may be more frequent and severe than in younger persons. More likely to itch around rectum and genitals.

Pregnancy:
No proven harm to unborn child. Avoid if possible.

Breast-feeding:
Drug passes into milk. Avoid drug or discontinue nursing until you finish medicine. Consult doctor for advice on maintaining milk supply.

Infants & children:
No special warnings.

Prolonged use:
Kills beneficial bacteria that protect body against other germs. Unchecked germs may cause secondary infections.

Skin & sunlight:
No problems expected.

Driving, piloting or hazardous work:
No problems expected.

Discontinuing:
Don't discontinue without doctor's advice until you complete prescribed dose, even though symptoms diminish or disappear.

Others:
No problems expected.

POSSIBLE INTERACTION WITH OTHER DRUGS

GENERIC NAME OR DRUG CLASS	COMBINED EFFECT
Anticoagulants	Increased anticoagulant effect.
Probenecid	Increased cephalexin effect.

POSSIBLE INTERACTION WITH OTHER SUBSTANCES

INTERACTS WITH	COMBINED EFFECT
Alcohol:	None expected.
Beverages:	None expected.
Cocaine:	None expected, but cocaine may slow body's recovery. Avoid.
Foods:	Slow absorption. Take with liquid 1 hour before or 2 hours after eating.
Marijuana:	None expected, but marijuana may slow body's recovery. Avoid.
Tobacco:	None expected.

CEPHRADINE

BRAND NAMES

Anspor   Velosef

BASIC INFORMATION

Habit forming? No
Prescription needed? Yes
Available as generic? No
Drug class: Antibiotic (cephalosporin)

 USES

Treatment of bacterial infections. Will not cure viral infections such as cold and flu.

 DOSAGE & USAGE INFORMATION

How to take:
- Tablet or capsule—Swallow with liquid. If you can't swallow whole, crumble tablet or open capsule and take with liquid or food.
- Liquid—Use measuring spoon.

When to take:
At same times each day, 1 hour before or 2 hours after eating.

If you forget a dose:
Take as soon as you remember or double next dose. Return to regular schedule.

What drug does:
Kills susceptible bacteria.

Time lapse before drug works:
May require several days to affect infection.

Don't take with:
See Interaction column and consult doctor.

 OVERDOSE

SYMPTOMS:
Abdominal cramps, nausea, vomiting, severe diarrhea with mucus or blood in stool.
WHAT TO DO:
Overdose unlikely to threaten life. If person takes much larger amount than prescribed, call doctor, poison-control center or hospital emergency room for instructions.

 POSSIBLE ADVERSE REACTIONS OR SIDE EFFECTS

SYMPTOMS	WHAT TO DO
Life-threatening:	
Hives, rash, intense itching, faintness soon after a dose (anaphylaxis).	Seek emergency treatment immediately.
Common:	
Rash, redness, itching.	Discontinue. Call doctor right away.
Infrequent:	
Rectal itching.	Continue. Call doctor when convenient.
Rare:	
Mild nausea, vomiting, cramps, severe diarrhea with mucus or blood in stool, unusual weakness, tiredness, weight loss, fever.	Discontinue. Call doctor right away.

CEPHRADINE

 WARNINGS & PRECAUTIONS

Don't take if:
You are allergic to any cephalosporin antibiotic.

Before you start, consult your doctor:
• If you are allergic to any penicillin antibiotic.
• If you have a kidney disorder.
• If you have colitis or enteritis.

Over age 60:
Adverse reactions and side effects may be more frequent and severe than in younger persons. More likely to itch around rectum and genitals.

Pregnancy:
No proven harm to unborn child. Avoid if possible.

Breast-feeding:
Drug passes into milk. Avoid drug or discontinue nursing until you finish medicine. Consult doctor for advice on maintaining milk supply.

Infants & children:
No special warnings.

Prolonged use:
Kills beneficial bacteria that protect body against other germs. Unchecked germs may cause secondary infections.

Skin & sunlight:
No problems expected.

Driving, piloting or hazardous work:
No problems expected.

Discontinuing:
Don't discontinue without doctor's advice until you complete prescribed dose, even though symptoms diminish or disappear.

Others:
No problems expected.

 POSSIBLE INTERACTION WITH OTHER DRUGS

GENERIC NAME OR DRUG CLASS	COMBINED EFFECT
Anticoagulants	Increased anticoagulant effect.
Probenecid	Increased cephradine effect.

 POSSIBLE INTERACTION WITH OTHER SUBSTANCES

INTERACTS WITH	COMBINED EFFECT
Alcohol:	None expected.
Beverages:	None expected.
Cocaine:	None expected, but cocaine may slow body's recovery. Avoid.
Foods:	Slow absorption. Take with liquid 1 hour before or 2 hours after eating.
Marijuana:	None expected, but marijuana may slow body's recovery. Avoid.
Tobacco:	None expected.

CHARCOAL, ACTIVATED

BRAND NAMES

Actidose-Aqua
Arm-a-Char
Charcoaid
Charcoalanti Dote

Charcocaps
Charcodote
Insta-Char
Liquid-Antidose

BASIC INFORMATION

Habit forming? No
Prescription needed? No
Available as generic? Yes
Drug class: Antidote (adsorbent)

 ## USES

- Treatment of poisonings from medication.
- Treatment (infrequent) for diarrhea or excessive gaseousness.

 ## DOSAGE & USAGE INFORMATION

How to take:
- Tablet or capsule—Swallow with liquid. If you can't swallow whole, crumble tablet or open capsule and take with liquid or food.
- Liquid—Take as directed on label.

When to take:
- For poisoning—Take immediately after poisoning. If your doctor or emergency poison control center has also recommended syrup of ipecac, don't take charcoal for 30 minutes or until vomiting from ipecac stops.
- For diarrhea or gas—Take at same times each day.

If you forget a dose:
- For poisonings—Not applicable.
- For diarrhea or gas—Take as soon as you remember up to 2 hours late. If more than 2 hours, wait for next scheduled dose (don't double this dose).

What drug does:
- Helps prevent poison from being absorbed from stomach and intestines.
- Helps absorb gas in intestinal tract.

Continued next column

 ## OVERDOSE

SYMPTOMS:
None expected.
WHAT TO DO:
Overdose unlikely to threaten life. If person takes much larger amount than prescribed, call doctor, poison-control center or hospital emergency room for instructions.

Time lapse before drug works:
Begins immediately.

Don't take with:
Ice cream or sherbet.

 ## POSSIBLE ADVERSE REACTIONS OR SIDE EFFECTS

SYMPTOMS	WHAT TO DO
Life-threatening: None expected.	
Always: Black bowel movements.	No action necessary.
Infrequent: None expected.	
Rare: None expected.	

WARNINGS & PRECAUTIONS

Don't take if:
The poison was lye or other strong alkali, strong acids (such as sulfuric acid), cyanide, iron, ethyl alcohol or methyl alcohol. Charcoal will not prevent these poisons from causing ill effects.

Before you start, consult your doctor:
If you are taking it as an antidote for poison.

Over age 60:
No problems expected.

Pregnancy:
No problems expected.

Breast-feeding:
No problems expected.

Infants & children:
Don't give to children for more than 3 or 4 days for diarrhea. Continuing for longer periods can interfere with normal nutrition.

Prolonged use:
No problems expected.

Skin & sunlight:
No problems expected.

Driving, piloting or hazardous work:
No problems expected.

Discontinuing:
No problems expected.

Others:
No problems expected.

POSSIBLE INTERACTION WITH OTHER DRUGS

GENERIC NAME OR DRUG CLASS	COMBINED EFFECT
Any medicine taken at the same time	May decrease absorption of medicine.

POSSIBLE INTERACTION WITH OTHER SUBSTANCES

INTERACTS WITH	COMBINED EFFECT
Alcohol:	None expected.
Beverages:	None expected.
Cocaine:	None expected.
Foods: Ice cream or sherbet.	Decreased charcoal effect.
Marijuana:	None expected.
Tobacco:	None expected.

CHLOPHEDIANOL

BRAND NAMES

Ulo   Ulone

BASIC INFORMATION

Habit forming? No
Prescription needed? Yes
Available as generic? No
Drug class: Cough suppressant

 USES

Reduces non-productive cough due to bronchial irritation.

 DOSAGE & USAGE INFORMATION

How to take:
Take syrup without diluting. Don't drink fluids immediately after medicine.

When to take:
3 or 4 times a day when needed. No more often than every 3 hours.

If you forget a dose:
Take as soon as you remember up to 2 hours late. If more than 2 hours, wait for next scheduled dose (don't double this dose).

What drug does:
Reduces cough reflex by direct effect on cough center in brain, and by local anesthetic action.

Time lapse before drug works:
30 minutes to 1 hour.

Don't take with:
- Alcohol or brain depressant or stimulant drugs.
- See Interaction column and consult doctor.

 OVERDOSE

SYMPTOMS:
Blurred vision, hallucinations, coma.
WHAT TO DO:
- Dial 0 (operator) or 911 (emergency) for an ambulance or medical help. Then give first aid immediately.
- If patient is unconscious and not breathing, give mouth-to-mouth breathing. If there is no heartbeat, use cardiac massage and mouth-to-mouth breathing (CPR). Don't try to make patient vomit. If you can't get help quickly, take patient to nearest emergency facility.
- See emergency information on inside covers.

 POSSIBLE ADVERSE REACTIONS OR SIDE EFFECTS

SYMPTOMS	WHAT TO DO
Life-threatening None expected.	
Common: Difficult urination in older men with enlarged prostate.	Continue. Call doctor when convenient.
Infrequent: None expected.	
Rare: • Hallucinations, drowsiness, rash or hives, nausea, vomiting, irregular heartbeat.	Discontinue. Call doctor right away.
• Nightmares, excitement or irritability, blurred vision, dry mouth.	Continue. Call doctor when convenient.

WARNINGS & PRECAUTIONS

Don't take if:
You are allergic to chlophedianol.

Before you start, consult your doctor:
- If medicine is for hyperactive child who takes medicine for treatment.
- If your cough brings up sputum (phlegm).
- If you have heart disease.
- If you will have surgery within 2 months, including dental surgery, requiring general or spinal anesthesia.

Over age 60:
Adverse reactions and side effects may be more frequent and severe than in younger persons.

Pregnancy:
Risk to unborn child outweighs drug benefits. Don't use.

Breast-feeding:
Unknown whether medicine filters into milk. Consult doctor.

Infants & children:
Not recommended for children under age 2.

Prolonged use:
Not recommended. If cough persists despite medicine, consult doctor.

Skin & sunlight:
No problems expected.

Driving, piloting or hazardous work:
Don't drive or pilot aircraft until you learn how medicine affects you. Don't work around dangerous machinery. Don't climb ladders or work in high places. Danger increases if you drink alcohol or take medicine affecting alertness and reflexes, such as antihistamines, tranquilizers, sedatives, pain medicine, narcotics and mind-altering drugs.

Discontinuing:
May be unnecessary to finish medicine. Follow doctor's instructions.

Others:
Consult doctor if cough persists despite medication for 7 days or if fever, skin rash or headache accompany cough.

POSSIBLE INTERACTION WITH OTHER DRUGS

GENERIC NAME OR DRUG CLASS	COMBINED EFFECT
Anticonvulsants	Interferes with actions of both.
Antidepressants (tricyclic)	Excess sedation.
Appetite suppressants	Excess stimulation.
Central-nervous-system depressants: antidepressants, antihistamines, muscle relaxants, narcotics, pain pills, sedatives, sleeping pills, tranquilizers.	Excess sedation.
MAO inhibitors	Excess sedation.
Sympathomimetics	Excess stimulation.

POSSIBLE INTERACTION WITH OTHER SUBSTANCES

INTERACTS WITH	COMBINED EFFECT
Alcohol:	Excess sedation. Avoid.
Beverages: Coffee, tea, cocoa, cola.	Excess stimulation. Avoid.
Cocaine:	Increased chance of toxic stimulation. Avoid.
Foods:	None expected.
Marijuana:	Increased chance of toxic stimulation. Avoid.
Tobacco:	Decreased effect of chlophedianol.

CHLORAL HYDRATE

BRAND NAMES

Aquachloral	Novochlorhydrate
Aquachloral	Oradrate
Supprettes	SK-Chloral Hydrate
Colidrate	
Noctec	

BASIC INFORMATION

Habit forming? Yes
Prescription needed? Yes
Available as generic? Yes
Drug class: Hypnotic

 USES

- Reduces anxiety.
- Relieves insomnia.

 DOSAGE & USAGE INFORMATION

How to take:
- Tablet or capsule—Swallow with milk or food to lessen stomach irritation.
- Drops—Dilute dose in beverage before swallowing.
- Suppositories—Remove wrapper and moisten suppository with water. Gently insert larger end into rectum. Push well into rectum with finger.

When to take:
At the same time each day.

If you forget a dose:
Take as soon as you remember up to 2 hours late. If more than 2 hours, wait for next scheduled dose (don't double this dose).

Continued next column

 OVERDOSE

SYMPTOMS:
Confusion, weakness, breathing difficulty, stagger, slow or irregular heartbeat.
WHAT TO DO:
- Dial 0 (operator) or 911 (emergency) for an ambulance or medical help. Then give first aid immediately.
- If patient is unconscious and not breathing, give mouth-to-mouth breathing. If there is no heartbeat, use cardiac massage and mouth-to-mouth breathing (CPR). Don't try to make patient vomit. If you can't get help quickly, take patient to nearest emergency facility.
- See emergency information on inside covers.

What drug does:
Affects brain centers that control wakefulness and alertness.

Time lapse before drug works:
30 to 60 minutes.

Don't take with:
See Interaction column and consult doctor.

 POSSIBLE ADVERSE REACTIONS OR SIDE EFFECTS

SYMPTOMS	WHAT TO DO
Life-threatening: None expected.	
Common: Nausea, stomach pain, vomiting.	Discontinue. Call doctor right away.
Infrequent: "Hangover" effect, clumsiness or unsteadiness, drowsiness, dizziness, lightheadedness.	Continue. Call doctor when convenient.
Rare:	
• Hallucinations, agitation, confusion.	Discontinue. Call doctor right away.
• Hives, rash.	Continue. Call doctor when convenient.

WARNINGS & PRECAUTIONS

Don't take if:
You are allergic to chloral hydrate.

Before you start, consult your doctor:
- If you have had liver, kidney or heart trouble.
- If you are prone to stomach upsets (if medicine is in oral form).
- If you have colitis or a rectal inflammation (if medicine is in suppository form).

Over age 60:
Adverse reactions and side effects may be more frequent and severe than in younger persons. More likely to have "hangover" effect.

Pregnancy:
Risk to unborn child outweighs drug benefits. Unborn child may become addicted to drug. Don't use.

Breast-feeding:
Drug filters into milk. May harm child. Avoid.

Infants & children:
Use only under medical supervision.

Prolonged use:
Addiction and possible kidney damage.

Skin & sunlight:
No problems expected.

Driving, piloting or hazardous work:
Don't drive or pilot aircraft until you learn how medicine affects you. Don't work around dangerous machinery. Don't climb ladders or work in high places. Danger increases if you drink alcohol or take medicine affecting alertness and reflexes, such as antihistamines, tranquilizers, sedatives, pain medicine, narcotics and mind-altering drugs.

Discontinuing:
Don't discontinue without consulting doctor. Dose may require gradual reduction if you have taken drug for a long time. Doses of other drugs may also require adjustment.

Others:
Frequent kidney-function tests recommended when drug is used for long time.

 ## POSSIBLE INTERACTION WITH OTHER DRUGS

GENERIC NAME OR DRUG CLASS	COMBINED EFFECT
Anticoagulants	Possible hemorrhaging.
Antidepressants	Increased chloral hydrate effect.
Antihistamines	Increased chloral hydrate effect.
Cortisone drugs	Decreased cortisone effect.
MAO inhibitors	Increased chloral hydrate effect.
Mind-altering drugs	Increased chloral hydrate effect.
Molindone	Increased tranquilizer effect.
Narcotics	Increased chloral hydrate effect.
Pain relievers	Increased chloral hydrate effect.
Phenothiazines	Increased chloral hydrate effect.
Sedatives	Increased chloral hydrate effect.
Sleep inducers	Increased chloral hydrate effect.
Tranquilizers	Increased chloral hydrate effect.

 ## POSSIBLE INTERACTION WITH OTHER SUBSTANCES

INTERACTS WITH	COMBINED EFFECT
Alcohol:	Increased sedative effect of both. Avoid.
Beverages:	None expected.
Cocaine:	Decreased chloral hydrate effect. Avoid.
Foods:	None expected.
Marijuana:	May severely impair mental and physical functioning. Avoid.
Tobacco:	None expected.

CHLORAMBUCIL

BRAND NAMES

Leukeran

BASIC INFORMATION

Habit forming? No
Prescription needed? Yes
Available as generic? No
Drug class: Antineoplastic,
                immunosuppressant

 USES

- Treatment for some kinds of cancer.
- Suppresses immune response after transplant and in immune disorders.

 DOSAGE & USAGE INFORMATION

How to take:
Tablet or capsule—Swallow with liquid after light meal. Don't drink fluids with meals. Drink extra fluids between meals. Avoid sweet or fatty foods.

When to take:
At the same time each day.

If you forget a dose:
Take as soon as you remember. Don't ever double dose.

What drug does:
Inhibits abnormal cell reproduction. May suppress immune system.

Time lapse before drug works:
Up to 6 weeks for full effect.

Continued next column

 OVERDOSE

SYMPTOMS:
Bleeding, chills, fever, collapse, stupor, seizure.
WHAT TO DO:
- Dial 0 (operator) or 911 (emergency) for an ambulance or medical help. Then give first aid immediately.
- If patient is unconscious and not breathing, give mouth-to-mouth breathing. If there is no heartbeat, use cardiac massage and mouth-to-mouth breathing (CPR). Don't try to make patient vomit. If you can't get help quickly, take patient to nearest emergency facility.
- See emergency information on inside covers.

Don't take with:
See Interaction column and consult doctor.

 POSSIBLE ADVERSE REACTIONS OR SIDE EFFECTS

SYMPTOMS	WHAT TO DO
Life-threatening: None expected.	
Common:	
• Unusual bleeding or bruising, mouth sores with sore throat, chills and fever, black stools, mouth and lip sores, menstrual irregularities.	Discontinue. Call doctor right away.
• Hair loss, joint pain.	Continue. Call doctor when convenient.
• Nausea, vomiting, diarrhea (unavoidable), tiredness, weakness.	Continue. Tell doctor at next visit.
Infrequent:	
• Mental confusion, shortness of breath; may increase chance of developing leukemia.	Continue. Call doctor when convenient.
• Cough.	Continue. Tell doctor at next visit.
Rare: Jaundice.	Discontinue. Call doctor right away.

WARNINGS & PRECAUTIONS

Don't take if:
- You have had hypersensitivity to alkylating antineoplastic drugs.
- Your physician has not explained serious nature of your medical problem and risks of taking this medicine.

Before you start, consult your doctor:
- If you have gout.
- If you have had kidney stones.
- If you have active infection.
- If you have impaired kidney or liver function.
- If you have taken other antineoplastic drugs or had radiation treatment in last 3 weeks.

Over age 60:
Adverse reactions and side effects may be more frequent and severe than in younger persons.

Pregnancy:
Consult doctor. Risk to child is significant.

Breast-feeding:
Drug passes into milk. Don't nurse.

Infants & children:
Use only under care of medical supervisors who are experienced in anticancer drugs.

Prolonged use:
Adverse reactions more likely the longer drug is required.

Skin & sunlight:
No problems expected.

Driving, piloting or hazardous work:
No problems expected.

Discontinuing:
Don't discontinue without doctor's advice until you complete prescribed dose, even though symptoms diminish or disappear. Some side effects may follow discontinuing. Report to doctor blurred vision, convulsions, confusion, persistent headache.

Others:
May cause sterility.

POSSIBLE INTERACTION WITH OTHER DRUGS

GENERIC NAME OR DRUG CLASS	COMBINED EFFECT
Antigout drugs	Decreased antigout effect.
Antineoplastic drugs (other)	Increased effect of all drugs, (may be beneficial).
Chloramphenicol	Increased likelihood of toxic effects of both drugs.

POSSIBLE INTERACTION WITH OTHER SUBSTANCES

INTERACTS WITH	COMBINED EFFECT
Alcohol:	May increase chance of intestinal bleeding.
Beverages:	No problems expected.
Cocaine:	Increases chance of toxicity.
Foods:	Reduces irritation in stomach.
Marijuana:	No problems expected.
Tobacco:	Increases lung toxicity.

CHLORAMPHENICOL

BRAND NAMES

Amphicol	Mychel
Antibiopto	Mychel-S
Chloromycetin	Nova-Phenicol
Chloroptic	Novochlorocap
Econochlor	Ophthochlor
Fenicol	Ophthocort
Isopto Fenicol	Pentamycetin
Minims	Sopamycetin

BASIC INFORMATION

Habit forming? No
Prescription needed? Yes
Available as generic? Yes
Drug class: Antibiotic

 ## USES

Treatment of infections susceptible to chloramphenicol.

 ## DOSAGE & USAGE INFORMATION

How to take:
- Tablet or capsule—Swallow with liquid.
- Eye solution or ointment, ear solution or cream—Follow label instructions.

When to take:
Tablet or capsule—1 hour before or 2 hours after eating.

If you forget a dose:
Take as soon as you remember up to 2 hours late. If more than 2 hours, wait for next scheduled dose (don't double this dose).

What drug does:
Prevents bacteria from growing and reproducing. Will not kill viruses.

Time lapse before drug works:
2 to 5 days, depending on type and severity of infection.

Don't take with:
See Interaction column and consult doctor.

 ## OVERDOSE

SYMPTOMS:
Nausea, vomiting, diarrhea.
WHAT TO DO:
Overdose unlikely to threaten life. If person takes much larger amount than prescribed, call doctor, poison-control center or hospital emergency room for instructions.

 ## POSSIBLE ADVERSE REACTIONS OR SIDE EFFECTS

SYMPTOMS	WHAT TO DO
Life-threatening:	
Hives, rash, intense itching, faintness soon after a dose (anaphylaxis).	Seek emergency treatment immediately.
Common:	
None expected.	
Infrequent:	
• Swollen face or extremities; diarrhea; nausea; vomiting; numbness, tingling, burning pain or weakness in hands and feet.	Discontinue. Call doctor right away.
• Headache, confusion.	Continue. Call doctor when convenient.
Rare:	
Pain, blurred vision, possible vision loss, sore throat, fever, jaundice, anemia.	Discontinue. Call doctor right away.

WARNINGS & PRECAUTIONS

Don't take if:
- You are allergic to chloramphenicol.
- It is prescribed for a minor disorder such as flu, cold or mild sore throat.

Before you start, consult your doctor:
- If you have had a blood disorder or bone-marrow disease.
- If you have had kidney or liver disease.
- If you have diabetes.

Over age 60:
Adverse reactions and side effects may be more frequent and severe than in younger persons, particularly skin irritation around rectum.

Pregnancy:
Risk to unborn child outweighs drug benefits. Don't use.

Breast-feeding:
Drug passes into milk. Avoid drug or discontinue nursing until you finish medicine. Consult doctor for advice on maintaining milk supply.

Infants & children:
Don't give to infants younger than 2.

Prolonged use:
You may become more susceptible to infections caused by germs not responsive to chloramphenicol.

Skin & sunlight:
No problems expected.

Driving, piloting or hazardous work:
Don't drive or pilot aircraft until you learn how medicine affects you. Don't work around dangerous machinery. Don't climb ladders or work in high places. Danger increases if you drink alcohol or take medicine affecting alertness and reflexes.

Discontinuing:
Don't discontinue without doctor's advice until you complete prescribed dose, even though symptoms diminish or disappear.

Others:
- Chloramphenicol can cause serious anemia. Frequent laboratory blood studies, liver and kidney tests recommended.
- Second medical opinion recommended before starting.

POSSIBLE INTERACTION WITH OTHER DRUGS

GENERIC NAME OR DRUG CLASS	COMBINED EFFECT
Anticoagulants	Increased anticoagulant effect.
Antidiabetics (oral)	Increased antidiabetic effect.
Cyclophosphamide	Decreased cyclophosphamide effect.
Flecainide	Possible decreased blood-cell production in bone marrow.
Penicillins	Decreased penicillin effect.
Phenytoin	Increased phenytoin effect.
Tocainide	Possible decreased blood-cell production in bone marrow.

POSSIBLE INTERACTION WITH OTHER SUBSTANCES

INTERACTS WITH	COMBINED EFFECT
Alcohol:	Possible liver problems. May cause disulfiram reaction (see Glossary).
Beverages:	None expected.
Cocaine:	No proven problems.
Foods:	None expected.
Marijuana:	None expected.
Tobacco:	None expected.

CHLORDIAZEPOXIDE

BRAND AND GENERIC NAMES

Apo-
  Chlordiazepoxide
CHLORDIAZEPOXIDE
Libritabs
Librium
Lipoxide
Medilium

Murcil
Novopoxide
Reposans
Sereen
SK-Lygen
Solium

BASIC INFORMATION

Habit forming? Yes
Prescription needed? Yes
Available as generic? Yes
Drug class: Tranquilizer (benzodiazepine)

USES

- Treatment for nervousness or tension.
- Treatment for muscle spasm.
- Treatment for convulsive disorders.

DOSAGE & USAGE INFORMATION

How to take:
Tablet or capsule—Swallow with liquid. If you can't swallow whole, crumble tablet or open capsule and take with liquid or food.

When to take:
At the same time each day, according to instructions on prescription label.

If you forget a dose:
Take as soon as you remember up to 2 hours late. If more than 2 hours, wait for next scheduled dose (don't double this dose).

Continued next column

OVERDOSE

SYMPTOMS:
Drowsiness, weakness, tremor, stupor, coma.
WHAT TO DO:
- **Dial 0 (operator) or 911 (emergency) for an ambulance or medical help. Then give first aid immediately.**
- **If patient is unconscious and not breathing, give mouth-to-mouth breathing. If there is no heartbeat, use cardiac massage and mouth-to-mouth breathing (CPR). Don't try to make patient vomit. If you can't get help quickly, take patient to nearest emergency facility.**
- **See emergency information on inside covers.**

What drug does:
Affects limbic system of brain—part that controls emotions.

Time lapse before drug works:
2 hours. May take 6 weeks for full benefit.

Don't take with:
See Interaction column and consult doctor.

POSSIBLE ADVERSE REACTIONS OR SIDE EFFECTS

SYMPTOMS	WHAT TO DO
Life-threatening:	
None expected.	
Common:	
Clumsiness, drowsiness, dizziness.	Continue. Call doctor when convenient.
Infrequent:	
• Hallucinations, confusion, depression, irritability, rash, itch, vision changes.	Discontinue. Call doctor right away.
• Constipation or diarrhea, nausea, vomiting, difficult urination.	Continue. Call doctor when convenient.
Rare:	
• Slow heartbeat, breathing difficulty.	Discontinue. Seek emergency treatment.
• Mouth, throat ulcers; jaundice.	Discontinue. Call doctor right away.

WARNINGS & PRECAUTIONS

Don't take if:
- You are allergic to any benzodiazepine.
- You have myasthenia gravis.
- You are active or recovering alcoholic.
- Patient is younger than 6 months.

Before you start, consult your doctor:
- If you have liver, kidney or lung disease.
- If you have diabetes, epilepsy or porphyria.

Over age 60:
Adverse reactions and side effects may be more frequent and severe than in younger persons. You need smaller doses for shorter periods of time. May develop agitation, rage or "hangover" effect.

Pregnancy:
Risk to unborn child outweighs drug benefits. Don't use.

Breast-feeding:
Drug passes into milk. Avoid drug or discontinue nursing until you finish medicine. Consult doctor for advice on maintaining milk supply.

Infants & children:
Use only under medical supervision for children older than 6 months.

Prolonged use:
May impair liver function.

Skin & sunlight:
No problems expected.

Driving, piloting or hazardous work:
Don't drive or pilot aircraft until you learn how medicine affects you. Don't work around dangerous machinery. Don't climb ladders or work in high places. Danger increases if you drink alcohol or take medicine affecting alertness and reflexes.

Discontinuing:
Don't discontinue without consulting doctor. Dose may require gradual reduction if you have taken drug for a long time. Doses of other drugs may also require adjustment.

Others:
- Hot weather, heavy exercise and profuse sweat may reduce excretion and cause overdose.
- Blood sugar may rise in diabetics, requiring insulin adjustment.

POSSIBLE INTERACTION WITH OTHER DRUGS

GENERIC NAME OR DRUG CLASS	COMBINED EFFECT
Anticonvulsants	Change in seizure frequency or severity.
Antidepressants	Increased sedative effect of both drugs.
Antihistamines	Increased sedative effect of both drugs.
Antihypertensives	Excessively low blood pressure.
Cimetidine	Excess sedation.
Disulfiram	Increased chlordiazepoxide effect.
Dronabinol	Increased effects of both drugs. Avoid.
MAO inhibitors	Convulsions, deep sedation, rage.
Molindone	Increased tranquilizer effect.
Narcotics	Increased sedative effect of both drugs.
Sedatives	Increased sedative effect of both drugs.
Sleep inducers	Increased sedative effect of both drugs.
Tranquilizers	Increased sedative effect of both drugs.

POSSIBLE INTERACTION WITH OTHER SUBSTANCES

INTERACTS WITH	COMBINED EFFECT
Alcohol:	Heavy sedation. Avoid.
Beverages:	None expected.
Cocaine:	Decreased chlordiazepoxide effect.
Foods:	None expected.
Marijuana:	Heavy sedation. Avoid.
Tobacco:	Decreased chlordiazepoxide effect.

CHLORDIAZEPOXIDE & AMITRIPTYLINE

BRAND NAMES

Limbitrol   Limbitrol DS

BASIC INFORMATION

Habit forming? Yes
Prescription needed? Yes
Available as generic? No
Drug class: Antidepressant, tranquilizer
(benzodiazepine)

 USES

- Treatment for nervousness or tension.
- Gradually relieves, but doesn't cure,
  symptoms of depression.

 DOSAGE & USAGE INFORMATION

How to take:
Tablet or capsule—Swallow with liquid. If you
can't swallow whole, crumble tablet or open
capsule and take with liquid or food.

When to take:
At the same time each day, according to
instructions on prescription label.

If you forget a dose:
Bedtime dose—If you forget your once-a-day
bedtime dose, don't take it more than 3 hours
late. If more than 3 hours, wait for next
scheduled dose (don't double this dose).

What drug does:
Affects limbic system of brain—part that
controls emotions.

Continued next column

 OVERDOSE

SYMPTOMS:
Drowsiness, weakness, tremor,
hallucinations, convulsions, stupor, coma.
WHAT TO DO:
- **Dial 0 (operator) or 911 (emergency) for an**
  ambulance or medical help. Then give first
  aid immediately.
- **If patient is unconscious and not**
  breathing, give mouth-to-mouth breathing.
  If there is no heartbeat, use cardiac
  massage and mouth-to-mouth breathing
  (CPR). Don't try to make patient vomit. If
  you can't get help quickly, take patient to
  nearest emergency facility.
- **See emergency information on inside**
  covers.

Time lapse before drug works:
Begins in 1 to 2 weeks. May require 4 to 6
weeks for maximum benefit.

Don't take with:
- Non-prescription drugs without consulting
  doctor.
- See Interaction column and consult doctor.

 POSSIBLE ADVERSE REACTIONS OR SIDE EFFECTS

SYMPTOMS	WHAT TO DO
Life-threatening:	
Slow heartbeat, irregular breathing.	Seek emergency treatment immediately.
Common:	
• Clumsiness, drowsiness, dizziness, headache, insomnia, dry mouth or unpleasant taste, constipation, fatigue, weakness.	Continue. Call doctor when convenient.
• "Sweet tooth."	Continue. Tell doctor at next visit.
Infrequent:	
• Hallucinations, confusion, depression, irritability, rash, itch, vision changes, jaundice, blurred vision, eye pain.	Discontinue. Call doctor right away.
• Constipation, diarrhea, nausea, vomiting, difficult urination, indigestion.	Continue. Call doctor when convenient.
Rare:	
Mouth or throat ulcers, fever.	Discontinue. Call doctor right away.

 WARNINGS & PRECAUTIONS

Don't take if:
- You are allergic to any benzodiazepine or
  tricyclic antidepressant.
- You have myasthenia gravis, glaucoma, taken
  MAO inhibitors within 2 weeks, had a heart
  attack within 6 weeks.
- You are active or recovering alcoholic.
- Patient is younger than 12.

Before you start, consult your doctor:
- If you have liver, kidney or lung disease,
  diabetes, epilepsy, porphyria, enlarged
  prostate, heart disease, high blood pressure,
  stomach or intestinal problems, overactive
  thyroid, asthma.

- If you will have surgery within 2 months, including dental surgery, requiring general or spinal anesthesia.

Over age 60:
More likely to develop urination difficulty and more side effects.

Pregnancy:
Risk to unborn child outweighs drug benefits. Don't use.

Breast-feeding:
Drug passes into milk. Avoid drug or discontinue nursing until you finish medicine. Consult doctor for advice on maintaining milk supply.

Infants & children:
Use only under medical supervision for children older than 6 months.

Prolonged use:
May impair liver function.

Skin & sunlight:
May cause rash or intensify sunburn in areas exposed to sun or sunlamp.

Driving, piloting or hazardous work:
Don't drive or pilot aircraft until you learn how medicine affects you. Don't work around dangerous machinery. Don't climb ladders or work in high places. Danger increases if you drink alcohol or take medicine affecting alertness and reflexes, such as antihistamines, tranquilizers, sedatives, pain medicine, narcotics and mind-altering drugs.

Discontinuing:
Don't discontinue without consulting doctor. Dose may require gradual reduction if you have taken drug for a long time. Doses of other drugs may also require adjustment.

Others:
- Hot weather, heavy exercise and profuse sweat may reduce excretion and cause overdose.
- Blood sugar may rise in diabetics, requiring insulin adjustment.

 POSSIBLE INTERACTION WITH OTHER DRUGS

GENERIC NAME OR DRUG CLASS	COMBINED EFFECT
Anticoagulants (oral)	Increased anticoagulant effect.
Anticonvulsants	Change in seizure frequency or severity.
Anticholinergics	Increased anticholinergic effect.
Antidepressants	Increased sedative effect of both drugs.

Antihistamines	Increased sedative effect of both drugs.
Antihypertensives	Excessively low blood pressure.
Barbiturates	Decreased antidepressant effect.
Cimetidine	Excess sedation.
Clonidine	Decreased clonidine effect.
Disulfiram	Increased chlordiazepoxide effect.
Diuretics	Increased antidepressant effect.
Dronabinol	Increased effect of both drugs.
Ethchlorvynol	Delirium.
Guanethidine	Decreased guanethidine effect.
MAO inhibitors	Convulsions, deep sedation, rage.
Methyldopa	Decreased methyldopa effect.
Narcotics	Dangerous oversedation.
Phenytoin	Decreased phenytoin effect.
Quinidine	Irregular heartbeat.
Sedatives	Dangerous oversedation.
Sleep inducers	Increased sedative effect of both drugs.
Sympathomimetics	Increased sympathomimetic effect.

Continued page 965

 POSSIBLE INTERACTION WITH OTHER SUBSTANCES

INTERACTS WITH	COMBINED EFFECT
Alcohol: Beverages or medicines with alcohol.	Excessive intoxication. Avoid.
Beverages:	None expected.
Cocaine:	Excessive intoxication. Avoid.
Foods:	None expected.
Marijuana:	Excessive drowsiness. Avoid.
Tobacco:	Decreased chlordiazepoxide effect.

179

CHLORDIAZEPOXIDE & CLIDINIUM

BRAND NAMES

See complete list of brand names in the *Brand Name Directory*, page 946.

BASIC INFORMATION

Habit forming? Yes
Prescription needed? Yes
Available as generic? No
Drug class: Tranquilizer (benzodiazepine), antispasmodic, anticholinergic

 USES

- Reduces spasms of digestive system, bladder and urethra.
- Treatment for nervousness or tension.
- Treatment for muscle spasm.

 DOSAGE & USAGE INFORMATION

How to take:
Tablet or capsule—Swallow with liquid. If you can't swallow whole, crumble tablet or open capsule and take with liquid or food.

When to take:
At the same time each day, according to instructions on prescription label.

If you forget a dose:
Take as soon as you remember up to 2 hours late. If more than 2 hours, wait for next scheduled dose (don't double this dose).

Continued next column

 OVERDOSE

SYMPTOMS:
Dilated pupils, rapid pulse and breathing, dizziness, drowsiness, weakness, tremor, stupor, fever, hallucinations, confusion, slurred speech, agitation, flushed face, convulsions, coma.
WHAT TO DO:
- Dial 0 (operator) or 911 (emergency) for an ambulance or medical help. Then give first aid immediately.
- If patient is unconscious and not breathing, give mouth-to-mouth breathing. If there is no heartbeat, use cardiac massage and mouth-to-mouth breathing (CPR). Don't try to make patient vomit. If you can't get help quickly, take patient to nearest emergency facility.
- See emergency information on inside covers.

What drug does:
- Blocks nerve impulses at parasympathetic nerve endings, preventing muscle contractions and gland secretions of organs involved.
- Affects limbic system of brain—part that controls emotions.

Time lapse before drug works:
15 to 30 minutes.

Don't take with:
See Interaction column and consult doctor.

 POSSIBLE ADVERSE REACTIONS OR SIDE EFFECTS

SYMPTOMS	WHAT TO DO
Life-threatening:	
Slow or rapid heartbeat, breathing difficulty.	Discontinue. Seek emergency treatment.
Common:	
• Clumsiness, drowsiness, dizziness, delirium.	Discontinue. Call doctor right away.
• Dry mouth, throat, nose.	Continue. Tell doctor at next visit.
Infrequent:	
• Hallucinations, confusion, depression, irritability, rash, itch, vision changes, vomiting.	Discontinue. Call doctor right away.
• Constipation, diarrhea, nausea, urination difficulty.	Continue. Call doctor when convenient.
Rare:	
Jaundice, rash or hives, eye pain, blurred vision.	Discontinue. Call doctor right away.

 WARNINGS & PRECAUTIONS

Don't take if:
- You are allergic to any anticholinergic or any benzodiazepine.
- You have trouble with stomach bloating, difficulty emptying your bladder completely, narrow-angle glaucoma, severe ulcerative colitis, myasthenia gravis.
- You are active or recovering alcoholic.
- Patient is younger than 6 months.

Before you start, consult your doctor:
- If you have open-angle glaucoma, angina, chronic bronchitis or asthma, hiatal hernia, enlarged prostate, myasthenia gravis, peptic ulcer, liver, kidney or lung disease, diabetes, epilepsy or porphyria.

- If you will have surgery within 2 months, including dental surgery, requiring general or spinal anesthesia.

Over age 60:
Adverse reactions and side effects may be more frequent and severe than in younger persons.

Pregnancy:
Risk to unborn child outweighs drug benefits. Don't use.

Breast-feeding:
Drug passes into milk. Avoid drug or discontinue nursing until you finish medicine. Consult doctor for advice on maintaining milk supply.

Infants & children:
Use only under medical supervision.

Prolonged use:
- Chronic constipation, possible fecal impaction.
- May impair liver function.

Skin & sunlight:
No problems expected.

Driving, piloting or hazardous work:
Don't drive or pilot aircraft until you learn how medicine affects you. Don't work around dangerous machinery. Don't climb ladders or work in high places. Danger increases if you drink alcohol or take medicine affecting alertness and reflexes, such as antihistamines, tranquilizers, sedatives, pain medicine, narcotics and mind-altering drugs.

Discontinuing:
Don't discontinue without consulting doctor. Dose may require gradual reduction if you have taken drug for a long time. Doses of other drugs may also require adjustment.

Others:
- Hot weather, heavy exercise and profuse sweat may reduce excretion and cause overdose.
- Blood sugar may rise in diabetics, requiring insulin adjustment.

POSSIBLE INTERACTION WITH OTHER DRUGS

GENERIC NAME OR DRUG CLASS	COMBINED EFFECT
Amantadine	Increased clidinium effect.
Antacids	Decreased clidinium effect.
Anticholinergics (other)	Increased clidinium effect.
Anticonvulsants	Change in seizure frequency or severity.
Antidepressants	Increased sedative effect of both drugs.
Antihistamines	Increased sedative effect of both drugs.
Antihypertensives	Excessively low blood pressure.
Cimetidine	Excess sedation.
Disulfiram	Increased chlordiazepoxide effect.
Dronabinol	Increased effects of both drugs. Avoid.
Haloperidol	Increased internal-eye pressure.
MAO inhibitors	Convulsions, deep sedation, rage.
Meperidine	Increased clidinium effect.
Methylphenidate	Increased clidinium effect.
Narcotics	Increased sedative effect of both drugs.
Nitrates	Increased internal-eye pressure.
Orphenadrine	Increased clidinium effect.
Phenothiazines	Increased clidinium effect.
Pilocarpine	Loss of pilocarpine effect in glaucoma treatment.
Potassium supplements	Possible intestinal ulcers with oral potassium tablets.

Continued page 965

POSSIBLE INTERACTION WITH OTHER SUBSTANCES

INTERACTS WITH	COMBINED EFFECT
Alcohol:	Heavy sedation. Avoid.
Beverages:	None expected.
Cocaine:	Excessively rapid heartbeat. Avoid.
Foods:	None expected.
Marijuana:	Drowsiness and dry mouth, heavy sedation. Avoid.
Tobacco:	Decreased chlordiazepoxide effect.

CHLOROQUINE

BRAND NAMES

Aralen

BASIC INFORMATION

Habit forming? No
Prescription needed? Yes
Available as generic? Yes
Drug class: Antiprotozoal, antirheumatic

 USES

- Treatment for protozoal infections, such as malaria and amebiasis.
- Treatment for some forms of arthritis and lupus.

 DOSAGE & USAGE INFORMATION

How to take:
Tablet—Swallow with food or milk to lessen stomach irritation.

When to take:
- Depends on condition. Is adjusted during treatment.
- Malaria prevention—Begin taking medicine 2 weeks before entering areas with malaria.

If you forget a dose:
- 1 or more doses a day—Take as soon as you remember up to 2 hours late. If more than 2 hours, wait for next scheduled dose (don't double this dose).
- 1 dose weekly—Take as soon as possible, then return to regular dosing schedule.

What drug does:
- Inhibits parasite multiplication.
- Decreases inflammatory response in diseased joint.

Time lapse before drug works:
1 to 2 hours.

Don't take with:
See Interaction column and consult doctor.

 OVERDOSE

SYMPTOMS:
Severe breathing difficulty, drowsiness, faintness.
WHAT TO DO:
- Dial 0 (operator) or 911 (emergency) for an ambulance or medical help. Then give first aid immediately.
- See emergency information on inside covers.

 POSSIBLE ADVERSE REACTIONS OR SIDE EFFECTS

SYMPTOMS	WHAT TO DO
Life-threatening: None expected.	
Common: Headache.	Continue. Tell doctor at next visit.
Infrequent:	
• Blurred or changed vision.	Discontinue. Call doctor right away.
• Rash or itch, diarrhea, nausea, vomiting.	Continue. Call doctor when convenient.
Rare:	
• Mood or mental changes, seizures, sore throat, fever, unusual bleeding or bruising, muscle weakness.	Discontinue. Call doctor right away.
• Ringing or buzzing in ears, hearing loss.	Continue. Call doctor when convenient.

WARNINGS & PRECAUTIONS

Don't take if:
You are allergic to chloroquine or hydroxychloroquine.

Before you start, consult your doctor:
- If you plan to become pregnant within the medication period.
- If you have blood disease.
- If you have eye or vision problems.
- If you have a G6PD deficiency.
- If you have liver disease.
- If you have nerve or brain disease (including seizure disorders).
- If you have porphyria.
- If you have psoriasis.
- If you have stomach or intestinal disease.
- If you drink more than 3 oz. of alcohol daily.

Over age 60:
Adverse reactions and side effects may be more frequent and severe than in younger persons.

Pregnancy:
Risk to unborn child outweighs drug benefits. Don't use.

Breast-feeding:
Drug passes into milk. Avoid drug or discontinue nursing.

Infants & children:
Not recommended. Dangerous.

Prolonged use:
Permanent damage to the retina (back part of the eye) or nerve deafness.

Skin & sunlight:
May cause rash or intensify sunburn in areas exposed to sun or sunlamp.

Driving, piloting or hazardous work:
Don't drive or pilot aircraft until you learn how medicine affects you. Don't work around dangerous machinery. Don't climb ladders or work in high places. Danger increases if you drink alcohol or take medicine affecting alertness and reflexes.

Discontinuing:
Don't discontinue without doctor's advice until you complete prescribed dose, even though symptoms diminish or disappear.

Others:
- Periodic physical and blood examinations recommended.
- If you are in a malaria area for a long time, you may need to change to another preventive drug every 2 years.

 POSSIBLE INTERACTION WITH OTHER DRUGS

GENERIC NAME OR DRUG CLASS	COMBINED EFFECT
Estrogens	Possible liver toxicity.
Gold compounds	Risk of severe rash and itch.
Oxyphenbutazone	Risk of severe rash and itch.
Penicillamine	Possible blood or kidney toxicity.
Phenylbutazone	Risk of severe rash and itch.
Sulfa drugs	Possible liver toxicity.

 POSSIBLE INTERACTION WITH OTHER SUBSTANCES

INTERACTS WITH	COMBINED EFFECT
Alcohol:	Possible liver toxicity. Avoid.
Beverages:	None expected.
Cocaine:	None expected.
Foods:	None expected.
Marijuana:	None expected.
Tobacco:	None expected.

CHLOROTHIAZIDE

BRAND NAMES

Aldoclor	Diuril
Chloroserpine	SK-Chlorothiazide
Diupres	

BASIC INFORMATION

Habit forming? No
Prescription needed? Yes
Available as generic? Yes
Drug class: Antihypertensive, diuretic
(thiazide)

 USES

- Controls, but doesn't cure, high blood pressure.
- Reduces fluid retention (edema) caused by conditions such as heart disorders and liver disease.

 DOSAGE & USAGE INFORMATION

How to take:
Tablet or capsule—Swallow with liquid. If you can't swallow whole, crumble tablet or open capsule and take with liquid or food. Don't exceed dose.

When to take:
At the same time each day.

If you forget a dose:
Take as soon as you remember up to 2 hours late. If more than 2 hours, wait for next scheduled dose (don't double this dose).

What drug does:
- Forces sodium and water excretion, reducing body fluid.
- Relaxes muscle cells of small arteries.
- Reduced body fluid and relaxed arteries lower blood pressure.

Continued next column

 OVERDOSE

SYMPTOMS:
Cramps, weakness, drowsiness, weak pulse, coma.
WHAT TO DO:
- **Dial 0 (operator) or 911 (emergency) for an ambulance or medical help. Then give first aid immediately.**
- **See emergency information on inside covers.**

Time lapse before drug works:
4 to 6 hours. May require several weeks to lower blood pressure.

Don't take with:
- See Interaction column and consult doctor.
- Non-prescription drugs without consulting doctor.

 POSSIBLE ADVERSE REACTIONS OR SIDE EFFECTS

SYMPTOMS	WHAT TO DO
Life-threatening: None expected.	
Common: None expected.	
Infrequent:	
• Blurred vision, severe abdominal pain, nausea, vomiting, irregular heartbeat, weak pulse.	Discontinue. Call doctor right away.
• Dizziness, mood changes, headaches, weakness, tiredness, weight changes.	Continue. Call doctor when convenient.
• Dry mouth, thirst.	Continue. Tell doctor at next visit.
Rare:	
• Rash or hives.	Discontinue. Seek emergency treatment.
• Jaundice.	Discontinue. Call doctor right away.
• Sore throat, fever.	Continue. Tell doctor at next visit.

 WARNINGS & PRECAUTIONS

Don't take if:
You are allergic to any thiazide diuretic drug.

Before you start, consult your doctor:
- If you are allergic to any sulfa drug.
- If you have gout.
- If you have liver, pancreas or kidney disorder.

Over age 60:
Adverse reactions and side effects may be more frequent and severe than in younger persons, especially dizziness and excessive potassium loss.

Pregnancy:
Risk to unborn child outweighs drug benefits. Don't use.

Breast-feeding:
Drug passes into milk. Avoid drug or discontinue nursing.

Infants & children:
No problems expected.

Prolonged use:
You may need medicine to treat high blood pressure for the rest of your life.

Skin & sunlight:
May cause rash or intensify sunburn in areas exposed to sun or sunlamp.

Driving, piloting or hazardous work:
Don't drive or pilot aircraft until you learn how medicine affects you. Don't work around dangerous machinery. Don't climb ladders or work in high places. Danger increases if you drink alcohol or take medicine affecting alertness and reflexes, such as antihistamines, tranquilizers, sedatives, pain medicine, narcotics and mind-altering drugs.

Discontinuing:
Don't discontinue without medical advice.

Others:
- Hot weather and fever may cause dehydration and drop in blood pressure. Dose may require temporary adjustment. Weigh daily and report any unexpected weight decreases to your doctor.
- May cause rise in uric acid, leading to gout.
- May cause blood-sugar rise in diabetics.

 POSSIBLE INTERACTION WITH OTHER DRUGS

GENERIC NAME OR DRUG CLASS	COMBINED EFFECT
Acebutolol	Increased antihypertensive effect. Dosages of both drugs may require adjustments.
Allopurinol	Decreased allopurinol effect.
Amiodarone	Increased risk of heartbeat irregularity due to low potassium.
Antidepressants (tricyclic)	Dangerous drop in blood pressure. Avoid combination unless under medical supervision.
Barbiturates	Increased chlorothiazide effect.
Calcium supplements	Increased calcium in blood.
Cholestyramine	Decreased chlorothiazide effect.

	COMBINED EFFECT
Cortisone drugs	Excessive potassium loss that causes dangerous heart rhythms.
Digitalis preparations	Excessive potassium loss that causes dangerous heart rhythms.
Diuretics (thiazide)	Increased effect of other thiazide diuretics.
Indapamide	Increased diuretic effect.
Labetolol	Increased antihypertensive effects.
Lithium	Increased effect of lithium.
MAO inhibitors	Increased chlorothiazide effect.
Nitrates	Excessive blood-pressure drop.
Oxprenolol	Increased antihypertensive effect. Dosages of both drugs may require adjustments.
Pentoxifylline	Increased antihypertensive effect.
Potassium supplements	Decreased potassium effect.
Probenecid	Decreased probenecid effect.

 POSSIBLE INTERACTION WITH OTHER SUBSTANCES

INTERACTS WITH	COMBINED EFFECT
Alcohol:	Dangerous blood-pressure drop.
Beverages:	None expected.
Cocaine:	None expected.
Foods: Licorice.	Excessive potassium loss that causes dangerous heart rhythms.
Marijuana:	May increase blood pressure.
Tobacco:	None expected.

CHLOROTRIANISENE

BRAND NAMES

TACE

BASIC INFORMATION

Habit forming? No
Prescription needed? Yes
Available as generic? Yes
Drug class: Female sex hormone (estrogen)

 USES

- Treatment for symptoms of menopause and menstrual-cycle irregularity.
- Replacement for female hormone deficiency.
- Treatment for cancer of prostate.

 DOSAGE & USAGE INFORMATION

How to take:
Capsule—Swallow with liquid. If you can't swallow whole, open capsule and take with liquid or food.

When to take:
At the same time each day.

If you forget a dose:
Take as soon as you remember up to 12 hours late. If more than 12 hours, wait for next scheduled dose (don't double this dose).

What drug does:
Restores normal estrogen level in tissues.

Time lapse before drug works:
10 to 20 days.

Don't take with:
See Interaction column and consult doctor.

 OVERDOSE

SYMPTOMS:
Nausea, vomiting, fluid retention, breast enlargement and discomfort, abnormal vaginal bleeding.
WHAT TO DO:
Overdose unlikely to threaten life. If person takes much larger amount than prescribed, call doctor, poison-control center or hospital emergency room for instructions.

 POSSIBLE ADVERSE REACTIONS OR SIDE EFFECTS

SYMPTOMS	WHAT TO DO
Life-threatening:	
None expected.	
Common:	
• Stomach cramps.	Discontinue. Call doctor right away.
• Appetite loss.	Continue. Call doctor when convenient.
• Swollen ankles or feet; swollen, tender breasts; nausea; diarrhea.	Continue. Tell doctor at next visit.
Infrequent:	
• Rash, stomach or side pain.	Discontinue. Call doctor right away.
• Depression, dizziness, irritability, vomiting, breast lumps.	Continue. Call doctor when convenient.
• Brown blotches on skin, hair loss, vaginal discharge or bleeding, changes in sex drive.	Continue. Tell doctor at next visit.
Rare:	
Jaundice.	Discontinue. Call doctor right away.

186

CHLOROTRIANISENE

WARNINGS & PRECAUTIONS

Don't take if:
- You are allergic to any estrogen-containing drugs.
- You have impaired liver function.
- You have had blood clots, stroke or heart attack.
- You have unexplained vaginal bleeding.

Before you start, consult your doctor:
- If you have had cancer of breast or reproductive organs, fibrocystic breast disease, fibroid tumors of the uterus or endometriosis.
- If you have had migraine headaches, epilepsy or porphyria.
- If you have diabetes, high blood pressure, asthma, congestive heart failure, kidney disease or gallstones.
- If you plan to become pregnant within 3 months.

Over age 60:
Controversial. You and your doctor must decide if drug risks outweigh benefits.

Pregnancy:
Risk to unborn child outweighs drug benefits. Don't use.

Breast-feeding:
Drug filters into milk. May harm child. Avoid.

Infants & children:
Not recommended.

Prolonged use:
Increased growth of fibroid tumors of uterus. Possible association with cancer of uterus.

Skin & sunlight:
May cause rash or intensify sunburn in areas exposed to sun or sunlamp.

Driving, piloting or hazardous work:
No problems expected.

Discontinuing:
You may need to discontinue chlorotrianisene periodically. Consult your doctor.

Others:
In rare instances, may cause blood clot in lung, brain or leg. Symptoms are *sudden* severe headache, coordination loss, vision change, chest pain, breathing difficulty, slurred speech, pain in legs or groin. Seek emergency treatment immediately.

POSSIBLE INTERACTION WITH OTHER DRUGS

GENERIC NAME OR DRUG CLASS	COMBINED EFFECT
Anticoagulants (oral)	Decreased anticoagulant effect.
Anticonvulsants (hydantoin)	Increased seizures.
Antidiabetics (oral)	Unpredictable increase or decrease in blood sugar.
Carbamazepine	Increased seizures.
Clofibrate	Decreased clofibrate effect.
Meprobamate	Increased chlorotrianisene effect.
Phenobarbital	Decreased chlorotrianisene effect.
Primidone	Decreased chlorotrianisene effect.
Rifampin	Decreased chlorotrianisene effect.
Thyroid hormones	Decreased thyroid effect.

POSSIBLE INTERACTION WITH OTHER SUBSTANCES

INTERACTS WITH	COMBINED EFFECT
Alcohol:	None expected.
Beverages:	None expected.
Cocaine:	No proven problems.
Foods:	None expected.
Marijuana:	Possible menstrual irregularities and bleeding between periods.
Tobacco:	Increased risk of blood clots leading to stroke or heart attack.

CHLORPHENESIN

BRAND NAMES

Maolate   Mycil

BASIC INFORMATION

Habit forming? No
Prescription needed? Yes
Available as generic? Yes
Drug class: Muscle relaxant (skeletal)

 USES

Treatment for sprains, strains and muscle spasms.

 DOSAGE & USAGE INFORMATION

How to take:
Tablet or capsule—Swallow with liquid.

When to take:
As needed, no more often than every 4 hours.

If you forget a dose:
Take as soon as you remember. Wait 4 hours for next dose.

What drug does:
Blocks body's pain messages to brain. May also sedate.

Time lapse before drug works:
60 minutes.

Don't take with:
See Interaction column and consult doctor.

 OVERDOSE

SYMPTOMS:
Nausea, vomiting, diarrhea, headache. May progress to severe weakness, difficult breathing, sensation of paralysis, coma.
WHAT TO DO:
- Dial 0 (operator) or 911 (emergency) for an ambulance or medical help. Then give first aid immediately.
- See emergency information on inside covers.

 POSSIBLE ADVERSE REACTIONS OR SIDE EFFECTS

SYMPTOMS	WHAT TO DO
Life-threatening:	
None expected.	
Common:	
• Drowsiness, fainting, dizziness.	Continue. Call doctor when convenient.
• Orange or red-purple urine.	No action necessary.
Infrequent:	
Agitation, constipation or diarrhea, nausea, cramps, vomiting, wheezing, shortness of breath.	Discontinue. Call doctor right away.
Rare:	
• Bloody or tarry, black stool.	Discontinue. Seek emergency treatment.
• Rash, hives or itch; sore throat, fever; jaundice; tiredness; weakness.	Discontinue. Call doctor right away.

WARNINGS & PRECAUTIONS

Don't take if:
- You are allergic to any skeletal-muscle relaxant.
- You have porphyria.

Before you start, consult your doctor:
- If you have had liver or kidney disease.
- If you plan pregnancy within medication period.
- If you will have surgery within 2 months, including dental surgery, requiring general or spinal anesthesia.

Over age 60:
Adverse reactions and side effects may be more frequent and severe than in younger persons.

Pregnancy:
No proven harm to unborn child. Avoid if possible.

Breast-feeding:
Drug passes into milk. Avoid drug or discontinue nursing until you finish medicine. Consult doctor for advice on maintaining milk supply.

Infants & children:
Not recommended.

Prolonged use:
Periodic liver-function tests recommended if you use this drug for a long time.

Skin & sunlight:
No problems expected.

Driving, piloting or hazardous work:
Don't drive or pilot aircraft until you learn how medicine affects you. Don't work around dangerous machinery. Don't climb ladders or work in high places. Danger increases if you drink alcohol or take medicine affecting alertness and reflexes, such as antihistamines, tranquilizers, sedatives, pain medicine, narcotics and mind-altering drugs.

Discontinuing:
Don't discontinue without doctor's advice until you complete prescribed dose, even though symptoms diminish or disappear.

Others:
No problems expected.

POSSIBLE INTERACTION WITH OTHER DRUGS

GENERIC NAME OR DRUG CLASS	COMBINED EFFECT
Antidepressants	Increased sedation.
Antihistamines	Increased sedation.
Dronabinol	Increased effects of dronabinol on central nervous system. Avoid combination.
Mind-altering drugs	Increased sedation.
Muscle relaxants (other)	Increased sedation.
Narcotics	Increased sedation.
Sedatives	Increased sedation.
Sleep inducers	Increased sedation.
Testosterone	Decreased metaxalone effect.
Tranquilizers	Increased sedation.

POSSIBLE INTERACTION WITH OTHER SUBSTANCES

INTERACTS WITH	COMBINED EFFECT
Alcohol:	Increased sedation. Avoid.
Beverages:	None expected.
Cocaine:	Lack of coordination, increased sedation. Avoid.
Foods:	None expected.
Marijuana:	Lack of coordination, drowsiness, fainting. Avoid.
Tobacco:	None expected.

CHLORPHENIRAMINE

BRAND NAMES

See complete list of brand names in the *Brand Name Directory,* page 946.

BASIC INFORMATION

Habit forming? No
Prescription needed? No
Available as generic? Yes
Drug class: Antihistamine

USES

- Reduces allergic symptoms such as hay fever, hives, rash or itching.
- Prevents motion sickness, nausea, vomiting.
- Induces sleep.

DOSAGE & USAGE INFORMATION

How to take:
- Tablet or syrup—Swallow with liquid or food to lessen stomach irritation.
- Extended-release tablets or capsules—Swallow each dose whole.

When to take:
Varies with form. Follow label directions.

If you forget a dose:
Take as soon as you remember up to 2 hours late. If more than 2 hours, wait for next scheduled dose (don't double this dose).

What drug does:
Blocks action of histamine after an allergic response triggers histamine release in sensitive cells.

Time lapse before drug works:
30 minutes.

Don't take with:
See Interaction column and consult doctor.

OVERDOSE

SYMPTOMS:
Convulsions, red face, hallucinations, coma.
WHAT TO DO:
- Dial 0 (operator) or 911 (emergency) for an ambulance or medical help. Then give first aid immediately.
- See emergency information on inside covers.

POSSIBLE ADVERSE REACTIONS OR SIDE EFFECTS

SYMPTOMS	WHAT TO DO
Life-threatening: None expected.	
Common: Drowsiness; dizziness; dry mouth, nose, throat; nausea.	Continue. Tell doctor at next visit.
Infrequent:	
• Vision changes.	Discontinue. Call doctor right away.
• Less tolerance for contact lenses, difficult urination.	Continue. Call doctor when convenient.
• Appetite loss.	Continue. Tell doctor at next visit.
Rare: Nightmares, agitation, irritability, sore throat, fever, rapid heartbeat, unusual bleeding or bruising, fatigue, weakness.	Discontinue. Call doctor right away.

WARNINGS & PRECAUTIONS

Don't take if:
You are allergic to any antihistamine.

Before you start, consult your doctor:
- If you have glaucoma.
- If you have enlarged prostate.
- If you have asthma.
- If you have kidney disease.
- If you have peptic ulcer.
- If you will have surgery within 2 months, including dental surgery, requiring general or spinal anesthesia.

Over age 60:
Don't exceed recommended dose. Adverse reactions and side effects may be more frequent and severe than in younger persons, especially urination difficulty, diminished alertness and other brain and nervous-system symptoms.

Pregnancy:
No proven harm to unborn child. Avoid if possible.

Breast-feeding:
Drug passes into milk. Avoid drug or discontinue nursing until you finish medicine. Consult doctor for advice on maintaining milk supply.

Infants & children:
Not recommended for premature or newborn infants. Otherwise, no problems expected.

Prolonged use:
Avoid. May damage bone marrow and nerve cells.

Skin & sunlight:
May cause rash or intensify sunburn in areas exposed to sun or sunlamp.

Driving, piloting or hazardous work:
Don't drive or pilot aircraft until you learn how medicine affects you. Don't work around dangerous machinery. Don't climb ladders or work in high places. Danger increases if you drink alcohol or take medicine affecting alertness and reflexes, such as antihistamines, tranquilizers, sedatives, pain medicine, narcotics and mind-altering drugs.

Discontinuing:
No problems expected.

Others:
May mask symptoms of hearing damage from aspirin, other salicylates, cisplatin, paromomycin, vancomycin or anticonvulsants. Consult doctor if you use these.

POSSIBLE INTERACTION WITH OTHER DRUGS

GENERIC NAME OR DRUG CLASS	COMBINED EFFECT
Anticholinergics	Increased anticholinergic effect.
Antidepressants	Excess sedation. Avoid.
Antihistamines (other)	Excess sedation. Avoid.
Dronabinol	Increased effects of both drugs. Avoid.
Hypnotics	Excess sedation. Avoid.
MAO inhibitors	Increased chlorpheniramine effect.
Mind-altering drugs	Excess sedation. Avoid.
Molindone	Increased antihistamine effect.
Narcotics	Excess sedation. Avoid.
Sedatives	Excess sedation. Avoid.
Sleep inducers	Excess sedation. Avoid.
Tranquilizers	Excess sedation. Avoid.

POSSIBLE INTERACTION WITH OTHER SUBSTANCES

INTERACTS WITH	COMBINED EFFECT
Alcohol:	Excess sedation. Avoid.
Beverages: Caffeine drinks.	Less chlorpheniramine sedation.
Cocaine:	Decreased chlorpheniramine effect. Avoid.
Foods:	None expected.
Marijuana:	Excess sedation. Avoid.
Tobacco:	None expected.

CHLORPROMAZINE

BRAND NAMES

Apo-Chlorpromazine	Ormazine
Chloramead	Promapar
Chlor-Promanyl	Promaz
Chlorprom	Promosol
Clorazine	Thorazine
Largactil	Thor-Prom
Novochlorpromazine	

BASIC INFORMATION

Habit forming? No
Prescription needed? Yes
Available as generic? Yes
Drug class: Tranquilizer, antiemetic
(phenothiazine)

 USES

- Stops nausea, vomiting.
- Reduces anxiety, agitation.

 DOSAGE & USAGE INFORMATION

How to take:
- Tablet or capsule—Swallow with liquid or food to lessen stomach irritation.
- Suppositories—Remove wrapper and moisten suppository with water. Gently insert into rectum, large end first.
- Drops or liquid—Dilute dose in beverage.

When to take:
- Nervous and mental disorders—Take at the same times each day.
- Nausea and vomiting—Take as needed, no more often than every 4 hours.

If you forget a dose:
- Nervous and mental disorders—Take up to 2 hours late. If more than 2 hours, wait for next scheduled dose (don't double this dose).
- Nausea and vomiting—Take as soon as you remember. Wait 4 hours for next dose.

Continued next column

 OVERDOSE

SYMPTOMS:
Stupor, convulsions, coma.
WHAT TO DO:
- Dial 0 (operator) or 911 (emergency) for an ambulance or medical help. Then give first aid immediately.
- See emergency information on inside covers.

What drug does:
- Suppresses brain's vomiting center.
- Suppresses brain centers that control abnormal emotions and behavior.

Time lapse before drug works:
- Nausea and vomiting—1 hour or less.
- Nervous and mental disorders—4-6 weeks.

Don't take with:
- Antacid or medicine for diarrhea.
- Non-prescription drug for cough, cold or allergy.
- See Interaction column and consult doctor.

 POSSIBLE ADVERSE REACTIONS OR SIDE EFFECTS

SYMPTOMS	WHAT TO DO
Life-threatening: None expected.	
Common:	
- Muscle spasms of face and neck, unsteady gait.	Discontinue. Seek emergency treatment.
- Restlessness, tremor, drowsiness.	Discontinue. Call doctor right away.
- Decreased sweating, dry mouth, stuffy nose, constipation.	Continue. Call doctor when convenient.
Infrequent:	
- Fainting.	Discontinue. Seek emergency treatment.
- Rash.	Discontinue. Call doctor right away.
- Difficult urination, diminished sex drive, swollen breasts, menstrual irregularities.	Continue. Call doctor when convenient.
Rare:	
Vision changes, sore throat, fever, jaundice.	Discontinue. Call doctor right away.

WARNINGS & PRECAUTIONS

Don't take if:
- You are allergic to any phenothiazine.
- You have a blood or bone-marrow disease.

Before you start, consult your doctor:
- If you will have surgery within 2 months, including dental surgery, requiring general or spinal anesthesia.
- If you have asthma, emphysema or other lung disorder.
- If you take non-prescription ulcer medicine, asthma medicine or amphetamines.

Over age 60:
Adverse reactions and side effects may be more frequent and severe than in younger persons. More likely to develop involuntary movement of jaws, lips, tongue, chewing. Report this to your doctor immediately. Early treatment can help.

Pregnancy:
Risk to unborn child outweighs drug benefits. Don't use.

Breast-feeding:
Drug passes into milk. Avoid drug or discontinue nursing until you finish medicine. Consult doctor for advice on maintaining milk supply.

Infants & children:
Don't give to children younger than 2.

Prolonged use:
May lead to tardive dyskinesia (involuntary movement of jaws, lips, tongue, chewing).

Skin & sunlight:
May cause rash or intensify sunburn in areas exposed to sun or sunlamp. Skin may remain sensitive for 3 months after discontinuing.

Driving, piloting or hazardous work:
Don't drive or pilot aircraft until you learn how medicine affects you. Don't work around dangerous machinery. Don't climb ladders or work in high places. Danger increases if you drink alcohol or take medicine affecting alertness and reflexes.

Discontinuing:
- Nervous and mental disorders—Don't discontinue without doctor's advice until you complete prescribed dose, even though symptoms diminish or disappear.
- Nausea and vomiting—May be unnecessary to finish medicine. Follow doctor's instructions.

Others:
No problems expected.

POSSIBLE INTERACTION WITH OTHER DRUGS

GENERIC NAME OR DRUG CLASS	COMBINED EFFECT
Anticholinergics	Increased anticholinergic effect.
Antidepressants (tricyclic)	Increased chlorpromazine effect.
Antihistamines	Increased antihistamine effect.
Appetite suppressants	Decreased suppressant effect.
Calcium supplements	Decreased chlorpromazine effect.
Dronabinol	Increased effects of both drugs. Avoid.
Levodopa	Decreased levodopa effect.
Mind-altering drugs	Increased effect of mind-altering drugs.
Molindone	Increased tranquilizer effect.
Narcotics	Increased narcotic effect.
Phenytoin	Increased phenytoin effect.
Quinidine	Impaired heart function. Dangerous mixture.
Sedatives	Increased sedative effect.
Tranquilizers (other)	Increased tranquilizer effect.

POSSIBLE INTERACTION WITH OTHER SUBSTANCES

INTERACTS WITH	COMBINED EFFECT
Alcohol:	Dangerous oversedation.
Beverages:	None expected.
Cocaine:	Decreased chlorpromazine effect. Avoid.
Foods:	None expected.
Marijuana:	Drowsiness. May increase antinausea effect.
Tobacco:	None expected.

CHLORPROPAMIDE

BRAND NAMES

Apo-Chlorpropamide
Chloromide
Chloronase
Diabinese
Glucamide
Novopropamide
Stabinol

BASIC INFORMATION

Habit forming? No
Prescription needed? Yes
Available as generic? Yes
Drug class: Antidiabetic (oral), sulfonurea

USES

Treatment for diabetes in adults who can't control blood sugar by diet, weight loss and exercise.

DOSAGE & USAGE INFORMATION

How to take:
Tablet—Swallow with liquid or food to lessen stomach irritation. If you can't swallow whole, crumble tablet and take with liquid or food.

When to take:
At the same times each day.

If you forget a dose:
Take as soon as you remember up to 2 hours late. If more than 2 hours, wait for next scheduled dose (don't double this dose).

What drug does:
Stimulates pancreas to produce more insulin. Insulin in blood forces cells to use sugar in blood.

Time lapse before drug works:
3 to 4 hours. May require 2 weeks for maximum benefit.

Don't take with:
See Interaction column and consult doctor.

OVERDOSE

SYMPTOMS:
Excessive hunger, nausea, anxiety, cool skin, cold sweats, drowsiness, rapid heartbeat, weakness, unconsciousness, coma.
WHAT TO DO:
● **Dial 0 (operator) or 911 (emergency) for an ambulance or medical help. Then give first aid immediately.**
● **See emergency information on inside covers.**

POSSIBLE ADVERSE REACTIONS OR SIDE EFFECTS

SYMPTOMS	WHAT TO DO
Life-threatening: None expected.	
Common:	
● Dizziness.	Discontinue. Call doctor right away.
● Diarrhea, appetite loss, nausea, stomach pain, heartburn.	Continue. Call doctor when convenient.
Infrequent: Low blood sugar (hunger, anxiety, cold sweats, rapid pulse).	Discontinue. Seek emergency treatment.
Rare: Fatigue, itching or rash, sore throat, fever, ringing in ears, unusual bleeding or bruising, jaundice.	Discontinue. Call doctor right away.

WARNINGS & PRECAUTIONS

Don't take if:
● You are allergic to any sulfonurea.
● You have impaired kidney or liver function.

Before you start, consult your doctor:
● If you have a severe infection.
● If you have thyroid disease.
● If you take insulin.
● If you have heart disease.

Over age 60:
Dose usually smaller than for younger adults. Avoid "low-blood-sugar" episodes because repeated ones can damage brain permanently.

Pregnancy:
No proven harm to unborn child. Avoid if possible.

Breast-feeding:
Drug filters into milk. May lower baby's blood sugar. Avoid.

Infants & children:
Don't give to infants or children.

Prolonged use:
None expected.

Skin & sunlight:
May cause rash or intensify sunburn in areas exposed to sun or sunlamp.

Driving, piloting or hazardous work:
No problems expected unless you develop hypoglycemia (low blood sugar). If so, avoid driving or hazardous activity.

Discontinuing:
Don't discontinue without consulting doctor. Dose may require gradual reduction if you have taken drug for a long time. Doses of other drugs may also require adjustment.

Others:
Don't exceed recommended dose. Hypoglycemia (low blood sugar) may occur, even with proper dose schedule. You must balance medicine, diet and exercise.

POSSIBLE INTERACTION WITH OTHER DRUGS

GENERIC NAME OR DRUG CLASS	COMBINED EFFECT
Acebutolol	Possible increased difficulty in regulating blood-sugar levels.
Androgens	Increased chlorpropamide effect.
Anticoagulants (oral)	Unpredictable prothrombin times (see Glossary).
Anticonvulsants (hydantoin)	Decreased chlorpropamide effect.
Anti-inflammatory drugs (non-steroidal)	Increased chlorpropamide effect.
Aspirin	Increased chlorpropamide effect.
Beta-adrenergic blockers	Increased chlorpropamide effect.
Chloramphenicol	Increased chlorpropamide effect.
Clofibrate	Increased chlorpropamide effect.
Contraceptives (oral)	Decreased chlorpropamide effect.
Cortisone drugs	Decreased chlorpropamide effect.
Diuretics (thiazide)	Decreased chlorpropamide effect.
Epinephrine	Decreased chlorpropamide effect.
Estrogens	Increased chlorpropamide effect.
Guanethidine	Unpredictable chlorpropamide effect.
Isoniazid	Decreased chlorpropamide effect.
Labetolol	Increased antidiabetic effect, may mask hypoglycemia.
MAO inhibitors	Increased chlorpropamide effect.
Oxyphenbutazone	Increased chlorpropamide effect.
Phenylbutazone	Increased chlorpropamide effect.
Phenyramidol	Increased chlorpropamide effect.
Probenecid	Increased chlorpropamide effect.
Pyrazinamide	Decreased chlorpropamide effect.
Sulfa drugs	Increased chlorpropamide effect.
Sulfaphenazole	Increased chlorpropamide effect.
Thyroid hormones	Decreased chlorpropamide effect.

POSSIBLE INTERACTION WITH OTHER SUBSTANCES

INTERACTS WITH	COMBINED EFFECT
Alcohol:	Disulfiram reaction (see Glossary). Avoid.
Beverages:	None expected.
Cocaine:	No proven problems.
Foods:	None expected.
Marijuana:	Decreased chlorpropamide effect. Avoid.
Tobacco:	None expected.

CHLORPROTHIXENE

BRAND NAMES

Taractan   Tarasan

BASIC INFORMATION

Habit forming? No
Prescription needed? Yes
Available as generic? No
Drug class: Tranquilizer (thioxanthine),
            antiemetic

 USES

- Reduces anxiety, agitation, psychosis.
- Stops vomiting.

 DOSAGE & USAGE INFORMATION

How to take:
- Tablet—Swallow with liquid. If you can't swallow whole, crumble tablet and take with liquid or food.
- Syrup—Dilute dose in beverage before swallowing.

When to take:
At the same time each day.

If you forget a dose:
Take as soon as you remember up to 2 hours late. If more than 2 hours, wait for next scheduled dose (don't double this dose).

What drug does:
Corrects imbalance of nerve impulses.

Continued next column

 OVERDOSE

SYMPTOMS:
Drowsiness, dizziness, weakness, muscle rigidity, twitching, tremors, confusion, dry mouth, blurred vision, rapid pulse, shallow breathing, low blood pressure, convulsions, coma.
WHAT TO DO:
- **Dial 0 (operator) or 911 (emergency) for an ambulance or medical help. Then give first aid immediately.**
- **If patient is unconscious and not breathing, give mouth-to-mouth breathing. If there is no heartbeat, use cardiac massage and mouth-to-mouth breathing (CPR). Don't try to make patient vomit. If you can't get help quickly, take patient to nearest emergency facility.**
- **See emergency information on inside covers.**

Time lapse before drug works:
3 weeks.
Don't take with:
See Interaction column and consult doctor.

 POSSIBLE ADVERSE REACTIONS OR SIDE EFFECTS

SYMPTOMS	WHAT TO DO
Life-threatening:	
None expected.	
Common:	
• Fainting; restlessness; jerky, involuntary, movements; blurred vision; rapid heartbeat.	Discontinue. Call doctor right away.
• Dizziness, drowsiness, constipation, muscle spasms, shuffling walk, decreased sweating.	Continue. Call doctor when convenient.
• Dry mouth, stuffy nose.	Continue. Tell doctor at next visit.
Infrequent:	
• Rash.	Discontinue. Call doctor right away.
• Less sexual ability, difficult urination.	Continue. Call doctor when convenient.
• Menstrual irregularities, swollen breasts.	Continue. Tell doctor at next visit.
Rare:	
Sore throat, fever, jaundice.	Discontinue. Call doctor right away.

 WARNINGS & PRECAUTIONS

Don't take if:
- You are allergic to any thioxanthine or phenothiazine tranquilizer.
- You have serious blood disorder.
- You have Parkinson's disease.
- Patient is younger than 12.

Before you start, consult your doctor:
- If you have had liver or kidney disease.
- If you have epilepsy or glaucoma.
- If you have high blood pressure or heart disease (especially angina).
- If you use alcohol daily.
- If you will have surgery within 2 months, including dental surgery, requiring general or spinal anesthesia.

Over age 60:
Adverse reactions and side effects may be more frequent and severe than in younger persons.

Pregnancy:
No proven harm to unborn child. Avoid if possible.

Breast-feeding:
Studies inconclusive. Consult your doctor.

Infants & children:
Not recommended.

Prolonged use:
• Pigment deposits in lens and retina of eye.
• Involuntary movements of jaws, lips, tongue (tardive dyskinesia).

Skin & sunlight:
May cause rash or intensify sunburn in areas exposed to sun or sunlamp.

Driving, piloting or hazardous work:
Don't drive or pilot aircraft until you learn how medicine affects you. Don't work around dangerous machinery. Don't climb ladders or work in high places. Danger increases if you drink alcohol or take medicine affecting alertness and reflexes.

Discontinuing:
Don't discontinue without consulting doctor. Dose may require gradual reduction if you have taken drug for a long time. Doses of other drugs may also require adjustment.

Others:
Hot temperatures increase chance of heat stroke.

POSSIBLE INTERACTION WITH OTHER DRUGS

GENERIC NAME OR DRUG CLASS	COMBINED EFFECT
Anticholinergics	Increased anticholinergic effect.
Anticonvulsants	Change in seizure pattern.
Antidepressants (tricyclic)	Increased chlorprothixene effect. Excessive sedation.
Antihistamines	Increased chlorprothixene effect. Excessive sedation.
Antihypertensives	Excessively low blood pressure.
Barbiturates	Increased chlorprothixene effect. Excessive sedation.

Bethanechol	Decreased bethanechol effect.
Dronabinol	Increased effects of both drugs. Avoid.
Guanethidine	Decreased guanethidine effect.
Levodopa	Decreased levodopa effect.
MAO inhibitors	Excessive sedation.
Mind-altering drugs	Increased chlorprothixene effect. Excessive sedation.
Narcotics	Increased chlorprothixene effect. Excessive sedation.
Sedatives	Increased chlorprothixene effect. Excessive sedation.
Sleep inducers	Increased chlorprothixene effect. Excessive sedation.
Tranquilizers	Increased chlorprothixene effect. Excessive sedation.

POSSIBLE INTERACTION WITH OTHER SUBSTANCES

INTERACTS WITH	COMBINED EFFECT
Alcohol:	Excessive brain depression. Avoid.
Beverages:	None expected.
Cocaine:	Decreased chlorprothixene effect. Avoid.
Foods:	None expected.
Marijuana:	Daily use—Fainting likely, possible psychosis.
Tobacco:	None expected.

CHLORTHALIDONE

BRAND NAMES

Apo-Chlorthalide	Regroton
Combipres	Tenoretic
Demi-Regroton	Thalitone
Hygroton	Uridon
Novothalidone	

BASIC INFORMATION

Habit forming? No
Prescription needed? Yes
Available as generic? Yes
Drug class: Antihypertensive, diuretic
(thiazide)

 USES

- Controls, but doesn't cure, high blood pressure.
- Reduces fluid retention (edema) caused by conditions such as heart disorders and liver disease.

 DOSAGE & USAGE INFORMATION

How to take:
Tablet or capsule—Swallow with liquid. If you can't swallow whole, crumble tablet or open capsule and take with liquid or food. Don't exceed dose.

When to take:
At the same time each day.

If you forget a dose:
Take as soon as you remember up to 2 hours late. If more than 2 hours, wait for next scheduled dose (don't double this dose).

What drug does:
- Forces sodium and water excretion, reducing body fluid.
- Relaxes muscle cells of small arteries.
- Reduced body fluid and relaxed arteries lower blood pressure.

Continued next column

 OVERDOSE

SYMPTOMS:
Cramps, weakness, drowsiness, weak pulse, coma.
WHAT TO DO:
- Dial 0 (operator) or 911 (emergency) for an ambulance or medical help. Then give first aid immediately.
- See emergency information on inside covers.

Time lapse before drug works:
4 to 6 hours. May require several weeks to lower blood pressure.

Don't take with:
- See Interaction column and consult doctor.
- Non-prescription drugs without consulting doctor.

 POSSIBLE ADVERSE REACTIONS OR SIDE EFFECTS

SYMPTOMS	WHAT TO DO
Life-threatening: None expected.	
Common: None expected.	
Infrequent:	
• Blurred vision, severe abdominal pain, nausea, vomiting, irregular heartbeat, weak pulse.	Discontinue. Call doctor right away.
• Dizziness, mood changes, headaches, weakness, tiredness, weight changes.	Continue. Call doctor when convenient.
• Dry mouth, thirst.	Continue. Tell doctor at next visit.
Rare:	
• Rash or hives.	Discontinue. Seek emergency treatment.
• Jaundice, sore throat, fever.	Discontinue. Call doctor right away.

 WARNINGS & PRECAUTIONS

Don't take if:
You are allergic to any thiazide diuretic drug.

Before you start, consult your doctor:
- If you are allergic to any sulfa drug.
- If you have gout.
- If you have liver, pancreas or kidney disorder.

Over age 60:
Adverse reactions and side effects may be more frequent and severe than in younger persons, especially dizziness and excessive potassium loss.

Pregnancy:
Risk to unborn child outweighs drug benefits. Don't use.

Breast-feeding:
Drug passes into milk. Avoid this medicine or discontinue nursing.

Infants & children:
No problems expected.

Prolonged use:
You may need medicine to treat high blood pressure for the rest of your life.

Skin & sunlight:
May cause rash or intensify sunburn in areas exposed to sun or sunlamp.

Driving, piloting or hazardous work:
Don't drive or pilot aircraft until you learn how medicine affects you. Don't work around dangerous machinery. Don't climb ladders or work in high places. Danger increases if you drink alcohol or take medicine affecting alertness and reflexes, such as antihistamines, tranquilizers, sedatives, pain medicine, narcotics and mind-altering drugs.

Discontinuing:
Don't discontinue without medical advice.

Others:
- Hot weather and fever may cause dehydration and drop in blood pressure. Dose may require temporary adjustment. Weigh daily and report any unexpected weight decreases to your doctor.
- May cause rise in uric acid, leading to gout.
- May cause blood-sugar rise in diabetics.

 POSSIBLE INTERACTION WITH OTHER DRUGS

GENERIC NAME OR DRUG CLASS	COMBINED EFFECT
Acebutolol	Increased antihypertensive effect. Dosages of both drugs may require adjustments.
Allopurinol	Decreased allopurinol effect.
Amiodarone	Increased risk of heartbeat irregularity due to low potassium.
Antidepressants (tricyclic)	Dangerous drop in blood pressure. Avoid combination unless under medical supervision.
Barbiturates	Increased chlorthalidone effect.
Calcium supplements	Increased calcium in blood.
Cholestyramine	Decreased chlorthalidone effect.
Cortisone drugs	Excessive potassium loss that causes dangerous heart rhythms.

Digitalis preparations	Excessive potassium loss that causes dangerous heart rhythms.
Diuretics (thiazide)	Increased effect of other thiazide diuretics.
Enalapril	Possible excessive potassium in blood.
Indapamide	Increased diuretic effect.
Labetolol	Increased antihypertensive effects.
Lithium	Increased effect of lithium.
MAO inhibitors	Increased chlorthalidone effect.
Nitrates	Excessive blood-pressure drop.
Oxprenolol	Increased antihypertensive effect. Dosages of both drugs may require adjustments.
Pentoxifylline	Increased antihypertensive effect.
Potassium supplements	Decreased potassium effect.
Probenecid	Decreased probenecid effect.

 POSSIBLE INTERACTION WITH OTHER SUBSTANCES

INTERACTS WITH	COMBINED EFFECT
Alcohol:	Dangerous blood-pressure drop.
Beverages:	None expected.
Cocaine:	None expected.
Foods: Licorice.	Excessive potassium loss that causes dangerous heart rhythms.
Marijuana:	May increase blood pressure.
Tobacco:	None expected.

CHLORZOXAZONE

BRAND NAMES

Algisin	Paraflex
Chlorzone Forte	Parafon Forte

BASIC INFORMATION

Habit forming? No
Prescription needed? Yes
Available as generic? Yes
Drug class: Muscle relaxant (skeletal)

 ## USES

Treatment for sprains, strains and muscle spasms.

 ## DOSAGE & USAGE INFORMATION

How to take:
Tablet or capsule—Swallow with liquid.

When to take:
As needed, no more often than every 4 hours.

If you forget a dose:
Take as soon as you remember. Wait 4 hours for next dose.

What drug does:
Blocks body's pain messages to brain. May also sedate.

Time lapse before drug works:
60 minutes.

Don't take with:
See Interaction column and consult doctor.

 ## OVERDOSE

SYMPTOMS:
Nausea, vomiting, diarrhea, headache, severe weakness, breathing difficulty, sensation of paralysis.
WHAT TO DO:
Overdose unlikely to threaten life. Depending on severity of symptoms and amount taken, call doctor, poison-control center or hospital emergency room for instructions.

 ## POSSIBLE ADVERSE REACTIONS OR SIDE EFFECTS

SYMPTOMS	WHAT TO DO
Life-threatening:	
None expected.	
Common:	
• Drowsiness, dizziness.	Continue. Call doctor when convenient.
• Orange or red-purple urine.	No action necessary.
Infrequent:	
Agitation, constipation or diarrhea, nausea, cramps, vomiting.	Discontinue. Call doctor right away.
Rare:	
• Bloody or tarry, black stool.	Discontinue. Seek emergency treatment.
• Rash or itch, sore throat, fever, jaundice, tiredness, weakness.	Discontinue. Call doctor right away.

WARNINGS & PRECAUTIONS

Don't take if:
You are allergic to any skeletal-muscle relaxant.

Before you start, consult your doctor:
- If you have had liver disease.
- If you plan pregnancy within medication period.

Over age 60:
Adverse reactions and side effects may be more frequent and severe than in younger persons.

Pregnancy:
No proven harm to unborn child. Avoid if possible.

Breast-feeding:
Drug passes into milk. Avoid drug or discontinue nursing until you finish medicine. Consult doctor for advice on maintaining milk supply.

Infants & children:
Not recommended.

Prolonged use:
No problems expected.

Skin & sunlight:
No problems expected.

Driving, piloting or hazardous work:
Don't drive or pilot aircraft until you learn how medicine affects you. Don't work around dangerous machinery. Don't climb ladders or work in high places. Danger increases if you drink alcohol or take medicine affecting alertness and reflexes, such as antihistamines, tranquilizers, sedatives, pain medicine, narcotics and mind-altering drugs.

Discontinuing:
Don't discontinue without doctor's advice until you complete prescribed dose, even though symptoms diminish or disappear.

Others:
Periodic liver-function tests recommended if you use this drug for a long time.

POSSIBLE INTERACTION WITH OTHER DRUGS

GENERIC NAME OR DRUG CLASS	COMBINED EFFECT
Antidepressants	Increased sedation.
Antihistamines	Increased sedation.
Dronabinol	Increased effect of dronabinol on central nervous system. Avoid combination.
MAO inhibitors	Increased effect of both drugs.
Mind-altering drugs	Increased sedation.
Muscle relaxants (others)	Increased sedation.
Narcotics	Increased sedation.
Sedatives	Increased sedation.
Sleep inducers	Increased sedation
Testosterone	Decreased chlorzoxazone effect.
Tranquilizers	Increased sedation.

POSSIBLE INTERACTION WITH OTHER SUBSTANCES

INTERACTS WITH	COMBINED EFFECT
Alcohol:	Increased sedation.
Beverages:	No problems expected.
Cocaine:	Lack of coordination.
Foods:	No problems expected.
Marijuana:	Lack of coordination, drowsiness, fainting.
Tobacco:	No problems expected.

CHLORZOXAZONE & ACETAMINOPHEN

BRAND NAMES

Blanex	Mus-Lax
Chlorofon-F	Paracet Forte
Chlorzone Forte	Parafon Forte
Flexaphen	Polyflex
Flexin	Zoxaphen
Lobac	

BASIC INFORMATION

Habit forming? No
Prescription needed? Yes
Available as generic? No
**Drug class: Muscle relaxant (skeletal),
analgesic, fever-reducer**

 ## USES

- Treatment for sprains, strains and muscle spasms.
- Treatment of mild to moderate pain and fever.

 ## DOSAGE & USAGE INFORMATION

How to take:
Tablet or capsule—Swallow with liquid.

When to take:
As needed, no more often than every 3 hours.

If you forget a dose:
Take as soon as you remember. Wait 3 hours for next dose.

Continued next column

 ## OVERDOSE

SYMPTOMS:
Nausea, vomiting, diarrhea, headache, severe weakness, unusual increase in sweating, fainting, breathing difficulty, irritability, convulsions, sensation of paralysis, coma.
WHAT TO DO:
- **Overdose unlikely to threaten life. Depending on severity of symptoms and amount taken, call doctor, poison-control center or hospital emergency room for instructions.**
- **Dial 0 (operator) or 911 (emergency) for an ambulance or medical help. Then give first aid immediately.**
- **See emergency information on inside covers.**

What drug does:
- Blocks body's pain messages to brain. May also sedate.
- May affect hypothalamus, the part of the brain that helps regulate body heat and receives body's pain messages.

Time lapse before drug works:
15 to 30 minutes. May last 4 hours.

Don't take with:
- Other drugs with acetaminophen. Too much acetaminophen can damage liver and kidneys.
- See Interaction column and consult doctor.

 ## POSSIBLE ADVERSE REACTIONS OR SIDE EFFECTS

SYMPTOMS	WHAT TO DO
Life-threatening: None expected.	
Common: Dizziness, lightheadedness, drowsiness.	Discontinue. Call doctor right away.
Infrequent: • Difficult or frequent urination.	Discontinue. Call doctor right away.
• Nervousness, restlessness, irritability, constipation, headache, indigestion.	Continue. Call doctor when convenient.
Rare: • Sudden decrease in urine output; swelling of lips, face or tongue.	Discontinue. Seek emergency treatment.
• Bloody or black stools, jaundice, unusual bleeding or bruising, sore mouth or throat, fever.	Discontinue. Call doctor right away.

WARNINGS & PRECAUTIONS

Don't take if:
- You are allergic to any skeletal-muscle relaxant or acetaminophen.
- Your symptoms don't improve after 2 days use. Call your doctor.

Before you start, consult your doctor:
- If you have had liver disease.
- If you have bronchial asthma, kidney disease or liver damage.
- If you plan pregnancy within medication period.

Over age 60:
- Adverse reactions and side effects may be more frequent and severe than in younger persons.
- Don't exceed recommended dose. You can't eliminate drug as efficiently as younger persons.

Pregnancy:
No proven harm to unborn child. Avoid if possible.

Breast-feeding:
Drug passes into milk. Avoid drug or discontinue nursing until you finish medicine. Consult doctor for advice on maintaining milk supply.

Infants & children:
Not recommended.

Prolonged use:
May affect blood system and cause anemia. Limit use to 5 days for children 12 and under, and 10 days for adults.

Skin & sunlight:
No problems expected.

Driving, piloting or hazardous work:
Don't drive or pilot aircraft until you learn how medicine affects you. Don't work around dangerous machinery. Don't climb ladders or work in high places. Danger increases if you drink alcohol or take medicine affecting alertness and reflexes, such as antihistamines, tranquilizers, sedatives, pain medicine, narcotics and mind-altering drugs.

Discontinuing:
Don't discontinue without consulting your doctor. Dose may require gradual reduction if you have taken drug for a long time. Doses of other drugs may also require adjustment.

Others:
Periodic liver-function tests recommended if you use this drug for a long time.

POSSIBLE INTERACTION WITH OTHER DRUGS

GENERIC NAME OR DRUG CLASS	COMBINED EFFECT
Anticoagulants (oral)	May increase anticoagulant effect. If combined frequently, prothrombin time should be monitored.
Antidepressants	Increased sedation.
Antihistamines	Increased sedation.
Dronabinol	Increased effect of dronabinol on central nervous system. Avoid combination.
MAO inhibitors	Increased effect (but safety not established) of both drugs.
Mind-altering drugs	Increased sedation.
Muscle relaxants (others)	Increased sedation.
Narcotics	Increased sedation.
Phenobarbital	Quicker elimination and decreased effects of acetaminophen.
Sedatives	Increased sedation.
Sleep inducers	Increased sedation.
Testosterone	Decreased chlorzoxazone effect.
Tetracyclines (effervescent granules or tablets)	May slow tetracycline absorption. Space doses 2 hours apart.
Tranquilizers	Increased sedation.

POSSIBLE INTERACTION WITH OTHER SUBSTANCES

INTERACTS WITH	COMBINED EFFECT
Alcohol:	Drowsiness, increased sedation.
Beverages:	No problems expected.
Cocaine:	Lack of coordination. May slow body's recovery. Avoid.
Foods:	No problems expected.
Marijuana:	Increased pain relief, lack of coordination, drowsiness, fainting. May slow body's recovery. Avoid.
Tobacco:	No problems expected.

CHOLESTYRAMINE

BRAND NAMES

Questran

BASIC INFORMATION

Habit forming? No
Prescription needed? Yes
Available as generic? No
Drug class: Antihyperlipidemic, antipruritic

 ## USES

- Removes excess bile acids that occur with some liver problems. Reduces persistent itch caused by bile acids.
- Lowers cholesterol level.

 ## DOSAGE & USAGE INFORMATION

How to take:
Powder, granules—Sprinkle into 8 oz. liquid. Let stand for 2 minutes, then mix with liquid before swallowing. Or mix with cereal, soup or pulpy fruit. Don't swallow dry.

When to take:
3 or 4 times a day on an empty stomach, 1 hour before or 2 hours after eating.

If you forget a dose:
Take as soon as you remember up to 2 hours late. If more than 2 hours, wait for next scheduled dose (don't double this dose).

What drug does:
Binds with bile acids to prevent their absorption.

Time lapse before drug works:
- Cholesterol reduction—1 day.
- Bile-acid reduction—3 to 4 weeks.

Don't take with:
- Any drug or vitamin simultaneously. Space doses 2 hours apart.
- See Interaction column and consult doctor.

 ## OVERDOSE

SYMPTOMS:
Increased side effects and adverse reactions.
WHAT TO DO:
Overdose unlikely to threaten life. Depending on severity of symptoms and amount taken, call doctor, poison-control center or hospital emergency room for instructions.

 ## POSSIBLE ADVERSE REACTIONS OR SIDE EFFECTS

SYMPTOMS	WHAT TO DO
Life-threatening:	
None expected.	
Common:	
Constipation.	Continue. Call doctor when convenient.
Infrequent:	
Belching, bloating, diarrhea, mild nausea, vomiting, stomach pain.	Discontinue. Call doctor right away.
Rare:	
• Severe stomach pain; nausea; vomiting; black, tarry stool.	Discontinue. Seek emergency treatment.
• Rash.	Discontinue. Call doctor right away.
• Sore tongue.	Continue. Call doctor when convenient.

WARNINGS & PRECAUTIONS

Don't take if:
You are allergic to cholestyramine.

Before you start, consult your doctor:
- If you plan to become pregnant within medication period.
- If you have angina, heart or blood-vessel disease.
- If you have stomach problems (including ulcer).
- If you have constipation or hemorrhoids.
- If you have kidney disease.

Over age 60:
Adverse reactions and side effects may be more frequent and severe than in younger persons.

Pregnancy:
No proven harm to unborn child. Avoid if possible.

Breast-feeding:
No problems expected, but consult doctor.

Infants & children:
Not recommended.

Prolonged use:
No problems expected.

Skin & sunlight:
No problems expected.

Driving, piloting or hazardous work:
No problems expected.

Discontinuing:
Don't discontinue without doctor's advice until you complete prescribed dose, even though symptoms diminish or disappear.

Others:
No problems expected.

POSSIBLE INTERACTION WITH OTHER DRUGS

GENERIC NAME OR DRUG CLASS	COMBINED EFFECT
Anticoagulants	Increased anticoagulant effect.
Digitalis preparations	Decreased digitalis effect.
Indapamide	Decreased indapamide effect.
Thyroid hormones	Decreased thyroid effect.
All other medicines	Decreased absorption, so dosages or dosage intervals may require adjustment.

POSSIBLE INTERACTION WITH OTHER SUBSTANCES

INTERACTS WITH	COMBINED EFFECT
Alcohol:	None expected.
Beverages:	None expected.
Cocaine:	None expected.
Foods:	Absorption of vitamins in foods decreased. Take vitamin supplements, particularly A, D, E & K.
Marijuana:	None expected.
Tobacco:	None expected.

CIMETIDINE

BRAND NAMES

Apo-Cimetidine
Novo-Cimetine

Peptol
Tagamet

BASIC INFORMATION

Habit forming? No
Prescription needed? Yes
Available as generic? No
Drug class: Histamine H-2 antagonist

 USES

Treatment for duodenal ulcers and other conditions in which stomach produces excess hydrochloric acid.

 DOSAGE & USAGE INFORMATION

How to take:
Tablet or capsule—Swallow with liquid.

When to take:
• 1 dose per day—Take at bedtime.
• 2 or more doses per day—Take at the same times each day.

If you forget a dose:
Take as soon as you remember up to 2 hours late. If more than 2 hours, wait for next scheduled dose (don't double this dose).

What drug does:
Blocks histamine release so stomach secretes less acid.

Time lapse before drug works:
Begins in 30 minutes. May require several days to relieve pain.

Don't take with:
See Interaction column and consult doctor.

 OVERDOSE

SYMPTOMS:
Confusion, slurred speech, breathing difficulty, rapid heartbeat, delirium.
WHAT TO DO:
Overdose unlikely to threaten life. If person takes much larger amount than prescribed, call doctor, poison-control center or hospital emergency room for instructions.

 POSSIBLE ADVERSE REACTIONS OR SIDE EFFECTS

SYMPTOMS	WHAT TO DO
Life-threatening: None expected.	
Common: None expected.	
Infrequent:	
• Dizziness or headache, diarrhea, decreased sperm production.	Continue. Call doctor when convenient.
• Diminished sex drive, breast swelling and soreness in males, unusual milk flow in females, hair loss.	Continue. Tell doctor at next visit.
Rare: Confusion; rash, hives; sore throat, fever; slow, fast or irregular heartbeat; unusual bleeding or bruising; muscle cramps or pain; fatigue; weakness.	Discontinue. Call doctor right away.

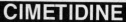

WARNINGS & PRECAUTIONS

Don't take if:
You are allergic to cimetidine or other histamine H-2 antagonist.

Before you start, consult your doctor:
- If you plan to become pregnant during medication period.
- If you take aspirin. Aspirin may irritate stomach.

Over age 60:
Adverse reactions and side effects may be more frequent and severe than in younger persons.

Pregnancy:
No proven harm to unborn child. Avoid if possible.

Breast-feeding:
No problems expected.

Infants & children:
Not recommended.

Prolonged use:
Possible liver damage.

Skin & sunlight:
No problems expected.

Driving, piloting or hazardous work:
Don't drive or pilot aircraft until you learn how medicine affects you. Don't work around dangerous machinery. Don't climb ladders or work in high places. Danger increases if you drink alcohol or take medicine affecting alertness and reflexes, such as antihistamines, tranquilizers, sedatives, pain medicine, narcotics and mind-altering drugs.

Discontinuing:
Don't discontinue without consulting doctor. Dose may require gradual reduction if you have taken drug for a long time. Doses of other drugs may also require adjustment.

Others:
Patients on kidney dialysis—Take at end of dialysis treatment.

POSSIBLE INTERACTION WITH OTHER DRUGS

GENERIC NAME OR DRUG CLASS	COMBINED EFFECT
Anticoagulants (oral)	Increased anticoagulant effect.
Anticholinergics	Decreased cimetidine effect.
Bethanechol	Increased cimetidine effect.
Carmustine (BCNU)	Severe impairment of red-blood-cell production; some interference with white-blood-cell formation.
Digitalis preparations	Increased digitalis effect.
Labetolol	Increased antihypertensive effects.
Penicillins	Increased penicillin effect.
Propranolol	May increase propranolol effect.
Quinidine	Increased quinidine effect.
Theophylline	Increased theophylline effect.

POSSIBLE INTERACTION WITH OTHER SUBSTANCES

INTERACTS WITH	COMBINED EFFECT
Alcohol:	No interactions expected, but alcohol may slow body's recovery. Avoid.
Beverages: Milk.	Enhanced effectiveness. Small amounts useful for taking medication.
Caffeine drinks.	May increase acid secretion and delay healing.
Cocaine:	Decreased cimetidine effect.
Foods:	Enhanced effectiveness. Protein-rich foods should be eaten in moderation to minimize secretion of stomach acid.
Marijuana:	Increased chance of low sperm count. Marijuana may slow body's recovery. Avoid.
Tobacco:	No interactions expected, but tobacco may slow body's recovery. Avoid.

CINOXACIN

BRAND NAMES

Azolinic Acid   Cinobactin
Cinobac

BASIC INFORMATION

Habit forming? No
Prescription needed? Yes
Available as generic? No
Drug class: Urinary anti-infective

 ## USES

Treatment for urinary-tract infections.

 ## DOSAGE & USAGE INFORMATION

How to take:
- Tablet—Swallow with food or milk to lessen stomach irritation. If you can't swallow whole, crumble tablet and take with liquid or food.
- Liquid—Take with liquid or food.

When to take:
At the same times each day.

If you forget a dose:
Take as soon as you remember up to 2 hours late. If more than 2 hours, wait for next scheduled dose (don't double this dose).

What drug does:
Destroys bacteria susceptible to cinoxacin.

Time lapse before drug works:
1 to 2 weeks.

Don't take with:
See Interaction column and consult doctor.

 ## OVERDOSE

SYMPTOMS:
Lethargy, stomach upset, behavioral changes, convulsions and stupor.
WHAT TO DO:
- Dial 0 (operator) or 911 (emergency) for an ambulance or medical help. Then give first aid immediately.
- If patient is unconscious and not breathing, give mouth-to-mouth breathing. If there is no heartbeat, use cardiac massage and mouth-to-mouth breathing (CPR). Don't try to make patient vomit. If you can't get help quickly, take patient to nearest emergency facility.
- See emergency information on inside covers.

 ## POSSIBLE ADVERSE REACTIONS OR SIDE EFFECTS

SYMPTOMS	WHAT TO DO
Life-threatening: None expected.	
Common: Rash, itch; decreased, blurred or double vision; halos around lights or excess brightness; changes in color vision; nausea, vomiting, diarrhea.	Discontinue. Call doctor right away.
Infrequent: Dizziness, drowsiness, headache, ringing in ears, insomnia.	Continue. Call doctor when convenient.
Rare: Severe stomach pain.	Discontinue. Call doctor right away.

WARNINGS & PRECAUTIONS

Don't take if:
- You are allergic to cinoxacin or nalidixic acid.
- You have a seizure disorder (epilepsy, convulsions).

Before you start, consult your doctor:
- If you plan to become pregnant during medication period.
- If you have or have had kidney or liver disease.
- If you have impaired circulation to the brain (hardened arteries).

Over age 60:
Adverse reactions and side effects may be more frequent and severe than in younger persons.

Pregnancy:
Risk to unborn child outweighs drug benefits. Don't use, especially during first 3 months.

Breast-feeding:
No problems expected, unless you have impaired kidney function. Consult doctor.

Infants & children:
Don't give to infants younger than 3 months.

Prolonged use:
No problems expected.

Skin & sunlight:
- May cause sunlight to hurt eyes.
- May cause rash or intensify sunburn in areas exposed to sun or sunlamp.

Driving, piloting or hazardous work:
Avoid if you feel drowsy, dizzy or have vision problems. Otherwise, no problems expected.

Discontinuing:
Don't discontinue without consulting doctor. Dose may require gradual reduction if you have taken drug for a long time. Doses of other drugs may also require adjustment.

Others:
Periodic blood counts, liver-function and kidney-function tests recommended.

POSSIBLE INTERACTION WITH OTHER DRUGS

GENERIC NAME OR DRUG CLASS	COMBINED EFFECT
None reported.	

POSSIBLE INTERACTION WITH OTHER SUBSTANCES

INTERACTS WITH	COMBINED EFFECT
Alcohol:	Impaired alertness, judgment and coordination.
Beverages:	None expected.
Cocaine:	Impaired judgment and coordination.
Foods:	None expected.
Marijuana:	Impaired alertness, judgment and coordination.
Tobacco:	None expected.

CITRATES

BRAND AND GENERIC NAMES

Albright's Solution
Bicitra
Citrolith
Modified Shohl's
    Solution
Oracit
Polycitra
Polycitra-K
POTASSIUM
    CITRATE

POTASSIUM
    CITRATE & CITRIC
    ACID
POTASSIUM
    CITRATE &
    SODIUM CITRATE
SODIUM CITRATE &
    CITRIC ACID
TRICITRATES
Urocit-K

BASIC INFORMATION

Habit forming? No
Prescription needed? Yes
Available as generic? No
Drug class: Urinary alkalizer, antiurolithic
(kidney stone)

 ## USES

- To make urine more alkaline (less acid).
- To treat or prevent recurrence of some types of kidney stones.

 ## DOSAGE & USAGE INFORMATION

How to take:
Tablets—Swallow whole with liquid. If tablets seem to stick in throat or esophagus, eat a banana to help ease it into the stomach.

When to take:
On full stomach, usually after meals or with food.

If you forget a dose:
Take as soon as you remember up to 2 hours late. If more than 2 hours, wait for next scheduled dose (don't double this dose).

Continued next column

 ## OVERDOSE

SYMPTOMS:
Convulsions, coma.
WHAT TO DO:
- **Dial 0 (operator) or 911 (emergency) for an ambulance or medical help. Then give first aid immediately.**
- **See emergency information on inside covers.**

What drug does:
Increases urinary alkalinity by excretion of bicarbonate ions.

Time lapse before drug works:
1 hour.

Don't take with:
- Any medicine that will decrease mental alertness or reflexes, such as alcohol, other mind-altering drugs, cough/cold medicines, antihistamines, allergy medicine, sedatives, tranquilizers (sleeping pills or "downers"), barbiturates, seizure medicine, narcotics, other prescription medicine for pain, muscle relaxants, anesthetics.
- See Interaction column and consult doctor.

 ## POSSIBLE ADVERSE REACTIONS OR SIDE EFFECTS

SYMPTOMS	WHAT TO DO
Life-threatening:	
Black, tarry stools; vomiting blood; severe abdominal cramps; irregular heartbeat; shortness of breath.	Discontinue. Seek emergency treatment.
Common:	
Nausea or vomiting.	Continue. Call doctor when convenient.
Infrequent:	
Confusion, dizziness, swollen feet and ankles, irritability, depression, muscle pain, nervousness, numbness or tingling in hands or feet, unpleasant taste, weakness.	Discontinue. Call doctor right away.
Rare:	
None expected.	

WARNINGS & PRECAUTIONS

Don't take if:
You are allergic to any citrate.

Before you start, consult your doctor:
- If you have any disease involving the adrenal glands, diabetes, chronic diarrhea, heart problems, hypertension, kidney disease, stomach ulcer or gastritis, urinary tract infection, toxemia of pregnancy.
- If you plan strenuous exercise.

Over age 60:
Adverse reactions and side effects may be more frequent and severe than in younger persons. Ask doctor about smaller doses.

Pregnancy:
Safety to unborn child unestablished. Avoid if possible.

Breast-feeding:
Safety during lactation not established. Consult doctor.

Infants & children:
Use only under close medical supervision.

Prolonged use:
Adverse reactions more likely.

Skin & sunlight:
No problems expected.

Driving, piloting or hazardous work:
Don't drive or pilot aircraft until you learn how medicine affects you. Don't work around dangerous machinery. Don't climb ladders or work in high places. Danger increases if you drink alcohol or take medicine affecting alertness and reflexes, such as antihistamines, tranquilizers, sedatives, pain medicine, narcotics and mind-altering drugs.

Discontinuing:
Don't discontinue without consulting doctor. Dose may require gradual reduction if you have taken drug for a long time. Doses of other drugs may also require adjustment.

Others:
- Drink at least 8 ounces of water or other liquid (except milk) every hour while awake.
- Liquid may be chilled (don't freeze) to improve taste.

POSSIBLE INTERACTION WITH OTHER DRUGS

GENERIC NAME OR DRUG CLASS	COMBINED EFFECT
Antacids	Toxic effect of citrates (alkalosis).
Calcium supplements	Increases risk of kidney stones.
Methenamine	Decreases effects of methenamine.
Mexiletine	May slow elimination of mexiletine and cause need to adjust dosage.
Quinidine	Prolongs citrate effect.

POSSIBLE INTERACTION WITH OTHER SUBSTANCES

INTERACTS WITH	COMBINED EFFECT
Alcohol:	Will decrease mental alertness.
Beverages: Salt-free milk.	May cause potassium toxicity.
Cocaine:	No proven problems.
Foods: Milk, cheese, ice cream, yogurt, buttermilk, salty foods, salt, salt substitutes.	May increase likelihood of kidney stones.
Marijuana:	No proven problems.
Tobacco:	Increases likelihood of stomach irritation.

CLEMASTINE

BRAND NAMES

Tavist

BASIC INFORMATION

Habit forming? No
Prescription needed? No
Available as generic? No
Drug class: Antihistamine

 USES

Reduces allergic symptoms such as hay fever, hives, rash or itching.

 DOSAGE & USAGE INFORMATION

How to take:
Tablet—Swallow with liquid or food to lessen stomach irritation.

When to take:
Varies with form. Follow label directions.

If you forget a dose:
Take as soon as you remember up to 2 hours late. If more than 2 hours, wait for next scheduled dose (don't double this dose).

What drug does:
Blocks action of histamine after an allergic response triggers histamine release in sensitive cells.

Time lapse before drug works:
30 minutes.

Don't take with:
See Interaction column and consult doctor.

 OVERDOSE

SYMPTOMS:
Convulsions, red face, hallucinations, coma.
WHAT TO DO:
- Dial 0 (operator) or 911 (emergency) for an ambulance or medical help. Then give first aid immediately.
- If patient is unconscious and not breathing, give mouth-to-mouth breathing. If there is no heartbeat, use cardiac massage and mouth-to-mouth breathing (CPR). Don't try to make patient vomit. If you can't get help quickly, take patient to nearest emergency facility.
- See emergency information on inside covers.

 POSSIBLE ADVERSE REACTIONS OR SIDE EFFECTS

SYMPTOMS	WHAT TO DO
Life-threatening:	
None expected.	
Common:	
Drowsiness; dizziness; dry mouth, nose, throat; nausea.	Continue. Tell doctor at next visit.
Infrequent:	
• Vision changes.	Discontinue. Call doctor right away.
• Less tolerance for contact lenses; difficult urination.	Continue. Call doctor when convenient.
• Appetite loss.	Continue. Tell doctor at next visit.
Rare:	
Nightmares, agitation, irritability; sore throat, fever; rapid heartbeat; unusual bleeding or bruising; fatigue, weakness.	Discontinue. Call doctor right away.

WARNINGS & PRECAUTIONS

Don't take if:
You are allergic to any antihistamine.

Before you start, consult your doctor:
- If you have glaucoma.
- If you have enlarged prostate.
- If you have asthma.
- If you have kidney disease.
- If you have peptic ulcer.
- If you will have surgery within 2 months, including dental surgery, requiring general or spinal anesthesia.

Over age 60:
Don't exceed recommended dose. Adverse reactions and side effects may be more frequent and severe than in younger persons, especially urination difficulty, diminished alertness and other brain and nervous-system symptoms.

Pregnancy:
No proven harm to unborn child. Avoid if possible.

Breast-feeding:
Drug passes into milk. Avoid drug or discontinue nursing until you finish medicine. Consult doctor for advice on maintaining milk supply.

Infants & children:
Not recommended for premature or newborn infants. Otherwise, no problems expected.

Prolonged use:
Avoid. May damage bone marrow and nerve cells.

Skin & sunlight:
May cause rash or intensify sunburn in areas exposed to sun or sunlamp.

Driving, piloting or hazardous work:
Don't drive or pilot aircraft until you learn how medicine affects you. Don't work around dangerous machinery. Don't climb ladders or work in high places. Danger increases if you drink alcohol or take medicine affecting alertness and reflexes, such as antihistamines, tranquilizers, sedatives, pain medicine, narcotics and mind-altering drugs.

Discontinuing:
No problems expected.

Others:
May mask symptoms of hearing damage from aspirin, other salicylates, cisplatin, paromomycin, vancomycin or anticonvulsants. Consult doctor if you use these.

POSSIBLE INTERACTION WITH OTHER DRUGS

GENERIC NAME OR DRUG CLASS	COMBINED EFFECT
Anticholinergics	Increased anticholinergic effect.
Antidepressants	Excess sedation. Avoid.
Antihistamines (other)	Excess sedation. Avoid.
Dronabinol	Increased effects of both drugs. Avoid.
Hypnotics	Excess sedation. Avoid.
MAO inhibitors	Increased clemastine effect.
Mind-altering drugs	Excess sedation. Avoid.
Molindone	Increased antihistamine effect.
Narcotics	Excess sedation. Avoid.
Sedatives	Excess sedation. Avoid.
Sleep inducers	Excess sedation. Avoid.
Tranquilizers	Excess sedation. Avoid.

POSSIBLE INTERACTION WITH OTHER SUBSTANCES

INTERACTS WITH	COMBINED EFFECT
Alcohol:	Excess sedation. Avoid.
Beverages: Caffeine drinks.	Less clemastine sedation.
Cocaine:	Decreased clemastine effect. Avoid.
Foods:	None expected.
Marijuana:	Excess sedation. Avoid.
Tobacco:	None expected.

CLIDINIUM

BRAND NAMES

Clipoxide   Quarzan
Librax

BASIC INFORMATION

Habit forming? No
Prescription needed?
  Low strength: No
  High strength: Yes
Available as generic? Yes
Drug class: Antispasmodic, anticholinergic

 USES

Reduces spasms of digestive system, bladder and urethra.

 DOSAGE & USAGE INFORMATION

How to take:
Capsule—Swallow with liquid or food to lessen stomach irritation.

When to take:
30 minutes before meals (unless directed otherwise by doctor).

If you forget a dose:
Take as soon as you remember up to 2 hours late. If more than 2 hours, wait for next scheduled dose (don't double this dose).

What drug does:
Blocks nerve impulses at parasympathetic nerve endings, preventing muscle contractions and gland secretions of organs involved.

Time lapse before drug works:
15 to 30 minutes.

Don't take with:
See Interaction column and consult doctor.

 OVERDOSE

SYMPTOMS:
Dilated pupils, rapid pulse and breathing, dizziness, fever, hallucinations, confusion, slurred speech, agitation, flushed face, convulsions, coma.
WHAT TO DO:
- **Dial 0 (operator) or 911 (emergency) for an ambulance or medical help. Then give first aid immediately.**
- **See emergency information on inside covers.**

 POSSIBLE ADVERSE REACTIONS OR SIDE EFFECTS

SYMPTOMS	WHAT TO DO
Life-threatening: None expected.	
Common:	
• Confusion, delirium, rapid heartbeat.	Discontinue. Call doctor right away.
• Nausea, vomiting, decreased sweating.	Continue. Call doctor when convenient.
• Constipation.	Continue. Tell doctor at next visit.
• Dryness in ears, nose, throat.	No action necessary.
Infrequent:	
• Nasal congestion, altered taste.	Discontinue. Call doctor right away.
• Difficult urination, headache.	Continue. Call doctor when convenient.
Rare:	
Rash or hives, pain, blurred vision.	Discontinue. Call doctor right away.

 WARNINGS & PRECAUTIONS

Don't take if:
- You are allergic to any anticholinergic.
- You have trouble with stomach bloating.
- You have difficulty emptying your bladder completely.
- You have narrow-angle glaucoma.
- You have severe ulcerative colitis.

Before you start, consult your doctor:
- If you have open-angle glaucoma.
- If you have angina.
- If you have chronic bronchitis or asthma.
- If you have hiatal hernia.
- If you have liver disease.
- If you have enlarged prostate.
- If you have myasthenia gravis.
- If you have peptic ulcer.
- If you will have surgery within 2 months, including dental surgery, requiring general or spinal anesthesia.

Over age 60:
Adverse reactions and side effects may be more frequent and severe than in younger persons.

Pregnancy:
Studies inconclusive on harm to unborn child. Animal studies show fetal abnormalities. Decide with your doctor whether drug benefits justify risk to unborn child.

Breast-feeding:
Drug passes into milk and decreases milk flow. Avoid drug or discontinue nursing until you finish medicine. Consult doctor for advice on maintaining milk supply.

Infants & children:
Use only under medical supervision.

Prolonged use:
Chronic constipation, possible fecal impaction. Consult doctor immediately.

Skin & sunlight:
No problems expected.

Driving, piloting or hazardous work:
Don't drive or pilot aircraft until you learn how medicine affects you. Don't work around dangerous machinery. Don't climb ladders or work in high places. Danger increases if you drink alcohol or take medicine affecting alertness and reflexes, such as antihistamines, tranquilizers, sedatives, pain medicine, narcotics, or mind-altering drugs.

Discontinuing:
May be unnecessary to finish medicine. Follow doctor's instructions.

Others:
No problems expected.

POSSIBLE INTERACTION WITH OTHER DRUGS

GENERIC NAME OR DRUG CLASS	COMBINED EFFECT
Amantadine	Increased clidinium effect.
Antacids	Decreased clidinium effect.
Anticholinergics (other)	Increased clidinium effect.
Antidepressants (tricyclic)	Increased clidinium effect. Increased sedation.
Antihistamines	Increased clidinium effect.
Haloperidol	Increased internal-eye pressure.
MAO inhibitors	Increased clidinium effect.
Meperidine	Increased clidinium effect.
Methylphenidate	Increased clidinium effect.
Molindone	Increased anticholinergic effect.
Nitrates	Increased internal-eye pressure.

Orphenadrine	Increased clidinium effect.
Phenothiazines	Increased clidinium effect.
Pilocarpine	Loss of pilocarpine effect in glaucoma treatment.
Potassium supplements	Possible intestinal ulcers with oral potassium tablets.
Tranquilizers	Decreased clidinium effect.
Vitamin C	Decreased clidinium effect. Avoid large doses of vitamin C.

POSSIBLE INTERACTION WITH OTHER SUBSTANCES

INTERACTS WITH	COMBINED EFFECT
Alcohol:	None expected.
Beverages:	None expected.
Cocaine:	Excessively rapid heartbeat. Avoid.
Foods:	None expected.
Marijuana:	Drowsiness and dry mouth.
Tobacco:	None expected.

CLINDAMYCIN

BRAND NAMES

Cleocin   Dalacin C
Cleocin-T

BASIC INFORMATION

Habit forming? No
Prescription needed? Yes
Available as generic? No
Drug class: Antibiotic (lincomycin)

 ## USES

Treatment of bacterial infections that are susceptible to clindamycin.

 ## DOSAGE & USAGE INFORMATION

How to take:
Capsule or liquid—Swallow with liquid 1 hour before or 2 hours after eating.

When to take:
At the same times each day.

If you forget a dose:
Take as soon as you remember up to 2 hours late. If more than 2 hours, wait for next scheduled dose (don't double this dose).

What drug does:
Destroys susceptible bacteria. Does not kill viruses.

Time lapse before drug works:
3 to 5 days.

Don't take with:
See Interaction column and consult doctor.

 ## OVERDOSE

SYMPTOMS:
Severe nausea, vomiting, diarrhea.
WHAT TO DO:
Overdose unlikely to threaten life. If person takes much larger amount than prescribed, call doctor, poison-control center or hospital emergency room for instructions.

 ## POSSIBLE ADVERSE REACTIONS OR SIDE EFFECTS

SYMPTOMS	WHAT TO DO
Life-threatening: None expected.	
Common: None expected.	
Infrequent:	
• Unusual thirst; vomiting; stomach cramps; severe and watery diarrhea with blood or mucus; painful, swollen joints; jaundice; fever; tiredness; weakness; weight loss.	Discontinue. Call doctor right away.
• White patches in mouth; rash, itch around groin, rectum or armpits; vaginal discharge, itching.	Continue. Call doctor when convenient.
Rare: None expected.	

216

WARNINGS & PRECAUTIONS

Don't take if:
- You are allergic to lincomycins.
- You have had ulcerative colitis.
- Prescribed for infant under 1 month old.

Before you start, consult your doctor:
- If you have had yeast infections of mouth, skin or vagina.
- If you will have surgery within 2 months, including dental surgery, requiring general or spinal anesthesia.
- If you have kidney or liver disease.
- If you have allergies of any kind.

Over age 60:
Adverse reactions and side effects may be more frequent and severe than in younger persons.

Pregnancy:
Risk to unborn child outweighs drug benefits. Don't use.

Breast-feeding:
Drug passes into milk. Avoid drug or discontinue nursing until you finish medicine. Consult doctor for advice on maintaining milk supply.

Infants & children:
Don't give to infants younger than 1 month. Use for children only under medical supervision.

Prolonged use:
- Severe colitis with diarrhea and bleeding.
- You may become more susceptible to infections caused by germs not responsive to clindamycin.

Skin & sunlight:
No problems expected.

Driving, piloting or hazardous work:
No problems expected.

Discontinuing:
Don't discontinue without doctor's advice until you complete prescribed dose, even though symptoms diminish or disappear.

Others:
No problems expected.

POSSIBLE INTERACTION WITH OTHER DRUGS

GENERIC NAME OR DRUG CLASS	COMBINED EFFECT
Antidiarrheal preparations	Decreased clindamycin effect.
Chloramphenicol	Decreased clindamycin effect.
Erythromycin	Decreased clindamycin effect.

POSSIBLE INTERACTION WITH OTHER SUBSTANCES

INTERACTS WITH	COMBINED EFFECT
Alcohol:	None expected.
Beverages:	None expected.
Cocaine:	None expected.
Foods:	None expected.
Marijuana:	None expected.
Tobacco:	None expected.

CLOFIBRATE

BRAND NAMES

Atromid-S
Claripex

Liprinal
Novofibrate

BASIC INFORMATION

Habit forming? No
Prescription needed? Yes
Available as generic? Yes
Drug class: Antihyperlipidemic

 USES

Reduces fatty substances in the blood (cholesterol and triglycerides).

 DOSAGE & USAGE INFORMATION

How to take:
Capsule—Swallow with liquid or food to lessen stomach irritation.

When to take:
At the same times each day.

If you forget a dose:
Take as soon as you remember up to 2 hours late. If more than 2 hours, wait for next scheduled dose (don't double this dose).

What drug does:
Inhibits formation of fatty substances.

Time lapse before drug works:
3 months or more.

Don't take with:
See Interaction column and consult doctor.

 OVERDOSE

SYMPTOMS:
Diarrhea, headache, muscle pain.
WHAT TO DO:
Overdose unlikely to threaten life. If person takes much larger amount than prescribed, call doctor, poison-control center or hospital emergency room for instructions.

 POSSIBLE ADVERSE REACTIONS OR SIDE EFFECTS

SYMPTOMS	WHAT TO DO
Life-threatening: None expected.	
Common: None expected.	
Infrequent:	
• Chest pain, shortness of breath, irregular heartbeat, gallstones.	Discontinue. Call doctor right away.
• Nausea, vomiting, diarrhea, stomach pain.	Continue. Call doctor when convenient.
Rare:	
• Rash, itch; mouth or lip sores; sore throat; swollen feet, legs; blood in urine; painful urination; fever; chills.	Discontinue. Call doctor right away.
• Dizziness, drowsiness, headache, muscle cramps, backache, diminished sex drive, dryness, hair loss.	Continue. Call doctor when convenient.

WARNINGS & PRECAUTIONS

Don't take if:
You are allergic to any antihyperlipidemic.

Before you start, consult your doctor:
- If you have had liver or kidney disease.
- If you have had peptic-ulcer disease.
- If you have diabetes.

Over age 60:
Adverse reactions and side effects may be more frequent and severe than in younger persons. May develop flu-like symptoms.

Pregnancy:
Risk to unborn child outweighs drug benefits. Don't use.

Breast-feeding:
May harm child. Avoid.

Infants & children:
Not recommended.

Prolonged use:
No problems expected.

Skin & sunlight:
No problems expected.

Driving, piloting or hazardous work:
Avoid if you feel drowsy or dizzy. Otherwise, no problems expected.

Discontinuing:
Don't discontinue without doctor's advice until you complete prescribed dose, even though symptoms diminish or disappear.

Others:
- Periodic blood-cell counts and liver-function studies recommended if you take clofibrate for a long time.
- Some studies question effectiveness. Many studies warn against toxicity.

POSSIBLE INTERACTION WITH OTHER DRUGS

GENERIC NAME OR DRUG CLASS	COMBINED EFFECT
Anticoagulants (oral)	Increased anticoagulant effect. Dose reduction of anticoagulant necessary.
Antidiabetics (oral)	Increased antidiabetic effect.
Contraceptives (oral)	Decreased clofibrate effect.
Estrogens	Decreased clofibrate effect.
Furosemide	Possible toxicity of both drugs.
Insulin	Increased insulin effect.
Thyroid hormones	Increased clofibrate effect.

POSSIBLE INTERACTION WITH OTHER SUBSTANCES

INTERACTS WITH	COMBINED EFFECT
Alcohol:	None expected.
Beverages:	None expected.
Cocaine:	None expected.
Foods: Fatty foods.	Decreased clofibrate effect.
Marijuana:	None expected.
Tobacco:	None expected.

CLOMIPHENE

BRAND NAMES

Clomid   Serophene

BASIC INFORMATION

Habit forming? No
Prescription needed? Yes
Available as generic? No
Drug class: Gonad stimulant

 USES

- Treatment for men with low sperm counts.
- Treatment for ovulatory failure in women who wish to become pregnant.

 DOSAGE & USAGE INFORMATION

How to take:
Tablet—Swallow with liquid.

When to take:
- Men—Take at the same time each day.
- Women—If you are to begin treatment on "Day 5," count your first menstrual day as "Day 1." Take a tablet each day for 5 days.

If you forget a dose:
Take as soon as you remember. If you forget a day, double next dose. If you miss 2 or more doses, consult doctor.

What drug does:
Antiestrogen effect stimulates ovulation and sperm production.

Time lapse before drug works:
Usually 3 to 6 months. Ovulation may occur 6 to 10 days after last day of treatment in any cycle.

Don't take with:
No restrictions.

 OVERDOSE

SYMPTOMS:
Increased severity of adverse reactions and side effects.
WHAT TO DO:
Overdose unlikely to threaten life. If person takes much larger amount than prescribed, call doctor, poison-control center or hospital emergency room for instructions.

 POSSIBLE ADVERSE REACTIONS OR SIDE EFFECTS

SYMPTOMS	WHAT TO DO
Life-threatening:	
None expected.	
Common:	
• Bloating, stomach pain, pelvic pain.	Discontinue. Call doctor right away.
• Hot flashes.	Continue. Tell doctor at next visit.
Infrequent:	
• Rash, itch, jaundice.	Discontinue. Call doctor right away.
• Constipation, diarrhea, increased appetite, heavy menstrual flow, frequent urination, breast discomfort, weight change, hair loss.	Continue. Call doctor when convenient.
Rare:	
• Vision changes.	Discontinue. Call doctor right away.
• Dizziness, headache, tiredness, depression, nervousness.	Continue. Call doctor when convenient.

WARNINGS & PRECAUTIONS

Don't take if:
You are allergic to clomiphene.

Before you start, consult your doctor:
- If you have an ovarian cyst, fibroid uterine tumors or unusual vaginal bleeding.
- If you have inflamed veins caused by blood clots.
- If you have liver disease.
- If you are depressed.

Over age 60:
Not recommended.

Pregnancy:
Stop taking at first sign of pregnancy.

Breast-feeding:
Not used.

Infants & children:
Not used.

Prolonged use:
Not recommended.

Skin & sunlight:
No problems expected.

Driving, piloting or hazardous work:
Avoid if you feel dizzy. Otherwise, no problems expected.

Discontinuing:
May be unnecessary to finish medicine. Follow doctor's instructions.

Others:
- Have a complete pelvic examination before treatment.
- If you become pregnant, twins or triplets are possible.

POSSIBLE INTERACTION WITH OTHER DRUGS

GENERIC NAME OR DRUG CLASS	COMBINED EFFECT
None	

POSSIBLE INTERACTION WITH OTHER SUBSTANCES

INTERACTS WITH	COMBINED EFFECT
Alcohol:	None expected.
Beverages:	None expected.
Cocaine:	None expected.
Foods:	None expected.
Marijuana:	None expected.
Tobacco:	None expected.

CLONIDINE

BRAND NAMES

Catapres   Combipres
Catapres-TTS

BASIC INFORMATION

Habit forming? No
Prescription needed? Yes
Available as generic? Yes
Drug class: Antihypertensive

 USES

- Treatment of high blood pressure.
- Prevention of vascular headaches.
- Treatment of dysmenorrhea and menopausal "hot flashes."
- Treatment of narcotic withdrawal syndrome.
- Treatment of congestive heart failure.

 DOSAGE & USAGE INFORMATION

How to take:
- Tablet or capsule—Swallow with liquid.
- Patches that attach to skin—Apply to clean, dry, hairless skin on arm or trunk.

When to take:
Daily dose at bedtime.

If you forget a dose:
Bedtime dose—If you forget your once-a-day dose, take it as soon as you remember. *Don't* double dose.

What drug does:
Relaxes and allows expansion of blood vessel walls.

Continued next column

 OVERDOSE

SYMPTOMS:
Difficult breathing, vomiting, fainting, slow heartbeat, coma, diminished reflexes.
WHAT TO DO:
- **Dial 0 (operator) or 911 (emergency) for an ambulance or medical help. Then give first aid immediately.**
- **If patient is unconscious and not breathing, give mouth-to-mouth breathing. If there is no heartbeat, use cardiac massage and mouth-to-mouth breathing (CPR). Don't try to make patient vomit. If you can't get help quickly, take patient to nearest emergency facility.**
- **See emergency information on inside covers.**

Time lapse before drug works:
1 to 3 hours.

Don't take with:
- Non-prescription medicines containing alcohol.
- See Interaction column and consult doctor.

 POSSIBLE ADVERSE REACTIONS OR SIDE EFFECTS

SYMPTOMS	WHAT TO DO
Life-threatening: None expected.	
Common:	
• Dizziness, drowsiness, weight gain, lightheadedness upon rising from sitting or lying, swollen breasts.	Continue. Call doctor when convenient.
• Dry mouth.	Continue. Tell doctor at next visit.
Infrequent:	
• Abnormal heart rhythm.	Discontinue. Call doctor right away.
• Headache; nightmares; painful glands in neck; nausea; vomiting; cold fingers and toes; dry, burning eyes.	Continue. Call doctor when convenient.
• Insomnia, constipation, appetite loss, diminished sex drive.	Continue. Tell doctor at next visit.
Rare:	
• Rash, itch.	Discontinue. Call doctor right away.
• Depression.	Continue. Call doctor when convenient.

 WARNINGS & PRECAUTIONS

Don't take if:
- You are allergic to any alpha-adrenergic blocker.
- You are under age 12.

Before you start, consult your doctor:
- If you will have surgery within 2 months, including dental surgery, requiring general or spinal anesthesia.
- If you have heart disease or chronic kidney disease.
- If you have a peripheral circulation disorder (intermittent claudication, Buerger's disease).
- If you have history of depression.

Over age 60:
Adverse reactions and side effects may be more frequent and severe than in younger persons.

Pregnancy:
Studies inconclusive on harm to unborn child. Animal studies show fetal abnormalities. Decide with your doctor whether drug benefits justify risk to unborn child.

Breast-feeding:
Unknown whether safe or not. Consult doctor.

Infants & children:
Use only under careful medical supervision after age 12. Avoid before age 12.

Prolonged use:
- Don't discontinue without consulting doctor. Dose may require gradual reduction if you have taken drug for a long time. Doses of other drugs may also require adjustment.
- Continued use may cause fluid retention, requiring addition of diuretic to treatment program.
- Request yearly eye examinations.

Skin & sunlight:
No problems expected.

Driving, piloting or hazardous work:
Don't drive or pilot aircraft until you learn how medicine affects you. Don't work around dangerous machinery. Don't climb ladders or work in high places. Danger increases if you drink alcohol or take medicine affecting alertness and reflexes.

Discontinuing:
Don't discontinue abruptly. May cause rebound high blood pressure, anxiety, chest pain, insomnia, headache, nausea, irregular heartbeat, flushed face, sweating.

Others:
No problems expected.

POSSIBLE INTERACTION WITH OTHER DRUGS

GENERIC NAME OR DRUG CLASS	COMBINED EFFECT
Acebutolol	Increased antihypertensive effect of each. Dosages may require adjustments.
Antidepressants (tricyclic)	Decreased clonidine effect.
Antihypertensives (other)	Excessive blood-pressure drop.
Appetite suppressants	Decreased clonidine effect.
Beta-blockers	Blood-pressure control impaired.
Diuretics	Excessive blood-pressure drop.
Enalapril	Possible excessive potassium in blood.
Fenfluramine	Possible increased clonidine effect.
Labetolol	May cause precipitous change in blood pressure if clonidine and labetolol are discontinued simultaneously.
Nitrates	Possible excessive blood-pressure drop.
Oxprenolol	May cause blood-pressure rise if clonidine is discontinued after simultaneous use with oxprenolol.
Pentoxifylline	Increased antihypertensive effect.

POSSIBLE INTERACTION WITH OTHER SUBSTANCES

INTERACTS WITH	COMBINED EFFECT
Alcohol:	Increased sensitivity to sedative effect of alcohol and very low blood pressure. Avoid.
Beverages: Caffeine-containing drinks.	Decreased clonidine effect.
Cocaine:	Blood pressure rise. Avoid.
Foods:	No problems expected.
Marijuana:	Weakness on standing.
Tobacco:	No problems expected.

CLONIDINE & CHLORTHALIDONE

BRAND NAMES

Combipres

BASIC INFORMATION

Habit forming? No
Prescription needed? Yes
Available as generic? No
Drug class: Antihypertensive

 USES

- Treatment of high blood pressure.
- Reduces fluid retention (edema) caused by conditions such as heart disorders and liver disease.

 DOSAGE & USAGE INFORMATION

How to take:
Tablet or capsule—Swallow with liquid. If you can't swallow whole, crumble tablet or open capsule and take with liquid or food. Don't exceed dose.

When to take:
At the same time each day.

If you forget a dose:
Take as soon as you remember up to 2 hours late. If more than 2 hours, wait for next scheduled dose (don't double this dose).

What drug does:
- Relaxes and allows expansion of blood vessel walls.

Continued next column

 OVERDOSE

SYMPTOMS:
Difficult breathing; vomiting; fainting; rapid, irregular, slow heartbeat; diminished reflexes; cramps; weakness; drowsiness; weak pulse; coma.
WHAT TO DO:
- **Dial 0 (operator) or 911 (emergency) for an ambulance or medical help. Then give first aid immediately.**
- **If patient is unconscious and not breathing, give mouth-to-mouth breathing. If there is no heartbeat, use cardiac massage and mouth-to-mouth breathing (CPR). Don't try to make patient vomit. If you can't get help quickly, take patient to nearest emergency facility.**
- **See emergency information on inside covers.**

- Forces sodium and water excretion, reducing body fluid.
- Reduced body fluid and relaxed arteries lower blood pressure.

Time lapse before drug works:
4 to 6 hours. May require several weeks to lower blood pressure.

Don't take with:
Any medicine that will decrease mental alertness such as alcohol, antihistamines, cold/cough medicines, sedatives, tranquilizers, narcotics, prescription pain medicine, barbiturates, seizure medicine, anesthetics.

 POSSIBLE ADVERSE REACTIONS OR SIDE EFFECTS

SYMPTOMS	WHAT TO DO
Life-threatening:	
Irregular heartbeat, weak pulse.	Discontinue. Seek emergency treatment.
Common:	
Dry mouth, increased thirst, muscle cramps, nausea or vomiting, mood changes, drowsiness.	Discontinue. Call doctor right away.
Infrequent:	
Vomiting, diminished sex desire and performance, insomnia, dizziness, diarrhea, constipaion, appetite loss.	Continue. Call doctor when convenient.
Rare:	
• Jaundice; easy bruising or bleeding; sore throat, fever, mouth ulcers; rash or hives; joint pain; flank pain; abdominal pain.	Discontinue. Call doctor right away.
• Cold fingers and toes, nightmares, vomiting.	Continue. Call doctor when convenient.

 WARNINGS & PRECAUTIONS

Don't take if:
- You are allergic to any thiazide diuretic drug or alpha-adrenergic blocker.
- You are under age 12.

Before you start, consult your doctor:
- If you are allergic to any sulfa drug.
- If you have gout, liver, pancreas or kidney disorder, a peripheral circulation disorder (intermittent claudication, Buerger's disease), history of depression, heart disease.

- If you will have surgery within 2 months, including dental surgery, requiring general or spinal anesthesia.

Over age 60:
Adverse reactions and side effects may be more frequent and severe than in younger persons, especially dizziness and excessive potassium loss.

Pregnancy:
Risk to unborn child outweighs drug benefits. Don't use.

Breast-feeding:
Drug passes into milk. Avoid drug or discontinue nursing until you finish medicine. Consult doctor for advice on maintaining milk supply.

Infants & children:
Use only after careful medical supervision after age 12. Avoid before age 12.

Prolonged use:
- Don't discontinue without consulting doctor. Dose may require gradual reduction if you have taken drug for a long time. Doses of other drugs may also require adjustment.
- Continued use may cause fluid retention, requiring addition of diuretic to treatment program.
- Request yearly eye examinations.

Skin & sunlight:
May cause rash or intensify sunburn in areas exposed to sun or sunlamp.

Driving, piloting or hazardous work:
Don't drive or pilot aircraft until you learn how medicine affects you. Don't work around dangerous machinery. Don't climb ladders or work in high places. Danger increases if you drink alcohol or take medicine affecting alertness and reflexes, such as antihistamines, tranquilizers, sedatives, pain medicine, narcotics and mind-altering drugs.

Discontinuing:
Don't discontinue abruptly. May cause rebound high blood pressure, anxiety, chest pain, insomnia, headache, nausea, irregular heartbeat, flushed face, sweating.

Others:
- Hot weather and fever may cause dehydration and drop in blood pressure. Dose may require temporary adjustment. Weigh daily and report any unexpected weight decreases to your doctor.
- May cause rise in uric acid, leading to gout.
- May cause blood-sugar rise in diabetics.

POSSIBLE INTERACTION WITH OTHER DRUGS

GENERIC NAME OR DRUG CLASS	COMBINED EFFECT
Acebutolol	Increased antihypertensive effect of each. Dosages may require adjustments.
Allopurinol	Decreased allopurinol effect.
Antidepressants (tricyclic)	Dangerous drop in blood pressure. Avoid combination unless under medical supervision.
Antihypertensives (other)	Excessive blood-pressure drop.
Appetite suppressants	Decreased clonidine effect.
Barbiturates	Increased chlorthalidone effect.
Beta-blockers	Blood-pressure control impaired.
Cholestyramine	Decreased chlorthalidone effect.
Cortisone drugs	Excessive potassium loss that causes dangerous heart rhythms.

Continued page 965

POSSIBLE INTERACTION WITH OTHER SUBSTANCES

INTERACTS WITH	COMBINED EFFECT
Alcohol:	Increased sensitivity to sedative effect of alcohol and very low blood pressure. Avoid.
Beverages: Caffeine-containing drinks.	Decreased clonidine effect.
Cocaine:	Blood pressure rise. Avoid.
Foods: Licorice.	Excessive potassium loss that causes dangerous heart rhythm.
Marijuana:	Weakness on standing. May increase blood pressure.
Tobacco:	None expected.

CLORAZEPATE

BRAND NAMES

Tranxene   Tranxene-SD

BASIC INFORMATION

Habit forming? Yes
Prescription needed? Yes
Available as generic? No
Drug class: Tranquilizer (benzodiazepine)

 USES

- Treatment for nervousness or tension.
- Treatment for convulsive disorders.

 DOSAGE & USAGE INFORMATION

How to take:
Tablet or capsule—Swallow with liquid. If you can't swallow whole, crumble tablet or open capsule and take with liquid or food.

When to take:
At the same time each day, according to instructions on prescription label.

If you forget a dose:
Take as soon as you remember up to 2 hours late. If more than 2 hours, wait for next scheduled dose (don't double this dose).

What drug does:
Affects limbic system of brain—part that controls emotions.

Time lapse before drug works:
2 hours. May take 6 weeks for full benefit.

Continued next column

 OVERDOSE

SYMPTOMS:
Drowsiness, weakness, tremor, stupor, coma.
WHAT TO DO:
- **Dial 0 (operator) or 911 (emergency) for an ambulance or medical help. Then give first aid immediately.**
- **If patient is unconscious and not breathing, give mouth-to-mouth breathing. If there is no heartbeat, use cardiac massage and mouth-to-mouth breathing (CPR). Don't try to make patient vomit. If you can't get help quickly, take patient to nearest emergency facility.**
- **See emergency information on inside covers.**

Don't take with:
See Interaction column and consult doctor.

 POSSIBLE ADVERSE REACTIONS OR SIDE EFFECTS

SYMPTOMS	WHAT TO DO
Life-threatening: None expected.	
Common: Clumsiness, drowsiness, dizziness.	Continue. Call doctor when convenient.
Infrequent:	
• Hallucinations, confusion, depression, irritability, rash, itch, vision changes.	Discontinue. Call doctor right away.
• Constipation or diarrhea, nausea, vomiting, difficult urination.	Continue. Call doctor when convenient.
Rare:	
• Slow heartbeat, breathing difficulty.	Discontinue. Seek emergency treatment.
• Mouth, throat ulcers; jaundice.	Discontinue. Call doctor right away.

WARNINGS & PRECAUTIONS

Don't take if:
- You are allergic to any benzodiazepine.
- You have myasthenia gravis.
- You are active or recovering alcoholic.
- Patient is younger than 6 months.

Before you start, consult your doctor:
- If you have liver, kidney or lung disease.
- If you have diabetes, epilepsy or porphyria.

Over age 60:
Adverse reactions and side effects may be more frequent and severe than in younger persons. You need smaller doses for shorter periods of time. May develop agitation, rage or "hangover" effect.

Pregnancy:
Risk to unborn child outweighs drug benefits. Don't use.

Breast-feeding:
Drug passes into milk. Avoid drug or discontinue nursing until you finish medicine. Consult doctor for advice on maintaining milk supply.

Infants & children:
Use only under medical supervision for children older than 6 months.

Prolonged use:
May impair liver function.

Skin & sunlight:
No problems expected.

Driving, piloting or hazardous work:
Don't drive or pilot aircraft until you learn how medicine affects you. Don't work around dangerous machinery. Don't climb ladders or work in high places. Danger increases if you drink alcohol or take medicine affecting alertness and reflexes.

Discontinuing:
Don't discontinue without consulting doctor. Dose may require gradual reduction if you have taken drug for a long time. Doses of other drugs may also require adjustment.

Others:
- Hot weather, heavy exercise and profuse sweat may reduce excretion and cause overdose.
- Blood sugar may rise in diabetics, requiring insulin adjustment.

POSSIBLE INTERACTION WITH OTHER DRUGS

GENERIC NAME OR DRUG CLASS	COMBINED EFFECT
Anticonvulsants	Change in seizure frequency or severity.
Antidepressants	Increased sedative effect of both drugs.
Antihistamines	Increased sedative effect of both drugs.
Antihypertensives	Excessively low blood pressure.
Cimetidine	Excess sedation.
Disulfiram	Increased clorazepate effect.
Dronabinol	Increased effects of both drugs. Avoid.
MAO inhibitors	Convulsions, deep sedation, rage.
Molindone	Increased tranquilizer effect.
Narcotics	Increased sedative effect of both drugs.
Sedatives	Increased sedative effect of both drugs.
Sleep inducers	Increased sedative effect of both drugs.
Tranquilizers	Increased sedative effect of both drugs.

POSSIBLE INTERACTION WITH OTHER SUBSTANCES

INTERACTS WITH	COMBINED EFFECT
Alcohol:	Heavy sedation. Avoid.
Beverages:	None expected.
Cocaine:	Decreased clorazepate effect.
Foods:	None expected.
Marijuana:	Heavy sedation. Avoid.
Tobacco:	Decreased clorazepate effect.

CLOXACILLIN

BRAND NAMES

Bactopen   Novocloxin
Cloxapen   Orbenin
Cloxilean   Tegopen

BASIC INFORMATION

Habit forming? No
Prescription needed? Yes
Available as generic? Yes
Drug class: Antibiotic (penicillin)

 USES

Treatment of bacterial infections that are
susceptible to cloxacillin.

 **DOSAGE & USAGE
INFORMATION**

How to take:
- Tablets or capsules—Swallow with liquid on
  an empty stomach 1 hour before or 2 hours
  after eating.
- Liquid—Take with cold beverage. Liquid form
  is perishable and effective for only 7 days at
  room temperature. Effective for 14 days if
  stored in refrigerator. Don't freeze.

When to take:
Follow instructions on prescription label or side
of package. Doses should be evenly spaced.
For example, 4 times a day means every 6
hours.

If you forget a dose:
Take as soon as you remember. Continue
regular schedule.

What drug does:
Destroys susceptible bacteria. Does not kill
viruses.

Time lapse before drug works:
May be several days before medicine affects
infection.

Don't take with:
See Interaction column and consult doctor.

 OVERDOSE

SYMPTOMS:
Severe diarrhea, nausea or vomiting.
WHAT TO DO:
**Overdose unlikely to threaten life. If person
takes much larger amount than prescribed,
call doctor, poison-control center or hospital
emergency room for instructions.**

 **POSSIBLE
ADVERSE REACTIONS
OR SIDE EFFECTS**

SYMPTOMS	WHAT TO DO
Life-threatening:	
Hives, rash, intense itching, faintness soon after a dose (anaphylaxis).	Seek emergency treatment immediately.
Common:	
Dark or discolored tongue.	Continue. Tell doctor at next visit.
Infrequent:	
Mild nausea, vomiting, diarrhea.	Continue. Call doctor when convenient.
Rare:	
Unexplained bleeding.	Discontinue. Call doctor right away.

WARNINGS & PRECAUTIONS

Don't take if:
You are allergic to cloxacillin, cephalosporin antibiotics, other penicillins or penicillamine. Life-threatening reaction may occur.

Before you start, consult your doctor:
If you are allergic to any substance or drug.

Over age 60:
You may have skin reactions, particularly around genitals and anus.

Pregnancy:
Studies inconclusive on harm to unborn child. Animal studies show fetal abnormalities. Decide with your doctor whether drug benefits justify risk to unborn child.

Breast-feeding:
Drug passes into milk. Child may become sensitive to penicillins and have allergic reactions to penicillin drugs. Avoid cloxacillin or discontinue nursing until you finish medicine. Consult doctor for advice on maintaining milk supply.

Infants & children:
No problems expected.

Prolonged use:
You may become more susceptible to infections caused by germs not responsive to cloxacillin.

Skin & sunlight:
No problems expected.

Driving, piloting or hazardous work:
Usually not dangerous. Most hazardous reactions likely to occur a few minutes after taking cloxacillin.

Discontinuing:
Don't discontinue without doctor's advice until you complete prescribed dose, even though symptoms diminish or disappear.

Others:
No problems expected.

POSSIBLE INTERACTION WITH OTHER DRUGS

GENERIC NAME OR DRUG CLASS	COMBINED EFFECT
Beta-adrenergic blockers	Increased chance of anaphylaxis (see emergency information on inside front cover).
Chloramphenicol	Decreased effect of both drugs.
Erythromycins	Decreased effect of both drugs.
Loperamide	Decreased cloxacillin effect.
Paromomycin	Decreased effect of both drugs.
Tetracyclines	Decreased effect of both drugs.
Troleandomycin	Decreased effect of both drugs.

POSSIBLE INTERACTION WITH OTHER SUBSTANCES

INTERACTS WITH	COMBINED EFFECT
Alcohol:	Occasional stomach irritation.
Beverages:	None expected.
Cocaine:	No proven problems.
Foods:	None expected.
Marijuana:	No proven problems.
Tobacco:	None expected.

COLCHICINE

BRAND NAMES

ColBenemid   Novocolchine
Col-Probenecid

BASIC INFORMATION

Habit forming? No
Prescription needed? Yes
Available as generic? Yes
Drug class: Antigout

 USES

Relieves joint pain, inflammation, swelling of gout.

 DOSAGE & USAGE INFORMATION

How to take:
- Tablet—Swallow with liquid or food to lessen stomach irritation.
- Granules—Dissolve in 3 oz. of fluid. Drink all fluid.

When to take:
As prescribed. Stop taking when pain stops or at first sign of digestive upset. Wait at least 3 days between treatments.

If you forget a dose:
Don't double next dose. Consult doctor.

What drug does:
Decreases acidity of joint tissues and prevents deposits of uric-acid crystals.

Time lapse before drug works:
12 to 48 hours.

Don't take with:
See Interaction column and consult doctor.

 OVERDOSE

SYMPTOMS:
Bloody urine, diarrhea, muscle weakness, fever, shortness of breath, stupor, convulsions, coma.
WHAT TO DO:
- Dial 0 (operator) or 911 (emergency) for an ambulance or medical help. Then give first aid immediately.
- See emergency information on inside covers.

 POSSIBLE ADVERSE REACTIONS OR SIDE EFFECTS

SYMPTOMS	WHAT TO DO
Life-threatening:	
Hives, rash, intense itching, faintness soon after a dose (anaphylaxis).	Seek emergency treatment immediately.
Common:	
Diarrhea, nausea, vomiting, abdominal pain.	Discontinue. Call doctor right away.
Infrequent:	
• Rash, itch, unusual bruising, blood in urine.	Discontinue. Call doctor right away.
• Numbness, tingling, pain or weakness in hands or feet; unusual tiredness or weakness; fever.	Continue. Call doctor when convenient.
Rare:	
Jaundice.	Discontinue. Call doctor right away.

WARNINGS & PRECAUTIONS

Don't take if:
You are allergic to colchicine.

Before you start, consult your doctor:
- If you have had peptic ulcers or ulcerative colitis.
- If you have heart, liver or kidney disease.
- If you will have surgery within 2 months, including dental surgery, requiring general or spinal anesthesia.

Over age 60:
Adverse reactions and side effects may be more frequent and severe than in younger persons. Colchicine has a narrow margin of safety for people in this age group.

Pregnancy:
Risk to unborn child outweighs drug benefits. Don't use.

Breast-feeding:
No problems expected, but consult doctor.

Infants & children:
Not recommended.

Prolonged use:
- Permanent hair loss.
- Anemia. Request blood counts.
- Numbness or tingling in hands and feet.

Skin & sunlight:
No problems expected.

Driving, piloting or hazardous work:
Don't drive or pilot aircraft until you learn how medicine affects you. Don't work around dangerous machinery. Don't climb ladders or work in high places. Danger increases if you drink alcohol or take medicine affecting alertness and reflexes, such as antihistamines, tranquilizers, sedatives, pain medicine, narcotics and mind-altering drugs.

Discontinuing:
- May be unnecessary to finish medicine. Follow doctor's instructions.
- Stop taking if digestive upsets occur before symptoms are relieved.

Others:
- Limit each course of treatment to 8 mg. Don't exceed 3 mg. per 24 hours.
- Possible sperm damage. May cause birth defects if child conceived while father taking colchicine.

POSSIBLE INTERACTION WITH OTHER DRUGS

GENERIC NAME OR DRUG CLASS	COMBINED EFFECT
Amphetamines	Increased amphetamine effect.
Anticoagulants	Decreased anticoagulant effect.
Antidepressants	Oversedation.
Antihistamines	Oversedation.
Antihypertensives	Decreased antihypertensive effect.
Appetite suppressants	Increased suppressant effect.
Mind-altering drugs	Oversedation.
Narcotics	Oversedation.
Sedatives	Oversedation.
Sleep inducers	Oversedation.
Tranquilizers	Oversedation.

POSSIBLE INTERACTION WITH OTHER SUBSTANCES

INTERACTS WITH	COMBINED EFFECT
Alcohol:	No proven problems.
Beverages: Herbal teas.	Increased colchicine effect. Avoid.
Cocaine:	Overstimulation. Avoid.
Foods:	No proven problems.
Marijuana:	Decreased colchicine effect.
Tobacco:	No proven problems.

COLESTIPOL

BRAND NAMES

Colestid

BASIC INFORMATION

Habit forming? No
Prescription needed? Yes
Available as generic? No
Drug class: Antihyperlipidemic

 USES

- Reduces cholesterol level in blood in patients with type IIa hyperlipidemia.
- Treats overdose of digitalis.
- Reduces skin itching associated with some forms of liver disease.
- Treats diarrhea after some surgical operations.

 DOSAGE & USAGE INFORMATION

How to take:
Mix well with 6 ounces or more or water or liquid, or in soups, pulpy fruits, with milk or in cereals. Will not dissolve.

When to take:
Before meals.

If you forget a dose:
Take as soon as you remember up to 2 hours late. If more than 2 hours, wait for next scheduled dose (don't double this dose).

What drug does:
Binds with bile acids in intestines, preventing reabsorption.

Time lapse before drug works:
3 to 12 months.

Don't take with:
See Interaction column and consult doctor.

 OVERDOSE

SYMPTOMS:
Fecal impaction.
WHAT TO DO:
Overdose unlikely to threaten life. If person takes much larger amount than prescribed, call doctor, poison-control center or hospital emergency room for instructions.

 POSSIBLE ADVERSE REACTIONS OR SIDE EFFECTS

SYMPTOMS	WHAT TO DO
Life-threatening: None expected.	
Common: None expected.	
Infrequent:	
• Black, tarry stools from gastrointestinal bleeding.	Discontinue. Seek emergency treatment.
• Severe abdominal pain.	Discontinue. Call doctor right away.
• Constipation, belching, diarrhea, nausea, unexpected weight loss.	Continue. Call doctor when convenient.
Rare: None expected.	

WARNINGS & PRECAUTIONS

Don't take if:
You are allergic to colestipol.

Before you start, consult your doctor:
- If you have liver disease such as cirrhosis.
- If you are jaundiced.
- If you will have surgery within 2 months, including dental surgery, requiring general or spinal anesthesia.
- If you are constipated.
- If you have peptic ulcer.
- If you have coronary artery disease.

Over age 60:
Constipation more likely. Other adverse effects more likely.

Pregnancy:
No proven harm to unborn child. Avoid if possible.

Breast-feeding:
No proven harm to child. Consult doctor.

Infants & children:
Only under expert medical supervision.

Prolonged use:
Request lab studies to determine serum cholesterol and serum triglycerides.

Skin & sunlight:
No problems expected.

Driving, piloting or hazardous work:
No problems expected.

Discontinuing:
Don't discontinue without consulting doctor. Dose may require gradual reduction if you have taken drug for a long time. Doses of other drugs may also require adjustment, particularly digitalis.

Others:
This medicine does not cure disorders, but helps to control them.

 POSSIBLE INTERACTION WITH OTHER DRUGS

GENERIC NAME OR DRUG CLASS	COMBINED EFFECT
Anticoagulants	Decreased anticoagulant effect.
Digitalis preparations	Decreased absorption.
Diuretics (thiazide)	Decreased absorption.
Penicillins	Decreased absorption.
Tetracyclines	Decreased absorption.
Vitamins	Decreased absorption of fat-soluble vitamins (A,D,E,K)
Other medicines	May delay or reduce absorption.

 POSSIBLE INTERACTION WITH OTHER SUBSTANCES

INTERACTS WITH	COMBINED EFFECT
Alcohol:	None expected.
Beverages:	None expected.
Cocaine:	None expected.
Foods:	Interferes with absorption of vitamins. Take supplements.
Marijuana:	None expected.
Tobacco:	None expected.

CONJUGATED ESTROGENS

BRAND NAMES

Premarin

BASIC INFORMATION

Habit forming? No
Prescription needed? Yes
Available as generic? Yes
Drug class: Female sex hormone (estrogen)

 USES

- Treatment for symptoms of menopause and menstrual-cycle irregularity.
- Replacement for female hormone deficiency.
- Treatment for estrogen-deficiency osteoporosis (bone softening from calcium loss).
- Treatment for cancer of prostate and breast.

 DOSAGE & USAGE INFORMATION

How to take:
- Tablet—Swallow with liquid. If you can't swallow whole, crumble tablet and take with liquid or food.
- Vaginal cream—Use as directed on label.

When to take:
At the same time each day.

If you forget a dose:
Take as soon as you remember up to 12 hours late. If more than 12 hours, wait for next scheduled dose (don't double this dose).

What drug does:
Restores normal estrogen level in tissues.

Time lapse before drug works:
10 to 20 days.

Don't take with:
See Interaction column and consult doctor.

 OVERDOSE

SYMPTOMS:
Nausea, vomiting, fluid retention, breast enlargement and discomfort, abnormal vaginal bleeding.
WHAT TO DO:
Overdose unlikely to threaten life. If person takes much larger amount than prescribed, call doctor, poison-control center or hospital emergency room for instructions.

 POSSIBLE ADVERSE REACTIONS OR SIDE EFFECTS

SYMPTOMS	WHAT TO DO
Life-threatening:	
None expected.	
Common:	
• Stomach cramps.	Discontinue. Call doctor right away.
• Appetite loss.	Continue. Call doctor when convenient.
• Nausea; diarrhea; swollen ankles or feet; swollen, tender breasts.	Continue. Tell doctor at next visit.
Infrequent:	
• Rash, stomach or side pain.	Discontinue. Call doctor right away.
• Depression, dizziness, irritability, vomiting, breast lumps.	Continue. Call doctor when convenient.
• Brown blotches on skin, hair loss, vaginal discharge or bleeding, changes in sex drive.	Continue. Tell doctor at next visit.
Rare:	
Jaundice.	Discontinue. Call doctor right away.

WARNINGS & PRECAUTIONS

Don't take if:
- You are allergic to any estrogen-containing drugs.
- You have impaired liver function.
- You have had blood clots, stroke or heart attack.
- You have unexplained vaginal bleeding.

Before you start, consult your doctor:
- If you have had cancer of breast or reproductive organs, fibrocystic breast disease, fibroid tumors of the uterus or endometriosis.
- If you have had migraine headaches, epilepsy or porphyria.
- If you have diabetes, high blood pressure, asthma, congestive heart failure, kidney disease or gallstones.
- If you plan to become pregnant within 3 months.

Over age 60:
Controversial. You and your doctor must decide if drug risks outweigh benefits.

Pregnancy:
Risk to unborn child outweighs drug benefits. Don't use.

Breast-feeding:
Drug filters into milk. May harm child. Avoid.

Infants & children:
Not recommended.

Prolonged use:
Increased growth of fibroid tumors of uterus. Possible association with cancer of uterus.

Skin & sunlight:
May cause rash or intensify sunburn in areas exposed to sun or sunlamp.

Driving, piloting or hazardous work:
No problems expected.

Discontinuing:
You may need to discontinue estrogen periodically. Consult your doctor.

Others:
In rare instances, may cause blood clot in lung, brain or leg. Symptoms are *sudden* severe headache, coordination loss, vision change, chest pain, breathing difficulty, slurred speech, pain in legs or groin. Seek emergency treatment immediately.

POSSIBLE INTERACTION WITH OTHER DRUGS

GENERIC NAME OR DRUG CLASS	COMBINED EFFECT
Anticoagulants (oral)	Decreased anticoagulant effect.
Anticonvulsants (hydantoin)	Increased seizures.
Antidiabetics (oral)	Unpredictable increase or decrease in blood sugar.
Carbamazepine	Increased seizures.
Clofibrate	Decreased clofibrate effect.
Meprobamate	Increased effect of conjugated estrogens.
Phenobarbital	Decreased effect of conjugated estrogens.
Primidone	Decreased effect of conjugated estrogens.
Rifampin	Decreased effect of conjugated estrogens.
Thyroid hormones	Decreased thyroid effect.

POSSIBLE INTERACTION WITH OTHER SUBSTANCES

INTERACTS WITH	COMBINED EFFECT
Alcohol:	None expected.
Beverages:	None expected.
Cocaine:	No proven problems.
Foods:	None expected.
Marijuana:	Possible menstrual irregularities and bleeding between periods.
Tobacco:	Increased risk of blood clots leading to stroke or heart attack.

CONTRACEPTIVES (ORAL)

BRAND NAMES

See complete list of brand names in the *Brand Name Directory*, page 947.

BASIC INFORMATION

Habit forming? No
Prescription needed? Yes
Available as generic? Yes
Drug class: Female sex hormone, contraceptive

 USES

- Prevents pregnancy.
- Regulates menstrual periods.

 DOSAGE & USAGE INFORMATION

How to take:
Tablet or capsule—Swallow with liquid or food to lessen stomach irritation.

When to take:
At same time each day according to prescribed instructions, usually for 21 days of 28-day cycle.

If you forget a dose:
Call doctor's office for advice about additional protection against pregnancy.

What drug does:
- Alters mucus at cervix entrance to prevent sperm entry.
- Alters uterus lining to resist implantation of fertilized egg.
- Creates same chemical atmosphere in blood that exists during pregnancy, suppressing pituitary hormones which stimulate ovulation.

Time lapse before drug works:
10 days or more to provide contraception.

Don't take with:
- Tobacco
- See Interaction column and consult doctor.

 OVERDOSE

SYMPTOMS:
Drowsiness
WHAT TO DO:
Overdose unlikely to threaten life. If person takes much larger amount than prescribed, call doctor, poison-control center or hospital emergency room for instructions.

 POSSIBLE ADVERSE REACTIONS OR SIDE EFFECTS

SYMPTOMS	WHAT TO DO
Life-threatening:	
Stroke, chest pain.	Seek emergency treatment immediately.
Common:	
Brown blotches on skin; vaginal discharge, itch; fluid retention.	Continue. Call doctor when convenient.
Infrequent:	
• Headache; depression; blood clots, pain, swelling in leg; muscle, joint pain.	Discontinue. Call doctor right away.
• Blue tinge to objects, lights; appetite change; nausea; bloating; vomiting; pain; changed sex drive.	Continue. Call doctor when convenient.
Rare:	
• Clotting tendency.	Discontinue. Seek emergency treatment.
• Jaundice, rash, hives, itch.	Discontinue. Call doctor right away.

 WARNINGS & PRECAUTIONS

Don't take if:
- You are allergic to any female hormone.
- You have had heart disease, blood clots or stroke.
- You have liver disease.
- You have cancer of breast, uterus or ovaries.
- You have unexplained vaginal bleeding.

Before you start, consult your doctor:
- If you have fibrocystic disease of breast.
- If you have migraine headaches.
- If you have fibroid tumors of uterus.
- If you have epilepsy.
- If you have asthma.
- If you have high blood pressure.
- If you will have surgery within 2 months, including dental surgery, requiring general or spinal anesthesia.
- If you have endometriosis.
- If you have diabetes.
- If you have sickle-cell anemia.
- If you smoke cigarettes.

Over age 60:
Not used.

Pregnancy:
May harm child. Discontinue at first sign of pregnancy.

Breast-feeding:
Drug passes into milk. Avoid drug or discontinue nursing.

Infants & children:
Not recommended.

Prolonged use:
- Gallstones.
- Gradual blood-pressure rise.
- Possible difficulty becoming pregnant after discontinuing.

Skin & sunlight:
May cause rash or intensify sunburn in areas exposed to sun or sunlamp.

Driving, piloting or hazardous work:
No problems expected.

Discontinuing:
Don't become pregnant for 6 months after discontinuing.

Others:
Failure to take oral contraceptives for 1 day may cancel pregnancy protection. If you forget a dose, use other contraceptive measures and call doctor for instructions on re-starting oral contraceptive.

POSSIBLE INTERACTION WITH OTHER DRUGS

GENERIC NAME OR DRUG CLASS	COMBINED EFFECT
Ampicillin	Decreased contraceptive effect.
Anticoagulants	Decreased anticoagulant effect.
Anticonvulsants (hydantoin)	Decreased contraceptive effect.
Antidiabetics	Decreased antidiabetic effect.
Antihistamines	Decreased contraceptive effect.
Anti-inflammatory drugs (non-steroid)	Decreased contraceptive effect.
Barbiturates	Decreased contraceptive effect.
Chloramphenicol	Decreased contraceptive effect.
Clofibrate	Decreased clofibrate effect.
Guanethidine	Decreased guanethidine effect.
Meperidine	Increased meperidine effect.
Meprobamate	Decreased contraceptive effect.
Mineral oil	Decreased contraceptive effect.
Phenothiazines	Increased phenothiazine effect.
Rifampin	Decreased contraceptive effect.
Tetracyclines	Decreased contraceptive effect.

POSSIBLE INTERACTION WITH OTHER SUBSTANCES

INTERACTS WITH	COMBINED EFFECT
Alcohol:	No proven problems.
Beverages:	No proven problems.
Cocaine:	No proven problems.
Foods: Salt.	Increased edema (fluid retention).
Marijuana:	Increased bleeding between periods. Avoid.
Tobacco:	Possible heart attack, blood clots and stroke.

CORTISONE

BRAND NAMES

Cortelan   Cortone
Cortistab

BASIC INFORMATION

Habit forming? No
Prescription needed? Yes
Available as generic? Yes
Drug class: Cortisone drug (adrenal corticosteroid)

USES

- Reduces inflammation caused by many different medical problems.
- Treatment for some allergic diseases, blood disorders, kidney diseases, asthma and emphysema.
- Replaces corticosteroid deficiencies.

DOSAGE & USAGE INFORMATION

How to take:
Tablet—Swallow with liquid or food to lessen stomach irritation. If you can't swallow whole, crumble tablet and take with liquid or food.

When to take:
At the same times each day. Take once-a-day or once-every-other-day doses in mornings.

If you forget a dose:
- Several-doses-per-day prescription—Take as soon as you remember up to 2 hours late. If more than 2 hours, wait for next scheduled dose (don't double this dose).
- Once-a-day dose or less—Wait for next dose. Double this dose.

What drug does:
Decreases inflammatory responses.

Time lapse before drug works:
2 to 4 days.

Don't take with:
See Interaction column and consult doctor.

OVERDOSE

SYMPTOMS:
Headache, convulsions, heart failure.
WHAT TO DO:
- Dial 0 (operator) or 911 (emergency) for an ambulance or medical help. Then give first aid immediately.
- See emergency information on inside covers.

POSSIBLE ADVERSE REACTIONS OR SIDE EFFECTS

SYMPTOMS	WHAT TO DO
Life-threatening: None expected.	
Common: Acne, thirst, indigestion, nausea, vomiting, poor wound healing.	Continue. Call doctor when convenient.
Infrequent:	
• Bloody or black, tarry stool.	Discontinue. Seek emergency treatment.
• Blurred vision; halos around lights; sore throat, fever; muscle cramps; swollen legs, feet.	Discontinue. Call doctor right away.
• Mood changes, insomnia, restlessness, frequent urination, weight gain, round face, fatigue, weakness, TB recurrence, irregular menstrual periods.	Continue. Call doctor when convenient.
Rare:	
• Irregular heartbeat.	Discontinue. Seek emergency treatment.
• Rash.	Discontinue. Call doctor right away.

WARNINGS & PRECAUTIONS

Don't take if:
- You are allergic to any cortisone drug.
- You have tuberculosis or fungus infection.
- You have herpes infection of eyes, lips or genitals.

Before you start, consult your doctor:
- If you have had tuberculosis.
- If you have congestive heart failure.
- If you have diabetes.
- If you have peptic ulcer.
- If you have glaucoma.
- If you have underactive thyroid.
- If you have high blood pressure.
- If you have myasthenia gravis.
- If you have blood clots in legs or lungs.

Over age 60:
Adverse reactions and side effects may be more frequent and severe than in younger persons. Likely to aggravate edema, diabetes or ulcers. Likely to cause cataracts and osteoporosis (softening of the bones).

Pregnancy:
Risk to unborn child outweighs drug benefits. Don't use.

Breast-feeding:
Drug passes into milk. Avoid drug or discontinue nursing until you finish medicine. Consult doctor for advice on maintaining milk supply.

Infants & children:
Use only under medical supervision.

Prolonged use:
- Retards growth in children.
- Possible glaucoma, cataracts, diabetes, fragile bones and thin skin.
- Functional dependence.

Skin & sunlight:
No problems expected.

Driving, piloting or hazardous work:
No problems expected.

Discontinuing:
- Don't discontinue without doctor's advice until you complete prescribed dose, even though symptoms diminish or disappear.
- Drug affects your response to surgery, illness, injury or stress for 2 years after discontinuing. Tell anyone who takes medical care of you within 2 years about drug.

Others:
Avoid immunizations if possible.

POSSIBLE INTERACTION WITH OTHER DRUGS

GENERIC NAME OR DRUG CLASS	COMBINED EFFECT
Amphoterecin B	Potassium depletion.
Anticholinergics	Possible glaucoma.
Anticoagulants (oral)	Decreased anticoagulant effect.
Anticonvulsants (hydantoin)	Decreased cortisone effect.
Antidiabetics (oral)	Decreased antidiabetic effect.
Antihistamines	Decreased cortisone effect.
Aspirin	Increased cortisone effect.
Barbiturates	Decreased cortisone effect. Oversedation.
Beta-adrenergic blockers	Decreased cortisone effect.
Chloral hydrate	Decreased cortisone effect.
Chlorthalidone	Potassium depletion.

Cholinergics	Decreased cholinergic effect.
Contraceptives (oral)	Increased cortisone effect.
Digitalis preparations	Dangerous potassium depletion. Possible digitalis toxicity.
Diuretics (thiazide)	Potassium depletion.
Ephedrine	Decreased cortisone effect.
Estrogens	Increased cortisone effect.
Ethacrynic acid	Potassium depletion.
Furosemide	Potassium depletion.
Glutethimide	Decreased cortisone effect.
Indapamide	Possible excessive potassium loss, causing dangerous heartbeat irregularity.
Indomethacin	Increased cortisone effect.
Insulin	Decreased insulin effect.
Isoniazid	Decreased isoniazid effect.
Ketoprofen	Increased risk of stomach ulcer and bleeding.
Oxyphenbutazone	Possible ulcers.
Phenylbutazone	Possible ulcers.
Potassium supplements	Decreased potassium effect.
Rifampin	Decreased cortisone effect.

Continued page 965

POSSIBLE INTERACTION WITH OTHER SUBSTANCES

INTERACTS WITH	COMBINED EFFECT
Alcohol:	Risk of stomach ulcers.
Beverages:	No proven problems.
Cocaine:	Overstimulation. Avoid.
Foods:	No proven problems.
Marijuana:	Decreased immunity.
Tobacco:	Increased cortisone effect. Possible toxicity.

CROMOLYN

BRAND NAMES

Fivent
Intal
Nalcrom
Nasalcrom

Opticrom
Rynacrom
Sodium
   Cromoblycate

BASIC INFORMATION

Habit forming? No
Prescription needed? Yes
Available as generic? No
Drug class: Antiasthmatic, anti-inflammatory

 USES

- Prevents asthma attacks. Will not stop an active asthma attack.
- Treatment for inflammation of covering to eye and cornea.
- Reduces nasal allergic symptoms.

 DOSAGE & USAGE INFORMATION

How to take:
- Inhaler—Follow instructions enclosed with inhaler. Don't swallow cartridges for inhaler. Gargle and rinse mouth after inhalations.
- Eye drops—Follow prescription instructions.
- Nasal solution—Follow prescription instructions.

When to take:
At the same times each day. If you also use a bronchodilator inhaler, use the bronchodilator before the cromolyn.

If you forget a dose:
Take as soon as you remember up to 2 hours late. If more than 2 hours, wait for next scheduled dose (don't double this dose).

What drug does:
Blocks histamine release from mast cells.

Time lapse before drug works:
- 4 weeks for prevention of asthma attacks.
- 1 to 2 weeks for nasal or eye symptoms.

Continued next column

 OVERDOSE

SYMPTOMS:
Increased side effects and adverse reactions listed.
WHAT TO DO:
Overdose unlikely to threaten life. If person inhales much larger amount than prescribed, call doctor, poison-control center or hospital emergency room for instructions.

Don't take with:
See Interaction column and consult doctor.

 POSSIBLE ADVERSE REACTIONS OR SIDE EFFECTS

SYMPTOMS	WHAT TO DO
Life-threatening:	
Hives, rash, intense itching, faintness soon after a dose (anaphylaxis).	Seek emergency treatment immediately.
Common:	
Hoarseness, cough.	Continue. Call doctor when convenient.
Infrequent:	
• Rash, hives, swallowing difficulty, nausea, vomiting, increased wheezing, joint pain or swelling, muscle pain, weakness, difficult or painful urination.	Discontinue. Call doctor right away.
• Drowsiness, dizziness, headache, watery eyes, stuffy nose, throat irritation.	Continue. Call doctor when convenient.
Rare:	
Nosebleed.	Continue. Call doctor when convenient.

WARNINGS & PRECAUTIONS

Don't take if:
You are allergic to cromolyn, lactose, milk or milk products.

Before you start, consult your doctor:
- If you plan to become pregnant within medication period.
- If you have kidney or liver disease.

Over age 60:
Adverse reactions and side effects may be more frequent and severe than in younger persons.

Pregnancy:
Risk to unborn child outweighs drug benefits. Don't use.

Breast-feeding:
Drug passes into milk. Avoid drug or discontinue nursing.

Infants & children:
Use only under medical supervision.

Prolonged use:
No problems expected.

Skin & sunlight:
No problems expected.

Driving, piloting or hazardous work:
No problems expected.

Discontinuing:
No problems expected.

Others:
- Inhaler must be cleaned and work well for drug to be effective.
- This treatment does not stop an acute asthma attack. It may aggravate it.
- Eye drops:
  Wash hands. Apply pressure to inside corner of eye with middle finger. Continue pressure for 1 minute after placing medicine in eye. Tilt head backward. Pull lower lid away from eye with index finger of the same hand. Drop eye drops into pouch and close eye. Don't blink. Keep eyes closed for 1 to 2 minutes. Don't touch applicator tip to any surface (including the eye). If you accidentally touch tip, clean with warm soap and water. Keep container tightly closed. Keep cool, but don't freeze. Wash hands immediately after using.

POSSIBLE INTERACTION WITH OTHER DRUGS

GENERIC NAME OR DRUG CLASS	COMBINED EFFECT
Cortisone drugs	Increased cortisone effect in treating asthma. Cortisone dose may be decreased.

POSSIBLE INTERACTION WITH OTHER SUBSTANCES

INTERACTS WITH	COMBINED EFFECT
Alcohol:	None expected.
Beverages:	None expected.
Cocaine:	None expected.
Foods:	None expected.
Marijuana:	None expected.
Tobacco:	None expected, but tobacco smoke aggravates asthma and eye irritation. Avoid.

CYCLACILLIN

BRAND NAMES

Cyclapen-W

BASIC INFORMATION

Habit forming? No
Prescription needed? Yes
Available as generic? Yes
Drug class: Antibiotic (penicillin)

 USES

Treatment of bacterial infections that are susceptible to cyclacillin.

 DOSAGE & USAGE INFORMATION

How to take:
- Tablets or capsules—Swallow with liquid on an empty stomach 1 hour before or 2 hours after eating.
- Liquid—Take with cold beverage. Liquid form is perishable and effective for only 7 days at room temperature. Effective for 14 days if stored in refrigerator. Don't freeze.

When to take:
Follow instructions on prescription label or side of package. Doses should be evenly spaced. For example, 4 times a day means every 6 hours.

If you forget a dose:
Take as soon as you remember. Continue regular schedule.

What drug does:
Destroys susceptible bacteria. Does not kill viruses.

Time lapse before drug works:
May be several days before medicine affects infection.

Don't take with:
See Interaction column and consult doctor.

 OVERDOSE

SYMPTOMS:
Severe diarrhea, nausea or vomiting.
WHAT TO DO:
Overdose unlikely to threaten life. If person takes much larger amount than prescribed, call doctor, poison-control center or hospital emergency room for instructions.

 POSSIBLE ADVERSE REACTIONS OR SIDE EFFECTS

SYMPTOMS	WHAT TO DO
Life-threatening:	
Hives, rash, intense itching, faintness soon after a dose (anaphylaxis).	Seek emergency treatment immediately.
Common:	
Dark or discolored tongue.	Continue. Tell doctor at next visit.
Infrequent:	
Mild nausea, vomiting, diarrhea.	Continue. Call doctor when convenient.
Rare:	
Unexplained bleeding.	Discontinue. Call doctor right away.

WARNINGS & PRECAUTIONS

Don't take if:
Your are allergic to cyclacillin, cephalosporin antibiotics, other penicillins or penicillamine. Life-threatening reaction may occur.

Before you start, consult your doctor:
If you are allergic to any substance or drug.

Over age 60:
You may have skin reactions, particularly around genitals and anus.

Pregnancy:
Studies inconclusive on harm to unborn child. Animal studies show fetal abnormalities. Decide with your doctor whether drug benefits justify risk to unborn child.

Breast-feeding:
Drug passes into milk. Child may become sensitive to penicillins and have allergic reactions to penicillin drugs. Avoid cyclacillin or discontinue nursing until you finish medicine. Consult doctor for advice on maintaining milk supply.

Infants & children:
No problems expected.

Prolonged use:
You may become more susceptible to infections caused by germs not responsive to cyclacillin.

Skin & sunlight:
No problems expected.

Driving, piloting or hazardous work:
Usually not dangerous. Most hazardous reactions likely to occur a few minutes after taking cyclacillin.

Discontinuing:
Don't discontinue without doctor's advice until you complete prescribed dose, even though symptoms diminish or disappear.

Others:
No problems expected.

 ## POSSIBLE INTERACTION WITH OTHER DRUGS

GENERIC NAME OR DRUG CLASS	COMBINED EFFECT
Beta-adrenergic blockers	Increased chance of anaphylaxis (see emergency information on inside front cover).
Chloramphenicol	Decreased effect of both drugs.
Erythromycins	Decreased effect of both drugs.
Loperamide	Decreased cyclacillin effect.
Paromomycin	Decreased effect of both drugs.
Tetracyclines	Decreased effect of both drugs.
Troleandomycin	Decreased effect of both drugs.

 ## POSSIBLE INTERACTION WITH OTHER SUBSTANCES

INTERACTS WITH	COMBINED EFFECT
Alcohol:	Occasional stomach irritation.
Beverages:	None expected.
Cocaine:	No proven problems.
Foods:	Decreased effect of cyclacillin.
Marijuana:	No proven problems.
Tobacco:	None expected.

CYCLANDELATE

BRAND NAMES

Cyclospasmol   Cyraso-400

BASIC INFORMATION

Habit forming? No
Prescription needed?
  U.S.: Yes
  Canada: No
Available as generic? Yes
Drug class: Vasodilator

 USES

Improves poor blood flow to brain and extremities.

 DOSAGE & USAGE INFORMATION

How to take:
Tablet or capsule—Swallow with liquid. If you can't swallow whole, crumble tablet or open capsule and take with liquid or food.

When to take:
At the same time each day.

If you forget a dose:
Take as soon as you remember up to 2 hours late. If more than 2 hours, wait for next scheduled dose (don't double this dose).

What drug does:
Increases blood flow by relaxing and expanding blood-vessel walls.

Time lapse before drug works:
3 weeks.

Don't take with:
See Interaction column and consult doctor.

 OVERDOSE

SYMPTOMS:
Severe headache, dizziness; nausea, vomiting; flushed, hot face.
WHAT TO DO:
Overdose unlikely to threaten life. If person takes much larger amount than prescribed, call doctor, poison-control center or hospital emergency room for instructions.

 POSSIBLE ADVERSE REACTIONS OR SIDE EFFECTS

SYMPTOMS	WHAT TO DO
Life-threatening:	
None expected.	
Common:	
None expected.	
Infrequent:	
● Rapid heartbeat.	Discontinue. Call doctor right away.
● Dizziness; headache; weakness; flushed face; tingling in face, fingers or toes; unusual sweating.	Continue. Call doctor when convenient.
● Belching, heartburn, nausea or stomach pain.	Continue. Tell doctor at next visit.
Rare:	
None expected.	

WARNINGS & PRECAUTIONS

Don't take if:
You have had allergic reaction to cyclandelate.

Before you start, consult your doctor:
• If you have glaucoma.
• If you have had heart attack or stroke.

Over age 60:
Adverse reactions and side effects may be more frequent and severe than in younger persons.

Pregnancy:
No proven harm to unborn child. Avoid if possible.

Breast-feeding:
No proven problems. Consult doctor.

Infants & children:
Not recommended.

Prolonged use:
No problems expected.

Skin & sunlight:
No problems expected.

Driving, piloting or hazardous work:
Avoid if you feel dizzy or weak. Otherwise, no problems expected.

Discontinuing:
Don't discontinue without doctor's advice until you complete prescribed dose, even though symptoms diminish or disappear.

Others:
Response to drug varies. If your symptoms don't improve after 3 weeks of use, consult doctor.

POSSIBLE INTERACTION WITH OTHER DRUGS

GENERIC NAME OR DRUG CLASS	COMBINED EFFECT
None	

POSSIBLE INTERACTION WITH OTHER SUBSTANCES

INTERACTS WITH	COMBINED EFFECT
Alcohol:	None expected.
Beverages:	None expected.
Cocaine:	Decreased cyclandelate effect. Avoid.
Foods:	None expected.
Marijuana:	None expected.
Tobacco:	May decrease cyclandelate effect.

CYCLIZINE

BRAND NAMES

Marezine   Marzine

BASIC INFORMATION

Habit forming? No
Prescription needed?
  U.S.: No
  Canada: Yes
Available as generic? No
Drug class: Antihistamine, antiemetic

 ## USES

Prevents motion sickness.

 ## DOSAGE & USAGE INFORMATION

How to take:
Tablet—Swallow with liquid or food to lessen stomach irritation. If you can't swallow whole, crumble tablet and chew or take with liquid or food.

When to take:
30 minutes to 1 hour before traveling.

If you forget a dose:
Take as soon as you remember. Wait 4 hours for next dose.

What drug does:
Reduces sensitivity of nerve endings in inner ear, blocking messages to brain's vomiting center.

Time lapse before drug works:
30 to 60 minutes.

Don't take with:
See Interaction column and consult doctor.

 ## OVERDOSE

SYMPTOMS:
Drowsiness, confusion, incoordination, stupor, coma, weak pulse, shallow breathing.
WHAT TO DO:
- Dial 0 (operator) or 911 (emergency) for an ambulance or medical help. Then give first aid immediately.
- See emergency information on inside covers.

 ## POSSIBLE ADVERSE REACTIONS OR SIDE EFFECTS

SYMPTOMS	WHAT TO DO
Life-threatening:	
None expected.	
Common:	
Drowsiness.	Continue. Tell doctor at next visit.
Infrequent:	
• Headache, diarrhea or constipation, fast heartbeat.	Continue. Call doctor when convenient.
• Dry mouth, nose, throat.	Continue. Tell doctor at next visit.
Rare:	
• Rash or hives, jaundice.	Discontinue. Call doctor right away.
• Restlessness, excitement, insomnia, blurred vision, frequent or difficult urination.	Continue. Call doctor when convenient.
• Appetite loss, nausea.	Continue. Tell doctor at next visit.

WARNINGS & PRECAUTIONS

Don't take if:
- You are allergic to meclizine, buclizine or cyclizine.
- You have taken MAO inhibitors in the past 2 weeks.

Before you start, consult your doctor:
- If you have glaucoma.
- If you have prostate enlargement.
- If you have reacted badly to any antihistamine.

Over age 60:
Adverse reactions and side effects may be more frequent and severe than in younger persons, especially impaired urination from enlarged prostate gland.

Pregnancy:
Studies inconclusive on harm to unborn child. Animal studies show fetal abnormalities. Decide with your doctor whether drug benefits justify risk to unborn child.

Breast-feeding:
Drug passes into milk. Avoid drug or discontinue nursing until you finish medicine. Consult doctor for advice on maintaining milk supply.

Infants & children:
No problems expected.

Prolonged use:
No problems expected.

Skin & sunlight:
No problems expected.

Driving, piloting or hazardous work:
Don't fly aircraft. Don't drive until you learn how medicine affects you. Don't work around dangerous machinery. Don't climb ladders or work in high places. Danger increases if you drink alcohol or take medicine affecting alertness and reflexes, such as antihistamines, tranquilizers, sedatives, pain medicine, narcotics and mind-altering drugs.

Discontinuing:
No problems expected.

Others:
No problems expected.

POSSIBLE INTERACTION WITH OTHER DRUGS

GENERIC NAME OR DRUG CLASS	COMBINED EFFECT
Amphetamines	May decrease drowsiness caused by cyclizine.
Anticholinergics	Increased effect of both drugs.
Antidepressants (tricyclic)	Increased effect of both drugs.
MAO inhibitors	Increased cyclizine effect.
Narcotics	Increased effect of both drugs.
Pain relievers	Increased effect of both drugs.
Sedatives	Increased effect of both drugs.
Sleep inducers	Increased effect of both drugs.
Tranquilizers	Increased effect of both drugs.

POSSIBLE INTERACTION WITH OTHER SUBSTANCES

INTERACTS WITH	COMBINED EFFECT
Alcohol:	Increased sedation. Avoid.
Beverages: Caffeine drinks.	May decrease drowsiness.
Cocaine:	None expected.
Foods:	None expected.
Marijuana:	Increased drowsiness, dry mouth.
Tobacco:	None expected.

CYCLOBENZAPRINE

BRAND NAMES

Flexeril

BASIC INFORMATION

Habit forming? No
Prescription needed? Yes
Available as generic? No
Drug class: Muscle relaxant (skeletal)

 USES

Treatment for pain and limited motion caused by spasms in voluntary muscles.

 DOSAGE & USAGE INFORMATION

How to take:
Tablet or capsule—Swallow with liquid.

When to take:
At the same time each day or according to label instructions.

If you forget a dose:
Take as soon as you remember. Wait 4 hours for next dose.

What drug does:
Blocks body's pain messages to brain. May also sedate.

Time lapse before drug works:
30 to 60 minutes.

Continued next column

 OVERDOSE

SYMPTOMS:
Drowsiness, confusion, difficulty concentrating, visual problems, vomiting, blood-pressure drop, low body temperature, weak and rapid pulse, convulsions, coma.
WHAT TO DO:
- **Dial 0 (operator) or 911 (emergency) for an ambulance or medical help. Then give first aid immediately.**
- **If patient is unconscious and not breathing, give mouth-to-mouth breathing. If there is no heartbeat, use cardiac massage and mouth-to-mouth breathing (CPR). Don't try to make patient vomit. If you can't get help quickly, take patient to nearest emergency facility.**
- **See emergency information on inside covers.**

Don't take with:
- Non-prescription drugs without consulting doctor.
- See Interaction column and consult doctor.

 POSSIBLE ADVERSE REACTIONS OR SIDE EFFECTS

SYMPTOMS	WHAT TO DO
Life-threatening:	
None expected.	
Common:	
Drowsiness, dizziness, dry mouth.	Continue. Call doctor when convenient.
Infrequent:	
• Blurred vision, fast heartbeat.	Discontinue. Call doctor right away.
• Insomnia, numbness in extremities, bad taste in mouth.	Continue. Call doctor when convenient.
Rare:	
• Unsteadiness, confusion, depression, hallucinations, rash, itch, swelling, breathing difficulty.	Discontinue. Call doctor right away.
• Difficult urination.	Continue. Call doctor when convenient.

WARNINGS & PRECAUTIONS

Don't take if:
- You are allergic to any skeletal-muscle relaxant.
- You have taken MAO inhibitors in last 2 weeks.
- You have had a heart attack within 6 weeks, or suffer from congestive heart failure.
- You have overactive thyroid.

Before you start, consult your doctor:
- If you have a heart problem.
- If you have reacted to tricyclic antidepressants.
- If you have glaucoma.
- If you have a prostate condition and urination difficulty.
- If you intend to pilot aircraft.

Over age 60:
Adverse reactions and side effects may be more frequent and severe than in younger persons. Avoid extremes of heat and cold.

Pregnancy:
Risk to unborn child outweighs drug benefits. Don't use.

Breast-feeding:
Drug passes into milk. Avoid drug or discontinue nursing until you finish medicine. Consult doctor for advice on maintaining milk supply.

Infants & children:
Don't use for children younger than 15.

Prolonged use:
No problems expected.

Skin & sunlight:
May cause rash or intensify sunburn in areas exposed to sun or sunlamp.

Driving, piloting or hazardous work:
Don't drive or pilot aircraft until you learn how medicine affects you. Don't work around dangerous machinery. Don't climb ladders or work in high places. Danger increases if you drink alcohol or take medicine affecting alertness and reflexes.

Discontinuing:
May be unnecessary to finish medicine. Follow doctor's instructions.

Others:
No problems expected.

POSSIBLE INTERACTION WITH OTHER DRUGS

GENERIC NAME OR DRUG CLASS	COMBINED EFFECT
Anticholinergics	Increased anticholinergic effect.
Antidepressants	Increased sedation.
Antihistamines	Increased antihistamine effect.
Clonidine	Decreased clonidine effect.
Dronabinol	Increased effect of dronabinol on central nervous system. Avoid combination.
Guanethidine	Decreased guanethidine effect.
MAO inhibitors	High fever, convulsions, possible death.
Mind-altering drugs	Increased mind-altering effect.
Narcotics	Increased sedation.
Pain relievers	Increased pain reliever effect.
Rauwolfia alkaloids	Decreased effect of rauwolfia alkaloids.
Sedatives	Increased sedative effect.
Sleep inducers	Increased sedation.
Tranquilizers	Increased tranquilizer effect.

POSSIBLE INTERACTION WITH OTHER SUBSTANCES

INTERACTS WITH	COMBINED EFFECT
Alcohol:	Depressed brain function. Avoid.
Beverages:	None expected.
Cocaine:	Decreased cyclobenzaprine effect.
Foods:	None expected.
Marijuana:	Occasional use—Drowsiness. Frequent use—Severe mental and physical impairment.
Tobacco:	None expected.

CYCLOPHOSPHAMIDE

BRAND NAMES

Cytoxan   Procytox
Neosar

BASIC INFORMATION

Habit forming? No
Available as generic? No
Prescription needed? Yes
Drug class: Immunosuppressant

 USES

- Treatment for cancer.
- Treatment for severe rheumatoid arthritis.
- Treatment for blood-vessel disease.
- Treatment for skin disease.

 DOSAGE & USAGE INFORMATION

How to take:
Tablet—Swallow with liquid. If you can't swallow whole, crumble tablet and take with liquid or food.

When to take:
Works best if taken first thing in morning. However, may take with food to lessen stomach irritation. Don't take at bedtime.

If you forget a dose:
Take as soon as you remember up to 12 hours late. If more than 12 hours, wait for next scheduled dose (don't double this dose).

What drug does:
- Kills cancer cells.
- Suppresses spread of cancer cells.
- Suppresses immune system.

Time lapse before drug works:
7 to 10 days continual use.

Don't take with:
See Interaction column and consult doctor.

 OVERDOSE

SYMPTOMS:
Bloody urine, water retention, weight gain, severe infection.
WHAT TO DO:
Overdose unlikely to threaten life. If person takes much larger amount than prescribed, call doctor, poison-control center or hospital emergency room for instructions.

 POSSIBLE ADVERSE REACTIONS OR SIDE EFFECTS

SYMPTOMS	WHAT TO DO
Life-threatening:	
None expected.	
Common:	
• Sore throat, fever.	Discontinue. Call doctor right away.
• Dark skin, nails; nausea; appetite loss; vomiting; missed period.	Continue. Call doctor when convenient.
Infrequent:	
• Rash, hives, itch; shortness of breath; rapid heartbeat; cough; blood in urine, painful urination; pain in side; bleeding, bruising; increased sweating.	Discontinue. Call doctor right away.
• Confusion, agitation, headache, dizziness, flushed face, stomach pain, joint pain, fatigue, weakness.	Continue. Call doctor when convenient.
Rare:	
• Mouth, lip sores; black stool; unusual thirst.	Discontinue. Call doctor right away.
• Blurred vision, increased urination.	Continue. Call doctor when convenient.

WARNINGS & PRECAUTIONS

Don't take if:
- You are allergic to any alkylating agent.
- You have an infection.
- You have bloody urine.
- You will have surgery within 2 months, including dental surgery, requiring general or spinal anesthesia.

Before you start, consult your doctor:
- If you have impaired liver or kidney function.
- If you have impaired bone-marrow or blood-cell production.
- If you have had chemotherapy or X-ray therapy.
- If you have taken cortisone drugs in the past year.

Over age 60:
Adverse reactions and side effects may be more frequent and severe than in younger persons. To reduce risk of chemical bladder inflammation, drink 8 to 10 glasses of water daily.

Pregnancy:
Risk to unborn child outweighs drug benefits. Don't use.

Breast-feeding:
Drug passes into milk. Avoid drug or discontinue nursing until you finish medicine. Consult doctor for advice on maintaining milk supply.

Infants & children:
Use only under medical supervision.

Prolonged use:
- Development of fibrous lung tissue.
- Possible jaundice.
- Swelling of feet, lower legs.

Skin & sunlight:
No problems expected.

Driving, piloting or hazardous work:
Avoid if you feel dizzy or have blurred vision. Otherwise, no problems expected.

Discontinuing:
Don't discontinue without consulting doctor. Dose may require gradual reduction if you have taken drug for a long time. Doses of other drugs may also require adjustment.

Others:
Frequently causes hair loss. After treatment ends, hair should grow back.

POSSIBLE INTERACTION WITH OTHER DRUGS

GENERIC NAME OR DRUG CLASS	COMBINED EFFECT
Allopurinol	Possible anemia.
Antidiabetics (oral)	Increased antidiabetic effect.
Insulin	Increased insulin effect.
Phenobarbital	Increased cyclophosphamide effect.

POSSIBLE INTERACTION WITH OTHER SUBSTANCES

INTERACTS WITH	COMBINED EFFECT
Alcohol:	No problems expected.
Beverages:	No problems expected. Drink at least 2 quarts fluid every day.
Cocaine:	None expected.
Foods:	None expected.
Marijuana:	Increased impairment of immunity.
Tobacco:	None expected.

CYCLOTHIAZIDE

BRAND NAMES

Anhydron   **Fluidil**

BASIC INFORMATION

Habit forming? No
Prescription needed? Yes
Available as generic? Yes
Drug class: Antihypertensive, diuretic
(thiazide)

USES

- Controls, but doesn't cure, high blood pressure.
- Reduces fluid retention (edema) caused by conditions such as heart disorders and liver disease.

DOSAGE & USAGE INFORMATION

How to take:
Tablet or capsule—Swallow with liquid. If you can't swallow whole, crumble tablet or open capsule and take with liquid or food.

When to take:
At the same time each day.

If you forget a dose:
Take as soon as you remember up to 2 hours late. If more than 2 hours, wait for next scheduled dose (don't double this dose).

What drug does:
- Forces sodium and water excretion, reducing body fluid.
- Relaxes muscle cells of small arteries.
- Reduced body fluid and relaxed arteries lower blood pressure.

Time lapse before drug works:
4 to 6 hours. May require several weeks to lower blood pressure.

Continued next column

OVERDOSE

SYMPTOMS:
Cramps, weakness, drowsiness, weak pulse, coma.
WHAT TO DO:
- **Dial 0 (operator) or 911 (emergency) for an ambulance or medical help. Then give first aid immediately.**
- **See emergency information on inside covers.**

Don't take with:
- See Interaction column and consult doctor.
- Non-prescription drugs without consulting doctor.

POSSIBLE ADVERSE REACTIONS OR SIDE EFFECTS

SYMPTOMS	WHAT TO DO
Life-threatening:	
None expected.	
Common:	
None expected.	
Infrequent:	
• Blurred vision, severe abdominal pain, nausea, vomiting, irregular heartbeat, weak pulse.	Discontinue. Call doctor right away.
• Dizziness, mood changes, headaches, weakness, tiredness, weight changes.	Continue. Call doctor when convenient.
• Dry mouth, thirst.	Continue. Tell doctor at next visit.
Rare:	
• Rash or hives.	Discontinue. Seek emergency treatment.
• Sore throat, fever, jaundice.	Discontinue. Call doctor right away.

WARNINGS & PRECAUTIONS

Don't take if:
You are allergic to any thiazide diuretic drugs.

Before you start, consult your doctor:
- If you are allergic to any sulfa drug.
- If you have gout.
- If you have liver, pancreas or kidney disorder.

Over age 60:
Adverse reactions and side effects may be more frequent and severe than in younger persons, especially dizziness and excessive potassium loss.

Pregnancy:
Risk to unborn child outweighs drug benefits. Don't use.

Breast-feeding:
Drug passes into milk. Avoid drug or discontinue nursing.

Infants & children:
No problems expected.

Prolonged use:
You may need medicine to treat high blood pressure for the rest of your life.

Skin & sunlight:
May cause rash or intensify sunburn in areas exposed to sun or sunlamp.

Driving, piloting or hazardous work:
Don't drive or pilot aircraft until you learn how medicine affects you. Don't work around dangerous machinery. Don't climb ladders or work in high places. Danger increases if you drink alcohol or take medicine affecting alertness and reflexes, such as antihistamines, tranquilizers, sedatives, pain medicine, narcotics and mind-altering drugs.

Discontinuing:
Don't discontinue without medical advice.

Others:
- Hot weather and fever may cause dehydration and drop in blood pressure. Dose may require temporary adjustment. Weigh daily and report any unexpected weight decreases to your doctor.
- May cause rise in uric acid, leading to gout.
- May cause blood-sugar rise in diabetics.

POSSIBLE INTERACTION WITH OTHER DRUGS

GENERIC NAME OR DRUG CLASS	COMBINED EFFECT
Acebutolol	Increased antihypertensive effect. Dosages of both drugs may require adjustments.
Allopurinol	Decreased allopurinol effect.
Amiodarone	Increased risk of heartbeat irregularity due to low potassium.
Antidepressants (tricyclic)	Dangerous drop in blood pressure. Avoid combination unless under medical supervision.
Barbiturates	Increased cyclothiazide effect.
Calcium supplements	Increased calcium in blood.
Cholestyramine	Decreased cyclothiazide effect.
Cortisone drugs	Excessive potassium loss that causes dangerous heart rhythms.
Digitalis preparations	Excessive potassium loss that causes dangerous heart rhythms.

Diuretics (thiazide)	Increased effect of other thiazide diuretics.
Indapamide	Increased diuretic effect.
Labetolol	Increased antihypertensive effects.
Lithium	Increased effect of lithium.
MAO inhibitors	Increased cyclothiazide effect.
Nitrates	Excessive blood-pressure drop.
Oxprenolol	Increased antihypertensive effect. Dosages of both drugs may require adjustments.
Pentoxifylline	Increased antihypertensive effect.
Potassium supplements	Decreased potassium effect.
Probenecid	Decreased probenecid effect.

POSSIBLE INTERACTION WITH OTHER SUBSTANCES

INTERACTS WITH	COMBINED EFFECT
Alcohol:	Dangerous blood-pressure drop.
Beverages:	None expected.
Cocaine:	None expected.
Foods: Licorice.	Excessive potassium loss that causes dangerous heart rhythms.
Marijuana:	May increase blood pressure.
Tobacco:	None expected.

CYCRIMINE

BRAND NAMES

Pagitane

BASIC INFORMATION

Habit forming? No
Prescription needed? Yes
Available as generic? No
Drug class: Antidyskinetic, antiparkinsonism

 USES

- Treatment of Parkinson's disease.
- Treatment of adverse effects of phenothiazines.

 DOSAGE & USAGE INFORMATION

How to take:
Tablets or capsules—Take with food to lessen stomach irritation.

When to take:
At the same times each day.

If you forget a dose:
Take as soon as you remember up to 2 hours late. If more than 2 hours, wait for next scheduled dose (don't double this dose).

What drug does:
- Balances chemical reactions necessary to send nerve impulses within base of brain.
- Improves muscle control and reduces stiffness.

Time lapse before drug works:
1 to 2 hours.

Continued next column

 OVERDOSE

SYMPTOMS:
Agitation, dilated pupils, hallucinations, dry mouth, rapid heartbeat, sleepiness.
WHAT TO DO:
- Dial 0 (operator) or 911 (emergency) for an ambulance or medical help. Then give first aid immediately.
- If patient is unconscious and not breathing, give mouth-to-mouth breathing. If there is no heartbeat, use cardiac massage and mouth-to-mouth breathing (CPR). Don't try to make patient vomit. If you can't get help quickly, take patient to nearest emergency facility.
- See emergency information on inside covers.

Don't take with:
- Non-prescription drugs for colds, cough or allergy.
- See Interaction column and consult doctor.

 POSSIBLE ADVERSE REACTIONS OR SIDE EFFECTS

SYMPTOMS	WHAT TO DO
Life-threatening: None expected.	
Common:	
• Blurred vision, light sensitivity, constipation, nausea, vomiting.	Continue. Call doctor when convenient.
• Difficult or painful urination.	Continue. Tell doctor at next visit.
Infrequent: None expected.	
Rare:	
• Rash, eye pain.	Discontinue. Call doctor right away.
• Confusion; dizziness; sore mouth or tongue; muscle cramps; numbness, weakness in hands or feet.	Continue. Call doctor when convenient.

WARNINGS & PRECAUTIONS

Don't take if:
You are allergic to any antidyskinetic.

Before you start, consult your doctor:
- If you have had glaucoma.
- If you have had high blood pressure or heart disease.
- If you have had impaired liver function.
- If you have had kidney disease or urination difficulty.

Over age 60:
More sensitive to drug. Aggravates symptoms of enlarged prostate. Causes impaired thinking, hallucinations, nightmares. Consult doctor about any of these.

Pregnancy:
Studies inconclusive on harm to unborn child. Animal studies show fetal abnormalities. Decide with your doctor whether drug benefits justify risk to unborn child.

Breast-feeding:
No problems expected.

Infants & children:
Not recommended for children 3 and younger. Use for older children only under doctor's supervision.

Prolonged use:
Possible glaucoma.

Skin & sunlight:
No problems expected.

Driving, piloting or hazardous work:
Don't drive or pilot aircraft until you learn how medicine affects you. Don't work around dangerous machinery. Don't climb ladders or work in high places. Danger increases if you drink alcohol or take medicine affecting alertness and reflexes, such as antihistamines, tranquilizers, sedatives, pain medicine, narcotics and mind-altering drugs.

Discontinuing:
Don't discontinue without consulting doctor. Dose may require gradual reduction if you have taken drug for a long time. Doses of other drugs may also require adjustment.

Others:
- Internal eye pressure should be measured regularly.
- Avoid becoming overheated.

POSSIBLE INTERACTION WITH OTHER DRUGS

GENERIC NAME OR DRUG CLASS	COMBINED EFFECT
Amantadine	Increased amantadine effect.
Antidepressants (tricyclic)	Increased cycrimine effect. May cause glaucoma.
Antihistamines	Increased cyrimine effect.
Levodopa	Increased levodopa effect. Improved results in treating Parkinson's disease.
Meperidine	Increased cyrimine effect.
MAO inhibitors	Increased cyrimine effect.
Orphenadrine	Increased cyrimine effect.
Phenothiazines	Behavior changes.
Primidone	Excessive sedation.
Procainamide	Increased procainamide effect.
Quinidine	Increased cyrimine effect.
Tranquilizers	Excessive sedation.

POSSIBLE INTERACTION WITH OTHER SUBSTANCES

INTERACTS WITH	COMBINED EFFECT
Alcohol:	None expected.
Beverages:	None expected.
Cocaine:	Decreased cyrimine effect. Avoid.
Foods:	None expected.
Marijuana:	None expected.
Tobacco:	None expected.

CYPROHEPTADINE

BRAND NAMES

Cyprodine   Vimicon
Periactin

BASIC INFORMATION

Habit forming? No
Prescription needed? Yes
Available as generic? Yes
Drug class: Antihistamine

 USES

- Reduces allergic symptoms such as hay fever, hives, rash or itching.
- Induces sleep.
- Reduces symptoms of cold urticaria.

 DOSAGE & USAGE INFORMATION

How to take:
Tablet or syrup—Swallow with liquid or food to lessen stomach irritation.

When to take:
Varies with form. Follow label directions.

If you forget a dose:
Take as soon as you remember up to 2 hours late. If more than 2 hours, wait for next scheduled dose (don't double this dose).

What drug does:
Blocks action of histamine after an allergic response triggers histamine release in sensitive cells.

Time lapse before drug works:
30 minutes.

Continued next column

 OVERDOSE

SYMPTOMS:
Convulsions, red face, hallucinations, coma.
WHAT TO DO:
- Dial 0 (operator) or 911 (emergency) for an ambulance or medical help. Then give first aid immediately.
- If patient is unconscious and not breathing, give mouth-to-mouth breathing. If there is no heartbeat, use cardiac massage and mouth-to-mouth breathing (CPR). Don't try to make patient vomit. If you can't get help quickly, take patient to nearest emergency facility.
- See emergency information on inside covers.

Don't take with:
See Interaction column and consult doctor.

 POSSIBLE ADVERSE REACTIONS OR SIDE EFFECTS

SYMPTOMS	WHAT TO DO
Life-threatening: None expected.	
Common: Drowsiness, dizziness, dry mouth, nose, throat, nausea.	Continue. Tell doctor at next visit.
Infrequent: • Vision changes.	Discontinue. Call doctor right away.
• Less tolerance for contact lenses, difficult urination.	Continue. Call doctor when convenient.
• Appetite loss.	Continue. Tell doctor at next visit.
Rare: Nightmares, agitation, irritability, sore throat, fever, rapid heartbeat, unusual bleeding or bruising, fatigue, weakness.	Discontinue. Call doctor right away.

WARNINGS & PRECAUTIONS

Don't take if:
You are allergic to any antihistamine.

Before you start, consult your doctor:
- If you have glaucoma.
- If you have enlarged prostate.
- If you have asthma.
- If you have kidney disease.
- If you have peptic ulcer.
- If you will have surgery within 2 months, including dental surgery, requiring general or spinal anesthesia.

Over age 60:
Don't exceed recommended dose. Adverse reactions and side effects may be more frequent and severe than in younger persons, especially urination difficulty, diminished alertness and other brain and nervous-system symptoms.

Pregnancy:
No proven harm to unborn child. Avoid if possible.

Breast-feeding:
Drug passes into milk. Avoid drug or discontinue nursing until you finish medicine. Consult doctor for advice on maintaining milk supply.

Infants & children:
Not recommended for premature or newborn infants. Otherwise, no problems expected.

Prolonged use:
Avoid. May damage bone marrow and nerve cells.

Skin & sunlight:
May cause rash or intensify sunburn in areas exposed to sun or sunlamp.

Driving, piloting or hazardous work:
Don't drive or pilot aircraft until you learn how medicine affects you. Don't work around dangerous machinery. Don't climb ladders or work in high places. Danger increases if you drink alcohol or take medicine affecting alertness and reflexes, such as antihistamines, tranquilizers, sedatives, pain medicine, narcotics and mind-altering drugs.

Discontinuing:
No problems expected.

Others:
May mask symptoms of hearing damage from aspirin, other salicylates, cisplatin, paromomycin, vancomycin or anticonvulsants. Consult doctor if you use these.

POSSIBLE INTERACTION WITH OTHER DRUGS

GENERIC NAME OR DRUG CLASS	COMBINED EFFECT
Anticholinergics	Increased anticholinergic effect.
Antidepressants	Excess sedation. Avoid.
Antihistamines (other)	Excess sedation. Avoid.
Dronabinol	Increased effects of both drugs. Avoid.
Hypnotics	Excess sedation. Avoid.
MAO inhibitors	Increased cyproheptadine effect.
Mind-altering drugs	Excess sedation. Avoid.
Molindone	Increased antihistamine effect.
Narcotics	Excess sedation. Avoid.
Sedatives	Excess sedation. Avoid.
Sleep inducers	Excess sedation. Avoid.
Tranquilizers	Excess sedation. Avoid.

POSSIBLE INTERACTION WITH OTHER SUBSTANCES

INTERACTS WITH	COMBINED EFFECT
Alcohol:	Excess sedation. Avoid.
Beverages: Caffeine drinks.	Less cyproheptadine sedation.
Cocaine:	Decreased cyproheptadine effect. Avoid.
Foods:	None expected.
Marijuana:	Excess sedation. Avoid.
Tobacco:	None expected.

DANAZOL

BRAND NAMES

Cyclomen   Danocrine

BASIC INFORMATION

Habit forming? No
Prescription needed? Yes
Available as generic? No
Drug class: Gonadotropin inhibitor

 USES

Treatment of endometriosis, fibrocystic breast disease, angioneurotic edema except in pregnant women, gynecomastia, infertility, excessive menstruation, precocious puberty.

 DOSAGE & USAGE INFORMATION

How to take:
Tablet or capsule—Swallow with liquid or food to lessen stomach irritation. If you can't swallow whole, crumble tablet or open capsule and take with liquid or food.

When to take:
At the same times each day.

If you forget a dose:
Take as soon as you remember (don't double dose).

What drug does:
Partially prevents output of pituitary follicle-stimulating hormone and lutenizing hormone reducing estrogen production.

Time lapse before drug works:
- 2 to 3 months to treat endometriosis.
- 1 to 2 months to treat other disorders.

Don't take with:
- Birth control pills.
- See Interaction column and consult doctor.

 OVERDOSE

SYMPTOMS:
None expected.
WHAT TO DO:
Overdose unlikely to threaten life. If person takes much larger amount than prescribed, call doctor, poison-control center or hospital emergency room for instructions.

 POSSIBLE ADVERSE REACTIONS OR SIDE EFFECTS

SYMPTOMS	WHAT TO DO
Life-threatening: None expected.	
Common: Menstrual irregularities.	Continue. Call doctor when convenient.
Infrequent:	
• Unnatural hair growth in women, nosebleeds.	Discontinue. Call doctor right away.
• Dizziness; hoarseness; voice deepens; flushed or red skin; muscle cramps; enlarged clitoris; decreased testicle size; vaginal burning, itch; swollen feet; decreased breast size.	Continue. Call doctor when convenient.
• Headache, acne, weight gain.	Continue. Tell doctor at next visit.
Rare: Jaundice.	Discontinue. Call doctor right away.

WARNINGS & PRECAUTIONS

Don't take if:
You become pregnant.

Before you start, consult your doctor:
- If you take birth control pills.
- If you have diabetes.
- If you have heart disease.
- If you have epilepsy.
- If you have kidney disease.
- If you have liver disease.
- If you have migraine headache.

Over age 60:
Adverse reactions and side effects may be more frequent and severe than in younger persons.

Pregnancy:
Risk to unborn child outweighs drug benefits. Don't use. Stop if you get pregnant.

Breast-feeding:
Unknown whether medicine filters into milk. Consult doctor.

Infants & children:
Not recommended.

Prolonged use:
Required for full effect. Don't discontinue without consulting doctor.

Skin & sunlight:
No problems expected.

Driving, piloting or hazardous work:
No problems expected.

Discontinuing:
Don't discontinue without consulting doctor. Menstrual periods may be absent for 2 to 3 months after discontinuation.

Others:
May alter blood-sugar levels in diabetic persons.

POSSIBLE INTERACTION WITH OTHER DRUGS

GENERIC NAME OR DRUG CLASS	COMBINED EFFECT
Anticoagulants (oral)	Increased anticoagulant effect.

POSSIBLE INTERACTION WITH OTHER SUBSTANCES

INTERACTS WITH	COMBINED EFFECT
Alcohol:	Excessive nervous system depression. Avoid.
Beverages: Caffeine.	Rapid, irregular heartbeat. Avoid.
Cocaine:	May interfere with expected action of danazol. Avoid.
Foods:	No problems expected.
Marijuana:	May interfere with expected action of danazol. Avoid.
Tobacco:	Rapid, irregular heartbeat. Avoid. Increased leg cramps.

DANTHRON

BRAND NAMES

AKshun	Doxidan
Dorbane	Modane
Dorbantyl L	Roydan

BASIC INFORMATION

Habit forming? No
Prescription needed? No
Available as generic? Yes
Drug class: Laxative (stimulant)

 ## USES

Constipation relief.

 ## DOSAGE & USAGE INFORMATION

How to take:
- Tablet—Swallow with liquid or food.
- Liquid—Drink 6 to 8 glasses of water each day, in addition to one taken with each dose.

When to take:
Usually at bedtime with a snack, unless directed otherwise.

If you forget a dose:
Take as soon as you remember.

What drug does:
Acts on smooth muscles of intestine wall to cause vigorous bowel movement.

Time lapse before drug works:
6 to 10 hours.

Don't take with:
- See Interaction column and consult doctor.
- Don't take within 2 hours of taking another medicine. Laxative interferes with medicine absorption.

 ## OVERDOSE

SYMPTOMS:
Vomiting, electrolyte depletion.
WHAT TO DO:
Overdose unlikely to threaten life. If person takes much larger amount than prescribed, call doctor, poison-control center or hospital emergency room for instructions.

 ## POSSIBLE ADVERSE REACTIONS OR SIDE EFFECTS

SYMPTOMS	WHAT TO DO
Life-threatening: None expected.	
Common: Rectal irritation.	Continue. Call doctor when convenient.
Infrequent:	
• Dangerous potassium loss.	Discontinue. Call doctor right away.
• Belching, cramps, nausea.	Continue. Call doctor when convenient.
Rare:	
• Irritability, confusion, headache, rash, breathing difficulty, irregular heartbeat, muscle cramps, unusual tiredness, weakness.	Discontinue. Call doctor right away.
• Burning on urination.	Continue. Call doctor when convenient.

WARNINGS & PRECAUTIONS

Don't take if:
- You have symptoms of appendicitis, inflamed bowel or intestinal blockage.
- You are allergic to a stimulant laxative.
- You have missed a bowel movement for only 1 or 2 days.

Before you start, consult your doctor:
- If you have a colostomy or ileostomy.
- If you have congestive heart disease.
- If you have diabetes.
- If you have high blood pressure.
- If you have a laxative habit.
- If you have rectal bleeding.
- If you take other laxatives.

Over age 60:
Adverse reactions and side effects may be more frequent and severe than in younger persons.

Pregnancy:
Risk to mother and unborn child outweighs drug benefits. Don't use.

Breast-feeding:
Drug passes into milk. Avoid drug or discontinue nursing until you finish medicine. Consult doctor for advice on maintaining milk supply.

Infants & children:
Use only under medical supervision.

Prolonged use:
Don't take for more than 1 week unless under a doctor's supervision. May cause laxative dependence.

Skin & sunlight:
No problems expected.

Driving, piloting or hazardous work:
No problems expected.

Discontinuing:
May be unnecessary to finish medicine. Follow doctor's instructions.

Others:
Don't take to "flush out" your system or as a "tonic."

POSSIBLE INTERACTION WITH OTHER DRUGS

GENERIC NAME OR DRUG CLASS	COMBINED EFFECT
Antihypertensives	May cause dangerous low potassium level.
Diuretics	May cause dangerous low potassium level.
Docusate calcium	Liver toxicity.
Docusate sodium	Liver toxicity.

POSSIBLE INTERACTION WITH OTHER SUBSTANCES

INTERACTS WITH	COMBINED EFFECT
Alcohol:	None expected.
Beverages:	None expected.
Cocaine:	None expected.
Foods:	None expected.
Marijuana:	None expected.
Tobacco:	None expected.

DANTROLENE

BRAND NAMES

Dantrium

BASIC INFORMATION

Habit forming? No
Prescription needed? Yes
Available as generic? No
Drug class: Muscle relaxant, antispastic

 USES

- Relieves muscle spasticity caused by diseases such as multiple sclerosis, cerebral palsy, stroke.
- Relieves muscle spasticity caused by injury to spinal cord.
- Relieves or prevents excess body temperature brought on by some surgical procedures.

 DOSAGE & USAGE INFORMATION

How to take:
Capsules—Swallow with liquid.

When to take:
Once a day for muscle spasticity during first 6 days. Later, every 6 hours. For excess temperature, follow label instructions.

If you forget a dose:
Take as soon as you remember up to 2 hours late. If more than 2 hours, wait for next scheduled dose (don't double this dose).

Continued next column

 OVERDOSE

SYMPTOMS:
Bloody stools, chest pain, convulsive seizures.
WHAT TO DO:
- **Dial 0 (operator) or 911 (emergency) for an ambulance or medical help. Then give first aid immediately.**
- **If patient is unconscious and not breathing, give mouth-to-mouth breathing. If there is no heartbeat, use cardiac massage and mouth-to-mouth breathing (CPR). Don't try to make patient vomit. If you can't get help quickly, take patient to nearest emergency facility.**
- **See emergency information on inside covers.**

What drug does:
Acts directly on muscles to prevent excess contractions.

Time lapse before drug works:
1 or more weeks.

Don't take with:
See Interaction column and consult doctor.

 POSSIBLE ADVERSE REACTIONS OR SIDE EFFECTS

SYMPTOMS	WHAT TO DO
Life-threatening:	
Seizure.	Seek emergency treatment immediately.
Common:	
None expected.	
Infrequent:	
• Rash, hives; black or bloody stools; chest pain; fast heartbeat; backache; blood in urine; painful, swollen feet; chills; fever.	Discontinue. Call doctor right away.
• Depression, confusion, headache, slurred speech, nervousness, insomnia, blurred vision, diarrhea, difficult swallowing, appetite loss, difficult urination, decreased sexual function in males.	Continue. Call doctor when convenient.
Rare:	
Jaundice.	Discontinue. Call doctor right away.

WARNINGS & PRECAUTIONS

Don't take if:
You are allergic to dantrolene or any muscle relaxant or antispastic medication.

Before you start, consult your doctor:
- If you have liver disease.
- If you have heart disease.
- If you have lung disease (especially emphysema).
- If you are over age 35.
- If you will have surgery within 2 months, including dental surgery, requiring general or spinal anesthesia.

Over age 60:
Adverse reactions and side effects may be more frequent and severe than in younger persons.

Pregnancy:
No proven harm to unborn child. Avoid if possible.

Breast-feeding:
Avoid nursing or discontinue until you finish drug.

Infants & children:
Only under close medical supervision.

Prolonged use:
Blood counts, G6PD tests before treatment begins in Negroes and Caucasians of Mediterranean heritage, liver function studies—all recommended periodically during prolonged use.

Skin & sunlight:
May cause rash or intensify sunburn in areas exposed to sun or sunlamp.

Driving, piloting or hazardous work:
Don't drive or pilot aircraft until you learn how medicine affects you. Don't work around dangerous machinery. Don't climb ladders or work in high places. Danger increases if you drink alcohol or take medicine affecting alertness and reflexes, such as antihistamines, tranquilizers, sedatives, pain medicine, narcotics and mind-altering drugs.

Discontinuing:
Don't discontinue without consulting doctor. Dose may require gradual reduction if you have taken drug for a long time. Doses of other drugs may also require adjustment.

Others:
No problems expected.

 ## POSSIBLE INTERACTION WITH OTHER DRUGS

GENERIC NAME OR DRUG CLASS	COMBINED EFFECT
Central nervous system depressants: Sedatives, sleeping pills, tranquilizers, antidepressants, antihistamines, narcotics, other muscle relaxants	Increased sedation, low blood pressure. Avoid.
Dronabinol	Increased effect of dronabinol on central nervous system. Avoid.

 ## POSSIBLE INTERACTION WITH OTHER SUBSTANCES

INTERACTS WITH	COMBINED EFFECT
Alcohol:	Increased sedation, low blood pressure. Avoid.
Beverages:	No problems expected.
Cocaine:	Increased spasticity. Avoid.
Foods:	No problems expected.
Marijuana:	Increased spasticity. Avoid.
Tobacco:	May interfere with absorption of medicine.

DAPSONE

BRAND NAMES

Avlosulfon   DDS

BASIC INFORMATION

Habit forming? No
Prescription needed? Yes
Available as generic? Yes
Drug class: Antibacterial (Antileprosy),
    Sulfone

 ## USES

- Treatment of dermatitis herpetiformis.
- Treatment of leprosy.

 ## DOSAGE & USAGE INFORMATION

How to take:
Tablet or capsule—Swallow with liquid or food
to lessen stomach irritation.

When to take:
Once a day at same time.

If you forget a dose:
Take as soon as you remember up to 2 hours
late. If more than 2 hours, wait for next
scheduled dose (don't double this dose).

What drug does:
Inhibits enzymes. Kills leprosy germs.

Time lapse before drug works:
- 3 years for leprosy.
- 1 to 2 weeks for dermatitis herpetiformis.

Don't take with:
See Interaction column and consult doctor.

 ## OVERDOSE

SYMPTOMS:
Bleeding, vomiting, coma.
WHAT TO DO:
- Dial 0 (operator) or 911 (emergency) for an
  ambulance or medical help. Then give first
  aid immediately.
- If patient is unconscious and not
  breathing, give mouth-to-mouth breathing.
  If there is no heartbeat, use cardiac
  massage and mouth-to-mouth breathing
  (CPR). Don't try to make patient vomit. If
  you can't get help quickly, take patient to
  nearest emergency facility.
- See emergency information on inside
  covers.

 ## POSSIBLE ADVERSE REACTIONS OR SIDE EFFECTS

SYMPTOMS	WHAT TO DO
Life-threatening:	
None expected.	
Common:	
• Rash.	Discontinue. Call doctor right away.
• Abdominal pain, appetite loss.	Continue. Call doctor when convenient.
Infrequent:	
Pale.	Discontinue. Call doctor right away.
Rare:	
• Dizziness; mental changes; sore throat; fever; difficult breathing; bleeding; jaundice; numbness, tingling, pain or burning in hands or feet.	Discontinue. Call doctor right away.
• Headache; itching; nausea; vomiting; blue fingernails, lips.	Continue. Call doctor when convenient.

WARNINGS & PRECAUTIONS

Don't take if:
- You have G6PD deficiency.
- You are allergic to furosemide, thiazide diuretics, sulfonureas, carbonic anhydrase inhibitors, sulfonamides.

Before you start, consult your doctor:
- If you are anemic.
- If you have liver or kidney disease.
- If you are Negro or Caucasian with Mediterranean heritage.
- If you will have surgery within 2 months, including dental surgery, requiring general or spinal anesthesia.

Over age 60:
Adverse reactions and side effects may be more frequent and severe than in younger persons.

Pregnancy:
No problems expected.

Breast-feeding:
Consult doctor.

Infants & children:
Under close medical supervision only.

Prolonged use:
Request blood counts, liver function studies.

Skin & sunlight:
No problems expected.

Driving, piloting or hazardous work:
Don't drive or pilot aircraft until you learn how medicine affects you. Don't work around dangerous machinery. Don't climb ladders or work in high places. Danger increases if you drink alcohol or take medicine affecting alertness and reflexes, such as antihistamines, tranquilizers, sedatives, pain medicine, narcotics and mind-altering drugs.

Discontinuing:
Don't discontinue without consulting doctor. Dose may require gradual reduction if you have taken drug for a long time. Doses of other drugs may also require adjustment.

Others:
No problems expected.

POSSIBLE INTERACTION WITH OTHER DRUGS

GENERIC NAME OR DRUG CLASS	COMBINED EFFECT
Aminobenzoic acid (PABA)	Decreased dapsone effect. Avoid.
Probenecid	Increased toxicity of dapsone.
Rifampin	Decreased effect of dapsone.

POSSIBLE INTERACTION WITH OTHER SUBSTANCES

INTERACTS WITH	COMBINED EFFECT
Alcohol:	Increased chance of toxicity to liver.
Beverages:	No problems expected.
Cocaine:	Increased chance of toxicity. Avoid.
Foods:	No problems expected.
Marijuana:	Increased chance of toxicity. Avoid.
Tobacco:	May interfere with absorption of medicine.

DEHYDROCHOLIC ACID

BRAND NAMES

Bilaz	G.B.S.
Cholan-DH	Hepahydrin
Cholan-HMB	Neocholan
Decholin	Neolax
Dycholium	Trilax

BASIC INFORMATION

Habit forming? No
Prescription needed? No
Available as generic? Yes
Drug class: Laxative (stimulant)

 ## USES

Constipation relief.

 ## DOSAGE & USAGE INFORMATION

How to take:
Tablet—Swallow with liquid.

When to take:
Usually at bedtime with a snack, unless directed otherwise.

If you forget a dose:
Take as soon as you remember.

What drug does:
Acts on smooth muscles of intestine wall to cause vigorous bowel movement.

Time lapse before drug works:
6 to 10 hours.

Don't take with:
- See Interaction column and consult doctor.
- Don't take within 2 hours of taking another medicine. Laxative interferes with medicine absorption.

 ## OVERDOSE

SYMPTOMS:
Vomiting, electrolyte depletion.
WHAT TO DO:
Overdose unlikely to threaten life. If person takes much larger amount than prescribed, call doctor, poison-control center or hospital emergency room for instructions.

 ## POSSIBLE ADVERSE REACTIONS OR SIDE EFFECTS

SYMPTOMS	WHAT TO DO
Life-threatening: None expected.	
Common: Rectal irritation.	Continue. Call doctor when convenient.
Infrequent:	
• Dangerous potassium loss.	Discontinue. Call doctor right away.
• Belching, cramps, nausea.	Continue. Call doctor when convenient.
Rare:	
• Irritability, confusion, headache, rash, breathing difficulty, irregular heartbeat, muscle cramps, unusual tiredness or weakness.	Discontinue. Call doctor right away.
• Burning on urination.	Continue. Call doctor when convenient.

266

WARNINGS & PRECAUTIONS

Don't take if:
- You have symptoms of appendicitis, inflamed bowel or intestinal blockage.
- You are allergic to a stimulant laxative.
- You have missed a bowel movement for only 1 or 2 days.
- You have liver disease.

Before you start, consult your doctor:
- If you have a colostomy or ileostomy.
- If you have congestive heart disease.
- If you have diabetes.
- If you have enlarged prostate.
- If you have a laxative habit.
- If you have rectal bleeding.
- If you take other laxatives.

Over age 60:
Adverse reactions and side effects may be more frequent and severe than in younger persons.

Pregnancy:
Risk to mother and unborn child outweighs drug benefits. Don't use.

Breast-feeding:
Drug passes into milk. Avoid drug or discontinue nursing until you finish medicine. Consult doctor for advice on maintaining milk supply.

Infants & children:
Use only under medical supervision.

Prolonged use:
Don't take for more than 1 week unless under a doctor's supervision. May cause laxative dependence.

Skin & sunlight:
No problems expected.

Driving, piloting or hazardous work:
No problems expected.

Discontinuing:
May be unnecessary to finish medicine. Follow doctor's instructions.

Others:
Don't take to "flush out" your system or as a "tonic."

 ## POSSIBLE INTERACTION WITH OTHER DRUGS

GENERIC NAME OR DRUG CLASS	COMBINED EFFECT
Antihypertensives	May cause dangerous low potassium level.
Diuretics	May cause dangerous low potassium level.

 ## POSSIBLE INTERACTION WITH OTHER SUBSTANCES

INTERACTS WITH	COMBINED EFFECT
Alcohol:	None expected.
Beverages:	None expected.
Cocaine:	None expected.
Foods:	None expected.
Marijuana:	None expected.
Tobacco:	None expected.

DEXAMETHASONE

BRAND NAMES

See complete list of brand names in the *Brand Name Directory*, page 947.

BASIC INFORMATION

Habit forming? No
Prescription needed? Yes
Available as generic? Yes
Drug class: Cortisone drug (adrenal corticosteroid)

USES

- Reduces inflammation caused by many different medical problems.
- Treatment for some allergic diseases, blood disorders, kidney diseases, asthma and emphysema.
- Replaces corticosteroid deficiencies.

DOSAGE & USAGE INFORMATION

How to take:
- Tablet or liquid—Swallow with liquid or food to lessen stomach irritation. If you can't swallow whole, crumble tablet and take with liquid or food.
- Inhaler—Follow label instructions.

When to take:
At the same times each day. Take once-a-day or once-every-other-day doses in mornings.

If you forget a dose:
- Several-doses-per-day prescription—Take as soon as you remember up to 2 hours late. If more than 2 hours, wait for next scheduled dose (don't double this dose).
- Once-a-day dose or less—Wait for next dose. Double this dose.

What drug does:
Decreases inflammatory responses.

Time lapse before drug works:
2 to 4 days.

Continued next column

OVERDOSE

SYMPTOMS:
Headache, convulsions, heart failure.
WHAT TO DO:
- Dial 0 (operator) or 911 (emergency) for an ambulance or medical help. Then give first aid immediately.
- See emergency information on inside covers.

Don't take with:
See Interaction column and consult doctor.

POSSIBLE ADVERSE REACTIONS OR SIDE EFFECTS

SYMPTOMS	WHAT TO DO
Life-threatening: None expected.	
Common: Poor wound healing, acne, thirst, indigestion, nausea, vomiting.	Continue. Call doctor when convenient.
Infrequent:	
• Bloody or black, tarry stool.	Discontinue. Seek emergency treatment.
• Blurred vision; halos around lights; sore throat, fever; muscle cramps; swollen legs, feet.	Discontinue. Call doctor right away.
• Mood changes, insomnia, restlessness, frequent urination, weight gain, round face, fatigue, weakness, TB recurrence, irregular menstrual periods.	Continue. Call doctor when convenient.
Rare:	
• Irregular heartbeat.	Discontinue. Seek emergency treatment.
• Rash.	Discontinue. Call doctor right away.

WARNINGS & PRECAUTIONS

Don't take if:
- You are allergic to any cortisone drug.
- You have tuberculosis or fungus infection.
- You have herpes infection of eyes, lips or genitals.

Before you start, consult your doctor:
- If you have had tuberculosis.
- If you have congestive heart failure.
- If you have diabetes.
- If you have peptic ulcer.
- If you have glaucoma.
- If you have underactive thyroid.
- If you have high blood pressure.
- If you have myasthenia gravis.
- If you have blood clots in legs or lungs.

Over age 60:
Adverse reactions and side effects may be more frequent and severe than in younger persons. Likely to aggravate edema, diabetes or ulcers. Likely to cause cataracts and osteoporosis (softening of the bones).

Pregnancy:
Risk to unborn child outweighs drug benefits. Don't use.

Breast-feeding:
Drug passes into milk. Avoid drug or discontinue nursing until you finish medicine. Consult doctor for advice on maintaining milk supply.

Infants & children:
Use only under medical supervision.

Prolonged use:
- Retards growth in children.
- Possible glaucoma, cataracts, diabetes, fragile bones and thin skin.
- Functional dependence.

Skin & sunlight:
No problems expected.

Driving, piloting or hazardous work:
No problems expected.

Discontinuing:
- Don't discontinue without doctor's advice until you complete prescribed dose, even though symptoms diminish or disappear.
- Drug affects your response to surgery, illness, injury or stress for 2 years after discontinuing. Tell anyone who takes medical care of you within 2 years about drug.

Others:
Avoid immunizations if possible.

POSSIBLE INTERACTION WITH OTHER DRUGS

GENERIC NAME OR DRUG CLASS	COMBINED EFFECT
Amphoterecin B	Potassium depletion.
Anticholinergics	Possible glaucoma.
Anticoagulants (oral)	Decreased anticoagulant effect.
Anticonvulsants (hydantoin)	Decreased dexamethasone effect.
Antidiabetics (oral)	Decreased antidiabetic effect.
Antihistamines	Decreased dexamethasone effect.
Aspirin	Increased dexamethasone effect.
Barbiturates	Decreased dexamethasone effect. Oversedation.

Beta-adrenergic blockers	Decreased dexamethasone effect.
Chloral hydrate	Decreased dexamethasone effect.
Chlorthalidone	Potassium depletion.
Cholinergics	Decreased cholinergic effect.
Contraceptives (oral)	Increased dexamethasone effect.
Digitalis preparations	Dangerous potassium depletion. Possible digitalis toxicity.
Diuretics (thiazide)	Potassium depletion.
Ephedrine	Decreased dexamethasone effect.
Estrogens	Increased dexamethasone effect.
Ethacrynic acid	Potassium depletion.
Furosemide	Potassium depletion.
Glutethimide	Decreased dexamethasone effect.
Indapamide	Possible excessive potassium loss, causing dangerous heartbeat irregularity.
Indomethacin	Increased dexamethasone effect.
Insulin	Decreased insulin effect.
Isoniazid	Decreased isoniazid effect.
Oxyphenbutazone	Possible ulcers.
Phenylbutazone	Possible ulcers.
Potassium supplements	Decreased potassium effect.

Continued page 965

POSSIBLE INTERACTION WITH OTHER SUBSTANCES

INTERACTS WITH	COMBINED EFFECT
Alcohol:	Risk of stomach ulcers.
Beverages:	No proven problems.
Cocaine:	Overstimulation. Avoid.
Foods:	No proven problems.
Marijuana:	Decreased immunity.
Tobacco:	Increased dexamethasone effect. Possible toxicity.

DEXCHLORPHENIRAMINE

BRAND NAMES

Dexchlor
Polaramine
Polaramine Repetabs

BASIC INFORMATION

Habit forming? No
Prescription needed? Yes
Available as generic? No
Drug class: Antihistamine

 USES

- Reduces allergic symptoms such as hay fever, hives, rash or itching.
- Induces sleep.

 DOSAGE & USAGE INFORMATION

How to take:
- Tablet or syrup—Swallow with liquid or food to lessen stomach irritation.
- Extended-release tablets or capsules—Swallow each dose whole. If you take regular tablets, you may chew or crush them.

When to take:
Varies with form. Follow label directions.

If you forget a dose:
Take as soon as you remember up to 2 hours late. If more than 2 hours, wait for next scheduled dose (don't double this dose).

What drug does:
Blocks action of histamine after an allergic response triggers histamine release in sensitive cells.

Continued next column

 OVERDOSE

SYMPTOMS:
Convulsions, red face, hallucinations, coma.
WHAT TO DO:
- **Dial 0 (operator) or 911 (emergency) for an ambulance or medical help. Then give first aid immediately.**
- **If patient is unconscious and not breathing, give mouth-to-mouth breathing. If there is no heartbeat, use cardiac massage and mouth-to-mouth breathing (CPR). Don't try to make patient vomit. If you can't get help quickly, take patient to nearest emergency facility.**
- **See emergency information on inside covers.**

Time lapse before drug works:
30 minutes.

Don't take with:
See Interaction column and consult doctor.

 POSSIBLE ADVERSE REACTIONS OR SIDE EFFECTS

SYMPTOMS	WHAT TO DO
Life-threatening: None expected.	
Common: Drowsiness; dizziness; dry mouth, nose, throat; nausea.	Continue. Tell doctor at next visit.
Infrequent:	
• Vision changes.	Discontinue. Call doctor right away.
• Less tolerance for contact lenses, difficult urination.	Continue. Call doctor when convenient.
• Appetite loss.	Continue. Tell doctor at next visit.
Rare: Nightmares, agitation, irritability, sore throat, fever, rapid heartbeat, unusual bleeding or bruising, fatigue, weakness.	Discontinue. Call doctor right away.

DEXCHLORPHENIRAMINE

WARNINGS & PRECAUTIONS

Don't take if:
You are allergic to any antihistamine.

Before you start, consult your doctor:
- If you have glaucoma.
- If you have enlarged prostate.
- If you have asthma.
- If you have kidney disease.
- If you have peptic ulcer.
- If you will have surgery within 2 months, including dental surgery, requiring general or spinal anesthesia.

Over age 60:
Don't exceed recommended dose. Adverse reactions and side effects may be more frequent and severe than in younger persons, especially urination difficulty, diminished alertness and other brain and nervous-system symptoms.

Pregnancy:
No proven harm to unborn child. Avoid if possible.

Breast-feeding:
Drug passes into milk. Avoid drug or discontinue nursing until you finish medicine. Consult doctor for advice on maintaining milk supply.

Infants & children:
Not recommended for premature or newborn infants. Otherwise, no problems expected.

Prolonged use:
Avoid. May damage bone marrow and nerve cells.

Skin & sunlight:
May cause rash or intensify sunburn in areas exposed to sun or sunlamp.

Driving, piloting or hazardous work:
Don't drive or pilot aircraft until you learn how medicine affects you. Don't work around dangerous machinery. Don't climb ladders or work in high places. Danger increases if you drink alcohol or take medicine affecting alertness and reflexes, such as antihistamines, tranquilizers, sedatives, pain medicine, narcotics and mind-altering drugs.

Discontinuing:
No problems expected.

Others:
May mask symptoms of hearing damage from aspirin, other salicylates, cisplatin, paromomycin, vancomycin or anticonvulsants. Consult doctor if you use these.

POSSIBLE INTERACTION WITH OTHER DRUGS

GENERIC NAME OR DRUG CLASS	COMBINED EFFECT
Anticholinergics	Increased anticholinergic effect.
Antidepressants	Excess sedation. Avoid.
Antihistamines (other)	Excess sedation. Avoid.
Dronabinol	Increased effects of both drugs. Avoid.
Hypnotics	Excess sedation. Avoid.
MAO inhibitors	Increased dexchlorpheniramine effect.
Mind-altering drugs	Excess sedation. Avoid.
Molindone	Increased antihistamine effect.
Narcotics	Excess sedation. Avoid.
Sedatives	Excess sedation. Avoid.
Sleep inducers	Excess sedation. Avoid.
Tranquilizers	Excess sedation. Avoid.

POSSIBLE INTERACTION WITH OTHER SUBSTANCES

INTERACTS WITH	COMBINED EFFECT
Alcohol:	Excess sedation. Avoid.
Beverages: Caffeine drinks.	Decreased dexchlorpheniramine effect.
Cocaine:	Decreased dexchlorpheniramine effect. Avoid.
Foods:	None expected.
Marijuana:	Excess sedation. Avoid.
Tobacco:	None expected.

DEXTROAMPHETAMINE

BRAND NAMES

Amphaplex	Ferndex
Biphetamine	Obetrol
Declobese	Obotan
Dexampex	Oxydess II
Dexedrine	Spancap No. 1
Eskatrol	

BASIC INFORMATION

Habit forming? Yes
Prescription needed? Yes
Available as generic? Yes
Drug class: Central-nervous-system
           stimulant (amphetamine)

 USES

- Prevents narcolepsy (attacks of uncontrollable sleepiness).
- Controls hyperactivity in children.

 DOSAGE & USAGE INFORMATION

How to take:
- Tablet or capsule—Swallow with liquid. If you can't swallow whole, crumble tablet or open capsule and take with liquid or food.
- Lozenges or syrups—Take as directed on label.

When to take:
- At the same times each day.
- Short-acting form—Don't take later than 6 hours before bedtime.
- Long-acting form—Take on awakening.

If you forget a dose:
- Short-acting form—Take up to 2 hours late. If more than 2 hours, wait for next dose (don't double this dose).
- Long-acting form—Take as soon as you remember. Wait 20 hours for next dose.

Continued next column

 OVERDOSE

SYMPTOMS:
Rapid heartbeat, hyperactivity, high fever, hallucinations, suicidal or homicidal feelings, convulsions, coma.
WHAT TO DO:
- **Dial 0 (operator) or 911 (emergency) for an ambulance or medical help. Then give first aid immediately.**
- **See emergency information on inside covers.**

What drug does:
- Narcolepsy—Apparently affects brain centers to decrease fatigue or sleepiness and increase alertness and motor activity.
- Hyperactive children—Calms children, opposite to effect on narcoleptic adults.

Time lapse before drug works:
15 to 30 minutes.

Don't take with:
See Interaction column and consult doctor.

 POSSIBLE ADVERSE REACTIONS OR SIDE EFFECTS

SYMPTOMS	WHAT TO DO
Life-threatening:	
None expected.	
Common:	
• Irritability, nervousness, insomnia.	Continue. Call doctor when convenient.
• Dry mouth.	Continue. Tell doctor at next visit.
Infrequent:	
• Dizziness; lack of alertness; blurred vision; fast, pounding heartbeat; unusual sweating.	Discontinue. Call doctor right away.
• Headache.	Continue. Call doctor when convenient.
• Diarrhea or constipation, appetite loss, stomach pain, nausea, vomiting, weight loss, diminished sex drive, impotence.	Continue. Tell doctor at next visit.
Rare:	
• Rash, hives; chest pain or irregular heartbeat; uncontrollable movements of head, neck, arms, legs.	Discontinue. Call doctor right away.
• Mood changes, enlarged breasts.	Continue. Call doctor when convenient.

DEXTROAMPHETAMINE

WARNINGS & PRECAUTIONS

Don't take if:
- You are allergic to any amphetamine or central-nervous-system stimulant.
- You will have surgery within 2 months, including dental surgery, requiring general or spinal anesthesia.

Before you start, consult your doctor:
- If you plan to become pregnant within medication period.
- If you have glaucoma.
- If you have heart or blood-vessel disease, or high blood pressure.
- If you have overactive thyroid, anxiety or tension.
- If you have a severe mental illness (especially children).

Over age 60:
Adverse reactions and side effects may be more frequent and severe than in younger persons.

Pregnancy:
Risk to unborn child outweighs drug benefits. Don't use.

Breast-feeding:
Drug passes into milk. Avoid drug or discontinue nursing.

Infants & children:
Not recommended for children under 12.

Prolonged use:
Habit forming.

Skin & sunlight:
No problems expected.

Driving, piloting or hazardous work:
Don't drive or pilot aircraft until you learn how medicine affects you. Don't work around dangerous machinery. Don't climb ladders or work in high places. Danger increases if you drink alcohol or take medicine affecting alertness and reflexes.

Discontinuing:
May be unnecessary to finish medicine. Follow doctor's instructions.

Others:
- This is a dangerous drug and must be closely supervised. Don't use for appetite control or depression. Potential for damage and abuse.
- During withdrawal phase, may cause prolonged sleep of several days.

POSSIBLE INTERACTION WITH OTHER DRUGS

GENERIC NAME OR DRUG CLASS	COMBINED EFFECT
Anesthesias (general)	Irregular heartbeat.
Antidepressants (tricyclic)	Decreased dextroamphetamine effect.
Antihypertensives	Decreased antihypertensive effect.
Carbonic anhydrase inhibitors	Increased dextroamphetamine effect.
Guanethidine	Decreased guanethidine effect.
Haloperidol	Decreased dextroamphetamine effect.
MAO inhibitors	May severely increase blood pressure.
Phenothiazines	Decreased dextroamphetamine effect.
Sodium bicarbonate	Increased dextroamphetamine effect.

POSSIBLE INTERACTION WITH OTHER SUBSTANCES

INTERACTS WITH	COMBINED EFFECT
Alcohol:	Decreased dextroamphetamine effect. Avoid.
Beverages: Caffeine drinks.	Overstimulation. Avoid.
Cocaine:	Dangerous stimulation of nervous system. Avoid.
Foods:	None expected.
Marijuana:	Frequent use— Severely impaired mental function.
Tobacco:	None expected.

DEXTROMETHORPHAN

BRAND NAMES

See complete list of brand names in the *Brand Name Directory*, page 948.

BASIC INFORMATION

Habit forming? No
Prescription needed? No
Available as generic? Yes
Drug class: Cough suppressant

 USES

Suppresses cough associated with allergies or infections such as colds, bronchitis, flu and lung disorders.

 DOSAGE & USAGE INFORMATION

How to take:
- Tablet or capsule—Swallow with liquid. If you can't swallow whole, crumble tablet or open capsule and take with liquid or food.
- Lozenges or syrups—Take as directed on label.

When to take:
As needed, no more often than every 3 hours.

If you forget a dose:
Take as soon as you remember. Wait 3 hours for next dose.

What drug does:
Reduces sensitivity of brain's cough-control center, suppressing urge to cough.

Time lapse before drug works:
15 to 30 minutes.

Don't take with:
See Interaction column and consult doctor.

 OVERDOSE

SYMPTOMS:
Euphoria, overactivity, sense of intoxication, visual and auditory hallucinations, lack of coordination, stagger, stupor, shallow breathing.
WHAT TO DO:
- **Dial 0 (operator) or 911 (emergency) for an ambulance or medical help. Then give first aid immediately.**
- **See emergency information on inside covers.**

 POSSIBLE ADVERSE REACTIONS OR SIDE EFFECTS

SYMPTOMS	WHAT TO DO
Life-threatening: None expected.	
Common: None expected.	
Infrequent: None expected.	
Rare: Dizziness, drowsiness, rash, diarrhea, nausea or vomiting, stomach pain.	Discontinue. Call doctor right away.

WARNINGS & PRECAUTIONS

Don't take if:
You are allergic to any cough syrup containing dextromethorphan.

Before you start, consult your doctor:
- If you have asthma attacks.
- If you have impaired liver function.

Over age 60:
May become constipated, excessively drowsy or unsteady. If drug is used for cough, other treatment may be necessary to liquefy thick mucus in bronchial tubes.

Pregnancy:
No proven harm to unborn child. Avoid if possible.

Breast-feeding:
No proven problems. Consult doctor.

Infants & children:
Use only as label directs.

Prolonged use:
No problems expected.

Skin & sunlight:
No problems expected.

Driving, piloting or hazardous work:
Don't drive or pilot aircraft until you learn how medicine affects you. Don't work around dangerous machinery. Don't climb ladders or work in high places. Danger increases if you drink alcohol or take medicine affecting alertness and reflexes, such as antihistamines, tranquilizers, sedatives, pain medicine, narcotics and mind-altering drugs.

Discontinuing:
May be unnecessary to finish medicine. Follow doctor's instructions.

Others:
- If cough persists or if you cough blood or brown-yellow, thick mucus, call your doctor.
- Excessive use may lead to functional dependence.

POSSIBLE INTERACTION WITH OTHER DRUGS

GENERIC NAME OR DRUG CLASS	COMBINED EFFECT
MAO inhibitors	Disorientation, high fever, drop in blood pressure and loss of consciousness.

POSSIBLE INTERACTION WITH OTHER SUBSTANCES

INTERACTS WITH	COMBINED EFFECT
Alcohol:	None expected.
Beverages:	None expected.
Cocaine:	Decreased dextromethorphan effect. Avoid.
Foods:	None expected.
Marijuana:	None expected.
Tobacco:	None expected.

DIAZEPAM

BRAND NAMES

Apo-Diazepam	Rival
D-Tran	Serenack
E-Pam	Stress-Pam
Meval	Valium
Neo-Calme	Valrelease
Novodipam	Vivol
Q-Pam	

BASIC INFORMATION

Habit forming? Yes
Prescription needed? Yes
Available as generic? Yes
Drug class: Tranquilizer (benzodiazepine)

 USES

- Treatment for nervousness or tension.
- Treatment for muscle spasm.
- Treatment for convulsive disorders.

 DOSAGE & USAGE INFORMATION

How to take:
Tablet or capsule—Swallow with liquid. If you can't swallow whole, crumble tablet or open capsule and take with liquid or food.

When to take:
At the same time each day, according to instructions on prescription label.

If you forget a dose:
Take as soon as you remember up to 2 hours late. If more than 2 hours, wait for next scheduled dose (don't double this dose).

Continued next column

 OVERDOSE

SYMPTOMS:
Drowsiness, weakness, tremor, stupor, coma.
WHAT TO DO:
- Dial 0 (operator) or 911 (emergency) for an ambulance or medical help. Then give first aid immediately.
- If patient is unconscious and not breathing, give mouth-to-mouth breathing. If there is no heartbeat, use cardiac massage and mouth-to-mouth breathing (CPR). Don't try to make patient vomit. If you can't get help quickly, take patient to nearest emergency facility.
- See emergency information on inside covers.

What drug does:
Affects limbic system of brain—part that controls emotions.

Time lapse before drug works:
2 hours. May take 6 weeks for full benefit.

Don't take with:
See Interaction column and consult doctor.

 POSSIBLE ADVERSE REACTIONS OR SIDE EFFECTS

SYMPTOMS	WHAT TO DO
Life-threatening: None expected.	
Common: Clumsiness, drowsiness, dizziness.	Continue. Call doctor when convenient.
Infrequent: • Hallucinations, confusion, depression, irritability, rash, itch, vision changes.	Discontinue. Call doctor right away.
• Constipation or diarrhea, nausea, vomiting, difficult urination.	Continue. Call doctor when convenient.
Rare: • Slow heartbeat, breathing difficulty.	Discontinue. Seek emergency treatment.
• Mouth, throat ulcers; jaundice.	Discontinue. Call doctor right away.

WARNINGS & PRECAUTIONS

Don't take if:
- You are allergic to any benzodiazepine.
- You have myasthenia gravis.
- You are active or recovering alcoholic.
- Patient is younger than 6 months.

Before you start, consult your doctor:
- If you have liver, kidney or lung disease.
- If you have diabetes, epilepsy or porphyria.

Over age 60:
Adverse reactions and side effects may be more frequent and severe than in younger persons. You need smaller doses for shorter periods of time. May develop agitation, rage or "hangover" effect.

Pregnancy:
Risk to unborn child outweighs drug benefits. Don't use.

Breast-feeding:
Drug passes into milk. Avoid drug or discontinue nursing until you finish medicine. Consult doctor for advice on maintaining milk supply.

Infants & children:
Use only under medical supervision for children older than 6 months.

Prolonged use:
May impair liver function.

Skin & sunlight:
No problems expected.

Driving, piloting or hazardous work:
Don't drive or pilot aircraft until you learn how medicine affects you. Don't work around dangerous machinery. Don't climb ladders or work in high places. Danger increases if you drink alcohol or take medicine affecting alertness and reflexes.

Discontinuing:
Don't discontinue without consulting doctor. Dose may require gradual reduction if you have taken drug for a long time. Doses of other drugs may also require adjustment.

Others:
- Hot weather, heavy exercise and profuse sweat may reduce excretion and cause overdose.
- Blood sugar may rise in diabetics, requiring insulin adjustment.

POSSIBLE INTERACTION WITH OTHER DRUGS

GENERIC NAME OR DRUG CLASS	COMBINED EFFECT
Anticonvulsants	Change in seizure frequency or severity.
Antidepressants	Increased sedative effect of both drugs.
Antihistamines	Increased sedative effect of both drugs.
Antihypertensives	Excessively low blood pressure.
Cimetidine	Excess sedation.
Disulfiram	Increased diazepam effect.
Dronabinol	Increased effects of both drugs. Avoid.
MAO inhibitors	Convulsions, deep sedation, rage.
Molindone	Increased tranquilizer effect.
Narcotics	Increased sedative effect of both drugs.
Sedatives	Increased sedative effect of both drugs.
Sleep inducers	Increased sedative effect of both drugs.
Tranquilizers	Increased sedative effect of both drugs.

POSSIBLE INTERACTION WITH OTHER SUBSTANCES

INTERACTS WITH	COMBINED EFFECT
Alcohol:	Heavy sedation. Avoid.
Beverages:	None expected.
Cocaine:	Decreased diazepam effect.
Foods:	None expected.
Marijuana:	Heavy sedation. Avoid.
Tobacco:	Decreased diazepam effect.

DICLOXACILLIN

BRAND NAMES

Dycill   Pathocil
Dynapen

BASIC INFORMATION

Habit forming? No
Prescription needed? Yes
Available as generic? Yes
Drug class: Antibiotic (penicillin)

USES

Treatment of bacterial infections that are susceptible to dicloxacillin.

DOSAGE & USAGE INFORMATION

How to take:
- Tablets or capsules—Swallow with liquid on an empty stomach 1 hour before or 2 hours after eating.
- Liquid—Take with cold beverage. Liquid form is perishable and effective for only 7 days at room temperature. Effective for 14 days if stored in refrigerator. Don't freeze.

When to take:
Follow instructions on prescription label or side of package. Doses should be evenly spaced. For example, 4 times a day means every 6 hours.

If you forget a dose:
Take as soon as you remember. Continue regular schedule.

What drug does:
Destroys susceptible bacteria. Does not kill viruses.

Time lapse before drug works:
May be several days before medicine affects infection.

Don't take with:
See Interaction column and consult doctor.

OVERDOSE

SYMPTOMS:
Severe diarrhea, nausea or vomiting.
WHAT TO DO:
Overdose unlikely to threaten life. If person takes much larger amount than prescribed, call doctor, poison-control center or hospital emergency room for instructions.

POSSIBLE ADVERSE REACTIONS OR SIDE EFFECTS

SYMPTOMS	WHAT TO DO
Life-threatening:	
Hives, rash, intense itching, faintness soon after a dose (anaphylaxis).	Seek emergency treatment immediately.
Common:	
Dark or discolored tongue.	Continue. Tell doctor at next visit.
Infrequent:	
Mild nausea, vomiting, diarrhea.	Continue. Call doctor when convenient.
Rare:	
Unexplained bleeding.	Discontinue. Call doctor right away.

WARNINGS & PRECAUTIONS

Don't take if:
You are allergic to dicloxacillin, cephalosporin antibiotics, other penicillins or penicillamine. Life-threatening reaction may occur.

Before you start, consult your doctor:
If you are allergic to any substance or drug.

Over age 60:
You may have skin reactions, particularly around genitals and anus.

Pregnancy:
Studies inconclusive on harm to unborn child. Animal studies show fetal abnormalities. Decide with your doctor whether drug benefits justify risk to unborn child.

Breast-feeding:
Drug passes into milk. Child may become sensitive to penicillins and have allergic reactions to penicillin drugs. Avoid dicloxacillin or discontinue nursing until you finish medicine. Consult doctor for advice on maintaining milk supply.

Infants & children:
No problems expected.

Prolonged use:
You may become more susceptible to infections caused by germs not responsive to dicloxacillin.

Skin & sunlight:
No problems expected.

Driving, piloting or hazardous work:
Usually not dangerous. Most hazardous reactions likely to occur a few minutes after taking dicloxacillin.

Discontinuing:
Don't discontinue without doctor's advice until you complete prescribed dose, even though symptoms diminish or disappear.

Others:
No problems expected.

POSSIBLE INTERACTION WITH OTHER DRUGS

GENERIC NAME OR DRUG CLASS	COMBINED EFFECT
Beta-adrenergic blockers	Increased chance of anaphylaxis (see emergency information on inside front cover).
Chloramphenicol	Decreased effect of both drugs.
Erythromycins	Decreased effect of both drugs.
Loperamide	Decreased dicloxacillin effect.
Paromomycin	Decreased effect of both drugs.
Tetracyclines	Decreased effect of both drugs.
Troleandomycin	Decreased effect of both drugs.

POSSIBLE INTERACTION WITH OTHER SUBSTANCES

INTERACTS WITH	COMBINED EFFECT
Alcohol:	Occasional stomach irritation.
Beverages:	None expected.
Cocaine:	No proven problems.
Foods:	None expected.
Marijuana:	No proven problems.
Tobacco:	None expected.

DICYCLOMINE

BRAND NAMES

See complete list of brand names in the
Brand Name Directory, page 948.

BASIC INFORMATION

Habit forming? No
Prescription needed?
 Low strength: No
 High strength: Yes
Available as generic? Yes
Drug class: Antispasmodic, anticholinergic

 USES

Reduces spasms of digestive system, bladder
and urethra.

DOSAGE & USAGE INFORMATION

How to take:
- Tablet, syrup or capsule—Swallow with liquid
  or food to lessen stomach irritation.
- Drops—Dilute dose in beverage before
  swallowing.

When to take:
30 minutes before meals (unless directed
otherwise by doctor).

If you forget a dose:
Take as soon as you remember up to 2 hours
late. If more than 2 hours, wait for next
scheduled dose (don't double this dose).

What drug does:
Blocks nerve impulses at parasympathetic nerve
endings, preventing muscle contractions and
gland secretions of organs involved.

Time lapse before drug works:
15 to 30 minutes.

Don't take with:
See Interaction column and consult doctor.

OVERDOSE

SYMPTOMS:
**Dilated pupils, rapid pulse and breathing,
dizziness, fever, hallucinations, confusion,
slurred speech, agitation, flushed face,
convulsions, coma.**
WHAT TO DO:
- **Dial 0 (operator) or 911 (emergency) for an
  ambulance or medical help. Then give first
  aid immediately.**
- **See emergency information on inside
  covers.**

POSSIBLE ADVERSE REACTIONS OR SIDE EFFECTS

SYMPTOMS	WHAT TO DO
Life-threatening:	
None expected.	
Common:	
• Confusion, delirium, rapid heartbeat.	Discontinue. Call doctor right away.
• Nausea, vomiting, decreased sweating.	Continue. Call doctor when convenient.
• Constipation.	Continue. Tell doctor at next visit.
• Dry ears, nose, throat.	No action necessary.
Infrequent:	
Headache, difficult urination.	Continue. Call doctor when convenient.
Rare:	
Rash or hives, pain, blurred vision.	Discontinue. Call doctor right away.

WARNINGS & PRECAUTIONS

Don't take if:
- You are allergic to any anticholinergic.
- You have trouble with stomach bloating.
- You have difficulty emptying your bladder
  completely.
- You have narrow-angle glaucoma.
- You have severe ulcerative colitis.

Before you start, consult your doctor:
- If you have open-angle glaucoma.
- If you have angina.
- If you have chronic bronchitis or asthma.
- If you have hiatal hernia.
- If you have liver disease.
- If you have enlarged prostate.
- If you have myasthenia gravis.
- If you have peptic ulcer.
- If you will have surgery within 2 months,
  including dental surgery, requiring general or
  spinal anesthesia.

Over age 60:
Adverse reactions and side effects may be
more frequent and severe than in younger
persons.

Pregnancy:
Studies inconclusive on harm to unborn child.
Animal studies show fetal abnormalities. Decide
with your doctor whether drug benefits justify
risk to unborn child.

Breast-feeding:
Drug passes into milk and decreases milk flow.
Avoid drug or discontinue nursing until you
finish medicine. Consult doctor for advice on
maintaining milk supply.

Infants & children:
Use only under medical supervision.

Prolonged use:
Chronic constipation, possible fecal impaction. Consult doctor immediately.

Skin & sunlight:
No problems expected.

Driving, piloting or hazardous work:
Use disqualifies you for piloting aircraft. Otherwise, no problems expected.

Discontinuing:
May be unnecessary to finish medicine. Follow doctor's instructions.

Others:
No problems expected.

POSSIBLE INTERACTION WITH OTHER DRUGS

GENERIC NAME OR DRUG CLASS	COMBINED EFFECT
Amantadine	Increased dicyclomine effect.
Anticholinergics (other)	Increased dicyclomine effect.
Antidepressants (tricyclic)	Increased dicyclomine effect. Increased sedation.
Antihistamines	Increased dicyclomine effect.
Cortisone drugs	Increased internal-eye pressure.
Haloperidol	Increased internal-eye pressure.
MAO inhibitors	Increased dicyclomine effect.
Meperidine	Increased dicyclomine effect.
Methylphenidate	Increased dicyclomine effect.
Nitrates	Increased internal-eye pressure.
Orphenadrine	Increased dicyclomine effect.
Phenothiazines	Increased dicyclomine effect.
Pilocarpine	Loss of pilocarpine effect in glaucoma treatment.

Potassium supplements	Possible intestinal ulcers with oral potassium tablets.
Vitamin C	Decreased dicyclomine effect. Avoid large doses of vitamin C.

POSSIBLE INTERACTION WITH OTHER SUBSTANCES

INTERACTS WITH	COMBINED EFFECT
Alcohol:	None expected.
Beverages:	None expected.
Cocaine:	Excessively rapid heartbeat. Avoid.
Foods:	None expected.
Marijuana:	Drowsiness and dry mouth.
Tobacco:	None expected.

DIETHYLSTILBESTROL

BRAND NAMES

DES
Honvol
Stilbestrol

Stilphostrol
Stilbilium

BASIC INFORMATION

Habit forming? No
Prescription needed? Yes
Available as generic? Yes
Drug class: Female sex hormone (estrogen)

 USES

- Treatment for symptoms of menopause and menstrual-cycle irregularity.
- Replacement for female hormone deficiency.
- Treatment for cancer of prostate and breast.

 DOSAGE & USAGE INFORMATION

How to take:
- Tablet—Swallow with liquid. If you can't swallow whole, crumble tablet and take with liquid or food.
- Vaginal suppositories—Use as directed on label.

When to take:
At the same time each day.

If you forget a dose:
Take as soon as you remember up to 12 hours late. If more than 12 hours, wait for next scheduled dose (don't double this dose).

What drug does:
Restores normal estrogen level in tissues.

Time lapse before drug works:
10 to 20 days.

Don't take with:
See Interaction column and consult doctor.

 OVERDOSE

SYMPTOMS:
Nausea, vomiting, fluid retention, breast enlargement and discomfort, abnormal vaginal bleeding.
WHAT TO DO:
Overdose unlikely to threaten life. If person takes much larger amount than prescribed, call doctor, poison-control center or hospital emergency room for instructions.

 POSSIBLE ADVERSE REACTIONS OR SIDE EFFECTS

SYMPTOMS	WHAT TO DO
Life-threatening: None expected.	
Common:	
• Stomach cramps.	Discontinue. Call doctor right away.
• Appetite loss.	Continue. Call doctor when convenient.
• Nausea; diarrhea; swollen ankles and feet; tender, swollen breasts.	Continue. Tell doctor at next visit.
Infrequent:	
• Rash, stomach or side pain.	Discontinue. Call doctor right away.
• Depression, dizziness, irritability, vomiting, breast lumps.	Continue. Call doctor when convenient.
• Brown blotches, hair loss, vaginal discharge or bleeding, changes in sex drive.	Continue. Tell doctor at next visit.
Rare:	
Jaundice.	Discontinue. Call doctor right away.

WARNINGS & PRECAUTIONS

Don't take if:
- You are allergic to any estrogen-containing drugs.
- You have impaired liver function.
- You have had blood clots, stroke or heart attack.
- You have unexplained vaginal bleeding.

Before you start, consult your doctor:
- If you have had cancer of breast or reproductive organs, fibrocystic breast disease, fibroid tumors of the uterus or endometriosis.
- If you have had migraine headaches, epilepsy or porphyria.
- If you have diabetes, high blood pressure, asthma, congestive heart failure, kidney disease or gallstones.
- If you plan to become pregnant within 3 months.

Over age 60:
Controversial. You and your doctor must decide if drug risks outweigh benefits.

Pregnancy:
Risk to unborn child outweighs drug benefits. Don't use.

Breast-feeding:
Drug filters into milk. May harm child. Avoid.

Infants & children:
Not recommended.

Prolonged use:
Increased growth of fibroid tumors of uterus. Possible association with cancer of uterus.

Skin & sunlight:
May cause rash or intensify sunburn in areas exposed to sun or sunlamp.

Driving, piloting or hazardous work:
No problems expected.

Discontinuing:
You may need to discontinue diethylstilbestrol periodically. Consult your doctor.

Others:
In rare instances, may cause blood clot in lung, brain or leg. Symptoms are *sudden* severe headache, coordination loss, vision change, chest pain, breathing difficulty, slurred speech, pain in legs or groin. Seek emergency treatment immediately.

POSSIBLE INTERACTION WITH OTHER DRUGS

GENERIC NAME OR DRUG CLASS	COMBINED EFFECT
Anticoagulants (oral)	Decreased anticoagulant effect.
Anticonvulsants (hydantoin)	Increased seizures.
Antidiabetics (oral)	Unpredictable increase or decrease in blood sugar.
Carbamazepine	Increased seizures.
Clofibrate	Decreased clofibrate effect.
Meprobamate	Increased diethylstilbestrol effect.
Phenobarbital	Decreased diethylstilbestrol effect.
Primidone	Decreased diethylstilbestrol effect.
Rifampin	Decreased diethylstilbestrol effect.
Thyroid hormones	Decreased thyroid effect.

POSSIBLE INTERACTION WITH OTHER SUBSTANCES

INTERACTS WITH	COMBINED EFFECT
Alcohol:	None expected.
Beverages:	None expected.
Cocaine:	No proven problems.
Foods:	None expected.
Marijuana:	Possible menstrual irregularities and bleeding between periods.
Tobacco:	Increased risk of blood clots leading to stroke or heart attack.

DIFENOXIN & ATROPINE

BRAND NAMES

Motofen

BASIC INFORMATION

Habit forming? No
Prescription needed? Yes
Available as generic? No
Drug class: Antidiarrheal

 USES

- Reduces spasms of digestive system.
- Treats severe diarrhea.

 DOSAGE & USAGE INFORMATION

How to take:
Tablet—Swallow with liquid or food to lessen stomach irritation.

When to take:
After each loose stool or every 3 to 4 hours. No more than 5 tablets in 12 hours.

If you forget a dose:
Take as soon as you remember. Don't double this dose.

What drug does:
- Blocks nerve impulses at parasympathetic nerve endings, preventing muscle contractions and gland secretions of organs involved.
- Acts on brain to decrease spasm of smooth muscle.

Time lapse before drug works:
40 to 60 minutes.

Continued next column

 OVERDOSE

SYMPTOMS:
Dilated pupils, rapid pulse and breathing, dizziness, fever, hallucinations, confusion, slurred speech, agitation, flushed face, convulsions, coma.
WHAT TO DO:
- **Dial 0 (operator) or 911 (emergency) for an ambulance or medical help. Then give first aid immediately.**
- **See emergency information on inside covers.**

Don't take with:
- Any medicine that will decrease mental alertness or reflexes, such as alcohol, other mind-altering drugs, cough/cold medicines, antihistamines, allergy medicine, sedatives, tranquilizers (sleeping pills or "downers") barbiturates, seizure medicine, narcotics, other prescription medicine for pain, muscle relaxants, anesthetics.
- See Interaction column and consult doctor.

 POSSIBLE ADVERSE REACTIONS OR SIDE EFFECTS

SYMPTOMS	WHAT TO DO
Life-threatening:	
Shortness of breath, agitation, nervousness.	Discontinue. Seek emergency treatment.
Common:	
Dizziness, drowsiness.	Continue. Call doctor when convenient.
Infrequent:	
• Bloating; constipation; appetite loss; abdominal pain; blurred vision; warm, flushed skin; fast heartbeat; dry mouth.	Discontinue. Call doctor right away.
• Frequent urination, lightheadedness, dry skin, headache, insomnia.	Continue. Call doctor when convenient.
Rare:	
Weakness, confusion, fever.	Continue. Call doctor when convenient.

 WARNINGS & PRECAUTIONS

Don't take if:
- You are allergic to any anticholinergic.
- You have trouble with stomach bloating, difficulty emptying your bladder completely, narrow-angle glaucoma, severe ulcerative colitis.
- You are dehydrated.

Before you start, consult your doctor:
- If you have open-angle glaucoma, angina, chronic bronchitis, asthma, liver disease, hiatal hernia, enlarged prostate, myasthenia gravis, peptic ulcer.
- If you will have surgery within 2 months, including dental surgery, requiring general or spinal anesthesia.

Over age 60:
Adverse reactions and side effects may be more frequent and severe than in younger persons.

Pregnancy:
Studies inconclusive on harm to unborn child. Animal studies show fetal abnormalities. Decide with your doctor whether drug benefits justify risk to unborn child.

Breast-feeding:
Drug passes into milk. Avoid drug or discontinue nursing until you finish medicine. Consult doctor for advice on maintaining milk supply.

Infants & children:
Use only under medical supervision.

Prolonged use:
Chronic constipation, possible fecal impaction. Consult doctor immediately.

Skin & sunlight:
No problems expected.

Driving, piloting or hazardous work:
Use disqualifies you for piloting aircraft. Otherwise, no problems expected.

Discontinuing:
May be unnecessary to finish medicine. Follow doctor's instructions.

Others:
Atropine included at doses below therapeutic level to prevent abuse.

POSSIBLE INTERACTION WITH OTHER DRUGS

GENERIC NAME OR DRUG CLASS	COMBINED EFFECT
Addictive substances (narcotics, others)	Increased chance of abuse.
Amantadine	Increased atropine effect.
Anticholinergics (other)	Increased atropine effect.
Antidepressants (tricyclic, see Glossary)	Increased atropine effect. Increased sedation.
Antihistamines	Increased atropine effect.
Antihypertensive medicines	Increased sedation.
Cortisone drugs	Increased internal-eye pressure.
Haloperidol	Increased internal-eye pressure.
MAO inhibitors	Increased atropine effect.
Meperidine	Increased atropine effect.
Methylphenidate	Increased atropine effect.

Nitrates	Increased internal-eye pressure.
Orphenadrine	Increased atropine effect.
Phenothiazines	Increased atropine effect.
Pilocarpine	Loss of pilocarpine effect in glaucoma treatment.
Potassium supplements	Possible intestinal ulcers with oral potassium tablets.
Procainamide	Increased atropine effect.
Vitamin C	Decreased atropine effect. Avoid large doses of vitamin C.

POSSIBLE INTERACTION WITH OTHER SUBSTANCES

INTERACTS WITH	COMBINED EFFECT
Alcohol:	Increased sedation Avoid.
Beverages:	None expected.
Cocaine:	Excessively rapid heartbeat. Avoid.
Foods:	None expected.
Marijuana:	Drowsiness and dry mouth.
Tobacco:	May increase diarrhea. Avoid.

DIFLUNISAL

BRAND NAMES

Dolobid

BASIC INFORMATION

Habit forming? No
Prescription needed? Yes
Available as generic? Yes
Drug class: Anti-inflammatory (non-steroid)

 USES

- Treatment for joint pain, stiffness, inflammation and swelling of arthritis and gout.
- Pain reliever.

 DOSAGE & USAGE INFORMATION

How to take:
Tablet or capsule—Swallow with liquid or food to lessen stomach irritation. If you can't swallow whole, crumble tablet or open capsule and take with liquid or food.

When to take:
At the same times each day.

If you forget a dose:
Take as soon as you remember up to 2 hours late. If more than 2 hours, wait for next scheduled dose (don't double this dose).

What drug does:
Reduces tissue concentration of prostaglandins (hormones which produce inflammation and pain).

Time lapse before drug works:
Begins in 4 to 24 hours. May require 3 weeks regular use for maximum benefit.

Don't take with:
See Interaction column and consult doctor.

 OVERDOSE

SYMPTOMS:
Confusion, agitation, incoherence, convulsions, possible hemorrhage from stomach or intestine, coma.
WHAT TO DO:
- **Dial 0 (operator) or 911 (emergency) for an ambulance or medical help. Then give first aid immediately.**
- **See emergency information on inside covers.**

 POSSIBLE ADVERSE REACTIONS OR SIDE EFFECTS

SYMPTOMS	WHAT TO DO
Life-threatening: None expected.	
Common: • Dizziness, nausea, pain.	Continue. Call doctor when convenient.
• Headache.	Continue. Tell doctor at next visit.
Infrequent: Depression; drowsiness; ringing in ears; constipation or diarrhea; vomiting; swollen feet, legs.	Continue. Call doctor when convenient.
Rare: • Convulsions; confusion; rash, hives, or itch; blurred vision; bloody or black, tarry stools; difficult breathing; tightness in chest; rapid heartbeat; unusual bleeding or bruising; blood in urine; jaundice.	Discontinue. Call doctor right away.
• Urgent, frequent, painful or difficult urination; fatigue; weakness.	Continue. Call doctor when convenient.

WARNINGS & PRECAUTIONS

Don't take if:
- You are allergic to aspirin or any non-steroid, anti-inflammatory drug.
- You have gastritis, peptic ulcer, enteritis, ileitis, ulcerative colitis, asthma, heart failure, high blood pressure or bleeding problems.
- Patient is younger than 15.

Before you start, consult your doctor:
- If you have epilepsy.
- If you have Parkinson's disease.
- If you have been mentally ill.
- If you have had kidney disease or impaired kidney function.

Over age 60:
Adverse reactions and side effects may be more frequent and severe than in younger persons.

Pregnancy:
Studies inconclusive on harm to unborn child. Animal studies show fetal abnormalities. Decide with your doctor whether drug benefits justify risk to unborn child.

Breast-feeding:
May harm child. Avoid.

Infants & children:
Not recommended for anyone younger than 15. Use only under medical supervision.

Prolonged use:
- Eye damage.
- Reduced hearing.
- Sore throat, fever.
- Weight gain.

Skin & sunlight:
No problems expected.

Driving, piloting or hazardous work:
Don't drive or pilot aircraft until you learn how medicine affects you. Don't work around dangerous machinery. Don't climb ladders or work in high places. Danger increases if you drink alcohol or take medicine affecting alertness and reflexes, such as antihistamines, tranquilizers, sedatives, pain medicine, narcotics and mind-altering drugs.

Discontinuing:
Don't discontinue without consulting doctor. Dose may require gradual reduction if you have taken drug for a long time. Doses of other drugs may also require adjustment.

Others:
No problems expected.

POSSIBLE INTERACTION WITH OTHER DRUGS

GENERIC NAME OR DRUG CLASS	COMBINED EFFECT
Acebutolol	Decreased antihypertensive effect of acebutolol.
Antacids	Decreased diflunisal effect.
Anticoagulants (oral)	Decreased effect of anticoagulant.
Aspirin, other anti-inflammatory drugs	Increased risk of stomach ulcer.
Cortisone drugs	Increased risk of stomach ulcer.
Furosemide	Decreased diuretic effect of furosemide.
Gold compounds	Possible increased likelihood of kidney damage.
Hydrochlorothiazide	Increased risk of severe blood-pressure drop.
Indomethacin	Increased possibility of intestinal hemorrhage.
Minoxidil	Decreased minoxidil effect.
Oxyphenbutazone	Possible stomach ulcer.
Oxprenolol	Decreased antihypertensive effect of oxprenolol.
Phenylbutazone	Possible stomach ulcer.
Probenecid	Increased diflunisal effect.
Thyroid hormones	Rapid heartbeat. Blood-pressure rise.

POSSIBLE INTERACTION WITH OTHER SUBSTANCES

INTERACTS WITH	COMBINED EFFECT
Alcohol:	Possible stomach ulcer or bleeding.
Beverages:	None expected.
Cocaine:	Increased cocaine toxicity. Avoid.
Foods:	None expected.
Marijuana:	Increased pain relief from diflunisal.
Tobacco:	Decreased absorption of diflunisal. Avoid.

DIGITALIS PREPARATIONS

BRAND AND GENERIC NAMES

Crystodigin
Crystogin
Digifortis
Digiglusin
DIGITALIS
DIGITOXIN
DIGOXIN

Gitaligen
GITALIN
Lanoxicaps
Lanoxin
Natigozine
Novodigoxin
Purodigin

BASIC INFORMATION

Habit forming? No
prescription needed? Yes
Available as generic? Yes
Drug class: Digitalis preparations

 USES

- Strengthens weak heart-muscle contractions to prevent congestive heart failure.
- Corrects irregular heartbeat.

 DOSAGE & USAGE INFORMATION

How to take:
- Tablet or capsule—Swallow with liquid. If you can't swallow whole, crumble tablet or open capsule and take with liquid or food.
- Liquid—Dilute dose in beverage before swallowing.

When to take:
At the same time each day.

If you forget a dose:
Take as soon as you remember up to 12 hours late. If more than 12 hours, wait for next scheduled dose (don't double this dose).

What drug does:
- Strengthens heart-muscle contraction.
- Delays nerve impulses to heart.

Continued next column

 OVERDOSE

SYMPTOMS:
Nausea, vomiting, diarrhea, vision disturbances with halos around lights, irregular heartbeat, confusion, hallucinations, convulsions.
WHAT TO DO:
- **Dial 0 (operator) or 911 (emergency) for an ambulance or medical help. Then give first aid immediately.**
- **See emergency information on inside covers.**

Time lapse before drug works:
May require regular use for a week or more.

Don't take with:
- Non-prescription drugs without consulting doctor.
- See Interaction column and consult doctor.

 POSSIBLE ADVERSE REACTIONS OR SIDE EFFECTS

SYMPTOMS	WHAT TO DO
Life-threatening: None expected.	
Common: Appetite loss, diarrhea.	Continue. Call doctor when convenient.
Infrequent: Drowsiness, lethargy, disorientation.	Discontinue. Call doctor right away.
Rare:	
• Rash, hives.	Discontinue. Call doctor right away.
• Double or yellow-green vision; enlarged, sensitive male breasts; tiredness; weakness.	Continue. Call doctor when convenient.

WARNINGS & PRECAUTIONS

Don't take if:
- You are allergic to any digitalis preparation.
- Your heartbeat is slower than 50 beats per minute.

Before you start, consult your doctor:
- If you have taken another digitalis preparation in past 2 weeks.
- If you have taken a diuretic within 2 weeks.
- If you have liver or kidney disease.
- If you have a thyroid disorder.
- If you will have surgery within 2 months, including dental surgery, requiring general or spinal anesthesia.

Over age 60:
Adverse reactions and side effects may be more frequent and severe than in younger persons.

Pregnancy:
Studies inconclusive on harm to unborn child. Consult your doctor.

Breast-feeding:
Drug filters into milk. May harm child. Avoid.

Infants & children:
Use only under medical supervision.

Prolonged use:
No problems expected.

Skin & sunlight:
No problems expected.

Driving, piloting or hazardous work:
Possible vision disturbances. Otherwise, no problems expected.

Discontinuing:
Don't stop without doctor's advice.

Others:
No problems expected.

POSSIBLE INTERACTION WITH OTHER DRUGS

GENERIC NAME OR DRUG CLASS	COMBINED EFFECT
Albuterol	Increased risk of heartbeat irregularity.
Amiodarone	Increased digitalis effect.
Antacids	Decreased digitalis effect.
Anticonvulsants (hydantoin)	Increased digitalis effect at first, then decreased.
Beta-adrenergic blockers	Increased digitalis effect.
Calcium supplements	Decreased digitalis effects.
Cortisone drugs	Digitalis toxicity.
Diuretics	Possible digitalis toxicity.
Ephedrine	Disturbed heart rhythm. Avoid.
Epinephrine	Disturbed heart rhythm. Avoid.
Flecainide	May increase digitalis blood level.
Guanethidine	Increased digitalis effect.
Indapamide	Excessive potassium loss that may cause irregular heartbeat.
Laxatives	Decreased digitalis effect.
Oxyphenbutazone	Decreased digitalis effect.
Phenobarbital	Decreased digitalis effect.
Phenylbutazone	Decreased digitalis effect.
Potassium supplements	Overdosage of either drug may cause severe heartbeat irregularity.
Quinidine	Increased digitalis effect.
Rauwolfia alkaloids	Increased digitalis effect.
Thyroid hormones	Digitalis toxicity.

POSSIBLE INTERACTION WITH OTHER SUBSTANCES

INTERACTS WITH	COMBINED EFFECT
Alcohol:	None expected.
Beverages: Caffeine drinks.	Irregular heartbeat. Avoid.
Cocaine:	Irregular heartbeat. Avoid.
Foods:	None expected.
Marijuana:	Decreased digitalis effect.
Tobacco:	Irregular heartbeat. Avoid.

DILTIAZEM

BRAND NAMES

Cardizem

BASIC INFORMATION

Habit forming? No
Prescription needed? Yes
Available as generic? No
Drug class: Calcium-channel blocker,
             antiarrhythmic, antianginal

 USES

- Prevents angina attacks.
- Stabilizes irregular heartbeat.

 DOSAGE & USAGE INFORMATION

How to take:
Tablet or capsule—Swallow with liquid.

When to take:
At the same times each day 1 hour before or 2 hours after eating.

If you forget a dose:
Take as soon as you remember up to 2 hours late. If more than 2 hours, wait for next scheduled dose (don't double this dose).

What drug does:
- Reduces work that heart must perform.
- Reduces normal artery pressure.
- Increases oxygen to heart muscle.

Time lapse before drug works:
1 to 2 hours.

Don't take with:
See Interaction column and consult doctor.

 OVERDOSE

SYMPTOMS:
Unusually fast or unusually slow heartbeat, loss of consciousness, cardiac arrest.
WHAT TO DO:
- Dial 0 (operator) or 911 (emergency) for an ambulance or medical help. Then give first aid immediately.
- See emergency information on inside covers.

 POSSIBLE ADVERSE REACTIONS OR SIDE EFFECTS

SYMPTOMS	WHAT TO DO
Life-threatening:	
None expected.	
Common:	
Tiredness.	Continue. Tell doctor at next visit.
Infrequent:	
• Unusually slow or fast heartbeat, wheezing, cough, shortness of breath.	Discontinue. Call doctor right away.
• Dizziness; numbness or tingling in hands or feet; swollen ankles, feet or legs; difficult urination.	Continue. Call doctor when convenient.
• Nausea, constipation or diarrhea, vomiting, indigestion.	Continue. Tell doctor at next visit.
Rare:	
• Fainting, rash, jaundice.	Discontinue. Call doctor right away.
• Headache.	Continue. Tell doctor at next visit.

WARNINGS & PRECAUTIONS

Don't take if:
You are allergic to any calcium-channel blocker.

Before you start, consult your doctor:
- If you have kidney or liver disease.
- If you have high or low blood pressure.
- If you have heart disease other than coronary artery disease.

Over age 60:
Adverse reactions and side effects may be more frequent and severe than in younger persons.

Pregnancy:
No proven harm to unborn child. Avoid if possible.

Breast-feeding:
No problems expected.

Infants & children:
Not recommended.

Prolonged use:
No problems expected.

Skin & sunlight:
May cause rash or intensify sunburn in areas exposed to sun or sunlamp.

Driving, piloting or hazardous work:
Avoid if you feel dizzy. Otherwise, no problems expected.

Discontinuing:
Don't discontinue without consulting doctor.

Others:
Learn to check your own pulse rate. If it drops to 50 beats per minute or lower, don't take diltiazem until your consult your doctor.

 ## POSSIBLE INTERACTION WITH OTHER DRUGS

GENERIC NAME OR DRUG CLASS	COMBINED EFFECT
Amiodarone	Increased likelihood of slow heartbeat.
Antihypertensives	Dangerous blood-pressure drop.
Beta-adrenergic blockers	Decreased angina attacks.
Diuretics	Dangerous blood-pressure drop.
Disopyramide	May cause dangerously slow, fast or irregular heartbeat.
Enalapril	Possible excessive potassium in blood.
Flecainide	Possible irregular heartbeat.
Nitrates	Reduced angina attacks.
Quinidine	Increased quinidine effect.
Tocainide	Increased likelihood of adverse reactions from either drug.

 ## POSSIBLE INTERACTION WITH OTHER SUBSTANCES

INTERACTS WITH	COMBINED EFFECT
Alcohol:	Dangerously low blood pressure.
Beverages:	None expected.
Cocaine:	Possible irregular heartbeat. Avoid.
Foods:	None expected.
Marijuana:	Possible irregular heartbeat. Avoid.
Tobacco:	Possible rapid heartbeat. Avoid.

DIMENHYDRINATE

BRAND NAMES

See complete list of brand names in the *Brand Name Directory,* page 948.

BASIC INFORMATION

Habit forming? No
Prescription needed?
  High strength: Yes
  Low strength: No
Available as generic? Yes
Drug class: Antihistamine

 ## USES

- Reduces allergic symptoms such as hay fever, hives, rash or itching.
- Prevents motion sickness, nausea, vomiting.
- Induces sleep.

 ## DOSAGE & USAGE INFORMATION

How to take:
Tablet or liquid—Swallow with liquid or food to lessen stomach irritation.

When to take:
Varies with form. Follow label directions.

If you forget a dose:
Take as soon as you remember up to 2 hours late. If more than 2 hours, wait for next scheduled dose (don't double this dose).

What drug does:
Blocks action of histamine after an allergic response triggers histamine release in sensitive cells.

Continued next column

 ## OVERDOSE

SYMPTOMS:
Convulsions, red face, hallucinations, coma.
WHAT TO DO:
- **Dial 0 (operator) or 911 (emergency) for an ambulance or medical help. Then give first aid immediately.**
- **If patient is unconscious and not breathing, give mouth-to-mouth breathing. If there is no heartbeat, use cardiac massage and mouth-to-mouth breathing (CPR). Don't try to make patient vomit. If you can't get help quickly, take patient to nearest emergency facility.**
- **See emergency information on inside covers.**

Time lapse before drug works:
30 minutes.

Don't take with:
See Interaction column and consult doctor.

 ## POSSIBLE ADVERSE REACTIONS OR SIDE EFFECTS

SYMPTOMS	WHAT TO DO
Life-threatening: None expected.	
Common: Drowsiness; dizziness; dry mouth, eyes and nose; nausea.	Continue. Tell doctor at next visit.
Infrequent:	
• Change in vision.	Discontinue. Call doctor right away.
• Less tolerance for contact lenses, frequent urination.	Continue. Call doctor when convenient.
• Appetite loss.	Continue. Tell doctor at next visit.
Rare: Nightmares, agitation, irritability, sore throat, fever, rapid heartbeat, unusual bleeding or bruising, fatigue, weakness.	Discontinue. Call doctor right away.

WARNINGS & PRECAUTIONS

Don't take if:
You are allergic to any antihistamine.

Before you start, consult your doctor:
- If you have glaucoma.
- If you have enlarged prostate.
- If you have asthma.
- If you have kidney disease.
- If you have peptic ulcer.
- If you will have surgery within 2 months, including dental surgery, requiring general or spinal anesthesia.

Over age 60:
Don't exceed recommended dose. Adverse reactions and side effects may be more frequent and severe than in younger persons, especially urination difficulty, diminished alertness and other brain and nervous-system symptoms.

Pregnancy:
No proven harm to unborn child. Avoid if possible.

Breast-feeding:
Drug passes into milk. Avoid drug or discontinue nursing until you finish medicine. Consult doctor for advice on maintaining milk supply.

Infants & children:
Not recommended for premature or newborn infants. Otherwise, no problems expected.

Prolonged use:
Avoid. May damage bone marrow and nerve cells.

Skin & sunlight:
May cause rash or intensify sunburn in areas exposed to sun or sunlamp.

Driving, piloting or hazardous work:
Don't drive or pilot aircraft until you learn how medicine affects you. Don't work around dangerous machinery. Don't climb ladders or work in high places. Danger increases if you drink alcohol or take medicine affecting alertness and reflexes, such as antihistamines, tranquilizers, sedatives, pain medicine, narcotics and mind-altering drugs.

Discontinuing:
No problems expected.

Others:
May mask symptoms of hearing damage from aspirin, other salicylates, cisplatin, paromomycin, vancomycin or anticonvulsants. Consult doctor if you use these.

POSSIBLE INTERACTION WITH OTHER DRUGS

GENERIC NAME OR DRUG CLASS	COMBINED EFFECT
Anticholinergics	Increased anticholinergic effect.
Antidepressants	Excess sedation. Avoid.
Antihistamines (other)	Excess sedation. Avoid.
Dronabinol	Increased effects of both drugs. Avoid.
Hypnotics	Excess sedation. Avoid.
MAO inhibitors	Increased dimenhydrinate effect.
Mind-altering drugs	Excess sedation. Avoid.
Molindone	Increased antihistamine effect.
Narcotics	Excess sedation. Avoid.
Sedatives	Excess sedation. Avoid.
Sleep inducers	Excess sedation. Avoid.
Tranquilizers	Excess sedation. Avoid.

POSSIBLE INTERACTION WITH OTHER SUBSTANCES

INTERACTS WITH	COMBINED EFFECT
Alcohol:	Excess sedation. Avoid.
Beverages: Caffeine drinks.	Less dimenhydrinate sedation.
Cocaine:	Decreased dimenhydrinate effect. Avoid.
Foods:	None expected.
Marijuana:	Excess sedation. Avoid.
Tobacco:	None expected.

DIMETHINDENE

BRAND NAMES

Forhistal   Triten Tab-In
Triten

BASIC INFORMATION

Habit forming? No
Prescription needed? Yes
Available as generic? Yes
Drug class: Antihistamine

 ## USES

- Reduces allergic symptoms such as hay fever, hives, rash or itching.
- Induces sleep.

 ## DOSAGE & USAGE INFORMATION

How to take:
Extended-release tablets or capsules—Take with liquid or food. Swallow each dose whole.

When to take:
Varies with form. Follow label directions.

If you forget a dose:
Take as soon as you remember up to 2 hours late. If more than 2 hours, wait for next scheduled dose (don't double this dose).

What drug does:
Blocks action of histamine after an allergic response triggers histamine release in sensitive cells.

Time lapse before drug works:
30 minutes.

Don't take with:
See Interaction column and consult doctor.

 ## OVERDOSE

SYMPTOMS:
Convulsions, red face, hallucinations, coma.
WHAT TO DO:
- Dial 0 (operator) or 911 (emergency) for an ambulance or medical help. Then give first aid immediately.
- If patient is unconscious and not breathing, give mouth-to-mouth breathing. If there is no heartbeat, use cardiac massage and mouth-to-mouth breathing (CPR). Don't try to make patient vomit. If you can't get help quickly, take patient to nearest emergency facility.
- See emergency information on inside covers.

 ## POSSIBLE ADVERSE REACTIONS OR SIDE EFFECTS

SYMPTOMS	WHAT TO DO
Life-threatening: None expected.	
Common: Drowsiness; dizziness; dry mouth, nose, throat; nausea.	Continue. Tell doctor at next visit.
Infrequent: • Change in vision.	Discontinue. Call doctor right away.
• Less tolerance for contact lenses, painful or difficult urination.	Continue. Call doctor when convenient.
• Appetite loss.	Continue. Tell doctor at next visit.
Rare: Nightmares, agitation, irritability, sore throat, fever, rapid heartbeat, unusual bleeding or bruising, fatigue, weakness.	Discontinue. Call doctor right away.

WARNINGS & PRECAUTIONS

Don't take if:
You are allergic to any antihistamine.

Before you start, consult your doctor:
- If you have glaucoma.
- If you have enlarged prostate.
- If you have asthma.
- If you have kidney disease.
- If you have peptic ulcer.
- If you will have surgery within 2 months, including dental surgery, requiring general or spinal anesthesia.

Over age 60:
Don't exceed recommended dose. Adverse reactions and side effects may be more frequent and severe than in younger persons, especially urination difficulty, diminished alertness and other brain and nervous-system symptoms.

Pregnancy:
No proven harm to unborn child. Avoid if possible.

Breast-feeding:
Drug passes into milk. Avoid drug or discontinue nursing until you finish medicine. Consult doctor for advice on maintaining milk supply.

Infants & children:
Not recommended for premature or newborn infants. Otherwise, no problems expected.

Prolonged use:
Avoid. May damage bone marrow and nerve cells.

Skin & sunlight:
May cause rash or intensify sunburn in areas exposed to sun or sunlamp.

Driving, piloting or hazardous work:
Don't drive or pilot aircraft until you learn how medicine affects you. Don't work around dangerous machinery. Don't climb ladders or work in high places. Danger increases if you drink alcohol or take medicine affecting alertness and reflexes, such as antihistamines, tranquilizers, sedatives, pain medicine, narcotics and mind-altering drugs.

Discontinuing:
No problems expected.

Others:
May mask symptoms of hearing damage from aspirin, other salicylates, cisplatin, paromomycin, vancomycin or anticonvulsants. Consult doctor if you use these.

POSSIBLE INTERACTION WITH OTHER DRUGS

GENERIC NAME OR DRUG CLASS	COMBINED EFFECT
Anticholinergics	Increased anticholinergic effect.
Antidepressants	Excess sedation. Avoid.
Antihistamines (other)	Excess sedation. Avoid.
Dronabinol	Increased effects of both drugs. Avoid.
Hypnotics	Excess sedation. Avoid.
MAO inhibitors	Increased dimethindene effect.
Mind-altering drugs	Excess sedation. Avoid.
Narcotics	Excess sedation. Avoid.
Sedatives	Excess sedation. Avoid.
Sleep inducers	Excess sedation. Avoid.
Tranquilizers	Excess sedation. Avoid.

POSSIBLE INTERACTION WITH OTHER SUBSTANCES

INTERACTS WITH	COMBINED EFFECT
Alcohol:	Excess sedation. Avoid.
Beverages: Caffeine drinks.	Less dimethindene sedation.
Cocaine:	Decreased dimethindene effect. Avoid.
Foods:	None expected.
Marijuana:	Excess sedation. Avoid.
Tobacco:	None expected.

DIPHENHYDRAMINE

BRAND NAMES

See complete list of brand names in the *Brand Name Directory,* page 948.

BASIC INFORMATION

Habit forming? No
Prescription needed?
  High strength: Yes
  Low strength: No
Available as generic? Yes
Drug class: Antihistamine

USES

- Reduces allergic symptoms such as hay fever, hives, rash or itching.
- Prevents motion sickness, nausea, vomiting.
- Induces sleep.
- Reduces stiffness and tremors of Parkinson's disease.

DOSAGE & USAGE INFORMATION

How to take:
- Tablet or capsule—Swallow with liquid or food to lessen stomach irritation.
- Extended-release tablets or capsules—Swallow each dose whole.
- Suppositories—Remove wrapper and moisten suppository with water. Gently insert larger end into rectum. Push well into rectum with finger.

When to take:
Varies with form. Follow label directions.

If you forget a dose:
Take as soon as you remember up to 2 hours late. If more than 2 hours, wait for next scheduled dose (don't double this dose).

What drug does:
Blocks action of histamine after an allergic response triggers histamine release in sensitive cells.

Continued next column

OVERDOSE

SYMPTOMS:
Convulsions, red face, hallucinations, coma.
WHAT TO DO:
- **Dial 0 (operator) or 911 (emergency) for an ambulance or medical help. Then give first aid immediately.**
- **See emergency information on inside covers.**

Time lapse before drug works:
30 minutes.

Don't take with:
See Interaction column and consult doctor.

POSSIBLE ADVERSE REACTIONS OR SIDE EFFECTS

SYMPTOMS	WHAT TO DO
Life-threatening: None expected.	
Common: Drowsiness; dizziness; dry mouth, nose, throat; nausea.	Continue. Tell doctor at next visit.
Infrequent: • Change in vision.	Discontinue. Call doctor right away.
• Less tolerance for contact lenses, painful or difficult urination.	Continue. Call doctor when convenient.
• Appetite loss.	Continue. Tell doctor at next visit.
Rare: Nightmares, agitation, irritability, sore throat, fever, rapid heartbeat, unusual bleeding or bruising, fatigue, weakness.	Discontinue. Call doctor right away.

WARNINGS & PRECAUTIONS

Don't take if:
You are allergic to any antihistamine.

Before you start, consult your doctor:
- If you have glaucoma.
- If you have enlarged prostate.
- If you have asthma.
- If you have kidney disease.
- If you have peptic ulcer.
- If you will have surgery within 2 months, including dental surgery, requiring general or spinal anesthesia.

Over age 60:
Don't exceed recommended dose. Adverse reactions and side effects may be more frequent and severe than in younger persons, especially urination difficulty, diminished alertness and other brain and nervous-system symptoms.

Pregnancy:
No proven harm to unborn child. Avoid if possible.

Breast-feeding:
Drug passes into milk. Avoid drug or discontinue nursing until you finish medicine. Consult doctor for advice on maintaining milk supply.

Infants & children:
Not recommended for premature or newborn infants. Otherwise, no problems expected.

Prolonged use:
Avoid. May damage bone marrow and nerve cells.

Skin & sunlight:
May cause rash or intensify sunburn in areas exposed to sun or sunlamp.

Driving, piloting or hazardous work:
Don't drive or pilot aircraft until you learn how medicine affects you. Don't work around dangerous machinery. Don't climb ladders or work in high places. Danger increases if you drink alcohol or take medicine affecting alertness and reflexes, such as antihistamines, tranquilizers, sedatives, pain medicine, narcotics and mind-altering drugs.

Discontinuing:
No problems expected.

Others:
May mask symptoms of hearing damage from aspirin, other salicylates, cisplatin, paromomycin, vancomycin or anticonvulsants. Consult doctor if you use these.

 ## POSSIBLE INTERACTION WITH OTHER DRUGS

GENERIC NAME OR DRUG CLASS	COMBINED EFFECT
Anticholinergics	Increased anticholinergic effect.
Antidepressants	Excess sedation. Avoid.
Antihistamines (other)	Excess sedation. Avoid.
Dronabinol	Increased effects of both drugs. Avoid.
Hypnotics	Excess sedation. Avoid.
MAO inhibitors	Increased diphenhydramine effect.
Mind-altering drugs	Excess sedation. Avoid.
Molindone	Increased sedative and antihistamine effect.
Narcotics	Excess sedation. Avoid.
Sedatives	Excess sedation. Avoid.
Sleep inducers	Excess sedation. Avoid.
Tranquilizers	Excess sedation. Avoid.

 ## POSSIBLE INTERACTION WITH OTHER SUBSTANCES

INTERACTS WITH	COMBINED EFFECT
Alcohol:	Excess sedation. Avoid.
Beverages: Caffeine drinks.	Less diphenhydramine sedation.
Cocaine:	Decreased diphenhydramine effect. Avoid.
Foods:	None expected.
Marijuana:	Excess sedation. Avoid.
Tobacco:	None expected.

DIPHENIDOL

BRAND NAMES

Vontrol

BASIC INFORMATION

Habit forming? No
Prescription needed? Yes
Available as generic? No
Drug class: Antiemetic, antivertigo

 ## USES

- Prevents motion sickness.
- Controls nausea and vomiting (do not use during pregnancy).

 ## DOSAGE & USAGE INFORMATION

How to take:
Tablet—Swallow with liquid or food to lessen stomach irritation. If you can't swallow whole, crumble tablet and chew or take with liquid or food.

When to take:
30 to 60 minutes before traveling.

If you forget a dose:
Take as soon as you remember. Wait 4 hours for next dose.

What drug does:
Reduces sensitivity of nerve endings in inner ear, blocking messages to brain's vomiting center.

Time lapse before drug works:
30 to 60 minutes.

Don't take with:
See Interaction column and consult doctor.

 ## OVERDOSE

SYMPTOMS:
Drowsiness, confusion, incoordination, weak pulse, shallow breathing, stupor, coma.
WHAT TO DO:
- Dial 0 (operator) or 911 (emergency) for an ambulance or medical help. Then give first aid immediately.
- See emergency information on inside covers.

 ## POSSIBLE ADVERSE REACTIONS OR SIDE EFFECTS

SYMPTOMS	WHAT TO DO
Life-threatening: None expected.	
Common: Drowsiness.	Continue. Tell doctor at next visit.
Infrequent: • Headache, diarrhea or constipation, fast heartbeat.	Continue. Call doctor when convenient.
• Dry mouth, nose, throat.	Continue. Tell doctor at next visit.
Rare: • Rash or hives.	Discontinue. Call doctor right away.
• Restlessness; excitement; insomnia; blurred vision; urgent, painful or difficult urination.	Continue. Call doctor when convenient.
• Appetite loss, nausea.	Continue. Tell doctor at next visit.

WARNINGS & PRECAUTIONS

Don't take if:
- You have severe kidney disease.
- You are allergic to diphenidol or meclizine.

Before you start, consult your doctor:
- If you have prostate enlargement.
- If you have glaucoma.
- If you have heart disease.
- If you have intestinal obstruction or ulcers in the gastrointestinal tract.
- If you have kidney disease.
- If you have low blood pressure.
- If you will have surgery within 2 months, including dental surgery, requiring general or spinal anesthesia.

Over age 60:
Adverse reactions and side effects may be more frequent and severe than in younger persons.

Pregnancy:
Animal studies show fetal abnormalities. Decide with your doctor whether drug benefits justify risk to unborn child.

Breast-feeding:
Drug passes into milk. Avoid drug or discontinue nursing until you finish medicine. Consult doctor for advice on maintaining milk supply.

Infants & children:
No problems expected.

Prolonged use:
No problems expected.

Skin & sunlight:
No problems expected.

Driving, piloting or hazardous work:
Don't fly aircraft. Don't drive until you learn how medicine affects you. Don't work around dangerous machinery. Don't climb ladders or work in high places. Danger increases if you drink alcohol or take medicine affecting alertness and reflexes, such as antihistamines, tranquilizers, sedatives, pain medicine, narcotics and mind-altering drugs.

Discontinuing:
No problems expected.

Others:
No problems expected.

POSSIBLE INTERACTION WITH OTHER DRUGS

GENERIC NAME OR DRUG CLASS	COMBINED EFFECT
Anticonvulsants	Increased effect of both drugs.
Antidepressants (tricyclic)	Increased sedative effect of both drugs.
Antihistamines	Increased sedative effect of both drugs.
Atropine	Increased chance of toxic effect of atropine and atropine-like medicines.
Narcotics	Increased sedative effect of both drugs.
Sedatives	Increased sedative effect of both drugs.
Tranquilizers	Increased sedative effect of both drugs.

POSSIBLE INTERACTION WITH OTHER SUBSTANCES

INTERACTS WITH	COMBINED EFFECT
Alcohol:	Increased sedation. Avoid.
Beverages: Caffeine.	May decrease drowsiness.
Cocaine:	Increased chance of toxic effects of cocaine. Avoid.
Foods:	None expected.
Marijuana:	Increased drowsiness, dry mouth.
Tobacco:	None expected.

DIPHENOXYLATE & ATROPINE

BRAND NAMES

Colonil	Lomotil
Diphenatol	Lonox
Enoxa	Lo-Trol
Latropine	Low-Quel
Lofene	Nor-Mil
Lomanate	SK-Diphenoxylate

BASIC INFORMATION

Habit forming? Yes
Prescription needed? Yes
Available as generic? Yes
Drug class: Antidiarrheal

 USES

Relieves diarrhea and intestinal cramps.

 DOSAGE & USAGE INFORMATION

How to take:
- Tablet or capsule—Swallow with liquid or food to lessen stomach irritation.
- Drops or liquid—Follow label instructions and use marked dropper.

When to take:
No more often than directed on label.

If you forget a dose:
Take as soon as you remember up to 2 hours late. If more than 2 hours, wait for next scheduled dose (don't double this dose).

What drug does:
Blocks digestive tract's nerve supply, which reduces propelling movements.

Continued next column

 OVERDOSE

SYMPTOMS:
Excitement, constricted pupils, shallow breathing, coma.
WHAT TO DO:
- Dial 0 (operator) or 911 (emergency) for an ambulance or medical help. Then give first aid immediately.
- If patient is unconscious and not breathing, give mouth-to-mouth breathing. If there is no heartbeat, use cardiac massage and mouth-to-mouth breathing (CPR). Don't try to make patient vomit. If you can't get help quickly, take patient to nearest emergency facility.
- See emergency information on inside covers.

Time lapse before drug works:
May require 12 to 24 hours of regular doses to control diarrhea.

Don't take with:
See Interaction column and consult doctor.

 POSSIBLE ADVERSE REACTIONS OR SIDE EFFECTS

SYMPTOMS	WHAT TO DO
Life-threatening: None expected.	
Common: None expected.	
Infrequent:	
• Dry mouth, swollen gums, rapid heartbeat.	Discontinue. Call doctor right away.
• Dizziness, depression, drowsiness, rash or itch, blurred vision, decreased urination.	Continue. Call doctor when convenient.
Rare: Restlessness, flush, fever, headache, stomach pain, nausea, vomiting, bloating, constipation, numbness of hands or feet.	Discontinue. Call doctor right away.

WARNINGS & PRECAUTIONS

Don't take if:
- You are allergic to diphenoxylate & atropine or any narcotic or anticholinergic.
- You have jaundice.
- Patient is younger than 2.

Before you start, consult your doctor:
- If you have had liver problems.
- If you have ulcerative colitis.
- If you plan to become pregnant within medication period.
- If you have any medical disorder.
- If you take any medication, including non-prescription drugs.

Over age 60:
Adverse reactions and side effects may be more frequent and severe than in younger persons.

Pregnancy:
No proven harm to unborn child. Avoid because of many side effects.

Breast-feeding:
Drug passes into milk. Avoid drug or discontinue nursing until you finish medicine. Consult doctor for advice on maintaining milk supply.

Infants & children:
Don't give to infants or toddlers. Use only under doctor's supervision for children older than 2.

Prolonged use:
Habit forming.

Skin & sunlight:
No problems expected.

Driving, piloting or hazardous work:
Don't drive or pilot aircraft until you learn how medicine affects you. Don't work around dangerous machinery. Don't climb ladders or work in high places. Danger increases if you drink alcohol or take medicine affecting alertness and reflexes.

Discontinuing:
- May be unnecessary to finish medicine. Follow doctor's instructions.
- After discontinuing, consult doctor if you experience muscle cramps, nausea, vomiting, trembling, stomach cramps or unusual sweating.

Others:
If diarrhea lasts longer than 4 days, discontinue and call doctor.

POSSIBLE INTERACTION WITH OTHER DRUGS

GENERIC NAME OR DRUG CLASS	COMBINED EFFECT
MAO inhibitors	May increase blood pressure excessively.
Sedatives	Increased effect of both drugs.
Tranquilizers	Increased effect of both drugs.

POSSIBLE INTERACTION WITH OTHER SUBSTANCES

INTERACTS WITH	COMBINED EFFECT
Alcohol:	Depressed brain function. Avoid.
Beverages:	None expected.
Cocaine:	Decreased effect of diphenoxylate and atropine.
Foods:	None expected.
Marijuana:	None expected.
Tobacco:	None expected.

DIPHENYLPYRALINE

BRAND NAMES

Diafen   Hispril

BASIC INFORMATION

Habit forming? No
Prescription needed?
  High strength: Yes
  Low strength: No
Available as generic? No
Drug class: Antihistamine

 ## USES

- Reduces allergic symptoms such as hay fever, hives, rash or itching.
- Induces sleep.

 ## DOSAGE & USAGE INFORMATION

How to take:
Extended-release capsules—Swallow each dose whole with liquid.

When to take:
Varies with form. Follow label directions.

If you forget a dose:
Take as soon as you remember up to 2 hours late. If more than 2 hours, wait for next scheduled dose (don't double this dose).

What drug does:
Blocks action of histamine after an allergic response triggers histamine release in sensitive cells.

Time lapse before drug works:
30 minutes.

Don't take with:
See Interaction column and consult doctor.

 ## OVERDOSE

SYMPTOMS:
Convulsions, red face, hallucinations, coma.
WHAT TO DO:
- **Dial 0 (operator) or 911 (emergency) for an ambulance or medical help. Then give first aid immediately.**
- **If patient is unconscious and not breathing, give mouth-to-mouth breathing. If there is no heartbeat, use cardiac massage and mouth-to-mouth breathing (CPR). Don't try to make patient vomit. If you can't get help quickly, take patient to nearest emergency facility.**
- **See emergency information on inside covers.**

 ## POSSIBLE ADVERSE REACTIONS OR SIDE EFFECTS

SYMPTOMS	WHAT TO DO
Life-threatening: None expected.	
Common: Drowsiness; dizziness; dry mouth, nose, throat; nausea.	Continue. Tell doctor at next visit.
Infrequent:	
• Change in vision.	Discontinue. Call doctor right away.
• Less tolerance for contact lenses, painful or difficult urination.	Continue. Call doctor when convenient.
• Appetite loss.	Continue. Tell doctor at next visit.
Rare: Nightmares, agitation, irritability, sore throat, fever, rapid heartbeat, unusual bleeding or bruising, fatigue, weakness.	Discontinue. Call doctor right away.

DIPHENYLPYRALINE

 ## WARNINGS & PRECAUTIONS

Don't take if:
You are allergic to any antihistamine.

Before you start, consult your doctor:
- If you have glaucoma.
- If you have enlarged prostate.
- If you have asthma.
- If you have kidney disease.
- If you have peptic ulcer.
- If you will have surgery within 2 months, including dental surgery, requiring general or spinal anesthesia.

Over age 60:
Don't exceed recommended dose. Adverse reactions and side effects may be more frequent and severe than in younger persons, especially urination difficulty, diminished alertness and other brain and nervous-system symptoms.

Pregnancy:
No proven harm to unborn child. Avoid if possible.

Breast-feeding:
Drug passes into milk. Avoid drug or discontinue nursing until you finish medicine. Consult doctor for advice on maintaining milk supply.

Infants & children:
Not recommended for premature or newborn infants. Otherwise, no problems expected.

Prolonged use:
Avoid. May damage bone marrow and nerve cells.

Skin & sunlight:
May cause rash or intensify sunburn in areas exposed to sun or sunlamp.

Driving, piloting or hazardous work:
Don't drive or pilot aircraft until you learn how medicine affects you. Don't work around dangerous machinery. Don't climb ladders or work in high places. Danger increases if you drink alcohol or take medicine affecting alertness and reflexes, such as antihistamines, tranquilizers, sedatives, pain medicine, narcotics and mind-altering drugs.

Discontinuing:
No problems expected.

Others:
May mask symptoms of hearing damage from aspirin, other salicylates, cisplatin, paromomycin, vancomycin or anticonvulsants. Consult doctor if you use these.

 ## POSSIBLE INTERACTION WITH OTHER DRUGS

GENERIC NAME OR DRUG CLASS	COMBINED EFFECT
Anticholinergics	Increased anticholinergic effect.
Antidepressants	Excess sedation. Avoid.
Antihistamines (other)	Excess sedation. Avoid.
Dronabinol	Increased effects of both drugs. Avoid.
Hypnotics	Excess sedation. Avoid.
MAO inhibitors	Increased diphenylpyraline effect.
Mind-altering drugs	Excess sedation. Avoid.
Molindone	Increased antihistamine effect.
Narcotics	Excess sedation. Avoid.
Sedatives	Excess sedation. Avoid.
Sleep inducers	Excess sedation. Avoid.
Tranquilizers	Excess sedation. Avoid.

POSSIBLE INTERACTION WITH OTHER SUBSTANCES

INTERACTS WITH	COMBINED EFFECT
Alcohol:	Excess sedation. Avoid.
Beverages: Caffeine drinks.	Less diphenylpyraline sedation.
Cocaine:	Decreased diphenylpyraline effect. Avoid.
Foods:	None expected.
Marijuana:	Excess sedation. Avoid.
Tobacco:	None expected.

303

DIPYRIDAMOLE

BRAND NAMES

Apo-Dipyridamole   Pyridamole
Persantine   SK-Dipyridamole

BASIC INFORMATION

Habit forming? No
Prescription needed?
  U.S.: Yes
  Canada: No
Available as generic? Yes
Drug class: Coronary vasodilator

USES

- Reduces frequency and intensity of angina attacks.
- Prevents blood clots after heart surgery.

DOSAGE & USAGE INFORMATION

How to take:
Tablet or capsule—Swallow with liquid. If you can't swallow whole, crumble tablet or open capsule and take with liquid.

When to take:
1 hour before meals.

If you forget a dose:
Take as soon as you remember up to 2 hours late. If more than 2 hours, wait for next scheduled dose (don't double this dose).

What drug does:
- Probably dilates blood vessels to increase oxygen to heart.
- Prevents platelet clumping, which causes blood clots.

Continued next column

OVERDOSE

SYMPTOMS:
Decreased blood pressure; weak, rapid pulse; cold, clammy skin; collapse.
WHAT TO DO:
- Dial 0 (operator) or 911 (emergency) for an ambulance or medical help. Then give first aid immediately.
- If patient is unconscious and not breathing, give mouth-to-mouth breathing. If there is no heartbeat, use cardiac massage and mouth-to-mouth breathing (CPR). Don't try to make patient vomit. If you can't get help quickly, take patient to nearest emergency facility.
- See emergency information on inside covers.

Time lapse before drug works:
3 months of continual use.

Don't take with:
See Interaction column and consult doctor.

POSSIBLE ADVERSE REACTIONS OR SIDE EFFECTS

SYMPTOMS	WHAT TO DO
Life-threatening: None expected.	
Common: None expected.	
Infrequent:	
• Dizziness, fainting, headache.	Discontinue. Call doctor right away.
• Red flush, rash, nausea, vomiting, cramps, weakness.	Continue. Call doctor when convenient.
Rare: None expected.	

WARNINGS & PRECAUTIONS

Don't take if:
- You are allergic to dipyridamole.
- You are recovering from a heart attack.

Before you start, consult your doctor:
- If you have low blood pressure.
- If you have liver disease.

Over age 60:
Begin treatment with small doses.

Pregnancy:
No proven harm to unborn child. Avoid if possible.

Breast-feeding:
No proven problems. Consult doctor.

Infants & children:
Not recommended.

Prolonged use:
No problems expected.

Skin & sunlight:
No problems expected.

Driving, piloting or hazardous work:
Avoid if you feel dizzy. Otherwise, no problems expected.

Discontinuing:
Don't discontinue without doctor's advice until you complete prescribed dose, even though symptoms diminish or disappear.

Others:
Drug increases your ability to be active without angina pain. Avoid excessive physical exertion that might injure heart.

POSSIBLE INTERACTION WITH OTHER DRUGS

GENERIC NAME OR DRUG CLASS	COMBINED EFFECT
Anticoagulants (oral)	Increased anticoagulant effect. Bleeding tendency.
Antihypertensives	Increased antihypertensive effect.
Aspirin	Increased dipyridamole effect. Dose may need adjustment.

POSSIBLE INTERACTION WITH OTHER SUBSTANCES

INTERACTS WITH	COMBINED EFFECT
Alcohol:	May lower blood pressure excessively.
Beverages:	None expected.
Cocaine:	No proven problems.
Foods:	Decreased dipyridamole absorption unless taken 1 hour before eating.
Marijuana:	Daily use—Decreased dipyridamole effect.
Tobacco: Nicotine.	May decrease dipyridamole effect.

DISOPYRAMIDE

BRAND NAMES

Norpace
Norpace CR

Rythmodan
Rythmodan-LA

BASIC INFORMATION

Habit forming? No
Prescription needed? Yes
Available as generic? Yes
Drug class: Antiarrhythmic

 USES

Corrects heart rhythm disorders.

 DOSAGE & USAGE INFORMATION

How to take:
Tablet or capsule—Swallow with liquid. If you can't swallow whole, crumble tablet or open capsule and take with liquid or food.

When to take:
At the same times each day.

If you forget a dose:
Take as soon as you remember up to 2 hours late. If more than 2 hours, wait for next scheduled dose (don't double this dose).

What drug does:
Delays nerve impulses to heart to regulate heartbeat.

Time lapse before drug works:
Begins in 30 to 60 minutes. Must use for 5 to 7 days to determine effectiveness.

Don't take with:
See Interaction column and consult doctor.

 OVERDOSE

SYMPTOMS:
Blood-pressure drop, irregular heartbeat.
WHAT TO DO:
- Dial 0 (operator) or 911 (emergency) for an ambulance or medical help. Then give first aid immediately.
- If patient is unconscious and not breathing, give mouth-to-mouth breathing. If there is no heartbeat, use cardiac massage and mouth-to-mouth breathing (CPR). Don't try to make patient vomit. If you can't get help quickly, take patient to nearest emergency facility.
- See emergency information on inside covers.

 POSSIBLE ADVERSE REACTIONS OR SIDE EFFECTS

SYMPTOMS	WHAT TO DO
Life-threatening: None expected.	
Common:	
● Hypoglycemia.	Discontinue. Call doctor right away.
● Dry mouth, constipation, painful or difficult urination, rapid weight gain.	Continue. Call doctor when convenient.
Infrequent:	
● Dizziness, fainting, confusion, nervousness, depression, chest pain, slow or fast heartbeat.	Discontinue. Call doctor right away.
● Swollen feet.	Continue. Call doctor when convenient.
Rare:	
● Sore throat with fever, jaundice.	Discontinue. Call doctor right away.
● Eye pain, diminished sex drive.	Continue. Call doctor when convenient.

WARNINGS & PRECAUTIONS

Don't take if:
- You are allergic to disopyramide or any antiarrhythmic.
- You have second- or third-degree heart block.

Before you start, consult your doctor:
- If you react unfavorably to other antiarrhythmic drugs.
- If you have had heart disease.
- If you have low blood pressure.
- If you have liver disease.
- If you have glaucoma.
- If you have enlarged prostate.
- If you have myasthenia gravis.
- If you take digitalis preparations or diuretics.

Over age 60:
- May require reduced dose.
- More likely to have difficulty urinating or be constipated.
- More likely to have blood-pressure drop.

Pregnancy:
No proven harm to unborn child. Avoid if possible.

Breast-feeding:
Drug passes into milk. Avoid drug or discontinue nursing until you finish medicine. Consult doctor for advice on maintaining milk supply.

Infants & children:
Safety not established. Don't use.

Prolonged use:
No problems expected.

Skin & sunlight:
No problems expected.

Driving, piloting or hazardous work:
Don't drive or pilot aircraft until you learn how medicine affects you. Don't work around dangerous machinery. Don't climb ladders or work in high places. Danger increases if you drink alcohol or take medicine affecting alertness and reflexes, such as antihistamines, tranquilizers, sedatives, pain medicine, narcotics, or mind-altering drugs.

Discontinuing:
Don't discontinue without doctor's advice until you complete prescribed dose, even though symptoms diminish or disappear.

Others:
If new illness, injury or surgery occurs, tell doctors of disopyramide use.

POSSIBLE INTERACTION WITH OTHER DRUGS

GENERIC NAME OR DRUG CLASS	COMBINED EFFECT
Ambenonium	Decreased ambenonium effect.
Anticholinergics	Increased anticholinergic effect.
Anticoagulants (oral)	Increased anticoagulant effect.
Antihypertensives	Increased antihypertensive effect.
Antimyasthenics	Decreased antimyasthenic effect.
Flecainide	Possible irregular heartbeat.
Tocainide	Increased likelihood of adverse reactions with either drug.

POSSIBLE INTERACTION WITH OTHER SUBSTANCES

INTERACTS WITH	COMBINED EFFECT
Alcohol:	Decreased blood pressure and blood sugar. Use caution.
Beverages:	None expected.
Cocaine:	Irregular heartbeat.
Foods:	None expected.
Marijuana:	Unpredictable. May decrease disopyramide effect.
Tobacco:	May decrease disopyramide effect.

307

DISULFIRAM

BRAND NAMES

Antabuse

BASIC INFORMATION

Habit forming? No
Prescription needed? Yes
Available as generic? Yes
Drug class: None

 USES

Treatment for alcoholism. Will not cure alcoholism, but is a powerful deterrent to drinking.

 DOSAGE & USAGE INFORMATION

How to take:
Tablet or capsule—Swallow with liquid.

When to take:
Morning or bedtime. Avoid if you have used *any* alcohol, tonics, cough syrups, fermented vinegar, after-shave lotion or backrub solutions within 12 hours.

If you forget a dose:
Take as soon as you remember up to 12 hours late. If more than 12 hours, wait for next scheduled dose (don't double this dose).

What drug does:
In combination with alcohol, produces a metabolic change that causes severe, temporary toxicity.

Time lapse before drug works:
Immediate.

Don't take with:
- See Interaction column and consult doctor.
- Non-prescription drugs that contain *any* alcohol.

 OVERDOSE

SYMPTOMS:
Memory loss, behavior disturbances, lethargy, confusion and headaches; nausea, vomiting, stomach pain and diarrhea; weakness and unsteady walk; temporary paralysis.
WHAT TO DO:
- **Dial 0 (operator) or 911 (emergency) for an ambulance or medical help. Then give first aid immediately.**
- **See emergency information on inside covers.**

 POSSIBLE ADVERSE REACTIONS OR SIDE EFFECTS

SYMPTOMS	WHAT TO DO
Life-threatening: None expected.	
Common: Drowsiness.	Continue. Tell doctor at next visit.
Infrequent: • Eye pain, vision changes, stomach discomfort, throbbing headache, numbness in hands and feet.	Continue. Call doctor when convenient.
• Mood change, decreased sexual ability in men, tiredness.	Continue. Tell doctor at next visit.
• Bad taste in mouth (metal or garlic).	No action necessary.
Rare: Rash, jaundice.	Discontinue. Call doctor right away.

WARNINGS & PRECAUTIONS

Don't take if:
- You are allergic to disulfiram (alcohol-disulfiram combination is not an allergic reaction).
- You have used alcohol in any form or amount within 12 hours.
- You have taken paraldehyde within 1 week.
- You have heart disease.

Before you start, consult your doctor:
- If you have allergies.
- If you plan to become pregnant within medication period.
- If no one has explained to you how disulfiram reacts.
- If you think you cannot avoid drinking.
- If you have diabetes, epilepsy, liver or kidney disease.
- If you take other drugs.

Over age 60:
Adverse reactions and side effects may be more frequent and severe than in younger persons.

Pregnancy:
Risk to unborn child outweighs drug benefits. Don't use.

Breast-feeding:
Studies inconclusive. Consult your doctor.

Infants & children:
Not recommended.

Prolonged use:
Periodic blood-cell counts and liver-function tests recommended if you take this drug a long time.

Skin & sunlight:
No problems expected.

Driving, piloting or hazardous work:
Avoid if you feel drowsy or have vision side effects. Otherwise, no restrictions.

Discontinuing:
Don't discontinue without consulting doctor. Dose may require gradual reduction if you have taken drug for a long time. Doses of other drugs may also require adjustment. Avoid alcohol at least 14 days following last dose.

Others:
No problems expected.

POSSIBLE INTERACTION WITH OTHER DRUGS

GENERIC NAME OR DRUG CLASS	COMBINED EFFECT
Anticoagulants	Possible unexplained bleeding.
Anticonvulsants	Excessive sedation.
Barbiturates	Excessive sedation.
Cephalosporins	Disulfiram reaction (see Glossary).
Isoniazid	Unsteady walk and disturbed behavior.
Metronidazole	Disulfiram reaction (see Glossary).
Sedatives	Excessive sedation.

POSSIBLE INTERACTION WITH OTHER SUBSTANCES

INTERACTS WITH	COMBINED EFFECT
Alcohol: *Any* form or amount.	Possible life-threatening toxicity. See disulfiram reaction in Glossary.
Beverages: Punch or fruit drink that may contain alcohol.	Disulfiram reaction.
Cocaine:	Increased disulfiram effect.
Foods: Sauces, fermented vinegar, marinades, desserts or other foods prepared with *any* alcohol.	Disulfiram reaction.
Marijuana:	None expected.
Tobacco:	None expected.

DIVALPOREX

BRAND NAMES

Depakote   Epival

BASIC INFORMATION

Habit forming? No
Prescription needed? Yes
Available as generic? No
Drug class: Anticonvulsant

 ## USES

Controls petit mal (absence) seizures in
treatment of epilepsy.

 ## DOSAGE & USAGE INFORMATION

How to take:
Tablet or capsule—Swallow with liquid or food
to lessen stomach irritation.

When to take:
Once a day.

If you forget a dose:
Take as soon as you remember. Don't ever
double dose.

What drug does:
Increases concentration of gamma aminobutyric
acid, which inhibits nerve transmission in parts
of brain.

Time lapse before drug works:
1 to 4 hours.

Don't take with:
See Interaction column and consult doctor.

 ## OVERDOSE

SYMPTOMS:
Coma.
WHAT TO DO:
- **Dial 0 (operator) or 911 (emergency) for an
  ambulance or medical help. Then give first
  aid immediately.**
- **If patient is unconscious and not
  breathing, give mouth-to-mouth breathing.
  If there is no heartbeat, use cardiac
  massage and mouth-to-mouth breathing
  (CPR). Don't try to make patient vomit. If
  you can't get help quickly, take patient to
  nearest emergency facility.**
- **See emergency information on inside
  covers.**

 ## POSSIBLE ADVERSE REACTIONS OR SIDE EFFECTS

SYMPTOMS	WHAT TO DO
Life-threatening: None expected.	
Common: Menstrual irregularities.	Continue. Call doctor when convenient.

Infrequent:
• Rash, bloody spots
  under skin, hair
  loss, bleeding,
  easy bruising.
	Discontinue. Call
	doctor right away.

• Drowsiness, weak-
  ness, easily upset
  emotionally,
  depression, psychic
  changes, headache,
  incoordination,
  nausea, vomiting,
  abdominal cramps,
  appetite change.
	Continue. Call doctor
	when convenient.

Rare:
• Double vision,
  unusual movements
  of eyes (nystagmus).
	Discontinue. Call
	doctor right away.

• Anemia.	Continue. Call doctor when convenient.

WARNINGS & PRECAUTIONS

Don't take if:
You are allergic to divalporex.

Before you start, consult your doctor:
- If you have blood, kidney or liver disease.
- If you will have surgery within 2 months, including dental surgery, requiring general or spinal anesthesia.

Over age 60:
Adverse reactions and side effects may be more frequent and severe than in younger persons.

Pregnancy:
No proven harm to unborn child. Avoid if possible.

Breast-feeding:
Unknown effect.

Infants & children:
Under close medical supervision only.

Prolonged use:
Request periodic blood tests, liver and kidney function tests.

Skin & sunlight:
No problems expected.

Driving, piloting or hazardous work:
Don't drive or pilot aircraft until you learn how medicine affects you. Don't work around dangerous machinery. Don't climb ladders or work in high places. Danger increases if you drink alcohol or take medicine affecting alertness and reflexes, such as antihistamines, tranquilizers, sedatives, pain medicine, narcotics and mind-altering drugs.

Discontinuing:
Don't discontinue without consulting doctor. Dose may require gradual reduction if you have taken drug for a long time. Doses of other drugs may also require adjustment.

Others:
No problems expected.

POSSIBLE INTERACTION WITH OTHER DRUGS

GENERIC NAME OR DRUG CLASS	COMBINED EFFECT
Anticoagulants	Increases chance of bleeding.
Aspirin	Increases chance of bleeding.
Central nervous system depressants: Antidepressants, antihistamines, narcotics, sedatives, sleeping pills, tranquilizers.	Increases sedative effect.
Clonazepam	May prolong seizure.
Dypiradamole	Increases chance of bleeding.
MAO inhibitors	Increases sedative effect.
Phenytoin	Unpredictable. May require increased or decreased dosage.
Primidone	Increases chance of toxicity.
Sulfinpyrazone	Increases chance of bleeding.

POSSIBLE INTERACTION WITH OTHER SUBSTANCES

INTERACTS WITH	COMBINED EFFECT
Alcohol:	Deep sedation. Avoid.
Beverages:	No problems expected.
Cocaine:	Increased brain sensitivity. Avoid.
Foods:	No problems expected.
Marijuana:	Increased brain sensitivity. Avoid.
Tobacco:	Increased brain sensitivity. Avoid.

DOCUSATE CALCIUM

BRAND NAMES

Dioctocal	Pro-Cal-Sof
Doxidan	Surfak
O-C-S	

BASIC INFORMATION

Habit forming? No
Prescription needed? No
Available as generic? Yes
Drug class: Laxative (emollient)

 USES

Constipation relief.

 DOSAGE & USAGE INFORMATION

How to take:
- Tablet or capsule—Swallow with liquid. Don't open capsules.
- Drops—Dilute dose in beverage before swallowing.
- Syrup—Take as directed on bottle.

When to take:
At the same time each day, preferably bedtime.

If you forget a dose:
Take as soon as you remember. Wait 12 hours for next dose. Return to regular schedule.

What drug does:
Makes stool hold fluid so it is easier to pass.

Time lapse before drug works:
2 to 3 days of continual use.

Don't take with:
- Other medicines at same time. Wait 2 hours.
- See Interaction column and consult doctor.

 OVERDOSE

SYMPTOMS:
Appetite loss, nausea, vomiting, diarrhea.
WHAT TO DO:
Overdose unlikely to threaten life. If person takes much larger amount than prescribed, call doctor, poison-control center or hospital emergency room for instructions.

 POSSIBLE ADVERSE REACTIONS OR SIDE EFFECTS

SYMPTOMS	WHAT TO DO
Life-threatening: None expected.	
Common: None expected.	
Infrequent: Throat irritation (liquid only), intestinal and stomach cramps.	Continue. Call doctor when convenient.
Rare: Rash.	Discontinue. Call doctor right away.

DOCUSATE CALCIUM

 ## WARNINGS & PRECAUTIONS

Don't take if:
- You are allergic to any emollient laxative.
- You have abdominal pain and fever that might be appendicitis.

Before you start, consult your doctor:
- If you are taking other laxatives.
- To be sure constipation isn't a sign of a serious disorder.

Over age 60:
You must drink 6 to 8 glasses of fluid every 24 hours for drug to work.

Pregnancy:
No problems expected. Consult doctor.

Breast-feeding:
No problems expected.

Infants & children:
No problems expected.

Prolonged use:
Avoid. Overuse of laxatives may damage intestine lining.

Skin & sunlight:
No problems expected.

Driving, piloting or hazardous work:
No problems expected.

Discontinuing:
May be unnecessary to finish medicine. Follow doctor's instructions.

Others:
No problems expected.

 ## POSSIBLE INTERACTION WITH OTHER DRUGS

GENERIC NAME OR DRUG CLASS	COMBINED EFFECT
Danthron	Possible liver damage.
Digitalis preparations	Toxic absorption of digitalis.
Mineral oil	Increased mineral oil absorption into bloodstream. Avoid.
Phenolphthalein	Increased phenolphthalein absorption. Possible toxicity.

 ## POSSIBLE INTERACTION WITH OTHER SUBSTANCES

INTERACTS WITH	COMBINED EFFECT
Alcohol:	None expected.
Beverages:	None expected.
Cocaine:	None expected.
Foods:	None expected.
Marijuana:	None expected.
Tobacco:	None expected.

DOCUSATE POTASSIUM

BRAND NAMES

Dialose	Pro-Cal-Sof
Kasof	Surfac

BASIC INFORMATION

Habit forming? No
Prescription needed? No
Available as generic? Yes
Drug class: Laxative (emollient)

 USES

Constipation relief.

 DOSAGE & USAGE INFORMATION

How to take:
- Tablet or capsule—Swallow with liquid. Don't open capsules.
- Drops—Dilute dose in beverage before swallowing.
- Syrup—Take as directed on bottle.

When to take:
At the same time each day, preferably bedtime.

If you forget a dose:
Take as soon as you remember. Wait 12 hours for next dose. Return to regular schedule.

What drug does:
Makes stool hold fluid so it is easier to pass.

Time lapse before drug works:
2 to 3 days of continual use.

Don't take with:
- Other medicines at same time. Wait 2 hours.
- See Interaction column and consult doctor.

 OVERDOSE

SYMPTOMS:
Appetite loss, nausea, vomiting, diarrhea.
WHAT TO DO:
Overdose unlikely to threaten life. If person takes much larger amount than prescribed, call doctor, poison-control center or hospital emergency room for instructions.

 POSSIBLE ADVERSE REACTIONS OR SIDE EFFECTS

SYMPTOMS	WHAT TO DO
Life-threatening: None expected.	
Common: None expected.	
Infrequent: Throat irritation (liquid only), intestinal and stomach cramps.	Continue. Call doctor when convenient.
Rare: Rash.	Discontinue. Call doctor right away.

DOCUSATE POTASSIUM

WARNINGS & PRECAUTIONS

Don't take if:
- You are allergic to any emollient laxative.
- You have abdominal pain and fever that might be appendicitis.

Before you start, consult your doctor:
- If you are taking other laxatives.
- To be sure constipation isn't a sign of a serious disorder.

Over age 60:
You must drink 6 to 8 glasses of fluid every 24 hours for drug to work.

Pregnancy:
No problems expected. Consult doctor.

Breast-feeding:
No problems expected.

Infants & children:
No problems expected.

Prolonged use:
Avoid. Overuse of laxatives may damage intestine lining.

Skin & sunlight:
No problems expected.

Driving, piloting or hazardous work:
No problems expected.

Discontinuing:
May be unnecessary to finish medicine. Follow doctor's instructions.

Others:
No problems expected.

POSSIBLE INTERACTION WITH OTHER DRUGS

GENERIC NAME OR DRUG CLASS	COMBINED EFFECT
Danthron	Possible liver damage.
Digitalis preparations	Toxic absorption of digitalis.
Mineral oil	Increased mineral oil absorption into bloodstream. Avoid.
Phenolphthalein	Increased phenolphthalein absorption. Possible toxicity.

POSSIBLE INTERACTION WITH OTHER SUBSTANCES

INTERACTS WITH	COMBINED EFFECT
Alcohol:	None expected.
Beverages:	None expected.
Cocaine:	None expected.
Foods:	None expected.
Marijuana:	None expected.
Tobacco:	None expected.

DOCUSATE SODIUM

BRAND NAMES

See complete list of brand names in the
Brand Name Directory, page 948.

BASIC INFORMATION

Habit forming? No
Prescription needed? No
Available as generic? Yes
Drug class: Laxative (emollient)

 USES

Constipation relief.

 DOSAGE & USAGE INFORMATION

How to take:
- Tablet or capsule—Swallow with liquid. Don't open capsules.
- Drops—Dilute dose in beverage before swallowing.
- Syrup—Take as directed on bottle.

When to take:
At the same time each day, preferably bedtime.

If you forget a dose:
Take as soon as you remember. Wait 12 hours for next dose. Return to regular schedule.

What drug does:
Makes stool hold fluid so it is easier to pass.

Time lapse before drug works:
2 to 3 days of continual use.

Don't take with:
- Other medicines at same time. Wait 2 hours.
- See Interaction column and consult doctor.

 OVERDOSE

SYMPTOMS:
Appetite loss, nausea, vomiting, diarrhea.
WHAT TO DO:
Overdose unlikely to threaten life. If person takes much larger amount than prescribed, call doctor, poison-control center or hospital emergency room for instructions.

 POSSIBLE ADVERSE REACTIONS OR SIDE EFFECTS

SYMPTOMS	WHAT TO DO
Life-threatening: None expected.	
Common: None expected.	
Infrequent: Throat irritation (liquid only), intestinal and stomach cramps.	Continue. Call doctor when convenient.
Rare: Rash.	Discontinue. Call doctor right away.

316

WARNINGS & PRECAUTIONS

Don't take if:
- You are allergic to any emollient laxative.
- You have abdominal pain and fever that might be appendicitis.

Before you start, consult your doctor:
- If you are taking other laxatives.
- To be sure constipation isn't a sign of a serious disorder.

Over age 60:
You must drink 6 to 8 glasses of fluid every 24 hours for drug to work.

Pregnancy:
No problems expected. Consult doctor.

Breast-feeding:
No problems expected.

Infants & children:
No problems expected.

Prolonged use:
Avoid. Overuse of laxatives may damage intestine lining.

Skin & sunlight:
No problems expected.

Driving, piloting or hazardous work:
No problems expected.

Discontinuing:
May be unnecessary to finish medicine. Follow doctor's instructions.

Others:
No problems expected.

POSSIBLE INTERACTION WITH OTHER DRUGS

GENERIC NAME OR DRUG CLASS	COMBINED EFFECT
Danthron	Possible liver damage.
Digitalis preparations	Toxic absorption of digitalis.
Mineral oil	Increased mineral oil absorption into bloodstream. Avoid.
Phenolphthalein	Increased phenolphthalein absorption. Possible toxicity.

POSSIBLE INTERACTION WITH OTHER SUBSTANCES

INTERACTS WITH	COMBINED EFFECT
Alcohol:	None expected.
Beverages:	None expected.
Cocaine:	None expected.
Foods:	None expected.
Marijuana:	None expected.
Tobacco:	None expected.

DOXYLAMINE

BRAND NAMES

Bendectin   Unisom Nighttime
Cremacoat 4   Sleep Aid
Decapryn

BASIC INFORMATION

Habit forming? No
Prescription needed? Yes
Available as generic? No
Drug class: Antihistamine

 USES

- Reduces allergic symptoms such as hay fever, hives, rash or itching.
- Prevents motion sickness, nausea, vomiting.
- Induces sleep.

 DOSAGE & USAGE INFORMATION

How to take:
Tablet or syrup—Swallow with liquid or food to lessen stomach irritation.

When to take:
Varies with form. Follow label directions.

If you forget a dose:
Take as soon as you remember up to 2 hours late. If more than 2 hours, wait for next scheduled dose (don't double this dose).

What drug does:
Blocks action of histamine after an allergic response triggers histamine release in sensitive cells.

Time lapse before drug works:
30 minutes.

Continued next column

 OVERDOSE

SYMPTOMS:
Convulsions, red face, hallucinations, coma.
WHAT TO DO:
- Dial 0 (operator) or 911 (emergency) for an ambulance or medical help. Then give first aid immediately.
- If patient is unconscious and not breathing, give mouth-to-mouth breathing. If there is no heartbeat, use cardiac massage and mouth-to-mouth breathing (CPR). Don't try to make patient vomit. If you can't get help quickly, take patient to nearest emergency facility.
- See emergency information on inside covers.

Don't take with:
See Interaction column and consult doctor.

 POSSIBLE ADVERSE REACTIONS OR SIDE EFFECTS

SYMPTOMS	WHAT TO DO
Life-threatening:	
None expected.	
Common:	
Drowsiness; dizziness; nausea; dry mouth, nose, throat.	Continue. Tell doctor at next visit.
Infrequent:	
• Change in vision.	Discontinue. Call doctor right away.
• Less tolerance for contact lenses, difficult urination.	Continue. Call doctor when convenient.
• Appetite loss.	Continue. Tell doctor at next visit.
Rare:	
Nightmares, agitation, irritability, sore throat, fever, rapid heartbeat, unusual bleeding or bruising, fatigue, weakness.	Discontinue. Call doctor right away.

WARNINGS & PRECAUTIONS

Don't take if:
You are allergic to any antihistamine.

Before you start, consult your doctor:
- If you have glaucoma.
- If you have enlarged prostate.
- If you have asthma.
- If you have kidney disease.
- If you have peptic ulcer.
- If you will have surgery within 2 months, including dental surgery, requiring general or spinal anesthesia.

Over age 60:
Don't exceed recommended dose. Adverse reactions and side effects may be more frequent and severe than in younger persons, especially urination difficulty, diminished alertness and other brain and nervous-system symptoms.

Pregnancy:
No proven harm to unborn child. Avoid if possible.

Breast-feeding:
Drug passes into milk. Avoid drug or discontinue nursing until you finish medicine. Consult doctor for advice on maintaining milk supply.

Infants & children:
Not recommended for premature or newborn infants. Otherwise, no problems expected.

Prolonged use:
Avoid. May damage bone marrow and nerve cells.

Skin & sunlight:
May cause rash or intensify sunburn in areas exposed to sun or sunlamp.

Driving, piloting or hazardous work:
Don't drive or pilot aircraft until you learn how medicine affects you. Don't work around dangerous machinery. Don't climb ladders or work in high places. Danger increases if you drink alcohol or take medicine affecting alertness and reflexes, such as antihistamines, tranquilizers, sedatives, pain medicine, narcotics and mind-altering drugs.

Discontinuing:
No problems expected.

Others:
May mask symptoms of hearing damage from aspirin, other salicylates, cisplatin, paromomycin, vancomycin or anticonvulsants. Consult doctor if you use these.

POSSIBLE INTERACTION WITH OTHER DRUGS

GENERIC NAME OR DRUG CLASS	COMBINED EFFECT
Anticholinergics	Increased anticholinergic effect.
Antidepressants	Excess sedation. Avoid.
Antihistamines (other)	Excess sedation. Avoid.
Dronabinol	Increased effects of both drugs. Avoid.
Hypnotics	Excess sedation. Avoid.
MAO inhibitors	Increased doxylamine effect.
Mind-altering drugs	Excess sedation. Avoid.
Molindone	Increased sedative and antihistamine effect.
Narcotics	Excess sedation. Avoid.
Sedatives	Excess sedation. Avoid.
Sleep inducers	Excess sedation. Avoid.
Tranquilizers	Excess sedation. Avoid.

POSSIBLE INTERACTION WITH OTHER SUBSTANCES

INTERACTS WITH	COMBINED EFFECT
Alcohol:	Excess sedation. Avoid.
Beverages: Caffeine drinks.	Less doxylamine sedation.
Cocaine:	Decreased doxylamine effect. Avoid.
Foods:	None expected.
Marijuana:	Excess sedation. Avoid.
Tobacco:	None expected.

DRONABINOL

BRAND NAMES

Marinol

BASIC INFORMATION

Habit forming? Yes
Prescription needed? Yes
Available as generic? No
Drug class: Antiemetic

 USES

Prevents nausea and vomiting that may accompany taking anticancer medication (cancer chemotherapy). Should not be used unless other antinausea medicines fail.

 DOSAGE & USAGE INFORMATION

How to take:
Capsule—Swallow with liquid.

When to take:
Under supervision, a total of no more than 4 to 6 doses per day, every 2 to 4 hours after cancer chemotherapy for prescribed number of days.

If you forget a dose:
Take as soon as you remember up to 2 hours late. If more than 2 hours, wait for next scheduled dose (don't double this dose).

What drug does:
Affects nausea and vomiting center in brain to make it less irritable following cancer chemotherapy. Exact mechanism is unknown.

Time lapse before drug works:
2 to 4 hours.

Don't take with:
- Non-prescription drugs without consulting doctor.
- Drugs in interaction column without consulting doctor.

 OVERDOSE

SYMPTOMS:
Pounding, rapid heart rate; high or low blood pressure; confusion; hallucinations; drastic mood changes; nervousness or anxiety.
WHAT TO DO:
Overdose unlikely to threaten life. If person takes much larger amount than prescribed, call doctor, poison-control center or hospital emergency room for instructions.

 POSSIBLE ADVERSE REACTIONS OR SIDE EFFECTS

SYMPTOMS	WHAT TO DO
Life-threatening:	
None expected.	
Common:	
• Rapid, pounding heartbeat.	Discontinue. Call doctor right away.
• Dizziness, drowsiness, decreased coordination, euphoria.	Continue. Call doctor when convenient.
• Red eyes, dry mouth.	No action necessary.
Infrequent:	
• Depression, nervousness, anxiety, hallucinations, dramatic mood changes.	Discontinue. Call doctor right away.
• Blurred or changed vision.	Continue. Call doctor when convenient.
Rare:	
None expected.	

WARNINGS & PRECAUTIONS

Don't take if:
- Your nausea and vomiting is caused by anything other than cancer chemotherapy.
- You are sensitive or allergic to any form of marijuana or sesame oil.
- Your cycle of chemotherapy is longer than 7 consecutive days. Harmful side effects may occur.

Before you start, consult your doctor:
- If you have heart disease or high blood pressure.
- If you are an alcoholic or drug addict.
- If you are pregnant or intend to become pregnant.
- If you are nursing an infant.
- If you have schizophrenia or a manic-depressive disorder.

Over age 60:
Adverse reactions and side effects may be more frequent and severe than in younger persons.

Pregnancy:
No studies in humans. Avoid if possible.

Breast-feeding:
No studies in humans. Avoid if possible.

Infants & children:
Not recommended.

Prolonged use:
Avoid. Habit forming.

Skin & sunlight:
No problems expected.

Driving, piloting or hazardous work:
Don't drive or pilot aircraft until you learn how medicine affects you. Don't work around dangerous machinery. Don't climb ladders or work in high places. Danger increases if you drink alcohol or take medicine affecting alertness and reflexes, such as antihistamines, tranquilizers, sedatives, pain medicine, narcotics and mind-altering drugs.

Discontinuing:
Withdrawal effects such as irritability, insomnia, restlessness, sweating, diarrhea, hiccoughs, loss of appetite and "hot flashes" may follow abrupt withdrawal within 12 hours. These symptoms, should they occur, will probably subside within 96 hours.

Others:
Store in refrigerator.

POSSIBLE INTERACTION WITH OTHER DRUGS

GENERIC NAME OR DRUG CLASS	COMBINED EFFECT
Anesthetics	Oversedation
Anticonvulsants	Oversedation
Antidepressants (tricyclics)	Oversedation
Antihistamines	Oversedation
Barbiturates	Oversedation
Molindone	Increased effects of both drugs. Avoid.
Muscle relaxants	Oversedation
Narcotics	Oversedation
Sedatives	Oversedation
Tranquilizers	Oversedation

POSSIBLE INTERACTION WITH OTHER SUBSTANCES

INTERACTS WITH	COMBINED EFFECT
Alcohol:	Oversedation
Beverages:	No problems expected.
Cocaine:	No problems expected.
Foods:	No problems expected.
Marijuana:	Oversedation
Tobacco:	No problems expected.

ENALAPRIL

BRAND NAMES

Vasotec

BASIC INFORMATION

Habit forming? No
Prescription needed? Yes
Available as generic? No
Drug class: Antihypertensive, A.C.E.
        inhibitor

 USES

Treatment for high blood pressure and congestive heart failure.

 DOSAGE & USAGE INFORMATION

How to take:
Tablets—Swallow with liquid. These are long-acting tablets. Food does not alter normal absorption from the gastrointestinal tract.

When to take:
Usually once a day, sometimes twice a day. Follow doctor's instructions.

If you forget a dose:
Take as soon as you remember up to 8 hours late. If more than 8 hours, wait for next scheduled dose (don't double this dose).

What drug does:
- Reduces resistance in arteries.
- Strengthens heartbeat.

Time lapse before drug works:
60 to 90 minutes.

Don't take with:
See Interaction column and consult doctor.

 OVERDOSE

SYMPTOMS:
Fever, chills, sore throat, fainting, convulsions, coma.
WHAT TO DO:
- Dial 0 (operator) or 911 (emergency) for an ambulance or medical help. Then give first aid immediately.
- See emergency information on inside covers.

 POSSIBLE ADVERSE REACTIONS OR SIDE EFFECTS

SYMPTOMS	WHAT TO DO
Life-threatening:	
None expected.	
Common:	
Rash, loss of taste.	Discontinue. Call doctor right away.
Infrequent:	
• Swelling of face, hands, mouth or feet.	Discontinue. Seek emergency treatment.
• Dizziness, fainting, chest pain, fast or irregular heartbeat.	Discontinue. Call doctor right away.
Rare:	
• Sore throat, cloudy urine, fever, chills.	Discontinue. Call doctor right away.
• Nausea, vomiting, indigestion, abdominal pain.	Continue. Call doctor when convenient.

WARNINGS & PRECAUTIONS

Don't take if:
- If you are allergic to enalapril or captopril.
- You have any autoimmune disease, including AIDS or lupus.
- You are receiving blood from a blood bank.
- You take drugs for cancer.
- You will have surgery within 2 months, including dental surgery, requiring general or spinal anesthesia.

Before you start, consult your doctor:
- If you have had a stroke.
- If you have angina, heart or blood-vessel disease, a high level of potassium in blood, kidney disease, lupus.
- If you are on severe salt-restricted diet.

Over age 60:
Adverse reactions and side effects may be more frequent and severe than in younger persons.

Pregnancy:
Risk to unborn child outweighs drug benefits. Don't use.

Breast-feeding:
Drug passes into milk. Avoid drug or discontinue nursing until you finish medicine. Consult doctor for advice on maintaining milk supply.

Infants & children:
Not recommended.

Prolonged use:
May decrease white cells in blood or cause protein loss in urine. Request periodic laboratory blood counts and urine tests.

Skin & sunlight:
No problems expected.

Driving, piloting or hazardous work:
Avoid if you become dizzy or faint. Otherwise, no problems expected.

Discontinuing:
Don't discontinue without consulting doctor. Dose may require gradual reduction if you have taken drug for a long time. Doses of other drugs may also require adjustment.

Others:
- Stop taking diuretics or increase salt intake 1 week before starting enalapril.
- Avoid exercising in hot weather.

POSSIBLE INTERACTION WITH OTHER DRUGS

GENERIC NAME OR DRUG CLASS	COMBINED EFFECT
Acebutolol	Increased antihypertensive effect. Dosage of each may require adjustment.
Amiloride	Possible excessive potassium in blood.
Antihypertensives (other)	Possible excessive blood-pressure drop.
Chloramphenicol	Possible blood disorders.
Diuretics	Possible severe blood-pressure drop with first dose.
Nitrates	Possible excessive blood-pressure drop.
Oxprenolol	Increased antihypertensive effect. Dosage of each may require adjustment.
Potassium supplements	Excessive potassium in blood.
Spironolactone	Possible excessive potassium in blood.
Triamterene	Possible excessive potassium in blood.

POSSIBLE INTERACTION WITH OTHER SUBSTANCES

INTERACTS WITH	COMBINED EFFECT
Alcohol:	Possible excessive blood-pressure drop.
Beverages: Low-salt milk.	Possible excessive potassium in blood.
Cocaine:	Increased dizziness and chest pain.
Foods: Salt substitutes.	Possible excessive potassium.
Marijuana:	Increased dizziness.
Tobacco:	May decrease enalapril effect.

ENALAPRIL & HYDROCHLOROTHIAZIDE

BRAND NAMES

Vaseretic

BASIC INFORMATION

Habit forming? No
Prescription needed? Yes
Available as generic? No
Drug class: Antihypertensive, diuretic, A.C.E.
    inhibitor

 USES

- Treatment for high blood pressure and congestive heart failure.
- Reduces fluid retention.

 DOSAGE & USAGE INFORMATION

How to take:
Tablets—Swallow with liquid. These tablets are long-acting. Food does not alter normal absorption from the gastrointestinal tract.

When to take:
Usually once a day.

If you forget a dose:
Take as soon as you remember up to 18 hours late. If more than 18 hours, wait for next scheduled dose (don't double this dose).

What drug does:
- Forces sodium and water excretion, reducing body fluid.
- Relaxes muscle cells of small arteries.
- Reduced body fluid and relaxed arteries lower blood pressure.
- Reduces resistance in arteries.
- Strengthens heartbeat.

Time lapse before drug works:
4 to 6 hours. May require several weeks to lower blood pressure.

Continued next column

 OVERDOSE

SYMPTOMS:
Cramps, weakness, drowsiness, weak pulse, fever, chills, sore throat, fainting, convulsions, coma.
WHAT TO DO:
- **Dial 0 (operator) or 911 (emergency) for an ambulance or medical help. Then give first aid immediately.**
- **See emergency information on inside covers.**

Don't take with:
- Non-prescription drugs without consulting doctor.
- See Interaction column and consult doctor.

 POSSIBLE ADVERSE REACTIONS OR SIDE EFFECTS

SYMPTOMS	WHAT TO DO
Life-threatening:	
Irregular heartbeat (fast or uneven).	Discontinue. Seek emergency treatment.
Common:	
• Dry mouth, thirst, tiredness, weakness, muscle cramps, vomiting, chest pain, skin rash.	Discontinue. Call doctor right away.
• Taste loss, dizziness.	Continue. Call doctor when convenient.
Infrequent:	
• Face, mouth, hands swelling.	Discontinue. Call doctor right away.
• Nausea, diarrhea.	Continue. Call doctor when convenient.
Rare:	
None expected.	

 WARNINGS & PRECAUTIONS

Don't take if:
- You are allergic to enalapril, captopril, or any thiazide diuretic drug.
- You have any autoimmune disease, including AIDS or lupus.
- You are receiving blood from a blood bank.
- You take drugs for cancer.
- If you will have surgery within 2 months, including dental surgery, requiring general or spinal anesthesia.

Before you start, consult your doctor:
- If you have had a stroke.
- If you have angina, heart or blood-vessel disease, a high level of potassium in blood, lupus, gout, liver, pancreas or kidney disorder.
- If you are on a severe salt-restricted diet.
- If you are allergic to any sulfa drug.

Over age 60:
Adverse reactions and side effects may be more frequent and severe than in younger persons, especially dizziness and excessive potassium loss.

Pregnancy:
Risk to unborn child outweighs drug benefits. Don't use.

Breast-feeding:
Drug passes into milk. Avoid drug or discontinue nursing until you finish medicine. Consult doctor for advice on maintaining milk supply.

Infants & children:
Not recommended.

Prolonged use:
May decrease white cells in blood or cause protein loss in urine. Request periodic laboratory blood counts and urine tests.

Skin & sunlight:
May cause rash or intensify sunburn in areas exposed to sun or sunlamp.

Driving, piloting or hazardous work:
Don't drive or pilot aircraft until you learn how medicine affects you. Don't work around dangerous machinery. Don't climb ladders or work in high places. Danger increases if you drink alcohol or take medicine affecting alertness and reflexes, such as antihistamines, tranquilizers, sedatives, pain medicine, narcotics and mind-altering drugs.

Discontinuing:
Don't discontinue without consulting doctor. Dose may require gradual reduction if you have taken drug for a long time. Doses of other drugs may also require adjustment.

Others:
- Hot weather and fever may cause dehydration and drop in blood pressure. Dose may require temporary adjustment. Weigh daily and report any unexpected weight decreases to your doctor.
- May cause rise in uric acid, leading to gout.
- May cause blood-sugar rise in diabetics.

POSSIBLE INTERACTION WITH OTHER DRUGS

GENERIC NAME OR DRUG CLASS	COMBINED EFFECT
Acebutolol	Increased antihypertensive effect Dosages of both drugs may require adjustments.
Allopurinol	Decreased allopurinol effect.
Amiloride	Possible excessive potassium in blood.
Antidepressants (tricyclic)	Dangerous drop in blood pressure. Avoid combination unless under medical supervision.
Antihypertensives (other)	Possible excessive blood-pressure drop.

Barbiturates	Increased hydrochlorothiazide effect.
Chloramphenicol	Possible blood disorders.
Cholestyramine	Decreased hydrochlorothiazide effect.
Cortisone drugs	Excessive potassium loss that causes dangerous heart rhythms.
Digitalis preparations	Excessive potassium loss that causes dangerous heart rhythms.
Diuretics (thiazide)	Increased effect of other thiazide diuretics.
Indapamide	Increased diuretic effect.
Lithium	Increased effect of lithium.
MAO inhibitors	Increased hydrochlorothiazide effect.
Nitrates	Excessive blood-pressure drop.
Oxprenolol	Increased antihypertensive effect. Dosages of both drugs may require adjustments.

Continued page 965

POSSIBLE INTERACTION WITH OTHER SUBSTANCES

INTERACTS WITH	COMBINED EFFECT
Alcohol:	Dangerous blood-pressure drop. Avoid.
Beverages: Low-salt milk.	Possible excessive potassium in blood.
Cocaine:	Increased dizziness, chest pain.
Foods: Salt substitutes.	Possible excessive potassium.
Marijuana:	Increased dizziness, may increase blood pressure.
Tobacco:	May decrease enalapril effect.

EPHEDRINE

BRAND NAMES

See complete list of brand names in the *Brand Name Directory*, page 948.

BASIC INFORMATION

Habit forming? No
Prescription needed?
  Low strength: No
  High strength: Yes
Available as generic? Yes
Drug class: Sympathomimetic

 USES

- Relieves bronchial asthma.
- Decreases congestion of breathing passages.
- Suppresses allergic reactions.

 DOSAGE & USAGE INFORMATION

How to take:
- Tablet or capsule—Swallow with liquid. You may chew or crush tablet.
- Extended-release tablets or capsules—Swallow each dose whole.
- Syrup—Take as directed on bottle.
- Drops—Dilute dose in beverage.

When to take:
As needed, no more often than every 4 hours.

If you forget a dose:
Take up to 2 hours late. If more than 2 hours, wait for next dose (don't double this dose).

What drug does:
- Prevents cells from releasing allergy-causing chemicals (histamines).
- Relaxes muscles of bronchial tubes.
- Decreases blood-vessel size and blood flow, thus causing decongestion.

Time lapse before drug works:
30 to 60 minutes.

Continued next column

 OVERDOSE

SYMPTOMS:
Severe anxiety, confusion, delirium, muscle tremors, rapid and irregular pulse.
WHAT TO DO:
- **Dial 0 (operator) or 911 (emergency) for an ambulance or medical help. Then give first aid immediately.**
- **See emergency information on inside covers.**

Don't take with:
- See Interaction column and consult doctor.
- Non-prescription drugs with ephedrine, pseudoephedrine or epinephrine.
- Non-prescription drugs for cough, cold, allergy or asthma without consulting doctor.

 POSSIBLE ADVERSE REACTIONS OR SIDE EFFECTS

SYMPTOMS	WHAT TO DO
Life-threatening: None expected.	
Common:	
• Nervousness, headache, paleness, rapid heartbeat.	Continue. Call doctor when convenient.
• Insomnia.	Continue. Tell doctor at next visit.
Infrequent:	
• Irregular heartbeat.	Discontinue. Call doctor right away.
• Dizziness, appetite loss, nausea, vomiting, painful or difficult urination.	Continue. Call doctor when convenient.
Rare: None expected.	

WARNINGS & PRECAUTIONS

Don't take if:
You are allergic to ephedrine or any sympathomimetic drug.

Before you start, consult your doctor:
- If you have high blood pressure.
- If you have diabetes.
- If you have overactive thyroid gland.
- If you have difficulty urinating.
- If you have taken any MAO inhibitor in past 2 weeks
- If you have taken digitalis preparations in the last 7 days.
- If you will have surgery within 2 months, including dental surgery, requiring general or spinal anesthesia.

Over age 60:
More likely to develop high blood pressure, heart-rhythm disturbances, angina and to feel drug's stimulant effects.

Pregnancy:
No proven harm to unborn child. Avoid if possible.

Breast-feeding:
Drug passes into milk. Avoid drug or discontinue nursing until you finish medicine. Consult doctor for advice on maintaining milk supply.

Infants & children:
No problems expected.

Prolonged use:
- Excessive doses—Rare toxic psychosis.
- Men with enlarged prostate gland may have more urination difficulty.

Skin & sunlight:
No problems expected.

Driving, piloting or hazardous work:
Avoid if you feel dizzy. Otherwise, no problems expected.

Discontinuing:
May be unnecessary to finish medicine. Follow doctor's instructions.

Others:
No problems expected.

POSSIBLE INTERACTION WITH OTHER DRUGS

GENERIC NAME OR DRUG CLASS	COMBINED EFFECT
Albuterol	Increased effect of both drugs, especially harmful side effects.
Antidepressants (tricyclic)	Increased effect of ephedrine. Excessive stimulation of heart and blood pressure.
Antihypertensives	Decreased antihypertensive effect.
Beta-adrenergic blockers	Decreased effects of both drugs.
Digitalis preparations	Serious heart-rhythm disturbances.
Epinephrine	Increased epinephrine effect.
Ergot preparations	Serious blood-pressure rise.
Guanethidine	Decreased effect of both drugs.
MAO inhibitors	Increased ephedrine effect. Dangerous blood-pressure rise.
Nitrates	Possible decreased effects of both drugs.
Pseudoephedrine	Increased pseudoephedrine effect.

POSSIBLE INTERACTION WITH OTHER SUBSTANCES

INTERACTS WITH	COMBINED EFFECT
Alcohol:	None expected.
Beverages: Caffeine drinks.	Nervousness or insomnia.
Cocaine:	Rapid heartbeat. Avoid.
Foods:	None expected.
Marijuana:	Rapid heartbeat, possible heart-rhythm disturbance.
Tobacco:	None expected.

EPINEPHRINE

BRAND NAMES

See complete list of brand names in the *Brand Name Directory,* page 948.

BASIC INFORMATION

Habit forming? No
Prescription needed? Yes
Available as generic?
  Nose drops, aerosol inhaler—No
  Eye drops, injection—Yes
Drug class: Sympathomimetic, antiglaucoma

 USES

- Relieves allergic symptoms of anaphylaxis.
- Eases symptoms of acute bronchial spasms.
- Relieves congestion of nose, sinuses and throat.
- Reduces internal eye pressure.

 DOSAGE & USAGE INFORMATION

How to take:
Eyedrops, nose drops, aerosol inhaler, injection—Use as directed on labels.

When to take:
As needed, no more often than label directs.

If you forget a dose:
If needed, take when you remember. Wait 3 hours for next dose.

What drug does:
- Contracts blood-vessel walls and raises blood pressure.
- Inhibits release of histamine.
- Dilates constricted bronchial tubes and decreases volume of blood in nasal tissue.
- Reduces fluid formation within the eye.

Time lapse before drug works:
1 to 2 minutes.

Continued next column

 OVERDOSE

SYMPTOMS:
Tremor, rapid breathing, palpitations, extreme rise in blood pressure, irregular heartbeat, breathing difficulty, convulsions, coma.
WHAT TO DO:
- **Dial 0 (operator) or 911 (emergency) for an ambulance or medical help. Then give first aid immediately.**
- **See emergency information on inside covers.**

Don't take with:
- Non-prescription drugs without consulting doctor.
- See Interaction column and consult doctor.

 POSSIBLE ADVERSE REACTIONS OR SIDE EFFECTS

SYMPTOMS	WHAT TO DO
Life-threatening: None expected.	
Common:	
• Headache, agitation, dizziness, insomnia, fast or pounding heartbeat.	Continue. Call doctor when convenient.
• Dry mouth and throat (inhaler only).	Continue. Tell doctor at next visit.
Infrequent:	
• Difficult breathing.	Discontinue. Call doctor right away.
• Shakiness, nausea, vomiting, cough or bronchial irritation (inhaler only), weakness, flushed face or redness.	Continue. Call doctor when convenient.
Rare: Chest pain, irregular heartbeat, sweating.	Discontinue. Call doctor right away.

 WARNINGS & PRECAUTIONS

Don't take if:
- You are allergic to any sympathomimetic.
- You have narrow-angle glaucoma.
- You have had a stroke or heart attack within 3 weeks.
- You have heart-rhythm disturbance.

Before you start, consult your doctor:
- If you have high blood pressure, heart disease or have had a stroke.
- If you have diabetes.
- If you have overactive thyroid.

Over age 60:
- Use with caution if you have hardening of the arteries.
- If you have enlarged prostate, drug may increase urination difficulty.
- If you have Parkinson's disease, drug may temporarily increase rigidity and tremor.
- If you see "floaters" in field of vision, tell your doctor.

Pregnancy:
No proven harm to unborn child. Avoid if possible.

Breast-feeding:
Drug passes into milk. Avoid drug or discontinue nursing until you finish medicine. Consult doctor for advice on maintaining milk supply.

Infants & children:
Use only under medical supervision.

Prolonged use:
- You may stop responding to drug.
- Drug may reduce blood volume.
- Drug may damage eye retina and impair vision.

Skin & sunlight:
No problems expected.

Driving, piloting or hazardous work:
No problems expected. Use caution if you feel dizzy or nervous.

Discontinuing:
- May be unnecessary to finish medicine. Follow doctor's instructions.
- If drug fails to provide relief after several doses, discontinue. Don't increase dose or frequency.

Others:
- May temporarily raise blood sugar in diabetics.
- Excessive use can cause sudden death.
- Discard medicine if cloudy or discolored.

POSSIBLE INTERACTION WITH OTHER DRUGS

GENERIC NAME OR DRUG CLASS	COMBINED EFFECT
Acebutolol	Decreased effects of both drugs.
Albuterol	Increased effect of both drugs, especially harmful side effects.
Antidepressants (tricyclic)	Increased epinephrine effect.
Antidiabetics (oral)	Decreased antidiabetic effect.
Antihistamines	Increased epinephrine effect.
Beta-adrenergic blockers	Decreased epinephrine effect.
Carbonic anhydrase inhibitors	Increased epinephrine effect.
Digitalis preparations	Possible irregular heartbeat.
Ephedrine	Increased ephedrine effect.
Guanethidine	Decreased guanethidine effect.

Insulin	Decreased insulin effect.
Isoproterenol	Dangerous to heart.
MAO inhibitors	Dangerous to heart.
Minoxidil	Decreased minoxidil effect.
Nitrates	Possible decreased effects of both drugs.
Oxprenolol	Decreased effects of both drugs.
Pilocarpine	Increased pilocarpine effect.
Rauwolfia alkaloids	Increased epinephrine effect.
Thyroid preparations	Increased epinephrine effect.

POSSIBLE INTERACTION WITH OTHER SUBSTANCES

INTERACTS WITH	COMBINED EFFECT
Alcohol:	May increase urinary excretion of drug and reduce effectiveness.
Beverages:	None expected.
Cocaine:	Dangerous overstimulation. Avoid.
Foods:	None expected.
Marijuana:	Increase in epinephrine's antiasthmatic effect.
Tobacco:	None expected.

ERGOLOID MESYLATES

BRAND NAMES

Circanol
Deapril-ST
Dihydrogenated
  Ergot Alkaloids
Hydergine
Hydergine LC
Trigot

BASIC INFORMATION

Habit forming? No
Prescription needed? Yes
Available as generic? No
Drug class: Ergot preparation

 USES

Treatment for reduced alertness, poor memory, confusion, depression or lack of motivation in the elderly.

 DOSAGE & USAGE INFORMATION

How to take:
- Tablet or capsule—Swallow with liquid. If you can't swallow whole, crumble tablet or open capsule and take with liquid or food.
- Liquid—Take as directed on label.
- Sublingual tablets—Dissolve tablet under tongue.

When to take:
At the same times each day.

If you forget a dose:
Take as soon as you remember up to 2 hours late. If more than 2 hours, wait for next scheduled dose (don't double this dose).

What drug does:
Stimulates brain-cell metabolism to increase use of oxygen and nutrients.

Time lapse before drug works:
Gradual improvements over 3 to 4 months.

Continued next column

 OVERDOSE

SYMPTOMS:
Headache, flushed face, nasal congestion, nausea, vomiting, blood-pressure drop, weakness, collapse, coma.
WHAT TO DO:
- **Dial 0 (operator) or 911 (emergency) for an ambulance or medical help. Then give first aid immediately.**
- **See emergency information on inside covers.**

Don't take with:
- Non-prescription drugs containing alcohol without consulting doctor.
- See Interaction column and consult doctor.

 POSSIBLE ADVERSE REACTIONS OR SIDE EFFECTS

SYMPTOMS	WHAT TO DO
Life-threatening: None expected.	
Common: Runny nose.	Continue. Tell doctor at next visit.
Infrequent:	
• Slow heartbeat, tingling fingers.	Discontinue. Call doctor right away.
• Nervousness, hostility, confusion, depression, blurred vision.	Continue. Call doctor when convenient.
Rare:	
• Fainting.	Discontinue. Seek emergency treatment.
• Rash, nausea, vomiting, stomach cramps.	Discontinue. Call doctor right away.
• Dizziness when getting up, drowsiness, soreness under tongue, appetite loss, fever.	Continue. Call doctor when convenient.

**WARNINGS &
PRECAUTIONS**

Don't use if:
- If you are allergic to any ergot preparation.
- Your heartbeat is less than 60 beats per minute.
- Your systolic blood pressure is consistently below 100.

Before you start, consult your doctor:
If you have had low blood pressure.

Over age 60:
Primarily used in persons older than 60. Results unpredictable, but many patients show improved brain function.

Pregnancy:
Not recommended.

Breast-feeding:
Risk to nursing child outweighs drug benefits. Don't use.

Infants & children:
Not recommended.

Prolonged use:
No problems expected.

Skin & sunlight:
No problems expected.

Driving, piloting or hazardous work:
Avoid if you feel dizzy, faint or have blurred vision. Otherwise, no problems expected.

Discontinuing:
No problems expected.

Others:
No problems expected.

 **POSSIBLE INTERACTION
WITH OTHER DRUGS**

GENERIC NAME OR DRUG CLASS	COMBINED EFFECT
Antihypertensives	Increased antihypertensive effect.
Beta-adrenergic blockers	Excessive decrease in heartbeat and/or blood pressure.
Digitalis preparations	Excessively slow heartbeat.

 **POSSIBLE INTERACTION
WITH OTHER SUBSTANCES**

INTERACTS WITH	COMBINED EFFECT
Alcohol:	Use caution. May drop blood pressure excessively.
Beverages:	None expected.
Cocaine:	Overstimulation. Avoid.
Foods:	None expected.
Marijuana:	Decreased effect of ergot alkaloids.
Tobacco:	None expected.

ERGONOVINE

BRAND NAMES

Ergometrine   Ergotrate

BASIC INFORMATION

Habit forming? No
Prescription needed? Yes
Available as generic? Yes
Drug class: Ergot preparation (uterine
      stimulant)

 ## USES

Retards excessive post-delivery bleeding.

 ## DOSAGE & USAGE INFORMATION

How to take:
Tablet—Swallow with liquid or food to lessen
stomach irritation.

When to take:
At the same times each day.

If you forget a dose:
Don't take missed dose and don't double next
one. Wait for next scheduled dose.

What drug does:
Causes smooth-muscle cells of uterine wall to
contract and surround bleeding blood vessels of
relaxed uterus.

Time lapse before drug works:
Tablets—20 to 30 minutes.

Don't take with:
See Interaction column and consult doctor.

 ## OVERDOSE

SYMPTOMS:
**Vomiting, diarrhea, weak pulse, low blood
pressure, convulsions.**
WHAT TO DO:
- **Dial 0 (operator) or 911 (emergency) for an
  ambulance or medical help. Then give first
  aid immediately.**
- **If patient is unconscious and not
  breathing, give mouth-to-mouth breathing.
  If there is no heartbeat, use cardiac
  massage and mouth-to-mouth breathing
  (CPR). Don't try to make patient vomit. If
  you can't get help quickly, take patient to
  nearest emergency facility.**
- **See emergency information on inside
  covers.**

 ## POSSIBLE ADVERSE REACTIONS OR SIDE EFFECTS

SYMPTOMS	WHAT TO DO
Life-threatening: None expected.	
Common: Nausea, vomiting.	Discontinue. Call doctor right away.
Infrequent: • Confusion, ringing in ears, diarrhea, muscle cramps.	Discontinue. Call doctor right away.
• Unusual sweating.	Continue. Call doctor when convenient.
Rare: Sudden, severe headache; shortness of breath; chest pain; numb, cold hands and feet.	Discontinue. Seek emergency treatment.

WARNINGS & PRECAUTIONS

Don't take if:
You are allergic to any ergot preparation.

Before you start, consult your doctor:
- If you have coronary-artery or blood-vessel disease.
- If you have liver or kidney disease.
- If you have high blood pressure.
- If you have postpartum infection.

Over age 60:
Not recommended.

Pregnancy:
Risk to unborn child outweighs drug benefits. Don't use.

Breast-feeding:
Drug passes into milk. Avoid drug or discontinue nursing until you finish medicine. Consult doctor for advice on maintaining milk supply.

Infants & children:
Not recommended.

Prolonged use:
Not recommended.

Skin & sunlight:
No problems expected.

Driving, piloting or hazardous work:
No problems expected.

Discontinuing:
May be unnecessary to finish medicine. Follow doctor's instructions.

Others:
Drug should be used for short time only following childbirth or miscarriage.

POSSIBLE INTERACTION WITH OTHER DRUGS

GENERIC NAME OR DRUG CLASS	COMBINED EFFECT
Ergot preparations (other)	Increased ergonovine effect.

POSSIBLE INTERACTION WITH OTHER SUBSTANCES

INTERACTS WITH	COMBINED EFFECT
Alcohol:	None expected.
Beverages:	None expected.
Cocaine:	None expected.
Foods:	None expected.
Marijuana:	None expected.
Tobacco:	None expected.

ERGOTAMINE

BRAND NAMES

Cafetrate-PB
Ergomar
Ergostat
Gynergen
Medihaler-Ergotamine
Migraine

Migral
Migrastat
Wigraine
Wigraine-PB
Wigrettes

BASIC INFORMATION

Habit forming? No
Prescription needed? Yes
Available as generic? Yes
Drug class: Vasoconstrictor,
ergot preparation

 ## USES

Relieves pain of migraines and other headaches caused by dilated blood vessels. Will not prevent headaches.

 ## DOSAGE & USAGE INFORMATION

How to take:
- Tablet or capsule—Swallow with liquid, or let dissolve under tongue. If you can't swallow whole, crumble tablet or open capsule and take with liquid or food.
- Suppositories—Remove wrapper and moisten suppository with water. Gently insert larger end into rectum. Push well into rectum with finger.
- Aerosol inhaler—Use only as directed on prescription label.
- Lie down in quiet, dark room after taking.

When to take:
At first sign of vascular or migraine headache.

Continued next column

 ## OVERDOSE

SYMPTOMS:
Tingling, cold extremities and muscle pain. Progresses to nausea, vomiting, diarrhea, cold skin, rapid and weak pulse, severe numbness of extremities, confusion, convulsions, coma.
WHAT TO DO:
- Dial 0 (operator) or 911 (emergency) for an ambulance or medical help. Then give first aid immediately.
- See emergency information on inside covers.

If you forget a dose:
Take as soon as you remember. Wait 4 hours for next dose.

What drug does:
Constricts blood vessels in the head.

Time lapse before drug works:
30 to 60 minutes.

Don't take with:
See Interaction column and consult doctor.

 ## POSSIBLE ADVERSE REACTIONS OR SIDE EFFECTS

SYMPTOMS	WHAT TO DO
Life-threatening: None expected.	
Common: Dizziness, nausea, diarrhea, vomiting.	Continue. Call doctor when convenient.
Infrequent: Itchy or swollen skin; cold, pale hands or feet; pain or weakness in arms, legs, back.	Discontinue. Call doctor right away.
Rare: Anxiety or confusion; red or purple blisters, especially on hands, feet; change in vision; extreme thirst; stomach pain or bloating; unusually fast or slow heartbeat; possible chest pain; numbness or tingling in face, fingers, toes.	Discontinue. Call doctor right away.

WARNINGS & PRECAUTIONS

Don't take if:
You are allergic to any ergot preparation.

Before you start, consult your doctor:
- If you plan to become pregnant within medication period.
- If you have an infection.
- If you have angina, heart problems, high blood pressure, hardening of the arteries or vein problems.
- If you have kidney or liver disease.
- If you are allergic to other spray inhalants.

Over age 60:
Adverse reactions and side effects may be more frequent and severe than in younger persons.

Pregnancy:
Risk to unborn child outweighs drug benefits. Don't use.

Breast-feeding:
Drug filters into milk. May harm child. Avoid.

Infants & children:
Studies inconclusive on harm to children. Consult your doctor.

Prolonged use:
Cold skin, muscle pain, gangrene of hands and feet. This medicine not intended for uninterrupted use.

Skin & sunlight:
No problems expected.

Driving, piloting or hazardous work:
Don't drive or pilot aircraft until you learn how medicine affects you. Don't work around dangerous machinery. Don't climb ladders or work in high places. Danger increases if you drink alcohol or take medicine affecting alertness and reflexes, such as antihistamines, tranquilizers, sedatives, pain medicine, narcotics and mind-altering drugs.

Discontinuing:
May be unnecessary to finish medicine. Follow doctor's instructions.

Others:
Impaired blood circulation can lead to gangrene in intestines or extremities. Never exceed recommended dose.

 ## POSSIBLE INTERACTION WITH OTHER DRUGS

GENERIC NAME OR DRUG CLASS	COMBINED EFFECT
Amphetamines	Dangerous blood-pressure rise.
Ephedrine	Dangerous blood-pressure rise.
Epinephrine	Dangerous blood-pressure rise.
Pseudoephedrine	Dangerous blood-pressure rise.
Troleandomycin	Increased adverse reactions of ergotamine.

 ## POSSIBLE INTERACTION WITH OTHER SUBSTANCES

INTERACTS WITH	COMBINED EFFECT
Alcohol:	Dilates blood vessels. Makes headache worse.
Beverages: Caffeine drinks.	May help relieve headache.
Cocaine:	Decreased ergotamine effect.
Foods: Any to which you are allergic.	May make headache worse. Avoid.
Marijuana:	Occasional use—Cool extremities. Regular use— Persistent chill.
Tobacco:	Decreased effect of ergotamine. Makes headache worse.

ERGOTAMINE, BELLADONNA & PHENOBARBITAL

BRAND NAMES

Bellergal   Bellergal-S

BASIC INFORMATION

Habit forming? Yes
Prescription needed? Yes
Available as generic? No
Drug class: Analgesic, antispasmodic,
vasoconstrictor

 ## USES

Reduces anxiety or nervous tension (low dose).

 ## DOSAGE & USAGE INFORMATION

How to take:
- Tablet or capsule—Swallow with liquid, or let dissolve under tongue. If you can't swallow whole, crumble tablet or open capsule and take with liquid or food.
- Suppositories—Remove wrapper and moisten suppository with water. Gently insert larger end into rectum. Push well into rectum with finger.
- Lie down in quiet, dark room after taking.

When to take:
At first sign of vascular or migraine headache.

If you forget a dose:
Take as soon as you remember. Wait 4 hours for next dose.

What drug does:
- Constricts blood vessels in the head.

Continued next column

 ## OVERDOSE

SYMPTOMS:
Tingling, cold extremities; muscle pain; nausea; vomiting; diarrhea; cold skin; rapid and weak pulse; severe numbness of extremities; confusion; dilated pupils; rapid pulse and breathing; dizziness; fever; hallucinations; slurred speech; agitation; flushed face; convulsions; coma.
WHAT TO DO:
- Dial 0 (operator) or 911 (emergency) for an ambulance or medical help. Then give first aid immediately.
- See emergency information on inside covers.

- Blocks nerve impulses at parasympathetic nerve endings, preventing muscle contractions and gland secretions of organs involved.

Time lapse before drug works:
15 to 30 minutes.

Don't take with:
Non-prescription drugs without consulting doctor.

 ## POSSIBLE ADVERSE REACTIONS OR SIDE EFFECTS

SYMPTOMS	WHAT TO DO
Life-threatening:	
Fast heartbeat, chest pain.	Discontinue. Seek emergency treatment.
Common:	
• Flushed skin, fever, drowsiness, depression, bloating, frequent urination.	Discontinue. Call doctor right away.
• Constipation, dizziness, drowsiness, "hangover" effect.	Continue. Call doctor when convenient.
Infrequent:	
Swollen feet and ankles, numbness or tingling in hands or feet, cold hands and feet, rash.	Discontinue. Call doctor right away.
Rare:	
Jaundice, weak legs, swallowing difficulty, dry mouth, increased sensitivity to sunlight, nausea, vomiting, decreased sweating.	Discontinue. Call doctor right away.

 ## WARNINGS & PRECAUTIONS

Don't take if:
- You are allergic to any barbiturate, anticholinergic or ergot preparation.
- You have porphyria, trouble with stomach bloating, difficulty emptying your bladder completely, narrow-angle glaucoma, severe ulcerative colitis.

ERGOTAMINE, BELLADONNA & PHENOBARBITAL

Before you start, consult your doctor:

- If you have epilepsy, kidney or liver damage, anemia, chronic pain, open-angle glaucoma, angina, heart problems, high blood pressure, hardening of the arteries, vein problems, chronic bronchitis, asthma, hiatal hernia, enlarged prostate, myasthenia gravis, peptic ulcer, an infection.
- If you plan to become pregnant within medication period.
- If you will have surgery within 2 months, including dental surgery, requiring general or spinal anesthesia.

Over age 60:
Adverse reactions and side effects may be more frequent and severe than in younger persons.

Pregnancy:
Risk to unborn child outweighs drug benefits. Don't use.

Breast-feeding:
Drug passes into milk. Avoid drug or discontinue nursing until you finish medicine. Consult doctor for advice on maintaining milk supply.

Infants & children:
Not recommended.

Prolonged use:
- May cause addiction, anemia, chronic intoxication.
- May lower body temperature, making exposure to cold temperatures hazardous.
- Chronic constipation, possible fecal impaction.
- Cold skin, muscle pain, gangrene of hands and feet. This medicine not intended for uninterrupted use.

Skin & sunlight:
May cause rash or intensify sunburn in areas exposed to sun or sunlamp.

Driving, piloting or hazardous work:
Don't drive or pilot aircraft until you learn how medicine affects you. Don't work around dangerous machinery. Don't climb ladders or work in high places. Danger increases if you drink alcohol or take medicine affecting alertness and reflexes, such as antihistamines, tranquilizers, sedatives, pain medicine, narcotics and mind-altering drugs.

Discontinuing:
May be unnecessary to finish medicine. Follow doctor's instructions. If you develop withdrawal symptoms of hallucinations, agitation or sleeplessness after discontinuing, call doctor right away.

Others:
Impaired blood circulation can lead to gangrene in intestines or extremities. Never exceed recommended dose.

POSSIBLE INTERACTION WITH OTHER DRUGS

GENERIC NAME OR DRUG CLASS	COMBINED EFFECT
Amantadine	Increased belladonna effect.
Amphetamines	Dangerous blood-pressure rise.
Anticholinergics (other)	Increased belladonna effect.
Anticoagulants (oral)	Decreased anticoagulant effect.
Anticonvulsants	Changed seizure patterns.
Antidepressants (tricyclics)	Decreased antidepressant effect. Possible dangerous oversedation.
Antidiabetics (oral)	Increased phenobarbital effect.
Antihistamines	Dangerous sedation. Avoid.
Anti-inflammatory drugs (non-steroidal)	Decreased anti-inflammatory effect.
Aspirin	Decreased aspirin effect.
Beta-adrenergic blockers	Decreased effect of beta-adrenergic blocker.

Continued page 965

POSSIBLE INTERACTION WITH OTHER SUBSTANCES

INTERACTS WITH	COMBINED EFFECT
Alcohol:	Possible fatal oversedation. Avoid.
Beverages:	None expected.
Cocaine:	Excessively rapid heartbeat. Avoid.
Foods:	None expected.
Marijuana:	Drowsiness and dry mouth, excessive sedation. Avoid.
Tobacco:	None expected.

ERGOTAMINE & CAFFEINE

BRAND NAMES

Cafergot	Ercaf
Cafertabs	Ercatabs
Cafetrate	Ergo-Caff

BASIC INFORMATION

Habit forming? No
Prescription needed? Yes
Available as generic? No
Drug class: Analgesic, stimulant (xanthine)
           vasoconstrictor

USES

Relieves pain of migraines and other headaches caused by dilated blood vessels. Will not prevent headaches.

DOSAGE & USAGE INFORMATION

How to take:
- Tablet or capsule—Swallow with liquid, or let dissolve under tongue. If you can't swallow whole, crumble tablet or open capsule and take with liquid or food.
- Suppositories—Remove wrapper and moisten suppository with water. Gently insert larger end into rectum. Push well into rectum with finger.
- Extended-release capsules—Swallow whole with liquid.
- Lie down in quiet, dark room after taking.

When to take:
At first sign of vascular or migraine headache.

If you forget a dose:
Take as soon as you remember up to 2 hours late. If more than 2 hours, wait for next scheduled dose (don't double this dose).

Continued next column

OVERDOSE

SYMPTOMS:
Tingling, cold extremities; muscle pain; nausea; vomiting; diarrhea; cold skin; severe numbness of extremities; confusion; excitement; rapid heartbeat; hallucinations; convulsions; coma.
WHAT TO DO:
- **Dial 0 (operator) or 911 (emergency) for an ambulance or medical help. Then give first aid immediately.**
- **See emergency information on inside covers.**

What drug does:
- Constricts blood vessels in the head.
- Constricts blood-vessel walls.
- Stimulates central nervous system.

Time lapse before drug works:
30 to 60 minutes.

Don't take with:
- Non-prescription drugs containing alcohol without consulting doctor.
- See Interaction column and consult doctor.

POSSIBLE ADVERSE REACTIONS OR SIDE EFFECTS

SYMPTOMS	WHAT TO DO
Life-threatening:	
Slow or fast heartbeat.	Discontinue. Seek emergency treatment.
Common:	
• Fast heartbeat.	Discontinue. Call doctor right away.
• Dizziness, nausea, diarrhea, vomiting, nervousness.	Continue. Call doctor when convenient.
Infrequent:	
Itchy skin; abdominal pain; cold hands and feet; weakness in arms, legs, back; confusion; irritability; indigestion; low blood sugar with weakness and trembling.	Discontinue. Call doctor right away.
Rare:	
Anxiety; red or purple blisters, especially on hands and feet; change in vision; extreme thirst; numbness or tingling in hands or feet.	Discontinue. Call doctor right away.

WARNINGS & PRECAUTIONS

Don't take if:
- You are allergic to any stimulant or any ergot preparation.
- You have heart disease.
- You have active peptic ulcer of stomach or duodenum.

Before you start, consult your doctor:
- If you have irregular heartbeat, angina, heart problems, high blood pressure, hardening of the arteries or vein problems.
- If you have hypoglycemia (low blood sugar), epilepsy, an infection, kidney or liver disease.
- If you are allergic to spray inhalants.
- If you plan to become pregnant within medication period.

Over age 60:
Adverse reactions and side effects may be more frequent and severe than in younger persons, especially dizziness and excessive potassium loss.

Pregnancy:
Risk to unborn child outweighs drug benefits. Don't use.

Breast-feeding:
Drug passes into milk. Avoid drug or discontinue nursing until you finish medicine. Consult doctor for advice on maintaining milk supply.

Infants & children:
Not recommended.

Prolonged use:
Cold skin, muscle pain, stomach ulcers, gangrene of hands and feet. This medicine not intended for uninterrupted use.

Skin & sunlight:
No problems expected.

Driving, piloting or hazardous work:
Don't drive or pilot aircraft until you learn how medicine affects you. Don't work around dangerous machinery. Don't climb ladders or work in high places. Danger increases if you drink alcohol or take medicine affecting alertness and reflexes, such as antihistamines, tranquilizers, sedatives, pain medicine, narcotics and mind-altering drugs.

Discontinuing:
Will cause withdrawal symptoms of headache, irritability, drowsiness. Discontinue gradually if you use caffeine for a month or more.

Others:
- May produce or aggravate fibrocystic breast disease in women.
- Impaired blood circulation can lead to gangrene in intestines or extremities. Never exceed recommended dose.

POSSIBLE INTERACTION WITH OTHER DRUGS

GENERIC NAME OR DRUG CLASS	COMBINED EFFECT
Amphetamines	Dangerous blood-pressure rise.
Contraceptives (oral)	Increased caffeine effect.
Ephedrine	Dangerous blood-pressure rise.
Epinephrine	Dangerous blood-pressure rise.
Isoniazid	Increased caffeine effect.

MAO inhibitors	Dangerous blood-pressure rise.
Pseudoephedrine	Dangerous blood-pressure rise.
Sedatives	Decreased sedative effect.
Sleep inducers	Decreased sedative effect.
Sympathomimetics	Overstimulation.
Thyroid hormones	Increased thyroid effect.
Tranquilizers	Decreased tranquilizer effect.
Troleandomycin	Increased adverse reactions of ergotamine.

POSSIBLE INTERACTION WITH OTHER SUBSTANCES

INTERACTS WITH	COMBINED EFFECT
Alcohol:	Dilates blood vessels. Makes headache worse.
Beverages: Caffeine drinks.	May help relieve headache.
Cocaine:	Overstimulation. Avoid.
Foods: Any to which you are allergic.	May make headache worse. Avoid.
Marijuana:	Occasional use—Cool extremities. Regular use—Persistent chill. Increased effect of both drugs. May lead to dangerous, rapid heartbeat. Avoid.
Tobacco:	Decreased effect of ergotamine. Makes headache worse. Avoid.

ERGOTAMINE, CAFFEINE, BELLADONNA & PENTOBARBITAL

BRAND NAMES

Cafergot-PB

BASIC INFORMATION

Habit forming? Yes
Prescription needed? Yes
Available as generic? No
Drug class: Vasoconstrictor, stimulant
(xanthine), sedative,
antispasmodic

 ## USES

- Relieves pain of migraines and other headaches caused by dilated blood vessels. Will not prevent headaches.
- Reduces anxiety or nervous tension (low dose).

 ## DOSAGE & USAGE INFORMATION

How to take:
- Tablet, elixir or capsule—Swallow with liquid or food to lessen stomach irritation.
- Tablet or capsule—Swallow with liquid, or let dissolve under tongue. If you can't swallow whole, crumble tablet or open capsule and take with liquid or food.
- Suppositories—Remove wrapper and moisen suppository with water. Gently insert larger end into rectum. Push well into rectum with finger.
- Lie down in quiet, dark room after taking.

When to take:
At first sign of vascular or migraine headache.

Continued next column

 ## OVERDOSE

SYMPTOMS:
Tingling, cold extremities and muscle pain.
Progresses to nausea, vomiting, diarrhea,
cold skin, rapid and weak pulse, severe
numbness of extremities, confusion,
convulsions, coma.
WHAT TO DO:
- **Dial 0 (operator) or 911 (emergency) for an ambulance or medical help. Then give first aid immediately.**
- **See emergency information on inside covers.**

If you forget a dose:
Take as soon as you remember up to 2 hours late. If more than 2 hours, wait for next scheduled dose (don't double this dose).

What drug does:
- Blocks nerve impulses at parasympathetic nerve endings, preventing muscle contractions and gland secretions of organs involved.
- May partially block nerve impulses at nerve-cell connections.
- Constricts blood-vessel walls.
- Stimulates central nervous system.

Time lapse before drug works:
15 to 30 minutes.

Don't take with:
- Non-prescription drugs without consulting doctor.
- See Interaction column and consult doctor.

 ## POSSIBLE ADVERSE REACTIONS OR SIDE EFFECTS

SYMPTOMS	WHAT TO DO
Life-threatening:	
Slow or fast heartbeat.	Discontinue. Seek emergency treatment.
Common:	
• Fast heartbeat.	Discontinue. Call doctor right away.
• Dizziness, nausea, diarrhea, vomiting, nervousness, "hangover" effect.	Continue. Call doctor when convenient.
Infrequent:	
Itchy skin; rash; abdominal pain; cold hands and feet; weakness in arms, back, legs; confusion; irritability; indigestion; low blood sugar with weakness and trembling.	Discontinue. Call doctor right away.
Rare:	
Anxiety; red or purple blisters, especially in hands and feet; change in vision; extreme thirst; numbness or tingling in hands or feet; jaundice.	Discontinue. Call doctor right away.

ERGOTAMINE, CAFFEINE, BELLADONNA & PENTOBARBITAL

WARNINGS & PRECAUTIONS

Don't take if:
- You are allergic to any stimulant, ergot preparation, barbiturate or anticholinergic.
- You have heart disease, peptic ulcer of stomach or duodenum, porphyria, trouble with stomach bloating, difficulty emptying your bladder completely, narrow-angle glaucoma, severe ulcerative colitis.

Before you start, consult your doctor:
- If you have hypoglycemia (low blood sugar), an infection, angina, heart problems, high blood pressure, hardening of the arteries, vein problems, kidney or liver disease, epilepsy, asthma, anemia, chronic pain, open-angle glaucoma, chronic bronchitis, hiatal hernia, enlarged prostate, myasthenia gravis, peptic ulcer.
- If you plan to become pregnant within medication period.
- If you will have surgery within 2 months, including dental surgery, requiring general or spinal anesthesia.

Over age 60:
Adverse reactions and side effects may be more frequent and severe than in younger persons, especially dizziness and excessive potassium loss.

Pregnancy:
Risk to unborn child outweighs drug benefits. Don't use.

Breast-feeding:
Drug filters into milk. May harm child. Avoid.

Infants & children:
Not recommended.

Prolonged use:
- Stomach ulcers.
- Cold skin, muscle pain, gangrene of hands and feet. This medicine not intended for uninterrupted use.
- May cause addiction, anemia, chronic intoxication.
- May lower body temperature, making exposure to cold temperatures hazardous.
- Chronic constipation, possible fecal impaction.

Skin & sunlight:
May cause rash or intensify sunburn in areas exposed to sun or sunlamp.

Driving, piloting or hazardous work:
Don't drive or pilot aircraft until you learn how medicine affects you. Don't work around dangerous machinery. Don't climb ladders or work in high places. Danger increases if you drink alcohol or take medicine affecting alertness and reflexes, such as antihistamines, tranquilizers, sedatives, pain medicine, narcotics and mind-altering drugs.

Discontinuing:
May be unnecessary to finish medicine. Follow doctor's instructions. If you develop withdrawal symptoms of hallucinations, headache, agitation or sleeplessness after discontinuing, call doctor right away.

Others:
- Great potential for abuse.
- May produce or aggravate fibrocystic breast disease in women.
- Impaired blood circulation can lead to gangrene in intestines or extremities. Never exceed recommended dose.

POSSIBLE INTERACTION WITH OTHER DRUGS

GENERIC NAME OR DRUG CLASS	COMBINED EFFECT
Amantadine	Increased belladonna effect.
Amphetamines	Dangerous blood-pressure rise.

Continued page 966

POSSIBLE INTERACTION WITH OTHER SUBSTANCES

INTERACTS WITH	COMBINED EFFECT
Alcohol:	Dilates blood vessels. Makes headache worse. Possible fatal oversedation. Avoid.
Beverages: Caffeine drinks.	May help relieve headache.
Cocaine:	Excessively rapid heartbeat. Avoid.
Foods: Any to which you are allergic.	May make headache worse. Avoid.
Marijuana:	Drowsiness and dry mouth, excessive sedation. Avoid. Occasional use—Cool extremities. Regular use—Persistent chill.
Tobacco:	Decreased effect of ergotamine. Makes headache worse.

BRAND AND GENERIC NAMES

See complete list of brand names in the *Brand Name Directory,* page 949.

BASIC INFORMATION

Habit forming? No
Prescription needed? Yes
Available as generic? Yes
Drug class: Antibiotic (erythromycin)

 USES

Treatment of infections responsive to erythromycin.

 DOSAGE & USAGE INFORMATION

How to take:
- Tablet or capsule—Swallow with liquid.
- Extended-release tablets or capsules—Swallow each dose whole. If you take regular tablets, you may chew or crush them.
- Liquid, drops, granules, skin ointment, eye ointment, skin solution—Follow prescription label directions.

When to take:
At the same times each day, 1 hour before or 2 hours after eating.

If you forget a dose:
- If you take 3 or more doses daily—Take as soon as you remember. Return to regular schedule.
- If you take 2 doses daily—Take as soon as you remember. Wait 5 to 6 hours for next dose. Return to regular schedule.

What drug does:
Prevents growth and reproduction of susceptible bacteria.

Time lapse before drug works:
2 to 5 days.

Continued next column

 OVERDOSE

SYMPTOMS:
Nausea, vomiting, abdominal discomfort, diarrhea.
WHAT TO DO:
Overdose unlikely to threaten life. If person takes much larger amount than prescribed, call doctor, poison-control center or hospital emergency room for instructions.

Don't take with:
See Interaction column and consult doctor.

 POSSIBLE ADVERSE REACTIONS OR SIDE EFFECTS

SYMPTOMS	WHAT TO DO
Life-threatening: None expected.	
Common: None expected.	
Infrequent:	
• Diarrhea, nausea, stomach cramps, discomfort, vomiting.	Discontinue. Call doctor right away.
• Skin dryness, irritation, itch, stinging with use of skin solution, sore mouth or tongue.	Continue. Call doctor when convenient.
Rare:	
• Jaundice in adults.	Discontinue. Call doctor right away.
• Unusual tiredness or weakness.	Continue. Call doctor when convenient.

WARNINGS & PRECAUTIONS

Don't take if:
- You are allergic to any erythromycin.
- You have had liver disease or impaired liver function.

Before you start, consult your doctor:
If you have taken erythromycin estolate in the past.

Over age 60:
Adverse reactions and side effects may be more frequent and severe than in younger persons, especially skin reactions around genitals and anus.

Pregnancy:
No proven harm to unborn child. Avoid if possible.

Breast-feeding:
Drug passes into milk. Avoid drug or discontinue nursing until you finish medicine. Consult doctor for advice on maintaining milk supply.

Infants & children:
Use only under medical supervision.

Prolonged use:
You may become more susceptible to infections caused by germs not responsive to erythromycin.

Skin & sunlight:
No problems expected.

Driving, piloting or hazardous work:
No problems expected.

Discontinuing:
You must take full dose at least 10 consecutive days for streptococcal or staphylococcal infections.

Others:
No problems expected.

POSSIBLE INTERACTION WITH OTHER DRUGS

GENERIC NAME OR DRUG CLASS	COMBINED EFFECT
Aminophylline	Increased effect of aminophylline in blood.
Lincomycins	Decreased lincomycin effect.
Oxtriphylline	Increased level of oxtriphylline in blood.
Penicillins	Decreased penicillin effect.
Theophylline	Increased level of theophylline in blood.

POSSIBLE INTERACTION WITH OTHER SUBSTANCES

INTERACTS WITH	COMBINED EFFECT
Alcohol:	Possible liver damage.
Beverages:	None expected.
Cocaine:	None expected.
Foods:	None expected.
Marijuana:	None expected.
Tobacco:	None expected.

ERYTHROMYCIN & SULFISOXAZOLE

BRAND NAMES

Pediazole

BASIC INFORMATION

Habit forming? No
Prescription needed? Yes
Available as generic? Yes
Drug class: Antibiotic (erythromycin), sulfa
        (sulfonamide)

USES

Treatment of infections responsive to
erythromycin and sulfa.

DOSAGE & USAGE INFORMATION

How to take:
Suspension—Swallow with liquid. Instructions to
take on empty stomach mean 1 hour before or
2 hours after eating. Shake carefully before
measuring.

When to take:
At the same times each day, 1 hour before or 2
hours after eating.

If you forget a dose:
Take as soon as you remember up to 2 hours
late. If more than 2 hours, wait for next
scheduled dose (don't double this dose).

What drug does:
Prevents growth and reproduction of susceptible
bacteria.

Time lapse before drug works:
2 to 5 days to affect infection.

Don't take with:
See Interaction column and consult doctor.

OVERDOSE

SYMPTOMS:
Less urine, bloody urine, nausea, vomiting,
abdominal discomfort, diarrhea, coma.
WHAT TO DO:
- **Dial 0 (operator) or 911 (emergency) for an**
  ambulance or medical help. Then give first
  aid immediately.
- **See emergency information on inside**
  covers.

POSSIBLE ADVERSE REACTIONS OR SIDE EFFECTS

SYMPTOMS	WHAT TO DO
Life-threatening: None expected.	
Common: Headache, dizziness, itchy skin, rash, appetite loss, vomiting.	Discontinue. Call doctor right away.
Infrequent: Dryness, irritation, itch, stinging with use of skin solution, mouth or tongue sore, diarrhea, nausea, abdominal cramps, vomiting, swallowing difficulty.	Continue. Call doctor when convenient.
Rare: • Jaundice, painful or difficult urination.	Discontinue. Call doctor right away.
• Weakness and unusual tiredness.	Continue. Call doctor when convenient.

WARNINGS & PRECAUTIONS

Don't take if:
- You are allergic to any sulfa drug or any
  erythromycin.
- You have had liver disease or impaired liver
  function.

Before you start, consult your doctor:
- If you are allergic to carbonic anhydrase
  inhibitors, oral antidiabetics or thiazide
  diuretics.
- If you are allergic by nature.
- If you have liver or kidney disease, porphyria,
  developed anemia from use of any drug,
  taken erythromycin estolate in the past.

Over age 60:
Adverse reactions and side effects may be
more frequent and severe than in younger
persons, especially skin reactions around
genitals and anus.

Pregnancy:
Risk to unborn child outweighs drug benefits.
Don't use.

Breast-feeding:
Drug passes into milk. Avoid drug or
discontinue nursing until you finish medicine.
Consult doctor for advice on maintaining milk
supply.

Infants & children:
Don't give to infants younger than 1 month.

Prolonged use:
- May enlarge thyroid gland.
- Request frequent blood counts, liver- and kidney-function studies.
- You may become more susceptible to infections caused by germs not responsive to erythromycin or sulfa.

Skin & sunlight:
May cause rash or intensify sunburn in areas exposed to sun or sunlamp.

Driving, piloting or hazardous work:
Avoid if you feel dizzy. Otherwise, no problems expected.

Discontinuing:
Don't discontinue without doctor's advice until you complete prescribed dose, even though symptoms diminish or disappear.

Others:
- Drink extra liquid each day to prevent adverse reactions.
- If you require surgery, tell anesthetist you take sulfa.

POSSIBLE INTERACTION WITH OTHER DRUGS

GENERIC NAME OR DRUG CLASS	COMBINED EFFECT
Aminobenzoate potassium	Possible decreased sulfisoxazole effect.
Aminophylline	Increased effect of aminophylline in blood.
Anticoagulants (oral)	Increased anticoagulant effect.
Anticonvulsants (hydantoin)	Toxic effect on brain.
Aspirin	Increased sulfa effect.
Flecainide	Possible decreased blood-cell production in bone marrow.
Isoniazid	Possible anemia.
Lincomycins	Decreased lincomycin effect.
Methenamine	Possible kidney blockage.
Methotrexate	Increased possibility of toxic side effects from methotrexate.
Oxtriphylline	Increased level of oxtriphylline in blood.
Oxyphenbutazone	Increased sulfa effect.
Para-aminosalicylic acid (PAS)	Decreased sulfa effect.

Penicillins	Decreased penicillin effect.
Phenylbutazone	Increased sulfa effect.
Probenecid	Increased sulfa effect.
Sulfinpyrazone	Increased sulfa effect.
Theophylline	Increased level of theophylline in blood.
Tocainide	Possible decreased blood-cell production in bone marrow.
Trimethoprim	Increased sulfa effect.

POSSIBLE INTERACTION WITH OTHER SUBSTANCES

INTERACTS WITH	COMBINED EFFECT
Alcohol:	Increased alcohol effect. Possible liver damage.
Beverages: Less than 2 quarts of fluid daily.	Kidney damage.
Cocaine:	None expected.
Foods:	None expected.
Marijuana:	None expected.
Tobacco:	None expected.

ESTERIFIED ESTROGENS

BRAND NAMES

Amnestrogen	Estromed
Climestrone	Evex
Estratab	Menest
Estratest	Neo-Estrone

BASIC INFORMATION

Habit forming? No
Prescription needed? Yes
Available as generic? Yes
Drug class: Female sex hormone (estrogen)

 ## USES

- Treatment for symptoms of menopause and menstrual-cycle irregularity.
- Replacement for female hormone deficiency.
- Treatment for cancer of prostate and breast.

 ## DOSAGE & USAGE INFORMATION

How to take:
Tablet—Swallow with liquid. If you can't swallow whole, crumble tablet and take with liquid or food.

When to take:
At the same time each day.

If you forget a dose:
Take as soon as you remember up to 12 hours late. If more than 12 hours, wait for next scheduled dose (don't double this dose).

What drug does:
Restores normal estrogen level in tissues.

Time lapse before drug works:
10 to 20 days.

Don't take with:
See Interaction column and consult doctor.

 ## OVERDOSE

SYMPTOMS:
Nausea, vomiting, fluid retention, breast enlargement and discomfort, abnormal vaginal bleeding.
WHAT TO DO:
Overdose unlikely to threaten life. If person takes much larger amount than prescribed, call doctor, poison-control center or hospital emergency room for instructions.

 ## POSSIBLE ADVERSE REACTIONS OR SIDE EFFECTS

SYMPTOMS	WHAT TO DO
Life-threatening:	
None expected.	
Common:	
● Stomach cramps.	Discontinue. Call doctor right away.
● Appetite loss.	Continue. Call doctor when convenient.
● Nausea; diarrhea; swollen feet and ankles; tender, swollen breasts.	Continue. Tell doctor at next visit.
Infrequent:	
● Rash, stomach or side pain.	Discontinue. Call doctor right away.
● Depression, dizziness, irritability, vomiting, breast lumps.	Continue. Call doctor when convenient.
● Brown blotches, hair loss, vaginal discharge or bleeding, changes in sex drive.	Continue. Tell doctor at next visit.
Rare:	
Jaundice.	Discontinue. Call doctor right away.

WARNINGS & PRECAUTIONS

Don't take if:
- You are allergic to any estrogen-containing drugs.
- You have impaired liver function.
- You have had blood clots, stroke or heart attack.
- You have unexplained vaginal bleeding.

Before you start, consult your doctor:
- If you have had cancer of breast or reproductive organs, fibrocystic breast disease, fibroid tumors of the uterus or endometriosis.
- If you have had migraine headaches, epilepsy or porphyria.
- If you have diabetes, high blood pressure, asthma, congestive heart failure, kidney disease or gallstones.
- If you plan to become pregnant within 3 months.

Over age 60:
Controversial. You and your doctor must decide if drug risks outweigh benefits.

Pregnancy:
Risk to unborn child outweighs drug benefits. Don't use.

Breast-feeding:
Drug filters into milk. May harm child. Avoid.

Infants & children:
Not recommended.

Prolonged use:
Increased growth of fibroid tumors of uterus. Possible association with cancer of uterus.

Skin & sunlight:
May cause rash or intensify sunburn in areas exposed to sun or sunlamp.

Driving, piloting or hazardous work:
No problems expected.

Discontinuing:
You may need to discontinue estrogen periodically. Consult your doctor.

Others:
In rare instances, may cause blood clot in lung, brain or leg. Symptoms are *sudden* severe headache, coordination loss, vision change, chest pain, breathing difficulty, slurred speech, pain in legs or groin. Seek emergency treatment immediately.

POSSIBLE INTERACTION WITH OTHER DRUGS

GENERIC NAME OR DRUG CLASS	COMBINED EFFECT
Anticoagulants (oral)	Decreased anticoagulant effect.
Anticonvulsants (hydantoin)	Increased seizures.
Antidiabetics (oral)	Unpredictable increase or decrease in blood sugar.
Carbamazepine	Increased seizures.
Clofibrate	Decreased clofibrate effect.
Meprobamate	Increased effect of esterified estrogens.
Phenobarbital	Decreased effect of esterified estrogens.
Primidone	Decreased effect of esterified estrogens.
Rifampin	Decreased effect of esterified estrogens.
Thyroid hormones	Decreased thyroid effect.

POSSIBLE INTERACTION WITH OTHER SUBSTANCES

INTERACTS WITH	COMBINED EFFECT
Alcohol:	None expected.
Beverages:	None expected.
Cocaine:	No proven problems.
Foods:	None expected.
Marijuana:	Possible menstrual irregularities and bleeding between periods.
Tobacco:	Increased risk of blood clots leading to stroke or heart attack.

ESTRADIOL

BRAND NAMES

Delestrogen   Estrace

BASIC INFORMATION

Habit forming? No
Prescription needed? Yes
Available as generic? Yes
Drug class: Female sex hormone (estrogen)

 USES

- Treatment for symptoms of menopause and menstrual-cycle irregularity.
- Replacement for female hormone deficiency.
- Treatment for cancer of prostate and breast.

 DOSAGE & USAGE INFORMATION

How to take:
Tablet—Swallow with liquid. If you can't swallow whole, crumble tablet and take with liquid or food.

When to take:
At the same time each day.

If you forget a dose:
Take as soon as you remember up to 12 hours late. If more than 12 hours, wait for next scheduled dose (don't double this dose).

What drug does:
Restores normal estrogen level in tissues.

Time lapse before drug works:
10 to 20 days.

Don't take with:
See Interaction column and consult doctor.

 OVERDOSE

SYMPTOMS:
Nausea, vomiting, fluid retention, breast enlargement and discomfort, abnormal vaginal bleeding.
WHAT TO DO:
Overdose unlikely to threaten life. If person takes much larger amount than prescribed, call doctor, poison-control center or hospital emergency room for instructions.

 POSSIBLE ADVERSE REACTIONS OR SIDE EFFECTS

SYMPTOMS	WHAT TO DO
Life-threatening:	
None expected.	
Common:	
• Stomach cramps.	Discontinue. Call doctor right away.
• Appetite loss.	Continue. Call doctor when convenient.
• Nausea; diarrhea; swollen feet and ankles; tender, swollen breasts.	Continue. Tell doctor at next visit.
Infrequent:	
• Rash, stomach or side pain.	Discontinue. Call doctor right away.
• Depression, dizziness, irritability, vomiting, breast lumps.	Continue. Call doctor when convenient.
• Brown blotches, hair loss, vaginal discharge or bleeding, changes in sex drive.	Continue. Tell doctor at next visit.
Rare:	
Jaundice.	Discontinue. Call doctor right away.

WARNINGS & PRECAUTIONS

Don't take if:
- You are allergic to any estrogen-containing drugs.
- You have impaired liver function.
- You have had blood clots, stroke or heart attack.
- You have unexplained vaginal bleeding.

Before you start, consult your doctor:
- If you have had cancer of breast or reproductive organs, fibrocystic breast disease, fibroid tumors of the uterus or endometriosis.
- If you have had migraine headaches, epilepsy or porphyria.
- If you have diabetes, high blood pressure, asthma, congestive heart failure, kidney disease or gallstones.
- If you plan to become pregnant within 3 months.

Over age 60:
Controversial. You and your doctor must decide if drug risks outweigh benefits.

Pregnancy:
Risk to unborn child outweighs drug benefits. Don't use.

Breast-feeding:
Drug filters into milk. May harm child. Avoid.

Infants & children:
Not recommended.

Prolonged use:
Increased growth of fibroid tumors of uterus. Possible association with cancer of uterus.

Skin & sunlight:
May cause rash or intensify sunburn in areas exposed to sun or sunlamp.

Driving, piloting or hazardous work:
No problems expected.

Discontinuing:
You may need to discontinue estradiol periodically. Consult your doctor.

Others:
In rare instances, may cause blood clot in lung, brain or leg. Symptoms are *sudden* severe headache, coordination loss, vision change, chest pain, breathing difficulty, slurred speech, pain in legs or groin. Seek emergency treatment immediately.

POSSIBLE INTERACTION WITH OTHER DRUGS

GENERIC NAME OR DRUG CLASS	COMBINED EFFECT
Anticoagulants (oral)	Decreased anticoagulant effect.
Anticonvulsants (hydantoin)	Increased seizures.
Antidiabetics (oral)	Unpredictable increase or decrease in blood sugar.
Carbamazepine	Increased seizures.
Clofibrate	Decreased clofibrate effect.
Meprobamate	Increased estradiol effect.
Phenobarbital	Decreased estradiol effect.
Primidone	Decreased estradiol effect.
Rifampin	Decreased estradiol effect.
Thyroid hormones	Decreased thyroid effect.

POSSIBLE INTERACTION WITH OTHER SUBSTANCES

INTERACTS WITH	COMBINED EFFECT
Alcohol:	None expected.
Beverages:	None expected.
Cocaine:	No proven problems.
Foods:	None expected.
Marijuana:	Possible menstrual irregularities and bleeding between periods.
Tobacco:	Increased risk of blood clots leading to stroke or heart attack.

ESTROGEN

BRAND NAMES

See complete list of brand names in the *Brand Name Directory,* page 949.

BASIC INFORMATION

Habit forming? No
Prescription needed? Yes
Available as generic? Yes
Drug class: Female sex hormone (estrogen)

 USES

- Treatment for symptoms of menopause and menstrual-cycle irregularity.
- Treatment for estrogen-deficiency osteoporosis (bone softening from calcium loss).
- Treatment for DES-induced cancer.
- Treatment for atrophic vaginitis.

 DOSAGE & USAGE INFORMATION

How to take:
- Tablet or capsule—Swallow with liquid. If you can't swallow whole, crumble tablet or open capsule and take with liquid or food.
- Vaginal cream or suppositories—Use as directed on label.

When to take:
At the same time each day.

If you forget a dose:
Take as soon as you remember up to 12 hours late. If more than 12 hours, wait for next scheduled dose (don't double this dose).

What drug does:
Restores normal estrogen level in tissues.

Time lapse before drug works:
10 to 20 days.

Don't take with:
See Interaction column and consult doctor.

 OVERDOSE

SYMPTOMS:
Nausea, vomiting, fluid retention, breast enlargement and discomfort, abnormal vaginal bleeding.
WHAT TO DO:
Overdose unlikely to threaten life. If person takes much larger amount than prescribed, call doctor, poison-control center or hospital emergency room for instructions.

 POSSIBLE ADVERSE REACTIONS OR SIDE EFFECTS

SYMPTOMS	WHAT TO DO
Life-threatening: None expected.	
Common:	
• Stomach cramps.	Discontinue. Call doctor right away.
• Appetite loss.	Continue. Call doctor when convenient.
• Nausea; diarrhea; swollen feet and ankles; tender, swollen breasts.	Continue. Tell doctor at next visit.
Infrequent:	
• Rash, stomach or side pain.	Discontinue. Call doctor right away.
• Depression, dizziness, irritability, vomiting, breast lumps.	Continue. Call doctor when convenient.
• Brown blotches, hair loss, vaginal discharge or bleeding, changes in sex drive.	Continue. Tell doctor at next visit.
Rare: Jaundice.	Discontinue. Call doctor right away.

WARNINGS & PRECAUTIONS

Don't take if:
- You are allergic to any estrogen-containing drugs.
- You have impaired liver function.
- You have had blood clots, stroke or heart attack.
- You have unexplained vaginal bleeding.

Before you start, consult your doctor:
- If you have had cancer of breast or reproductive organs, fibrocystic breast disease, fibroid tumors of the uterus or endometriosis.
- If you have had migraine headaches, epilepsy or porphyria.
- If you have diabetes, high blood pressure, asthma, congestive heart failure, kidney disease or gallstones.
- If you plan to become pregnant within 3 months.

Over age 60:
Controversial. You and your doctor must decide if drug risks outweigh benefits.

Pregnancy:
Risk to unborn child outweighs drug benefits. Don't use.

Breast-feeding:
Drug filters into milk. May harm child. Avoid.

Infants & children:
Not recommended.

Prolonged use:
Increased growth of fibroid tumors of uterus. Possible association with cancer of uterus.

Skin & sunlight:
May cause rash or intensify sunburn in areas exposed to sun or sunlamp.

Driving, piloting or hazardous work:
No problems expected.

Discontinuing:
You may need to discontinue estrogens periodically. Consult your doctor.

Others:
- In rare instances, may cause blood clot in lung, brain or leg. Symptoms are *sudden* severe headache, coordination loss, vision change, chest pain, breathing difficulty, slurred speech, pain in legs or groin. Seek emergency treatment immediately.
- Carefully read the paper called "Information for the Patient" that was given to you with your prescription. If you lose it, ask your pharmacist for a copy.

POSSIBLE INTERACTION WITH OTHER DRUGS

GENERIC NAME OR DRUG CLASS	COMBINED EFFECT
Anticoagulants (oral)	Decreased anticoagulant effect.
Anticonvulsants (hydantoin)	Increased seizures.
Antidiabetics (oral)	Unpredictable increase or decrease in blood sugar.
Carbamazepine	Increased seizures.
Clofibrate	Decreased clofibrate effect.
Meprobamate	Increased estrogen effect.
Phenobarbital	Decreased estrogen effect.
Primidone	Decreased estrogen effect.
Rifampin	Decreased estrogen effect.
Thyroid hormones	Decreased thyroid effect.

POSSIBLE INTERACTION WITH OTHER SUBSTANCES

INTERACTS WITH	COMBINED EFFECT
Alcohol:	None expected.
Beverages:	None expected.
Cocaine:	No proven problems.
Foods:	None expected.
Marijuana:	Possible menstrual irregularities and bleeding between periods.
Tobacco:	Increased risk of blood clots leading to stroke or heart attack.

ESTRONE

BRAND NAMES

Besterone	Kestrin
Estaqua	Kestrin Aqueous
Estrofol	Kestrone
Estroject	Natural Estrogenic
Estrone-A	Substance
Estronol	Ogen
Femogen	Theelin
Foygen Aqueous	Theogen
Gynogen	Unigen
Hormogen-A	Wehgen

BASIC INFORMATION

Habit forming? No
Prescription needed? Yes
Available as generic? Yes
Drug class: Female sex hormone (estrogen)

 USES

- Treatment for symptoms of menopause and menstrual-cycle irregularity.
- Replacement for female hormone deficiency.
- Treatment for cancer of prostate.

 DOSAGE & USAGE INFORMATION

How to take:
By injection under medical supervision.

When to take:
Varies according to doctor's instructions.

If you forget an injection:
Consult doctor.

What drug does:
Restores normal estrogen level in tissues.

Time lapse before drug works:
10 to 20 days.

Don't take with:
See Interaction column and consult doctor.

 OVERDOSE

SYMPTOMS:
Nausea, vomiting, fluid retention, breast enlargement and discomfort, abnormal vaginal bleeding.
WHAT TO DO:
Overdose unlikely to threaten life. If person takes much larger amount than prescribed, call doctor, poison-control center or hospital emergency room for instructions.

 POSSIBLE ADVERSE REACTIONS OR SIDE EFFECTS

SYMPTOMS	WHAT TO DO
Life-threatening: None expected.	
Common:	
• Stomach cramps.	Discontinue. Call doctor right away.
• Appetite loss.	Continue. Call doctor when convenient.
• Nausea; diarrhea; swollen feet and ankles; tender, swollen breasts.	Continue. Tell doctor at next visit.
Infrequent:	
• Rash, stomach or side pain.	Discontinue. Call doctor right away.
• Depression, dizziness, irritability, vomiting, breast lumps.	Continue. Call doctor when convenient.
• Brown blotches, hair loss, vaginal discharge or bleeding, changes in sex drive.	Continue. Tell doctor at next visit.
Rare: Jaundice.	Discontinue. Call doctor right away.

WARNINGS & PRECAUTIONS

Don't take if:
- You are allergic to any estrogen-containing drugs.
- You have impaired liver function.
- You have had blood clots, stroke or heart attack.
- You have unexplained vaginal bleeding.

Before you start, consult your doctor:
- If you have had cancer of breast or reproductive organs, fibrocystic breast disease, fibroid tumors of the uterus or endometriosis.
- If you have had migraine headaches, epilepsy or porphyria.
- If you have diabetes, high blood pressure, asthma, congestive heart failure, kidney disease or gallstones.
- If you plan to become pregnant within 3 months.

Over age 60:
Controversial. You and your doctor must decide if drug risks outweigh benefits.

Pregnancy:
Risk to unborn child outweighs drug benefits. Don't use.

Breast-feeding:
Drug filters into milk. May harm child. Avoid.

Infants & children:
Not recommended.

Prolonged use:
Increased growth of fibroid tumors of uterus. Possible association with cancer of uterus.

Skin & sunlight:
May cause rash or intensify sunburn in areas exposed to sun or sunlamp.

Driving, piloting or hazardous work:
No problems expected.

Discontinuing:
You may need to discontinue estrone periodically. Consult your doctor.

Others:
In rare instances, may cause blood clot in lung, brain or leg. Symptoms are *sudden* severe headache, coordination loss, vision change, chest pain, breathing difficulty, slurred speech, pain in legs or groin. Seek emergency treatment immediately.

POSSIBLE INTERACTION WITH OTHER DRUGS

GENERIC NAME OR DRUG CLASS	COMBINED EFFECT
Anticoagulants (oral)	Decreased anticoagulant effect.
Anticonvulsants (hydantoin)	Increased seizures.
Antidiabetics (oral)	Unpredictable increase or decrease in blood sugar.
Carbamazepine	Increased seizures.
Clofibrate	Decreased clofibrate effect.
Meprobamate	Increased estrone effect.
Phenobarbital	Decreased estrone effect.
Primidone	Decreased estrone effect.
Rifampin	Decreased estrone effect.
Thyroid hormones	Decreased thyroid effect.

POSSIBLE INTERACTION WITH OTHER SUBSTANCES

INTERACTS WITH	COMBINED EFFECT
Alcohol:	None expected.
Beverages:	None expected.
Cocaine:	No proven problems.
Foods:	None expected.
Marijuana:	Possible menstrual irregularities and bleeding between periods.
Tobacco:	Increased risk of blood clots leading to stroke or heart attack.

ESTROPIPATE

BRAND NAMES

Ogen

Piperazine Estrone
Sulfate

BASIC INFORMATION

Habit forming? No
Prescription needed? Yes
Available as generic? Yes
Drug class: Female sex hormone (estrogen)

 USES

- Treatment for symptoms of menopause and menstrual-cycle irregularity.
- Replacement for female hormone deficiency.

 DOSAGE & USAGE INFORMATION

How to take:
- Tablet—Swallow with liquid. If you can't swallow whole, crumble tablet and take with liquid or food.
- Vaginal cream—Use as directed on label.

When to take:
At the same time each day.

If you forget a dose:
Take as soon as you remember up to 12 hours late. If more than 12 hours, wait for next scheduled dose (don't double this dose).

What drug does:
Restores normal estrogen level in tissues.

Time lapse before drug works:
10 to 20 days.

Don't take with:
See Interaction column and consult doctor.

 OVERDOSE

SYMPTOMS:
Nausea, vomiting, fluid retention, breast enlargement and discomfort, abnormal vaginal bleeding.
WHAT TO DO:
Overdose unlikely to threaten life. If person takes much larger amount than prescribed, call doctor, poison-control center or hospital emergency room for instructions.

 POSSIBLE ADVERSE REACTIONS OR SIDE EFFECTS

SYMPTOMS	WHAT TO DO
Life-threatening:	
None expected.	
Common:	
• Stomach cramps.	Discontinue. Call doctor right away.
• Appetite loss.	Continue. Call doctor when convenient.
• Nausea; diarrhea; swollen feet and ankles; tender, swollen breasts.	Continue. Tell doctor at next visit.
Infrequent:	
• Rash, stomach or side pain.	Discontinue. Call doctor right away.
• Depression, dizziness, irritability, vomiting, breast lumps.	Continue. Call doctor when convenient.
• Brown blotches, hair loss, vaginal discharge or bleeding, changes in sex drive.	Continue. Tell doctor at next visit.
Rare:	
Jaundice.	Discontinue. Call doctor right away.

WARNINGS & PRECAUTIONS

Don't take if:
- You are allergic to any estrogen-containing drugs.
- You have impaired liver function.
- You have had blood clots, stroke or heart attack.
- You have unexplained vaginal bleeding.

Before you start, consult your doctor:
- If you have had cancer of breast or reproductive organs, fibrocystic breast disease, fibroid tumors of the uterus or endometriosis.
- If you have had migraine headaches, epilepsy or porphyria.
- If you have diabetes, high blood pressure, asthma, congestive heart failure, kidney disease or gallstones.
- If you plan to become pregnant within 3 months.

Over age 60:
Controversial. You and your doctor must decide if drug risks outweigh benefits.

Pregnancy:
Risk to unborn child outweighs drug benefits. Don't use.

Breast-feeding:
Drug filters into milk. May harm child. Avoid.

Infants & children:
Not recommended.

Prolonged use:
Increased growth of fibroid tumors of uterus. Possible association with cancer of uterus.

Skin & sunlight:
May cause rash or intensify sunburn in areas exposed to sun or sunlamp.

Driving, piloting or hazardous work:
No problems expected.

Discontinuing:
You may need to discontinue estropipate periodically. Consult your doctor.

Others:
In rare instances, may cause blood clot in lung, brain or leg. Symptoms are *sudden* severe headache, coordination loss, vision change, chest pain, breathing difficulty, slurred speech, pain in legs or groin. Seek emergency treatment immediately.

POSSIBLE INTERACTION WITH OTHER DRUGS

GENERIC NAME OR DRUG CLASS	COMBINED EFFECT
Anticoagulants (oral)	Decreased anticoagulant effect.
Anticonvulsants (hydantoin)	Increased seizures.
Antidiabetics (oral)	Unpredictable increase or decrease in blood sugar.
Carbamazepine	Increased seizures.
Clofibrate	Decreased clofibrate effect.
Meprobamate	Increased estropipate effect.
Phenobarbital	Decreased estropipate effect.
Primidone	Decreased estropipate effect.
Rifampin	Decreased estropipate effect.
Thyroid hormones	Decreased thyroid effect.

POSSIBLE INTERACTION WITH OTHER SUBSTANCES

INTERACTS WITH	COMBINED EFFECT
Alcohol:	None expected.
Beverages:	None expected.
Cocaine:	No proven problems.
Foods:	None expected.
Marijuana:	Possible menstrual irregularities and bleeding between periods.
Tobacco:	Increased risk of blood clots leading to stroke or heart attack.

ETHACRYNIC ACID

BRAND NAMES

Edecrin

BASIC INFORMATION

Habit forming? No
Prescription needed? Yes
Available as generic? No
Drug class: Diuretic (loop diuretic);
 antihypertensive

 USES

- Lowers blood pressure.
- Decreases fluid retention.

 DOSAGE & USAGE INFORMATION

How to take:
Tablet or capsule—Swallow with liquid or food to lessen stomach irritation. If you can't swallow whole, crumble tablet or open capsule and take with liquid or food.

When to take:
- 1 dose a day—Take after breakfast.
- More than 1 dose a day—Take last dose no later than 6 p.m. unless otherwise directed.

If you forget a dose:
- 1 dose a day—Take as soon as you remember up to 12 hours late. If more than 12 hours, wait for next scheduled dose (don't double this dose).
- More than 1 dose a day—Take as soon as you remember up to 2 hours late. If more than 2 hours, wait for next scheduled dose (don't double this dose).

What drug does:
Increases elimination of sodium and water from body. Decreased body fluid reduces blood pressure.

Continued next column

 OVERDOSE

SYMPTOMS:
Weakness, lethargy, dizziness, confusion, nausea, vomiting, leg-muscle cramps, thirst, stupor, deep sleep, weak and rapid pulse, cardiac arrest.
WHAT TO DO:
- **Dial 0 (operator) or 911 (emergency) for an ambulance or medical help. Then give first aid immediately.**
- **See emergency information on inside covers.**

Time lapse before drug works:
1 hour to increase water loss. Requires 2 to 3 weeks to lower blood pressure.

Don't take with:
- Non-prescription drugs with aspirin.
- See Interaction column and consult doctor.

 POSSIBLE ADVERSE REACTIONS OR SIDE EFFECTS

SYMPTOMS	WHAT TO DO
Life-threatening: None expected.	
Common: Dizziness.	Continue. Call doctor when convenient.
Infrequent: Mood change, appetite loss, diarrhea, irregular heartbeat, muscle cramps, fatigue, weakness.	Discontinue. Call doctor right away.
Rare: Rash or hives, yellow vision, ringing in ears, hearing loss, sore throat, fever, dry mouth, thirst, side or stomach pain, nausea, vomiting, unusual bleeding or bruising, joint pain, jaundice.	Discontinue. Call doctor right away.

 WARNINGS & PRECAUTIONS

Don't take if:
You are allergic to ethacrynic acid.

Before you start, consult your doctor:
- If you are allergic to any sulfa drug.
- If you have liver or kidney disease.
- If you have gout.
- If you have diabetes.
- If you have impaired hearing.
- If you will have surgery within 2 months, including dental surgery, requiring general or spinal anesthesia.

Over age 60:
Adverse reactions and side effects may be more frequent and severe than in younger persons. Hot weather may cause need to reduce dosage.

Pregnancy:
Risk to unborn child outweighs drug benefits. Don't use.

Breast-feeding:
Drug filters into milk. May harm child. Avoid.

Infants & children:
Use only under medical supervision.

Prolonged use:
- Impaired balance of water, salt and potassium in blood and body tissues.
- Possible diabetes.

Skin & sunlight:
May cause rash or intensify sunburn in areas exposed to sun or sunlamp.

Driving, piloting or hazardous work:
No problems expected.

Discontinuing:
Don't discontinue without doctor's advice until you complete prescribed dose, even though symptoms diminish or disappear.

Others:
Frequent laboratory studies to monitor potassium level in blood recommended. Eat foods rich in potassium or take potassium supplements. Consult doctor.

 POSSIBLE INTERACTION WITH OTHER DRUGS

GENERIC NAME OR DRUG CLASS	COMBINED EFFECT
Acebutolol	Increased antihypertensive effect of each. Dosages may require adjustments.
Allopurinol	Decreased allopurinol effect.
Amiodarone	Increased risk of heartbeat irregularity due to low potassium.
Anticoagulants	Abnormal clotting.
Antidepressants (tricyclic)	Excessive blood-pressure drop.
Antidiabetics (oral)	Decreased antidiabetic effect.
Antihypertensives	Increased antihypertensive effect.
Anti-inflammatory drugs (non-steroid)	Decreased ethacrynic acid effect.
Barbiturates	Low blood pressure.
Calcium supplements	Increased calcium in blood.
Cortisone drugs	Excessive potassium loss.
Digitalis preparations	Serious heart-rhythm disorders.
Insulin	Decreased insulin effect.
Labetolol	Increased antihypertensive effects.
Lithium	Increased lithium toxicity.
MAO inhibitors	Increased ethacrynic acid effect.
Narcotics	Dangerous low blood pressure. Avoid.
Nitrates	Excessive blood-pressure drop.
Oxprenolol	Increased antihypertensive effect of each. Dosages may require adjustments.
Phenothiazines	Increased phenothiazine effect.
Potassium supplements	Decreased potassium effect.
Probenecid	Decreased probenecid effect.
Salicylates (including aspirin)	Dangerous salicylate retention.
Sedatives	Increased ethacrynic acid effect.

 POSSIBLE INTERACTION WITH OTHER SUBSTANCES

INTERACTS WITH	COMBINED EFFECT
Alcohol:	Blood-pressure drop. Avoid.
Beverages:	None expected.
Cocaine:	Dangerous blood-pressure drop. Avoid.
Foods:	None expected.
Marijuana:	Increased thirst and urinary frequency, fainting.
Tobacco:	Decreased ethacrynic acid effect.

ETHCHLORVYNOL

BRAND NAMES

Placidyl

BASIC INFORMATION

Habit forming? Yes
Prescription needed? Yes
Available as generic? No
Drug class: Sleep inducer (hypnotic)

 USES

Treatment of insomnia.

 DOSAGE & USAGE INFORMATION

How to take:
With food or milk to lessen side effects.

When to take:
At or near bedtime.

If you forget a dose:
Bedtime dose—If you forget your once-a-day bedtime dose, don't take it more than 3 hours late.

What drug does:
Affects brain centers that control waking and sleeping.

Time lapse before drug works:
30 to 60 minutes.

Don't take with:
See Interaction column and consult doctor.

 OVERDOSE

SYMPTOMS:
Excitement, delirium, incoordination, excessive drowsiness, deep coma.
WHAT TO DO:
- Dial 0 (operator) or 911 (emergency) for an ambulance or medical help. Then give first aid immediately.
- If patient is unconscious and not breathing, give mouth-to-mouth breathing. If there is no heartbeat, use cardiac massage and mouth-to-mouth breathing (CPR). Don't try to make patient vomit. If you can't get help quickly, take patient to nearest emergency facility.
- See emergency information on inside covers.

 POSSIBLE ADVERSE REACTIONS OR SIDE EFFECTS

SYMPTOMS	WHAT TO DO
Life-threatening: None expected.	
Common:	
• Indigestion, nausea, vomiting, stomach pain.	Discontinue. Call doctor right away.
• Blurred vision, dizziness.	Continue. Call doctor when convenient.
• Unpleasant taste in mouth, fatigue, weakness.	Continue. Tell doctor at next visit.
Infrequent: Jitters, clumsiness, unsteadiness, drowsiness, confusion, rash, hives, unusual bleeding or bruising.	Discontinue. Call doctor right away.
Rare: Slow heartbeat, difficult breathing, jaundice.	Discontinue. Call doctor right away.

WARNINGS & PRECAUTIONS

Don't take if:
- You are allergic to any hypnotic.
- You have porphyria.
- Patient is younger than 12.

Before you start, consult your doctor:
- If you plan to become pregnant within medication period.
- If you have kidney or liver disease.

Over age 60:
Adverse reactions and side effects, especially a "hangover" effect, may be more frequent and severe than in younger persons.

Pregnancy:
Risk to unborn child outweighs drug benefits. Don't use.

Breast-feeding:
No problems expected, but observe child and ask doctor for guidance.

Infants & children:
Not recommended.

Prolonged use:
Impaired vision.

Skin & sunlight:
No problems expected.

Driving, piloting or hazardous work:
Don't drive or pilot aircraft until you learn how medicine affects you. Don't work around dangerous machinery. Don't climb ladders or work in high places. Danger increases if you drink alcohol or take medicine affecting alertness and reflexes.

Discontinuing:
- Don't discontinue without consulting doctor. Dose may require gradual reduction if you have taken drug for a long time. Doses of other drugs may also require adjustment.
- Many side effects may occur when you stop taking this drug, including irritability, muscle twitching, hallucinations or seizures. Consult your doctor.

Others:
No problems expected.

POSSIBLE INTERACTION WITH OTHER DRUGS

GENERIC NAME OR DRUG CLASS	COMBINED EFFECT
Anticoagulants (oral)	Decreased anticoagulant effect.
Antidepressants (tricyclic)	Delirium and deep sedation.
Antihistamines	Increased antihistamine effect.
Molindone	Increased sedative effect.
Narcotics	Increased narcotic effect.
Pain relievers	Increased effect of pain reliever.
Sedatives	Increased sedative effect.
Tranquilizers	Increased tranquilizer effect.

POSSIBLE INTERACTION WITH OTHER SUBSTANCES

INTERACTS WITH	COMBINED EFFECT
Alcohol:	Excessive depressant and sedative effect. Avoid.
Beverages:	None expected.
Cocaine:	Decreased ethchlorvynol effect.
Foods:	None expected.
Marijuana:	Occasional use— Drowsiness, unsteadiness, depressed function. Frequent use—Severe drowsiness, impaired physical and mental function.
Tobacco:	None expected.

ETHINYL ESTRADIOL

BRAND NAMES

Brevicon	Norette
Demulen	Norinyl
Estinyl	Norlestrin
Feminone	Ortho-Novum
Loestrin	Ovcon
Lo-Ovral	Ovral
Modicon	Tri-Norinyl

BASIC INFORMATION

Habit forming? No
Prescription needed? Yes
Available as generic? Yes
Drug class: Female sex hormone (estrogen)

USES

- Treatment for symptoms of menopause and menstrual-cycle irregularity.
- Replacement for female hormone deficiency.
- Prevention of pregnancy.
- Treatment for cancer of breast and prostate.

DOSAGE & USAGE INFORMATION

How to take:
Tablet—Swallow with liquid. If you can't swallow whole, crumble tablet and take with liquid or food.

When to take:
At the same time each day.

If you forget a dose:
Take as soon as you remember up to 12 hours late. If more than 12 hours, wait for next scheduled dose (don't double this dose).

What drug does:
- Restores normal estrogen level in tissues.
- Prevents pituitary gland from secreting hormone that causes ovary to ripen and release egg.

Continued next column

OVERDOSE

SYMPTOMS:
Nausea, vomiting, fluid retention, breast enlargement and discomfort, abnormal vaginal bleeding.
WHAT TO DO:
Overdose unlikely to threaten life. If person takes much larger amount than prescribed, call doctor, poison-control center or hospital emergency room for instructions.

Time lapse before drug works:
10 to 20 days.

Don't take with:
See Interaction column and consult doctor.

POSSIBLE ADVERSE REACTIONS OR SIDE EFFECTS

SYMPTOMS	WHAT TO DO
Life-threatening: None expected.	
Common:	
• Stomach cramps.	Discontinue. Call doctor right away.
• Appetite loss.	Continue. Call doctor when convenient.
• Nausea; diarrhea; swollen feet and ankles; tender, swollen breasts.	Continue. Tell doctor at next visit.
Infrequent:	
• Rash, stomach or side pain.	Discontinue. Call doctor right away.
• Depression, dizziness, irritability, vomiting, breast lumps.	Continue. Call doctor when convenient.
• Brown blotches, hair loss, vaginal discharge or bleeding, changes in sex drive.	Continue. Tell doctor at next visit.
Rare:	
Jaundice.	Discontinue. Call doctor right away.

WARNINGS & PRECAUTIONS

Don't take if:
- You are allergic to any estrogen-containing drugs.
- You have impaired liver function.
- You have had blood clots, stroke or heart attack.
- You have unexplained vaginal bleeding.

Before you start, consult your doctor:
- If you have had cancer of breast or reproductive organs, fibrocystic breast disease, fibroid tumors of the uterus or endometriosis.
- If you have had migraine headaches, epilepsy or porphyria.
- If you have diabetes, high blood pressure, asthma, congestive heart failure, kidney disease or gallstones.
- If you plan to become pregnant within 3 months.

Over age 60:
Controversial. You and your doctor must decide if drug risks outweigh benefits.

Pregnancy:
Risk to unborn child outweighs drug benefits. Don't use.

Breast-feeding:
Drug filters into milk. May harm child. Avoid.

Infants & children:
Not recommended.

Prolonged use:
Increased growth of fibroid tumors of uterus. Possible association with cancer of uterus.

Skin & sunlight:
May cause rash or intensify sunburn in areas exposed to sun or sunlamp.

Driving, piloting or hazardous work:
No problems expected.

Discontinuing:
You may need to discontinue ethinyl estradiol periodically. Consult your doctor.

Others:
In rare instances, may cause blood clot in lung, brain or leg. Symptoms are *sudden* severe headache, coordination loss, vision change, chest pain, breathing difficulty, slurred speech, pain in legs or groin. Seek emergency treatment immediately.

POSSIBLE INTERACTION WITH OTHER DRUGS

GENERIC NAME OR DRUG CLASS	COMBINED EFFECT
Anticoagulants (oral)	Decreased anticoagulant effect.
Anticonvulsants (hydantoin)	Increased seizures.
Antidiabetics (oral)	Unpredictable increase or decrease in blood sugar.
Carbamazepine	Increased seizures.
Clofibrate	Decreased clofibrate effect.
Meprobamate	Increased effect of ethinyl estradiol.
Phenobarbital	Decreased effect of ethinyl estradiol.
Primidone	Decreased effect of ethinyl estradiol.
Rifampin	Decreased effect of ethinyl estradiol.
Thyroid hormones	Decreased thyroid effect.

POSSIBLE INTERACTION WITH OTHER SUBSTANCES

INTERACTS WITH	COMBINED EFFECT
Alcohol:	None expected.
Beverages:	None expected.
Cocaine:	No proven problems.
Foods:	None expected.
Marijuana:	Possible menstrual irregularities and bleeding between periods.
Tobacco:	Increased risk of blood clots leading to stroke or heart attack.

ETHOPROPAZINE

BRAND NAMES

Parsidol   Parsitan

BASIC INFORMATION

Habit forming? No
Prescription needed? Yes
Available as generic? No
Drug class: Antidyskinetic, antiparkinsonism

 USES

- Treatment of Parkinson's disease.
- Treatment of adverse effects of phenothiazines.

 DOSAGE & USAGE INFORMATION

How to take:
Tablets or capsules—Take with food to lessen stomach irritation.

When to take:
At the same times each day.

If you forget a dose:
Take as soon as you remember up to 2 hours late. If more than 2 hours, wait for next scheduled dose (don't double this dose).

What drug does:
- Balances chemical reactions necessary to send nerve impulses within base of brain.
- Improves muscle control and reduces stiffness.

Time lapse before drug works:
1 to 2 hours.

Continued next column

 OVERDOSE

SYMPTOMS:
Agitation, dilated pupils, hallucinations, dry mouth, rapid heartbeat, sleepiness.
WHAT TO DO:
- **Dial 0 (operator) or 911 (emergency) for an ambulance or medical help. Then give first aid immediately.**
- **If patient is unconscious and not breathing, give mouth-to-mouth breathing. If there is no heartbeat, use cardiac massage and mouth-to-mouth breathing (CPR). Don't try to make patient vomit. If you can't get help quickly, take patient to nearest emergency facility.**
- **See emergency information on inside covers.**

Don't take with:
- Non-prescription drugs for colds, cough or allergy.
- See Interaction column and consult doctor.

 POSSIBLE ADVERSE REACTIONS OR SIDE EFFECTS

SYMPTOMS	WHAT TO DO
Life-threatening: None expected.	
Common:	
• Blurred vision, light sensitivity, constipation, nausea, vomiting.	Continue. Call doctor when convenient.
• Painful or difficult urination.	Continue. Tell doctor at next visit.
Infrequent: None expected.	
Rare:	
• Rash, eye pain.	Discontinue. Call doctor right away.
• Confusion; dizziness; sore mouth or tongue; muscle cramps; numbness, weakness in hands or feet.	Continue. Call doctor when convenient.

WARNINGS & PRECAUTIONS

Don't take if:
You are allergic to any antidyskinetic.

Before you start, consult your doctor:
- If you have had glaucoma.
- If you have had high blood pressure or heart disease.
- If you have had impaired liver function.
- If you have had kidney disease or urination difficulty.

Over age 60:
More sensitive to drug. Aggravates symptoms of enlarged prostate. Causes impaired thinking, hallucinations, nightmares. Consult doctor about any of these.

Pregnancy:
Studies inconclusive on harm to unborn child. Animal studies show fetal abnormalities. Decide with your doctor whether drug benefits justify risk to unborn child.

Breast-feeding:
No problems expected.

Infants & children:
Not recommended for children 3 and younger. Use for older children only under doctor's supervision.

Prolonged use:
Possible glaucoma.

Skin & sunlight:
No problems expected.

Driving, piloting or hazardous work:
Don't drive or pilot aircraft until you learn how medicine affects you. Don't work around dangerous machinery. Don't climb ladders or work in high places. Danger increases if you drink alcohol or take medicine affecting alertness and reflexes, such as antihistamines, tranquilizers, sedatives, pain medicine, narcotics and mind-altering drugs.

Discontinuing:
Don't discontinue without consulting doctor. Dose may require gradual reduction if you have taken drug for a long time. Doses of other drugs may also require adjustment.

Others:
- Internal eye pressure should be measured regularly.
- Avoid becoming overheated.

POSSIBLE INTERACTION WITH OTHER DRUGS

GENERIC NAME OR DRUG CLASS	COMBINED EFFECT
Amantadine	Increased amantadine effect.
Antidepressants (tricyclic)	Increased ethopropazine effect. May cause glaucoma.
Antihistamines	Increased ethopropazine effect.
Levodopa	Increased levodopa effect. Improved results in treating Parkinson's disease.
MAO inhibitors	Increased ethopropazine effect.
Meperidine	Increased ethopropazine effect.
Orphenadrine	Increased ethopropazine effect.
Phenothiazines	Behavior changes.
Primidone	Excessive sedation.
Procainamide	Increased procainamide effect.
Quinidine	Increased ethopropazine effect.
Tranquilizers	Excessive sedation.

POSSIBLE INTERACTION WITH OTHER SUBSTANCES

INTERACTS WITH	COMBINED EFFECT
Alcohol:	None expected.
Beverages:	None expected.
Cocaine:	Decreased ethopropazine effect. Avoid.
Foods:	None expected.
Marijuana:	None expected.
Tobacco:	None expected.

ETHOSUXIMIDE

BRAND NAMES

Zarontin

BASIC INFORMATION

Habit forming? No
Prescription needed? Yes
Available as generic? No
Drug class: Anticonvulsant (succinimide)

 ## USES

Controls seizures in treatment of epilepsy.

 ## DOSAGE & USAGE INFORMATION

How to take:
Capsule—Swallow with liquid or food to lessen stomach irritation.

When to take:
Every day in regularly-spaced doses, according to prescription.

If you forget a dose:
Take as soon as you remember up to 2 hours late. If more than 2 hours, wait for next scheduled dose (don't double this dose).

What drug does:
Depresses nerve transmissions in part of brain that controls muscles.

Time lapse before drug works:
3 hours.

Don't take with:
See Interaction column and consult doctor.

 ## OVERDOSE

SYMPTOMS:
Coma
WHAT TO DO:
- Dial 0 (operator) or 911 (emergency) for an ambulance or medical help. Then give first aid immediately.
- If patient is unconscious and not breathing, give mouth-to-mouth breathing. If there is no heartbeat, use cardiac massage and mouth-to-mouth breathing (CPR). Don't try to make patient vomit. If you can't get help quickly, take patient to nearest emergency facility.
- See emergency information on inside covers.

 ## POSSIBLE ADVERSE REACTIONS OR SIDE EFFECTS

SYMPTOMS	WHAT TO DO
Life-threatening: None expected.	
Common: Nausea, vomiting, stomach cramps, appetite loss.	Continue. Call doctor when convenient.
Infrequent: Dizziness, drowsiness, headache, irritability, mood change.	Continue. Call doctor when convenient.
Rare: • Sore throat, fever, rash, unusual bleeding or bruising.	Discontinue. Call doctor right away.
• Swollen lymph glands.	Continue. Call doctor when convenient.

ETHOSUXIMIDE

WARNINGS & PRECAUTIONS

Don't take if:
You are allergic to any succinimide anticonvulsant.

Before you start, consult your doctor:
- If you plan to become pregnant within medication period.
- If you take other anticonvulsants.
- If you have blood disease.
- If you have kidney or liver disease.

Over age 60:
Adverse reactions and side effects may be more frequent and severe than in younger persons.

Pregnancy:
Risk to unborn child outweighs drug benefits. Don't use.

Breast-feeding:
Drug passes into milk. Avoid drug or discontinue nursing.

Infants & children:
Use only under medical supervision.

Prolonged use:
No problems expected.

Skin & sunlight:
No problems expected.

Driving, piloting or hazardous work:
Don't drive or pilot aircraft until you learn how medicine affects you. Don't work around dangerous machinery. Don't climb ladders or work in high places. Danger increases if you drink alcohol or take medicine affecting alertness and reflexes, such as antihistamines, tranquilizers, sedatives, pain medicine, narcotics and mind-altering drugs.

Discontinuing:
Don't discontinue without doctor's advice until you complete prescribed dose, even though symptoms diminish or disappear.

Others:
- Your response to medicine should be checked regularly by your doctor. Dose and schedule may have to be altered frequently to fit individual needs.
- Periodic blood-cell counts, kidney- and liver-function studies recommended.

POSSIBLE INTERACTION WITH OTHER DRUGS

GENERIC NAME OR DRUG CLASS	COMBINED EFFECT
Anticonvulsants (other)	Increased effect of both drugs.
Antidepressants (tricyclic)	May provoke seizures.
Antipsychotics	May provoke seizures.

POSSIBLE INTERACTION WITH OTHER SUBSTANCES

INTERACTS WITH	COMBINED EFFECT
Alcohol:	May provoke seizures.
Beverages:	None expected.
Cocaine:	May provoke seizures.
Foods:	None expected.
Marijuana:	May provoke seizures.
Tobacco:	None expected.

ETHOTOIN

BRAND NAMES

Peganone

BASIC INFORMATION

Habit forming? No
Prescription needed? Yes
Available as generic? Yes
Drug class: Anticonvulsant (hydantoin)

 USES

- Prevents epileptic seizures.
- Stabilizes irregular heartbeat.

 DOSAGE & USAGE INFORMATION

How to take:
- Tablet or capsule—Swallow with liquid.
- Extended-release tablets or capsules—Swallow each dose whole. If you take regular tablets, you may chew or crush them.

When to take:
At the same time each day.

If you forget a dose:
- If drug taken 1 time per day—Take as soon as you remember up to 12 hours late. If more than 12 hours, wait for next scheduled dose (don't double this dose).
- If taken several times per day—Take as soon as possible, then return to regular schedule.

What drug does:
Promotes sodium loss from nerve fibers. This lessens excitability and inhibits spread of nerve impulses.

Time lapse before drug works:
7 to 10 days continual use.

Don't take with:
See Interaction column and consult doctor.

 OVERDOSE

SYMPTOMS:
Jerky eye movements; stagger; slurred speech; imbalance; drowsiness; blood-pressure drop; slow, shallow breathing; coma.
WHAT TO DO:
- **Dial 0 (operator) or 911 (emergency) for an ambulance or medical help. Then give first aid immediately.**
- **See emergency information on inside covers.**

 POSSIBLE ADVERSE REACTIONS OR SIDE EFFECTS

SYMPTOMS	WHAT TO DO
Life-threatening: None expected.	
Common: Mild dizziness, drowsiness, constipation, nausea, vomiting.	Continue. Call doctor when convenient.
Infrequent: • Hallucinations, confusion, slurred speech, stagger, rash, change in vision.	Discontinue. Call doctor right away.
• Headache, sleeplessness, diarrhea, muscle twitching.	Continue. Call doctor when convenient.
• Increased body and facial hair.	Continue. Tell doctor at next visit.
Rare: Sore throat, fever, unusual bleeding or bruising, stomach pain, jaundice.	Discontinue. Call doctor right away.

 WARNINGS & PRECAUTIONS

Don't take if:
You are allergic to any hydantoin anticonvulsant.

Before you start, consult your doctor:
- If you have had impaired liver function or disease.
- If you will have surgery within 2 months, including dental surgery, requiring general or spinal anesthesia.

Over age 60:
Adverse reactions and side effects may be more frequent and severe than in younger persons.

Pregnancy:
Risk to unborn child outweighs drug benefits. Don't use.

Breast-feeding:
Drug passes into milk. Avoid drug or discontinue nursing until you finish medicine. Consult doctor for advice on maintaining milk supply.

Infants & children:
Use only under medical supervision.

Prolonged use:
- Weakened bones.
- Lymph gland enlargement.
- Possible liver damage.

- Numbness and tingling of hands and feet.
- Continual back-and-forth eye movements.
- Bleeding, swollen or tender gums.

Skin & sunlight:
May cause rash or intensify sunburn in areas exposed to sun or sunlamp.

Driving, piloting or hazardous work:
Don't drive or pilot aircraft until you learn how medicine affects you. Don't work around dangerous machinery. Don't climb ladders or work in high places. Danger increases if you drink alcohol or take medicine affecting alertness and reflexes.

Discontinuing:
Don't discontinue without consulting doctor. Dose may require gradual reduction if you have taken drug for a long time. Doses of other drugs may also require adjustment.

Others:
No problems expected.

 POSSIBLE INTERACTION WITH OTHER DRUGS

GENERIC NAME OR DRUG CLASS	COMBINED EFFECT
Anticoagulants	Increased effect of both drugs.
Antidepressants (tricyclic)	Need to adjust ethotoin dose.
Antihypertensives	Increased effect of antihypertensive.
Aspirin	Increased ethotoin effect.
Barbiturates	Changed seizure pattern.
Carbonic anhydrase inhibitors	Increased chance of bone disease.
Chloramphenicol	Increased ethotoin effect.
Contraceptives (oral)	Increased seizures.
Cortisone drugs	Decreased cortisone effect.
Digitalis preparations	Decreased digitalis effect.
Disulfiram	Increased ethotoin effect.
Estrogens	Increased ethotoin effect.
Furosemide	Decreased furosemide effect.
Glutethimide	Decreased ethotoin effect.

Griseofulvin	Increased griseofulvin effect.
Isoniazid	Increased ethotoin effect.
Methadone	Decreased methadone effect.
Methotrexate	Increased methotrexate effect.
Methylphenidate	Increased ethotoin effect.
Oxyphenbutazone	Increased ethotoin effect.
Para-aminosalicylic acid (PAS)	Increased ethotoin effect.
Phenothiazines	Increased ethotoin effect.
Phenylbutazone	Increased ethotoin effect.
Propranolol	Increased propranolol effect.
Quinidine	Increased quinidine effect.
Sedatives	Increased sedative effect.
Sulfa drugs	Increased ethotoin effect.
Theophylline	Reduced anticonvulsant effect.

 POSSIBLE INTERACTION WITH OTHER SUBSTANCES

INTERACTS WITH	COMBINED EFFECT
Alcohol:	Possible decreased anticonvulsant effect. Use with caution.
Beverages:	None expected.
Cocaine:	Possible seizures.
Foods:	None expected.
Marijuana:	Drowsiness, unsteadiness, decreased anticonvulsant effect.
Tobacco:	None expected.

FENOPROFEN

BRAND NAMES

Fenopron   Progesic
Nalfon

BASIC INFORMATION

Habit forming? No
Available as generic? No
Prescription needed? Yes
Drug class: Anti-inflammatory (non-steroid)

USES

- Treatment for joint pain, stiffness, inflammation and swelling of arthritis and gout.
- Pain reliever.
- Treatment for dysmenorrhea (painful or difficult menstruation).

DOSAGE & USAGE INFORMATION

How to take:
Tablet or capsule—Swallow with liquid or food to lessen stomach irritation. If you can't swallow whole, crumble tablet or open capsule and take with liquid or food.

When to take:
At the same times each day.

If you forget a dose:
Take as soon as you remember up to 2 hours late. If more than 2 hours, wait for next scheduled dose (don't double this dose).

What drug does:
Reduces tissue concentration of prostaglandins (hormones which produce inflammation and pain).

Time lapse before drug works:
Begins in 4 to 24 hours. May require 3 weeks regular use for maximum benefit.

Continued next column

OVERDOSE

SYMPTOMS:
Confusion, agitation, incoherence, convulsions, possible hemorrhage from stomach or intestine, coma.
WHAT TO DO:
- **Dial 0 (operator) or 911 (emergency) for an ambulance or medical help. Then give first aid immediately.**
- **See emergency information on inside covers.**

Don't take with:
See Interaction column and consult doctor.

POSSIBLE ADVERSE REACTIONS OR SIDE EFFECTS

SYMPTOMS	WHAT TO DO
Life-threatening:	
None expected.	
Common:	
• Dizziness, nausea, pain.	Continue. Call doctor when convenient.
• Headache.	Continue. Tell doctor at next visit.
Infrequent:	
Depression; drowsiness; ringing in ears; swollen feet, legs; constipation or diarrhea; vomiting.	Continue. Call doctor when convenient.
Rare:	
• Convulsions; confusion, rash, hives or itch; black or bloody, tarry stools; difficult breathing; tightness in chest; blurred vision; rapid heartbeat; unusual bleeding or bruising; blood in urine; jaundice.	Discontinue. Call doctor right away.
• Urgent, frequent or painful urination; fatigue; weakness.	Continue. Call doctor when convenient.

WARNINGS & PRECAUTIONS

Don't take if:
- You are allergic to aspirin or any non-steroid, anti-inflammatory drug.
- You have gastritis, peptic ulcer, enteritis, ileitis, ulcerative colitis, asthma, heart failure, high blood pressure or bleeding problems.
- Patient is younger than 15.

Before you start, consult your doctor:
- If you have epilepsy.
- If you have Parkinson's disease.
- If you have been mentally ill.
- If you have had kidney disease or impaired kidney function.

Over age 60:
Adverse reactions and side effects may be more frequent and severe than in younger persons.

Pregnancy:
Studies inconclusive on harm to unborn child. Decide with your doctor whether drug benefits justify risk to unborn child.

Breast-feeding:
May harm child. Avoid.

Infants & children:
Not recommended for anyone younger than 15. Use only under medical supervision.

Prolonged use:
- Eye damage.
- Reduced hearing.
- Sore throat, fever.
- Weight gain.

Skin & sunlight:
No problems expected.

Driving, piloting or hazardous work:
Don't drive or pilot aircraft until you learn how medicine affects you. Don't work around dangerous machinery. Don't climb ladders or work in high places. Danger increases if you drink alcohol or take medicine affecting alertness and reflexes, such as antihistamines, tranquilizers, sedatives, pain medicine, narcotics and mind-altering drugs.

Discontinuing:
Don't discontinue without consulting doctor. Dose may require gradual reduction if you have taken drug for a long time. Doses of other drugs may also require adjustment.

Others:
No problems expected.

 POSSIBLE INTERACTION WITH OTHER DRUGS

GENERIC NAME OR DRUG CLASS	COMBINED EFFECT
Anticoagulants (oral)	Increased risk of bleeding.
Aspirin	Increased risk of stomach ulcer.
Cortisone drugs	Increased risk of stomach ulcer.
Furosemide	Decreased diuretic effect of furosemide.
Ketoprofen	Increased possibility of internal bleeding.
Oxyphenbutazone	Possible stomach ulcer.
Phenylbutazone	Possible stomach ulcer.
Probenecid	Increased fenoprofen effect.
Thyroid hormones	Rapid heartbeat, blood-pressure rise.

 POSSIBLE INTERACTION WITH OTHER SUBSTANCES

INTERACTS WITH	COMBINED EFFECT
Alcohol:	Possible stomach ulcer or bleeding.
Beverages:	None expected.
Cocaine:	None expected.
Foods:	None expected.
Marijuana:	Increased pain relief from fenoprofen.
Tobacco:	None expected.

FERROUS FUMARATE

BRAND NAMES

See complete list of brand names in the *Brand Name Directory,* page 949.

BASIC INFORMATION

Habit forming? No
Prescription needed?
　With folic acid: Yes
　Without folic acid: No
Available as generic? Yes
Drug class: Mineral supplement (iron)

 ## USES

Treatment for dietary iron deficiency or iron-deficiency anemia from other causes.

 ## DOSAGE & USAGE INFORMATION

How to take:
- Tablet, capsule or liquid—Swallow with liquid or food to lessen stomach irritation. If you can't swallow whole, crumble tablet or open capsule and take with liquid or food. Place medicine far back on tongue to avoid staining teeth.
- Drops—Dilute dose in beverage before swallowing and drink through a straw.

When to take:
1 hour before or 2 hours after meals.

If you forget a dose:
Take up to 2 hours late. If more than 2 hours, wait for next dose (don't double this dose).

What drug does:
Stimulates bone-marrow production of hemoglobin (red-blood-cell pigment that carries oxygen to body cells).

Time lapse before drug works:
3 to 7 days. May require 3 weeks for maximum benefit.

Continued next column

 ## OVERDOSE

SYMPTOMS:
Weakness, collapse; pallor, blue lips, hands and fingernails; weak, rapid heartbeat; shallow breathing; convulsions; coma.
WHAT TO DO:
- **Dial 0 (operator) or 911 (emergency) for an ambulance or medical help. Then give first aid immediately.**
- **See emergency information on inside covers.**

Don't take with:
- Multiple vitamin and mineral supplements.
- See Interaction column and consult doctor.

 ## POSSIBLE ADVERSE REACTIONS OR SIDE EFFECTS

SYMPTOMS	WHAT TO DO
Life-threatening:	
Weak, rapid heartbeat.	Seek emergency treatment immediately.
Always:	
Gray or black stool.	No action necessary.
Common:	
Stained teeth with liquid iron.	No action necessary.
Infrequent:	
• Constipation or diarrhea, heartburn, nausea, vomiting.	Discontinue. Call doctor right away.
• Fatigue, weakness.	Continue. Call doctor when convenient.
• Dark urine.	Continue. Tell doctor at next visit.
Rare:	
• Throat or chest pain on swallowing, pain, cramps, blood in stool.	Discontinue. Call doctor right away.
• Drowsiness.	Continue. Call doctor when convenient.

WARNINGS & PRECAUTIONS

Don't take if:
- You are allergic to any iron supplement.
- You take iron injections.
- Your daily iron intake is high.
- You plan to take this supplement for a long time.
- You have acute hepatitis.
- You have hemosiderosis or hemochromatosis (conditions involving excess iron in body).
- You have hemolytic anemia.

Before you start, consult your doctor:
- If you plan to become pregnant within medication period.
- If you have had stomach surgery.
- If you have had peptic ulcer disease, enteritis or colitis.
- If you have had pancreatitis or hepatitis.

Over age 60:
May cause hemochromatosis (iron storage disease) with bronze skin, liver damage, diabetes, heart problems and impotence.

Pregnancy:
No proven harm to unborn child. Avoid if possible. Take only if your doctor prescribes supplement during last half of pregnancy.

Breast-feeding:
No problems expected. Take only if your doctor confirms you have a dietary deficiency or an iron-deficiency anemia.

Infants & children:
Use only under medical supervision. Overdose common and dangerous. Keep out of children's reach.

Prolonged use:
May cause hemochromatosis (iron storage disease) with bronze skin, liver damage, diabetes, heart problems and impotence.

Skin & sunlight:
No problems expected.

Driving, piloting or hazardous work:
No problems expected.

Discontinuing:
May be unnecessary to finish medicine. Follow doctor's instructions.

Others:
Liquid form stains teeth. Mix with water or juice to lessen the effect. Brush with baking soda or hydrogen peroxide to help remove stain.

POSSIBLE INTERACTION WITH OTHER DRUGS

GENERIC NAME OR DRUG CLASS	COMBINED EFFECT
Acetohydroxamic acid	Decreased effects of both drugs.
Allopurinol	Possible excess iron storage in liver.
Antacids	Poor iron absorption.
Chloramphenicol	Decreased effect of iron. Interferes with red-blood-cell and hemoglobin formation.
Cholestyramine	Decreased iron effect.
Iron supplements (other)	Possible excess iron storage in liver.
Penicillamine	Decreased penicillamine effect.
Sulfasalazine	Decreased iron effect.
Tetracyclines	Decreased tetracycline effect. Take iron 3 hours before or 2 hours after taking tetracycline.
Vitamin C	Increased iron effect. Contributes to red-blood-cell and hemoglobin formation.
Vitamin E	Decreased iron effect.

POSSIBLE INTERACTION WITH OTHER SUBSTANCES

INTERACTS WITH	COMBINED EFFECT
Alcohol:	Increased iron absorption. May cause organ damage. Avoid or use in moderation.
Beverages: Milk, tea.	Decreased iron effect.
Cocaine:	None expected.
Foods: Dairy foods, eggs, whole-grain bread and cereal.	Decreased iron effect.
Marijuana:	None expected.
Tobacco:	None expected.

FERROUS GLUCONATE

BRAND NAMES

Apo-Ferrous
  Gluconate
Fergon
Ferralet
Ferralet Plus
Ferrous-G
Fertinic
Fosfree

Glytinic
I.L.X. B-12
Iromin-G
Megadose
Mission
Novoferrogluc
Simron

BASIC INFORMATION

Habit forming? No
Prescription needed?
  With folic acid: Yes
  Without folic acid: No
Available as generic? Yes
Drug class: Mineral supplement (iron)

 ## USES

Treatment for dietary iron deficiency or
iron-deficiency anemia from other causes.

 ## DOSAGE & USAGE INFORMATION

How to take:
- Tablet or capsule—Swallow with liquid or
food to lessen stomach irritation. If you can't
swallow whole, crumble tablet or open
capsule and take with liquid or food. Place
medicine far back on tongue to avoid staining
teeth.
- Drops—Dilute dose in beverage before
swallowing and drink through a straw.

When to take:
1 hour before or 2 hours after eating.

If you forget a dose:
Take up to 2 hours late. If more than 2 hours,
wait for next dose (don't double this dose).

Continued next column

 ## OVERDOSE

SYMPTOMS:
- Moderate overdose—Stomach pain,
vomiting, diarrhea, black stools, lethargy.
- Serious overdose—Weakness and
collapse; pallor, weak and rapid heartbeat;
shallow breathing; convulsions and coma.

WHAT TO DO:
- Dial 0 (operator) or 911 (emergency) for an
ambulance or medical help. Then give first
aid immediately.
- See emergency information on inside
covers.

What drug does:
Stimulates bone-marrow production of
hemoglobin (red-blood-cell pigment that carries
oxygen to body cells).

Time lapse before drug works:
3 to 7 days. May require 3 weeks for maximum
benefit.

Don't take with:
- Multiple vitamin and mineral supplements.
- See Interaction column and consult doctor.

 ## POSSIBLE ADVERSE REACTIONS OR SIDE EFFECTS

SYMPTOMS	WHAT TO DO
Life-threatening: Weak, rapid heartbeat.	Seek emergency treatment immediately.
Always: Gray or black stool.	No action necessary.
Common: Stained teeth with liquid iron.	No action necessary.
Infrequent: • Constipation or diarrhea, heartburn, nausea, vomiting.	Discontinue. Call doctor right away.
• Fatigue, weakness.	Continue. Call doctor when convenient.
Rare: • Blue lips, fingernails, palms of hands; pale, clammy skin.	Discontinue. Seek emergency treatment.
• Throat pain on swallowing, pain, cramps, blood in stool.	Discontinue. Call doctor right away.
• Drowsiness.	Continue. Call doctor when convenient.

WARNINGS & PRECAUTIONS

Don't take if:
- You are allergic to any iron supplement.
- You take iron injections.
- You have acute hepatitis, hemosiderosis or hemochromatosis (conditions involving excess iron in body).
- You have hemolytic anemia.

Before you start, consult your doctor:
- If you plan to become pregnant within medication period.
- If you have had stomach surgery.
- If you have had peptic ulcer, enteritis or colitis.

Over age 60:
May cause hemochromatosis (iron storage disease) with bronze skin, liver damage, diabetes, heart problems and impotence.

Pregnancy:
No proven harm to unborn child. Avoid if possible. Take only if your doctor advises supplement during last half of pregnancy.

Breast-feeding:
No problems expected. Take only if your doctor confirms you have a dietary deficiency or an iron-deficiency anemia.

Infants & children:
Use only under medical supervision. Overdose common and dangerous. Keep out of children's reach.

Prolonged use:
May cause hemochromatosis (iron storage disease) with bronze skin, liver damage, diabetes, heart problems and impotence.

Skin & sunlight:
No problems expected.

Driving, piloting or hazardous work:
No problems expected.

Discontinuing:
May be unnecessary to finish medicine. Follow doctor's instructions.

Others:
Liquid form stains teeth. Mix with water or juice to lessen the effect. Brush with baking soda or hydrogen peroxide to help remove.

POSSIBLE INTERACTION WITH OTHER DRUGS

GENERIC NAME OR DRUG CLASS	COMBINED EFFECT
Acetohydroxamic acid	Decreased effects of both drugs.
Allopurinol	Possible excess iron storage in liver.
Antacids	Poor iron absorption.
Chloramphenicol	Decreased effect of iron. Interferes with red-blood-cell and hemoglobin formation.
Cholestyramine	Decreased iron effect.
Iron supplements (other)	Possible excess iron storage in liver.
Sulfasalazine	Decreased iron effect.
Tetracyclines	Decreased tetracycline effect. Take iron 3 hours before or 2 hours after taking tetracycline.
Vitamin C	Increased iron effect. Contributes to red-blood-cell and hemoglobin formation.
Vitamin E	Decreased iron effect.

POSSIBLE INTERACTION WITH OTHER SUBSTANCES

INTERACTS WITH	COMBINED EFFECT
Alcohol:	Increased iron absorption. May cause organ damage. Avoid or use in moderation.
Beverages: Milk, tea.	Decreased iron effect.
Cocaine:	None expected.
Foods: Dairy foods, eggs, whole-grain bread and cereal.	Decreased iron effect.
Marijuana:	None expected.
Tobacco:	None expected.

FERROUS SULFATE

BRAND NAMES

See complete list of brand names in the *Brand Name Directory,* page 949.

BASIC INFORMATION

Habit forming? No
Prescription needed?
   With folic acid: Yes
   Without folic acid: No
Available as generic? Yes
Drug class: Mineral supplement (iron)

USES

Treatment for dietary iron deficiency or iron-deficiency anemia from other causes.

DOSAGE & USAGE INFORMATION

How to take:
- Tablet, capsule, or liquid—Swallow with liquid or food to lessen stomach irritation. Place medicine far back on tongue to avoid staining teeth.
- Drops—Dilute dose in beverage before swallowing and drink through a straw.
- Extended release tablet or capsule—Swallow whole with liquid.

When to take:
1 hour before or 2 hours after meals.

If you forget a dose:
Take up to 2 hours late. If more than 2 hours, wait for next dose (don't double this dose).

What drug does:
Stimulates bone-marrow production of hemoglobin (red-blood-cell pigment that carries oxygen to body cells).

Time lapse before drug works:
3 to 7 days. May require 3 weeks for maximum benefit.

Continued next column

OVERDOSE

SYMPTOMS:
Weakness, collapse; pallor, blue lips, hands and fingernails; weak, rapid heartbeat; shallow breathing; convulsions; coma.
WHAT TO DO:
- **Dial 0 (operator) or 911 (emergency) for an ambulance or medical help. Then give first aid immediately.**
- **See emergency information on inside covers.**

Don't take with:
- Multiple vitamin and mineral supplements.
- See Interaction column and consult doctor.

POSSIBLE ADVERSE REACTIONS OR SIDE EFFECTS

SYMPTOMS	WHAT TO DO
Life-threatening:	
Weak, rapid heartbeat.	Seek emergency treatment immediately.
Always:	
Gray or black stool.	No action necessary.
Common:	
Stained teeth with liquid iron.	No action necessary.
Infrequent:	
• Constipation or diarrhea, heartburn, nausea, vomiting.	Discontinue. Call doctor right away.
• Fatigue, weakness.	Continue. Call doctor when convenient.
• Dark urine.	Continue. Tell doctor at next visit.
Rare:	
• Throat or chest pain on swallowing, pain, cramps, blood in stool.	Discontinue. Call doctor right away.
• Drowsiness.	Continue. Call doctor when convenient.

WARNINGS & PRECAUTIONS

Don't take if:
- You are allergic to any iron supplement.
- You take iron injections.
- Your daily iron intake is high.
- You plan to take this supplement for a long time.
- You have acute hepatitis.
- You have hemosiderosis or hemochromatosis (conditions involving excess iron in body).
- You have hemolytic anemia.

Before you start, consult your doctor:
- If you plan to become pregnant within medication period.
- If you have had stomach surgery.
- If you have had peptic ulcer disease, enteritis or colitis.
- If you have had pancreatitis or hepatitis.

Over age 60:
May cause hemochromatosis (iron storage disease) with bronze skin, liver damage, diabetes, heart problems and impotence.

Pregnancy:
No proven harm to unborn child. Avoid if possible. Take only if your doctor prescribes supplement during last half of pregnancy.

Breast-feeding:
No problems expected. Take only if your doctor confirms you have a dietary deficiency or an iron-deficiency anemia.

Infants & children:
Use only under medical supervision. Overdose common and dangerous. Keep out of children's reach.

Prolonged use:
May cause hemochromatosis (iron storage disease) with bronze skin, liver damage, diabetes, heart problems and impotence.

Skin & sunlight:
No problems expected.

Driving, piloting or hazardous work:
No problems expected.

Discontinuing:
May be unnecessary to finish medicine. Follow doctor's instructions.

Others:
Liquid form stains teeth. Mix with water or juice to lessen the effect. Brush with baking soda or hydrogen peroxide to help remove stain.

POSSIBLE INTERACTION WITH OTHER DRUGS

GENERIC NAME OR DRUG CLASS	COMBINED EFFECT
Acetohydroxamic acid	Decreased effects of both drugs.
Allopurinol	Possible excess iron storage in liver.
Antacids	Poor iron absorption.
Chloramphenicol	Decreased effect of iron. Interferes with red-blood-cell and hemoglobin formation.
Cholestyramine	Decreased iron effect.
Iron supplements (other)	Possible excess iron storage in liver.
Penicillamine	Decreased penicillamine effect.
Sulfasalazine	Decreased iron effect.
Tetracyclines	Decreased tetracycline effect. Take iron 3 hours before or 2 hours after taking tetracycline.
Vitamin C	Increased iron effect. Contributes to red-blood-cell and hemoglobin formation.
Vitamin E	Decreased iron effect.

POSSIBLE INTERACTION WITH OTHER SUBSTANCES

INTERACTS WITH	COMBINED EFFECT
Alcohol:	Increased iron absorption. May cause organ damage. Avoid or use in moderation.
Beverages: Milk, tea.	Decreased iron effect.
Cocaine:	None expected.
Foods: Dairy foods, eggs, whole-grain bread and cereal.	Decreased iron effect.
Marijuana:	None expected.
Tobacco:	None expected.

FLAVOXATE

BRAND NAMES

Urispas

BASIC INFORMATION

Habit forming? No
Prescription needed? Yes
Available as generic? No
Drug class: Smooth-muscle relaxant,
anticholinergic

 ## USES

Relieves urinary pain, urgency, nighttime
urination, unusual frequency of urination
associated with urinary system disorders.

 ## DOSAGE & USAGE INFORMATION

How to take:
Tablet or capsule—Swallow with liquid or food
to lessen stomach irritation.

When to take:
30 minutes before meals (unless directed
otherwise by doctor).

If you forget a dose:
Take as soon as you remember up to 2 hours
late. If more than 2 hours, wait for next
scheduled dose (don't double this dose).

What drug does:
Blocks nerve impulses at smooth muscle nerve
endings, preventing muscle contractions and
gland secretions of organs involved.

Time lapse before drug works:
15 to 30 minutes.

Don't take with:
See Interaction column and consult doctor.

 ## OVERDOSE

SYMPTOMS:
Dilated pupils, rapid pulse and breathing,
dizziness, fever, hallucinations, confusion,
slurred speech, agitation, flushed face,
convulsions, coma.
WHAT TO DO:
- **Dial 0 (operator) or 911 (emergency) for an**
  ambulance or medical help. Then give first
  aid immediately.
- **See emergency information on inside**
  covers.

 ## POSSIBLE ADVERSE REACTIONS OR SIDE EFFECTS

SYMPTOMS	WHAT TO DO
Life-threatening:	
None expected.	
Common:	
• Confusion, delirium, rapid heartbeat.	Discontinue. Call doctor right away.
• Nausea, vomiting, less perspiration.	Continue. Call doctor when convenient.
• Constipation.	Continue. Tell doctor at next visit.
• Dry ears, nose, throat.	No action necessary.
Infrequent:	
• Unusual excitement, irritability, restlessness.	Discontinue. Call doctor right away.
• Headache, increased sensitivity to light, painful or difficult urination.	Continue. Call doctor when convenient.
Rare:	
• Shortness of breath.	Discontinue. Seek emergency treatment.
• Rash or hives; pain; blurred vision; sore throat, fever, mouth sores.	Discontinue. Call doctor right away.

WARNINGS & PRECAUTIONS

Don't take if:
- You are allergic to any anticholinergic.
- You have trouble with stomach bloating.
- You have difficulty emptying your bladder completely.
- You have narrow-angle glaucoma.
- You have severe ulcerative colitis.

Before you start, consult your doctor:
- If you have open-angle glaucoma.
- If you have angina.
- If you have chronic bronchitis or asthma.
- If you have liver disease.
- If you have hiatal hernia.
- If you have enlarged prostate.
- If you have myasthenia gravis.
- If you have peptic ulcer.
- If you will have surgery within 2 months, including dental surgery, requiring general or spinal anesthesia.

Over age 60:
Adverse reactions and side effects, particularly mental confusion, may be more frequent and severe than in younger persons.

Pregnancy:
Studies inconclusive on harm to unborn child. Animal studies show fetal abnormalities. Decide with your doctor whether drug benefits justify risk to unborn child.

Breast-feeding:
Drug passes into milk. Avoid drug or discontinue nursing until you finish medicine. Consult doctor for advice on maintaining milk supply.

Infants & children:
Use only under medical supervision.

Prolonged use:
Chronic constipation, possible fecal impaction. Consult doctor immediately.

Skin & sunlight:
No problems expected.

Driving, piloting or hazardous work:
Use disqualifies you for piloting aircraft. Otherwise, no problems expected.

Discontinuing:
May be unnecessary to finish medicine. Follow doctor's instructions.

Others:
No problems expected.

POSSIBLE INTERACTION WITH OTHER DRUGS

GENERIC NAME OR DRUG CLASS	COMBINED EFFECT
Amantadine	Increased flavoxate effect.
Anticholinergics (other)	Increased flavoxate effect.
Antidepressants (tricyclic)	Increased flavoxate effect. Increased sedation.
Antihistamines	Increased flavoxate effect.
Atropine	Increased effect of both drugs.
Cortisone drugs	Increased internal-eye pressure.
Haloperidol	Increased internal-eye pressure.
MAO inhibitors	Increased flavoxate effect.
Meperidine	Increased flavoxate effect.
Nitrates	Increased internal-eye pressure.
Orphenadrine	Increased flavoxate effect.
Phenothiazines	Increased flavoxate effect.
Pilocarpine	Loss of pilocarpine effect in glaucoma treatment.
Potassium supplements	Increased possibility of intestinal ulcers with oral potassium tablets.
Vitamin C	Decreased flavoxate effect. Avoid large doses of vitamin C.

POSSIBLE INTERACTION WITH OTHER SUBSTANCES

INTERACTS WITH	COMBINED EFFECT
Alcohol:	None expected.
Beverages:	None expected.
Cocaine:	Excessively rapid heartbeat. Avoid.
Foods:	None expected.
Marijuana:	Drowsiness, dry mouth.
Tobacco:	None expected.

FLECAINIDE ACETATE

BRAND NAMES

Tambocor

BASIC INFORMATION

Habit forming? No
Prescription needed? Yes
Available as generic? No
Drug class: Antiarrhythmic

 ## USES

Stabilizes irregular heartbeat.

 ## DOSAGE & USAGE INFORMATION

How to take:
Tablet or capsule—Swallow with liquid. If you can't swallow whole, crumble tablet or open capsule and take with liquid or food.

When to take:
At the same time each day, according to instructions on prescription label. Take tablets approximately 12 hours apart.

If you forget a dose:
Take as soon as you remember up to 4 hours late. If more than 4 hours, wait for next scheduled dose (don't double this dose).

What drug does:
Decreases conduction of abnormal electrical activity in the heart muscle or its regulating systems.

Time lapse before drug works:
1 to 6 hours. May need doses daily for 2 to 3 days for maximum effect.

Continued next column

 ## OVERDOSE

SYMPTOMS:
Low blood pressure or unconsciousness, irregular or rapid heartbeat.
WHAT TO DO:
- Dial 0 (operator) or 911 (emergency) for an ambulance or medical help. Then give first aid immediately.
- If patient is unconscious and not breathing, give mouth-to-mouth breathing. If there is no heartbeat, use cardiac massage and mouth-to-mouth breathing (CPR). Don't try to make patient vomit. If you can't get help quickly, take patient to nearest emergency facility.
- See emergency information on inside covers.

Don't take with:
See Interaction column and consult doctor.

 ## POSSIBLE ADVERSE REACTIONS OR SIDE EFFECTS

SYMPTOMS	WHAT TO DO
Life-threatening: None expected.	
Common: Blurred vision.	Continue. Call doctor when convenient.
Infrequent: • Chest pain, irregular heartbeat.	Discontinue. Seek emergency treatment.
• Shakiness, dizziness, rash, nausea, vomiting.	Discontinue. Call doctor right away.
• Anxiety; depression; weakness; headache; appetite loss; weakness in muscles, bones, joints; swollen feet, ankles or legs.	Continue. Call doctor when convenient.
• Constipation.	Continue. Tell doctor at next visit.
Rare: Unusual bleeding or bruising, sore throat, jaundice, fever, chills.	Discontinue. Call doctor right away.

WARNINGS & PRECAUTIONS

Don't take if:
You are allergic to flecainide or a local anesthetic such as novocaine, xylocaine or other drug whose generic name ends with "caine."

Before you start, consult your doctor:
- If you have kidney disease.
- If you have liver disease.
- If you have had a heart attack in past 3 weeks.
- If you have a pacemaker.

Over age 60:
Adverse reactions and side effects may be more frequent and severe than in younger persons.

Pregnancy:
Studies inconclusive on harm to unborn child. Animal studies show fetal abnormalities. Decide with your doctor whether drug benefits justify risk to unborn child.

Breast-feeding:
No proven problems.

Infants & children:
Not recommended. Safety and dosage have not been established.

Prolonged use:
No proven problems.

Skin & sunlight:
No problems expected.

Driving, piloting or hazardous work:
Don't drive or pilot aircraft until you learn how medicine affects you. Don't work around dangerous machinery. Don't climb ladders or work in high places. Danger increases if you drink alcohol or take medicine affecting alertness and reflexes, such as antihistamines, tranquilizers, sedatives, pain medicine, narcotics and mind-altering drugs.

Discontinuing:
Don't discontinue without consulting doctor. Dose may require gradual reduction if you have taken drug for a long time. Doses of other drugs may also require adjustment.

Others:
Wear identification bracelet or carry an identification card with inscription of medicine you take.

POSSIBLE INTERACTION WITH OTHER DRUGS

GENERIC NAME OR DRUG CLASS	COMBINED EFFECT
Antiarrhythmics (other)	Possible irregular heartbeat.
Beta-adrenergic blockers	Possible decreased efficiency of heart-muscle contraction, leading to congestive heart failure.
Digitalis preparations	Increased digitalis effect. Possible irregular heartbeat.
Drugs that depress bone-marrow function, such as anticancer drugs, antithyroid drugs, azathioprine, carbamazepine, chloramphenicol, flucytosine, penicillamine, phenylbutazone, primaquine, pyrimethamine, rifampin, sulfa drugs, tocainide, trimethoprim, valproic acid.	Possible decreased production of blood cells in bone marrow.

POSSIBLE INTERACTION WITH OTHER SUBSTANCES

INTERACTS WITH	COMBINED EFFECT
Alcohol:	May further depress normal heart function.
Beverages: Caffeine-containing beverages.	Possible decreased flecainide effect.
Cocaine:	Possible decreased flecainide effect.
Foods:	None expected.
Marijuana:	Possible decreased flecainide effect.
Tobacco:	Possible decreased flecainide effect.

FLUPHENAZINE

BRAND NAMES

Apo-Fluphenazine	Permitil
Modecate	Prolixin
Moditen	Prolixin Decanoate
Moditen Etanthate	Prolixin Enanthate

BASIC INFORMATION

Habit forming? No
Prescription needed? Yes
Available as generic? Yes
Drug class: Tranquilizer, antiemetic (phenothiazine)

USES

- Stops nausea, vomiting.
- Reduces anxiety, agitation.

DOSAGE & USAGE INFORMATION

How to take:
- Tablet or capsule—Swallow with liquid or food to lessen stomach irritation.
- Suppositories—Remove wrapper and moisten suppository with water. Gently insert into rectum, large end first.
- Drops or liquid—Dilute dose in beverage.

When to take:
- Nervous and mental disorders—Take at the same times each day.
- Nausea and vomiting—Take as needed, no more often than every 4 hours.

If you forget a dose:
- Nervous and mental disorders—Take up to 2 hours late. If more than 2 hours, wait for next scheduled dose (don't double this dose).
- Nausea and vomiting—Take as soon as you remember. Wait 4 hours for next dose.

What drug does:
- Suppresses brain's vomiting center.
- Suppresses brain centers that control abnormal emotions and behavior.

Continued next column

OVERDOSE

SYMPTOMS:
Stupor, convulsions, coma.
WHAT TO DO:
- Dial 0 (operator) or 911 (emergency) for an ambulance or medical help. Then give first aid immediately.
- See emergency information on inside covers.

Time lapse before drug works:
- Nausea and vomiting—1 hour or less.
- Nervous and mental disorders—4-6 weeks.

Don't take with:
- Antacid or medicine for diarrhea.
- Non-prescription drug for cough, cold or allergy.
- See Interaction column and consult doctor.

POSSIBLE ADVERSE REACTIONS OR SIDE EFFECTS

SYMPTOMS	WHAT TO DO
Life-threatening: None expected.	
Common:	
- Muscle spasms of face and neck, unsteady gait.	Discontinue. Seek emergency treatment.
- Restlessness, tremor, drowsiness.	Discontinue. Call doctor right away.
- Decreased sweating, dry mouth, runny nose, constipation.	Continue. Call doctor when convenient.
Infrequent:	
- Fainting.	Discontinue. Seek emergency treatment.
- Rash.	Discontinue. Call doctor right away.
- Painful or difficult urination, diminished sex drive, swollen breasts, menstrual irregularities.	Continue. Call doctor when convenient.
Rare: Change in vision, sore throat, fever, jaundice.	Discontinue. Call doctor right away.

WARNINGS & PRECAUTIONS

Don't take if:
- You are allergic to any phenothiazine.
- You have a blood or bone-marrow disease.

Before you start, consult your doctor:
- If you will have surgery within 2 months, including dental surgery, requiring general or spinal anesthesia.
- If you have asthma, emphysema or other lung disorder.
- If you take non-prescription ulcer medicine, asthma medicine or amphetamines.

Over age 60:
Adverse reactions and side effects may be more frequent and severe than in younger persons. More likely to develop involuntary movement of jaws, lips, tongue, chewing. Report this to your doctor immediately. Early treatment can help.

Pregnancy:
Risk to unborn child outweighs drug benefits. Don't use.

Breast-feeding:
Drug passes into milk. Avoid drug or discontinue nursing until you finish medicine. Consult doctor for advice on maintaining milk supply.

Infants & children:
Don't give to children younger than 2.

Prolonged use:
May lead to tardive dyskinesia (involuntary movement of jaws, lips, tongue, chewing).

Skin & sunlight:
May cause rash or intensify sunburn in areas exposed to sun or sunlamp. Skin may remain sensitive for 3 months after discontinuing.

Driving, piloting or hazardous work:
Don't drive or pilot aircraft until you learn how medicine affects you. Don't work around dangerous machinery. Don't climb ladders or work in high places. Danger increases if you drink alcohol or take medicine affecting alertness and reflexes.

Discontinuing:
- Nervous and mental disorders—Don't discontinue without doctor's advice until you complete prescribed dose, even though symptoms diminish or disappear.
- Nausea and vomiting—May be unnecessary to finish medicine. Follow doctor's instructions.

Others:
No problems expected.

POSSIBLE INTERACTION WITH OTHER DRUGS

GENERIC NAME OR DRUG CLASS	COMBINED EFFECT
Anticholinergics	Increased anticholinergic effect.
Antidepressants (tricyclic)	Increased fluphenazine effect.
Antihistamines	Increased antihistamine effect.
Appetite suppressants	Decreased suppressant effect.
Dronabinol	Increased effects of both drugs. Avoid.
Levodopa	Decreased levodopa effect.
Mind-altering drugs	Increased effect of mind-altering drugs.
Molindone	Increased tranquilizer effect.
Narcotics	Increased narcotic effect.
Phenytoin	Increased phenytoin effect.
Quinidine	Impaired heart function. Dangerous mixture.
Sedatives	Increased sedative effect.
Tranquilizers (other)	Increased tranquilizer effect.

POSSIBLE INTERACTION WITH OTHER SUBSTANCES

INTERACTS WITH	COMBINED EFFECT
Alcohol:	Dangerous oversedation.
Beverages:	None expected.
Cocaine:	Decreased fluphenazine effect. Avoid.
Foods:	None expected.
Marijuana:	Drowsiness. May increase antinausea effect.
Tobacco:	None expected.

FLUPREDNISOLONE

BRAND NAMES

Alphadrol

BASIC INFORMATION

Habit forming? No
Prescription needed? Yes
Available as generic? No
Drug class: Cortisone drug (adrenal corticosteroid)

 ## USES

- Reduces inflammation caused by many different medical problems.
- Treatment for some allergic diseases, blood disorders, kidney diseases, asthma and emphysema.
- Replaces corticosteroid deficiencies.

 ## DOSAGE & USAGE INFORMATION

How to take:
Tablet—Swallow with liquid or food to lessen stomach irritation. If you can't swallow whole, crumble tablet.

When to take:
At the same times each day. Take once-a-day or once-every-other-day doses in mornings.

If you forget a dose:
- Several-doses-per-day prescription—Take as soon as you remember up to 2 hours late. If more than 2 hours, wait for next scheduled dose (don't double this dose).
- Once-a-day dose or less—Wait for next dose. Double this dose.

What drug does:
Decreases inflammatory responses.

Time lapse before drug works:
2 to 4 days.

Don't take with:
See Interaction column and consult doctor.

 ## OVERDOSE

SYMPTOMS:
Headache, convulsions, heart failure.
WHAT TO DO:
- **Dial 0 (operator) or 911 (emergency) for an ambulance or medical help. Then give first aid immediately.**
- **See emergency information on inside covers.**

 ## POSSIBLE ADVERSE REACTIONS OR SIDE EFFECTS

SYMPTOMS	WHAT TO DO
Life-threatening: None expected.	
Common: Acne, poor wound healing, thirst, indigestion, nausea, vomiting.	Continue. Call doctor when convenient.
Infrequent:	
• Black, bloody or tarry stools.	Discontinue. Seek emergency treatment.
• Blurred vision; halos around lights; sore throat; fever; muscle cramps; swollen legs, feet.	Discontinue. Call doctor right away.
• Mood changes, insomnia, restlessness, frequent urination, weight gain, round face, fatigue, weakness, TB recurrence, menstrual irregularities.	Continue. Call doctor when convenient.
Rare:	
• Irregular heartbeat.	Discontinue. Seek emergency treatment.
• Rash.	Discontinue. Call doctor right away.

 ## WARNINGS & PRECAUTIONS

Don't take if:
- You are allergic to any cortisone drug.
- You have tuberculosis or fungus infection.
- You have herpes infection of eyes, lips or genitals.

Before you start, consult your doctor:
- If you have had tuberculosis.
- If you have congestive heart failure.
- If you have diabetes.
- If you have peptic ulcer.
- If you have glaucoma.
- If you have underactive thyroid.
- If you have high blood pressure.
- If you have myasthenia gravis.
- If you have blood clots in legs or lungs.

Over age 60:
Adverse reactions and side effects may be more frequent and severe than in younger persons. Likely to aggravate edema, diabetes or ulcers. Likely to cause cataracts and osteoporosis (softening of the bones).

Pregnancy:
Risk to unborn child outweighs drug benefits. Don't use.

Breast-feeding:
Drug passes into milk. Avoid drug or discontinue nursing until you finish medicine. Consult doctor for advice on maintaining milk supply.

Infants & children:
Use only under medical supervision.

Prolonged use:
- Retards growth in children.
- Possible glaucoma, cataracts, diabetes, fragile bones and thin skin.
- Functional dependence.

Skin & sunlight:
No problems expected.

Driving, piloting or hazardous work:
No problems expected.

Discontinuing:
- Don't discontinue without doctor's advice until you complete prescribed dose, even though symptoms diminish or disappear.
- Drug affects your response to surgery, illness, injury or stress for 2 years after discontinuing. Tell anyone who takes medical care of you about this drug for 2 years after discontinuing.

Others:
Avoid immunizations if possible.

 ## POSSIBLE INTERACTION WITH OTHER DRUGS

GENERIC NAME OR DRUG CLASS	COMBINED EFFECT
Amphoterecin B	Potassium depletion.
Anticholinergics	Possible glaucoma.
Anticoagulants (oral)	Decreased anticoagulant effect.
Anticonvulsants (hydantoin)	Decreased fluprednisolone effect.
Antidiabetics (oral)	Decreased antidiabetic effect.
Antihistamines	Decreased fluprednisolone effect.
Aspirin	Increased fluprednisolone effect.
Barbiturates	Decreased fluprednisolone effect. Oversedation.
Beta-adrenergic blockers	Decreased fluprednisolone effect.
Chloral hydrate	Decreased fluprednisolone effect.
Chlorthalidone	Potassium depletion.
Cholinergics	Decreased cholinergic effect.
Contraceptives (oral)	Increased fluprednisolone effect.
Digitalis preparations	Dangerous potassium depletion. Possible digitalis toxicity.
Diuretics (thiazide)	Potassium depletion.
Ephedrine	Decreased fluprednisolone effect.
Estrogens	Increased fluprednisolone effect.
Ethacrynic acid	Potassium depletion.
Furosemide	Potassium depletion.
Glutethimide	Decreased fluprednisolone effect.
Indapamide	Possible excessive potassium loss, causing dangerous heartbeat irregularity.
Indomethacin	Increased fluprednisolone effect.
Insulin	Decreased insulin effect.
Isoniazid	Decreased isoniazid effect.
Oxyphenbutazone	Possible ulcers.
Phenylbutazone	Possible ulcers.
Potassium supplements	Decreased potassium effect.
Rifampin	Decreased fluprednisolone effect.
Sympathomimetics	Possible glaucoma.

 ## POSSIBLE INTERACTION WITH OTHER SUBSTANCES

INTERACTS WITH	COMBINED EFFECT
Alcohol:	Risk of stomach ulcers.
Beverages:	No proven problems.
Cocaine:	Overstimulation. Avoid.
Foods:	No proven problems.
Marijuana:	Decreased immunity.
Tobacco:	Increased fluprednisolone effect. Possible toxicity.

FLURAZEPAM

BRAND NAMES

Apo-Flurazepam   Somnal
Dalmane   Som-Pam
Novoflupam

BASIC INFORMATION

Habit forming? Yes
Prescription needed? Yes
Available as generic? Yes
Drug class: Tranquilizer (benzodiazepine)

USES

Treatment for insomnia and tension.

DOSAGE & USAGE INFORMATION

How to take:
Tablet or capsule—Swallow with liquid. If you can't swallow whole, crumble tablet or open capsule and take with liquid or food.

When to take:
At the same time each day, according to instructions on prescription label.

If you forget a dose:
Take as soon as you remember up to 2 hours late. If more than 2 hours, wait for next scheduled dose (don't double this dose).

What drug does:
Affects limbic system of brain—part that controls emotions. Induces near-normal sleep pattern.

Time lapse before drug works:
30 minutes.

Continued next column

OVERDOSE

SYMPTOMS:
Drowsiness, weakness, tremor, stupor, coma.
WHAT TO DO:
- Dial 0 (operator) or 911 (emergency) for an ambulance or medical help. Then give first aid immediately.
- If patient is unconscious and not breathing, give mouth-to-mouth breathing. If there is no heartbeat, use cardiac massage and mouth-to-mouth breathing (CPR). Don't try to make patient vomit. If you can't get help quickly, take patient to nearest emergency facility.
- See emergency information on inside covers.

Don't take with:
See Interaction column and consult doctor.

POSSIBLE ADVERSE REACTIONS OR SIDE EFFECTS

SYMPTOMS	WHAT TO DO
Life-threatening:	
None expected.	
Common:	
Clumsiness, drowsiness, dizziness.	Continue. Call doctor when convenient.
Infrequent:	
● Hallucinations, confusion, depression, irritability, rash, itch, change in vision.	Discontinue. Call doctor right away.
● Constipation or diarrhea, nausea, vomiting, painful or difficult urination.	Continue. Call doctor when convenient.
Rare:	
● Slow heartbeat, difficult breathing.	Discontinue. Seek emergency treatment.
● Mouth, throat ulcers, jaundice.	Discontinue. Call doctor right away.

WARNINGS & PRECAUTIONS

Don't take if:
- You are allergic to any benzodiazepine.
- You have myasthenia gravis.
- You are active or recovering alcoholic.
- Patient is younger than 6 months.

Before you start, consult your doctor:
- If you have liver, kidney or lung disease.
- If you have diabetes, epilepsy or porphyria.

Over age 60:
Adverse reactions and side effects may be more frequent and severe than in younger persons. May develop agitation, rage or "hangover" effect.

Pregnancy:
Risk to unborn child outweighs drug benefits. Don't use.

Breast-feeding:
Drug passes into milk. Avoid drug or discontinue nursing until you finish medicine. Consult doctor for advice on maintaining milk supply.

Infants & children:
Use only under medical supervision for children older than 6 months.

Prolonged use:
May impair liver function.

Skin & sunlight:
No problems expected.

Driving, piloting or hazardous work:
Don't drive or pilot aircraft until you learn how medicine affects you. Don't work around dangerous machinery. Don't climb ladders or work in high places. Danger increases if you drink alcohol or take medicine affecting alertness and reflexes.

Discontinuing:
Don't discontinue without doctor's advice until you complete prescribed dose, even though symptoms diminish or disappear.

Others:
- Hot weather, heavy exercise and profuse sweat may reduce excretion and cause overdose.
- "Hangover" effect may occur.
- Blood sugar may rise in diabetics, requiring insulin adjustment.

POSSIBLE INTERACTION WITH OTHER DRUGS

GENERIC NAME OR DRUG CLASS	COMBINED EFFECT
Anticonvulsants	Change in seizure frequency or severity.
Antidepressants	Increased sedative effect of both drugs.
Antihistamines	Increased sedative effect of both drugs.
Antihypertensives	Excessively low blood pressure.
Cimetidine	Excess sedation.
Disulfiram	Increased flurazepam effect.
Dronabinol	Increased effects of both drugs. Avoid.
MAO inhibitors	Convulsions, deep sedation, rage.
Molindone	Increased sedative effect.
Narcotics	Increased sedative effect of both drugs.
Sedatives	Increased sedative effect of both drugs.
Sleep inducers	Increased sedative effect of both drugs.
Tranquilizers	Increased sedative effect of both drugs.

POSSIBLE INTERACTION WITH OTHER SUBSTANCES

INTERACTS WITH	COMBINED EFFECT
Alcohol:	Heavy sedation. Avoid.
Beverages:	None expected.
Cocaine:	Decreased flurazepam effect.
Foods:	None expected.
Marijuana:	Heavy sedation. Avoid.
Tobacco:	Decreased flurazepam effect.

FOLIC ACID (VITAMIN B-9)

BRAND NAMES

Apo-Folic
Folvite
Novofolacid

Numerous other
multiple
vitamin-mineral
supplements.

BASIC INFORMATION

Habit forming? No
Prescription needed?
  High strength: Yes
  Vitamin mixtures: No
Available as generic? Yes
Drug class: Vitamin supplement

 ## USES

- Dietary supplement to promote normal growth, development and good health.
- Treatment for anemias due to folic-acid deficiency occurring from alcoholism, liver disease, hemolytic anemia, sprue, infants on artificial formula, pregnancy, breast-feeding and oral-contraceptive use.

 ## DOSAGE & USAGE INFORMATION

How to take:
Tablet—Swallow with liquid or food to lessen stomach irritation. If you can't swallow whole, crumble tablet and take with liquid or food.

When to take:
At the same time each day.

If you forget a dose:
Take when you remember. Don't double next dose. Resume regular schedule.

What drug does:
Essential to normal red-blood-cell formation.

Time lapse before drug works:
Not determined.

Don't take with:
See Interaction column and consult doctor.

 ## OVERDOSE

SYMPTOMS:
None expected.
WHAT TO DO:
Overdose unlikely to threaten life.

 ## POSSIBLE ADVERSE REACTIONS OR SIDE EFFECTS

SYMPTOMS	WHAT TO DO
Life-threatening: None expected.	
Common: Large dose may produce yellow urine.	Continue. Tell doctor at next visit.
Infrequent: None expected.	
Rare: None expected.	

WARNINGS & PRECAUTIONS

Don't take if:
You are allergic to any B vitamin.

Before you start, consult your doctor:
• If you have liver disease.
• If you have pernicious anemia. (Folic acid corrects anemia, but nerve damage of pernicious anemia continues.)

Over age 60:
No problems expected.

Pregnancy:
No problems expected.

Breast-feeding:
No problems expected.

Infants & children:
No problems expected.

Prolonged use:
No problems expected.

Skin & sunlight:
No problems expected.

Driving, piloting or hazardous work:
No problems expected.

Discontinuing:
Don't discontinue without doctor's advice until you complete prescribed dose, even though symptoms diminish or disappear.

Others:
• Folic acid removed by kidney dialysis. Dialysis patients should increase intake to 300% of RDA.
• A balanced diet should provide all the folic acid a healthy person needs and make supplements unnecessary. Best sources are green, leafy vegetables, fruits, liver and kidney.

POSSIBLE INTERACTION WITH OTHER DRUGS

GENERIC NAME OR DRUG CLASS	COMBINED EFFECT
Analgesics	Decreased effect of folic acid.
Anticonvulsants	Decreased effect of folic acid.
Contraceptives (oral)	Decreased effect of folic acid.
Cortisone drugs	Decreased effect of folic acid.
Methotrexate	Decreased effect of folic acid.
Pyrimethamine	Decreased effect of folic acid.
Quinine	Decreased effect of folic acid.
Sulfasalazine	Decreased dietary absorption of folic acid.
Triamterene	Decreased effect of folic acid.
Trimethoprim	Decreased effect of folic acid.
Zinc	Decreased zinc effect.

POSSIBLE INTERACTION WITH OTHER SUBSTANCES

INTERACTS WITH	COMBINED EFFECT
Alcohol:	None expected.
Beverages:	None expected.
Cocaine:	None expected.
Foods:	None expected.
Marijuana:	None expected.
Tobacco:	None expected.

FUROSEMIDE

BRAND NAMES

Apo-Furosemide	Novosemide
Furoside	SK-Furosemide
Lasix	Uritol
Neo-Renal	

BASIC INFORMATION

Habit forming? No
Prescription needed? Yes
Available as generic? Yes
Drug class: Diuretic, antihypertensive

USES

- Lowers high blood pressure.
- Decreases fluid retention.

DOSAGE & USAGE INFORMATION

How to take:
Tablet, liquid or capsule—Swallow with liquid. If you can't swallow whole, crumble tablet or open capsule and take with liquid or food.

When to take:
- 1 dose a day—Take after breakfast.
- More than 1 dose a day—Take last dose no later than 6 p.m. unless otherwise directed.

If you forget a dose:
- 1 dose a day—Take as soon as you remember up to 12 hours late. If more than 12 hours, wait for next scheduled dose (don't double this dose).
- More than 1 dose a day—Take as soon as you remember up to 2 hours late. If more than 2 hours, wait for next scheduled dose (don't double this dose).

What drug does:
Increases elimination of sodium and water from body. Decreased body fluid reduces blood pressure.

Continued next column

OVERDOSE

SYMPTOMS:
Weakness, lethargy, dizziness, confusion, nausea, vomiting, leg-muscle cramps, thirst, stupor, deep sleep, weak and rapid pulse, cardiac arrest.
WHAT TO DO:
- **Dial 0 (operator) or 911 (emergency) for an ambulance or medical help. Then give first aid immediately.**
- **See emergency information on inside covers.**

Time lapse before drug works:
1 hour to increase water loss. Requires 2 to 3 weeks to lower blood pressure.

Don't take with:
- Non-prescription drugs with aspirin.
- See Interaction column and consult doctor.

POSSIBLE ADVERSE REACTIONS OR SIDE EFFECTS

SYMPTOMS	WHAT TO DO
Life-threatening: None expected.	
Common: Dizziness.	Continue. Call doctor when convenient.
Infrequent: Mood change, appetite loss, diarrhea, irregular heartbeat, muscle cramps, fatigue, weakness.	Discontinue. Call doctor right away.
Rare: Rash or hives, yellow vision, ringing in ears, hearing loss, sore throat, fever, dry mouth, thirst, side or stomach pain, nausea, vomiting, unusual bleeding or bruising, joint pain, jaundice.	Discontinue. Call doctor right away.

WARNINGS & PRECAUTIONS

Don't take if:
You are allergic to furosemide.

Before you start, consult your doctor:
- If you are allergic to any sulfa drug.
- If you have liver or kidney disease.
- If you have gout.
- If you have diabetes.
- If you have impaired hearing.
- If you will have surgery within 2 months, including dental surgery, requiring general or spinal anesthesia.

Over age 60:
Adverse reactions and side effects may be more frequent and severe than in younger persons.

Pregnancy:
Risk to unborn child outweighs drug benefits. Don't use.

Breast-feeding:
Drug filters into milk. May harm child. Avoid.

Infants & children:
Use only under medical supervision.

Prolonged use:
- Impaired balance of water, salt and potassium in blood and body tissues.
- Possible diabetes.

Skin & sunlight:
May cause rash or intensify sunburn in areas exposed to sun or sunlamp.

Driving, piloting or hazardous work:
No problems expected.

Discontinuing:
Don't discontinue without doctor's advice until you complete prescribed dose, even though symptoms diminish or disappear.

Others:
Frequent laboratory studies to monitor potassium level in blood recommended. Eat foods rich in potassium or take potassium supplements. Consult doctor.

POSSIBLE INTERACTION WITH OTHER DRUGS

GENERIC NAME OR DRUG CLASS	COMBINED EFFECT
Acebutolol	Increased antihypertensive effect. Dosages may require adjustment.
Allopurinol	Decreased allopurinol effect.
Amiodarone	Increased risk of heartbeat irregularity due to low potassium.
Anticoagulants	Abnormal clotting.
Antidepressants (tricyclic)	Excessive blood-pressure drop.
Antidiabetics (oral)	Decreased antidiabetic effect.
Anti-inflammatory drugs (non-steroid)	Decreased furosemide effect.
Antihypertensives	Increased antihypertensive effect.
Barbiturates	Low blood pressure.
Calcium supplements	Increased calcium in blood.
Cortisone drugs	Excessive potassium loss.
Digitalis preparations	Serious heart-rhythm disorders.
Indapamide	Increased diuretic effect.

Insulin	Decreased insulin effect.
Ketoprofen	Decreased diuretic effect of furosemide.
Labetolol	Increased antihypertensive effects.
Lithium	Increased lithium toxicity.
MAO inhibitors	Increased furosemide effect.
Narcotics	Dangerous low blood pressure. Avoid.
Nitrates	Excessive blood-pressure drop.
Oxprenolol	Increased antihypertensive effect. Dosages may require adjustment.
Phenothiazines	Increased phenothiazine effect.
Potassium supplements	Decreased potassium effect.
Probenecid	Decreased probenecid effect.
Salicylates (including aspirin)	Dangerous salicylate retention.
Sedatives	Increased furosemide effect.
Suprofen	Decreased diuretic effect of furosemide.

POSSIBLE INTERACTION WITH OTHER SUBSTANCES

INTERACTS WITH	COMBINED EFFECT
Alcohol:	Blood-pressure drop. Avoid.
Beverages:	None expected.
Cocaine:	Dangerous blood-pressure drop. Avoid.
Foods:	None expected.
Marijuana:	Increased thirst and urinary frequency, fainting.
Tobacco:	Decreased furosemide effect.

GALLBLADDER X-RAY TEST DRUGS (CHOLECYSTOGRAPHIC AGENTS)

BRAND AND GENERIC NAMES

Bilivist	IPODATE
Bilopaque	Oragrafin Calcium
Cholebrine	Oragrafin Sodium
IOCETAMIC ACID	Telepaque
IOPANOIC ACID	TYROPANOATE

BASIC INFORMATION

Habit forming? No
Prescription needed? Yes
Available as generic? No
Drug class: Diagnostic aid, radiopaque

USES

To check for problems with the gallbladder or the bile ducts.

DOSAGE & USAGE INFORMATION

How to take:
- Take tablets or liquid as directed after the evening meal on the evening before special x-rays will be taken.
- Don't eat or drink anything (except water) after taking.

When to take:
As directed.

If you forget a dose:
Take as soon as you remember.

What drug does:
These are organic iodine compounds which get absorbed into the blood stream, get concentrated in a healthy gallbladder and make the gallbladder and gallstones (if present) visible on special x-rays.

Time lapse before drug works:
10 to 15 hours.

Continued next column

OVERDOSE

SYMPTOMS:
Severe diarrhea, nausea or vomiting; difficult urination.
WHAT TO DO:
Not life-threatening. Discontinue and call doctor right away.

Don't take with:
- Other medicines unless directed by your doctor or x-ray specialist.
- If you take cholestyramine, discontinue it for 48 hours before taking the radiopaque drug.

POSSIBLE ADVERSE REACTIONS OR SIDE EFFECTS

SYMPTOMS	WHAT TO DO
Life-threatening: None expected.	
Common: None expected.	
Infrequent: Abdominal cramps, diarrhea, dizziness, headache, indigestion, vomiting.	Discontinue. Call doctor right away.
Rare: Itching, unusual bleeding or bruising, hives or rash.	Discontinue. Call doctor right away.

GALLBLADDER X-RAY TEST DRUGS (CHOLECYSTOGRAPHIC AGENTS)

WARNINGS & PRECAUTIONS

Don't take if:
You are allergic to any iodine compound or other radiopaque chemicals.

Before you start, consult your doctor:
If you are allergic to anything, including shellfish, cabbage, kale, turnips, iodized salt.

Over age 60:
Adverse reactions and side effects may be more frequent and severe than in younger persons. Ask doctor about smaller doses.

Pregnancy:
X-rays should not be taken unless absolutely necessary during pregnancy.

Breast-feeding:
No problems expected, but ask doctor.

Infants & children:
No problems expected, but ask doctor.

Prolonged use:
Not intended for prolonged use.

Skin & sunlight:
No problems expected.

Driving, piloting or hazardous work:
Don't drive or pilot aircraft until you learn how medicine affects you. Don't work around dangerous machinery. Don't climb ladders or work in high places. Danger increases if you drink alcohol or take medicine affecting alertness and reflexes, such as antihistamines, tranquilizers, sedatives, pain medicine, narcotics and mind-altering drugs.

Discontinuing:
No problems expected.

Others:
- Special diets and laxatives or enemas before x-rays may be ordered. Follow instructions.
- Tests on your thyroid gland may be made inaccurate for 8 weeks because of the iodine contained in radiopaque substances. Keep this in mind if your doctor orders thyroid tests.

POSSIBLE INTERACTION WITH OTHER DRUGS

GENERIC NAME OR DRUG CLASS	COMBINED EFFECT
None expected.	

POSSIBLE INTERACTION WITH OTHER SUBSTANCES

INTERACTS WITH	COMBINED EFFECT
Alcohol:	None expected.
Beverages:	None expected.
Cocaine:	None expected.
Foods:	None expected.
Marijuana:	None expected.
Tobacco:	None expected.

GEMFIBROZIL

BRAND NAMES

Lopid

BASIC INFORMATION

Habit forming? No
Prescription needed? Yes
Available as generic? No
Drug class: Antihyperlipidemic

 USES

Reduces fatty substances in the blood (cholesterol and triglycerides).

 DOSAGE & USAGE INFORMATION

How to take:
Capsule—Swallow with liquid or food to lessen stomach irritation.

When to take:
At the same times each day.

If you forget a dose:
Take as soon as you remember up to 2 hours late. If more than 2 hours, wait for next scheduled dose (don't double this dose).

What drug does:
Inhibits formation of fatty substances.

Time lapse before drug works:
3 months or more.

Don't take with:
See Interaction column and consult doctor.

 OVERDOSE

SYMPTOMS:
Diarrhea, headache, muscle pain.
WHAT TO DO:
Overdose unlikely to threaten life. If person takes much larger amount than prescribed, call doctor, poison-control center or hospital emergency room for instructions.

 POSSIBLE ADVERSE REACTIONS OR SIDE EFFECTS

SYMPTOMS	WHAT TO DO
Life-threatening: None expected.	
Common: None expected.	
Infrequent:	
• Chest pain, shortness of breath, irregular heartbeat, gallstones.	Discontinue. Call doctor right away.
• Nausea, vomiting, diarrhea, stomach pain.	Continue. Call doctor when convenient.
Rare:	
• Rash, itch; sores in mouth, on lips; sore throat; swollen feet, legs; blood in urine; painful urination; fever; chills.	Discontinue. Call doctor right away.
• Dizziness, drowsiness, headache, dryness (skin), hair loss, muscle cramps, backache, diminished sex drive.	Continue. Call doctor when convenient.

WARNINGS & PRECAUTIONS

Don't take if:
You are allergic to any antihyperlipidemic.

Before you start, consult your doctor:
• If you have had liver or kidney disease.
• If you have had peptic-ulcer disease.
• If you have diabetes.

Over age 60:
Adverse reactions and side effects may be more frequent and severe than in younger persons.

Pregnancy:
Risk to unborn child outweighs drug benefits. Don't use.

Breast-feeding:
May harm child. Avoid.

Infants & children:
Not recommended.

Prolonged use:
Periodic blood-cell counts and liver-function studies recommended if you take gemfibrozil for a long time.

Skin & sunlight:
No problems expected.

Driving, piloting or hazardous work:
Avoid if you feel drowsy or dizzy. Otherwise, no problems expected.

Discontinuing:
Don't discontinue without doctor's advice until you complete prescribed dose, even though symptoms diminish or disappear.

Others:
Some studies question effectiveness. Many studies warn against toxicity.

POSSIBLE INTERACTION WITH OTHER DRUGS

GENERIC NAME OR DRUG CLASS	COMBINED EFFECT
Anticoagulants (oral)	Increased anticoagulant effect. Dose reduction of anticoagulant necessary.
Antidiabetics (oral)	Increased antidiabetic effect.
Contraceptives (oral)	Decreased gemfibrozil effect.
Estrogens	Decreased gemfibrozil effect.
Furosemide	Possible toxicity of both drugs.
Insulin	Increased insulin effect.
Thyroid hormones	Increased gemfibrozil effect.

POSSIBLE INTERACTION WITH OTHER SUBSTANCES

INTERACTS WITH	COMBINED EFFECT
Alcohol:	None expected.
Beverages:	None expected.
Cocaine:	Decreased effect of gemfibrozil. Avoid cocaine.
Foods: Fatty foods.	Decreased gemfibrozil effect.
Marijuana:	None expected.
Tobacco:	Decreased gemfibrozil absorption. Avoid.

GLIPIZIDE

BRAND NAMES

Glucotrol

BASIC INFORMATION

Habit forming? No
Prescription needed? Yes
Available as generic? No
Drug class: Antidiabetic (oral), sulfonurea

 USES

Treatment for diabetes in adults who can't control blood sugar by diet, weight loss and exercise.

 DOSAGE & USAGE INFORMATION

How to take:
Tablet—Swallow with liquid or food to lessen stomach irritation. If you can't swallow whole, crumble tablet and take with liquid or food.

When to take:
At the same times each day.

If you forget a dose:
Take as soon as you remember up to 2 hours late. If more than 2 hours, wait for next scheduled dose (don't double this dose).

What drug does:
Stimulates pancreas to produce more insulin. Insulin in blood forces cells to use sugar in blood.

Time lapse before drug works:
3 to 4 hours. May require 2 weeks for maximum benefit.

Don't take with:
See Interaction column and consult doctor.

 OVERDOSE

SYMPTOMS:
Excessive hunger, nausea, anxiety, cool skin, cold sweats, drowsiness, rapid heartbeat, weakness, unconsciousness, coma.
WHAT TO DO:
- **Dial 0 (operator) or 911 (emergency) for an ambulance or medical help. Then give first aid immediately.**
- **See emergency information on inside covers.**

 POSSIBLE ADVERSE REACTIONS OR SIDE EFFECTS

SYMPTOMS	WHAT TO DO
Life-threatening: None expected.	
Common:	
• Dizziness.	Discontinue. Call doctor right away.
• Diarrhea, appetite loss, nausea, stomach pain, heartburn.	Continue. Call doctor when convenient.
Infrequent: Low blood sugar (hunger, anxiety, cold sweats, rapid pulse), drowsiness, nervousness, headache, weakness.	Discontinue. Seek emergency treatment.
Rare: Itching or rash, sore throat, fever, ringing in ears, unusual bleeding or bruising, fatigue, jaundice.	Discontinue. Call doctor right away.

WARNINGS & PRECAUTIONS

Don't take if:
- You are allergic to any sulfonurea.
- You have impaired kidney or liver function.

Before you start, consult your doctor:
- If you have a severe infection.
- If you have thyroid disease.
- If you take insulin.
- If you have heart disease.

Over age 60:
Dose usually smaller than for younger adults. Avoid "low-blood-sugar" episodes because repeated ones can damage brain permanently.

Pregnancy:
No proven harm to unborn child. Avoid if possible.

Breast-feeding:
Drug filters into milk. May lower baby's blood sugar. Avoid.

Infants & children:
Don't give to infants or children.

Prolonged use:
None expected.

Skin & sunlight:
May cause rash or intensify sunburn in areas exposed to sun or sunlamp.

Driving, piloting or hazardous work:
No problems expected unless you develop hypoglycemia (low blood sugar). If so, avoid driving or hazardous activity.

Discontinuing:
Don't discontinue without consulting doctor. Dose may require gradual reduction if you have taken drug for a long time. Doses of other drugs may also require adjustment.

Others:
Don't exceed recommended dose. Hypoglycemia (low blood sugar) may occur, even with proper dose schedule. You must balance medicine, diet and exercise.

POSSIBLE INTERACTION WITH OTHER DRUGS

GENERIC NAME OR DRUG CLASS	COMBINED EFFECT
Androgens	Increased glipizide effect.
Anticoagulants (oral)	Unpredictable prothrombin times (see Glossary).
Anticonvulsants (hydantoin)	Decreased glipizide effect.
Anti-inflammatory drugs (non-steroidal)	Increased glipizide effect.
Aspirin	Increased glipizide effect.
Beta-adrenergic blockers	Increased glipizide effect. May increase difficulty in regulating blood sugar.
Chloramphenicol	Increased glipizide effect.
Clofibrate	Increased glipizide effect.
Contraceptives (oral)	Decreased glipizide effect.
Cortisone drugs	Decreased glipizide effect.
Diuretics (thiazide)	Decreased glipizide effect.
Epinephrine	Decreased glipizide effect.
Estrogens	Increased glipizide effect.
Guanethidine	Unpredictable glipizide effect.
Labetolol	Increased antidiabetic effect, may mask hypoglycemia.

POSSIBLE INTERACTION WITH OTHER SUBSTANCES

INTERACTS WITH	COMBINED EFFECT
Alcohol:	Disulfiram reaction (see Glossary). Avoid.
Beverages:	None expected.
Cocaine:	No proven problems.
Foods:	None expected.
Marijuana:	Decreased glipizide effect. Avoid.
Tobacco:	None expected.

GLYBURIDE

BRAND NAMES

DiaBeta
Euglucon

Glibenclamide
Micronase

BASIC INFORMATION

Habit forming? No
Prescription needed? Yes
Available as generic? No
Drug class: Antidiabetic (oral), sulfonurea

USES

Treatment for diabetes in adults who can't
control blood sugar by diet, weight loss and
exercise.

DOSAGE & USAGE INFORMATION

How to take:
Tablet—Swallow with liquid or food to lessen
stomach irritation. If you can't swallow whole,
crumble tablet and take with liquid or food.

When to take:
At the same times each day.

If you forget a dose:
Take as soon as you remember up to 2 hours
late. If more than 2 hours, wait for next
scheduled dose (don't double this dose).

What drug does:
Stimulates pancreas to produce more insulin.
Insulin in blood forces cells to use sugar in
blood.

Time lapse before drug works:
3 to 4 hours. May require 2 weeks for maximum
benefit.

Don't take with:
See Interaction column and consult doctor.

OVERDOSE

SYMPTOMS:
Excessive hunger, nausea, anxiety, cool
skin, cold sweats, drowsiness, rapid
heartbeat, weakness, unconsciousness,
coma.
WHAT TO DO:
- Dial 0 (operator) or 911 (emergency) for an
  ambulance or medical help. Then give first
  aid immediately.
- See emergency information on inside
  covers.

POSSIBLE ADVERSE REACTIONS OR SIDE EFFECTS

SYMPTOMS	WHAT TO DO
Life-threatening: None expected.	
Common:	
• Dizziness.	Discontinue. Call doctor right away.
• Diarrhea, appetite loss, nausea, stomach pain, heartburn.	Continue. Call doctor when convenient.
Infrequent: Low blood sugar (hunger, anxiety, cold sweats, rapid pulse), drowsiness, nervousness, headache, weakness, rapid heartbeat.	Discontinue. Seek emergency treatment.
Rare: Itching or rash, sore throat, fever, ringing in ears, unusual bleeding or bruising, fatigue, jaundice.	Discontinue. Call doctor right away.

WARNINGS & PRECAUTIONS

Don't take if:
- You are allergic to any sulfonurea.
- You have impaired kidney or liver function.

Before you start, consult your doctor:
- If you have a severe infection.
- If you have thyroid disease.
- If you take insulin.
- If you have heart disease.

Over age 60:
Dose usually smaller than for younger adults. Avoid "low-blood-sugar" episodes because repeated ones can damage brain permanently.

Pregnancy:
No proven harm to unborn child. Avoid if possible.

Breast-feeding:
Drug filters into milk. May lower baby's blood sugar. Avoid.

Infants & children:
Don't give to infants or children.

Prolonged use:
None expected.

Skin & sunlight:
May cause rash or intensify sunburn in areas exposed to sun or sunlamp.

Driving, piloting or hazardous work:
No problems expected unless you develop hypoglycemia (low blood sugar). If so, avoid driving or hazardous activity.

Discontinuing:
Don't discontinue without consulting doctor. Dose may require gradual reduction if you have taken drug for a long time. Doses of other drugs may also require adjustment.

Others:
Don't exceed recommended dose. Hypoglycemia (low blood sugar) may occur, even with proper dose schedule. You must balance medicine, diet and exercise.

POSSIBLE INTERACTION WITH OTHER DRUGS

GENERIC NAME OR DRUG CLASS	COMBINED EFFECT
Androgens	Increased glyburide effect.
Anticoagulants (oral)	Unpredictable prothrombin times.
Anticonvulsants (hydantoin)	Decreased glyburide effect.
Anti-inflammatory drugs (non-steroidal)	Increased glyburide effect.
Aspirin	Increased glyburide effect.
Beta-adrenergic blockers	Increased glyburide effect. Possible increased difficulty in regulating blood-sugar levels.
Chloramphenicol	Increased glyburide effect.
Clofibrate	Increased glyburide effect.
Contraceptives (oral)	Decreased glyburide effect.
Cortisone drugs	Decreased glyburide effect.
Diuretics (thiazide)	Decreased glyburide effect.
Epinephrine	Decreased glyburide effect.
Estrogens	Increased glyburide effect.
Guanethidine	Unpredictable glyburide effect.
Labetolol	Increased antidiabetic effect, may mask hypoglycemia.

POSSIBLE INTERACTION WITH OTHER SUBSTANCES

INTERACTS WITH	COMBINED EFFECT
Alcohol:	Disulfiram reaction (see Glossary). Avoid.
Beverages:	None expected.
Cocaine:	No proven problems.
Foods:	None expected.
Marijuana:	Decreased glyburide effect. Avoid.
Tobacco:	None expected.

GLYCOPYRROLATE

BRAND NAMES

Robinul   Robinul Forte

BASIC INFORMATION

Habit forming? No
Prescription needed? Yes
Available as generic? Yes
Drug class: Antispasmodic, anticholinergic

 USES

- Reduces spasms of digestive system.
- Reduces production of saliva during dental procedures.

 DOSAGE & USAGE INFORMATION

How to take:
Tablet or capsule—Swallow with liquid. If you can't swallow whole, crumble tablet or open capsule and take with small amount of liquid or food.

When to take:
30 minutes before meals (unless directed otherwise by doctor).

If you forget a dose:
Wait for next scheduled dose (don't double this dose).

What drug does:
Blocks nerve impulses at parasympathetic nerve endings, preventing smooth (involuntary) muscle contractions and gland secretions of organs involved.

Time lapse before drug works:
15 to 30 minutes.

Don't take with:
See Interaction column and consult doctor.

 OVERDOSE

SYMPTOMS:
Dry mouth, low blood pressure, decreased breathing rate, rapid heartbeat, flushed skin, drowsiness.
WHAT TO DO:
- **Dial 0 (operator) or 911 (emergency) for an ambulance or medical help. Then give first aid immediately.**
- **See emergency information on inside covers.**

 POSSIBLE ADVERSE REACTIONS OR SIDE EFFECTS

SYMPTOMS	WHAT TO DO
Life-threatening: None expected.	
Common: Dry mouth, constipation, difficult urination.	Continue. Call doctor when convenient.
Infrequent: • Confusion; dizziness; drowsiness; headache; sleep disturbance such as nightmares, frequent waking; rash; pain in eyes; nausea; vomiting; rapid heartbeat.	Discontinue. Call doctor right away.
• Insomnia, blurred vision, diminished sex drive, decreased sweating.	Continue. Call doctor when convenient.
Rare: None expected.	

 WARNINGS & PRECAUTIONS

Don't take if:
- You are allergic to any anticholinergic.
- You have trouble with stomach bloating.
- You have difficulty emptying your bladder completely.
- You have narrow-angle glaucoma.
- You have severe ulcerative colitis.

Before you start, consult your doctor:
- If you have open-angle glaucoma.
- If you have angina.
- If you have chronic bronchitis or asthma.
- If you have liver disease.
- If you have hiatal hernia.
- If you have enlarged prostate.
- If you have myasthenia gravis.
- If you have peptic ulcer.
- If you will have surgery within 2 months, including dental surgery, requiring general or spinal anesthesia.

Over age 60:
Adverse reactions and side effects may be more frequent and severe than in younger persons.

Pregnancy:
Studies inconclusive on harm to unborn child. Animal studies show fetal abnormalities. Decide with your doctor whether drug benefits justify risk to unborn child.

Breast-feeding:
Drug passes into milk and decreases milk flow. Avoid drug or discontinue nursing until you finish medicine. Consult doctor for advice on maintaining milk supply.

Infants & children:
Use only under medical supervision.

Prolonged use:
Chronic constipation, possible fecal impaction. Consult doctor immediately.

Skin & sunlight:
No problems expected.

Driving, piloting or hazardous work:
Use disqualifies you for piloting aircraft. Otherwise, no problems expected.

Discontinuing:
May be unnecessary to finish medicine. Follow doctor's instructions.

Others:
Heatstroke more likely if you become overheated during exertion.

 POSSIBLE INTERACTION WITH OTHER DRUGS

GENERIC NAME OR DRUG CLASS	COMBINED EFFECT
Amantadine	Increased glycopyrrolate effect.
Anticholinergics (other)	Increased glycopyrrolate effect.
Antidepressants (tricyclics)	Increased glycopyrrolate effect.
Cortisone drugs	Increased internal-eye pressure.
Haloperidol	Increased internal-eye pressure.
MAO inhibitors	Increased glycopyrrolate effect.
Meperidine	Increased glycopyrrolate effect.
Methylphenidate	Increased glycopyrrolate effect.
Molindone	Increased anticholinergic effect.
Orphenadrine	Increased glycopyrrolate effect.
Phenothiazines	Increased glycopyrrolate effect.
Pilocarpine	Increased glycopyrrolate effect. Loss of pilocarpine effect in glaucoma treatment.

Potassium chloride tabs	Increased side effects of potassium tablets.
Retocunazole	Decreased absorption of both.
Vitamin C	Increased glycopyrrolate effect. Avoid large doses of vitamin C.

 POSSIBLE INTERACTION WITH OTHER SUBSTANCES

INTERACTS WITH	COMBINED EFFECT
Alcohol:	None expected.
Beverages:	None expected.
Cocaine:	Excessively rapid heartbeat. Avoid.
Foods:	None expected.
Marijuana:	Drowsiness and dry mouth.
Tobacco:	None expected.

GOLD COMPOUNDS

BRAND AND GENERIC NAMES

AURANOFIN—oral
Aurothioglucose—
  injection
Gold Sodium
  Thiomalate
Myochrysine—
  injection

Myocrisin
Ridaura—oral
SODIUM
  AUROTHIOMALATE
SOLGANAL—
  injection

BASIC INFORMATION

Habit forming? No
Prescription needed? Yes
Available as generic? No
Drug class: Gold compounds

USES

Treatment for rheumatoid arthritis.

DOSAGE & USAGE INFORMATION

How to take:
Swallow with full glass of fluid. Follow prescription directions. Taking too much can cause serious adverse reactions.

When to take:
Once or twice daily, morning and night.

If you forget a dose:
Take as soon as you remember up to 6 hours late, then go back to usual schedule.

What drug does:
Modifies disease activity of rheumatoid arthritis by mechanisms not yet understood.

Time lapse before drug works:
3 to 6 months.

Don't take with:
See Interaction column and consult doctor.

OVERDOSE

SYMPTOMS:
Confusion, delirium, numbness and tingling in feet and hands.
WHAT TO DO:
- Induce vomiting with syrup of ipecac if available.
- Dial 0 (operator) or 911 (emergency) for an ambulance or medical help. Then give first aid immediately.
- See emergency information on inside covers.

POSSIBLE ADVERSE REACTIONS OR SIDE EFFECTS

SYMPTOMS	WHAT TO DO
Life-threatening:	
None expected.	
Common:	
• Itch; rash or hives; sores or white spots in mouth, throat; appetite loss; diarrhea; vomiting; protein in urine; skin rashes; fever.	Discontinue. Call doctor right away.
• Abdominal cramps.	Continue. Call doctor when convenient.
Infrequent:	
• Excessive fatigue; sore tongue, mouth or gums; metallic or odd taste; unusual bleeding or bruising; blood in urine; changes in white blood cells, platelets.	Discontinue. Call doctor right away.
• Hair loss; pain in muscles, bones and joints (with injections).	Continue. Call doctor when convenient.
Rare:	
• Blood in stool, difficult breathing, coughing.	Discontinue. Seek emergency treatment.
• Abdominal pain, jaundice.	Discontinue. Call doctor right away.
• "Pink eye."	Continue. Call doctor when convenient.

WARNINGS & PRECAUTIONS

Don't take if:
- You have history of allergy to gold or other metals.
- You have any blood disorder.
- You have kidney disease.

Before you start, consult your doctor:
- If you are pregnant or may become pregnant.
- If you have lupus erythematosus.
- If you have Schogren's syndrome.
- If you have chronic skin disease.

Over age 60:
Adverse reactions and side effects may be more frequent and severe than in younger persons.

Pregnancy:
Avoid if possible. Animal studies show that gold compounds can cause birth defects.

Breast-feeding:
Drug may filter into milk, causing side effects in infants. Avoid.

Infants & children:
Not recommended. Safety and dosage have not been established.

Prolonged use:
Request periodic laboratory studies of blood counts, urine and liver function. These should be done before use and at least once a month during treatment.

Skin & sunlight:
No problems expected.

Driving, piloting or hazardous work:
Avoid if you have serious adverse reactions or side effects. Otherwise, no problems expected.

Discontinuing:
Don't discontinue without doctor's advice until you complete prescribed dose.

Others:
- Side effects and adverse reactions may appear during treatment or for many months after discontinuing.
- Gold has been shown to cause kidney tumors and kidney cancer in animals given excessive doses.

POSSIBLE INTERACTION WITH OTHER DRUGS

GENERIC NAME OR DRUG CLASS	COMBINED EFFECT
Ketoprofen	Increased likelihood of kidney damage.
Non-steroidal anti-inflammatory drugs	Possible increased likelihood of kidney damage.
Penicillamine	Possible increased likelihood of kidney damage.
Phenytoin	Increased phenytoin blood levels. Phenytoin dosage may require adjustment.
Suprofen	Increased likelihood of kidney damage.

POSSIBLE INTERACTION WITH OTHER SUBSTANCES

INTERACTS WITH	COMBINED EFFECT
Alcohol:	None expected.
Beverages:	None expected.
Cocaine:	None expected.
Foods:	None expected.
Marijuana:	None expected.
Tobacco:	None expected.

GRISEOFULVIN

BRAND NAMES

Fulvicin P/G	Grisactin
Fulvicin U/F	Grisactin Ultra
Grifulvin V	Grisovin-FP
Gris-PEG	grisOwen

BASIC INFORMATION

Habit forming? No
Prescription needed? Yes
Available as generic? Yes
Drug class: Antibiotic (antifungal)

USES

Treatment for fungal infections susceptible to griseofulvin.

DOSAGE & USAGE INFORMATION

How to take:
- Tablet or capsule—Swallow with liquid or food to lessen stomach irritation. If you can't swallow whole, crumble tablet or open capsule and take with liquid or food.
- Liquid—Follow label instructions.

When to take:
With or immediately after meals.

If you forget a dose:
Take as soon as you remember up to 2 hours late. If more than 2 hours, wait for next scheduled dose (don't double this dose).

What drug does:
Prevents fungi from growing and reproducing.

Time lapse before drug works:
2 to 10 days for skin infections. 2 to 4 weeks for infections of fingernails or toenails. Complete cure of either may require several months.

Don't take with:
See Interaction column and consult doctor.

OVERDOSE

SYMPTOMS:
Nausea, vomiting, diarrhea. In sensitive individuals, severe diarrhea may occur without overdosing.
WHAT TO DO:
Overdose unlikely to threaten life. If person takes much larger amount than prescribed, call doctor, poison-control center or hospital emergency room for instructions.

POSSIBLE ADVERSE REACTIONS OR SIDE EFFECTS

SYMPTOMS	WHAT TO DO
Life-threatening: None expected.	
Common: Headache.	Continue. Tell doctor at next visit.
Infrequent: • Confusion; rash, hives, itch; mouth or tongue irritation; soreness; nausea; vomiting; diarrhea; stomach pain.	Discontinue. Call doctor right away.
• Insomnia, tiredness.	Continue. Call doctor when convenient.
Rare: Sore throat, fever, numbness or tingling in hands or feet.	Discontinue. Call doctor right away.

WARNINGS & PRECAUTIONS

Don't take if:
- You are allergic to any antifungal medicine.
- You have liver disease.
- You have porphyria.
- The infection is minor and will respond to less-potent drugs.

Before you start, consult your doctor:
- If you plan to become pregnant within medication period.
- If you have liver disease.
- If you have lupus.

Over age 60:
Adverse reactions and side effects may be more frequent and severe than in younger persons.

Pregnancy:
Risk to unborn child outweighs drug benefits. Don't use.

Breast-feeding:
No problems expected, but consult your doctor.

Infants & children:
Not recommended for children younger than 2.

Prolonged use:
You may become susceptible to infections caused by germs not responsive to griseofulvin.

Skin & sunlight:
May cause rash or intensify sunburn in areas exposed to sun or sunlamp.

Driving, piloting or hazardous work:
- Don't drive if you feel dizzy or have vision problems.
- Don't pilot aircraft.

Discontinuing:
Don't discontinue without doctor's advice until you complete prescribed dose, even though symptoms diminish or disappear.

Others:
Periodic laboratory blood studies and liver- and kidney-function tests recommended.

POSSIBLE INTERACTION WITH OTHER DRUGS

GENERIC NAME OR DRUG CLASS	COMBINED EFFECT
Anticoagulants (oral)	Decreased anticoagulant effect.
Barbiturates	Decreased griseofulvin effect.
Contraceptives (oral)	Decreased contraceptive effect.

POSSIBLE INTERACTION WITH OTHER SUBSTANCES

INTERACTS WITH	COMBINED EFFECT
Alcohol:	Increased intoxication. Possible disulfiram reaction (see Glossary).
Beverages:	None expected.
Cocaine:	None expected.
Foods:	None expected, but foods high in fat will improve drug absorption.
Marijuana:	None expected.
Tobacco:	None expected.

GUAIFENESIN

BRAND NAMES

See complete list of brand names in the *Brand Name Directory,* page 949.

BASIC INFORMATION

Habit forming? No
Prescription needed? No
Available as generic? Yes
Drug class: Cough/cold preparation

 ## USES

Loosens mucus in respiratory passages from allergies and infections (hay fever, cough, cold).

 ## DOSAGE & USAGE INFORMATION

How to take:
- Tablet or capsule—Swallow with liquid. If you can't swallow whole, crumble tablet or open capsule and take with liquid or food.
- Syrup or lozenge—Take as directed on label. Follow with 8 oz. water.

When to take:
As needed, no more often than every 3 hours.

If you forget a dose:
Take as soon as you remember. Wait 3 hours for next dose.

What drug does:
Increases production of watery fluids to thin mucus so it can be coughed out or absorbed.

Time lapse before drug works:
15 to 30 minutes. Regular use for 5 to 7 days necessary for maximum benefit.

Don't take with:
See Interaction column and consult doctor.

 ## OVERDOSE

SYMPTOMS:
Drowsiness, mild weakness, nausea, vomiting.
WHAT TO DO:
Overdose unlikely to threaten life. If person takes much larger amount than prescribed, call doctor, poison-control center or hospital emergency room for instructions.

 ## POSSIBLE ADVERSE REACTIONS OR SIDE EFFECTS

SYMPTOMS	WHAT TO DO
Life-threatening:	
None expected.	
Common:	
None expected.	
Infrequent:	
• Rash, stomach pain, diarrhea, nausea, vomiting.	Discontinue. Call doctor right away.
• Drowsiness.	Continue. Call doctor when convenient.
Rare:	
None expected.	

WARNINGS & PRECAUTIONS

Don't take if:
You are allergic to any cough or cold preparation containing guaifenesin.

Before you start, consult your doctor:
See Interaction column and consult doctor.

Over age 60:
Adverse reactions and side effects may be more frequent and severe than in younger persons. For drug to work, you must drink 8 to 10 glasses of fluid per day.

Pregnancy:
No proven harm to unborn child. Avoid if possible.

Breast-feeding:
No proven problems. Consult your doctor.

Infants & children:
No problems expected.

Prolonged use:
No problems expected.

Skin & sunlight:
No problems expected.

Driving, piloting or hazardous work:
Avoid if you feel drowsy. Otherwise, no problems expected.

Discontinuing:
May be unnecessary to finish medicine. Discontinue when symptoms disappear. If symptoms persist more than 1 week, consult doctor.

Others:
No problems expected.

POSSIBLE INTERACTION WITH OTHER DRUGS

GENERIC NAME OR DRUG CLASS	COMBINED EFFECT
Anticoagulants	Risk of bleeding.

POSSIBLE INTERACTION WITH OTHER SUBSTANCES

INTERACTS WITH	COMBINED EFFECT
Alcohol:	No proven problems.
Beverages:	You must drink 8 to 10 glasses of fluid per day for drug to work.
Cocaine:	No proven problems.
Foods:	None expected.
Marijuana:	No proven problems.
Tobacco:	No proven problems.

GUANABENZ

BRAND NAMES

Wytensin

BASIC INFORMATION

Habit forming? No
Prescription needed? Yes
Available as generic? No
Drug class: Antihypertensive (alpha
adrenergic stimulant)

 USES

Controls, but doesn't cure, high blood pressure.

 DOSAGE & USAGE INFORMATION

How to take:
Tablet—Swallow with liquid or food to lessen
stomach irritation. If you can't swallow whole,
crumble tablet and take with liquid or food.

When to take:
At the same times each day.

If you forget a dose:
Take as soon as you remember up to 2 hours
late. If more than 2 hours, wait for next
scheduled dose (don't double this dose).

What drug does:
● Relaxes muscle cells of small arteries.
● Slows heartbeat.

Time lapse before drug works:
1 hour.

Don't take with:
See Interaction column and consult doctor.

 OVERDOSE

SYMPTOMS:
Severe dizziness, slow heartbeat, pinpoint
pupils, fainting, coma.
WHAT TO DO:
● **Dial 0 (operator) or 911 (emergency) for an**
ambulance or medical help. Then give first
aid immediately.
● **If patient is unconscious and not**
breathing, give mouth-to-mouth breathing.
If there is no heartbeat, use cardiac
massage and mouth-to-mouth breathing
(CPR). Don't try to make patient vomit. If
you can't get help quickly, take patient to
nearest emergency facility.
● **See emergency information on inside**
covers.

 POSSIBLE ADVERSE REACTIONS OR SIDE EFFECTS

SYMPTOMS	WHAT TO DO
Life-threatening: None expected.	
Common:	
● Nervousness, headache, paleness, dry mouth, rapid heartbeat.	Continue. Call doctor when convenient.
● Insomnia.	Continue. Tell doctor at next visit.
Infrequent:	
● Irregular heartbeat, shakiness in hands.	Discontinue. Call doctor right away.
● Dizziness, appetite loss, nausea, vomiting, painful or difficult urination, diminished sex drive.	Continue. Call doctor when convenient.
Rare: None expected.	

WARNINGS & PRECAUTIONS

Don't take if:
You are allergic to any sympathomimetic drug.

Before you start, consult your doctor:
- If you have blood disease.
- If you have heart disease.
- If you have liver disease.
- If you have diabetes or overactive thyroid.
- If you will have surgery within 2 months, including dental surgery, requiring general or spinal anesthesia.

Over age 60:
Adverse reactions and side effects may be more frequent and severe than in younger persons. Hot weather may cause need to reduce dosage.

Pregnancy:
Risk to unborn child outweighs drug benefits. Don't use.

Breast-feeding:
Avoid nursing.

Infants & children:
Not recommended.

Prolonged use:
Side effects tend to diminish. Request uric-acid and kidney-function studies periodically.

Skin & sunlight:
No problems expected.

Driving, piloting or hazardous work:
Avoid if you feel dizzy; otherwise, no problems expected.

Discontinuing:
Don't discontinue without consulting doctor. Dose may require gradual reduction if you have taken drug for a long time. Doses of other drugs may also require adjustment. Abrupt discontinuing may cause anxiety, chest pain, salivation, headache, abdominal cramps, fast heartbeat.

Others:
Stay away from high sodium foods. Lose weight if you are overweight.

POSSIBLE INTERACTION WITH OTHER DRUGS

GENERIC NAME OR DRUG CLASS	COMBINED EFFECT
Antihypertensives (other)	Decreases blood pressure more than either alone. May be beneficial, but requires dosage adjustment.
Brain depressants: Sedatives, sleeping pills, tranquilizers, antidepressants, narcotics	Increased brain depression. Avoid.
Diuretics	Decreases blood pressure more than either alone. May be beneficial, but requires dosage adjustment.
Enalapril	Possible excessive potassium in blood.

POSSIBLE INTERACTION WITH OTHER SUBSTANCES

INTERACTS WITH	COMBINED EFFECT
Alcohol:	Oversedation. Avoid.
Beverages: Caffeine.	Overstimulation. Avoid.
Cocaine:	Overstimulation. Avoid.
Foods: Salt.	Decrease salt intake to increase beneficial effects of guanabenz.
Marijuana:	Overstimulation. Avoid.
Tobacco:	Decreased guanabenz effect.

GUANADREL

BRAND NAMES

Hylorel

BASIC INFORMATION

Habit forming? No
Prescription needed? Yes
Available as generic? No
Drug class: Antihypertensive

 USES

Controls, but doesn't cure, high blood pressure.

 DOSAGE & USAGE INFORMATION

How to take:
Tablet or capsule—Swallow with liquid or food to lessen stomach irritation. If you can't swallow whole, crumble tablet or open capsule and take with liquid or food.

When to take:
At the same time each day.

If you forget a dose:
Take as soon as you remember up to 2 hours late. If more than 2 hours, wait for next scheduled dose (don't double this dose).

What drug does:
Relaxes muscle cells of small arteries.

Time lapse before drug works:
4 to 6 hours. May need to take for lifetime.

Don't take with:
See Interaction column and consult doctor.

 OVERDOSE

SYMPTOMS:
Severe blood-pressure drop; fainting; slow, weak pulse; cold, sweaty skin; loss of consciousness.
WHAT TO DO:
- Dial 0 (operator) or 911 (emergency) for an ambulance or medical help. Then give first aid immediately.
- See emergency information on inside covers.

 POSSIBLE ADVERSE REACTIONS OR SIDE EFFECTS

SYMPTOMS	WHAT TO DO
Life-threatening:	
None expected.	
Common:	
• Diarrhea, more bowel movements, fatigue, weakness.	Continue. Call doctor when convenient.
• Dizziness, headache, lower sex drive.	Continue. Tell doctor at next visit.
• Stuffy nose, dry mouth.	No action necessary.
Infrequent:	
• Rash, blurred vision, drooping eyelids, chest pain or shortness of breath, muscle pain or tremor.	Discontinue. Call doctor right away.
• Nausea or vomiting.	Continue. Call doctor when convenient.
• Impotence, nighttime urination.	Continue. Tell doctor at next visit.
Rare:	
None expected.	

WARNINGS & PRECAUTIONS

Don't take if:
- You are allergic to guanadrel.
- You have taken MAO inhibitors within 2 weeks.

Before you start, consult your doctor:
- If you have stroke or heart disease.
- If you have asthma.
- If you have had kidney disease.
- If you have peptic ulcer or chronic acid indigestion.
- If you will have surgery within 2 months, including dental surgery, requiring general or spinal anesthesia.

Over age 60:
Adverse reactions and side effects may be more frequent and severe than in younger persons. Start with small doses and monitor blood pressure frequently.

Pregnancy:
No proven harm to unborn child. Avoid if possible.

Breast-feeding:
No proven harm to nursing infant. Avoid if possible.

Infants & children:
Not recommended.

Prolonged use:
Due to drug's cumulative effect, dose will require adjustment to prevent wide fluctuations in blood pressure.

Skin & sunlight:
No problems expected.

Driving, piloting or hazardous work:
Don't drive or pilot aircraft until you learn how medicine affects you. Don't work around dangerous machinery. Don't climb ladders or work in high places. Danger increases if you drink alcohol or take medicine affecting alertness and reflexes, such as antihistamines, tranquilizers, sedatives, pain medicine, narcotics and mind-altering drugs.

Discontinuing:
Don't discontinue without consulting doctor. Dose may require gradual reduction if you have taken drug for a long time. Doses of other drugs may also require adjustment.

Others:
Hot weather further lowers blood pressure, particularly in patients over 60.

POSSIBLE INTERACTION WITH OTHER DRUGS

GENERIC NAME OR DRUG CLASS	COMBINED EFFECT
Antidepressants (tricyclic)	Decreased effect of guanadrel.
Antihypertensives (other)	Increased effect of guanadrel.
Beta blockers	Increased likelihood of dizziness and fainting.
CNS depressants: Anticonvulsants, antihistamines, muscle relaxants, narcotics, sedatives, tranquilizers.	Decreased effect of guanadrel.
Diuretics	Increased likelihood of dizziness and fainting.
Enalapril	Possible excessive potassium in blood.
MAO inhibitors	Severe high blood pressure. Avoid.
Phenothiazines	Decreased effect of guanadrel.
Rauwolfia alkaloids	Increased likelihood of dizziness and fainting.
Sympathomimetics	Decreased effect of guanadrel.

POSSIBLE INTERACTION WITH OTHER SUBSTANCES

INTERACTS WITH	COMBINED EFFECT
Alcohol:	Decreased effect of guanadrel. Avoid.
Beverages: Caffeine.	Decreased effect of guanadrel.
Cocaine:	Higher blood pressure. Avoid.
Foods:	No problems expected.
Marijuana:	Higher blood pressure. Avoid.
Tobacco:	Higher blood pressure. Avoid.

GUANETHIDINE

BRAND NAMES

Apo-Guanethidine   Ismelin
Esimil   Ismelin-Esidrix

BASIC INFORMATION

Habit forming? No
Prescription needed? Yes
Available as generic? Yes
Drug class: Antihypertensive

 ## USES

Reduces high blood pressure.

 ## DOSAGE & USAGE INFORMATION

How to take:
Tablet or capsule—Swallow with liquid. If you can't swallow tablet or capsule whole, crumble or open and take with liquid or food.

When to take:
At the same time each day.

If you forget a dose:
Take as soon as you remember up to 2 hours late. If more than 2 hours, wait for next scheduled dose (don't double this dose).

What drug does:
Displaces norepinephrine—hormone necessary to maintain small blood-vessel tone. Blood vessels relax and high blood pressure drops.

Time lapse before drug works:
Regular use for several weeks may be necessary to determine effectiveness.

Don't take with:
- Non-prescription drugs containing alcohol without consulting doctor.
- See Interaction column and consult doctor.

 ## OVERDOSE

SYMPTOMS:
Severe blood-pressure drop; fainting; slow, weak pulse; cold, sweaty skin; loss of consciousness.
WHAT TO DO:
- **Dial 0 (operator) or 911 (emergency) for an ambulance or medical help. Then give first aid immediately.**
- **See emergency information on inside covers.**

 ## POSSIBLE ADVERSE REACTIONS OR SIDE EFFECTS

SYMPTOMS	WHAT TO DO
Life-threatening:	
None expected.	
Common:	
• Unusually slow heartbeat.	Discontinue. Call doctor right away.
• Diarrhea; more bowel movements; swollen feet, legs; fatigue, weakness.	Continue. Call doctor when convenient.
• Dizziness, headache, lower sex drive.	Continue. Tell doctor at next visit.
• Stuffy nose, dry mouth.	No action necessary.
Infrequent:	
• Rash, blurred vision, drooping eyelids, chest pain or shortness of breath, muscle pain or tremor.	Discontinue. Call doctor right away.
• Nausea or vomiting.	Continue. Call doctor when convenient.
• Impotence, nighttime urination.	Continue. Tell doctor at next visit.
Rare:	
None expected.	

 ## WARNINGS & PRECAUTIONS

Don't take if:
- You are allergic to guanethidine.
- You have taken MAO inhibitors within 2 weeks.

Before you start, consult your doctor:
- If you have had stroke or heart disease.
- If you have asthma.
- If you have had kidney disease.
- If you have peptic ulcer or chronic acid indigestion.
- If you will have surgery within 2 months, including dental surgery, requiring general or spinal anesthesia.

Over age 60:
Adverse reactions and side effects may be more frequent and severe than in younger persons. Start with small doses and monitor blood pressure frequently.

Pregnancy:
No proven harm to unborn child. Avoid if possible.

Breast-feeding:
No proven harm to nursing infant. Avoid if possible.

Infants & children:
Not recommended.

Prolonged use:
Due to drug's cumulative effect, dose will require adjustment to prevent wide fluctuations in blood pressure.

Skin & sunlight:
No problems expected.

Driving, piloting or hazardous work:
Don't drive or pilot aircraft until you learn how medicine affects you. Don't work around dangerous machinery. Don't climb ladders or work in high places. Danger increases if you drink alcohol or take medicine affecting alertness and reflexes, such as antihistamines, tranquilizers, sedatives, pain medicine, narcotics and mind-altering drugs.

Discontinuing:
Don't discontinue without consulting doctor. Dose may require gradual reduction if you have taken drug for a long time. Doses of other drugs may also require adjustment.

Others:
Hot weather further lowers blood pressure.

 POSSIBLE INTERACTION WITH OTHER DRUGS

GENERIC NAME OR DRUG CLASS	COMBINED EFFECT
Amphetamines	Decreased guanethidine effect.
Antidepressants (tricyclic)	Decreased guanethidine effect.
Antihistamines	Decreased guanethidine effect.
Contraceptives (oral)	Decreased guanethidine effect.
Digitalis preparations	Slower heartbeat.
Diuretics (thiazide)	Increased guanethidine effect.
Enalapril	Possible excessive potassium in blood.
Indapamide	Possible increased effects of both drugs. When monitored carefully, combination may be beneficial in controlling hypertension.
Minoxidil	Dosage adjustments may be necessary to keep blood pressure at proper level.

Pentoxifylline	Increased antihypertensive effect.
Rauwolfia alkaloids	Increased guanethidine effect.

 POSSIBLE INTERACTION WITH OTHER SUBSTANCES

INTERACTS WITH	COMBINED EFFECT
Alcohol:	Use caution. Decreases blood pressure.
Beverages: Carbonated drinks.	Use sparingly. Sodium content increases blood pressure.
Cocaine:	Raises blood pressure. Avoid.
Foods: Spicy or acid foods.	Avoid if subject to indigestion or peptic ulcer.
Marijuana:	Excessively low blood pressure. Avoid.
Tobacco:	Possible blood-pressure rise. Avoid.

GUANETHIDINE & HYDROCHLOROTHIAZIDE

BRAND NAMES

Esimil

BASIC INFORMATION

Habit forming? No
Prescription needed? Yes
Available as generic? No
Drug class: Antihypertensive-diuretic

USES

- Controls, but doesn't cure, high blood pressure.
- Reduces fluid retention (edema).

DOSAGE & USAGE INFORMATION

How to take:
Tablet or capsule—Swallow with liquid. If you can't swallow whole, crumble tablet or open capsule and take with liquid or food.

When to take:
At the same time each day.

If you forget a dose:
Take as soon as you remember up to 2 hours late. If more than 2 hours, wait for next scheduled dose (don't double this dose).

What drug does:
- Forces sodium and water secretion, reducing body fluid.
- Displaces norepinephrine—hormone necessary to maintain small blood-vessel tone. Blood vessels relax and high blood pressure drops.

Time lapse before drug works:
Regular use for several weeks may be necessary to determine effectiveness.

Continued next column

OVERDOSE

SYMPTOMS:
Cramps, weakness, drowsiness, weak pulse, severe blood-pressure drop, fainting, cold and sweaty skin, loss of consciousness, coma.
WHAT TO DO:
- **Dial 0 (operator) or 911 (emergency) for an ambulance or medical help. Then give first aid immediately.**
- **See emergency information on inside covers.**

Don't take with:
- Non-prescription drugs containing alcohol without consulting doctor.
- See Interaction column and consult doctor.

POSSIBLE ADVERSE REACTIONS OR SIDE EFFECTS

SYMPTOMS	WHAT TO DO
Life-threatening:	
Chest pain, shortness of breath, irregular heartbeat.	Discontinue. Seek emergency treatment.
Common:	
• Slow heartbeat, swollen feet and ankles, fatigue, weakness.	Discontinue. Call doctor right away.
• Dizziness, headache, stuffy nose, dry mouth, diarrhea, diminished sex drive.	Continue. Call doctor when convenient.
Infrequent:	
• Mood change, rash or hives, blurred vision, drooping eyelids, muscle pain or tremors.	Discontinue. Call doctor right away.
• Increased nighttime urination, abdominal pain, vomiting, nausea, weakness.	Continue. Call doctor when convenient.
• Impotence.	Continue. Tell doctor at next visit.
Rare:	
• Sore throat, jaundice.	Discontinue. Call doctor right away.
• Weight gain or loss.	Continue. Call doctor when convenient.

WARNINGS & PRECAUTIONS

Don't take if:
- You are allergic to any thiazide diuretic drug or guanethidine.
- You have taken MAO inhibitors within 2 weeks.

Before you start, consult your doctor:
- If you are allergic to any sulfa drug.
- If you have gout, asthma, liver, pancreas or kidney disorder, peptic ulcer or chronic acid indigestion.
- If you have had stroke or heart disease.
- If you will have surgery within 2 months, including dental surgery, requiring general or spinal anesthesia.

Over age 60:
Adverse reactions and side effects may be more frequent and severe than in younger persons, especially dizziness and excessive potassium loss.

Pregnancy:
Risk to unborn child outweighs drug benefits. Don't use.

Breast-feeding:
Drug passes into milk. Avoid drug or discontinue nursing until you finish medicine. Consult doctor for advice on maintaining milk supply.

Infants & children:
Not recommended.

Prolonged use:
Due to drug's cumulative effect, dose will require adjustment to prevent wide fluctuations in blood pressure.

Skin & sunlight:
May cause rash or intensify sunburn in areas exposed to sun or sunlamp.

Driving, piloting or hazardous work:
Don't drive or pilot aircraft until you learn how medicine affects you. Don't work around dangerous machinery. Don't climb ladders or work in high places. Danger increases if you drink alcohol or take medicine affecting alertness and reflexes, such as antihistamines, tranquilizers, sedatives, pain medicine, narcotics and mind-altering drugs.

Discontinuing:
Don't discontinue without consulting doctor. Dose may require gradual reduction if you have taken drug for a long time. Doses of other drugs may also require adjustment.

Others:
- Hot weather and fever may cause dehydration and drop in blood pressure. Dose may require temporary adjustment. Weigh daily and report any unexpected weight decreases to your doctor.
- May cause rise in uric acid, leading to gout.
- May cause blood-sugar rise in diabetics.

 POSSIBLE INTERACTION WITH OTHER DRUGS

GENERIC NAME OR DRUG CLASS	COMBINED EFFECT
Acebutolol	Increased antihypertensive effect. Dosages of both drugs may require adjustments.
Allopurinol	Decreased allopurinol effect.

Amphetamines	Decreased guanethidine effect.
Antidepressants (tricyclic)	Dangerous drop in blood pressure. Avoid combination unless under medical supervision.
Antihistamines	Decreased guanethidine effect.
Barbiturates	Increased hydrochlorothiazide effect.
Cholestyramine	Decreased hydrochlorothiazide effect.
Contraceptives (oral)	Decreased guanethidine effect.
Cortisone drugs	Excessive potassium loss that causes dangerous heart rhythms.
Digitalis preparations	Excessive potassium loss that causes dangerous heart rhythms.
Diuretics (thiazide)	Increased thiazide and guanethidine effect.

Continued page 967

 POSSIBLE INTERACTION WITH OTHER SUBSTANCES

INTERACTS WITH	COMBINED EFFECT
Alcohol:	Use caution. Decreases blood pressure.
Beverages: Carbonated drinks.	Use sparingly. Sodium content increases blood pressure.
Cocaine:	Raises blood pressure. Avoid.
Foods: Spicy or acid foods.	Avoid if subject to indigestion or peptic ulcer.
Licorice.	Excessive potassium loss that causes dangerous heart rhythms.
Marijuana:	Effect on blood pressure unpredictable.
Tobacco:	Possible blood-pressure rise. Avoid.

HALAZEPAM

BRAND NAMES

Paxipam

BASIC INFORMATION

Habit forming? Yes
Prescription needed? Yes
Available as generic? No
Drug class: Tranquilizer (benzodiazepine)

 ## USES

Treatment for nervousness or tension.

 ## DOSAGE & USAGE INFORMATION

How to take:
Tablet or capsule—Swallow with liquid. If you can't swallow whole, crumble tablet or open capsule and take with liquid or food.

When to take:
At the same time each day, according to instructions on prescription label.

If you forget a dose:
Take as soon as you remember up to 2 hours late. If more than 2 hours, wait for next scheduled dose (don't double this dose).

What drug does:
Affects limbic system of brain—part that controls emotions.

Time lapse before drug works:
2 hours. May take 6 weeks for full benefit.

Don't take with:
See Interaction column and consult doctor.

 ## OVERDOSE

SYMPTOMS:
Drowsiness, weakness, tremor, stupor, coma.
WHAT TO DO:
- **Dial 0 (operator) or 911 (emergency) for an ambulance or medical help. Then give first aid immediately.**
- **If patient is unconscious and not breathing, give mouth-to-mouth breathing. If there is no heartbeat, use cardiac massage and mouth-to-mouth breathing (CPR). Don't try to make patient vomit. If you can't get help quickly, take patient to nearest emergency facility.**
- **See emergency information on inside covers.**

 ## POSSIBLE ADVERSE REACTIONS OR SIDE EFFECTS

SYMPTOMS	WHAT TO DO
Life-threatening: None expected.	
Common: Clumsiness, drowsiness, dizziness.	Continue. Call doctor when convenient.
Infrequent:	
• Hallucinations, confusion, depression, irritability, rash, itch, change in vision.	Discontinue. Call doctor right away.
• Constipation or diarrhea, nausea, vomiting, painful or difficult urination.	Continue. Call doctor when convenient.
Rare:	
• Slow heartbeat, difficult breathing.	Discontinue. Seek emergency treatment.
• Mouth, throat ulcers; jaundice.	Discontinue. Call doctor right away.

WARNINGS & PRECAUTIONS

Don't take if:
- You are allergic to any benzodiazepine.
- You have myasthenia gravis.
- You are active or recovering alcoholic.
- Patient is younger than 6 months.

Before you start, consult your doctor:
- If you have liver, kidney or lung disease.
- If you have diabetes, epilepsy or porphyria.

Over age 60:
Adverse reactions and side effects may be more frequent and severe than in younger persons. You need smaller doses for shorter periods of time. May develop agitation, rage or "hangover" effect.

Pregnancy:
Risk to unborn child outweighs drug benefits. Don't use.

Breast-feeding:
Drug passes into milk. Avoid drug or discontinue nursing until you finish medicine. Consult doctor for advice on maintaining milk supply.

Infants & children:
Use only under medical supervision for children older than 6 months.

Prolonged use:
May impair liver function.

Skin & sunlight:
No problems expected.

Driving, piloting or hazardous work:
Don't drive or pilot aircraft until you learn how medicine affects you. Don't work around dangerous machinery. Don't climb ladders or work in high places. Danger increases if you drink alcohol or take medicine affecting alertness and reflexes.

Discontinuing:
Don't discontinue without consulting doctor. Dose may require gradual reduction if you have taken drug for a long time. Doses of other drugs may also require adjustment.

Others:
- Hot weather, heavy exercise and profuse sweat may reduce excretion and cause overdose.
- Blood sugar may rise in diabetics, requiring insulin adjustment.

POSSIBLE INTERACTION WITH OTHER DRUGS

GENERIC NAME OR DRUG CLASS	COMBINED EFFECT
Anticonvulsants	Change in seizure frequency or severity.
Antidepressants	Increased sedative effect of both drugs.
Antihistamines	Increased sedative effect of both drugs.
Antihypertensives	Excessively low blood pressure.
Cimetidine	Excess sedation.
Disulfiram	Increased halazepam effect.
Dronabinol	Increased effects of both drugs. Avoid.
MAO inhibitors	Convulsions, deep sedation, rage.
Molindone	Increased tranquilizer effect.
Narcotics	Increased sedative effect of both drugs.
Sedatives	Increased sedative effect of both drugs.
Sleep inducers	Increased sedative effect of both drugs.
Tranquilizers	Increased sedative effect of both drugs.

POSSIBLE INTERACTION WITH OTHER SUBSTANCES

INTERACTS WITH	COMBINED EFFECT
Alcohol:	Heavy sedation. Avoid.
Beverages:	None expected.
Cocaine:	Decreased halazepam effect.
Foods:	None expected.
Marijuana:	Heavy sedation. Avoid.
Tobacco:	Decreased halazepam effect.

HALOPERIDOL

BRAND NAMES

Apo-Haloperidol	Haldol LA
Haldol	Novoperidol
Haldol Decanoate	Peridol

BASIC INFORMATION

Habit forming? No
Prescription needed? Yes
Available as generic? Yes
Drug class: Tranquilizer (antipsychotic)

 ## USES

Reduces severe anxiety, agitation and psychotic behavior.

 ## DOSAGE & USAGE INFORMATION

How to take:
- Tablet or capsule—Swallow with liquid. If you can't swallow whole, crumble tablet or open capsule and take with liquid or food.
- Drops—Dilute dose in beverage before swallowing.

When to take:
At the same times each day.

If you forget a dose:
Take as soon as you remember up to 2 hours late. If more than 2 hours, wait for next scheduled dose (don't double this dose).

What drug does:
Corrects an imbalance in nerve impulses from brain.

Continued next column

 ## OVERDOSE

SYMPTOMS:
Weak, rapid pulse; shallow, slow breathing; very low blood pressure; convulsions; deep sleep ending in coma.
WHAT TO DO:
- **Dial 0 (operator) or 911 (emergency) for an ambulance or medical help. Then give first aid immediately.**
- **If patient is unconscious and not breathing, give mouth-to-mouth breathing. If there is no heartbeat, use cardiac massage and mouth-to-mouth breathing (CPR). Don't try to make patient vomit. If you can't get help quickly, take patient to nearest emergency facility.**
- **See emergency information on inside covers.**

Time lapse before drug works:
3 weeks to 2 months for maximum benefit.

Don't take with:
- Non-prescription drugs without consulting doctor.
- See Interaction column and consult doctor.

 ## POSSIBLE ADVERSE REACTIONS OR SIDE EFFECTS

SYMPTOMS	WHAT TO DO
Life-threatening: None expected.	
Common:	
• Blurred vision.	Discontinue. Call doctor right away.
• Shuffling, stiffness, jerkiness, shakiness, constipation.	Continue. Call doctor when convenient.
• Dry mouth.	No action necessary.
Infrequent:	
• Rash, circling motions of tongue.	Discontinue. Call doctor right away.
• Dizziness, faintness, drowsiness, difficult urination, decreased sexual ability, nausea or vomiting.	Continue. Call doctor when convenient.
Rare: Sore throat, fever, jaundice.	Discontinue. Call doctor right away.

WARNINGS & PRECAUTIONS

Don't take if:
- You have ever been allergic to haloperidol.
- You are depressed.
- You have Parkinson's disease.
- Patient is younger than 3 years old.

Before you start, consult your doctor:
- If you take sedatives, sleeping pills, tranquilizers, antidepressants, antihistamines, narcotics or mind-altering drugs.
- If you have a history of mental depression.
- If you have had kidney or liver problems.
- If you have diabetes, epilepsy, glaucoma, high blood pressure or heart disease.
- If you drink alcoholic beverages frequently.

Over age 60:
Adverse reactions and side effects may be more frequent and severe than in younger persons.

Pregnancy:
Risk to unborn child outweighs drug benefits. Don't use.

Breast-feeding:
No proven harm to nursing infant. Avoid if possible.

Infants & children:
Not recommended.

Prolonged use:
May develop tardive dyskinesia (involuntary movements of jaws, lips and tongue).

Skin & sunlight:
May cause rash or intensify sunburn in areas exposed to sun or sunlamp.

Driving, piloting or hazardous work:
Don't drive or pilot aircraft until you learn how medicine affects you. Don't work around dangerous machinery. Don't climb ladders or work in high places. Danger increases if you drink alcohol or take medicine affecting alertness and reflexes.

Discontinuing:
Don't discontinue without consulting doctor. Dose may require gradual reduction if you have taken drug for a long time. Doses of other drugs may also require adjustment.

Others:
No problems expected.

POSSIBLE INTERACTION WITH OTHER DRUGS

GENERIC NAME OR DRUG CLASS	COMBINED EFFECT
Anticholinergics	Increased anticholinergic effect. May cause pressure within the eye.
Anticoagulants (oral)	Decreased anticoagulant effect.
Anticonvulsants	Changed seizure pattern.
Antidepressants	Excessive sedation.
Antihistamines	Excessive sedation.
Antihypertensives	May cause severe blood-pressure drop.
Barbiturates	Excessive sedation.
Bethanidine	Decreased bethanidine effect.
Dronabinol	Increased effects of both drugs. Avoid.
Guanethidine	Decreased guanethidine effect.
Levodopa	Decreased levodopa effect.
Methyldopa	Possible psychosis.
Narcotics	Excessive sedation.
Sedatives	Excessive sedation.
Tranquilizers	Excessive sedation.

POSSIBLE INTERACTION WITH OTHER SUBSTANCES

INTERACTS WITH	COMBINED EFFECT
Alcohol:	Excessive sedation and depressed brain function. Avoid.
Beverages:	None expected.
Cocaine:	Decreased effect of haloperidol. Avoid.
Foods:	None expected.
Marijuana:	Occasional use—Increased sedation. Frequent use—Possible toxic psychosis.
Tobacco:	None expected.

HETACILLIN

BRAND NAMES

Versapen   Versapen-K

BASIC INFORMATION

Habit forming? No
Prescription needed? Yes
Available as generic? Yes
Drug class: Antibiotic (penicillin)

 USES

Treatment of bacterial infections that are susceptible to hetacillin.

 DOSAGE & USAGE INFORMATION

How to take:
- Tablets or capsules—Swallow with liquid on an empty stomach 1 hour before or 2 hours after eating.
- Liquid—Take with cold beverage. Liquid form is perishable and effective for only 7 days at room temperature. Effective for 14 days if stored in refrigerator. Don't freeze.

When to take:
Follow instructions on prescription label or side of package. Doses should be evenly spaced. For example, 4 times a day means every 6 hours.

If you forget a dose:
Take as soon as you remember. Continue regular schedule.

What drug does:
Destroys susceptible bacteria. Does not kill viruses.

Time lapse before drug works:
May be several days before medicine affects infection.

Don't take with:
See Interaction column and consult doctor.

 OVERDOSE

SYMPTOMS:
Severe diarrhea, nausea or vomiting.
WHAT TO DO:
Overdose unlikely to threaten life. If person takes much larger amount than prescribed, call doctor, poison-control center or hospital emergency room for instructions.

 POSSIBLE ADVERSE REACTIONS OR SIDE EFFECTS

SYMPTOMS	WHAT TO DO
Life-threatening: Hives, rash, intense itching, faintness soon after a dose (anaphylaxis).	Seek emergency treatment immediately.
Common: Dark or discolored tongue.	Continue. Tell doctor at next visit.
Infrequent: Nausea, vomiting, diarrhea.	Continue. Call doctor when convenient.
Rare: Unexplained bleeding.	Discontinue. Call doctor right away.

WARNINGS & PRECAUTIONS

Don't take if:
You are allergic to hetacillin, cephalosporin antibiotics, other penicillins or penicillamine. Life-threatening reaction may occur.

Before you start, consult your doctor:
If you are allergic to any substance or drug.

Over age 60:
You may have skin reactions, particularly around genitals and anus.

Pregnancy:
Studies inconclusive on harm to unborn child. Animal studies show fetal abnormalities. Decide with your doctor whether drug benefits justify risk to unborn child.

Breast-feeding:
Drug passes into milk. Child may become sensitive to penicillins and have allergic reactions to penicillin drugs. Avoid hetacillin or discontinue nursing until you finish medicine. Consult doctor for advice on maintaining milk supply.

Infants & children:
No problems expected.

Prolonged use:
You may become more susceptible to infections caused by germs not responsive to hetacillin.

Skin & sunlight:
No problems expected.

Driving, piloting or hazardous work:
Usually not dangerous. Most hazardous reactions likely to occur a few minutes after taking hetacillin.

Discontinuing:
Don't discontinue without doctor's advice until you complete prescribed dose, even though symptoms diminish or disappear.

Others:
Urine sugar test for diabetes may show false positive result.

POSSIBLE INTERACTION WITH OTHER DRUGS

GENERIC NAME OR DRUG CLASS	COMBINED EFFECT
Beta-adrenergic blockers	Increased chance of anaphylaxis (see emergency information on inside front cover).
Chloramphenicol	Decreased effect of both drugs.
Erythromycins	Decreased effect of both drugs.
Loperamide	Decreased hetacillin effect.
Paromomycin	Decreased effect of both drugs.
Tetracyclines	Decreased effect of both drugs.
Troleandomycin	Decreased effect of both drugs.

POSSIBLE INTERACTION WITH OTHER SUBSTANCES

INTERACTS WITH	COMBINED EFFECT
Alcohol:	Occasional stomach irritation.
Beverages:	None expected.
Cocaine:	No proven problems.
Foods:	None expected.
Marijuana:	No proven problems.
Tobacco:	None expected.

HEXOBARBITAL

BRAND NAMES

Sombulex

BASIC INFORMATION

Habit forming? Yes
Prescription needed? Yes
Available as generic? Yes
Drug class: Sedative, hypnotic (barbiturate)

 ## USES

- Reduces anxiety or nervous tension (low dose).
- Relieves insomnia (higher bedtime dose).

 ## DOSAGE & USAGE INFORMATION

How to take:
Tablet—Swallow with liquid or food to lessen stomach irritation. If you can't swallow whole, crumble tablet and take with liquid or food.

When to take:
At the same times each day.

If you forget a dose:
Take as soon as you remember up to 2 hours late. If more than 2 hours, wait for next scheduled dose (don't double this dose).

What drug does:
May partially block nerve impulses at nerve-cell connections.

Time lapse before drug works:
60 minutes.

Don't take with:
- Non-prescription drugs without consulting doctor.
- See Interaction column and consult doctor.

 ## OVERDOSE

SYMPTOMS:
Deep sleep, weak pulse, coma.
WHAT TO DO:
- **Dial 0 (operator) or 911 (emergency) for an ambulance or medical help. Then give first aid immediately.**
- **If patient is unconscious and not breathing, give mouth-to-mouth breathing. If there is no heartbeat use cardiac massage and mouth-to-mouth breathing (CPR). Don't try to make patient vomit. If you can't get help quickly, take patient to nearest emergency facility.**
- **See emergency information on inside covers.**

 ## POSSIBLE ADVERSE REACTIONS OR SIDE EFFECTS

SYMPTOMS	WHAT TO DO
Life-threatening: None expected.	
Common: Dizziness, drowsiness, "hangover" effect.	Continue. Call doctor when convenient.
Infrequent:	
• Rash or hives; face, lip swelling; swollen eyelids; sore throat; fever.	Discontinue. Call doctor right away.
• Depression, confusion, slurred speech, diarrhea, nausea, vomiting, joint or muscle pain.	Continue. Call doctor when convenient.
Rare:	
• Agitation, slow heartbeat, difficult breathing, jaundice.	Discontinue. Call doctor right away.
• Unusual bleeding or bruising.	Continue. Call doctor when convenient.

 ## WARNINGS & PRECAUTIONS

Don't take if:
- You are allergic to any barbiturate.
- You have porphyria.

Before you start, consult your doctor:
- If you have epilepsy.
- If you have kidney or liver damage.
- If you have asthma.
- If you have anemia.
- If you have chronic pain.
- If you will have surgery within 2 months, including dental surgery, requiring general or spinal anesthesia.

Over age 60:
Adverse reactions and side effects may be more frequent and severe than in younger persons. Use small doses.

Pregnancy:
Risk to unborn child outweighs drug benefits. Don't use.

Breast-feeding:
Drug passes into milk. Avoid drug or discontinue nursing until you finish medicine. Consult doctor for advice on maintaining milk supply.

Infants & children:
Use only under doctor's supervision.

Prolonged use:
- May cause addiction, anemia, chronic intoxication.
- May lower body temperature, making exposure to cold temperatures hazardous.

Skin & sunlight:
May cause rash or intensify sunburn in areas exposed to sun or sunlamp.

Driving, piloting or hazardous work:
Don't drive or pilot aircraft until you learn how medicine affects you. Don't work around dangerous machinery. Don't climb ladders or work in high places. Danger increases if you drink alcohol or take medicine affecting alertness and reflexes.

Discontinuing:
May be unnecessary to finish medicine. Follow doctor's instructions. If you develop withdrawal symptoms of hallucinations, agitation or sleeplessness after discontinuing, call doctor right away.

Others:
No problems expected.

POSSIBLE INTERACTION WITH OTHER DRUGS

GENERIC NAME OR DRUG CLASS	COMBINED EFFECT
Anticoagulants (oral)	Decreased anticoagulant effect.
Anticonvulsants	Changed seizure patterns.
Antidepressants (tricyclics)	Decreased antidepressant effect. Possible dangerous oversedation.
Antidiabetics (oral)	Increased hexobarbital effect.
Antihistamines	Dangerous sedation. Avoid.
Anti-inflammatory drugs (non-steroidal)	Decreased anti-inflammatory effect.
Aspirin	Decreased aspirin effect.
Beta-adrenergic blockers	Decreased effect of beta-adrenergic blocker.
Contraceptives (oral)	Decreased contraceptive effect.
Cortisone drugs	Decreased cortisone effect.

Digitoxin	Decreased digitoxin effect.
Doxycycline	Decreased doxycycline effect.
Dronabinol	Increased effects of both drugs. Avoid.
Griseofulvin	Decreased griseofulvin effect.
Indapamide	Increased indapamide effect.
MAO inhibitors	Increased hexobarbital effect.
Mind-altering drugs	Dangerous sedation. Avoid.
Narcotics	Dangerous sedation. Avoid.
Pain relievers	Dangerous sedation. Avoid.
Sedatives	Dangerous sedation. Avoid.
Sleep inducers	Dangerous sedation. Avoid.
Tranquilizers	Dangerous sedation. Avoid.
Valproic acid	Increased hexobarbital effect.

POSSIBLE INTERACTION WITH OTHER SUBSTANCES

INTERACTS WITH	COMBINED EFFECT
Alcohol:	Possible fatal oversedation. Avoid.
Beverages:	None expected.
Cocaine:	Decreased hexobarbital effect.
Foods:	None expected.
Marijuana:	Excessive sedation. Avoid.
Tobacco:	None expected.

HYDRALAZINE

BRAND NAMES

Apresoline
Dralzine
H-H-R
Hydralazide
Rolazine

Ser-Ap-Es
Serpasil-Apresoline
Unipes
Uniserp

BASIC INFORMATION

Habit forming? No
Prescription needed? Yes
Available as generic? Yes
Drug class: Antihypertensive

 USES

Treatment for high blood pressure and
congestive heart failure.

 DOSAGE & USAGE INFORMATION

How to take:
Tablet or capsule—Swallow with liquid. If you
can't swallow whole, crumble tablet or open
capsule and take with liquid or food.

When to take:
At the same time each day.

If you forget a dose:
Take as soon as you remember up to 2 hours
late. If more than 2 hours, wait for next
scheduled dose (don't double this dose).

What drug does:
Relaxes and expands blood-vessel walls,
lowering blood pressure.

Continued next column

 OVERDOSE

SYMPTOMS:
**Rapid and weak heartbeat, fainting, extreme
weakness, cold and sweaty skin.**
WHAT TO DO:
- **Dial 0 (operator) or 911 (emergency) for an
  ambulance or medical help. Then give first
  aid immediately.**
- **If patient is unconscious and not
  breathing, give mouth-to-mouth breathing.
  If there is no heartbeat, use cardiac
  massage and mouth-to-mouth breathing
  (CPR). Don't try to make patient vomit. If
  you can't get help quickly, take patient to
  nearest emergency facility.**
- **See emergency information on inside
  covers.**

Time lapse before drug works:
Regular use for several weeks may be
necessary to determine drug's effectiveness.

Don't take with:
- Non-prescription drugs containing alcohol
  without consulting doctor.
- See Interaction column and consult doctor.

 POSSIBLE ADVERSE REACTIONS OR SIDE EFFECTS

SYMPTOMS	WHAT TO DO
Life-threatening: None expected.	
Common:	
• Nausea or vomiting, rapid or irregular heartbeat.	Discontinue. Call doctor right away.
• Headache, diarrhea, appetite loss, painful or difficult urination.	Continue. Tell doctor at next visit.
Infrequent:	
• Hives or rash, flushed face, sore throat, fever, chest pain, swelling of lymph gland.	Discontinue. Call doctor right away.
• Confusion, dizziness, joint pain, general discomfort or weakness.	Continue. Call doctor when convenient.
• Watery eyes and irritation, constipation.	Continue. Tell doctor at next visit.
Rare: Jaundice.	Discontinue. Call doctor right away.

WARNINGS & PRECAUTIONS

Don't take if:
- You are allergic to hydralazine.
- You have history of coronary-artery disease or rheumatic heart disease.

Before you start, consult your doctor:
- If you feel pain in chest, neck or arms on physical exertion.
- If you have had lupus.
- If you have had a stroke.
- If you have had kidney disease or impaired kidney function.
- If you will have surgery within 2 months, including dental surgery, requiring general or spinal anesthesia.

Over age 60:
Adverse reactions and side effects may be more frequent and severe than in younger persons.

Pregnancy:
Risk to unborn child outweighs drug benefits. Don't use.

Breast-feeding:
Drug filters into milk. May harm child. Avoid.

Infants & children:
Not recommended.

Prolonged use:
- May cause lupus (arthritis-like illness).
- Possible psychosis.
- May cause numbness, tingling in hands or feet.

Skin & sunlight:
No problems expected.

Driving, piloting or hazardous work:
Don't drive or pilot aircraft until you learn how medicine affects you. Don't work around dangerous machinery. Don't climb ladders or work in high places. Danger increases if you drink alcohol or take medicine affecting alertness and reflexes, such as antihistamines, tranquilizers, sedatives, pain medicine, narcotics and mind-altering drugs.

Discontinuing:
Don't discontinue without doctor's advice until you complete prescribed dose, even though symptoms diminish or disappear.

Others:
Vitamin B-6 diet supplement may be advisable. Consult doctor.

POSSIBLE INTERACTION WITH OTHER DRUGS

GENERIC NAME OR DRUG CLASS	COMBINED EFFECT
Albuterol	Decreased hydralazine effect.
Amphetamines	Decreased hydralazine effect.
Antidepressants (tricyclic)	Increased hydralazine effect.
Antihypertensives (other)	Increased antihypertensive effect.
Diuretics (oral)	Increased effects of both drugs. When monitored carefully, combination may be beneficial in controlling hypertension.
Enalapril	Possible excessive potassium in blood.
MAO inhibitors	Increased hydralazine effect.
Pentoxifylline	Increased antihypertensive effect.

POSSIBLE INTERACTION WITH OTHER SUBSTANCES

INTERACTS WITH	COMBINED EFFECT
Alcohol:	May lower blood pressure excessively. Use extreme caution.
Beverages:	None expected.
Cocaine:	Dangerous blood-pressure rise. Avoid.
Foods:	Increased hydralazine absorption.
Marijuana:	Weakness on standing.
Tobacco:	Possible angina attacks.

HYDRALAZINE & HYDROCHLOROTHIAZIDE

BRAND NAMES

Apresazide	Apresoline-Esidrix
Apresodez	Hydral

BASIC INFORMATION

Habit forming? No
Prescription needed? Yes
Available as generic? Yes
Drug class: Antihypertensive-diuretic

 ## USES

- Controls, but doesn't cure, high blood pressure.
- Reduces fluid retention (edema).

 ## DOSAGE & USAGE INFORMATION

How to take:
Tablet or capsule—Swallow with liquid. If you can't swallow whole, crumble tablet or open capsule and take with liquid or food.

When to take:
At the same time each day.

If you forget a dose:
Take as soon as you remember up to 2 hours late. If more than 2 hours, wait for next scheduled dose (don't double this dose).

What drug does:
- Forces sodium and water excretion, reducing body fluid.
- Relaxes and expands blood-vessel walls, lowering blood pressure.

Continued next column

 ## OVERDOSE

SYMPTOMS:
Cramps, drowsiness, weak pulse, rapid and weak heartbeat, fainting, extreme weakness, cold and sweaty skin, coma.
WHAT TO DO:
- **Dial 0 (operator) or 911 (emergency) for an ambulance or medical help. Then give first aid immediately.**
- **If patient is unconscious and not breathing, give mouth-to-mouth breathing. If there is no heartbeat, use cardiac massage and mouth-to-mouth breathing (CPR). Don't try to make patient vomit. If you can't get help quickly, take patient to nearest emergency facility.**
- **See emergency information on inside covers.**

- Reduced body fluid and relaxed arteries lower blood pressure.

Time lapse before drug works:
Regular use for several weeks may be necessary to determine drug's effectiveness.

Don't take with:
- Non-prescription drugs containing alcohol without consulting doctor.
- See Interaction column and consult doctor.

 ## POSSIBLE ADVERSE REACTIONS OR SIDE EFFECTS

SYMPTOMS	WHAT TO DO
Life-threatening:	
Chest pain, irregular and fast heartbeat, weak pulse.	Discontinue. Seek emergency treatment.
Common:	
• Nausea, vomiting.	Discontinue. Call doctor right away.
• Headache, diarrhea, appetite loss, frequent urination, dry mouth, thirst.	Continue. Call doctor when convenient.
Infrequent:	
• Rash; black, bloody or tarry stool; red or flushed face; sore throat, fever, mouth sores; constipation; lymph glands swelling; blurred vision.	Discontinue. Call doctor right away.
• Dizziness, confusion, watery eyes, joint pain, weight gain or loss.	Continue. Call doctor when convenient.
Rare:	
Jaundice.	Discontinue. Call doctor right away.

 ## WARNINGS & PRECAUTIONS

Don't take if:
- You are allergic to hydralazine or any thiazide diuretic drug.
- You have history of coronary-artery disease or rheumatic heart disease.

Before you start, consult your doctor:
- If you feel pain in chest, neck or arms on physical exertion.
- If you are allergic to any sulfa drug.
- If you have had lupus or a stroke.
- If you have gout, liver, pancreas or kidney disorder.

- If you will have surgery within 2 months, including dental surgery, requiring general or spinal anesthesia.

Over age 60:
Adverse reactions and side effects may be more frequent and severe than in younger persons, especially dizziness and excessive potassium loss.

Pregnancy:
Risk to unborn child outweighs drug benefits. Don't use.

Breast-feeding:
Drug passes into milk. Avoid drug or discontinue nursing until you finish medicine. Consult doctor for advice on maintaining milk supply.

Infants & children:
Not recommended.

Prolonged use:
- May cause lupus (arthritis-like illness).
- Possible psychosis.
- May cause numbness, tingling in hands or feet.

Skin & sunlight:
May cause rash or intensify sunburn in areas exposed to sun or sunlamp.

Driving, piloting or hazardous work:
Don't drive or pilot aircraft until you learn how medicine affects you. Don't work around dangerous machinery. Don't climb ladders or work in high places. Danger increases if you drink alcohol or take medicine affecting alertness and reflexes, such as antihistamines, tranquilizers, sedatives, pain medicine, narcotics and mind-altering drugs.

Discontinuing:
Don't discontinue without consulting doctor's advice until you complete prescribed dose, even though symptoms diminish or disappear.

Others:
- Vitamin B-6 diet supplement may be advisable. Consult doctor.
- Hot weather and fever may cause dehydration and drop in blood pressure. Dose may require temporary adjustment. Weigh daily and report any unexpected weight decreases to your doctor.
- May cause rise in uric acid, leading to gout.
- May cause blood-sugar rise in diabetics.

POSSIBLE INTERACTION WITH OTHER DRUGS

GENERIC NAME OR DRUG CLASS	COMBINED EFFECT
Acebutolol	Decreased antihypertensive effect of acebutolol.
Allopurinol	Decreased allopurinol effect.
Amphetamines	Decreased hydralazine effect.
Antidepressants (tricyclic)	Dangerous drop in blood pressure. Avoid combination unless under medical supervision.
Antihypertensives (other)	Increased antihypertensive effect.
Barbiturates	Increased hydrochlorothiazide effect.
Cholestyramine	Decreased hydrochlorothiazide effect.
Cortisone drugs	Excessive potassium loss that causes dangerous heart rhythms.
Digitalis preparations	Excessive potassium loss that causes dangerous heart rhythms.
Diuretics (oral)	Increased effect of both drugs. When monitored carefully, combination may be beneficial in controlling hypertension.
Indapamide	Increased diuretic effect.

Continued page 967

POSSIBLE INTERACTION WITH OTHER SUBSTANCES

INTERACTS WITH	COMBINED EFFECT
Alcohol:	May lower blood pressure excessively. Use extreme caution.
Beverages:	None expected.
Cocaine:	Dangerous blood-pressure rise. Avoid.
Foods: Licorice.	Excessive potassium loss that causes dangerous heart rhythms.
Marijuana:	Weakness on standing. May increase blood pressure.
Tobacco:	Possible angina attacks.

HYDROCHLOROTHIAZIDE

BRAND NAMES

See complete list of brand names in the *Brand Name Directory*, page 950.

BASIC INFORMATION

Habit forming? No
Prescription needed? Yes
Available as generic? Yes
Drug class: Antihypertensive, diuretic (thiazide)

 USES

- Controls, but doesn't cure, high blood pressure.
- Reduces fluid retention (edema).

 DOSAGE & USAGE INFORMATION

How to take:
Tablet or capsule—Swallow with liquid. If you can't swallow whole, crumble tablet or open capsule and take with liquid or food.

When to take:
At the same time each day.

If you forget a dose:
Take as soon as you remember up to 2 hours late. If more than 2 hours, wait for next scheduled dose (don't double this dose).

What drug does:
- Forces sodium and water excretion, reducing body fluid.
- Relaxes muscle cells of small arteries.
- Reduced body fluid and relaxed arteries lower blood pressure.

Time lapse before drug works:
4 to 6 hours. May require several weeks to lower blood pressure.

Continued next column

 OVERDOSE

SYMPTOMS:
Cramps, weakness, drowsiness, weak pulse, coma.
WHAT TO DO:
- **Dial 0 (operator) or 911 (emergency) for an ambulance or medical help. Then give first aid immediately.**
- **See emergency information on inside covers.**

Don't take with:
- See Interaction column and consult doctor.
- Non-prescription drugs without consulting doctor.

 POSSIBLE ADVERSE REACTIONS OR SIDE EFFECTS

SYMPTOMS	WHAT TO DO
Life-threatening: None expected.	
Common: None expected.	
Infrequent:	
• Blurred vision, severe abdominal pain, nausea, vomiting, irregular heartbeat, weak pulse.	Discontinue. Call doctor right away.
• Dizziness, mood change, headache, weakness, tiredness, weight changes.	Continue. Call doctor when convenient.
• Dry mouth, thirst.	Continue. Tell doctor at next visit.
Rare:	
• Rash or hives.	Discontinue. Seek emergency treatment.
• Sore throat, fever, jaundice.	Discontinue. Call doctor right away.

 WARNINGS & PRECAUTIONS

Don't take if:
You are allergic to any thiazide diuretic drug.

Before you start, consult your doctor:
- If you are allergic to any sulfa drug.
- If you have gout.
- If you have liver, pancreas or kidney disorder.

Over age 60:
Adverse reactions and side effects may be more frequent and severe than in younger persons, especially dizziness and excessive potassium loss.

Pregnancy:
Risk to unborn child outweighs drug benefits. Don't use.

Breast-feeding:
Drug passes into milk. Avoid drug or discontinue nursing.

Infants & children:
No problems expected.

Prolonged use:
You may need medicine to treat high blood pressure for the rest of your life.

Skin & sunlight:
May cause rash or intensify sunburn in areas exposed to sun or sunlamp.

Driving, piloting or hazardous work:
Don't drive or pilot aircraft until you learn how medicine affects you. Don't work around dangerous machinery. Don't climb ladders or work in high places. Danger increases if you drink alcohol or take medicine affecting alertness and reflexes, such as antihistamines, tranquilizers, sedatives, pain medicine, narcotics and mind-altering drugs.

Discontinuing:
Don't discontinue without medical advice.

Others:
- Hot weather and fever may cause dehydration and drop in blood pressure. Dose may require temporary adjustment. Weigh daily and report any unexpected weight decreases to your doctor.
- May cause rise in uric acid, leading to gout.
- May cause blood-sugar rise in diabetics.

 ## POSSIBLE INTERACTION WITH OTHER DRUGS

GENERIC NAME OR DRUG CLASS	COMBINED EFFECT
Acebutolol	Increased antihypertensive effect. Dosages of both drugs may require adjustments.
Allopurinol	Decreased allopurinol effect.
Amiodarone	Increased risk of heartbeat irregularity due to low potassium.
Antidepressants (tricyclic)	Dangerous drop in blood pressure. Avoid combination unless under medical supervision.
Barbiturates	Increased hydrochlorothiazide effect.
Calcium supplements	Increased calcium in blood.
Cholestyramine	Decreased hydrochlorothiazide effect.
Cortisone drugs	Excessive potassium loss that causes dangerous heart rhythms.

Digitalis preparations	Excessive potassium loss that causes dangerous heart rhythms.
Diuretics (thiazide)	Increased effect of other thiazide diuretics.
Indapamide	Increased diuretic effect.
Labetolol	Increased antihypertensive effects.
Lithium	Increased effect of lithium.
MAO inhibitors	Increased hydrochlorothiazide effect.
Nitrates	Excessive blood-pressure drop.
Oxprenolol	Increased antihypertensive effect. Dosages of both drugs may require adjustments.
Potassium supplements	Decreased potassium effect.
Probenecid	Decreased probenecid effect.

 ## POSSIBLE INTERACTION WITH OTHER SUBSTANCES

INTERACTS WITH	COMBINED EFFECT
Alcohol:	Dangerous blood-pressure drop.
Beverages:	None expected.
Cocaine:	None expected.
Foods: Licorice.	Excessive potassium loss that causes dangerous heart rhythms.
Marijuana:	May increase blood pressure.
Tobacco:	None expected.

HYDROCORTISONE (CORTISOL)

BRAND NAMES

See complete list of brand names in the *Brand Name Directory,* page 950.

BASIC INFORMATION

Habit forming? No
Prescription needed? Yes
Available as generic? Yes
Drug class: Cortisone drug (adrenal corticosteroid)

USES

- Reduces inflammation caused by many different medical problems.
- Treatment for some allergic diseases, blood disorders, kidney diseases, asthma and emphysema.
- Replaces corticosteroid deficiencies.

DOSAGE & USAGE INFORMATION

How to take:
- Tablet or liquid—Swallow with liquid or food to lessen stomach irritation. If you can't swallow whole, crumble tablet.
- Other forms—Follow label instructions.

When to take:
At the same times each day. Take once-a-day or once-every-other-day doses in mornings.

If you forget a dose:
- Several-doses-per-day prescription—Take as soon as you remember up to 2 hours late. If more than 2 hours, wait for next scheduled dose (don't double this dose).
- Once-a-day dose or less—Wait for next dose. Double this dose.

What drug does:
Decreases inflammatory responses.

Time lapse before drug works:
2 to 4 days.

Don't take with:
See Interaction column and consult doctor.

OVERDOSE

SYMPTOMS:
Headache, convulsions, heart failure.
WHAT TO DO:
- **Dial 0 (operator) or 911 (emergency) for an ambulance or medical help. Then give first aid immediately.**
- **See emergency information on inside covers.**

POSSIBLE ADVERSE REACTIONS OR SIDE EFFECTS

SYMPTOMS	WHAT TO DO
Life-threatening: None expected.	
Common: Acne, poor wound healing, thirst, indigestion, nausea, vomiting.	Continue. Call doctor when convenient.
Infrequent:	
• Black, bloody or tarry stools.	Discontinue. Seek emergency treatment.
• Blurred vision; halos around lights; sore throat; fever; muscle cramps; swollen legs, feet.	Discontinue. Call doctor right away.
• Mood change, insomnia, restlessness, frequent urination, weight gain, round face, fatigue, weakness, TB recurrence, irregular menstrual periods.	Continue. Tell doctor at next visit.
Rare:	
• Irregular heartbeat.	Discontinue. Seek emergency treatment.
• Rash.	Discontinue. Call doctor right away.

WARNINGS & PRECAUTIONS

Don't take if:
- You are allergic to any cortisone drug.
- You have tuberculosis or fungus infection.
- You have herpes infection of eyes, lips or genitals.

Before you start, consult your doctor:
- If you have had tuberculosis.
- If you have congestive heart failure.
- If you have diabetes.
- If you have peptic ulcer.
- If you have glaucoma.
- If you have underactive thyroid.
- If you have high blood pressure.
- If you have myasthenia gravis.
- If you have blood clots in legs or lungs.

Over age 60:
Adverse reactions and side effects may be more frequent and severe than in younger persons. Likely to aggravate edema, diabetes or ulcers. Likely to cause cataracts and osteoporosis (softening of the bones).

Pregnancy:
Risk to unborn child outweighs drug benefits.
Don't use.

Breast-feeding:
Drug passes into milk. Avoid drug or
discontinue nursing until you finish medicine.
Consult doctor for advice on maintaining milk
supply.

Infants & children:
Use only under medical supervision.

Prolonged use:
- Retards growth in children.
- Possible glaucoma, cataracts, diabetes,
  fragile bones and thin skin.
- Functional dependence.

Skin & sunlight:
No problems expected.

Driving, piloting or hazardous work:
No problems expected.

Discontinuing:
- Don't discontinue without doctor's advice until
  you complete prescribed dose, even though
  symptoms diminish or disappear.
- Drug affects your response to surgery, illness,
  injury or stress for 2 years after discontinuing.
  Tell anyone who takes medical care of you
  about the drug for up to 2 years after
  discontinuing.

Others:
Avoid immunizations if possible.

POSSIBLE INTERACTION WITH OTHER DRUGS

GENERIC NAME OR DRUG CLASS	COMBINED EFFECT
Amphoterecin B	Potassium depletion.
Anticholinergics	Possible glaucoma.
Anticoagulants (oral)	Decreased anticoagulant effect.
Anticonvulsants (hydantoin)	Decreased hydrocortisone effect.
Antidiabetics (oral)	Decreased antidiabetic effect.
Antihistamines	Decreased hydrocortisone effect.
Aspirin	Increased hydrocortisone effect.
Barbiturates	Decreased hydrocortisone effect. Oversedation.
Beta-adrenergic blockers	Decreased hydrocortisone effect.
Chloral hydrate	Decreased hydrocortisone effect.
Chlorthalidone	Potassium depletion.
Cholinergics	Decreased cholinergic effect.
Contraceptives (oral)	Increased hydrocortisone effect.
Digitalis preparations	Dangerous potassium depletion. Possible digitalis toxicity.
Diuretics (thiazide)	Potassium depletion.
Ephedrine	Decreased hydrocortisone effect.
Estrogens	Increased hydrocortisone effect.
Ethacrynic acid	Potassium depletion.
Furosemide	Potassium depletion.
Glutethimide	Decreased hydrocortisone effect.
Indapamide	Possible excessive potassium loss, causing dangerous heartbeat irregularity.
Indomethacin	Increased hydrocortisone effect.
Insulin	Decreased insulin effect.
Isoniazid	Decreased isoniazid effect.
Oxyphenbutazone	Possible ulcers.
Phenylbutazone	Possible ulcers.
Potassium supplements	Decreased potassium effect.
Rifampin	Decreased hydrocortisone effect.
Sympathomimetics	Possible glaucoma.

POSSIBLE INTERACTION WITH OTHER SUBSTANCES

INTERACTS WITH	COMBINED EFFECT
Alcohol:	Risk of stomach ulcers.
Beverages:	No proven problems.
Cocaine:	Overstimulation. Avoid.
Foods:	No proven problems.
Marijuana:	Decreased immunity.
Tobacco:	Increased hydrocortisone effect. Possible toxicity.

HYDROFLUMETHIAZIDE

BRAND NAMES

Diucardin	Saluron
Hydro-Fluserpine	Salutensin
#1 & #2	

BASIC INFORMATION

Habit forming? No
Prescription needed? Yes
Available as generic? Yes
Drug class: Antihypertensive, diuretic
(thiazide)

USES

- Controls, but doesn't cure, high blood pressure.
- Reduces fluid retention (edema) caused by conditions such as heart disorders and liver disease.

DOSAGE & USAGE INFORMATION

How to take:
Tablet or capsule—Swallow with liquid. If you can't swallow whole, crumble tablet or open capsule and take with liquid or food.
Don't exceed dose.

When to take:
At the same time each day.

If you forget a dose:
Take as soon as you remember up to 2 hours late. If more than 2 hours, wait for next scheduled dose (don't double this dose).

What drug does:
- Forces sodium and water excretion, reducing body fluid.
- Relaxes muscle cells of small arteries.
- Reduced body fluid and relaxed arteries lower blood pressure.

Continued next column

OVERDOSE

SYMPTOMS:
Cramps, weakness, drowsiness, weak pulse, coma.
WHAT TO DO:
- Dial 0 (operator) or 911 (emergency) for an ambulance or medical help. Then give first aid immediately.
- See emergency information on inside covers.

Time lapse before drug works:
4 to 6 hours. May require several weeks to lower blood pressure.

Don't take with:
- See Interaction column and consult doctor.
- Non-prescription drugs without consulting doctor.

POSSIBLE ADVERSE REACTIONS OR SIDE EFFECTS

SYMPTOMS	WHAT TO DO
Life-threatening: None expected.	
Common: None expected.	
Infrequent:	
• Blurred vision, severe abdominal pain, nausea, vomiting, irregular heartbeat, weak pulse.	Discontinue. Call doctor right away.
• Dizziness, mood change, headache, weakness, tiredness, weight changes.	Continue. Call doctor when convenient.
• Dry mouth, thirst.	Continue. Tell doctor at next visit.
Rare:	
• Rash or hives.	Discontinue. Seek emergency treatment.
• Sore throat, fever, jaundice.	Discontinue. Call doctor right away.

WARNINGS & PRECAUTIONS

Don't take if:
You are allergic to any thiazide diuretic drug.

Before you start, consult your doctor:
- If you are allergic to any sulfa drug.
- If you have gout.
- If you have liver, pancreas or kidney disorder.

Over age 60:
Adverse reactions and side effects may be more frequent and severe than in younger persons, especially dizziness and excessive potassium loss.

Pregnancy:
Risk to unborn child outweighs drug benefits. Don't use.

Breast-feeding:
Drug passes into milk. Avoid drug or discontinue nursing.

Infants & children:
No problems expected.

Prolonged use:
You may need medicine to treat high blood pressure for the rest of your life.

Skin & sunlight:
May cause rash or intensify sunburn in areas exposed to sun or sunlamp.

Driving, piloting or hazardous work:
Don't drive or pilot aircraft until you learn how medicine affects you. Don't work around dangerous machinery. Don't climb ladders or work in high places. Danger increases if you drink alcohol or take medicine affecting alertness and reflexes, such as antihistamines, tranquilizers, sedatives, pain medicine, narcotics and mind-altering drugs.

Discontinuing:
Don't discontinue without medical advice.

Others:
- Hot weather and fever may cause dehydration and drop in blood pressure. Dose may require temporary adjustment. Weigh daily and report any unexpected weight decreases to your doctor.
- May cause rise in uric acid, leading to gout.
- May cause blood-sugar rise in diabetics.

POSSIBLE INTERACTION WITH OTHER DRUGS

GENERIC NAME OR DRUG CLASS	COMBINED EFFECT
Acebutolol	Increased antihypertensive effect. Dosages of both drugs may require adjustments.
Allopurinol	Decreased allopurinol effect.
Amiodarone	Increased risk of heartbeat irregularity due to low potassium.
Antidepressants (tricyclic)	Dangerous drop in blood pressure. Avoid combination unless under medical supervision.
Barbiturates	Increased hydroflumethiazide effect.
Calcium supplements	Increased calcium in blood.
Cholestyramine	Decreased hydroflumethiazide effect.
Cortisone drugs	Excessive potassium loss that causes dangerous heart rhythms.

Digitalis preparations	Excessive potassium loss that causes dangerous heart rhythms.
Diuretics (thiazide)	Increased effect of other thiazide diuretics.
Indapamide	Increased diuretic effect.
Labetolol	Increased antihypertensive effects.
Lithium	Increased effect of lithium.
MAO inhibitors	Increased hydroflumethiazide effect.
Nitrates	Excessive blood-pressure drop.
Oxprenolol	Increased antihypertensive effect. Dosages of both drugs may require adjustments.
Potassium supplements	Decreased potassium effect.
Probenecid	Decreased probenecid effect.

POSSIBLE INTERACTION WITH OTHER SUBSTANCES

INTERACTS WITH	COMBINED EFFECT
Alcohol:	Dangerous blood-pressure drop.
Beverages:	None expected.
Cocaine:	None expected.
Foods: Licorice.	Excessive potassium loss that causes dangerous heart rhythms.
Marijuana:	May increase blood pressure.
Tobacco:	None expected.

HYDROXYCHLOROQUINE

BRAND NAMES

Plaquenil

BASIC INFORMATION

Habit forming? No
Prescription needed? Yes
Available as generic? Yes
Drug class: Antiprotozoal, antirheumatic

USES

- Treatment for protozoal infections, such as malaria and amebiasis.
- Treatment for some forms of arthritis and lupus.

DOSAGE & USAGE INFORMATION

How to take:
Tablet—Swallow with food or milk to lessen stomach irritation.

When to take:
- Depends on condition. Is adjusted during treatment.
- Malaria prevention—Begin taking medicine 2 weeks before entering areas with malaria.

If you forget a dose:
- 1 or more doses a day—Take as soon as you remember up to 2 hours late. If more than 2 hours, wait for next scheduled dose (don't double this dose).
- 1 dose weekly—Take as soon as possible, then return to regular dosing schedule.

What drug does:
- Inhibits parasite multiplication.
- Decreases inflammatory response in diseased joint.

Time lapse before drug works:
1 to 2 hours.

Don't take with:
See Interaction column and consult doctor.

OVERDOSE

SYMPTOMS:
Severe breathing difficulty, drowsiness, faintness.
WHAT TO DO:
- **Dial 0 (operator) or 911 (emergency) for an ambulance or medical help. Then give first aid immediately.**
- **See emergency information on inside covers.**

POSSIBLE ADVERSE REACTIONS OR SIDE EFFECTS

SYMPTOMS	WHAT TO DO
Life-threatening:	
None expected.	
Common:	
Headache.	Continue. Tell doctor at next visit.
Infrequent:	
• Blurred vision, changes in vision.	Discontinue. Call doctor right away.
• Rash or itch, diarrhea, nausea, vomiting.	Continue. Call doctor when convenient.
Rare:	
• Mood or mental changes, seizures, sore throat, fever, unusual bleeding or bruising, muscle weakness.	Discontinue. Call doctor right away.
• Ringing or buzzing in ears, hearing loss.	Continue. Call doctor when convenient.

WARNINGS & PRECAUTIONS

Don't take if:
You are allergic to chloroquine or hydroxychloroquine.

Before you start, consult your doctor:
- If you plan to become pregnant within the medication period.
- If you have blood disease.
- If you have eye or vision problems.
- If you have a G6PD deficiency.
- If you have liver disease.
- If you have nerve or brain disease (including seizure disorders).
- If you have porphyria.
- If you have psoriasis.
- If you have stomach or intestinal disease.
- If you drink more than 3 oz. of alcohol daily.

Over age 60:
Adverse reactions and side effects may be more frequent and severe than in younger persons.

Pregnancy:
Risk to unborn child outweighs drug benefits. Don't use.

Breast-feeding:
Drug passes into milk. Avoid drug or discontinue nursing.

Infants & children:
Not recommended. Dangerous.

Prolonged use:
Permanent damage to the retina (back part of the eye) or nerve deafness.

Skin & sunlight:
May cause rash or intensify sunburn in areas exposed to sun or sunlamp.

Driving, piloting or hazardous work:
Don't drive or pilot aircraft until you learn how medicine affects you. Don't work around dangerous machinery. Don't climb ladders or work in high places. Danger increases if you drink alcohol or take medicine affecting alertness and reflexes.

Discontinuing:
Don't discontinue without doctor's advice until you complete prescribed dose, even though symptoms diminish or disappear.

Others:
- Periodic physical and blood examinations recommended.
- If you are in a malaria area for a long time, you may need to change to another preventive drug every 2 years.

POSSIBLE INTERACTION WITH OTHER DRUGS

GENERIC NAME OR DRUG CLASS	COMBINED EFFECT
Estrogens	Possible liver toxicity.
Gold compounds	Risk of severe rash and itch.
Oxyphenbutazone	Risk of severe rash and itch.
Penicillamine	Possible blood or kidney toxicity.
Phenylbutazone	Risk of severe rash and itch.
Sulfa drugs	Possible liver toxicity.

POSSIBLE INTERACTION WITH OTHER SUBSTANCES

INTERACTS WITH	COMBINED EFFECT
Alcohol:	Possible liver toxicity. Avoid.
Beverages:	None expected.
Cocaine:	None expected.
Foods:	None expected.
Marijuana:	None expected.
Tobacco:	None expected.

HYDROXYZINE

BRAND NAMES

See complete list of brand names in the *Brand Name Directory,* page 950.

BASIC INFORMATION

Habit forming? No
Prescription needed? Yes
Available as generic? Yes
Drug class: Tranquilizer, antihistamine

 USES

- Treatment for anxiety, tension and agitation.
- Relieves itching from allergic reactions.

 DOSAGE & USAGE INFORMATION

How to take:
- Tablet or capsule—Swallow with liquid. If you can't swallow whole, crumble tablet or open capsule and take with liquid or food.
- Liquid—If desired, dilute dose in beverage before swallowing.

When to take:
At the same times each day.

If you forget a dose:
Take as soon as you remember up to 2 hours late. If more than 2 hours, wait for next scheduled dose (don't double this dose).

What drug does:
May reduce activity in areas of the brain that influence emotional stability.

Time lapse before drug works:
15 to 30 minutes.

Don't take with:
- Non-prescription drugs without consulting doctor.
- See Interaction column and consult doctor.

 OVERDOSE

SYMPTOMS:
Drowsiness, unsteadiness, agitation, purposeless movements, tremor, convulsions.
WHAT TO DO:
- **Dial 0 (operator) or 911 (emergency) for an ambulance or medical help. Then give first aid immediately.**
- **See emergency information on inside covers.**

 POSSIBLE ADVERSE REACTIONS OR SIDE EFFECTS

SYMPTOMS	WHAT TO DO
Life-threatening:	
None expected.	
Common:	
Drowsiness, difficult urination, dry mouth.	Continue. Tell doctor at next visit.
Infrequent:	
Headache.	Continue. Tell doctor at next visit.
Rare:	
Tremor, rash.	Discontinue. Call doctor right away.

HYDROXYZINE

WARNINGS & PRECAUTIONS

Don't take if:
You are allergic to any antihistamine.

Before you start, consult your doctor:
- If you have epilepsy.
- If you will have surgery within 2 months, including dental surgery, requiring general or spinal anesthesia.

Over age 60:
Adverse reactions and side effects may be more frequent and severe than in younger persons. Drug likely to increase urination difficulty caused by enlarged prostate gland.

Pregnancy:
Studies inconclusive on harm to unborn child. Animal studies show fetal abnormalities. Decide with your doctor whether drug benefits justify risk to unborn child.

Breast-feeding:
Drug passes into milk. Avoid drug or discontinue nursing until you finish medicine. Consult doctor for advice on maintaining milk supply.

Infants & children:
Use only under medical supervision.

Prolonged use:
Tolerance develops and reduces effectiveness.

Skin & sunlight:
No problems expected.

Driving, piloting or hazardous work:
Don't drive or pilot aircraft until you learn how medicine affects you. Don't work around dangerous machinery. Don't climb ladders or work in high places. Danger increases if you drink alcohol or take medicine affecting alertness and reflexes, such as antihistamines, tranquilizers, sedatives, pain medicine, narcotics and mind-altering drugs.

Discontinuing:
Don't discontinue without consulting doctor. Dose may require gradual reduction if you have taken drug for a long time. Doses of other drugs may also require adjustment.

Others:
No problems expected.

POSSIBLE INTERACTION WITH OTHER DRUGS

GENERIC NAME OR DRUG CLASS	COMBINED EFFECT
Anticoagulants (oral)	Increased anticoagulant effect.
Anticonvulsants (hydantoin)	Decreased anticonvulsant effect.
Antidepressants (tricyclic)	Increased effect of both drugs.
Antihistamines	Increased hydroxyzine effect.
Dronabinol	Increased effects of both drugs. Avoid.
Molindone	Increased tranquilizer and antihistamine effect.
Narcotics	Increased effect of both drugs.
Pain relievers	Increased effect of both drugs.
Sedatives	Increased effect of both drugs.
Sleep inducers	Increased effect of both drugs.
Tranquilizers	Increased effect of both drugs.

POSSIBLE INTERACTION WITH OTHER SUBSTANCES

INTERACTS WITH	COMBINED EFFECT
Alcohol:	Increased sedation and intoxication. Use with caution.
Beverages: Caffeine drinks.	Decreased tranquilizer effect of hydroxyzine.
Cocaine:	Decreased hydroxyzine effect. Avoid.
Foods:	None expected.
Marijuana:	None expected.
Tobacco:	None expected.

HYOSCYAMINE

BRAND NAMES

See complete list of brand names in the *Brand Name Directory*, page 950.

BASIC INFORMATION

Habit forming? No
Prescription needed?
  Low strength: No
  High strength: Yes
Available as generic? Yes
Drug class: Antispasmodic, anticholinergic

 ## USES

Reduces spasms of digestive system, bladder and urethra.

 ## DOSAGE & USAGE INFORMATION

How to take:
- Tablet or liquid—Swallow with liquid or food to lessen stomach irritation.
- Extended-release tablets or capsules—Swallow each dose whole. If you take regular tablets, you may chew or crush them.
- Drops—Dilute dose in beverage before swallowing.

When to take:
30 minutes before meals (unless directed otherwise by doctor).

If you forget a dose:
Take as soon as you remember up to 2 hours late. If more than 2 hours, wait for next scheduled dose (don't double this dose).

What drug does:
Blocks nerve impulses at parasympathetic nerve endings, preventing muscle contractions and gland secretions of organs involved.

Continued next column

 ## OVERDOSE

SYMPTOMS:
Dilated pupils, rapid pulse and breathing, dizziness, fever, hallucinations, confusion, slurred speech, agitation, flushed face, convulsions, coma.
WHAT TO DO:
- Dial 0 (operator) or 911 (emergency) for an ambulance or medical help. Then give first aid immediately.
- See emergency information on inside covers.

Time lapse before drug works:
15 to 30 minutes.

Don't take with:
See Interaction column and consult doctor.

 ## POSSIBLE ADVERSE REACTIONS OR SIDE EFFECTS

SYMPTOMS	WHAT TO DO
Life-threatening: None expected.	
Common:	
● Confusion, delirium, rapid heartbeat.	Discontinue. Call doctor right away.
● Nausea, vomiting, decreased sweating.	Continue. Call doctor when convenient.
● Constipation.	Continue. Tell doctor at next visit.
● Dryness in ears, nose, throat.	No action necessary.
Infrequent: Headache, painful or difficult urination.	Continue. Call doctor when convenient.
Rare: Rash or hives, pain, blurred vision.	Discontinue. Call doctor right away.

WARNINGS & PRECAUTIONS

Don't take if:
- You are allergic to any anticholinergic.
- You have trouble with stomach bloating.
- You have difficulty emptying your bladder completely.
- You have narrow-angle glaucoma.
- You have severe ulcerative colitis.

Before you start, consult your doctor:
- If you have open-angle glaucoma.
- If you have angina.
- If you have chronic bronchitis or asthma.
- If you have hiatal hernia.
- If you have liver disease.
- If you have enlarged prostate.
- If you have myasthenia gravis.
- If you have peptic ulcer.
- If you will have surgery within 2 months, including dental surgery, requiring general or spinal anesthesia.

Over age 60:
Adverse reactions and side effects may be more frequent and severe than in younger persons.

Pregnancy:
Studies inconclusive on harm to unborn child. Animal studies show fetal abnormalities. Decide with your doctor whether drug benefits justify risk to unborn child.

Breast-feeding:
Drug passes into milk and decreases milk flow. Avoid drug or discontinue nursing until you finish medicine. Consult doctor for advice on maintaining milk supply.

Infants & children:
Use only under medical supervision.

Prolonged use:
Chronic constipation, possible fecal impaction. Consult doctor immediately.

Skin & sunlight:
No problems expected.

Driving, piloting or hazardous work:
Use disqualifies you for piloting aircraft. Otherwise, no problems expected.

Discontinuing:
May be unnecessary to finish medicine. Follow doctor's instructions.

Others:
No problems expected.

POSSIBLE INTERACTION WITH OTHER DRUGS

GENERIC NAME OR DRUG CLASS	COMBINED EFFECT
Amantadine	Increased hyoscyamine effect.
Anticholinergics (other)	Increased hyoscyamine effect.
Antidepressants (tricyclic)	Increased hyoscyamine effect.
Antihistamines	Increased hyoscyamine effect.
Cortisone drugs	Increased internal-eye pressure.
Haloperidol	Increased internal-eye pressure.
MAO inhibitors	Increased hyoscyamine effect.
Meperidine	Increased hyoscyamine effect.
Methylphenidate	Increased hyoscyamine effect.
Molindone	Increased anticholinergic effect.
Orphenadrine	Increased hyoscyamine effect.
Phenothiazines	Increased hyoscyamine effect.
Pilocarpine	Loss of pilocarpine effect in glaucoma treatment.
Vitamin C	Decreased hyoscyamine effect. Avoid large doses of vitamin C.

POSSIBLE INTERACTION WITH OTHER SUBSTANCES

INTERACTS WITH	COMBINED EFFECT
Alcohol:	None expected.
Beverages:	None expected.
Cocaine:	Excessively rapid heartbeat. Avoid.
Foods:	None expected.
Marijuana:	Drowsiness and dry mouth.
Tobacco:	None expected.

IBUPROFEN

BRAND NAMES

Advil	Haltran
Amersol	Medipren
Apo-Ibuprofen	Motrin
Apsifen	Novoprofen
Apsifen-F	Nuprin
Brufen	Rufen

BASIC INFORMATION

Habit forming? No
Prescription needed? No
Available as generic? Yes
Drug class: Anti-inflammatory (non-steroid)

 ## USES

- Treatment for joint pain, stiffness, inflammation and swelling of arthritis and gout.
- Pain reliever.
- Treatment for dysmenorrhea (painful or difficult menstruation).

 ## DOSAGE & USAGE INFORMATION

How to take:
Tablet—Swallow with liquid or food to lessen stomach irritation. If you can't swallow whole, crumble tablet and take with liquid or food.

When to take:
At the same times each day.

If you forget a dose:
Take as soon as you remember up to 2 hours late. If more than 2 hours, wait for next scheduled dose (don't double this dose).

What drug does:
Reduces tissue concentration of prostaglandins (hormones which produce inflammation and pain).

Continued next column

 ## OVERDOSE

SYMPTOMS:
Confusion, agitation, incoherence, convulsions, possible hemorrhage from stomach or intestine, coma.
WHAT TO DO:
- Dial 0 (operator) or 911 (emergency) for an ambulance or medical help. Then give first aid immediately.
- See emergency information on inside covers.

Time lapse before drug works:
Begins in 4 to 24 hours. May require 3 weeks regular use for maximum benefit.

Don't take with:
See Interaction column and consult doctor.

 ## POSSIBLE ADVERSE REACTIONS OR SIDE EFFECTS

SYMPTOMS	WHAT TO DO
Life-threatening: None expected.	
Common:	
• Dizziness, nausea, pain.	Continue. Call doctor when convenient.
• Headache.	Continue. Tell doctor at next visit.
Infrequent: Depression; drowsiness; ringing in ears; swollen feet, legs; constipation or diarrhea; vomiting.	Continue. Call doctor when convenient.
Rare:	
• Convulsions; confusion; rash, hives or itch; blurred vision; black, bloody, tarry stool; difficult breathing; tightness in chest; rapid heartbeat; unusual bleeding or bruising; blood in urine; jaundice.	Discontinue. Call doctor right away.
• Frequent, painful, or difficult urination; fatigue; weakness.	Continue. Call doctor when convenient.

WARNINGS & PRECAUTIONS

Don't take if:
- You are allergic to aspirin or any non-steroid, anti-inflammatory drug.
- You have gastritis, peptic ulcer, enteritis, ileitis, ulcerative colitis, asthma, heart failure, high blood pressure or bleeding problems.
- Patient is younger than 15.

Before you start, consult your doctor:
- If you have epilepsy.
- If you have Parkinson's disease.
- If you have been mentally ill.
- If you have had kidney disease or impaired kidney function.

Over age 60:
Adverse reactions and side effects may be more frequent and severe than in younger persons.

Pregnancy:
Studies inconclusive on harm to unborn child. Decide with your doctor whether drug benefits justify risk to unborn child.

Breast-feeding:
May harm child. Avoid.

Infants & children:
Not recommended for anyone younger than 15. Use only under medical supervision.

Prolonged use:
- Eye damage.
- Reduced hearing.
- Sore throat, fever.
- Weight gain.

Skin & sunlight:
No problems expected.

Driving, piloting or hazardous work:
Don't drive or pilot aircraft until you learn how medicine affects you. Don't work around dangerous machinery. Don't climb ladders or work in high places. Danger increases if you drink alcohol or take medicine affecting alertness and reflexes, such as antihistamines, tranquilizers, sedatives, pain medicine, narcotics and mind-altering drugs.

Discontinuing:
Don't discontinue without consulting doctor. Dose may require gradual reduction if you have taken drug for a long time. Doses of other drugs may also require adjustment.

Others:
No problems expected.

POSSIBLE INTERACTION WITH OTHER DRUGS

GENERIC NAME OR DRUG CLASS	COMBINED EFFECT
Acebutolol	Decreased antihypertensive effect of acebutolol.
Anticoagulants (oral)	Increased risk of bleeding.
Aspirin	Increased risk of stomach ulcer.
Cortisone drugs	Increased risk of stomach ulcer.
Furosemide	Decreased diuretic effect of furosemide.
Gold compounds	Possible increased likelihood of kidney damage.
Ketoprofen	Increased possibility of internal bleeding.
Minoxidil	Decreased minoxidil effect.
Oxprenolol	Decreased antihypertensive effect of oxprenolol.
Oxyphenbutazone	Possible stomach ulcer.
Phenylbutazone	Possible stomach ulcer.
Probenecid	Increased ibuprofen effect.
Thyroid hormones	Rapid heartbeat, blood-pressure rise.

POSSIBLE INTERACTION WITH OTHER SUBSTANCES

INTERACTS WITH	COMBINED EFFECT
Alcohol:	Possible stomach ulcer or bleeding.
Beverages:	None expected.
Cocaine:	None expected.
Foods:	None expected.
Marijuana:	Increased pain relief from ibuprofen.
Tobacco:	None expected.

INDAPAMIDE

BRAND NAMES

Lozide   Lozol

BASIC INFORMATION

Habit forming? No
Prescription needed? Yes
Available as generic? No
Drug class: Antihypertensive, diuretic

 USES

- Controls, but doesn't cure, high blood pressure.
- Reduces fluid retention (edema) caused by conditions such as heart disorders.

 DOSAGE & USAGE INFORMATION

How to take:
Tablet or capsule—Swallow with liquid or food to lessen stomach irritation.

When to take:
At the same times each day, usually at bedtime.

If you forget a dose:
Bedtime dose—If you forget your once-a-day bedtime dose, don't take it more than 3 hours late. Never double dose.

What drug does:
Forces kidney to excrete more sodium and causes excess salt and fluid to be excreted.

Time lapse before drug works:
2 hours for effect to begin. May require 1 to 4 weeks for full effects.

Continued next column

 OVERDOSE

SYMPTOMS:
Nausea, vomiting, diarrhea, very dry mouth, thirst, weakness, excessive fatigue, very rapid heart rate, weak pulse.
WHAT TO DO:
- **Dial 0 (operator) or 911 (emergency) for an ambulance or medical help. Then give first aid immediately.**
- **If patient is unconscious and not breathing, give mouth-to-mouth breathing. If there is no heartbeat, use cardiac massage and mouth-to-mouth breathing (CPR). Don't try to make patient vomit. If you can't get help quickly, take patient to nearest emergency facility.**
- **See emergency information on inside covers.**

Don't take with:
See Interaction column and consult doctor.

 POSSIBLE ADVERSE REACTIONS OR SIDE EFFECTS

SYMPTOMS	WHAT TO DO
Life-threatening:	
None expected.	
Common:	
• Excessive tiredness or weakness, muscle cramps.	Discontinue. Call doctor right away.
• Frequent urination.	Continue. Tell doctor at next visit.
Infrequent:	
• Gouty arthritis.	Discontinue. Call doctor right away.
• Insomnia, mood change, dizziness on changing position, headache, excessive thirst, diarrhea, appetite loss, nausea.	Continue. Call doctor when convenient.
Rare:	
• Weak pulse.	Discontinue. Seek emergency treatment.
• Itching, rash, hives, irregular heartbeat.	Discontinue. Call doctor right away.

 WARNINGS & PRECAUTIONS

Don't take if:
- You are allergic to indapamide or to any sulfa drug or thiazide diuretic (see index).
- You have severe kidney disease.

Before you start, consult your doctor:
- If you have severe kidney disease.
- If you have diabetes.
- If you have gout.
- If you have liver disease.
- If you will have surgery within 2 months, including dental surgery, requiring general or spinal anesthesia.
- If you have lupus erythematosus.
- If you are pregnant or plan to become pregnant.

Over age 60:
Adverse reactions and side effects may be more frequent and severe than in younger persons.

Pregnancy:
Risk to unborn child outweighs drug benefits. Don't use.

Breast-feeding:
Unknown effect on child. Consult doctor.

Infants & children:
Use only under close medical supervision.

Prolonged use:
Request laboratory studies for blood sugar, BUN, uric acid and serum electrolytes (potassium and sodium).

Skin & sunlight:
May cause rash or intensify sunburn in areas exposed to sun or sunlamp.

Driving, piloting or hazardous work:
Don't drive or pilot aircraft until you learn how medicine affects you. Don't work around dangerous machinery. Don't climb ladders or work in high places. Danger increases if you drink alcohol or take medicine affecting alertness and reflexes, such as antihistamines, tranquilizers, sedatives, pain medicine, narcotics and mind-altering drugs.

Discontinuing:
Don't discontinue without consulting doctor. Dose may require gradual reduction if you have taken drug for a long time. Doses of other drugs may also require adjustment.

Others:
No problems expected.

POSSIBLE INTERACTION WITH OTHER DRUGS

GENERIC NAME OR DRUG CLASS	COMBINED EFFECT
Antihypertensives (other)	Increased antihypertensive effect.
Allopurinol	Decreased allopurinol effect.
Amiodarone	Increased risk of heartbeat irregularity due to low potassium.
Antidepressants (tricyclic)	Dangerous drop in blood pressure.
Barbiturates	Increased indapamide effect.
Calcium supplements	Increased calcium in blood.
Cholestyramine	Decreased indapamide effect.
Cortisone drugs	Excessive potassium loss that may cause dangerous heart rhythms.
Digitalis preparations	Excessive potassium loss that may cause dangerous heart rhythms.
Diuretics (thiazide)	Increased effect of thiazide diuretics.

Enalapril	Possible excessive potassium in blood.
Labetolol	Increased antihypertensive effects.
Lithium	High risk of lithium toxicity.
MAO inhibitors	Increased indapamide effect.
Probenecid	Decreased probenecid effect.

POSSIBLE INTERACTION WITH OTHER SUBSTANCES

INTERACTS WITH	COMBINED EFFECT
Alcohol:	Dangerous blood-pressure drop. Avoid.
Beverages:	No problems expected.
Cocaine:	Reduced effectiveness of indapamide. Avoid.
Foods: Licorice.	Excessive potassium loss that may cause dangerous heart rhythms.
Marijuana:	Reduced effectiveness of indapamide. Avoid.
Tobacco:	Reduced effectiveness of indapamide. Avoid.

INDOMETHACIN

BRAND NAMES

Apo-Indomethacin
Imbrilon
Indocid
Indocid R
Indocid-SR
Indocin

Indocin-SR
Indolar SR
Indo-Lemmon
Indometacin
Novomethacin
Zendole

BASIC INFORMATION

Habit forming? No
Prescription needed? Yes
Available as generic? Yes
Drug class: Anti-inflammatory (non-steroid)

USES

- Treatment for joint pain, stiffness, inflammation and swelling of arthritis and gout.
- Pain reliever.
- Treatment for dysmenorrhea (painful or difficult menstruation).

DOSAGE & USAGE INFORMATION

How to take:
- Tablet or capsule—Swallow with liquid or food to lessen stomach irritation. If you can't swallow whole, crumble tablet or open capsule and take with liquid or food.
- Extended release tablets or capsules—Swallow whole with liquid or food to lessen stomach irritation.

When to take:
At the same times each day.

If you forget a dose:
Take as soon as you remember up to 2 hours late. If more than 2 hours, wait for next scheduled dose (don't double this dose).

Continued next column

OVERDOSE

SYMPTOMS:
Confusion, agitation, incoherence, convulsions, possible hemorrhage from stomach or intestine, coma.
WHAT TO DO:
- Dial 0 (operator) or 911 (emergency) for an ambulance or medical help. Then give first aid immediately.
- See emergency information on inside covers.

What drug does:
Reduces tissue concentration of prostaglandins (hormones which produce inflammation and pain).

Time lapse before drug works:
Begins in 4 to 24 hours. May require 3 weeks regular use for maximum benefit.

Don't take with:
See Interaction column and consult doctor.

POSSIBLE ADVERSE REACTIONS OR SIDE EFFECTS

SYMPTOMS	WHAT TO DO
Life-threatening: None expected.	
Common: • Dizziness, nausea, pain.	Continue. Call doctor when convenient.
• Headache.	Continue. Tell doctor at next visit.
Infrequent: Depression; drowsiness; ringing in ears; constipation or diarrhea; vomiting; swollen feet, legs.	Continue. Call doctor when convenient.
Rare: • Convulsions; confusion; rash, hives or itch; blurred vision; black, bloody, tarry stool; difficult breathing; tightness in chest; rapid heartbeat; unusual bleeding or bruising; blood in urine; jaundice.	Discontinue. Call doctor right away.
• Frequent, painful or difficult urination; fatigue; weakness.	Continue. Call doctor when convenient.

WARNINGS & PRECAUTIONS

Don't take if:
- You are allergic to aspirin or any non-steroid, anti-inflammatory drug.
- You have gastritis, peptic ulcer, enteritis, ileitis, ulcerative colitis, asthma, heart failure, high blood pressure or bleeding problems.
- Patient is younger than 15.

Before you start, consult your doctor:
- If you have epilepsy.
- If you have Parkinson's disease.
- If you have been mentally ill.
- If you have had kidney disease or impaired kidney function.

Over age 60:
Adverse reactions and side effects may be more frequent and severe than in younger persons.

Pregnancy:
Studies inconclusive on harm to unborn child. Decide with your doctor whether drug benefits justify risk to unborn child.

Breast-feeding:
May harm child. Avoid.

Infants & children:
Not recommended for anyone younger than 15. Use only under medical supervision.

Prolonged use:
- Eye damage.
- Reduced hearing.
- Sore throat, fever.
- Weight gain.

Skin & sunlight:
No problems expected.

Driving, piloting or hazardous work:
Don't drive or pilot aircraft until you learn how medicine affects you. Don't work around dangerous machinery. Don't climb ladders or work in high places. Danger increases if you drink alcohol or take medicine affecting alertness and reflexes, such as antihistamines, tranquilizers, sedatives, pain medicine, narcotics and mind-altering drugs.

Discontinuing:
Don't discontinue without consulting doctor. Dose may require gradual reduction if you have taken drug for a long time. Doses of other drugs may also require adjustment.

Others:
No problems expected.

 POSSIBLE INTERACTION WITH OTHER DRUGS

GENERIC NAME OR DRUG CLASS	COMBINED EFFECT
Acebutolol	Decreased antihypertensive effect of acebutolol.
Anticoagulants (oral)	Increased risk of bleeding.
Aspirin	Increased risk of stomach ulcer.
Cortisone drugs	Increased risk of stomach ulcer.
Furosemide	Decreased diuretic effect of furosemide.
Gold compounds	Possible increased likelihood of kidney damage.
Ketoprofen	Increased possibility of internal bleeding.
Lithium	Increased lithium effect.
Minoxidil	Reduced minoxidil effect.
Oxprenolol	Decreased antihypertensive effect of oxprenolol.
Oxyphenbutazone	Possible stomach ulcer.
Phenylbutazone	Possible stomach ulcer.
Probenecid	Increased indomethacin effect.
Thyroid hormones	Rapid heartbeat, blood-pressure rise.

 POSSIBLE INTERACTION WITH OTHER SUBSTANCES

INTERACTS WITH	COMBINED EFFECT
Alcohol:	Possible stomach ulcer or bleeding.
Beverages:	None expected.
Cocaine:	None expected.
Foods:	None expected.
Marijuana:	Increased pain relief from indomethacin.
Tobacco:	None expected.

INSULIN

BRAND NAMES

See complete list of brand names in the *Brand Name Directory,* page 951.

BASIC INFORMATION

Habit forming? No
Prescription needed? No
Available as generic? Yes
Drug class: Antidiabetic

 ## USES

Controls diabetes, a complex metabolic disorder, in which the body does not manufacture insulin.

 ## DOSAGE & USAGE INFORMATION

How to take:
Must be taken by injection under the skin. Use disposable, sterile needles. Rotate injection sites.

When to take:
At the same time each day.

If you forget a dose:
Take as soon as you remember. Wait at least 4 hours for next dose. Resume regular schedule.

What drug does:
Facilitates passage of blood sugar through cell membranes so sugar is usable.

Continued next column

 ## OVERDOSE

SYMPTOMS:
Low blood sugar (hypoglycemia)—Anxiety; chills, cold sweats, pale skin; drowsiness; excess hunger; headache; nausea; nervousness; fast heartbeat; shakiness; unusual tiredness or weakness.
WHAT TO DO:
- Eat some type of sugar immediately, such as orange juice, honey, sugar cubes, crackers, sandwich.
- If patient loses consciousness, give glucagon if you have it and know how to use it.
- Otherwise, dial 0 (operator) or 911 (emergency) for an ambulance or medical help. Then give first aid immediately.
- See emergency information on inside covers.

Time lapse before drug works:
30 minutes to 8 hours, depending on type of insulin used.

Don't take with:
See Interaction column and consult doctor.

 ## POSSIBLE ADVERSE REACTIONS OR SIDE EFFECTS

SYMPTOMS	WHAT TO DO
Life-threatening:	
Hives, rash, intense itching, faintness soon after a dose (anaphylaxis).	Seek emergency treatment immediately.
Common:	
None expected.	
Infrequent:	
• Hives.	Discontinue. Call doctor right away.
• Swelling, redness, itch at injection site.	Continue. Call doctor when convenient.
Rare:	
None expected.	

WARNINGS & PRECAUTIONS

Don't take if:
- Your diagnosis and dose schedule is not established.
- You don't know how to deal with overdose emergencies.

Before you start, consult your doctor:
- If you are allergic to insulin.
- If you take MAO inhibitors.
- If you have liver or kidney disease or low thyroid function.

Over age 60:
Guard against hypoglycemia. Repeated episodes can cause permanent confusion and abnormal behavior.

Pregnancy:
Possible drug benefits outweigh risk to unborn child. Adhere rigidly to diabetes treatment program.

Breast-feeding:
No problems expected.

Infants & children:
Use only under medical supervision.

Prolonged use:
No problems expected.

Skin & sunlight:
No problems expected.

Driving, piloting or hazardous work:
No problems expected after dose is established.

Discontinuing:
Don't discontinue without doctor's advice until you complete prescribed dose, even though symptoms diminish or disappear.

Others:
- Diet and exercise affect how much insulin you need. Work with your doctor to determine accurate dose.
- Notify your doctor if you skip a dose, overeat, have fever or infection.
- Notify doctor if you develop symptoms of high blood sugar: drowsiness, dry skin, orange fruit-like odor to breath, increased urination, appetite loss, unusual thirst.

POSSIBLE INTERACTION WITH OTHER DRUGS

GENERIC NAME OR DRUG CLASS	COMBINED EFFECT
Anticoagulants (oral)	Increased anticoagulant effect.
Anticonvulsants (hydantoin)	Decreased insulin effect.
Antidiabetics (oral)	Increased antibiabetic effect.
Beta-adrenergic blockers	Possible increased difficulty in regulating blood-sugar levels.
Contraceptives (oral)	Decreased insulin effect.
Cortisone drugs	Decreased insulin effect.
Diuretics	Decreased insulin effect.
Furosemide	Decreased insulin effect.
MAO inhibitors	Increased insulin effect.
Oxyphenbutazone	Increased insulin effect.
Phenylbutazone	Increased insulin effect.
Salicylates	Increased insulin effect.
Sulfa drugs	Increased insulin effect.
Tetracyclines	Increased insulin effect.
Thyroid hormones	Decreased insulin effect.

POSSIBLE INTERACTION WITH OTHER SUBSTANCES

INTERACTS WITH	COMBINED EFFECT
Alcohol:	Increased insulin effect. May cause hypoglycemia and brain damage.
Beverages:	None expected.
Cocaine:	May cause brain damage.
Foods:	None expected.
Marijuana:	Possible increase in blood sugar.
Tobacco:	None expected.

IODOQUINOL

BRAND NAMES

Diiodohydroxyquin	Diquinol
Diodoquin	Yodoxin

BASIC INFORMATION

Habit forming? No
Prescription needed? Yes
Available as generic? Yes
Drug class: Antiprotozoal

 ## USES

Treatment for intestinal amebiasis.

 ## DOSAGE & USAGE INFORMATION

How to take:
Tablets—Mix with applesauce or chocolate syrup if unable to swallow tablets.

When to take:
Three times daily after meals for 20 days. Treatment may be repeated after 2 to 3 weeks.

If you forget a dose:
Take as soon as you remember up to 2 hours late. If more than 2 hours, wait for next scheduled dose (don't double this dose).

What drug does:
Kills amoeba (microscopic parasites) in intestinal tract.

Time lapse before drug works:
May require full course of treatment (20 days) to cure.

Don't take with:
See Interaction column and consult doctor.

 ## OVERDOSE

SYMPTOMS:
- **Prolonged dosing at high level may produce blurred vision, muscle pain, eye pain, numbness and tingling in hands or feet.**
- **Single overdosage unlikely to threaten life.**
WHAT TO DO:
If person takes much larger amount than prescribed, call doctor, poison-control center or hospital emergency room for instructions.

 ## POSSIBLE ADVERSE REACTIONS OR SIDE EFFECTS

SYMPTOMS	WHAT TO DO
Life-threatening:	
None expected.	
Common:	
• Diarrhea, nausea, vomiting, stomach pain.	Discontinue. Call doctor right away.
• Dizziness, headache.	Continue. Call doctor when convenient.
Infrequent:	
Clumsiness, rash, hives, itching, blurred vision, muscle pain, numbness or tingling in hands or feet, chills, fever, weakness.	Discontinue. Call doctor right away.
Rare:	
None expected.	

WARNINGS & PRECAUTIONS

Don't take if:
You have kidney or liver disease.

Before you start, consult your doctor:
If you have optic atrophy thyroid disease.

Over age 60:
Adverse reactions and side effects may be more frequent and severe than in younger persons.

Pregnancy:
No proven problems, but avoid if possible.

Breast-feeding:
No proven problems, but avoid if possible. Discontinue nursing until you finish medicine. Consult doctor for advice on maintaining milk supply.

Infants & children:
Not recommended. Safety and dosage has not been established.

Prolonged use:
Not recommended.

Skin & sunlight:
No problems expected.

Driving, piloting or hazardous work:
No problems expected.

Discontinuing:
Don't discontinue without consulting doctor.

Others:
Thyroid tests may be inaccurate for as long as 6 months after discontinuing iodoquinol treatment.

POSSIBLE INTERACTION WITH OTHER DRUGS

GENERIC NAME OR DRUG CLASS	COMBINED EFFECT
None expected.	

POSSIBLE INTERACTION WITH OTHER SUBSTANCES

INTERACTS WITH	COMBINED EFFECT
Alcohol:	None expected.
Beverages:	None expected.
Cocaine:	None expected.
Foods:	Taking with food may decrease gastrointestinal side effects.
Marijuana:	None expected.
Tobacco:	None expected.

IRON-POLYSACCHARIDE

BRAND NAMES

Hytinic   Nu-Iron
Niferex

BASIC INFORMATION

Habit forming? No
Prescription needed?
  With folic acid: Yes
  Without folic acid: No
Available as generic? Yes
Drug class: Mineral supplement (iron)

USES

Treatment for dietary iron deficiency or
iron-deficiency anemia from other causes.

DOSAGE & USAGE INFORMATION

How to take:
Tablet, capsule or liquid—Swallow with liquid or
food to lessen stomach irritation. If you can't
swallow whole, crumble tablet or open capsule
and take with liquid or food. Place medicine far
back on tongue to avoid staining teeth.

When to take:
1 hour before or 2 hours after meals.

If you forget a dose:
Take up to 2 hours late. If more than 2 hours,
wait for next dose (don't double this dose).

What drug does:
Stimulates bone-marrow production of
hemoglobin (red-blood-cell pigment that carries
oxygen to body cells).

Time lapse before drug works:
3 to 7 days. May require 3 weeks for maximum
benefit.

Don't take with:
- Multiple vitamin and mineral supplements.
- See Interaction column and consult doctor.

OVERDOSE

SYMPTOMS:
**Weakness, collapse; pallor, blue lips, hands
and fingernails; weak, rapid heartbeat;
shallow breathing; convulsions; coma.**
WHAT TO DO:
- **Dial 0 (operator) or 911 (emergency) for an
  ambulance or medical help. Then give first
  aid immediately.**
- **See emergency information on inside
  covers.**

POSSIBLE ADVERSE REACTIONS OR SIDE EFFECTS

SYMPTOMS	WHAT TO DO
Life-threatening: Weak, rapid heartbeat.	Seek emergency treatment immediately.
Common: Stained teeth with liquid iron.	No action necessary.
Always: Gray or black stool.	No action necessary.
Infrequent: • Constipation or diarrhea, heartburn, nausea, vomiting.	Discontinue. Call doctor right away.
• Fatigue, weakness.	Continue. Call doctor when convenient.
• Dark urine.	Continue. Tell doctor at next visit.
Rare: • Throat or chest pain on swallowing, pain, cramps, blood in stool.	Discontinue. Call doctor right away.
• Drowsiness.	Continue. Call doctor when convenient.

WARNINGS & PRECAUTIONS

Don't take if:
- You are allergic to any iron supplement.
- You take iron injections.
- Your daily iron intake is high.
- You plan to take this supplement for a long time.
- You have acute hepatitis.
- You have hemosiderosis or hemochromatosis (conditions involving excess iron in body).
- You have hemolytic anemia.

Before you start, consult your doctor:
- If you plan to become pregnant within medication period.
- If you have had stomach surgery.
- If you have had peptic ulcer disease, enteritis or colitis.
- If you have had pancreatitis or hepatitis.

Over age 60:
May cause hemochromatosis (iron storage disease) with bronze skin, liver damage, diabetes, heart problems and impotence.

Pregnancy:
No proven harm to unborn child. Avoid if possible. Take only if your doctor prescribes supplement during last half of pregnancy.

Breast-feeding:
No problems expected. Take only if your doctor confirms you have a dietary deficiency or an iron-deficiency anemia.

Infants & children:
Use only under medical supervision. Overdose common and dangerous. Keep out of children's reach.

Prolonged use:
May cause hemochromatosis (iron storage disease) with bronze skin, liver damage, diabetes, heart problems and impotence.

Skin & sunlight:
No problems expected.

Driving, piloting or hazardous work:
No problems expected.

Discontinuing:
May be unnecessary to finish medicine. Follow doctor's instructions.

Others:
Liquid form stains teeth. Mix with water or juice to lessen the effect. Brush with baking soda or hydrogen peroxide to help remove stain.

POSSIBLE INTERACTION WITH OTHER DRUGS

GENERIC NAME OR DRUG CLASS	COMBINED EFFECT
Allopurinol	Possible excess iron storage in liver.
Antacids	Poor iron absorption.
Calcium supplements	Decreased iron effect.
Chloramphenicol	Decreased effect of iron. Interferes with red-blood-cell and hemoglobin formation.
Cholestyramine	Decreased iron effect.
Iron supplements (other)	Possible excess iron storage in liver.
Penicillamine	Decreased penicillamine effect.
Sulfasalazine	Decreased iron effect.
Tetracyclines	Decreased tetracycline effect. Take iron 3 hours before or 2 hours after taking tetracycline.
Vitamin C	Increased iron effect. Contributes to red-blood-cell and hemoglobin formation.
Vitamin E	Decreased iron effect.

POSSIBLE INTERACTION WITH OTHER SUBSTANCES

INTERACTS WITH	COMBINED EFFECT
Alcohol:	Increased iron absorption. May cause organ damage. Avoid or use in moderation.
Beverages: Milk, tea.	Decreased iron effect.
Cocaine:	None expected.
Foods: Dairy foods, eggs, whole-grain bread and cereal.	Decreased iron effect.
Marijuana:	None expected.
Tobacco:	None expected.

ISOETHARINE

BRAND NAMES

Arm-a-Med
  Isoetharine
Beta-2
Bronkometer
Bronkosol
Dey-Dose Isoetharine

Dey-Lute Isoetharine
Dilabron
Disorine
Dispos-a Med
  Isoetharine

BASIC INFORMATION

Habit forming? No
Prescription needed? Yes
Available as generic? Yes
Drug class: Sympathomimetic
         (bronchodilator)

 USES

Eases breathing difficulty from bronchial asthma attacks, bronchitis and emphysema.

 DOSAGE & USAGE INFORMATION

How to take:
Aerosol—Use only as directed on label. Don't inhale medicine more than twice per dose unless otherwise directed by doctor.

When to take:
As needed, no more often than every 3 hours.

If you forget a dose:
Take as soon as you remember if you need it. Never double dose.

What drug does:
Dilates constricted bronchial tubes so air can pass.

Continued next column

 OVERDOSE

SYMPTOMS:
Nervousness, anxiety, dizziness, palpitations, tremor, rapid heartbeat, spasm of bronchial tubes, cardiac arrest.
WHAT TO DO:
• Dial 0 (operator) or 911 (emergency) for an ambulance or medical help. Then give first aid immediately.
• If patient is unconscious and not breathing, give mouth-to-mouth breathing. If there is no heartbeat, use cardiac massage and mouth-to-mouth breathing (CPR). Don't try to make patient vomit. If you can't get help quickly, take patient to nearest emergency facility.
• See emergency information on inside covers.

Time lapse before drug works:
1 to 2 minutes.

Don't take with:
• Non-prescription drugs containing caffeine without consulting doctor.
• See Interaction column and consult doctor.

 POSSIBLE ADVERSE REACTIONS OR SIDE EFFECTS

SYMPTOMS	WHAT TO DO
Life-threatening: None expected.	
Common: Dizziness, agitation, headache, insomnia, nausea, fast or pounding heartbeat.	Continue. Call doctor when convenient.
Infrequent: • Constriction of bronchial tubes, particularly after overuse.	Discontinue. Call doctor right away.
• Weakness.	Continue. Call doctor when convenient.
Rare: None expected.	

WARNINGS & PRECAUTIONS

Don't take if:
- You are allergic to any sympathomimetic drug.
- You have a heart-rhythm disorder.
- You have taken MAO inhibitors in past 2 weeks.

Before you start, consult your doctor:
- If you use epinephrine for asthma.
- If you have diabetes.
- If you have an overactive thyroid gland.
- If you take a digitalis preparation, have high blood pressure or heart disease.

Over age 60:
- If you have hardening of the arteries, use with caution.
- If you have enlarged prostate gland, drug may increase urination difficulty.
- If you have Parkinson's disease, drug may temporarily increase rigidity and tremor in extremities.

Pregnancy:
No proven harm to unborn child. Avoid if possible.

Breast-feeding:
No problems expected, but consult doctor.

Infants & children:
Don't give to infants younger than 2. For older children, use only under medical supervision.

Prolonged use:
No problems expected.

Skin & sunlight:
No problems expected.

Driving, piloting or hazardous work:
No problems expected. Use caution if you feel nervous or dizzy.

Discontinuing:
Discontinue if drug fails to provide relief. Don't increase dose or frequency.

Others:
May increase blood- and urine-sugar levels, particularly in diabetics.

POSSIBLE INTERACTION WITH OTHER DRUGS

GENERIC NAME OR DRUG CLASS	COMBINED EFFECT
Antidepressants (tricyclic)	Increased isoetharine effect.
Beta-adrenergic blockers	Decreased effects of both drugs.
Ephedrine	Increased ephedrine effect. Excessive heart stimulation.
Epinephrine	Excessive heart stimulation.
Isoproterenol	Excessive heart stimulation.
MAO inhibitors	Dangerous mixture. Avoid.
Minoxidil	Decreased minoxidil effect.
Nitrates	Possible decreased effects of both drugs.

POSSIBLE INTERACTION WITH OTHER SUBSTANCES

INTERACTS WITH	COMBINED EFFECT
Alcohol:	None expected.
Beverages: Caffeine drinks.	May cause irregular or fast heartbeat.
Cocaine:	Excessive stimulation. Avoid.
Foods: Chocolates.	May cause irregular or fast heartbeat.
Marijuana:	Improves drug's antiasthmatic effect.
Tobacco:	None expected.

ISOMETHAPRINE, DICHLORALPHENAZONE & ACETAMINOPHEN

BRAND NAMES

Midrin

BASIC INFORMATION

Habit forming? No
Prescription needed? Yes
Available as generic? No
Drug class: Analgesic, sedative

 USES

Treatment of vascular (throbbing or migraine type) and tension headaches.

 DOSAGE & USAGE INFORMATION

How to take:
Capsules—Take with fluid. Usual dose—2 capsules at start, then 1 every hour until fully relieved. Don't exceed 5 capsules in 12 hours.

When to take:
At first sign of headache.

If you forget a dose:
Use as soon as you remember.

What drug does:
Causes blood vessels in head to constrict or become narrower. Acetaminophen relieves pain by effects on hypothalamus—the part of the brain that helps regulate body heat and receives body's pain messages.

Time lapse before drug works:
30-60 minutes.

Continued next column

 OVERDOSE

SYMPTOMS:
Stomach upsets, irritability, convulsions, coma.
WHAT TO DO:
- **Dial 0 (operator) or 911 (emergency) for an ambulance or medical help. Then give first aid immediately.**
- **See emergency information on inside covers.**

Don't take with:
- Any medicine that will decrease mental alertness or reflexes, such as alcohol, other mind-altering drugs, cough/cold medicines, antihistamines, allergy medicine, sedatives, tranquilizers (sleeping pills or "downers") barbiturates, seizure medicine, narcotics, other prescription medicine for pain, muscle relaxants, anesthetics.
- See Interaction column and consult doctor.

 POSSIBLE ADVERSE REACTIONS OR SIDE EFFECTS

SYMPTOMS	WHAT TO DO
Life-threatening:	
Fast heartbeat.	Discontinue. Seek emergency treatment.
Common:	
Dizziness.	Continue. Call doctor when convenient.
Infrequent:	
Diarrhea, vomiting, nausea, abdominal cramps.	Discontinue. Call doctor right away.
Rare:	
Rash; itchy skin; sore throat, fever, mouth sores; unusual bleeding or bruising; weakness; jaundice.	Discontinue. Call doctor right away.

ISOMETHAPRINE, DICHLORALPHENAZONE & ACETAMINOPHEN

WARNINGS & PRECAUTIONS

Don't take if:
- You are allergic to acetaminophen or any other component of this combination medicine.
- Your symptoms don't improve after 2 days use. Call your doctor.

Before you start, consult your doctor:
If you have bronchial asthma, kidney disease, liver damage, glaucoma, heart or blood vessel disorder, hypertension.

Over age 60:
Don't exceed recommended dose. You can't eliminate drug as efficiently as younger persons.

Pregnancy:
No proven harm to unborn child. Avoid if possible.

Breast-feeding:
No proven harm to nursing infant.

Infants & children:
Not recommended.

Prolonged use:
May affect blood system and cause anemia. Limit use to 5 days for children 12 and under, and 10 days for adults.

Skin & sunlight:
No problems expected.

Driving, piloting or hazardous work:
Avoid if you feel drowsy. Otherwise, no restrictions.

Discontinuing:
Discontinue in 2 days if symptoms don't improve.

Others:
No problems expected.

POSSIBLE INTERACTION WITH OTHER DRUGS

GENERIC NAME OR DRUG CLASS	COMBINED EFFECT
Anticoagulants (oral)	May increase anticoagulant effect. If combined frequently, prothrombin time should be monitored.
Anti-inflammatory agents (non-steroidal)	Long-term combined effect (3 years or longer) increases chance of damage to kidney, including malignancy.
Aspirin or other salicylates	Long-term combined effect (3 years or longer) increases chance of damage to kidney, including malignancy.
MAO inhibitors	Sudden increase in blood pressure.
Phenacetin	Long-term combined effect (3 years or longer) increases chance of damage to kidney, including malignancy.
Phenobarbital	Quicker elimination and decreased effect of acetaminophen.
Tetracyclines (effervescent granules or tablets)	May slow tetracycline absorption. Space doses 2 hours apart.

POSSIBLE INTERACTION WITH OTHER SUBSTANCES

INTERACTS WITH	COMBINED EFFECT
Alcohol:	Drowsiness. Toxicity to liver.
Beverages:	None expected.
Cocaine:	None expected. However, cocaine may slow body's recovery. Avoid.
Foods:	None expected.
Marijuana:	Increased pain relief. However, marijuana may slow body's recovery. Avoid.
Tobacco:	May decrease effectiveness of Midrin.

ISONIAZID

BRAND NAMES

DOW-Isoniazid
Ethionamide
INH
Isotamine
Laniazid
Laniazid C.P.

Nydrazid
PMS Isoniazid
Rifamate
Rimifon
Trecator-SC

BASIC INFORMATION

Habit forming? No
Prescription needed? Yes
Available as generic? Yes
Drug class: Antitubercular (antimicrobial)

USES

Kills tuberculosis germs.

DOSAGE & USAGE INFORMATION

How to take:
- Tablet or capsule—Swallow with liquid to lessen stomach irritation.
- Syrup—Follow label directions.

When to take:
At the same time each day.

If you forget a dose:
Take as soon as you remember up to 12 hours late. If more than 12 hours, wait for next scheduled dose (don't double this dose).

What drug does:
Interferes with TB germ metabolism. Eventually destroys the germ.

Continued next column

OVERDOSE

SYMPTOMS:
Difficult breathing, convulsions, coma.
WHAT TO DO:
- Dial 0 (operator) or 911 (emergency) for an ambulance or medical help. Then give first aid immediately.
- If patient is unconscious and not breathing, give mouth-to-mouth breathing. If there is no heartbeat, use cardiac massage and mouth-to-mouth breathing (CPR). Don't try to make patient vomit. If you can't get help quickly, take patient to nearest emergency facility.
- See emergency information on inside covers.

Time lapse before drug works:
3 to 6 months. You may need to take drug as long as 2 years.

Don't take with:
See Interaction column and consult doctor.

POSSIBLE ADVERSE REACTIONS OR SIDE EFFECTS

SYMPTOMS	WHAT TO DO
Life-threatening:	
None expected.	
Common:	
• Muscle pain and pain in joints, tingling or numbness in extremities, jaundice.	Discontinue. Call doctor right away.
• Confusion, unsteady walk.	Continue. Call doctor when convenient.
Infrequent:	
• Swollen glands, nausea, indigestion, vomiting, appetite loss.	Discontinue. Call doctor right away.
• Dizziness, increase in blood sugar.	Continue. Call doctor when convenient.
Rare:	
• Rash, fever, impaired vision, anemia with fatigue, weakness, fever, sore throat, unusual bleeding or bruising.	Discontinue. Call doctor right away.
• Breast enlargement or discomfort.	Continue. Tell doctor at next visit.

WARNINGS & PRECAUTIONS

Don't take if:
You are allergic to isoniazid.

Before you start, consult your doctor:
- If you plan to become pregnant within medication period.
- If you are allergic to athionamide, pyrazinamide or nicotinic acid.
- If you drink alcohol.
- If you have liver or kidney disease.
- If you have epilepsy, diabetes or lupus.

Over age 60:
Adverse reactions and side effects, especially jaundice, may be more frequent and severe than in younger persons. Kidneys may be less efficient.

Pregnancy:
No proven harm to unborn child. Avoid if possible, especially in the first 6 months of pregnancy. Consult doctor about use in last 3 months.

Breast-feeding:
Drug passes into milk. Avoid drug or discontinue nursing until you finish medicine. Consult doctor for advice on maintaining milk supply.

Infants & children:
Use only under medical supervision.

Prolonged use:
Numbness and tingling of hands and feet.

Skin & sunlight:
No problems expected.

Driving, piloting or hazardous work:
Avoid if you feel dizzy. Otherwise, no problems expected.

Discontinuing:
Don't discontinue without doctor's advice until you complete prescribed dose, even though symptoms diminish or disappear.

Others:
- Diabetic patients may have false blood-sugar tests.
- Periodic liver-function tests and laboratory blood studies recommended.
- Prescription for vitamin B-6 (pyridoxine) recommended to prevent nerve damage.

POSSIBLE INTERACTION WITH OTHER DRUGS

GENERIC NAME OR DRUG CLASS	COMBINED EFFECT
Antacids	Decreased absorption of isoniazid.
Anticholinergics	May increase pressure within eyeball.
Anticoagulants	Increased anticoagulant effect.
Antidiabetics	Increased antidiabetic effect.
Antihypertensives	Increased antihypertensive effect.
Disulfiram	Increased effect of disulfiram.
Laxatives	Decreased absorption and effect of isoniazid.
Narcotics	Increased narcotic effect.
Phenytoin	Increased phenytoin effect.
Pyridoxine (Vitamin B-6)	Decreased chance of nerve damage in extremities.
Rifampin	Increased isoniazid toxicity to liver.
Sedatives	Increased sedative effect.
Stimulants	Increased stimulant effect.

POSSIBLE INTERACTION WITH OTHER SUBSTANCES

INTERACTS WITH	COMBINED EFFECT
Alcohol:	Decreased isoniazid effect. Avoid.
Beverages:	None expected.
Cocaine:	None expected.
Foods:	Decreased absorption of isoniazid.
Marijuana:	No interactions expected, but marijuana may slow body's recovery.
Tobacco:	No interactions expected, but tobacco may slow body's recovery.

ISOPROPAMIDE

BRAND NAMES

Allergine	Oraminic
Allernade	Ornade
Capade	Prochlor-Iso
Combid	Pro-Iso
Darbid	

BASIC INFORMATION

Habit forming? No
Prescription needed?
  Low strength: No
  High strength: Yes
Available as generic? Yes
Drug class: Antispasmodic, anticholinergic

 USES

Reduces spasms of digestive system, bladder and urethra.

 DOSAGE & USAGE INFORMATION

How to take:
- Tablet or capsule—Swallow with liquid or food to lessen stomach irritation.
- Extended-release tablets or capsules—Swallow each dose whole. If you take regular tablets, you may chew or crush them.

When to take:
30 minutes before meals (unless directed otherwise by doctor).

If you forget a dose:
Take as soon as you remember up to 2 hours late. If more than 2 hours, wait for next scheduled dose (don't double this dose).

What drug does:
Blocks nerve impulses at parasympathetic nerve endings, preventing muscle contractions and gland secretions of organs involved.

Continued next column

 OVERDOSE

SYMPTOMS:
Dilated pupils, rapid pulse and breathing, dizziness, fever, hallucinations, confusion, slurred speech, agitation, flushed face, convulsions, coma.
WHAT TO DO:
- **Dial 0 (operator) or 911 (emergency) for an ambulance or medical help. Then give first aid immediately.**
- **See emergency information on inside covers.**

Time lapse before drug works:
15 to 30 minutes.

Don't take with:
See Interaction column and consult doctor.

 POSSIBLE ADVERSE REACTIONS OR SIDE EFFECTS

SYMPTOMS	WHAT TO DO
Life-threatening:	
None expected.	
Common:	
• Confusion, delirium, rapid heartbeat.	Discontinue. Call doctor right away.
• Nausea, vomiting, decreased sweating.	Continue. Call doctor when convenient.
• Constipation.	Continue. Tell doctor at next visit.
• Dryness in ears, nose, throat.	No action necessary.
Infrequent:	
Headache, difficult urination.	Continue. Call doctor when convenient.
Rare:	
Rash or hives, pain, blurred vision.	Discontinue. Call doctor right away.

WARNINGS & PRECAUTIONS

Don't take if:
- You are allergic to any anticholinergic.
- You have trouble with stomach bloating.
- You have difficulty emptying your bladder completely.
- You have narrow-angle glaucoma.
- You have severe ulcerative colitis.

Before you start, consult your doctor:
- If you have open-angle glaucoma.
- If you have angina.
- If you have chronic bronchitis or asthma.
- If you have hiatal hernia.
- If you have liver disease.
- If you have enlarged prostate.
- If you have myasthenia gravis.
- If you have peptic ulcer.
- If you will have surgery within 2 months, including dental surgery, requiring general or spinal anesthesia.

Over age 60:
Adverse reactions and side effects may be more frequent and severe than in younger persons.

Pregnancy:
Studies inconclusive on harm to unborn child. Animal studies show fetal abnormalities. Decide with your doctor whether drug benefits justify risk to unborn child.

Breast-feeding:
Drug passes into milk and decreases milk flow. Avoid drug or discontinue nursing until you finish medicine. Consult doctor for advice on maintaining milk supply.

Infants & children:
Use only under medical supervision.

Prolonged use:
Chronic constipation, possible fecal impaction. Consult doctor immediately.

Skin & sunlight:
No problems expected.

Driving, piloting or hazardous work:
Use disqualifies you for piloting aircraft. Otherwise, no problems expected.

Discontinuing:
May be unnecessary to finish medicine. Follow doctor's instructions.

Others:
No problems expected.

POSSIBLE INTERACTION WITH OTHER DRUGS

GENERIC NAME OR DRUG CLASS	COMBINED EFFECT
Amantadine	Increased isopropamide effect.
Anticholinergics (other)	Increased isopropamide effect
Antidepressants (tricyclic)	Increased atropine effect. Increased sedation.
Antihistamines	Increased isopropamide effect.
Cortisone drugs	Increased internal-eye pressure.
Haloperidol	Increased internal-eye pressure.
MAO inhibitors	Increased isopropamide effect.
Meperidine	Increased isopropamide effect.
Methylphenidate	Increased isopropamide effect.
Nitrates	Increased internal-eye pressure.
Orphenadrine	Increased isopropamide effect.
Phenothiazines	Increased isopropamide effect.
Pilocarpine	Loss of pilocarpine effect in glaucoma treatment.
Potassium supplements	Possible intestinal ulcers with oral potassium tablets.
Vitamin C	Decreased isopropamide effect. Avoid large doses of vitamin C.

POSSIBLE INTERACTION WITH OTHER SUBSTANCES

INTERACTS WITH	COMBINED EFFECT
Alcohol:	None expected.
Beverages:	None expected.
Cocaine:	Excessively rapid heartbeat. Avoid.
Foods:	None expected.
Marijuana:	Drowsiness and dry mouth.
Tobacco:	None expected.

ISOPROTERENOL

BRAND NAMES

Aerolone	Medihaler-Iso
Brondilate	Norisodrine
Duo-Medihaler	Norisodrine Aerotrol
Iprenol	Proternol
Isuprel	Vapo-Iso

BASIC INFORMATION

Habit forming? No
Prescription needed? Yes
Available as generic? Yes
Drug class: Sympathomimetic,
**   bronchodilator**

USES

Treatment for breathing difficulty from acute asthma, bronchitis and emphysema.

DOSAGE & USAGE INFORMATION

How to take:
- Tablet—Swallow with liquid or food to lessen stomach irritation.
- Extended-release tablets—Swallow each dose whole.
- Sublingual tablets—Dissolve under tongue.
- Aerosol inhaler—Don't inhale more than twice per dose.

When to take:
As needed, no more often than every 4 hours.

If you forget a dose:
Take as soon as you remember. Wait 4 hours for next dose.

What drug does:
- Dilates constricted bronchial tubes, improving air flow.
- Stimulates heart muscle and dilates blood vessels.

Continued next column

OVERDOSE

SYMPTOMS:
Nervousness, rapid or irregular heartbeat, fainting, sweating, headache, tremor, vomiting, chest pain, blood-pressure drop.
WHAT TO DO:
- **Dial 0 (operator) or 911 (emergency) for an ambulance or medical help. Then give first aid immediately.**
- **See emergency information on inside covers.**

Time lapse before drug works:
2 to 4 minutes.

Don't take with:
See Interaction column and consult doctor.

POSSIBLE ADVERSE REACTIONS OR SIDE EFFECTS

SYMPTOMS	WHAT TO DO
Life-threatening:	
None expected.	
Common:	
• Nervousness, insomnia.	Continue. Call doctor when convenient.
• Dry mouth, dry throat.	Continue. Tell doctor at next visit.
Infrequent:	
• Chest pain; irregular, fast or pounding heartbeat; unusual sweating.	Discontinue. Call doctor right away.
• Dizziness, headache, shakiness, weakness, flushed face, nausea, vomiting.	Continue. Call doctor when convenient.
Rare:	
None expected.	

ISOPROTERENOL

WARNINGS & PRECAUTIONS

Don't take if:
- You are allergic to any sympathomimetic, including some diet pills.
- You have serious heart-rhythm disorder.
- You have taken MAO inhibitors in past 2 weeks.

Before you start, consult your doctor:
- If you are sensitive to sympathomimetics.
- If you use epinephrine.
- If you have high blood pressure, heart disease, or take a digitalis preparation.
- If you have diabetes.
- If you have overactive thyroid.
- If your heartbeat is faster than 100 beats per minute.

Over age 60:
You may be more sensitive to drug's stimulant effects. Use with caution if you have hardening of the arteries.

Pregnancy:
Studies inconclusive on harm to unborn child. Animal studies show fetal abnormalities. Decide with your doctor whether drug benefits justify risk to unborn child.

Breast-feeding:
Drug does not appear in milk. Consult doctor.

Infants & children:
Not recommended.

Prolonged use:
- Salivary glands may swell.
- Mouth ulcers (sublingual tablets).

Skin & sunlight:
No problems expected.

Driving, piloting or hazardous work:
Use caution if you feel dizzy or nervous.

Discontinuing:
Discontinue if drug fails to provide relief after 2 or 3 days. Consult doctor.

Others:
No problems expected.

POSSIBLE INTERACTION WITH OTHER DRUGS

GENERIC NAME OR DRUG CLASS	COMBINED EFFECT
Albuterol	Increased effect of both drugs, especially harmful side effects.
Antidepressants (tricyclic)	Increased effect of both drugs.
Beta-adrenergic blockers	Decreased effects of both drugs.
Ephedrine	Increased ephedrine effect.
Epinephrine	Increased chance of serious heart disturbances.
Minoxidil	Decreased minoxidil effect.
Nitrates	Possible decreased effects of both drugs.
Sympathomimetics (other)	Increased effect of both drugs, especially harmful side effects.

POSSIBLE INTERACTION WITH OTHER SUBSTANCES

INTERACTS WITH	COMBINED EFFECT
Alcohol:	Decreased isoproterenol effect.
Beverages: Caffeine drinks.	Overstimulation. Avoid.
Cocaine:	Overstimulation of brain and heart. Avoid.
Foods:	None expected.
Marijuana:	Increased antiasthmatic effect of isoproterenol.
Tobacco:	None expected.

BRAND NAMES

Duo-Medihaler

BASIC INFORMATION

Habit forming? No
Prescription needed? Yes
Available as generic? No
Drug class: Sympathomimetic,
        bronchodilator

 USES

- Temporary relief of congestion of nose, sinuses and throat caused by allergies, colds or sinusitis.
- Treatment for breathing difficulty from acute asthma, bronchitis and emphysema.

 DOSAGE & USAGE INFORMATION

How to take:
Aerosol inhaler—Don't inhale more than twice per dose. Follow package instructions.

When to take:
As needed, no more often than every 4 hours.

If you forget a dose:
Take as soon as you remember. Wait 4 hours for next dose. Don't double this dose.

What drug does:
- Dilates constricted bronchial tubes, improving air flow.
- Stimulates heart muscle and dilates blood vessels.

Time lapse before drug works:
2 to 4 minutes.

Continued next column

 OVERDOSE

SYMPTOMS:
Headache, blood-pressure rise, slow and forceful pulse, nervousness, rapid or irregular heartbeat, fainting, sweating, tremor, vomiting, chest pain, convulsions, coma.
WHAT TO DO:
- **Dial 0 (operator) or 911 (emergency) for an ambulance or medical help. Then give first aid immediately.**
- **See emergency information on inside covers.**

Don't take with:
Non-prescription drugs for asthma, cough, cold, allergy, appetite suppressants, sleeping pills or drugs containing caffeine without consulting doctor.

 POSSIBLE ADVERSE REACTIONS OR SIDE EFFECTS

SYMPTOMS	WHAT TO DO
Life-threatening:	
None expected.	
Common:	
Chest pain; irregular, fast heartbeat; dry mouth.	Discontinue. Call doctor right away.
Infrequent:	
• Increased sweating.	Discontinue. Call doctor right away.
• Nervousness, insomnia, dizziness, headache, shakiness, weakness, red or flushed face, vomiting, nausea, pale skin.	Continue. Call doctor when convenient.
Rare:	
None expected.	

ISOPROTERENOL & PHENYLEPHRINE

WARNINGS & PRECAUTIONS

Don't take if:
- You are allergic to any sympathomimetic, including some diet pills.
- You have serious heart-rhythm disorder.
- You have taken MAO inhibitors in past 2 weeks.

Before you start, consult your doctor:
- If you have high blood pressure, heart disease, or take a digitalis preparation.
- If you have diabetes or overactive thyroid.
- If you have taken MAO inhibitors in past 2 weeks.
- If you are sensitive to sympathomimetics.
- If you use epinephrine.
- If your heartbeat is faster than 100 beats per minute.

Over age 60:
You may be more sensitive to drug's stimulant effects. Use with caution if you have hardening of the arteries.

Pregnancy:
Risk to unborn child outweighs drug benefits. Don't use.

Breast-feeding:
Drug passes into milk. Avoid drug or discontinue nursing until you finish medicine. Consult doctor for advice on maintaining milk supply.

Infants & children:
Use only under close supervision.

Prolonged use:
- May cause functional dependence.
- Salivary glands may swell.

Skin & sunlight:
No problems expected.

Driving, piloting or hazardous work:
Use caution if you feel dizzy or nervous.

Discontinuing:
Discontinue if drug fails to provide relief after 2 or 3 days. Consult doctor.

Others:
No problems expected.

POSSIBLE INTERACTION WITH OTHER DRUGS

GENERIC NAME OR DRUG CLASS	COMBINED EFFECT
Acebutolol	Decreased effect of both drugs.
Amphetamines	Increased nervousness.
Antiasthmatics	Nervous stimulation.
Antidepressants	Increased effect of both drugs.
Antihypertensives	Increased antihypertensive effect.
Beta-adrenergic blockers	Decreased effect of both drugs.
Ephedrine	Increased ephedrine effect.
Epinephrine	Increased chance of serious heart disturbances.
MAO inhibitors	Dangerous blood-pressure rise.
Minoxidil	Increased minoxidil effect.
Nitrates	Possible decreased effect of both drugs.
Oxprenolol	Decreased effect of both drugs.
Sedatives	Decreased sedative effect.
Sympathomimetics (other)	Increased effect of both drugs, especially harmful side effects.
Tranquilizers	Decreased tranquilizer effect.

POSSIBLE INTERACTION WITH OTHER SUBSTANCES

INTERACTS WITH	COMBINED EFFECT
Alcohol:	Decreased isoproterenol effect.
Beverages: Caffeine drinks.	Overstimulation. Avoid.
Cocaine:	Overstimulation of brain and heart. Avoid.
Foods:	None expected.
Marijuana:	Increased antiasthmatic effect of isoproterenol.
Tobacco:	None expected.

461

ISOTRETINOIN

BRAND NAMES

Accutane

BASIC INFORMATION

Habit forming? No
Prescription needed? Yes
Available as generic? No
Drug classification: Antiacne

 USES

- Decreases cystic acne formation in severe cases.
- Certain other skin disorders involving an overabundance of outer skin layer.

 DOSAGE & USAGE INFORMATION

How to take:
Tablet or capsule—Swallow with liquid or food to lessen stomach irritation. If you can't swallow whole, crumble tablet or open capsule and take with liquid or food.

When to take:
Twice a day. Follow prescription directions.

If you forget a dose:
Take as soon as you remember up to 2 hours late. If more than 2 hours, wait for next scheduled dose and double dose.

What drug does:
Reduces sebaceous gland activity and size.

Time lapse before drug works:
May require 15 to 20 weeks to experience full benefit.

Don't take with:
Vitamin A or supplements containing Vitamin A.

 OVERDOSE

SYMPTOMS:
None reported.
WHAT TO DO:
Overdose unlikely to threaten life. If person takes much larger amount than prescribed, call doctor, poison-control center or hospital emergency room for instructions.

 POSSIBLE ADVERSE REACTIONS OR SIDE EFFECTS

SYMPTOMS	WHAT TO DO
Life-threatening: None expected.	
Common:	
• Burning, red, itching eyes; lip scaling; burning pain.	Discontinue. Call doctor right away.
• Itchy skin.	Continue. Call doctor when convenient.
Frequent: Dry mouth.	Continue. Tell doctor at next visit. (Suck ice or chew gum.)
Infrequent:	
• Rash, infection, nausea, vomiting.	Discontinue. Call doctor right away.
• Headache; pain in muscles, bones, joints; hair thinning; tiredness.	Continue. Call doctor when convenient.
Rare: None expected.	

WARNINGS & PRECAUTIONS

Don't take if:
- You are allergic to isotretinoin.
- You are pregnant or plan pregnancy.

Before you start, consult your doctor:
- If you have diabetes.
- If you or any member of family have high triglyceride levels in blood.

Over age 60:
Adverse reactions and side effects may be more frequent and severe than in younger persons.

Pregnancy:
Risk to unborn child outweighs drug benefits. Don't use.

Breast-feeding:
Drug filters into milk. May harm child. Avoid.

Infants & children:
Not recommended.

Prolonged use:
Possible damage to cornea.

Skin & sunlight:
May cause rash or intensify sunburn in areas exposed to sun or sunlamp.

Driving, piloting or hazardous work:
No problems expected.

Discontinuing:
Single course of treatment usually all needed. If second course required, wait 8 weeks after completing first course.

Others:
Use only for severe cases of cystic acne that have not responded to less hazardous forms of acne treatment.

POSSIBLE INTERACTION WITH OTHER DRUGS

GENERIC NAME OR DRUG CLASS	COMBINED EFFECT
Vitamin A	Additive toxic effect of each. Avoid.

POSSIBLE INTERACTION WITH OTHER SUBSTANCES

INTERACTS WITH	COMBINED EFFECT
Alcohol:	Significant increase in triglycerides in blood. Avoid.
Beverages:	No problems expected.
Cocaine:	Increased chance of toxicity of isotretinoin. Avoid.
Foods:	No problems expected.
Marijuana:	Increased chance of toxicity of isotretinoin. Avoid.
Tobacco:	May decrease absorption of medicine. Avoid tobacco while in treatment.

ISOXSUPRINE

BRAND NAMES

Vasodilan   Vasoprine

BASIC INFORMATION

Habit forming? No
Prescription needed? Yes
Available as generic? Yes
Drug class: Vasodilator

USES

Improves poor blood circulation.

DOSAGE & USAGE INFORMATION

How to take:
Tablet—Swallow with liquid or food to lessen stomach irritation. If you can't swallow whole, crumble tablet and take with liquid or food.

When to take:
At the same times each day.

If you forget a dose:
Take as soon as you remember up to 2 hours late. If more than 2 hours, wait for next scheduled dose (don't double this dose).

What drug does:
Expands blood vessels, increasing flow and permitting distribution of oxygen and nutrients.

Time lapse before drug works:
1 hour.

Don't take with:
See Interaction column and consult doctor.

OVERDOSE

SYMPTOMS:
Headache, dizziness, flush, vomiting, weakness, sweating, fainting, shortness of breath, coma.
WHAT TO DO:
- Dial 0 (operator) or 911 (emergency) for an ambulance or medical help. Then give first aid immediately.
- If patient is unconscious and not breathing, give mouth-to-mouth breathing. If there is no heartbeat, use cardiac massage and mouth-to-mouth breathing (CPR). Don't try to make patient vomit. If you can't get help quickly, take patient to nearest emergency facility.
- See emergency information on inside covers.

POSSIBLE ADVERSE REACTIONS OR SIDE EFFECTS

SYMPTOMS	WHAT TO DO
Life-threatening:	
None expected.	
Common:	
• Appetite loss, nausea, vomiting.	Discontinue. Call doctor right away.
• Dizziness, faintness.	Continue. Call doctor when convenient.
• Weakness, lethargy.	Continue. Tell doctor at next visit.
Infrequent:	
Rash.	Discontinue. Call doctor right away.
Rare:	
Rapid or irregular heartbeat.	Discontinue. Call doctor right away.

WARNINGS & PRECAUTIONS

Don't take if:
- You are allergic to any vasodilator.
- You have any bleeding disease.

Before you start, consult your doctor:
- If you have high blood pressure, hardening of the arteries or heart disease.
- If you plan to become pregnant within medication period.
- If you have glaucoma.

Over age 60:
Adverse reactions and side effects may be more frequent and severe than in younger persons.

Pregnancy:
Studies inconclusive on harm to unborn child. Decide with your doctor whether drug benefits justify risk to unborn child.

Breast-feeding:
No problems expected, but consult doctor.

Infants & children:
Not recommended.

Prolonged use:
No problems expected.

Skin & sunlight:
No problems expected.

Driving, piloting or hazardous work:
Avoid if you feel dizzy or faint. Otherwise, no problems expected.

Discontinuing:
Don't discontinue without doctor's advice until you complete prescribed dose, even though symptoms diminish or disappear.

Others:
Be cautious when arising from lying or sitting position, when climbing stairs, or if dizziness occurs.

POSSIBLE INTERACTION WITH OTHER DRUGS

GENERIC NAME OR DRUG CLASS	COMBINED EFFECT
None	

POSSIBLE INTERACTION WITH OTHER SUBSTANCES

INTERACTS WITH	COMBINED EFFECT
Alcohol:	None expected.
Beverages: Milk.	Decreased stomach irritation.
Cocaine:	Decreased blood circulation to extremities. Avoid.
Foods:	None expected.
Marijuana:	Rapid heartbeat.
Tobacco:	Decreased isoxsuprine effect.

KAOLIN & PECTIN

BRAND NAMES

Donnagel-MB	K-C
Donnagel-PG	K-P
Kao-Con	K-Pek
Kaopectate	Parepectolin
Kapectolin	Pecto Kay
Kaypectol	

BASIC INFORMATION

Habit forming? No
Prescription needed? No
Available as generic? Yes
Drug class: Antidiarrheal

USES

Reduces intestinal cramps and diarrhea.

DOSAGE & USAGE INFORMATION

How to take:
Liquid—Swallow prescribed dosage (without diluting) after each loose bowel movement.

When to take:
After each loose bowel movement.

If you forget a dose:
Take when you remember.

What drug does:
Makes loose stools less watery, but may not prevent loss of fluids.

Time lapse before drug works:
15 to 30 minutes.

Don't take with:
See Interaction column and consult doctor.

OVERDOSE

SYMPTOMS:
Fecal impaction.
WHAT TO DO:
Overdose unlikely to threaten life. If person takes much larger amount than prescribed, call doctor, poison-control center or hospital emergency room for instructions.

POSSIBLE ADVERSE REACTIONS OR SIDE EFFECTS

SYMPTOMS	WHAT TO DO
Life-threatening: None expected.	
Common: None expected.	
Infrequent: None expected.	
Rare: Constipation (mild).	Continue. Call doctor when convenient.

WARNINGS & PRECAUTIONS

Don't take if:
You are allergic to kaolin or pectin.

Before you start, consult your doctor:
- If patient is child or infant.
- If you have any chronic medical problem with heart disease, peptic ulcer, asthma or others.
- If you have fever over 101F.

Over age 60:
Fluid loss caused by diarrhea, especially if taking other medicines, may lead to serious disability. Consult doctor.

Pregnancy:
No problems expected.

Breast-feeding:
No problems expected.

Infants & children:
Fluid loss caused by diarrhea in infants and children can cause serious dehydration. Consult doctor before giving any medicine for diarrhea.

Prolonged use:
Not recommended.

Skin & sunlight:
No problems expected.

Driving, piloting or hazardous work:
No problems expected.

Discontinuing:
May be unnecessary to finish medicine. Follow doctor's instructions.

Others:
Consult doctor about fluids, diet and rest.

POSSIBLE INTERACTION WITH OTHER DRUGS

GENERIC NAME OR DRUG CLASS	COMBINED EFFECT
Digoxin	Decreases absorption of digoxin. Separate doses by at least 2 hours.
Lincomycin	Decreases absorption of lincomycin. Separate doses by at least 2 hours.
All other oral medicines.	Decreases absorption of other medicines. Separate doses by at least 2 hours.

POSSIBLE INTERACTION WITH OTHER SUBSTANCES

INTERACTS WITH	COMBINED EFFECT
Alcohol:	Increased diarrhea. Prevents action of kaolin and pectin.
Beverages:	No problems expected.
Cocaine:	Aggravates underlying disease. Avoid.
Foods:	No problems expected.
Marijuana:	Aggravates underlying disease. Avoid.
Tobacco:	Aggravates underlying disease. Avoid.

KAOLIN, PECTIN, BELLADONNA & OPIUM

BRAND NAMES

Donnagel-PG

BASIC INFORMATION

Habit forming? Yes
Prescription needed? Yes
Available as generic? No
Drug class: Narcotic, antidiarrheal,
           antispasmodic

 ## USES

Reduces intestinal cramps and diarrhea.

 ## DOSAGE & USAGE INFORMATION

How to take:
Liquid—Swallow prescribed dosage (without diluting) after each loose bowel movement.

When to take:
As needed for diarrhea, no more often than every 4 hours.

If you forget a dose:
Take when you remember.

What drug does:
- Blocks nerve impulses at parasympathetic nerve endings, preventing muscle contractions and gland secretions of organs involved.
- Makes loose stools less watery, but may not prevent loss of fluids.

Continued next column

 ## OVERDOSE

SYMPTOMS:
Fecal impaction, rapid pulse, dizziness, fever, hallucinations, confusion, slurred speech, agitation, flushed face, convulsions, deep sleep, slow breathing, slow pulse, warm skin, constricted pupils, coma.
WHAT TO DO:
- **Dial 0 (operator) or 911 (emergency) for an ambulance or medical help. Then give first aid immediately.**
- **If patient is unconscious and not breathing, give mouth-to-mouth breathing. If there is no heartbeat, use cardiac massage and mouth-to-mouth breathing (CPR). Don't try to make patient vomit. If you can't get help quickly, take patient to nearest emergency facility.**
- **See emergency information on inside covers.**

- Anesthetizes surface membranes of intestines and blocks nerve impulses.

Time lapse before drug works:
15 to 30 minutes.

Don't take with:
See Interaction column and consult doctor.

 ## POSSIBLE ADVERSE REACTIONS OR SIDE EFFECTS

SYMPTOMS	WHAT TO DO
Life-threatening: Unusually rapid heartbeat (over 100), difficult breathing, slow heartbeat (under 50/minute).	Discontinue. Seek emergency treatment.
Common: (with large dosage) Weakness, increased sweating, red or flushed face, lightheadedness, headache, dry mouth, dry skin, drowsiness, dizziness, frequent urination, decreased sweating, constipation, confusion.	Continue. Call doctor when convenient.
Infrequent: • Taste sense reduced, nervousness, sunlight hurts eyes, blurred vision.	Discontinue. Call doctor right away.
• Diminished sex drive.	Continue. Call doctor when convenient.
Rare: Bloating, abdominal cramps and vomiting, eye pain, hallucinations, shortness of breath, rash, itchy skin.	Discontinue. Call doctor right away.

 ## WARNINGS & PRECAUTIONS

Don't take if:
- You are allergic to any anticholinergic, narcotic, kaolin or pectin.
- You have trouble with stomach bloating, difficulty emptying your bladder completely, narrow-angle glaucoma, severe ulcerative colitis.

Before you start, consult your doctor:
- If you have open-angle glaucoma, angina, chronic bronchitis or asthma, hiatal hernia, liver disease, enlarged prostate, myasthenia gravis, peptic ulcer, impaired liver or kidney function, fever over 101F, any chronic medical problem with heart disease, peptic ulcer, asthma or others.
- If patient is child or infant.
- If you will have surgery within 2 months, including dental surgery, requiring general or spinal anesthesia.

Over age 60:
- Adverse reactions and side effects may be more frequent and severe than in younger persons.
- More likely to be drowsy, dizzy, unsteady or constipated.
- Fluid loss caused by diarrhea, especially if taking other medicines, may lead to serious disability. Consult doctor.

Pregnancy:
No proven harm to unborn child. Avoid if possible.

Breast-feeding:
Drug passes into milk. Avoid drug or discontinue nursing until you finish medicine. Consult doctor for advice on maintaining milk supply.

Infants & children:
Fluid loss caused by diarrhea in infants and children can cause serious dehydration. Consult doctor before giving any medicine for diarrhea.

Prolonged use:
Causes psychological and physical dependence. Not recommended.

Skin & sunlight:
No problems expected.

Driving, piloting or hazardous work:
Don't drive or pilot aircraft until you learn how medicine affects you. Don't work around dangerous machinery. Don't climb ladders or work in high places. Danger increases if you drink alcohol or take medicine affecting alertness and reflexes, such as antihistamines, tranquilizers, sedatives, pain medicine, narcotics and mind-altering drugs.

Discontinuing:
May be unnecessary to finish medicine. Follow doctor's instructions.

Others:
- Great potential for abuse.
- Consult doctor about fluids, diet and rest.

POSSIBLE INTERACTION WITH OTHER DRUGS

GENERIC NAME OR DRUG CLASS	COMBINED EFFECT
Amantadine	Increased belladonna effect.
Analgesics	Increased analgesic effect.
Antidepressants	Increased sedative effect.
Antihistamines	Increased sedative effect.
Cortisone drugs	Increased internal-eye pressure.
Digoxin	Decreases absorption of digoxin. Separate doses by at least 2 hours.
Haloperidol	Increased internal-eye pressure.
Lincomycin	Decreases absorption of lincomycin. Separate doses by at least 2 hours.
MAO inhibitors	Increased belladonna effect.
Meperidine	Increased belladonna effect.
Methylphenidate	Increased belladonna effect.

Continued page 968

POSSIBLE INTERACTION WITH OTHER SUBSTANCES

INTERACTS WITH	COMBINED EFFECT
Alcohol:	Increases alcohol's intoxicating effect, increased diarrhea, prevents action of kaolin and pectin. Avoid.
Beverages:	No problems expected.
Cocaine:	Aggravates underlying disease. Avoid.
Foods:	No problems expected.
Marijuana:	Impairs physical and mental performance, aggravates underlying disease. Avoid.
Tobacco:	Aggravates underlying disease. Avoid.

KAOLIN, PECTIN & PAREGORIC

BRAND NAMES

Parepectolin

BASIC INFORMATION

Habit forming? Yes
Prescription needed? Yes
Available as generic? Yes
Drug class: Narcotic, antidiarrheal,
antispasmodic

 USES

- Reduces intestinal cramps and diarrhea.
- Relieves pain.

 DOSAGE & USAGE INFORMATION

How to take:
Liquid—Swallow prescribed dosage (without diluting) after each loose bowel movement.

When to take:
After each loose bowel movement. No more often then every 4 hours.

If you forget a dose:
Take when you remember.

What drug does:
Makes loose stools less watery, but may not prevent loss of fluids.

Time lapse before drug works:
15 to 30 minutes.

Don't take with:
See Interaction column and consult doctor.

 OVERDOSE

SYMPTOMS:
Deep sleep; slow breathing; slow pulse; flushed, warm skin.
WHAT TO DO:

- **Dial 0 (operator) or 911 (emergency) for an ambulance or medical help. Then give first aid immediately.**
- **If patient is unconscious and not breathing, give mouth-to-mouth breathing. If there is no heartbeat, use cardiac massage and mouth-to-mouth breathing (CPR). Don't try to make patient vomit. If you can't get help quickly, take patient to nearest emergency facility.**
- **See emergency information on inside covers.**

 POSSIBLE ADVERSE REACTIONS OR SIDE EFFECTS

SYMPTOMS	WHAT TO DO
Life-threatening: Unusually rapid heartbeat (over 100), difficult breathing, slow heartbeat (under 50/minute).	Discontinue. Seek emergency treatment.
Common: (with large dosage) Weakness, increased sweating, red or flushed face, lightheadedness, headache, dry mouth, dry skin, drowsiness, dizziness, frequent urination, decreased sweating, constipation, confusion.	Continue. Call doctor when convenient.
Infrequent: • Taste sense reduced, nervousness, sunlight hurts eyes, blurred vision.	Discontinue. Call doctor right away.
• Diminished sex drive.	Continue. Call doctor when convenient.
Rare: Bloating, abdominal cramps and vomiting, eye pain, hallucinations, shortness of breath, rash, itchy skin.	Discontinue. Call doctor right away.

WARNINGS & PRECAUTIONS

Don't take if:
You are allergic to any narcotic, kaolin or pectin.

Before you start, consult your doctor:
- If you have impaired liver or kidney function, chronic medical problem with heart disease, peptic ulcer, asthma or others, fever over 101F.
- If patient is child or infant.
- If you will have surgery within 2 months, including dental surgery, requiring general or spinal anesthesia.

Over age 60:
Fluid loss caused by diarrhea, especially if taking other medicines, may lead to serious disability. Consult doctor.

Pregnancy:
Abuse by pregnant woman will result in addicted newborn. Withdrawal of newborn can be life-threatening.

Breast-feeding:
Drug filters into milk. May harm child. Avoid.

Infants & children:
Fluid loss caused by diarrhea in infants and children can cause serious dehydration. Consult doctor before giving any medicine for diarrhea.

Prolonged use:
Causes psychological and physical dependence. Not recommended.

Skin & sunlight:
May cause rash or intensify sunburn in areas exposed to sun or sunlamp.

Driving, piloting or hazardous work:
Don't drive or pilot aircraft until you learn how medicine affects you. Don't work around dangerous machinery. Don't climb ladders or work in high places. Danger increases if you drink alcohol or take medicine affecting alertness and reflexes, such as antihistamines, tranquilizers, sedatives, pain medicine, narcotics and mind-altering drugs.

Discontinuing:
May be unnecessary to finish medicine. Follow doctor's instructions.

Others:
Consult doctor about fluids, diet and rest.

POSSIBLE INTERACTION WITH OTHER DRUGS

GENERIC NAME OR DRUG CLASS	COMBINED EFFECT
Analgesics (other)	Increased analgesic effect.
Anticholinergics	Increased anticholinergic effect.
Antidepressants	Increased sedative effect.
Antihistamines	Increased sedative effect.
Digoxin	Decreases absorption of digoxin. Separate doses by at least 2 hours.
Lincomycin	Decreases absorption of lincomycin. Separate doses by at least 2 hours.
Mind-altering drugs	Increased sedative effect.
Narcotics (other)	Increased narcotic effect.
Phenothiazines	Increased phenothiazine effect.
Sedatives	Increased sedative effect.
Sleep inducers	Increased sedative effect.
Terfenadine	Possible oversedation.
Tranquilizers	Increased sedative effect.
All other oral medicines	Decreases absorption of other medicines. Separate doses by at least 2 hours.

POSSIBLE INTERACTION WITH OTHER SUBSTANCES

INTERACTS WITH	COMBINED EFFECT
Alcohol:	Increases alcohol's intoxicating effect, increased diarrhea, prevents action of kaolin and pectin. Avoid.
Beverages:	No problems expected.
Cocaine:	Increased cocaine toxic effects, aggravates underlying disease. Avoid.
Foods:	No problems expected.
Marijuana:	Aggravates underlying disease. Avoid.
Tobacco:	Aggravates underlying disease. Avoid.

KETOCONAZOLE

BRAND NAMES

Nizoral

BASIC INFORMATION

Habit forming? No
Prescription needed? Yes
Available as generic? No
Drug class: Antifungal

 USES

Treatment of fungus infections susceptible to ketoconazole.

 DOSAGE & USAGE INFORMATION

How to take:
Tablet or capsule—Swallow with liquid or food to lessen stomach irritation. If you can't swallow whole, crumble tablet or open capsule and take with liquid or food.

When to take:
At same time once a day.

If you forget a dose:
Take as soon as you remember up to 2 hours late. If more than 2 hours, wait for next scheduled dose (don't double this dose).

What drug does:
Prevents fungi from growing and reproducing.

Time lapse before drug works:
8 to 10 months or longer.

Don't take with:
See Interaction column and consult doctor.

 OVERDOSE

SYMPTOMS:
Nausea, vomiting, diarrhea.
WHAT TO DO:
Overdose unlikely to threaten life. If person takes much larger amount than prescribed, call doctor, poison-control center or hospital emergency room for instructions.

 POSSIBLE ADVERSE REACTIONS OR SIDE EFFECTS

SYMPTOMS	WHAT TO DO
Life-threatening:	
None expected.	
Common:	
Nausea or vomiting.	Discontinue. Call doctor right away.
Infrequent:	
• Rash or itchy skin, increased sensitivity to light.	Discontinue. Call doctor right away.
• Drowsiness, insomnia, diarrhea.	Continue. Call doctor when convenient.
Rare:	
• Pale stools, abdominal pain, dark or amber urine.	Discontinue. Call doctor right away.
• Diminished sex drive in males, tiredness, weakness.	Continue. Call doctor when convenient.

WARNINGS & PRECAUTIONS

Don't take if:
You are allergic to ketoconazole.

Before you start, consult your doctor:
- If you have absence of stomach acid (achlorhydria).
- If you have liver disease.

Over age 60:
Adverse reactions and side effects may be more frequent and severe than in younger persons.

Pregnancy:
Risk to unborn child outweighs drug benefits. Don't use.

Breast-feeding:
Drug passes into milk. Avoid drug or discontinue nursing until you finish medicine. Consult doctor for advice on maintaining milk supply.

Infants & children:
Only under close medical supervision.

Prolonged use:
Request liver-function studies.

Skin & sunlight:
No problems expected.

Driving, piloting or hazardous work:
Don't drive or pilot aircraft until you learn how medicine affects you. Don't work around dangerous machinery. Don't climb ladders or work in high places. Danger increases if you drink alcohol or take medicine affecting alertness and reflexes, such as antihistamines, tranquilizers, sedatives, pain medicine, narcotics and mind-altering drugs.

Discontinuing:
May be unnecessary to finish medicine. Follow doctor's instructions.

Others:
No problems expected.

 ## POSSIBLE INTERACTION WITH OTHER DRUGS

GENERIC NAME OR DRUG CLASS	COMBINED EFFECT
Antacids	Decreased absorption of ketoconazole.
Anticholinergics	Decreased absorption of ketoconazole.
Atropine	Decreased absorption of ketoconazole.
Belladonna	Decreased absorption of ketoconazole.
Cimetidine	Decreased absorption of ketoconazole.
Clidinium	Decreased absorption of ketoconazole.
Glycopyrrolate	Decreased absorption of ketoconazole.
Hyoscyamine	Decreased absorption of ketoconazole.
Methscopolamine	Decreased absorption of ketoconazole.
Propantheline	Decreased absorption of ketoconazole.
Ranitidine	Decreased absorption of ketoconazole.
Scopolamine	Decreased absorption of ketoconazole.

 ## POSSIBLE INTERACTION WITH OTHER SUBSTANCES

INTERACTS WITH	COMBINED EFFECT
Alcohol:	Increased chance of liver damage.
Beverages:	No problems expected.
Cocaine:	Decreased ketoconazole effect. Avoid cocaine.
Foods:	No problems expected.
Marijuana:	Decreased ketoconazole effect. Avoid marijuana.
Tobacco:	Decreased ketoconazole effect. Avoid tobacco.

KETOPROFEN

BRAND NAMES

Alrheumat	Orudis-E
Orudis	Profenid

BASIC INFORMATION

Habit forming? No
Prescription needed? Yes
Available as generic? No
Drug class: Analgesic, antidysmenorreal (non-steroidal anti-inflammatory analgesic [NSAIA])

 USES

- Treatment of pain.
- Treatment of soft-tissue athletic injuries.
- Treats dysmenorrhea.

 DOSAGE & USAGE INFORMATION

How to take:
- Extended-release tablets or capsules—Swallow dose whole. If you take regular tablets, you may chew or crush them.
- Tablets or capsules—Swallow whole with liquid or food to lessen stomach irritation.
- Suppositories—Remove wrapper and moisten suppository with water. Gently insert into rectum, large end first. If suppository is too soft, chill in refrigerator or cool water before removing wrapper.
- Capsule—Take with full glass of water while sitting or standing upright. Take on any empty stomach either 1/2 hour before or 2 hours after meals. If stomach irritation occurs, may take with food or aluminum hydroxide or magnesium hydroxide antacids.

When to take:
At the same times each day.

If you forget a dose:
Take as soon as you remember up to 2 hours late. If more than 2 hours, wait for next scheduled dose (don't double this dose).

Continued next column

 OVERDOSE

SYMPTOMS:
Confusion, agitation, incoherence, convulsions, possible hemorrhage from stomach or intestine, coma.
WHAT TO DO:
- **Dial 0 (operator) or 911 (emergency) for an ambulance or medical help. Then give first aid immediately.**
- **See emergency information on inside covers.**

What drug does:
Reduces tissue concentration of prostaglandins (hormones which produce inflammation and pain).

Time lapse before drug works:
Begins in 4 to 24 hours. May require 3 weeks regular use for maximum benefit.

Don't take with:
- Large doses of acetaminophen. Combination increases possibility of kidney damage.
- See Interaction column and consult doctor.

 POSSIBLE ADVERSE REACTIONS OR SIDE EFFECTS

SYMPTOMS	WHAT TO DO
Life-threatening:	
Hives, rash, intense itching, faintness soon after a dose (anaphylaxis); breathing difficulty; tightness in chest; rapid heartbeat.	Discontinue. Seek emergency treatment.
Common:	
Dizziness, headache, nausea, pain, depression, drowsiness, ringing in ears.	Continue. Call doctor when convenient.
Infrequent:	
• Flank pain.	Discontinue. Call doctor right away.
• Constipation or diarrhea, vomiting.	Continue. Call doctor when convenient.
Rare:	
• Bloody or black, tarry stools; convulsions; confusion; rash, hives or itch; blurred vision; unusual bleeding or bruising; jaundice; blood in urine; difficult, painful or frequent urination.	Discontinue. Call doctor right away.
• Fatigue, weakness.	Continue. Call doctor when convenient.

 WARNINGS & PRECAUTIONS

Don't take if:
- You are allergic to ketoprofen, aspirin or any non-steroid, anti-inflammatory drug.
- You have gastritis, peptic ulcer, enteritis, ileitis, ulcerative colitis, asthma, heart failure, high blood pressure or bleeding problems.
- Patient is younger than 15.

Before you start, consult your doctor:
- If you have epilepsy or Parkinson's disease.
- If you have been mentally ill.
- If you have had kidney disease or impaired kidney function.

Over age 60:
Adverse reactions and side effects may be more frequent and severe than in younger persons.

Pregnancy:
Studies inconclusive on harm to unborn child. Decide with your doctor whether drug benefits justify risk to unborn child.

Breast-feeding:
May harm child. Avoid.

Infants & children:
Not recommended for anyone younger than 15. Use only under medical supervision.

Prolonged use:
- Eye damage.
- Reduced hearing.
- Sore throat, fever.
- Weight gain.

Skin & sunlight:
No problems expected.

Driving, piloting or hazardous work:
Don't drive or pilot aircraft until you learn how medicine affects you. Don't work around dangerous machinery. Don't climb ladders or work in high places. Danger increases if you drink alcohol or take medicine affecting alertness and reflexes, such as antihistamines, tranquilizers, sedatives, pain medicine, narcotics and mind-altering drugs.

Discontinuing:
Don't discontinue without consulting doctor. Dose may require gradual reduction if you have taken drug for a long time. Doses of other drugs may also require adjustment.

Others:
No problems expected.

POSSIBLE INTERACTION WITH OTHER DRUGS

GENERIC NAME OR DRUG CLASS	COMBINED EFFECT
Acebutolol	Decreased antihypertensive effect of acebutolol.
Anticoagulants (oral)	Increased risk of bleeding.
Any other non-steroidal anti-inflammatory analgesic, such as: fenoprofen, ibuprofen, indomethacin, meclofenamate, naproxen, oxyphenbutazone, phenylbutazone, salicylates, sulindac, tolmetin	Increased possibility of internal bleeding.
Aspirin	Increased risk of stomach ulcer.
Cortisone drugs	Increased risk of stomach ulcer and bleeding.
Furosemide	Decreased diuretic effect of furosemide.
Gold compounds	Possible increased likelihood of kidney damage.
Lithium	May increase lithium in blood.
Minoxidil	Decreased minoxidil effect.
Nifedipine	Increases chance of nifedipine toxicity.
Oxprenolol	Increased antihypertensive effect of oxprenolol.
Oxyphenbutazone	Possible stomach ulcer.
Phenylbutazone	Possible stomach ulcer.
Probenecid	Increased ketoprofen effect.
Thyroid hormones	Rapid heartbeat, blood-pressure rise.
Verapamil	Increases chance of verapamil toxicity.

POSSIBLE INTERACTION WITH OTHER SUBSTANCES

INTERACTS WITH	COMBINED EFFECT
Alcohol:	Possible stomach ulcer or bleeding. Avoid.
Beverages:	None expected.
Cocaine:	None expected.
Foods:	None expected.
Marijuana:	Increased pain relief from ketoprofen.
Tobacco:	None expected.

LABETOLOL

BRAND NAMES

Normodyne   **Trandate**

BASIC INFORMATION

Habit forming? No
Prescription needed? Yes
Available as generic? No
Drug class: Antihypertensive (beta- and
                alpha-adrenergic blocker)

 ## USES

Controls, but doesn't cure, high blood pressure.

 ## DOSAGE & USAGE INFORMATION

How to take:
Tablets or capsules—Swallow whole with liquid
or food to lessen stomach irritation.

When to take:
With meals or milk at same times each day.

If you forget a dose:
Take as soon as you remember up to 3 hours
late. If more than 3 hours, wait for next
scheduled dose (don't double this dose).

What drug does:
- Blocks transmission of impulses in
  sympathetic nervous system.
- Slows nerve impulses through heart.

Time lapse before drug works:
1 to 4 hours.

Don't take with:
See Interaction column and consult doctor.

 ## OVERDOSE

SYMPTOMS:
Fainting, convulsions, coma.
WHAT TO DO:
- Dial 0 (operator) or 911 (emergency) for an
  ambulance or medical help. Then give first
  aid immediately.
- See emergency information on inside
  covers.

 ## POSSIBLE ADVERSE REACTIONS OR SIDE EFFECTS

SYMPTOMS	WHAT TO DO
Life-threatening:
Congestive heart failure (weight gain, rapid pulse, breathlessness on exertion, swelling of feet and abdomen).	Discontinue. Seek emergency treatment.
Common:
None expected.	
Infrequent:
Taste change, diminished sex drive, dizziness, drowsiness, headache, itchy skin, skin and scalp numbness and tingling, abdominal pain, stuffy nose, vomiting.	Discontinue. Call doctor right away.
Rare:
Jaundice.	Discontinue. Call doctor right away.

WARNINGS & PRECAUTIONS

Don't take if:
- You are allergic to any alpha- or beta-blocking agent.
- You have asthma, congestive heart failure, heart block.

Before you start, consult your doctor:
- If you have allergies, coronary artery disease, liver disease, overactive thyroid function, chronic kidney disease.
- If you will have surgery within 2 months, including dental surgery, requiring general or spinal anesthesia.

Over age 60:
Adverse reactions and side effects may be more frequent and severe than in younger persons. Ask doctor about smaller doses.

Pregnancy:
Risk to unborn child outweighs drug benefits. Don't use.

Breast-feeding:
Risk to unborn child outweighs drug benefits. Don't use.

Infants & children:
Use only under close medical supervision.

Prolonged use:
Weakens heart muscle contractions.

Skin & sunlight:
No problems expected.

Driving, piloting or hazardous work:
Don't drive or pilot aircraft until you learn how medicine affects you. Don't work around dangerous machinery. Don't climb ladders or work in high places. Danger increases if you drink alcohol or take medicine affecting alertness and reflexes, such as antihistamines, tranquilizers, sedatives, pain medicine, narcotics and mind-altering drugs.

Discontinuing:
- Don't discontinue without consulting doctor. Dose may require gradual reduction if you have taken drug for a long time. Doses of other drugs may also require adjustment.
- These symptoms may occur if you stop taking labetolol abruptly—Chest pain, headache, sweating, weakness, trembling, fast or irregular heartbeat.

Others:
- You may need to take some form of antihypertensive treatment for the remainder of your life.
- May mask hypoglycemia.
- Get up slowly after sitting or lying to prevent fainting or dizziness.

POSSIBLE INTERACTION WITH OTHER DRUGS

GENERIC NAME OR DRUG CLASS	COMBINED EFFECT
Antidiabetics	Increased antidiabetic effect, may mask hypoglycemia.
Cimetidine	Increased antihypertensive effect of labetolol.
Clonidine	May cause precipitous change in blood pressure if clonidine and labetolol are discontinued simultaneously.
Diuretics	Increased antihypertensive effect.
Insulin	Increased antidiabetic effect, may mask hypoglycemia.
Nitroglycerin	Increased antihypertensive effect.
Phentolamine	Increased antihypertensive effect.

POSSIBLE INTERACTION WITH OTHER SUBSTANCES

INTERACTS WITH	COMBINED EFFECT
Alcohol:	Excessive blood pressure drop. Avoid.
Beverages:	No problems expected.
Cocaine:	Irregular heartbeat, unusual anxiety. Avoid.
Foods:	No problems expected.
Marijuana:	Daily use—Impaired circulation to hands and feet.
Tobacco:	Irregular heartbeat. Avoid.

LACTULOSE

BRAND NAMES

Cephalac   Chronulac

BASIC INFORMATION

Habit forming? No
Prescription needed? No
Available as generic? No
Drug class: Laxative (hyperosmotic)

 USES

Constipation relief.

 DOSAGE & USAGE INFORMATION

How to take:
Liquid—Dilute dose in beverage before swallowing.

When to take:
Usually once a day, preferably in the morning.

If you forget a dose:
Take as soon as you remember up to 8 hours before bedtime. If later, wait for next scheduled dose (don't double this dose). Don't take at bedtime.

What drug does:
Draws water into bowel from other body tissues. Causes distention through fluid accumulation, which promotes soft stool and accelerates bowel motion.

Time lapse before drug works:
30 minutes to 3 hours.

Don't take with:
Another medicine. Space 2 hours apart.

 OVERDOSE

SYMPTOMS:
Fluid depletion, weakness, vomiting, fainting.
WHAT TO DO:
Overdose unlikely to threaten life. If person takes much larger amount than prescribed, call doctor, poison-control center or hospital emergency room for instructions.

 POSSIBLE ADVERSE REACTIONS OR SIDE EFFECTS

SYMPTOMS	WHAT TO DO
Life-threatening: None expected.	
Common: None expected.	
Infrequent:	
• Irregular heartbeat.	Discontinue. Call doctor right away.
• Increased thirst, cramps, nausea, diarrhea, gaseousness.	Continue. Tell doctor at next visit.
Rare: Dizziness, confusion, fatigue, weakness.	Continue. Call doctor when convenient.

WARNINGS & PRECAUTIONS

Don't take if:
- You are allergic to any hyperosmotic laxative.
- You have symptoms of appendicitis, inflamed bowel or intestinal blockage.
- You have missed a bowel movement for only 1 or 2 days.

Before you start, consult your doctor:
- If you have congestive heart disease.
- If you have diabetes.
- If you have high blood pressure.
- If you have a colostomy or ileostomy.
- If you have kidney disease.
- If you have a laxative habit.
- If you have rectal bleeding.
- If you take another laxative.
- If you require a low-galactose diet.

Over age 60:
Adverse reactions and side effects may be more frequent and severe than in younger persons.

Pregnancy:
No proven problems. Avoid if possible.

Breast-feeding:
No problems expected.

Infants & children:
Use only under medical supervision.

Prolonged use:
Don't take for more than 1 week unless under a doctor's supervision. May cause laxative dependence.

Skin & sunlight:
No problems expected.

Driving, piloting or hazardous work:
No problems expected.

Discontinuing:
May be unnecessary to finish medicine. Follow doctor's instructions.

Others:
Don't take to "flush out" your system or as a "tonic."

POSSIBLE INTERACTION WITH OTHER DRUGS

GENERIC NAME OR DRUG CLASS	COMBINED EFFECT
None	

POSSIBLE INTERACTION WITH OTHER SUBSTANCES

INTERACTS WITH	COMBINED EFFECT
Alcohol:	None expected.
Beverages:	None expected.
Cocaine:	None expected.
Foods:	None expected.
Marijuana:	None expected.
Tobacco:	None expected.

LEVODOPA

BRAND NAMES

Bendopa	Levopa
Dopar	Sinemet
Larodopa	

BASIC INFORMATION

Habit forming? No
Prescription needed? Yes
Available as generic? Yes
Drug class: Antiparkinsonism

 USES

Controls Parkinson's disease symptoms such as rigidity, tremor and unsteady gait.

 DOSAGE & USAGE INFORMATION

How to take:
Tablet or capsule—Swallow with liquid or food to lessen stomach irritation. If you can't swallow whole, crumble tablet or open capsule and take with liquid or food.

When to take:
At the same times each day.

If you forget a dose:
Take as soon as you remember up to 2 hours late. If more than 2 hours, wait for next scheduled dose (don't double this dose).

What drug does:
Restores chemical balance necessary for normal nerve impulses.

Continued next column

 OVERDOSE

SYMPTOMS:
Muscle twitch, spastic eyelid closure, nausea, vomiting, diarrhea, irregular and rapid pulse, weakness, fainting, confusion, agitation, hallucination, coma.
WHAT TO DO:
- **Dial 0 (operator) or 911 (emergency) for an ambulance or medical help. Then give first aid immediately.**
- **If patient is unconscious and not breathing, give mouth-to-mouth breathing. If there is no heartbeat, use cardiac massage and mouth-to-mouth breathing (CPR). Don't try to make patient vomit. If you can't get help quickly, take patient to nearest emergency facility.**
- **See emergency information on inside covers.**

Time lapse before drug works:
2 to 3 weeks to improve; 6 weeks or longer for maximum benefit.

Don't take with:
See Interaction column and consult doctor.

 POSSIBLE ADVERSE REACTIONS OR SIDE EFFECTS

SYMPTOMS	WHAT TO DO
Life-threatening:	
None expected.	
Common:	
• Mood change, uncontrollable body movements, diarrhea.	Continue. Call doctor when convenient.
• Dry mouth, body odor.	No action necessary.
Infrequent:	
• Fainting, severe dizziness, headache, insomnia, nightmares, itchy skin, rash, nausea, vomiting, irregular heartbeat.	Discontinue. Call doctor right away.
• Flushed face, muscle twitching, discolored or dark urine, difficult urination, blurred vision.	Continue. Call doctor when convenient.
• Constipation, tiredness.	Continue. Tell doctor at next visit.
Rare:	
• High blood pressure.	Discontinue. Call doctor right away.
• Duodenal ulcer, anemia.	Continue. Call doctor when convenient.

WARNINGS & PRECAUTIONS

Don't take if:
- You are allergic to levodopa or carbidopa.
- You have taken MAO inhibitors in past 2 weeks.
- You have glaucoma (narrow-angle type).

Before you start, consult your doctor:
- If you have diabetes or epilepsy.
- If you have had high blood pressure, heart or lung disease.
- If you have had liver or kidney disease.
- If you have a peptic ulcer.
- If you have malignant melanoma.
- If you will have surgery within 2 months, including dental surgery, requiring general or spinal anesthesia.

Over age 60:
Adverse reactions and side effects may be more frequent and severe than in younger persons.

Pregnancy:
Risk to unborn child outweighs drug benefits. Don't use.

Breast-feeding:
Drug filters into milk. May harm child. Avoid.

Infants & children:
Not recommended.

Prolonged use:
May lead to uncontrolled movements of head, face, mouth, tongue, arms or legs.

Skin & sunlight:
No problems expected.

Driving, piloting or hazardous work:
Don't drive or pilot aircraft until you learn how medicine affects you. Don't work around dangerous machinery. Don't climb ladders or work in high places. Danger increases if you drink alcohol or take medicine affecting alertness and reflexes, such as antihistamines, tranquilizers, sedatives, pain medicine, narcotics and mind-altering drugs.

Discontinuing:
Don't discontinue without doctor's advice until you complete prescribed dose, even though symptoms diminish or disappear.

Others:
Expect to start with small dose and increase gradually to lessen frequency and severity of adverse reactions.

POSSIBLE INTERACTION WITH OTHER DRUGS

GENERIC NAME OR DRUG CLASS	COMBINED EFFECT
Albuterol	Increased risk of heartbeat irregularity.
Antiparkinsonism drugs (other)	Increased levodopa effect.
Haloperidol	Decreased levodopa effect.
MAO inhibitors	Dangerous rise in blood pressure.
Methyldopa	Decreased levodopa effect.
Molindone	Decreased levodopa effect.
Papaverine	Decreased levodopa effect.
Phenothiazines	Decreased levodopa effect.
Pyridoxine (Vitamin B-6)	Decreased levodopa effect.
Rauwolfia alkaloids	Decreased levodopa effect.

POSSIBLE INTERACTION WITH OTHER SUBSTANCES

INTERACTS WITH	COMBINED EFFECT
Alcohol:	None expected.
Beverages:	None expected.
Cocaine:	Decreased levodopa effect.
Foods:	None expected.
Marijuana:	Increased fatigue, lethargy, fainting.
Tobacco:	None expected.

LINCOMYCIN

BRAND AND GENERIC NAMES

Cleocin
CLINDAYCIN
Dalacin C

Lincocin
LINCOMYCIN

BASIC INFORMATION

Habit forming? No
Prescription needed? Yes
Available as generic? No
Drug class: Antibiotic (lincomycin)

 USES

Treatment of bacterial infections that are susceptible to lincomycin.

 DOSAGE & USAGE INFORMATION

How to take:
Capsule or liquid—Swallow with liquid 1 hour before or 2 hours after eating.

When to take:
At the same times each day.

If you forget a dose:
Take as soon as you remember up to 2 hours late. If more than 2 hours, wait for next scheduled dose (don't double this dose).

What drug does:
Destroys susceptible bacteria. Does not kill viruses.

Time lapse before drug works:
3 to 5 days.

Don't take with:
See Interaction column and consult doctor.

 OVERDOSE

SYMPTOMS:
Severe nausea, vomiting, diarrhea.
WHAT TO DO:
Overdose unlikely to threaten life. If person takes much larger amount than prescribed, call doctor, poison-control center or hospital emergency room for instructions.

 POSSIBLE ADVERSE REACTIONS OR SIDE EFFECTS

SYMPTOMS	WHAT TO DO
Life-threatening: None expected.	
Common: None expected.	
Infrequent: Unusual thirst; vomiting; stomach cramps; severe and watery diarrhea with blood or mucus; painful, swollen joints; jaundice; fever; tiredness; weakness; weight loss; rash; itch around groin, rectum or armpits; white patches in mouth; vaginal discharge, itching.	Discontinue. Call doctor right away.
Rare: None expected.	

WARNINGS &
PRECAUTIONS

Don't take if:
- You are allergic to lincomycins.
- You have had ulcerative colitis.
- Prescribed for infant under 1 month old.

Before you start, consult your doctor:
- If you have had yeast infections of mouth, skin or vagina.
- If you will have surgery within 2 months, including dental surgery, requiring general or spinal anesthesia.
- If you have kidney or liver disease.
- If you have allergies of any kind.

Over age 60:
Adverse reactions and side effects may be more frequent and severe than in younger persons.

Pregnancy:
Risk to unborn child outweighs drug benefits. Don't use.

Breast-feeding:
Drug passes into milk. Avoid drug or discontinue nursing until you finish medicine. Consult doctor for advice on maintaining milk supply.

Infants & children:
Don't give to infants younger than 1 month. Use for children only under medical supervision.

Prolonged use:
- Severe colitis with diarrhea and bleeding.
- You may become more susceptible to infections caused by germs not responsive to lincomycin.

Skin & sunlight:
No problems expected.

Driving, piloting or hazardous work:
No problems expected.

Discontinuing:
Don't discontinue without doctor's advice until you complete prescribed dose, even though symptoms diminish or disappear.

Others:
No problems expected.

 ## POSSIBLE INTERACTION
WITH OTHER DRUGS

GENERIC NAME OR DRUG CLASS	COMBINED EFFECT
Antidiarrheal preparations	Decreased lincomycin effect.
Chloramphenicol	Decreased lincomycin effect.
Erythromycin	Decreased lincomycin effect.
Loperamide	May delay removal of toxins from colon in cases of diarrhea caused by side effects of lincomycin.

 ## POSSIBLE INTERACTION
WITH OTHER SUBSTANCES

INTERACTS WITH	COMBINED EFFECT
Alcohol:	None expected.
Beverages:	None expected.
Cocaine:	None expected.
Foods:	None expected.
Marijuana:	None expected.
Tobacco:	None expected.

LIOTHYRONINE

BRAND NAMES

Cytomel   Tertroxin
Ro-Thyronine

BASIC INFORMATION

Habit forming? No
Prescription needed? Yes
Available as generic? Yes
Drug class: Thyroid hormone

 USES

Replacement for thyroid hormone deficiency.

 DOSAGE & USAGE INFORMATION

How to take:
- Tablet or capsule—Swallow with liquid.
- Extended-release tablets or capsules—Swallow each dose whole. If you take regular tablets, you may chew or crush them.

When to take:
At the same time each day before a meal or on awakening.

If you forget a dose:
Take as soon as you remember up to 12 hours late. If more than 12 hours, wait for next scheduled dose (don't double this dose).

What drug does:
Increases cell metabolism rate.

Time lapse before drug works:
48 hours.

Don't take with:
See Interaction column and consult doctor.

 OVERDOSE

SYMPTOMS:
"Hot" feeling, heart palpitations, nervousness, sweating, hand tremors, insomnia, rapid and irregular pulse, headache, irritability, diarrhea, weight loss, muscle cramps.
WHAT TO DO:
Overdose unlikely to threaten life. If person takes much larger amount than prescribed, call doctor, poison-control center or hospital emergency room for instructions.

 POSSIBLE ADVERSE REACTIONS OR SIDE EFFECTS

SYMPTOMS	WHAT TO DO
Life-threatening: None expected.	
Common:	
• Tremor, headache, irritability, insomnia.	Discontinue. Call doctor right away.
• Appetite change, diarrhea, leg cramps, menstrual irregularities, fever, heat sensitivity, unusual sweating, weight loss.	Continue. Call doctor when convenient.
Infrequent: Hives, rash, chest pain, rapid and irregular heartbeat, shortness of breath, vomiting.	Discontinue. Call doctor right away.
Rare: None expected.	

WARNINGS & PRECAUTIONS

Don't take if:
- You have had a heart attack within 6 weeks.
- You have no thyroid deficiency, but use this to lose weight.

Before you start, consult your doctor:
- If you have heart disease or high blood pressure.
- If you have diabetes.
- If you have Addison's disease, have had adrenal gland deficiency or use epinephrine, ephedrine or isoproterenol for asthma.

Over age 60:
More sensitive to thyroid hormone. May need smaller doses.

Pregnancy:
Considered safe if for thyroid deficiency only.

Breast-feeding:
Present in milk. Considered safe if dose is correct.

Infants & children:
Use only under medical supervision.

Prolonged use:
No problems expected, if dose is correct.

Skin & sunlight:
No problems expected.

Driving, piloting or hazardous work:
No problems expected.

Discontinuing:
Don't discontinue without consulting doctor. Dose may require gradual reduction if you have taken drug for a long time. Doses of other drugs may also require adjustment.

Others:
Digestive upsets, tremors, cramps, nervousness, insomnia or diarrhea may indicate need for dose adjustment.

POSSIBLE INTERACTION WITH OTHER DRUGS

GENERIC NAME OR DRUG CLASS	COMBINED EFFECT
Amphetamines	Increased amphetamine effect.
Anticoagulants (oral)	Increased anticoagulant effect.
Antidepressants (tricyclic)	Irregular heartbeat.
Antidiabetics	Antidiabetic may require adjustment.
Aspirin (large doses, continuous use)	Increased liothyronine effect.
Barbiturates	Decreased barbiturate effect.
Cholestyramine	Decreased liothyronine effect.
Contraceptives (oral)	Decreased liothyronine effect.
Cortisone drugs	Requires dose adjustment to prevent cortisone deficiency.
Digitalis preparations	Increased digitalis effect.
Ephedrine	Increased ephedrine effect.
Epinephrine	Increased epinephrine effect.
Methylphenidate	Increased methylphenidate effect.
Phenytoin	Increased liothyronine effect.

POSSIBLE INTERACTION WITH OTHER SUBSTANCES

INTERACTS WITH	COMBINED EFFECT
Alcohol:	None expected.
Beverages:	None expected.
Cocaine:	Excess stimulation. Avoid.
Foods: Soybeans.	Heavy consumption interferes with thyroid function.
Marijuana:	None expected.
Tobacco:	None expected.

LIOTRIX

BRAND NAMES

Euthroid   **Thyrolar**

BASIC INFORMATION

Habit forming? No
Prescription needed? Yes
Available as generic? Yes
Drug class: Thyroid hormone

 USES

Replacement for thyroid hormone deficiency.

 DOSAGE & USAGE INFORMATION

How to take:
- Tablet or capsule—Swallow with liquid.
- Extended-release tablets or capsules—Swallow each dose whole. If you take regular tablets, you may chew or crush them.

When to take:
At the same time each day before a meal or on awakening.

If you forget a dose:
Take as soon as you remember up to 12 hours late. If more than 12 hours, wait for next scheduled dose (don't double this dose).

What drug does:
Increases cell metabolism rate.

Time lapse before drug works:
48 hours.

Don't take with:
See Interaction column and consult doctor.

 OVERDOSE

SYMPTOMS:
"Hot" feeling, heart palpitations, nervousness, sweating, hand tremors, insomnia, rapid and irregular pulse, headache, irritability, diarrhea, weight loss, muscle cramps.
WHAT TO DO:
Overdose unlikely to threaten life. If person takes much larger amount than prescribed, call doctor, poison-control center or hospital emergency room for instructions.

 POSSIBLE ADVERSE REACTIONS OR SIDE EFFECTS

SYMPTOMS	WHAT TO DO
Life-threatening:	
None expected.	
Common:	
• Tremor, headache, irritability, insomnia.	Discontinue. Call doctor right away.
• Appetite change, diarrhea, leg cramps, menstrual irregularities, fever, heat sensitivity, unusual sweating, weight loss.	Continue. Call doctor when convenient.
Infrequent:	
Hives, itchy skin, vomiting, chest pain, rapid and irregular heartbeat, shortness of breath.	Discontinue. Call doctor right away.
Rare:	
None expected.	

WARNINGS & PRECAUTIONS

Don't take if:
- You have had a heart attack within 6 weeks.
- You have no thyroid deficiency, but use this to lose weight.

Before you start, consult your doctor:
- If you have heart disease or high blood pressure.
- If you have diabetes.
- If you have Addison's disease, have had adrenal gland deficiency or use epinephrine, ephedrine or isoproterenol for asthma.

Over age 60:
More sensitive to thyroid hormone. May need smaller doses.

Pregnancy:
Considered safe if for thyroid deficiency only.

Breast-feeding:
Present in milk. Considered safe if dose is correct.

Infants & children:
Use only under medical supervision.

Prolonged use:
No problems expected, if dose is correct.

Skin & sunlight:
No problems expected.

Driving, piloting or hazardous work:
No problems expected.

Discontinuing:
Don't discontinue without consulting doctor. Dose may require gradual reduction if you have taken drug for a long time. Doses of other drugs may also require adjustment.

Others:
Digestive upsets, tremors, cramps, nervousness, insomnia or diarrhea may indicate need for dose adjustment.

POSSIBLE INTERACTION WITH OTHER DRUGS

GENERIC NAME OR DRUG CLASS	COMBINED EFFECT
Amphetamines	Increased amphetamine effect.
Anticoagulants (oral)	Increased anticoagulant effect.
Antidepressants (tricyclic)	Irregular heartbeat.
Antidiabetics	Antidiabetic may require adjustment.
Aspirin (large doses, continuous use)	Increased liotrix effect.
Barbiturates	Decreased barbiturate effect.
Cholestyramine	Decreased liotrix effect.
Contraceptives (oral)	Decreased liotrix effect.
Cortisone drugs	Requires dose adjustment to prevent cortisone deficiency.
Digitalis preparations	Increased digitalis effect.
Ephedrine	Increased ephedrine effect.
Epinephrine	Increased epinephrine effect.
Methylphenidate	Increased methylphenidate effect.
Phenytoin	Increased liotrix effect.

POSSIBLE INTERACTION WITH OTHER SUBSTANCES

INTERACTS WITH	COMBINED EFFECT
Alcohol:	None expected.
Beverages:	None expected.
Cocaine:	Excess stimulation. Avoid.
Foods: Soybeans.	Heavy consumption interferes with thyroid function.
Marijuana:	None expected.
Tobacco:	None expected.

LITHIUM

BRAND NAMES

Carbolith
Cibalith-S
Duralith
Eskalith
Eskalith CR
Lithane

Lithizine
Lithobid
Lithonate
Lithotabs
Pfi-Lithium

BASIC INFORMATION

Habit forming? No
Prescription needed? Yes
Available as generic? Yes
Drug class: Tranquilizer

 USES

Normalizes mood and behavior in manic-depressive illness.

 DOSAGE & USAGE INFORMATION

How to take:
- Tablet or capsule—Swallow with liquid or food to lessen stomach irritation. If you can't swallow whole, crumble tablet or open capsule and take with liquid or food. Drink 2 or 3 quarts liquid per day.
- Extended-release tablets or capsules—Swallow each dose whole.
- Syrup—Take at mealtime. Follow with 8 oz. water.

When to take:
At the same times each day, preferably mealtime.

If you forget a dose:
Take as soon as you remember up to 2 hours late. If more than 2 hours, wait for next scheduled dose (don't double this dose).

Continued next column

 OVERDOSE

SYMPTOMS:
Moderate overdose increases some side effects. Large overdose may cause convulsions, stupor and coma.
WHAT TO DO:
- **Dial 0 (operator) or 911 (emergency) for an ambulance or medical help. Then give first aid immediately.**
- **See emergency information on inside covers.**

What drug does:
May correct chemical imbalance in brain's transmission of nerve impulses that influence mood and behavior.

Time lapse before drug works:
1 to 3 weeks. May require 3 months before depressive phase of illness improves.

Don't take with:
See Interaction column and consult doctor.

 POSSIBLE ADVERSE REACTIONS OR SIDE EFFECTS

SYMPTOMS	WHAT TO DO
Life-threatening: None expected.	
Common:	
• Dizziness, diarrhea, nausea, vomiting, shakiness, tremor.	Continue. Call doctor when convenient.
• Dry mouth, thirst, decreased sexual ability, increased urination.	Continue. Tell doctor at next visit.
Infrequent:	
• Rash, stomach pain.	Discontinue. Call doctor right away.
• Swollen hands, feet; slurred speech; thyroid impairment (coldness, dry, puffy skin); muscle aches; headache; weight gain; fatigue; menstrual irregularities.	Continue. Call doctor when convenient.
• Drowsiness, confusion, weakness.	Continue. Tell doctor at next visit.
Rare:	
• Blurred vision.	Discontinue. Call doctor right away.
• Jerking of arms and legs.	Continue. Call doctor when convenient.

WARNINGS & PRECAUTIONS

Don't take if:
- You are allergic to lithium.
- You have kidney or heart disease.
- Patient is younger than 12.

Before you start, consult your doctor:
- About all medications you take.
- If you plan to become pregnant within medication period.
- If you have diabetes, low thyroid function, epilepsy or any significant medical problem.
- If you are on a low-salt diet or drink more than 4 cups of coffee per day.
- If you plan surgery within 2 months.

Over age 60:
Adverse reactions and side effects may be more frequent and severe than in younger persons.

Pregnancy:
Risk to unborn child outweighs drug benefits. Don't use.

Breast-feeding:
Drug passes into milk. Avoid drug or discontinue nursing until you finish medicine. Consult doctor for advice on maintaining milk supply.

Infants & children:
Don't give to children younger than 12.

Prolonged use:
Enlarged thyroid with possible impaired function.

Skin & sunlight:
No problems expected.

Driving, piloting or hazardous work:
Don't drive or pilot aircraft until you learn how medicine affects you. Don't work around dangerous machinery. Don't climb ladders or work in high places. Danger increases if you drink alcohol or take medicine affecting alertness and reflexes.

Discontinuing:
Don't discontinue without consulting doctor. Dose may require gradual reduction if you have taken drug for a long time. Doses of other drugs may also require adjustment.

Others:
- Regular checkups, periodic blood tests, and tests of lithium levels and thyroid function recommended.
- Avoid exercise in hot weather and other activities that cause heavy sweating. This contributes to lithium poisoning.

POSSIBLE INTERACTION WITH OTHER DRUGS

GENERIC NAME OR DRUG CLASS	COMBINED EFFECT
Acetazolamide	Decreased lithium effect.
Aminophylline	Decreased lithium effect.
Diuretics	Increased lithium effect.
Dronabinol	Increased effects of both drugs. Avoid.
Haloperidol	Increased toxicity of both drugs.
Indomethacin	Increased lithium effect.
Ketoprofen	May increase lithium in blood.
Methyldopa	Increased lithium effect.
Muscle relaxants (skeletal)	Increased skeletal-muscle relaxation.
Oxyphenbutazone	Increased lithium effect.
Phenothiazines	Decreased lithium effect.
Phentyoin	Increased lithium effect.
Phenylbutazone	Increased lithium effect.
Potassium iodide	Increased potassium iodide effect.
Sodium bicarbonate	Decreased lithium effect.
Suprofen	May increase lithium in blood.
Terfenadine	Possible excessive sedation.
Tetracyclines	Increased lithium effect.

POSSIBLE INTERACTION WITH OTHER SUBSTANCES

INTERACTS WITH	COMBINED EFFECT
Alcohol:	Possible lithium poisoning.
Beverages: Caffeine drinks.	Increased lithium effect.
Cocaine:	Possible psychosis.
Foods: Salt.	*Don't* restrict intake.
Marijuana:	Increased tremor and possible psychosis.
Tobacco:	None expected.

LOPERAMIDE

BRAND NAMES

Imodium

BASIC INFORMATION

Habit forming? No, unless taken in high
doses for long periods.
Prescription needed? Yes
Available as generic? No
Drug class: Antidiarrheal

 USES

Relieves diarrhea and reduces volume of
discharge from ileostomies and colostomies.

 DOSAGE & USAGE INFORMATION

How to take:
- Tablet or capsule—Swallow with food to
lessen stomach irritation.
- Liquid—Follow label instructions and use
marked dropper.

When to take:
No more often than directed on label.

If you forget a dose:
Take as soon as you remember up to 2 hours
late. If more than 2 hours, wait for next
scheduled dose (don't double this dose).

What drug does:
Blocks digestive tract's nerve supply, which
reduces irritability and contractions in intestinal
tract.

Time lapse before drug works:
1 to 2 hours.

Don't take with:
See Interaction column and consult doctor.

 OVERDOSE

SYMPTOMS:
**Constipation, lethargy, drowsiness or
unconsciousness.**
WHAT TO DO:
**Overdose unlikely to threaten life. If person
takes much larger amount than prescribed,
call doctor, poison-control center or hospital
emergency room for instructions.**

 POSSIBLE ADVERSE REACTIONS OR SIDE EFFECTS

SYMPTOMS	WHAT TO DO
Life-threatening: None expected.	
Common: None expected.	
Infrequent:	
• Rash.	Discontinue. Call doctor right away.
• Drowsiness, dry mouth, bloating, constipation, appetite loss, stomach pain.	Continue. Call doctor when convenient.
Rare: Unexplained fever.	Discontinue. Call doctor right away.

WARNINGS & PRECAUTION

Don't take if:
- You have severe colitis.
- You have colitis resulting from antibiotic treatment.

Before you start, consult your doctor:
- If you are dehydrated from fluid loss caused by diarrhea.
- If you have liver disease.

Over age 60:
Adverse reactions and side effects may be more frequent and severe than in younger persons.

Pregnancy:
No proven harm. Avoid if possible.

Breast-feeding:
No proven problems, but avoid if possible or discontinue nursing until you finish medicine. Consult doctor for advice on maintaining milk supply.

Infants & children:
Don't give to infants or toddlers. Use only under doctor's supervision for children older than 2.

Prolonged use:
Habit forming at high dose.

Skin & sunlight:
No problems expected.

Driving, piloting or hazardous work:
Don't drive or pilot aircraft until you learn how medicine affects you. Don't work around dangerous machinery. Don't climb ladders or work in high places. Danger increases if you drink alcohol or take medicine affecting alertness and reflexes.

Discontinuing:
- May be unnecessary to finish medicine. Follow doctor's instructions.
- After discontinuing, consult doctor if you experience muscle cramps, nausea, vomiting, trembling, stomach cramps or unusual sweating.

Others:
If acute diarrhea lasts longer than 48 hours, discontinue and call doctor. In chronic diarrhea, loperamide is unlikely to be effective if diarrhea doesn't improve in 10 days.

POSSIBLE INTERACTION WITH OTHER DRUGS

GENERIC NAME OR DRUG CLASS	COMBINED EFFECT
Antibiotics (cephalosporins, clindamycin, lincomycins, penicillins).	May delay removal of toxins from colon in cases of diarrhea caused by side effects of these antibiotics.

POSSIBLE INTERACTION WITH OTHER SUBSTANCES

INTERACTS WITH	COMBINED EFFECT
Alcohol:	Depressed brain function. Avoid.
Beverages:	None expected.
Cocaine:	Decreased loperamide effect.
Foods:	None expected.
Marijuana:	None expected.
Tobacco:	None expected.

LORAZEPAM

BRAND NAMES

Apo-Lorazepam	Loraz
Ativan	Novolorazem

BASIC INFORMATION

Habit forming? Yes
Prescription needed? Yes
Available as generic? Yes
Drug class: Tranquilizer (benzodiazepine)

USES

Treatment for nervousness or tension.

DOSAGE & USAGE INFORMATION

How to take:
Tablet or capsule—Swallow with liquid. If you can't swallow whole, crumble tablet or open capsule and take with liquid or food.

When to take:
At the same time each day, according to instructions on prescription label.

If you forget a dose:
Take as soon as you remember up to 2 hours late. If more than 2 hours, wait for next scheduled dose (don't double this dose).

What drug does:
Affects limbic system of brain—part that controls emotions.

Time lapse before drug works:
2 hours. May take 6 weeks for full benefit.

Don't take with:
See Interaction column and consult doctor.

OVERDOSE

SYMPTOMS:
Drowsiness, weakness, tremor, stupor, coma.
WHAT TO DO:
- **Dial 0 (operator) or 911 (emergency) for an ambulance or medical help. Then give first aid immediately.**
- **If patient is unconscious and not breathing, give mouth-to-mouth breathing. If there is no heartbeat, use cardiac massage and mouth-to-mouth breathing (CPR). Don't try to make patient vomit. If you can't get help quickly, take patient to nearest emergency facility.**
- **See emergency information on inside covers.**

POSSIBLE ADVERSE REACTIONS OR SIDE EFFECTS

SYMPTOMS	WHAT TO DO
Life-threatening: None expected.	
Common: Clumsiness, drowsiness, dizziness.	Continue. Call doctor when convenient.
Infrequent: • Hallucinations, confusion, depression, irritability, itchy skin, rash, change in vision.	Discontinue. Call doctor right away.
• Constipation or diarrhea, nausea, vomiting, difficult urination.	Continue. Call doctor when convenient.
Rare: • Slow heartbeat, difficult breathing.	Discontinue. Seek emergency treatment.
• Mouth, throat ulcers; jaundice.	Discontinue. Call doctor right away.

WARNINGS & PRECAUTIONS

Don't take if:
- You are allergic to any benzodiazepine.
- You have myasthenia gravis.
- You are active or recovering alcoholic.
- Patient is younger than 6 months.

Before you start, consult your doctor:
- If you have liver, kidney or lung disease.
- If you have diabetes, epilepsy or porphyria.

Over age 60:
Adverse reactions and side effects may be more frequent and severe than in younger persons. You need smaller doses for shorter periods of time. May develop agitation, rage or "hangover" effect.

Pregnancy:
Risk to unborn child outweighs drug benefits. Don't use.

Breast-feeding:
Drug passes into milk. Avoid drug or discontinue nursing until you finish medicine. Consult doctor for advice on maintaining milk supply.

Infants & children:
Use only under medical supervision for children older than 6 months.

Prolonged use:
May impair liver function.

Skin & sunlight:
No problems expected.

Driving, piloting or hazardous work:
Don't drive or pilot aircraft until you learn how medicine affects you. Don't work around dangerous machinery. Don't climb ladders or work in high places. Danger increases if you drink alcohol or take medicine affecting alertness and reflexes.

Discontinuing:
Don't discontinue without consulting doctor. Dose may require gradual reduction if you have taken drug for a long time. Doses of other drugs may also require adjustment.

Others:
- Hot weather, heavy exercise and profuse sweat may reduce excretion and cause overdose.
- Blood sugar may rise in diabetics, requiring insulin adjustment.

POSSIBLE INTERACTION WITH OTHER DRUGS

GENERIC NAME OR DRUG CLASS	COMBINED EFFECT
Anticonvulsants	Change in seizure frequency or severity.
Antidepressants	Increased sedative effect of both drugs.
Antihistamines	Increased sedative effect of both drugs.
Antihypertensives	Excessively low blood pressure.
Cimetidine	Excess sedation.
Disulfiram	Increased lorazepam effect.
Dronabinol	Increased effects of both drugs. Avoid.
MAO inhibitors	Convulsions, deep sedation, rage.
Molindone	Increased tranquilizer effect.
Narcotics	Increased sedative effect of both drugs.
Sedatives	Increased sedative effect of both drugs.
Sleep inducers	Increased sedative effect of both drugs.
Tranquilizers	Increased sedative effect of both drugs.

POSSIBLE INTERACTION WITH OTHER SUBSTANCES

INTERACTS WITH	COMBINED EFFECT
Alcohol:	Heavy sedation. Avoid.
Beverages:	None expected.
Cocaine:	Decreased lorazepam effect.
Foods:	None expected.
Marijuana:	Heavy sedation. Avoid.
Tobacco:	Decreased lorazepam effect.

MAGNESIUM CARBONATE

BRAND NAMES

Alkets	Gaviscon
Bisodol	Magnagel
De Witt's	Marblen
Di-Gel	Osti-Derm
Estomul-M	Silain-Gel

BASIC INFORMATION

Habit forming? No
Prescription needed? No
Available as generic? Yes
Drug class: Antacid, laxative

USES

- Treatment for hyperacidity in upper gastrointestinal tract, including stomach and esophagus. Symptoms may be heartburn or acid indigestion. Diseases include peptic ulcer, gastritis, esophagitis, hiatal hernia.
- Constipation relief.

DOSAGE & USAGE INFORMATION

How to take:
- Tablet or capsule—Swallow with liquid.
- Chewable tablets or wafers—Chew well before swallowing.
- Liquid—Shake well and take undiluted.
- Powder—Mix with water and drink all liquid.

When to take:
1 to 3 hours after meals unless directed otherwise by your doctor.

If you forget a dose:
Take as soon as you remember.

What drug does:
- Neutralizes some of the hydrochloric acid in the stomach.
- Reduces action of pepsin, a digestive enzyme.
- Stimulates muscles in lower bowel wall.

Continued next column

OVERDOSE

SYMPTOMS:
Dry mouth, diarrhea, shallow breathing, stupor.
WHAT TO DO:
- Dial 0 (operator) or 911 (emergency) for an ambulance or medical help. Then give first aid immediately.
- See emergency information on inside covers.

Time lapse before drug works:
15 minutes.

Don't take with:
Other medicines at the same time. Decreases absorption of other drugs.

POSSIBLE ADVERSE REACTIONS OR SIDE EFFECTS

SYMPTOMS	WHAT TO DO
Life-threatening: None expected.	
Common: Constipation, appetite loss.	Continue. Call doctor when convenient.
Infrequent:	
• Lower abdominal pain and swelling, bone pain, muscle weakness, swollen wrists or ankles.	Discontinue. Call doctor right away.
• Weight loss, mood change, nausea, vomiting.	Continue. Call doctor when convenient.
Rare: Unusual weakness or tiredness.	Discontinue. Call doctor right away.

MAGNESIUM CARBONATE

WARNINGS & PRECAUTIONS

Don't take if:
You are allergic to any antacid.

Before you start, consult your doctor:
- If you have kidney disease.
- If you have chronic constipation, colitis or diarrhea.
- If you have symptoms of appendicitis.
- If you have stomach or intestinal bleeding.

Over age 60:
Adverse reactions and side effects may be more frequent and severe than in younger persons. Diarrhea or constipation particularly likely.

Pregnancy:
Risk to unborn child outweighs drug benefits. Don't use.

Breast-feeding:
Drug passes into milk. Avoid drug or discontinue nursing until you finish medicine. Consult doctor for advice on maintaining milk supply.

Infants & children:
Use only under medical supervision.

Prolonged use:
No problems expected.

Skin & sunlight:
No problems expected.

Driving, piloting or hazardous work:
No problems expected.

Discontinuing:
May be unnecessary to finish medicine. Follow doctor's instructions.

Others:
Don't take longer than 2 weeks unless under medical supervision.

POSSIBLE INTERACTION WITH OTHER DRUGS

GENERIC NAME OR DRUG CLASS	COMBINED EFFECT
Anticoagulants	Decreased anticoagulant effect.
Chlorpromazine	Decreased chlorpromazine effect.
Digitalis preparations	Decreased digitalis effect.
Iron supplements	Decreased iron effect.
Isoniazid	Decreased isoniazid effect.
Levodopa	Increased levodopa effect.
Meperidine	Increased meperidine effect.
Mexiletine	May slow elimination of mexiletine and cause need to adjust dosage.
Nalidixic acid	Decreased effect of nalidixic acid.
Oxyphenbutazone	Decreased oxyphenbutazone effect.
Para-aminosalicylic acid (PAS)	Decreased PAS effect.
Penicillins	Decreased penicillin effect.
Pentobarbital	Decreased pentobarbital effect.
Phenylbutazone	Decreased phenylbutazone effect.
Pseudoephedrine	Increased pseudoephedrine effect.
Sulfa drugs	Decreased sulfa effect.
Tetracyclines	Decreased tetracycline effect.
Vitamins A and C	Decreased vitamin effect.
Vitamin D	Too much calcium in blood.

POSSIBLE INTERACTION WITH OTHER SUBSTANCES

INTERACTS WITH	COMBINED EFFECT
Alcohol:	Decreased antacid effect.
Beverages:	No proven problems.
Cocaine:	No proven problems.
Foods:	Decreased antacid effect if taken with food. Wait 1 hour after eating.
Marijuana:	No proven problems.
Tobacco:	Decreased antacid effect.

MAGNESIUM CITRATE

BRAND NAMES

Citrate of Magnesia
Citro-Mag
Citro-Nesia
Citroma

Evac-Q-Kit
Evac-Q-Kwik
National

BASIC INFORMATION

Habit forming? No
Prescription needed? No
Available as generic? Yes
Drug class: Laxative (hyperosmotic)

 USES

Constipation relief.

 DOSAGE & USAGE INFORMATION

How to take:
Liquid—Dilute dose in beverage before swallowing.

When to take:
Usually once a day, preferably in the morning.

If you forget a dose:
Take as soon as you remember up to 8 hours before bedtime. If later, wait for next scheduled dose (don't double this dose). Don't take at bedtime.

What drug does:
Draws water into bowel from other body tissues. Causes distention through fluid accumulation, which promotes soft stool and accelerates bowel motion.

Time lapse before drug works:
30 minutes to 3 hours.

Don't take with:
See Interaction column and consult doctor.

 OVERDOSE

SYMPTOMS:
Fluid depletion, weakness, vomiting, fainting.
WHAT TO DO:
Overdose unlikely to threaten life. If person takes much larger amount than prescribed, call doctor, poison-control center or hospital emergency room for instructions.

 POSSIBLE ADVERSE REACTIONS OR SIDE EFFECTS

SYMPTOMS	WHAT TO DO
Life-threatening: None expected.	
Common: None expected.	
Infrequent:	
• Irregular heartbeat.	Discontinue. Call doctor right away.
• Increased thirst, cramps, nausea, diarrhea, gaseousness.	Continue. Tell doctor at next visit.
Rare: Dizziness, confusion, tiredness or weakness.	Continue. Call doctor when convenient.

WARNINGS & PRECAUTIONS

Don't take if:
- You are allergic to any hyperosmotic laxative.
- You have symptoms of appendicitis, inflamed bowel or intestinal blockage.
- You have missed a bowel movement for only 1 or 2 days.

Before you start, consult your doctor:
- If you have congestive heart disease.
- If you have diabetes.
- If you have high blood pressure.
- If you have a colostomy or ileostomy.
- If you have kidney disease.
- If you have a laxative habit.
- If you have rectal bleeding.
- If you take another laxative.

Over age 60:
Adverse reactions and side effects may be more frequent and severe than in younger persons.

Pregnancy:
Salt content may cause fluid retention and swelling. Avoid if possible.

Breast-feeding:
No problems expected.

Infants & children:
Use only under medical supervision.

Prolonged use:
Don't take for more than 1 week unless under a doctor's supervision. May cause laxative dependence.

Skin & sunlight:
No problems expected.

Driving, piloting or hazardous work:
No problems expected.

Discontinuing:
May be unnecessary to finish medicine. Follow doctor's instructions.

Others:
- Don't take to "flush out" your system or as a "tonic."
- Don't take within 2 hours of taking another medicine.

POSSIBLE INTERACTION WITH OTHER DRUGS

GENERIC NAME OR DRUG CLASS	COMBINED EFFECT
Chlordiazepoxide	Decreased chlordiazepoxide effect.
Chlorpromazine	Decreased chlorpromazine effect.
Dicumarol	Decreased dicumarol effect.
Digoxin	Decreased digoxin effect.
Isoniazid	Decreased isoniazid effect.
Mexiletine	May slow elimination of mexiletine and cause need to adjust dosage.
Tetracyclines	Possible intestinal blockage.

POSSIBLE INTERACTION WITH OTHER SUBSTANCES

INTERACTS WITH	COMBINED EFFECT
Alcohol:	None expected.
Beverages:	None expected.
Cocaine:	None expected.
Foods:	None expected.
Marijuana:	None expected.
Tobacco:	None expected.

MAGNESIUM HYDROXIDE

BRAND NAMES

See complete list of brand names in the *Brand Name Directory,* page 951.

BASIC INFORMATION

Habit forming? No
Prescription needed? No
Available as generic? Yes
Drug class: Antacid, laxative

USES

- Treatment for hyperacidity in upper gastrointestinal tract, including stomach and esophagus. Symptoms may be heartburn or acid indigestion. Diseases include peptic ulcer, gastritis, esophagitis, hiatal hernia.
- Constipation relief.

DOSAGE & USAGE INFORMATION

How to take:
- Tablet—Swallow with liquid.
- Liquid—Shake well and take undiluted.

When to take:
1 to 3 hours after meals unless directed otherwise by your doctor.

If you forget a dose:
Take as soon as you remember.

What drug does:
- Neutralizes some of the hydrochloric acid in the stomach.
- Reduces action of pepsin, a digestive enzyme.
- Stimulates muscles in lower bowel wall.

Time lapse before drug works:
15 minutes.

Don't take with:
Other medicines at the same time. Decreases absorption of other drugs.

OVERDOSE

SYMPTOMS:
Dry mouth, shallow breathing, diarrhea, stupor.
WHAT TO DO:
- Dial 0 (operator) or 911 (emergency) for an ambulance or medical help. Then give first aid immediately.
- See emergency information on inside covers.

POSSIBLE ADVERSE REACTIONS OR SIDE EFFECTS

SYMPTOMS	WHAT TO DO
Life-threatening: None expected.	
Common: Constipation, appetite loss.	Continue. Call doctor when convenient.
Infrequent: • Lower abdominal pain and swelling, bone pain, muscle weakness, swollen wrists or ankles.	Discontinue. Call doctor right away.
• Mood change, nausea, vomiting, weight loss.	Continue. Call doctor when convenient.
Rare: None expected.	

WARNINGS & PRECAUTIONS

Don't take if:
You are allergic to any antacid.

Before you start, consult your doctor:
- If you have kidney disease.
- If you have chronic constipation, colitis or diarrhea.
- If you have symptoms of appendicitis.
- If you have stomach or intestinal bleeding.

Over age 60:
Adverse reactions and side effects may be more frequent and severe than in younger persons. Diarrhea or constipation particularly likely.

Pregnancy:
Risk to unborn child outweighs drug benefits. Don't use.

Breast-feeding:
Drug passes into milk. Avoid drug or discontinue nursing until you finish medicine. Consult doctor for advice on maintaining milk supply.

Infants & children:
Use only under medical supervision.

Prolonged use:
No problems expected.

Skin & sunlight:
No problems expected.

Driving, piloting or hazardous work:
No problems expected.

Discontinuing:
May be unnecessary to finish medicine. Follow doctor's instructions.

Others:
Don't take longer than 2 weeks unless under medical supervision.

POSSIBLE INTERACTION WITH OTHER DRUGS

GENERIC NAME OR DRUG CLASS	COMBINED EFFECT
Anticoagulants	Decreased anticoagulant effect.
Chlorpromazine	Decreased chlorpromazine effect.
Digitalis preparations	Decreased digitalis effect.
Iron supplements	Decreased iron effect.
Isoniazid	Decreased isoniazid effect.
Levodopa	Increased levodopa effect.
Meperidine	Increased meperidine effect.
Mexiletine	May slow elimination of mexiletine and cause need to adjust dosage.
Nalidixic acid	Decreased effect of nalidixic acid.
Oxyphenbutazone	Decreased oxyphenbutazone effect.
Para-aminosalicylic acid (PAS)	Decreased PAS effect.
Penicillins	Decreased penicillin effect.
Pentobarbital	Decreased pentobarbital effect.
Phenylbutazone	Decreased phenylbutazone effect.
Pseudoephedrine	Increased pseudoephedrine effect.
Sulfa drugs	Decreased sulfa effect.
Tetracyclines	Decreased tetracycline effect.
Vitamins A and C	Decreased vitamin effect.
Vitamin D	Too much calcium in blood.

POSSIBLE INTERACTION WITH OTHER SUBSTANCES

INTERACTS WITH	COMBINED EFFECT
Alcohol:	Decreased antacid effect.
Beverages:	No proven problems.
Cocaine:	No proven problems.
Foods:	Decreased antacid effect if taken with food. Wait 1 hour after eating.
Marijuana:	No proven problems.
Tobacco:	Decreased antacid effect.

MAGNESIUM SULFATE

BRAND NAMES

Bilagog
Eldercaps
Eldertonic

Epsom Salts
Glutofac
Vicon

BASIC INFORMATION

Habit forming? No
Prescription needed? No
Available as generic? Yes
Drug class: Laxative (hyperosmotic)

 USES

Constipation relief.

 DOSAGE & USAGE INFORMATION

How to take:
Powder or solid form—Dilute dose in beverage before swallowing. Solid form must be dissolved.

When to take:
Usually once a day, preferably in the morning.

If you forget a dose:
Take as soon as you remember up to 8 hours before bedtime. If later, wait for next scheduled dose (don't double this dose). Don't take at bedtime.

What drug does:
Draws water into bowel from other body tissues. Causes distention through fluid accumulation, which promotes soft stool and accelerates bowel motion.

Time lapse before drug works:
30 minutes to 3 hours.

Don't take with:
See Interaction column and consult doctor.

 OVERDOSE

SYMPTOMS:
Fluid depletion, weakness, vomiting, fainting.
WHAT TO DO:
Overdose unlikely to threaten life. If person takes much larger amount than prescribed, call doctor, poison-control center or hospital emergency room for instructions.

 POSSIBLE ADVERSE REACTIONS OR SIDE EFFECTS

SYMPTOMS	WHAT TO DO
Life-threatening:	
None expected.	
Common:	
None expected.	
Infrequent:	
● Irregular heartbeat.	Discontinue. Call doctor right away.
● Increased thirst, cramps, nausea, diarrhea, gaseousness.	Continue. Tell doctor at next visit.
Rare:	
Dizziness, confusion, tiredness or weakness.	Continue. Call doctor when convenient.

WARNINGS & PRECAUTIONS

Don't take if:
- You are allergic to any hyperosmotic laxative.
- You have symptoms of appendicitis, inflamed bowel or intestinal blockage.
- You have missed a bowel movement for only 1 or 2 days.

Before you start, consult your doctor:
- If you have congestive heart disease.
- If you have diabetes.
- If you have high blood pressure.
- If you have a colostomy or ileostomy.
- If you have kidney disease.
- If you have a laxative habit.
- If you have rectal bleeding.
- If you take another laxative.

Over age 60:
Adverse reactions and side effects may be more frequent and severe than in younger persons.

Pregnancy:
Salt content may cause fluid retention and swelling. Avoid if possible.

Breast-feeding:
No problems expected.

Infants & children:
Use only under medical supervision.

Prolonged use:
Don't take for more than 1 week unless under a doctor's supervision. May cause laxative dependence.

Skin & sunlight:
No problems expected.

Driving, piloting or hazardous work:
No problems expected.

Discontinuing:
May be unnecessary to finish medicine. Follow doctor's instructions.

Others:
- Don't take to "flush out" your system or as a "tonic."
- Don't take within 2 hours of taking another medicine.

POSSIBLE INTERACTION WITH OTHER DRUGS

GENERIC NAME OR DRUG CLASS	COMBINED EFFECT
Chlordiazepoxide	Decreased chlordiazepoxide effect.
Chlorpromazine	Decreased chlorpromazine effect.
Dicumarol	Decreased dicumarol effect.
Digoxin	Decreased digoxin effect.
Isoniazid	Decreased isoniazid effect.
Mexiletine	May slow elimination of mexiletine and cause need to adjust dosage.
Tetracyclines	Possible intestinal blockage.

POSSIBLE INTERACTION WITH OTHER SUBSTANCES

INTERACTS WITH	COMBINED EFFECT
Alcohol:	None expected.
Beverages:	None expected.
Cocaine:	None expected.
Foods:	None expected.
Marijuana:	None expected.
Tobacco:	None expected.

MAGNESIUM TRISILICATE

BRAND NAMES

A-M-T	Magnatril
Alma-Mag	Mucotin
Gaviscon	Neutrocomp
Gelusil	Sterazolidin
Gelusil-M	Trisogel

BASIC INFORMATION

Habit forming? No
Prescription needed? No
Available as generic? Yes
Drug class: Antacid, laxative

USES

- Treatment for hyperacidity in upper gastrointestinal tract, including stomach and esophagus. Symptoms may be heartburn or acid indigestion. Diseases include peptic ulcer, gastritis, esophagitis, hiatal hernia.
- Constipation relief.

DOSAGE & USAGE INFORMATION

How to take:
- Tablet or capsule—Swallow with liquid.
- Chewable tablets or wafers—Chew well before swallowing.
- Liquid—Shake well and take undiluted.

When to take:
1 to 3 hours after meals unless directed otherwise by your doctor.

If you forget a dose:
Take as soon as you remember.

What drug does:
- Neutralizes some of the hydrochloric acid in the stomach.
- Reduces action of pepsin, a digestive enzyme.
- Stimulates muscles in lower bowel wall.

Continued next column

OVERDOSE

SYMPTOMS:
Dry mouth, diarrhea, shallow breathing, stupor.
WHAT TO DO:
- Dial 0 (operator) or 911 (emergency) for an ambulance or medical help. Then give first aid immediately.
- See emergency information on inside covers.

Time lapse before drug works:
15 minutes.

Don't take with:
Other medicines at the same time. Decreases absorption of other drugs.

POSSIBLE ADVERSE REACTIONS OR SIDE EFFECTS

SYMPTOMS	WHAT TO DO
Life-threatening:	
None expected.	
Common:	
Constipation, appetite loss.	Continue. Call doctor when convenient.
Infrequent:	
• Lower abdominal pain and swelling, bone pain, muscle weakness, swollen wrists or ankles.	Discontinue. Call doctor right away.
• Mood change, nausea, vomiting, weight loss.	Continue. Call doctor when convenient.
Rare:	
None expected.	

WARNINGS & PRECAUTIONS

Don't take if:
You are allergic to any antacid.

Before you start, consult your doctor:
- If you have kidney disease.
- If you have chronic constipation, colitis or diarrhea.
- If you have symptoms of appendicitis.
- If you have stomach or intestinal bleeding.

Over age 60:
Adverse reactions and side effects may be more frequent and severe than in younger persons. Diarrhea or constipation particularly likely.

Pregnancy:
Risk to unborn child outweighs drug benefits. Don't use.

Breast-feeding:
Drug passes into milk. Avoid drug or discontinue nursing until you finish medicine. Consult doctor for advice on maintaining milk supply.

Infants & children:
Use only under medical supervision.

Prolonged use:
No problems expected.

Skin & sunlight:
No problems expected.

Driving, piloting or hazardous work:
No problems expected.

Discontinuing:
May be unnecessary to finish medicine. Follow doctor's instructions.

Others:
Don't take longer than 2 weeks unless under medical supervision.

POSSIBLE INTERACTION WITH OTHER DRUGS

GENERIC NAME OR DRUG CLASS	COMBINED EFFECT
Anticoagulants	Decreased anticoagulant effect.
Chlorpromazine	Decreased chlorpromazine effect.
Digitalis preparations	Decreased digitalis effect.
Iron supplements	Decreased iron effect.
Isoniazid	Decreased isoniazid effect.
Levodopa	Increased levodopa effect.
Meperidine	Increased meperidine effect.
Mexiletine	May slow elimination of mexiletine and cause need to adjust dosage.
Nalidixic acid	Decreased effect of nalidixic acid.
Oxyphenbutazone	Decreased oxyphenbutazone effect.
Para-aminosalicylic acid (PAS)	Decreased PAS effect.
Penicillins	Decreased penicillin effect.
Pentobarbital	Decreased pentobarbital effect.
Phenylbutazone	Decreased phenylbutazone effect.
Pseudoephedrine	Increased pseudoephedrine effect.
Sulfa drugs	Decreased sulfa effect.
Tetracyclines	Decreased tetracycline effect.
Vitamins A and C	Decreased vitamin effect.
Vitamin D	Too much calcium in blood.

POSSIBLE INTERACTION WITH OTHER SUBSTANCES

INTERACTS WITH	COMBINED EFFECT
Alcohol:	Decreased antacid effect.
Beverages:	No proven problems.
Cocaine:	No proven problems.
Foods:	Decreased antacid effect if taken with food. Wait 1 hour after eating.
Marijuana:	No proven problems.
Tobacco:	Decreased antacid effect.

MALT SOUP EXTRACT

BRAND NAMES

Maltsupex

BASIC INFORMATION

Habit forming? No
Prescription needed? No
Available as generic? Yes
Drug class: Laxative (bulk-forming)

 USES

Relieves constipation and prevents straining for bowel movement.

 DOSAGE & USAGE INFORMATION

How to take:
- Liquid or powder—Dilute dose in 8 oz. cold water or fruit juice.
- Tablets—Swallow with 8 oz. cold liquid. Drink 6 to 8 glasses of water each day in addition to the one with each dose.

When to take:
At the same time each day, preferably morning.

If you forget a dose:
Take as soon as you remember. Resume regular schedule.

What drug does:
Absorbs water, stimulating the bowel to form a soft, bulky stool.

Time lapse before drug works:
May require 2 or 3 days to begin, then works in 12 to 24 hours.

Don't take with:
- See Interaction column and consult doctor.
- Don't take within 2 hours of taking another medicine.

 OVERDOSE

SYMPTOMS:
None expected.
WHAT TO DO:
Overdose unlikely to threaten life. If person takes much larger amount than prescribed, call doctor, poison-control center or hospital emergency room for instructions.

 POSSIBLE ADVERSE REACTIONS OR SIDE EFFECTS

SYMPTOMS	WHAT TO DO
Life-threatening: None expected.	
Common: None expected.	
Infrequent: Swallowing difficulty, "lump in throat" sensation, nausea, vomiting, diarrhea.	Continue. Call doctor when convenient.
Rare: Itchy skin, rash, asthma, intestinal blockage.	Discontinue. Call doctor right away.

WARNINGS & PRECAUTIONS

Don't take if:
- You are allergic to any bulk-forming laxative.
- You have symptoms of appendicitis, inflamed bowel or intestinal blockage.
- You have missed a bowel movement for only 1 or 2 days.

Before you start, consult your doctor:
- If you have diabetes.
- If you have a laxative habit.
- If you have rectal bleeding.
- If you have difficulty swallowing.
- If you take other laxatives.

Over age 60:
Adverse reactions and side effects may be more frequent and severe than in younger persons.

Pregnancy:
Most bulk-forming laxatives contain sodium or sugars which may cause fluid retention. Avoid if possible.

Breast-feeding:
No problems expected.

Infants & children:
Use only under medical supervision.

Prolonged use:
Don't take for more than 1 week unless under a doctor's supervision. May cause laxative dependence.

Skin & sunlight:
No problems expected.

Driving, piloting or hazardous work:
No problems expected.

Discontinuing:
May be unnecessary to finish medicine. Follow doctor's instructions.

Others:
Don't take to "flush out" your system or as a "tonic."

POSSIBLE INTERACTION WITH OTHER DRUGS

GENERIC NAME OR DRUG CLASS	COMBINED EFFECT
Antibiotics	Decreased antibiotic effect.
Anticoagulants	Decreased anticoagulant effect.
Digitalis preparations	Decreased digitalis effect.
Salicylates (including aspirin)	Decreased salicylate effect.

POSSIBLE INTERACTION WITH OTHER SUBSTANCES

INTERACTS WITH	COMBINED EFFECT
Alcohol:	None expected.
Beverages:	None expected.
Cocaine:	None expected.
Foods:	None expected.
Marijuana:	None expected.
Tobacco:	None expected.

MAPROTILINE

BRAND NAMES

Ludiomil

BASIC INFORMATION

Habit forming? No
Prescription needed? Yes
Available as generic? No
Drug class: Antidepressant

 USES

Treatment for depression or anxiety associated with depression.

 DOSAGE & USAGE INFORMATION

How to take:
Tablet or capsule—Swallow with liquid.

When to take:
At the same time each day, usually bedtime.

If you forget a dose:
Bedtime dose—If you forget your once-a-day bedtime dose, don't take it more than 3 hours late. If more than 3 hours, wait for next scheduled dose. Don't double this dose.

What drug does:
Probably affects part of brain that controls messages between nerve cells.

Time lapse before drug works:
Begins in 1 to 2 weeks. May require 4 to 6 weeks for maximum benefit.

Don't take with:
- Non-prescription drugs without consulting doctor.
- See Interaction column and consult doctor.

 OVERDOSE

SYMPTOMS:
Hallucinations, convulsions, coma.
WHAT TO DO:
- **Dial 0 (operator) or 911 (emergency) for an ambulance or medical help. Then give first aid immediately.**
- **If patient is unconscious and not breathing, give mouth-to-mouth breathing. If there is no heartbeat, use cardiac massage and mouth-to-mouth breathing (CPR). Don't try to make patient vomit. If you can't get help quickly, take patient to nearest emergency facility.**
- **See emergency information on inside covers.**

 POSSIBLE ADVERSE REACTIONS OR SIDE EFFECTS

SYMPTOMS	WHAT TO DO
Life-threatening:	
Seizures.	Seek emergency treatment immediately.
Common:	
• Headache, dry mouth or unpleasant taste, constipation or diarrhea, nausea, indigestion, fatigue, weakness.	Continue. Call doctor when convenient.
• Insomnia, craving sweets.	Continue. Tell doctor at next visit.
Infrequent:	
• Hallucinations, shakiness, dizziness, fainting, blurred vision, eye pain, vomiting, irregular heartbeat or slow pulse.	Discontinue. Call doctor right away.
• Painful or difficult urination.	Continue. Call doctor when convenient.
Rare:	
Itchy skin, rash, sore throat, jaundice, fever.	Discontinue. Call doctor right away.

 WARNINGS & PRECAUTIONS

Don't take if:
- You are allergic to any tricyclic antidepressant.
- You drink alcohol.
- You have had a heart attack within 6 weeks.
- You have glaucoma.
- You have taken MAO inhibitors within 2 weeks.
- Patient is younger than 12.

Before you start, consult your doctor:
- If you will have surgery within 2 months, including dental surgery, requiring general or spinal anesthesia.
- If you have an enlarged prostate.
- If you have heart disease or high blood pressure.
- If you have stomach or intestinal problems.
- If you have overactive thyroid.
- If you have asthma.
- If you have liver disease.

Over age 60:
More likely to develop urination difficulty and side effects such as hallucinations, shakiness, dizziness, fainting, headache or insomnia.

MAPROTILINE

Pregnancy:
Studies inconclusive on harm to unborn child. Animal studies show fetal abnormalities. Decide with your doctor whether drug benefits justify risk to unborn child.

Breast-feeding:
Drug passes into milk. Avoid drug or discontinue nursing until you finish medicine. Consult doctor for advice on maintaining milk supply.

Infants & children:
Don't give to children younger than 12.

Prolonged use:
Request blood cell counts, liver-function studies, monitor blood pressure closely.

Skin & sunlight:
May cause rash or intensify sunburn in areas exposed to sun or sunlamp.

Driving, piloting or hazardous work:
Don't drive or pilot aircraft until you learn how medicine affects you. Don't work around dangerous machinery. Don't climb ladders or work in high places. Danger increases if you drink alcohol or take medicine affecting alertness and reflexes.

Discontinuing:
Don't discontinue without consulting doctor. Dose may require gradual reduction if you have taken drug for a long time. Doses of other drugs may also require adjustment.

Others:
No problems expected.

 POSSIBLE INTERACTION WITH OTHER DRUGS

GENERIC NAME OR DRUG CLASS	COMBINED EFFECT
Anticoagulants	Increased anticoagulant effect.
Anticholinergics	Increased sedation.
Antihistamines	Increased antihistamine effect.
Barbiturates	Decreased antidepressant effect.
Clonidine	Decreased clonidine effect.
Ethchlorvynol	Delirium.
Guanethidine	Decreased guanethidine effect.
MAO inhibitors	Fever, delirium, convulsions.
Methyldopa	Decreased methyldopa effect.

Molindone	Increased tranquilizer effect.
Narcotics	Dangerous oversedation.
Phenytoin	Decreased phenytoin effect.
Quinidine	Irregular heartbeat.
Sedatives	Dangerous oversedation.
Sympathomimetics	Increased sympathomimetic effect.
Thiazide diuretics	Increased maprotiline effect.
Thyroid hormones	Irregular heartbeat.

 POSSIBLE INTERACTION WITH OTHER SUBSTANCES

INTERACTS WITH	COMBINED EFFECT
Alcohol: Beverages or medicines with alcohol.	Excessive intoxication. Avoid.
Beverages:	None expected.
Cocaine:	Excessive intoxication. Avoid.
Foods:	None expected.
Marijuana:	Excessive drowsiness. Avoid.
Tobacco:	May decrease absorption of maprotiline. Avoid.

MECLIZINE

BRAND NAMES

Antivert	Motion Cure
Bonamine	Ru-Vert-M
Bonine	Wehvert

BASIC INFORMATION

Habit forming? No
Prescription needed?
  U.S.—Tablets: No
          Liquid: Yes
  Canada: Yes
Available as generic? Yes
Drug class: Antihistamine, antiemetic

 USES

Prevents motion sickness.

 DOSAGE & USAGE INFORMATION

How to take:
Tablet—Swallow with liquid or food to lessen stomach irritation. If you can't swallow whole, crumble tablet and chew or take with liquid or food.

When to take:
30 minutes to 1 hour before traveling.

If you forget a dose:
Take as soon as you remember. Wait 4 hours for next dose.

What drug does:
Reduces sensitivity of nerve endings in inner ear, blocking messages to brain's vomiting center.

Time lapse before drug works:
30 to 60 minutes.

Don't take with:
See Interaction column and consult doctor.

 OVERDOSE

SYMPTOMS:
Drowsiness, confusion, incoordination, stupor, coma, weak pulse, shallow breathing.
WHAT TO DO:
● **Dial 0 (operator) or 911 (emergency) for an ambulance or medical help. Then give first aid immediately.**
● **See emergency information on inside covers.**

 POSSIBLE ADVERSE REACTIONS OR SIDE EFFECTS

SYMPTOMS	WHAT TO DO
Life-threatening: None expected.	
Common: Drowsiness.	Continue. Tell doctor at next visit.
Infrequent: ● Headache, diarrhea or constipation, fast heartbeat.	Continue. Call doctor when convenient.
● Dry mouth, nose, throat.	Continue. Tell doctor at next visit.
Rare: ● Rash, hives.	Discontinue. Call doctor right away.
● Restlessness, excitement, insomnia, blurred vision, frequent and difficult urination.	Continue. Call doctor when convenient.
● Appetite loss, nausea.	Continue. Tell doctor at next visit.

WARNINGS & PRECAUTIONS

Don't take if:
- You are allergic to meclizine, buclizine or cyclizine.
- You have taken MAO inhibitors in the past 2 weeks.

Before you start, consult your doctor:
- If you have glaucoma.
- If you have prostate enlargement.
- If you have reacted badly to any antihistamine.

Over age 60:
Adverse reactions and side effects may be more frequent and severe than in younger persons, especially impaired urination from enlarged prostate gland.

Pregnancy:
Studies inconclusive on harm to unborn child. Animal studies show fetal abnormalities. Decide with your doctor whether drug benefits justify risk to unborn child.

Breast-feeding:
Drug passes into milk. Avoid drug or discontinue nursing until you finish medicine. Consult doctor for advice on maintaining milk supply.

Infants & children:
No problems expected.

Prolonged use:
No problems expected.

Skin & sunlight:
No problems expected.

Driving, piloting or hazardous work:
Don't fly aircraft. Don't drive until you learn how medicine affects you. Don't work around dangerous machinery. Don't climb ladders or work in high places. Danger increases if you drink alcohol or take medicine affecting alertness and reflexes, such as antihistamines, tranquilizers, sedatives, pain medicine, narcotics and mind-altering drugs.

Discontinuing:
No problems expected.

Others:
No problems expected.

 ## POSSIBLE INTERACTION WITH OTHER DRUGS

GENERIC NAME OR DRUG CLASS	COMBINED EFFECT
Amphetamines	May decrease drowsiness caused by meclizine.
Anticholinergics	Increased effect of both drugs.
Antidepressants (tricyclic)	Increased effect of both drugs.
MAO inhibitors	Increased meclizine effect.
Narcotics	Increased effect of both drugs.
Pain relievers	Increased effect of both drugs.
Sedatives	Increased effect of both drugs.
Sleep inducers	Increased effect of both drugs.
Tranquilizers	Increased effect of both drugs.

 ## POSSIBLE INTERACTION WITH OTHER SUBSTANCES

INTERACTS WITH	COMBINED EFFECT
Alcohol:	Increased sedation. Avoid.
Beverages: Caffeine drinks.	May decrease drowsiness.
Cocaine:	None expected.
Foods:	None expected.
Marijuana:	Increased drowsiness, dry mouth.
Tobacco:	None expected.

MECLOFENAMATE

BRAND NAMES

Meclomen

BASIC INFORMATION

Habit forming? No
Prescription needed? Yes
Available as generic? No
Drug class: Anti-inflammatory (non-steroid)

 ## USES

Treatment for joint pain, stiffness, inflammation and swelling of arthritis and gout.

 ## DOSAGE & USAGE INFORMATION

How to take:
Capsule—Swallow with liquid or food to lessen stomach irritation. If you can't swallow whole, open capsule and take with liquid or food.

When to take:
At the same times each day.

If you forget a dose:
Take as soon as you remember up to 2 hours late. If more than 2 hours, wait for next scheduled dose (don't double this dose).

What drug does:
Reduces tissue concentration of prostaglandins (hormones which produce inflammation and pain).

Time lapse before drug works:
Begins in 4 to 24 hours. May require 3 weeks regular use for maximum benefit.

Don't take with:
See Interaction column and consult doctor.

 ## OVERDOSE

SYMPTOMS:
Confusion, agitation, incoherence, convulsions, possible hemorrhage from stomach or intestine, coma.
WHAT TO DO:
- **Dial 0 (operator) or 911 (emergency) for an ambulance or medical help. Then give first aid immediately.**
- **See emergency information on inside covers.**

 ## POSSIBLE ADVERSE REACTIONS OR SIDE EFFECTS

SYMPTOMS	WHAT TO DO
Life-threatening: None expected.	
Common: • Dizziness, nausea, pain.	Continue. Call doctor when convenient.
• Headache.	Continue. Tell doctor at next visit.
Infrequent: Depression; drowsiness; ringing in ears; constipation or diarrhea; vomiting; swollen feet, legs.	Continue. Call doctor when convenient.
Rare: • Convulsions; confusion; rash, hives or itchy skin; blurred vision; black, bloody or tarry stool; difficult breathing; tightness in chest; rapid heartbeat; unusual bleeding or bruising; blood in urine; jaundice.	Discontinue. Call doctor right away.
• Frequent, painful or difficult urination; fatigue, weakness.	Continue. Call doctor when convenient.

WARNINGS & PRECAUTIONS

Don't take if:
- You are allergic to aspirin or any non-steroid, anti-inflammatory drug.
- You have gastritis, peptic ulcer, enteritis, ileitis, ulcerative colitis, asthma, heart failure, high blood pressure or bleeding problems.
- Patient is younger than 15.

Before you start, consult your doctor:
- If you have epilepsy.
- If you have Parkinson's disease.
- If you have been mentally ill.
- If you have had kidney disease or impaired kidney function.

Over age 60:
Adverse reactions and side effects may be more frequent and severe than in younger persons.

Pregnancy:
Studies inconclusive on harm to unborn child. Decide with your doctor whether drug benefits justify risk to unborn child.

Breast-feeding:
May harm child. Avoid.

Infants & children:
Not recommended for anyone younger than 15. Use only under medical supervision.

Prolonged use:
- Eye damage.
- Reduced hearing.
- Sore throat, fever.
- Weight gain.

Skin & sunlight:
No problems expected.

Driving, piloting or hazardous work:
Don't drive or pilot aircraft until you learn how medicine affects you. Don't work around dangerous machinery. Don't climb ladders or work in high places. Danger increases if you drink alcohol or take medicine affecting alertness and reflexes, such as antihistamines, tranquilizers, sedatives, pain medicine, narcotics and mind-altering drugs.

Discontinuing:
Don't discontinue without consulting doctor. Dose may require gradual reduction if you have taken drug for a long time. Doses of other drugs may also require adjustment.

Others:
No problems expected.

POSSIBLE INTERACTION WITH OTHER DRUGS

GENERIC NAME OR DRUG CLASS	COMBINED EFFECT
Acebutolol	Decreased antihypertensive effect of acebutolol.
Anticoagulants (oral)	Increased risk of bleeding.
Aspirin	Increased risk of stomach ulcer.
Cortisone drugs	Increased risk of stomach ulcer.
Furosemide	Decreased diuretic effect of furosemide.
Gold compounds	Possible increased likelihood of kidney damage.
Ketoprofen	Increased possibility of internal bleeding.
Minoxidil	Decreased minoxidil effect.
Oxprenolol	Decreased antihypertensive effect of oxprenolol.
Oxyphenbutazone	Possible stomach ulcer.
Phenylbutazone	Possible stomach ulcer.
Probenecid	Increased meclofenamate effect.
Thyroid hormones	Rapid heartbeat, blood-pressure rise.

POSSIBLE INTERACTION WITH OTHER SUBSTANCES

INTERACTS WITH	COMBINED EFFECT
Alcohol:	Possible stomach ulcer or bleeding.
Beverages:	None expected.
Cocaine:	None expected.
Foods:	None expected.
Marijuana:	Increased pain relief from meclofenamate.
Tobacco:	None expected.

MEDROXYPROGESTERONE

BRAND NAMES

Amen
Curretab

Depo-Provera
Provera

BASIC INFORMATION

Habit forming? No
Prescription needed? Yes
Available as generic? Yes
Drug class: Female sex hormone (progestin)

 ## USES

- Treatment for menstrual or uterine disorders caused by progestin imbalance.
- Contraceptive.
- Treatment for cancer of breast and uterus.

 ## DOSAGE & USAGE INFORMATION

How to take:
- Tablet or capsule—Swallow with liquid or food to lessen stomach irritation. You may crumble tablet or open capsule.
- Injection—Take under doctor's supervision.

When to take:
Tablet, capsule—At the same time each day.

If you forget a dose:
- Menstrual disorders—Take up to 2 hours late. If more than 2 hours, wait for next dose (don't double this dose).
- Contraceptive—Consult your doctor. You may need to use another birth-control method until next period.

What drug does:
- Creates a uterine lining similar to pregnancy that prevents bleeding.
- Suppresses a pituitary gland hormone responsible for ovulation.
- Stimulates cervical mucus, which stops sperm penetration and prevents pregnancy.

Continued next column

 ## OVERDOSE

SYMPTOMS:
Nausea, vomiting, fluid retention, breast discomfort or enlargement, vaginal bleeding.
WHAT TO DO:
Overdose unlikely to threaten life. If person takes much larger amount than prescribed, call doctor, poison-control center or hospital emergency room for instructions.

Time lapse before drug works:
- Menstrual disorders—24 to 48 hours.
- Contraception—3 weeks.
- Cancer—May require 2 to 3 months regular use for maximum benefit.

Don't take with:
See Interaction column and consult doctor.

 ## POSSIBLE ADVERSE REACTIONS OR SIDE EFFECTS

SYMPTOMS	WHAT TO DO
Life-threatening: Blood clot in leg, brain or lung.	Seek emergency treatment immediately.
Common: Appetite or weight changes, swollen feet or ankles, unusual tiredness or weakness.	Continue. Tell doctor at next visit.
Infrequent: • Prolonged vaginal bleeding.	Discontinue. Call doctor right away.
• Depression.	Continue. Call doctor when convenient.
• Acne, increased facial or body hair, nausea, tender breasts.	Continue. Tell doctor at next visit.
Rare: Rash, stomach or side pain, jaundice.	Discontinue. Call doctor right away.

512

MEDROXYPROGESTERONE

WARNINGS & PRECAUTIONS

Don't take if:
- You are allergic to any progestin hormone.
- You may be pregnant.
- You have liver or gallbladder disease.
- You have had thrombophlebitis, embolism or stroke.
- You have unexplained vaginal bleeding.
- You have had breast or uterine cancer.

Before you start, consult your doctor:
- If you have heart or kidney disease.
- If you have diabetes.
- If you have a seizure disorder.
- If you suffer migraines.
- If you are easily depressed.

Over age 60:
Not recommended.

Pregnancy:
May harm child. Discontinue at first sign of pregnancy.

Breast-feeding:
Drug passes into milk. Avoid drug or discontinue nursing until you finish medicine. Consult doctor for advice on maintaining milk supply.

Infants & children:
Use only for female children under medical supervision.

Prolonged use:
No problems expected.

Skin & sunlight:
No problems expected.

Driving, piloting or hazardous work:
No problems expected.

Discontinuing:
Consult doctor. This medicine stays in the body and causes fetal abnormalities. Wait at least 3 months before becoming pregnant.

Others:
- Patients with diabetes must be monitored closely.
- Symptoms of blood clot in leg, brain or lung are: chest, groin, leg pain; sudden, severe headache; loss of coordination; vision change; shortness of breath; slurred speech.

POSSIBLE INTERACTION WITH OTHER DRUGS

GENERIC NAME OR DRUG CLASS	COMBINED EFFECT
Antihistamines	Decreased medroxyprogesterone effect.
Oxyphenbutazone	Decreased medroxyprogesterone effect.
Phenobarbital	Decreased medroxyprogesterone effect.
Phenothiazines	Increased phenothiazine effect.
Phenylbutazone	Decreased medroxyprogesterone effect.
Rifampin	Decreased contraceptive effect.

POSSIBLE INTERACTION WITH OTHER SUBSTANCES

INTERACTS WITH	COMBINED EFFECT
Alcohol:	None expected.
Beverages:	None expected.
Cocaine:	Decreased medroxyprogesterone effect.
Foods: Salt.	Fluid retention.
Marijuana:	Possible menstrual irregularities or bleeding between periods.
Tobacco: All forms.	Possible blood clots in lung, brain, legs. Avoid.

MEFENAMIC ACID

BRAND NAMES

Ponstan   Ponstel

BASIC INFORMATION

Habit forming? No
Prescription needed? Yes
Available as generic? No
Drug class: Anti-inflammatory (non-steroid)

USES

- Pain reliever.
- Treatment for dysmenorrhea (painful or difficult menstruation).

DOSAGE & USAGE INFORMATION

How to take:
Capsule—Swallow with liquid or food to lessen stomach irritation. If you can't swallow whole, open capsule and take with liquid or food.

When to take:
At the same times each day.

If you forget a dose:
Take as soon as you remember up to 2 hours late. If more than 2 hours, wait for next scheduled dose (don't double this dose).

What drug does:
Reduces tissue concentration of prostaglandins (hormones which produce inflammation and pain).

Time lapse before drug works:
Begins in 4 to 24 hours. May require 3 weeks regular use for maximum benefit.

Don't take with:
See Interaction column and consult doctor.

OVERDOSE

SYMPTOMS:
Confusion, agitation, incoherence, convulsions, possible hemorrhage from stomach or intestine, coma.
WHAT TO DO:
- **Dial 0 (operator) or 911 (emergency) for an ambulance or medical help. Then give first aid immediately.**
- **See emergency information on inside covers.**

POSSIBLE ADVERSE REACTIONS OR SIDE EFFECTS

SYMPTOMS	WHAT TO DO
Life-threatening: None expected.	
Common: • Dizziness, nausea, pain.	Continue. Call doctor when convenient.
• Headache.	Continue. Tell doctor at next visit.
Infrequent: Depression, drowsiness, ringing in ears, constipation or diarrhea, vomiting, swollen feet or legs.	Continue. Call doctor when convenient.
Rare: • Convulsions; confusion; rash, hives or itchy skin; blurred vision; black, bloody or tarry stool; difficult breathing; tightness in chest; rapid heartbeat; unusual bleeding or bruising; blood in urine; jaundice.	Discontinue. Call doctor right away.
• Frequent, painful or difficult urination; fatigue, weakness.	Continue. Call doctor when convenient.

WARNINGS & PRECAUTIONS

Don't take if:
- You are allergic to aspirin or any non-steroid, anti-inflammatory drug.
- You have gastritis, peptic ulcer, enteritis, ileitis, ulcerative colitis, asthma, heart failure, high blood pressure or bleeding problems.
- Patient is younger than 15.

Before you start, consult your doctor:
- If you have epilepsy.
- If you have Parkinson's disease.
- If you have been mentally ill.
- If you have had kidney disease or impaired kidney function.

Over age 60:
Adverse reactions and side effects may be more frequent and severe than in younger persons.

Pregnancy:
Studies inconclusive on harm to unborn child. Decide with your doctor whether drug benefits justify risk to unborn child.

Breast-feeding:
May harm child. Avoid.

Infants & children:
Not recommended for anyone younger than 15. Use only under medical supervision.

Prolonged use:
- Eye damage.
- Reduced hearing.
- Sore throat, fever.
- Weight gain.

Skin & sunlight:
No problems expected.

Driving, piloting or hazardous work:
Don't drive or pilot aircraft until you learn how medicine affects you. Don't work around dangerous machinery. Don't climb ladders or work in high places. Danger increases if you drink alcohol or take medicine affecting alertness and reflexes, such as antihistamines, tranquilizers, sedatives, pain medicine, narcotics and mind-altering drugs.

Discontinuing:
Don't discontinue without consulting doctor. Dose may require gradual reduction if you have taken drug for a long time. Doses of other drugs may also require adjustment.

Others:
Don't take for more than 1 week.

POSSIBLE INTERACTION WITH OTHER DRUGS

GENERIC NAME OR DRUG CLASS	COMBINED EFFECT
Acebutolol	Decreased antihypertensive effect of acebutolol.
Anticoagulants (oral)	Increased risk of bleeding.
Aspirin	Increased risk of stomach ulcer.
Cortisone drugs	Increased risk of stomach ulcer.
Furosemide	Decreased diuretic effect of furosemide.
Gold compounds	Possible increased likelihood of kidney damage.
Minoxidil	Decreased minoxidil effect.
Oxprenolol	Decreased antihypertensive effect of oxprenolol.
Oxyphenbutazone	Possible stomach ulcer.
Phenylbutazone	Possible stomach ulcer.
Probenecid	Increased effect of mefenamic acid.
Thyroid hormones	Rapid heartbeat, blood-pressure rise.

POSSIBLE INTERACTION WITH OTHER SUBSTANCES

INTERACTS WITH	COMBINED EFFECT
Alcohol:	Possible stomach ulcer or bleeding.
Beverages:	None expected.
Cocaine:	None expected.
Foods:	None expected.
Marijuana:	Increased pain relief from mefenamic acid.
Tobacco:	None expected.

MELPHALAN (PAM, L-PAM, PHENYLALANINE MUSTARD)

BRAND NAMES

Alkeran
L-PAM

Phenylalanine
Mustard

BASIC INFORMATION

Habit forming? No
Prescription needed? Yes
Available as generic? No
Drug class: Antineoplastic, immunosuppressant

 USES

- Treatment for some kinds of cancer.
- Suppresses immune response after transplant and in immune disorders.

 DOSAGE & USAGE INFORMATION

How to take:
Tablet or capsule—Swallow with liquid after light meal. Don't drink fluids with meals. Drink extra fluids between meals. Avoid sweet or fatty foods.

When to take:
At the same time each day.

If you forget a dose:
Take as soon as you remember. Don't ever double dose.

What drug does:
Inhibits abnormal cell reproduction. May suppress immune system.

Continued next column

 OVERDOSE

SYMPTOMS:
Bleeding, chills, fever, collapse, stupor, seizure.
WHAT TO DO:
- Dial 0 (operator) or 911 (emergency) for an ambulance or medical help. Then give first aid immediately.
- If patient is unconscious and not breathing, give mouth-to-mouth breathing. If there is no heartbeat, use cardiac massage and mouth-to-mouth breathing (CPR). Don't try to make patient vomit. If you can't get help quickly, take patient to nearest emergency facility.
- See emergency information on inside covers.

Time lapse before drug works:
Up to 6 weeks for full effect.

Don't take with:
See Interaction column and consult doctor.

 POSSIBLE ADVERSE REACTIONS OR SIDE EFFECTS

SYMPTOMS	WHAT TO DO
Life-threatening: None expected.	
Common:	
• Unusual bleeding or bruising, mouth sores with sore throat, chills and fever, black stools, sores in mouth and lips, menstrual irregularities.	Discontinue. Call doctor right away.
• Hair loss, joint pain.	Continue. Call doctor when convenient.
• Nausea, vomiting, diarrhea (unavoidable), tiredness, weakness.	Continue. Tell doctor at next visit.
Infrequent:	
• Mental confusion, shortness of breath, may increase chance of developing leukemia.	Continue. Call doctor when convenient.
• Cough.	Continue. Tell doctor at next visit.
Rare:	
Jaundice.	Discontinue. Call doctor right away.

WARNINGS & PRECAUTIONS

Don't take if:
- You have had hypersensitivity to alkylating antineoplastic drugs.
- Your physician has not explained serious nature of your medical problem and risks of taking this medicine.

Before you start, consult your doctor:
- If you have gout.
- If you have had kidney stones.
- If you have active infection.
- If you have impaired kidney or liver function.
- If you have taken other antineoplastic drugs or had radiation treatment in last 3 weeks.

Over age 60:
Adverse reactions and side effects may be more frequent and severe than in younger persons.

Pregnancy:
Consult doctor. Risk to child is significant.

Breast-feeding:
Drug passes into milk. Don't nurse.

Infants & children:
Use only under special medical supervision at center experienced in anticancer drugs.

Prolonged use:
Adverse reactions more likely the longer drug is required.

Skin & sunlight:
No problems expected.

Driving, piloting or hazardous work:
No problems expected.

Discontinuing:
Don't discontinue without doctor's advice until you complete prescribed dose, even though symptoms diminish or disappear. Some side effects may follow discontinuing. Report to doctor blurred vision, convulsions, confusion, persistent headache.

Others:
May cause sterility.

POSSIBLE INTERACTION WITH OTHER DRUGS

GENERIC NAME OR DRUG CLASS	COMBINED EFFECT
Antigout drugs	Decreased antigout effect.
Antineoplastic drugs (other)	Increased effect of all drugs (may be beneficial).
Chloramphenicol	Increased likelihood of toxic effects of both drugs.

POSSIBLE INTERACTION WITH OTHER SUBSTANCES

INTERACTS WITH	COMBINED EFFECT
Alcohol:	May increase chance of intestinal bleeding.
Beverages:	No problems expected.
Cocaine:	Increases chance of toxicity.
Foods:	Reduces irritation in stomach.
Marijuana:	No problems expected.
Tobacco:	Increases lung toxicity.

MEPHENYTOIN

BRAND NAMES

Mesantoin   Methoin

BASIC INFORMATION

Habit forming? No
Prescription needed? Yes
Available as generic? Yes
Drug class: Anticonvulsant (hydantoin)

USES

- Prevents epileptic seizures.
- Stabilizes irregular heartbeat.

DOSAGE & USAGE INFORMATION

How to take:
- Tablet or capsule—Swallow with liquid.
- Extended-release tablets or capsules—Swallow each dose whole. If you take regular tablets, you may chew or crush them.

When to take:
At the same time each day.

If you forget a dose:
- If drug taken 1 time per day—Take as soon as you remember up to 12 hours late. If more than 12 hours, wait for next scheduled dose (don't double this dose).
- If taken several times per day—Take as soon as possible, then return to regular schedule.

What drug does:
Promotes sodium loss from nerve fibers. This lessens excitability and inhibits spread of nerve impulses.

Time lapse before drug works:
7 to 10 days continual use.

Don't take with:
See Interaction column and consult doctor.

OVERDOSE

SYMPTOMS:
Jerky eye movements; stagger; slurred speech; imbalance; drowsiness; blood-pressure drop; slow, shallow breathing; coma.
WHAT TO DO:
- **Dial 0 (operator) or 911 (emergency) for an ambulance or medical help. Then give first aid immediately.**
- **See emergency information on inside covers.**

POSSIBLE ADVERSE REACTIONS OR SIDE EFFECTS

SYMPTOMS	WHAT TO DO
Life-threatening: None expected.	
Common: Mild dizziness, drowsiness, constipation, nausea, vomiting.	Continue. Call doctor when convenient.
Infrequent: • Hallucinations, confusion, slurred speech, stagger, rash, change in vision.	Discontinue. Call doctor right away.
• Headache, sleeplessness, diarrhea, muscle twitching.	Continue. Call doctor when convenient.
• Increased body and facial hair.	Continue. Tell doctor at next visit.
Rare: Sore throat, fever, stomach pain, unusual bleeding or bruising, jaundice.	Discontinue. Call doctor right away.

WARNINGS & PRECAUTIONS

Don't take if:
You are allergic to any hydantoin anticonvulsant.

Before you start, consult your doctor:
- If you have had impaired liver function or disease.
- If you will have surgery within 2 months, including dental surgery, requiring general or spinal anesthesia.

Over age 60:
Adverse reactions and side effects may be more frequent and severe than in younger persons.

Pregnancy:
Risk to unborn child outweighs drug benefits. Don't use.

Breast-feeding:
Drug passes into milk. Avoid drug or discontinue nursing until you finish medicine. Consult doctor for advice on maintaining milk supply.

Infants & children:
Use only under medical supervision.

Prolonged use:
- Weakened bones.
- Lymph gland enlargement.
- Possible liver damage.
- Numbness and tingling of hands and feet.
- Continual back-and-forth eye movements.
- Bleeding, swollen or tender gums.

Skin & sunlight:
May cause rash or intensify sunburn in areas exposed to sun or sunlamp.

Driving, piloting or hazardous work:
Don't drive or pilot aircraft until you learn how medicine affects you. Don't work around dangerous machinery. Don't climb ladders or work in high places. Danger increases if you drink alcohol or take medicine affecting alertness and reflexes.

Discontinuing:
Don't discontinue without consulting doctor. Dose may require gradual reduction if you have taken drug for a long time. Doses of other drugs may also require adjustment.

Others:
No problems expected.

POSSIBLE INTERACTION WITH OTHER DRUGS

GENERIC NAME OR DRUG CLASS	COMBINED EFFECT
Anticoagulants	Increased effect of both drugs.
Antidepressants (tricyclic)	Need to adjust mephenytoin dose.
Antihypertensives	Increased effect of antihypertensive.
Aspirin	Increased mephenytoin effect.
Barbiturates	Changed seizure pattern.
Carbonic anhydrase inhibitors	Increased chance of bone disease.
Chloramphenicol	Increased mephenytoin effect.
Contraceptives (oral)	Increased seizures.
Cortisone drugs	Decreased cortisone effect.
Digitalis preparations	Decreased digitalis effect.
Disulfiram	Increased mephenytoin effect.
Estrogens	Increased mephenytoin effect.
Furosemide	Decreased furosemide effect.
Glutethimide	Decreased mephenytoin effect.
Griseofulvin	Increased griseofulvin effect.
Isoniazid	Increased mephenytoin effect.
Methadone	Decreased methadone effect.
Methotrexate	Increased methotrexate effect.
Methylphenidate	Increased mephenytoin effect.
Oxyphenbutazone	Increased mephenytoin effect.
Para-aminosalicylic acid (PAS)	Increased mephenytoin effect.
Phenothiazines	Increased mephenytoin effect.
Phenylbutazone	Increased mephenytoin effect.
Propranolol	Increased propranolol effect.
Quinidine	Increased quinidine effect.
Sedatives	Increased sedative effect.
Sulfa drugs	Increased mephenytoin effect.
Theophylline	Reduced anticonvulsant effect.

POSSIBLE INTERACTION WITH OTHER SUBSTANCES

INTERACTS WITH	COMBINED EFFECT
Alcohol:	Possible decreased anticonvulsant effect. Use with caution.
Beverages:	None expected.
Cocaine:	Possible seizures.
Foods:	None expected.
Marijuana:	Drowsiness, unsteadiness, decreased anticonvulsant effect.
Tobacco:	None expected.

MEPHOBARBITAL

BRAND NAMES

Mebaral

BASIC INFORMATION

Habit forming? Yes
Prescription needed? Yes
Available as generic? Yes
Drug class: Sedative, hypnotic (barbiturate)

 USES

- Reduces anxiety or nervous tension (low dose).
- Relieves insomnia (higher bedtime dose).
- Prevents seizures in epilepsy.

 DOSAGE & USAGE INFORMATION

How to take:
Tablet—Swallow with liquid or food to lessen stomach irritation. If you can't swallow whole, crumble tablet and take with liquid or food.

When to take:
At the same times each day.

If you forget a dose:
Take as soon as you remember up to 2 hours late. If more than 2 hours, wait for next scheduled dose (don't double this dose).

What drug does:
May partially block nerve impulses at nerve-cell connections.

Time lapse before drug works:
60 minutes.

Continued next column

 OVERDOSE

SYMPTOMS:
Deep sleep, weak pulse, coma.
WHAT TO DO:
- **Dial 0 (operator) or 911 (emergency) for an ambulance or medical help. Then give first aid immediately.**
- **If patient is unconscious and not breathing, give mouth-to-mouth breathing. If there is no heartbeat use cardiac massage and mouth-to-mouth breathing (CPR). Don't try to make patient vomit. If you can't get help quickly, take patient to nearest emergency facility.**
- **See emergency information on inside covers.**

Don't take with:
- Non-prescription drugs without consulting doctor.
- See Interaction column and consult doctor.

 POSSIBLE ADVERSE REACTIONS OR SIDE EFFECTS

SYMPTOMS	WHAT TO DO
Life-threatening: None expected.	
Common: Dizziness, drowsiness, "hangover" effect.	Continue. Call doctor when convenient.
Infrequent: • Rash or hives; face, lip or eyelid swelling; sore throat; fever.	Discontinue. Call doctor right away.
• Depression, confusion, diarrhea, nausea, vomiting, joint or muscle pain, slurred speech.	Continue. Call doctor when convenient.
Rare: • Agitation, slow heartbeat, difficult breathing, jaundice.	Discontinue. Call doctor right away.
• Unexplained bleeding or bruising.	Continue. Call doctor when convenient.

 WARNINGS & PRECAUTIONS

Don't take if:
- You are allergic to any barbiturate.
- You have porphyria.

Before you start, consult your doctor:
- If you have epilepsy.
- If you have kidney or liver damage.
- If you have asthma.
- If you have anemia.
- If you have chronic pain.
- If you will have surgery within 2 months, including dental surgery, requiring general or spinal anesthesia.

Over age 60:
Adverse reactions and side effects may be more frequent and severe than in younger persons. Use small doses.

Pregnancy:
Risk to unborn child outweighs drug benefits. Don't use.

Breast-feeding:
Drug passes into milk. Avoid drug or discontinue nursing until you finish medicine. Consult doctor for advice on maintaining milk supply.

Infants & children:
Use only under doctor's supervision.

Prolonged use:
- May cause addiction, anemia, chronic intoxication.
- May lower body temperature, making exposure to cold temperatures hazardous.

Skin & sunlight:
May cause rash or intensify sunburn in areas exposed to sun or sunlamp.

Driving, piloting or hazardous work:
Don't drive or pilot aircraft until you learn how medicine affects you. Don't work around dangerous machinery. Don't climb ladders or work in high places. Danger increases if you drink alcohol or take medicine affecting alertness and reflexes.

Discontinuing:
May be unnecessary to finish medicine. Follow doctor's instructions. If you develop withdrawal symptoms of hallucinations, agitation or sleeplessness after discontinuing, call doctor right away.

Others:
No problems expected.

POSSIBLE INTERACTION WITH OTHER DRUGS

GENERIC NAME OR DRUG CLASS	COMBINED EFFECT
Anticoagulants (oral)	Decreased effect of anticoagulant.
Anticonvulsants	Changed seizure patterns.
Antidepressants (tricyclics)	Decreased antidepressant effect. Possible dangerous oversedation.
Antidiabetics (oral)	Increased effect of mephobarbital.
Antihistamines	Dangerous sedation. Avoid.
Anti-inflammatory drugs (non-steroidal)	Decreased anti-inflammatory effect.
Aspirin	Decreased aspirin effect.
Beta-adrenergic blockers	Decreased effect of beta-adrenergic blocker.
Contraceptives (oral)	Decreased contraceptive effect.
Cortisone drugs	Decreased cortisone effect.

Digitoxin	Decreased digitoxin effect.
Doxycycline	Decreased doxycycline effect.
Dronabinol	Increased effects of both drugs. Avoid.
Griseofulvin	Decreased griseofulvin effect.
Indapamide	Increased indapamide effect.
MAO inhibitors	Increased mephobarbital effect.
Mind-altering drugs	Dangerous sedation. Avoid.
Molindone	Increased sedative effect.
Narcotics	Dangerous sedation. Avoid.
Pain relievers	Dangerous sedation. Avoid.
Sedatives	Dangerous sedation. Avoid.
Sleep inducers	Dangerous sedation. Avoid.
Tranquilizers	Dangerous sedation. Avoid.
Valproic acid	Increased mephobarbital effect.

POSSIBLE INTERACTION WITH OTHER SUBSTANCES

INTERACTS WITH	COMBINED EFFECT
Alcohol:	Possible fatal oversedation. Avoid.
Beverages:	None expected.
Cocaine:	Decreased mephobarbital effect.
Foods:	None expected.
Marijuana:	Excessive sedation. Avoid.
Tobacco:	None expected.

MEPROBAMATE

BRAND NAMES

See complete list of brand names in the *Brand Name Directory,* page 951.

BASIC INFORMATION

Habit forming? Yes
Prescription needed? Yes
Available as generic? Yes
Drug class: Tranquilizer

 ## USES

Reduces mild anxiety, tension and insomnia.

 ## DOSAGE & USAGE INFORMATION

How to take:
- Tablet or capsule—Swallow with liquid.
- Extended-release tablets or capsules—Swallow each dose whole. If you take regular tablets, you may chew or crush them.
- Liquid—Take as directed on label.

When to take:
At the same time each day.

If you forget a dose:
Take as soon as you remember up to 2 hours late. If more than 2 hours, wait for next scheduled dose (don't double this dose).

What drug does:
Sedates brain centers which control behavior and emotions.

Time lapse before drug works:
1 to 2 hours.

Don't take with:
- Non-prescription drugs containing alcohol or caffeine without consulting doctor.
- See Interaction column and consult doctor.

 ## OVERDOSE

SYMPTOMS:
Dizziness, slurred speech, stagger, depressed breathing and heart function, stupor, coma.
WHAT TO DO:
- **Dial 0 (operator) or 911 (emergency) for an ambulance or medical help. Then give first aid immediately.**
- **See emergency information on inside covers.**

 ## POSSIBLE ADVERSE REACTIONS OR SIDE EFFECTS

SYMPTOMS	WHAT TO DO
Life-threatening: None expected.	
Common: Dizziness, confusion, agitation, drowsiness, unsteadiness, fatigue, weakness.	Continue. Tell doctor at next visit.
Infrequent: • Rash, hives, itchy skin; change in vision; diarrhea, nausea or vomiting.	Discontinue. Call doctor right away.
• False sense of well-being, headache, slurred speech.	Continue. Call doctor when convenient.
Rare: Sore throat; fever; rapid, pounding, unusually slow or irregular heartbeat; difficult breathing; unusual bleeding or bruising.	Discontinue. Call doctor right away.

WARNINGS & PRECAUTIONS

Don't take if:
- You are allergic to meprobamate, tybanate, carbromal or carisoprodol.
- You have had porphyria.
- Patient is younger than 6.

Before you start, consult your doctor:
- If you have epilepsy.
- If you have impaired liver or kidney function.

Over age 60:
Adverse reactions and side effects may be more frequent and severe than in younger persons.

Pregnancy:
Risk to unborn child outweighs drug benefits. Don't use.

Breast-feeding:
Drug filters into milk. May harm child. Avoid.

Infants & children:
Not recommended.

Prolonged use:
- Habit forming.
- May impair blood-cell production.

Skin & sunlight:
No problems expected.

Driving, piloting or hazardous work:
Don't drive or pilot aircraft until you learn how medicine affects you. Don't work around dangerous machinery. Don't climb ladders or work in high places. Danger increases if you drink alcohol or take medicine affecting alertness and reflexes, such as antihistamines, tranquilizers, sedatives, pain medicine, narcotics and mind-altering drugs.

Discontinuing:
Don't discontinue without consulting doctor. Dose may require gradual reduction if you have taken drug for a long time. Doses of other drugs may also require adjustment.

Others:
No problems expected.

 POSSIBLE INTERACTION WITH OTHER DRUGS

GENERIC NAME OR DRUG CLASS	COMBINED EFFECT
Anticoagulants	Decreased anticoagulant effect.
Anticonvulsants	Change in seizure pattern.
Antidepressants	Increased antidepressant effect.
Contraceptives (oral)	Decreased contraceptive effect.
Dronabinol	Increased effects of both drugs. Avoid.
Estrogens	Decreased estrogen effect.
MAO inhibitors	Increased meprobamate effect.
Molindone	Increased tranquilizer effect.
Narcotics	Increased narcotic effect.
Sedatives	Increased sedative effect.
Sleep inducers	Increased effect of sleep inducer.
Terfenadine	Possible excessive sedation.
Tranquilizers	Increased tranquilizer effect.

 POSSIBLE INTERACTION WITH OTHER SUBSTANCES

INTERACTS WITH	COMBINED EFFECT
Alcohol:	Dangerous increased effect of meprobamate.
Beverages: Caffeine drinks.	Decreased calming effect of meprobamate.
Cocaine:	Decreased meprobamate effect.
Foods:	None expected.
Marijuana:	Increased sedative effect of meprobamate.
Tobacco:	None expected.

MEPROBAMATE & ASPIRIN

BRAND NAMES

Equagesic   Micrainin

BASIC INFORMATION

Habit forming? Yes
Prescription needed? Yes
Available as generic? No
Drug class: Anti-inflammatory, analgesic,
    tranquilizer

USES

- Reduces mild anxiety, tension and insomnia.
- Reduces pain, fever, inflammation.
- Relieves swelling, stiffness, joint pain.

DOSAGE & USAGE INFORMATION

How to take:
- Tablet or capsule—Swallow with liquid.
- Extended-release tablets or capsules—Swallow each dose whole. If you take regular tablets, you may chew or crush them.
- Liquid—Take as directed on label.

When to take:
Pain, fever, inflammation—As needed, no more often than every 4 hours.

If you forget a dose:
Take as soon as you remember up to 2 hours late. If more than 2 hours, wait for next scheduled dose (don't double this dose).

What drug does:
- Sedates brain centers which control behavior and emotions.
- Affects hypothalamus, the part of the brain which regulates temperature by dilating small blood vessels in skin.

Continued next column

OVERDOSE

SYMPTOMS:
Dizziness; slurred speech; stagger; depressed heart function; ringing in ears; nausea; vomiting; fever; deep, rapid breathing; hallucinations; convulsions; stupor; coma.
WHAT TO DO:
- **Dial 0 (operator) or 911 (emergency) for an ambulance or medical help. Then give first aid immediately.**
- **See emergency information on inside covers.**

- Prevents clumping of platelets (small blood cells) so blood vessels remain open.
- Decreases prostaglandin effect.
- Suppresses body's pain messages.

Time lapse before drug works:
1 to 2 hours.

Don't take with:
- Tetracyclines.
- Non-prescription drugs containing alcohol or caffeine without consulting doctor.
- See Interaction column and consult doctor.

POSSIBLE ADVERSE REACTIONS OR SIDE EFFECTS

SYMPTOMS	WHAT TO DO
Life-threatening:	
Hives, rash, intense itching, faintness soon after a dose (anaphylaxis).	Seek emergency treatment immediately.
Common:	
• Nausea, vomiting.	Discontinue. Call doctor right away.
• Dizziness, confusion, agitation, drowsiness, unsteadiness, fatigue, weakness, ears ringing, heartburn, indigestion.	Continue. Call doctor when convenient.
Infrequent:	
None expected.	
Rare:	
• Black, bloody or tarry stool; vomiting blood or black material; blood in urine.	Discontinue. Seek emergency treatment.
• Rash, hives, itchy skin, change in vision, fever, jaundice.	Discontinue. Call doctor right away.

WARNINGS & PRECAUTIONS

Don't take if:
- You are allergic to meprobamate, tybanate, carbromal or carisoprodol.
- You have had porphyria.
- You have a peptic ulcer of stomach or duodenum or a bleeding disorder.
- Patient is younger than 6.

Before you start, consult your doctor:
- If you have epilepsy, impaired liver or kidney function, asthma or nasal polyps.
- If you have had gout, stomach or duodenal ulcers.

Over age 60:
Adverse reactions and side effects may be more frequent and severe than in younger

persons. More likely to cause hidden bleeding in stomach or intestines. Watch for dark stools.

Pregnancy:
Risk to unborn child outweighs drug benefits. Don't use.

Breast-feeding:
Drug passes into milk. Avoid drug or discontinue nursing until you finish medicine. Consult doctor for advice on maintaining milk supply.

Infants & children:
Not recommended.

Prolonged use:
- Habit forming.
- May impair blood-cell production.
- Kidney damage. Periodic kidney-function test recommended.

Skin & sunlight:
Aspirin combined with sunscreen may decrease sunburn.

Driving, piloting or hazardous work:
Don't drive or pilot aircraft until you learn how medicine affects you. Don't work around dangerous machinery. Don't climb ladders or work in high places. Danger increases if you drink alcohol or take medicine affecting alertness and reflexes, such as antihistamines, tranquilizers, sedatives, pain medicine, narcotics and mind-altering drugs.

Discontinuing:
Don't discontinue without consulting doctor. Dose may require gradual reduction if you have taken drug for a long time. Doses of other drugs may also require adjustment.

Others:
- Aspirin can complicate surgery, pregnancy, labor and delivery, and illness.
- Urine tests for blood sugar may be inaccurate.

POSSIBLE INTERACTION WITH OTHER DRUGS

GENERIC NAME OR DRUG CLASS	COMBINED EFFECT
Acebutolol	Decreased antihypertensive effect of acebutolol.
Allopurinol	Decreased allopurinol effect.
Antacids	Decreased aspirin effect.
Anticoagulants	Increased anticoagulant effect. Abnormal bleeding.
Anticonvulsants	Change in seizure pattern.

Antidepressants	Increased antidepressant effect.
Antidiabetics (oral)	Low blood sugar.
Anti-inflammatory drugs (non-steroid)	Risk of stomach bleeding and ulcers.
Aspirin (other)	Likely aspirin toxicity.
Contraceptives (oral)	Decreased contraceptive effect.
Cortisone drugs	Increased cortisone effect. Risk of ulcers and stomach bleeding.
Dronabinol	Increased effect of both drugs.
Estrogens	Decreased estrogen effect.
Furosemide	Possible aspirin toxicity.
Gold compounds	Increased likelihood of kidney damage.
Indomethacin	Risk of stomach bleeding and ulcers.
MAO inhibitors	Increased meprobamate effect.
Methotrexate	Increased methotrexate effect.
Minoxidil	Decreased minoxidil effect.
Narcotics	Increased narcotic effect.
Oxprenolol	Decreased antihypertensive effect of oxprenolol.

Continued page 968

POSSIBLE INTERACTION WITH OTHER SUBSTANCES

INTERACTS WITH	COMBINED EFFECT
Alcohol:	Possible stomach irritation and bleeding. Dangerous increased effect of meprobamate. Avoid.
Beverages: Caffeine drinks.	Decreased calming effect of meprobamate.
Cocaine:	Decreased meprobamate effect.
Foods:	None expected.
Marijuana:	Possible increased pain relief, but marijuana may slow body's recovery. Avoid.
Tobacco:	None expected.

525

MERCAPTOPURINE

BRAND NAMES

Purinethol

BASIC INFORMATION

Habit forming? No
Prescription needed? Yes
Available as generic? Yes
Drug class: Antineoplastic,
immunosuppressant

 USES

- Treatment for some kinds of cancer.
- Treatment for regional enteritis and ulcerative colitis and other immune disorders.

 DOSAGE & USAGE INFORMATION

How to take:
Tablet—Swallow with liquid.

When to take:
At the same time each day.

If you forget a dose:
Skip the missed dose. Don't double the next dose.

What drug does:
Inhibits abnormal-cell reproduction.

Time lapse before drug works:
May require 6 weeks for maximum effect.

Don't take with:
See Interaction column and consult doctor.

 OVERDOSE

SYMPTOMS:
Headache, stupor, seizures.
WHAT TO DO:
- Dial 0 (operator) or 911 (emergency) for an ambulance or medical help. Then give first aid immediately.
- If patient is unconscious and not breathing, give mouth-to-mouth breathing. If there is no heartbeat, use cardiac massage and mouth-to-mouth breathing (CPR). Don't try to make patient vomit. If you can't get help quickly, take patient to nearest emergency facility.
- See emergency information on inside covers.

 POSSIBLE ADVERSE REACTIONS OR SIDE EFFECTS

SYMPTOMS	WHAT TO DO
Life-threatening:	
None expected.	
Common:	
• Black stools or bloody vomit.	Discontinue. Seek emergency treatment.
• Mouth sores, sore throat, fever, chills, unusual bleeding or bruising.	Discontinue. Call doctor right away.
• Stomach pain, nausea, vomiting.	Continue. Call doctor when convenient.
Infrequent:	
• Seizures.	Discontinue. Seek emergency treatment.
• Dizziness, drowsiness, head-ache, confusion, blurred vision, shortness of breath, joint pain, blood in urine, jaundice.	Discontinue. Call doctor right away.
• Cough.	Continue. Call doctor when convenient.
• Acne, boils, hair loss, itchy skin.	Continue. Tell doctor at next visit.
Rare:	
None expected.	

WARNINGS & PRECAUTIONS

Don't take if:
You are allergic to any antineoplastic.

Before you start, consult your doctor:
- If you are alcoholic.
- If you have blood, liver or kidney disease.
- If you have colitis or peptic ulcer.
- If you have gout.
- If you have an infection.
- If you plan to become pregnant within 3 months.

Over age 60:
Adverse reactions and side effects may be more frequent and severe than in younger persons.

Pregnancy:
Consult doctor.

Breast-feeding:
Drug passes into milk. Avoid drug or discontinue nursing.

Infants & children:
Use only under special medical supervision.

Prolonged use:
Adverse reactions more likely the longer drug is required.

Skin & sunlight:
No problems expected.

Driving, piloting or hazardous work:
Avoid if you feel dizzy, drowsy or confused. Otherwise, no problems expected.

Discontinuing:
Don't discontinue without doctor's advice until you complete prescribed dose, even though symptoms diminish or disappear. Some side effects may follow discontinuing. Report to doctor blurred vision, convulsions, confusion, persistent headache.

Others:
- Drink more water than usual to cause frequent urination.
- Don't give this medicine to anyone else for any purpose. It is a strong drug that requires close medical supervision.
- Report for frequent medical follow-up and laboratory studies.

POSSIBLE INTERACTION WITH OTHER DRUGS

GENERIC NAME OR DRUG CLASS	COMBINED EFFECT
Acetaminophen	Increased likelihood of liver toxicity.
Allopurinol	Increased toxic effect of mercaptopurine.
Antineoplastic drugs (other)	Increased effect of both (may be desirable) or increase toxicity of each.
Chloramphenicol	Increased toxicity of each.
Isoniazid	Increased likelihood of liver toxicity.

POSSIBLE INTERACTION WITH OTHER SUBSTANCES

INTERACTS WITH	COMBINED EFFECT
Alcohol:	May increase chance of intestinal bleeding.
Beverages:	No problems expected.
Cocaine:	Increases chance of toxicity.
Foods:	Reduced irritation in stomach.
Marijuana:	No problems expected.
Tobacco:	Increases lung toxicity.

MESORIDAZINE

BRAND NAMES

Serentil

BASIC INFORMATION

Habit forming? No
Prescription needed? Yes
Available as generic? Yes
Drug class: Tranquilizer, antiemetic
(phenothiazine)

 USES

- Stops nausea, vomiting.
- Reduces anxiety, agitation.

 DOSAGE & USAGE INFORMATION

How to take:
- Tablet or capsule—Swallow with liquid or food to lessen stomach irritation.
- Suppositories—Remove wrapper and moisten suppository with water. Gently insert into rectum, large end first.
- Drops or liquid—Dilute dose in beverage.

When to take:
- Nervous and mental disorders—Take at the same times each day.
- Nausea and vomiting—Take as needed, no more often than every 4 hours.

If you forget a dose:
- Nervous and mental disorders—Take up to 2 hours late. If more than 2 hours, wait for next scheduled dose (don't double this dose).
- Nausea and vomiting—Take as soon as you remember. Wait 4 hours for next dose.

What drug does:
- Suppresses brain's vomiting center.
- Suppresses brain centers that control abnormal emotions and behavior.

Time lapse before drug works:
- Nausea and vomiting—1 hour or less.
- Nervous and mental disorders—4-6 weeks.

Continued next column

 OVERDOSE

SYMPTOMS:
Stupor, convulsions, coma.
WHAT TO DO:
- Dial 0 (operator) or 911 (emergency) for an ambulance or medical help. Then give first aid immediately.
- See emergency information on inside covers.

Don't take with:
- Antacid or medicine for diarrhea.
- Non-prescription drug for cough, cold or allergy.
- See Interaction column and consult doctor.

 POSSIBLE ADVERSE REACTIONS OR SIDE EFFECTS

SYMPTOMS	WHAT TO DO
Life-threatening:	
None expected.	
Common:	
• Muscle spasms of face and neck, unsteady gait.	Discontinue. Seek emergency treatment.
• Restlessness, tremor, drowsiness.	Discontinue. Call doctor right away.
• Decreased sweating, dry mouth, runny nose, constipation.	Continue. Call doctor when convenient.
Infrequent:	
• Fainting.	Discontinue. Seek emergency treatment.
• Rash.	Discontinue. Call doctor right away.
• Difficult urination, diminished sex drive, swollen breasts, menstrual irregularities.	Continue. Call doctor when convenient.
Rare:	
Change in vision, jaundice, sore throat, fever.	Discontinue. Call doctor right away.

WARNINGS & PRECAUTIONS

Don't take if:
- You are allergic to any phenothiazine.
- You have a blood or bone-marrow disease.

Before you start, consult your doctor:
- If you will have surgery within 2 months, including dental surgery, requiring general or spinal anesthesia.
- If you have asthma, emphysema or other lung disorder.
- If you take non-prescription ulcer medicine, asthma medicine or amphetamines.

Over age 60:
Adverse reactions and side effects may be more frequent and severe than in younger persons. More likely to develop involuntary movement of jaws, lips, tongue, chewing. Report this to your doctor immediately. Early treatment can help.

Pregnancy:
Risk to unborn child outweighs drug benefits. Don't use.

Breast-feeding:
Drug passes into milk. Avoid drug or discontinue nursing until you finish medicine. Consult doctor for advice on maintaining milk supply.

Infants & children:
Don't give to children younger than 2.

Prolonged use:
May lead to tardive dyskinesia (involuntary movement of jaws, lips, tongue, chewing).

Skin & sunlight:
May cause rash or intensify sunburn in areas exposed to sun or sunlamp. Skin may remain sensitive for 3 months after discontinuing.

Driving, piloting or hazardous work:
Don't drive or pilot aircraft until you learn how medicine affects you. Don't work around dangerous machinery. Don't climb ladders or work in high places. Danger increases if you drink alcohol or take medicine affecting alertness and reflexes.

Discontinuing:
- Nervous and mental disorders—Don't discontinue without doctor's advice until you complete prescribed dose, even though symptoms diminish or disappear.
- Nausea and vomiting—May be unnecessary to finish medicine. Follow doctor's instructions.

Others:
No problems expected.

POSSIBLE INTERACTION WITH OTHER DRUGS

GENERIC NAME OR DRUG CLASS	COMBINED EFFECT
Anticholinergics	Increased anticholinergic effect.
Antidepressants (tricyclic)	Increased mesoridazine effect.
Antihistamines	Increased antihistamine effect.
Appetite suppressants	Decreased suppressant effect.
Dronabinol	Increased effects of both drugs. Avoid.
Levodopa	Decreased levodopa effect.
Mind-altering drugs	Increased effect of mind-altering drugs.
Molindone	Increased tranquilizer effect.
Narcotics	Increased narcotic effect.
Phenytoin	Increased phenytoin effect.
Quinidine	Impaired heart function. Dangerous mixture.
Sedatives	Increased sedative effect.
Tranquilizers (other)	Increased tranquilizer effect.

POSSIBLE INTERACTION WITH OTHER SUBSTANCES

INTERACTS WITH	COMBINED EFFECT
Alcohol:	Dangerous oversedation.
Beverages:	None expected.
Cocaine:	Decreased effect of mesoridazine. Avoid.
Foods:	None expected.
Marijuana:	Drowsiness. May increase antinausea effect.
Tobacco:	None expected.

METAPROTERENOL

BRAND NAMES

Alupent   Metaprel

BASIC INFORMATION

Habit forming? No
Prescription needed? Yes
Available as generic? No
Drug class: Bronchodilator,
           sympathomimetic

 ## USES

Relieves wheezing and shortness of breath in
bronchial asthma attacks, bronchitis and
emphysema.

 ## DOSAGE & USAGE INFORMATION

How to take:
- Tablet or liquid—Swallow with liquid or food
  to lessen stomach irritation.
- Inhaler—Follow instructions on package.

When to take:
When needed, according to doctor's
instructions. Don't take more than 2 doses 1
hour apart.

If you forget a dose:
Take when you remember. Wait 2 hours for
next dose.

What drug does:
Relaxes smooth muscles to relieve constriction
of bronchial tubes.

Time lapse before drug works:
5 to 30 minutes.

Don't take with:
See Interaction column and consult doctor.

 ## OVERDOSE

SYMPTOMS:
**Chest pain, irregular heartbeat, convulsions,
coma.**
WHAT TO DO:
- **Dial 0 (operator) or 911 (emergency) for an
  ambulance or medical help. Then give first
  aid immediately.**
- **If patient is unconscious and not
  breathing, give mouth-to-mouth breathing.
  If there is no heartbeat, use cardiac
  massage and mouth-to-mouth breathing
  (CPR). Don't try to make patient vomit. If
  you can't get help quickly, take patient to
  nearest emergency facility.**
- **See emergency information on inside
  covers.**

 ## POSSIBLE ADVERSE REACTIONS OR SIDE EFFECTS

SYMPTOMS	WHAT TO DO
Life-threatening:	
None expected.	
Common:	
• Rapid or pounding heartbeat.	Discontinue. Call doctor right away.
• Nervousness, restlessness, dizziness, weakness, headache, shakiness.	Continue. Call doctor when convenient.
Infrequent:	
Chest pain; muscle cramps in arms, hands, legs; unusual sweating; paleness; bad taste in mouth; nausea or vomiting.	Discontinue. Call doctor right away.
Rare:	
None expected.	

WARNINGS & PRECAUTIONS

Don't take if:
You are allergic to any sympathomimetic.

Before you start, consult your doctor:
- If you have irregular or rapid heartbeat, congestive heart failure, coronary-artery disease or high blood pressure.
- If you have diabetes.
- If you have overactive thyroid.

Over age 60:
Adverse reactions and side effects may be more frequent and severe than in younger persons.

Pregnancy:
Risk to unborn child outweighs drug benefits. Don't use.

Breast-feeding:
Drug passes into milk. Avoid drug or discontinue nursing until you finish medicine. Consult doctor for advice on maintaining milk supply.

Infants & children:
Use only under medical supervision.

Prolonged use:
No problems expected.

Skin & sunlight:
No problems expected.

Driving, piloting or hazardous work:
Don't drive or pilot aircraft until you learn how medicine affects you. Don't work around dangerous machinery. Don't climb ladders or work in high places. Danger increases if you drink alcohol or take medicine affecting alertness and reflexes, such as antihistamines, tranquilizers, sedatives, pain medicine, narcotics and mind-altering drugs.

Discontinuing:
No problems expected.

Others:
Consult doctor immediately if breathing difficulty continues or worsens after using metaproterenol.

POSSIBLE INTERACTION WITH OTHER DRUGS

GENERIC NAME OR DRUG CLASS	COMBINED EFFECT
Albuterol	Increased effect of both drugs, especially harmful side effects.
Antidepressants (tricyclic)	Increased effect of both drugs.
Beta-adrenergic blockers	Decreased effects of both drugs.
Hydralazine	Decreased hydralazine effect.
Minoxidil	Decreased minoxidil effect.
Nitrates	Possible decreased effects of both drugs.
Sympathomimetics (other)	Increased effect of both drugs, especially harmful side effects.

POSSIBLE INTERACTION WITH OTHER SUBSTANCES

INTERACTS WITH	COMBINED EFFECT
Alcohol:	Decreased metaproterenol effect.
Beverages:	None expected.
Cocaine:	Possible metaproterenol toxicity.
Foods:	None expected.
Marijuana:	Overstimulation. Avoid.
Tobacco:	No proven problems.

METAXALONE

BRAND NAMES

Skelaxin

BASIC INFORMATION

Habit forming? No
Prescription needed? Yes
Available as generic? Yes
Drug class: Muscle relaxant (skeletal)

 USES

Treatment for sprains, strains and muscle spasms.

 DOSAGE & USAGE INFORMATION

How to take:
Tablet or capsule—Swallow with liquid.

When to take:
As needed, no more often than every 4 hours.

If you forget a dose:
Take as soon as you remember. Wait 4 hours for next dose.

What drug does:
Blocks body's pain messages to brain. May also sedate.

Time lapse before drug works:
60 minutes.

Don't take with:
See Interaction column and consult doctor.

 OVERDOSE

SYMPTOMS:
Nausea, vomiting, diarrhea, headache. May progress to severe weakness, difficult breathing, sensation of paralysis, coma.
WHAT TO DO:
- **Dial 0 (operator) or 911 (emergency) for an ambulance or medical help. Then give first aid immediately.**
- **If patient is unconscious and not breathing, give mouth-to-mouth breathing. If there is no heartbeat, use cardiac massage and mouth-to-mouth breathing (CPR). Don't try to make patient vomit. If you can't get help quickly, take patient to nearest emergency facility.**
- **See emergency information on inside covers.**

 POSSIBLE ADVERSE REACTIONS OR SIDE EFFECTS

SYMPTOMS	WHAT TO DO
Life-threatening: None expected.	
Common:	
• Drowsiness, fainting, dizziness.	Continue. Call doctor when convenient.
• Orange or red-purple urine.	No action necessary.
Infrequent: Agitation, constipation or diarrhea, nausea, cramps, vomiting, wheezing, shortness of breath.	Discontinue. Call doctor right away.
Rare:	
• Black, bloody or tarry stools.	Discontinue. Seek emergency treatment.
• Rash, hives or itch; sore throat; fever; jaundice; tiredness; weakness.	Discontinue. Call doctor right away.

WARNINGS & PRECAUTIONS

Don't take if:
- You are allergic to any skeletal-muscle relaxant.
- You have porphyria.

Before you start, consult your doctor:
- If you have had liver or kidney disease.
- If you plan pregnancy within medication period.

Over age 60:
Adverse reactions and side effects may be more frequent and severe than in younger persons.

Pregnancy:
No proven harm to unborn child. Avoid if possible.

Breast-feeding:
Drug passes into milk. Avoid drug or discontinue nursing until you finish medicine. Consult doctor for advice on maintaining milk supply.

Infants & children:
Not recommended.

Prolonged use:
Periodic liver-function tests recommended if you use this drug for a long time.

Skin & sunlight:
No problems expected.

Driving, piloting or hazardous work:
Don't drive or pilot aircraft until you learn how medicine affects you. Don't work around dangerous machinery. Don't climb ladders or work in high places. Danger increases if you drink alcohol or take medicine affecting alertness and reflexes, such as antihistamines, tranquilizers, sedatives, pain medicine, narcotics and mind-altering drugs.

Discontinuing:
Don't discontinue without doctor's advice until you complete prescribed dose, even though symptoms diminish or disappear.

Others:
No problems expected.

POSSIBLE INTERACTION WITH OTHER DRUGS

GENERIC NAME OR DRUG CLASS	COMBINED EFFECT
Antidepressants	Increased sedation.
Antihistamines	Increased sedation.
Dronabinol	Increased effect of dronabinol on central nervous system. Avoid combination.
Mind-altering drugs	Increased sedation.
Muscle relaxants (other)	Increased sedation.
Narcotics	Increased sedation.
Sedatives	Increased sedation.
Sleep inducers	Increased sedation.
Testosterone	Decreased metaxalone effect.
Tranquilizers	Increased sedation.

POSSIBLE INTERACTION WITH OTHER SUBSTANCES

INTERACTS WITH	COMBINED EFFECT
Alcohol:	Increased sedation.
Beverages:	None expected.
Cocaine:	Lack of coordination, increased sedation.
Foods:	None expected.
Marijuana:	Lack of coordination, drowsiness, fainting.
Tobacco:	None expected.

METHAMPHETAMINE

BRAND NAMES

Desoxyn   Methampex

BASIC INFORMATION

Habit forming? Yes
Prescription needed? Yes
Available as generic? Yes
Drug class: Central-nervous-system
stimulant (amphetamine)

 USES

- Prevents narcolepsy (attacks of uncontrollable sleepiness).
- Controls hyperactivity in children.

 DOSAGE & USAGE INFORMATION

How to take:
- Tablet—Swallow with liquid.
- Extended-release tablets—Swallow each dose whole with liquid.

When to take:
- At the same times each day.
- Short-acting form—Don't take later than 6 hours before bedtime.
- Long-acting form—Take on awakening.

If you forget a dose:
- Short-acting form—Take up to 2 hours late. If more than 2 hours, wait for next dose (don't double this dose).
- Long-acting form—Take as soon as you remember. Wait 20 hours for next dose.

What drug does:
- Narcolepsy—Apparently affects brain centers to decrease fatigue or sleepiness and increase alertness and motor activity.
- Hyperactive children—Calms children, opposite to effect on narcoleptic adults.

Continued next column

 OVERDOSE

SYMPTOMS:
Rapid heartbeat, hyperactivity, high fever, hallucinations, suicidal or homicidal feelings, convulsions, coma.
WHAT TO DO:
- **Dial 0 (operator) or 911 (emergency) for an ambulance or medical help. Then give first aid immediately.**
- **See emergency information on inside covers.**

Time lapse before drug works:
15 to 30 minutes.

Don't take with:
See Interaction column and consult doctor.

 POSSIBLE ADVERSE REACTIONS OR SIDE EFFECTS

SYMPTOMS	WHAT TO DO
Life-threatening: None expected.	
Common:	
• Irritability, nervousness, insomnia.	Continue. Call doctor when convenient.
• Dry mouth.	Continue. Tell doctor at next visit.
Infrequent:	
• Dizziness; lack of alertness; blurred vision; fast, pounding heartbeat; unusual sweating.	Discontinue. Call doctor right away.
• Headache.	Continue. Call doctor when convenient.
• Diarrhea or constipation, appetite loss, stomach pain, nausea, vomiting, weight loss, diminished sex drive, impotence.	Continue. Tell doctor at next visit.
Rare:	
• Rash; hives; chest pain or irregular heartbeat; uncontrollable movements of head, neck, arms, legs.	Discontinue. Call doctor right away.
• Swollen breasts, mood change.	Continue. Call doctor when convenient.

WARNINGS & PRECAUTIONS

Don't take if:
- You are allergic to any methamphetamine.
- You will have surgery within 2 months, including dental surgery, requiring general or spinal anesthesia.

Before you start, consult your doctor:
- If you plan to become pregnant within medication period.
- If you have glaucoma.
- If you have heart or blood-vessel disease, or high blood pressure.
- If you have overactive thyroid, anxiety or tension.
- If you have a severe mental illness (especially children).

Over age 60:
Adverse reactions and side effects may be more frequent and severe than in younger persons.

Pregnancy:
Risk to unborn child outweighs drug benefits. Don't use.

Breast-feeding:
Drug passes into milk. Avoid drug or discontinue nursing.

Infants & children:
Not recommended for children under 12.

Prolonged use:
Habit forming.

Skin & sunlight:
No problems expected.

Driving, piloting or hazardous work:
Don't drive or pilot aircraft until you learn how medicine affects you. Don't work around dangerous machinery. Don't climb ladders or work in high places. Danger increases if you drink alcohol or take medicine affecting alertness and reflexes.

Discontinuing:
May be unnecessary to finish medicine. Follow doctor's instructions.

Others:
- This is a dangerous drug and must be closely supervised. Don't use for appetite control or depression. Potential for damage and abuse.
- During withdrawal phase, may cause prolonged sleep of several days.

POSSIBLE INTERACTION WITH OTHER DRUGS

GENERIC NAME OR DRUG CLASS	COMBINED EFFECT
Anesthesias (general)	Irregular heartbeat.
Antidepressants (tricyclic)	Decreased methamphetamine effect.
Antihypertensives	Decreased antihypertensive effect.
Carbonic anhydrase inhibitors	Increased methamphetamine effect.
Guanethidine	Decreased guanethidine effect.
Haloperidol	Decreased methamphetamine effect.
MAO inhibitors	May severely increase blood pressure.
Phenothiazines	Decreased methamphetamine effect.
Sodium bicarbonate	Increased methamphetamine effect.

POSSIBLE INTERACTION WITH OTHER SUBSTANCES

INTERACTS WITH	COMBINED EFFECT
Alcohol:	Decreased methamphetamine effect. Avoid.
Beverages: Caffeine drinks.	Overstimulation. Avoid.
Cocaine:	Dangerous stimulation of nervous system. Avoid.
Foods:	None expected.
Marijuana:	Frequent use— Severely impaired mental function.
Tobacco:	None expected.

METHAQUALONE

BRAND NAMES

Mandrax	Sedalone
Mequelon	Sopor
Mequin	Triador
Methadorm	Tualone
Parest	Tualone-300
Quaalude	Vitalone
Rouqualone-300	

BASIC INFORMATION

Habit forming? Yes
Prescription needed? Yes
Available as generic? No
Drug class: Hypnotic

 USES

Decreases anxiety, tension or insomnia.

 DOSAGE & USAGE INFORMATION

How to take:
Tablet or capsule—Swallow with liquid. If you can't swallow whole, crumble tablet or open capsule and take with liquid or food.

When to take:
At the same time each day.

If you forget a dose:
Don't take missed dose. Wait for next scheduled dose. Don't double this dose.

What drug does:
Undetermined.

Continued next column

 OVERDOSE

SYMPTOMS:
Drowsiness, confusion, delirium, incoordination, vomiting, convulsions, abnormal bleeding, stupor, coma.
WHAT TO DO:
- Dial 0 (operator) or 911 (emergency) for an ambulance or medical help. Then give first aid immediately.
- If patient is unconscious and not breathing, give mouth-to-mouth breathing. If there is no heartbeat, use cardiac massage and mouth-to-mouth breathing (CPR). Don't try to make patient vomit. If you can't get help quickly, take patient to nearest emergency facility.
- See emergency information on inside covers.

Time lapse before drug works:
20 to 30 minutes.

Don't take with:
- Alcohol or mind-altering drugs. Combinations can be fatal.
- Non-prescription drugs without consulting doctor.
- See Interaction column and consult doctor.

 POSSIBLE ADVERSE REACTIONS OR SIDE EFFECTS

SYMPTOMS	WHAT TO DO
Life-threatening: None expected.	
Common:	
• Diarrhea, nausea, vomiting, stomach pain.	Discontinue. Call doctor right away.
• Drowsiness.	Continue. Call doctor when convenient.
• Tiredness or weakness.	Continue. Tell doctor at next visit.
• "Hangover" effect.	No action necessary.
Infrequent:	
• Unusually slow heartbeat, difficult breathing.	Discontinue. Seek emergency treatment.
• Agitation; skin rash or hives; numbness, tingling, pain or weakness in hands or feet; sweating.	Discontinue. Call doctor right away.
Rare: None expected.	

WARNINGS & PRECAUTIONS

Don't take if:
- You are allergic to any hypnotic drug.
- You plan to become pregnant within medication period.
- Patient is younger than 12.

Before you start, consult your doctor:
- If you have had liver disease or impaired liver function.
- If you will have surgery within 2 months, including dental surgery, requiring general or spinal anesthesia.

Over age 60:
Adverse reactions and side effects may be more frequent and severe than in younger persons.

Pregnancy:
Risk to unborn child outweighs drug benefits. Don't use.

Breast-feeding:
Drug may filter into milk and harm child. Don't use.

Infants & children:
Not recommended.

Prolonged use:
Psychological and physical dependence.

Skin & sunlight:
No problems expected.

Driving, piloting or hazardous work:
Don't drive or pilot aircraft until you learn how medicine affects you. Don't work around dangerous machinery. Don't climb ladders or work in high places. Danger increases if you drink alcohol or take medicine affecting alertness and reflexes, such as antihistamines, tranquilizers, sedatives, pain medicine, narcotics and mind-altering drugs.

Discontinuing:
Don't discontinue without consulting doctor. Dose may require gradual reduction if you have taken drug for a long time. Doses of other drugs may also require adjustment.

Others:
No problems expected.

POSSIBLE INTERACTION WITH OTHER DRUGS

GENERIC NAME OR DRUG CLASS	COMBINED EFFECT
Anticoagulants	Decreased anticoagulant effect.
Antihistamines	Increased sedation.
Narcotics	Increased narcotic effect.
Pain relievers	Increased effect of pain reliever.
Sedatives	Increased sedative effect.
Sleep inducers	Increased effect of sleep inducer.
Tranquilizers	Increased tranquilizer effect.

POSSIBLE INTERACTION WITH OTHER SUBSTANCES

INTERACTS WITH	COMBINED EFFECT
Alcohol:	Dangerous depression of brain function. Avoid.
Beverages:	None expected.
Cocaine:	Decreased effect of both drugs. Avoid.
Foods:	None expected.
Marijuana:	Impairs physical performance. Avoid.
Tobacco:	None expected.

METHARBITAL

BRAND NAMES

Gemonil

BASIC INFORMATION

Habit forming? Yes
Prescription needed? Yes
Available as generic? Yes
Drug class: Sedative, hypnotic (barbiturate)

 USES

Prevents convulsions.

 DOSAGE & USAGE INFORMATION

How to take:
Tablet—Swallow with liquid or food to lessen stomach irritation. If you can't swallow whole, crumble tablet and take with liquid or food.

When to take:
At the same times each day.

If you forget a dose:
Take as soon as you remember up to 2 hours late. If more than 2 hours, wait for next scheduled dose (don't double this dose).

What drug does:
May partially block nerve impulses at nerve-cell connections.

Time lapse before drug works:
60 minutes.

Don't take with:
- Non-prescription drugs without consulting doctor.
- See Interaction column and consult doctor.

 OVERDOSE

SYMPTOMS:
Deep sleep, weak pulse, coma.
WHAT TO DO:
- **Dial 0 (operator) or 911 (emergency) for an ambulance or medical help. Then give first aid immediately.**
- **If patient is unconscious and not breathing, give mouth-to-mouth breathing. If there is no heartbeat use cardiac massage and mouth-to-mouth breathing (CPR). Don't try to make patient vomit. If you can't get help quickly, take patient to nearest emergency facility.**
- **See emergency information on inside covers.**

 POSSIBLE ADVERSE REACTIONS OR SIDE EFFECTS

SYMPTOMS	WHAT TO DO
Life-threatening: None expected.	
Common: Dizziness, drowsiness, "hangover" effect.	Continue. Call doctor when convenient.
Infrequent: • Rash or hives; face, lip or eyelid swelling; sore throat; fever.	Discontinue. Call doctor right away.
• Depression, confusion, slurred speech, diarrhea, nausea, vomiting, joint or muscle pain.	Continue. Call doctor when convenient.
Rare: • Agitation, slow heartbeat, difficult breathing, jaundice.	Discontinue. Call doctor right away.
• Unusual bleeding or bruising.	Continue. Call doctor when convenient.

 WARNINGS & PRECAUTIONS

Don't take if:
- You are allergic to any barbiturate.
- You have porphyria.

Before you start, consult your doctor:
- If you have epilepsy.
- If you have kidney or liver damage.
- If you have asthma.
- If you have anemia.
- If you have chronic pain.
- If you will have surgery within 2 months, including dental surgery, requiring general or spinal anesthesia.

Over age 60:
Adverse reactions and side effects may be more frequent and severe than in younger persons. Use small doses.

Pregnancy:
Risk to unborn child outweighs drug benefits. Don't use.

Breast-feeding:
Drug passes into milk. Avoid drug or discontinue nursing until you finish medicine. Consult doctor for advice on maintaining milk supply.

Infants & children:
Use only under doctor's supervision.

Prolonged use:
- May cause addiction, anemia, chronic intoxication.
- May lower body temperature, making exposure to cold temperatures hazardous.

Skin & sunlight:
May cause rash or intensify sunburn in areas exposed to sun or sunlamp.

Driving, piloting or hazardous work:
Don't drive or pilot aircraft until you learn how medicine affects you. Don't work around dangerous machinery. Don't climb ladders or work in high places. Danger increases if you drink alcohol or take medicine affecting alertness and reflexes.

Discontinuing:
May be unnecessary to finish medicine. Follow doctor's instructions. If you develop withdrawal symptoms of hallucinations, agitation or sleeplessness after discontinuing, call doctor right away.

Others:
Great potential for abuse.

POSSIBLE INTERACTION WITH OTHER DRUGS

GENERIC NAME OR DRUG CLASS	COMBINED EFFECT
Anticoagulants (oral)	Decreased anticoagulant effect.
Anticonvulsants	Changed seizure patterns.
Antidepressants (tricyclics)	Decreased antidepressant effect. Possible dangerous oversedation.
Antidiabetics (oral)	Increased metharbital effect.
Antihistamines	Dangerous sedation. Avoid.
Anti-inflammatory drugs (non-steroidal)	Decreased anti-inflammatory effect.
Aspirin	Decreased aspirin effect.
Beta-adrenergic blockers	Decreased effect of beta-adrenergic blocker.

Contraceptives (oral)	Decreased contraceptive effect.
Cortisone drugs	Decreased cortisone effect.
Digitoxin	Decreased digitoxin effect.
Doxycycline	Decreased doxycycline effect.
Dronabinol	Increased effects of both drugs. Avoid.
Griseofulvin	Decreased griseofulvin effect.
Indapamide	Increased indapamide effect.
MAO inhibitors	Increased metharbital effect.
Mind-altering drugs	Dangerous sedation. Avoid.
Narcotics	Dangerous sedation. Avoid.
Pain relievers	Dangerous sedation. Avoid.
Sedatives	Dangerous sedation. Avoid.
Sleep inducers	Dangerous sedation. Avoid.
Tranquilizers	Dangerous sedation. Avoid.
Valproic acid	Increased metharbital effect.

POSSIBLE INTERACTION WITH OTHER SUBSTANCES

INTERACTS WITH	COMBINED EFFECT
Alcohol:	Possible fatal oversedation. Avoid.
Beverages:	None expected.
Cocaine:	Decreased metharbital effect.
Foods:	None expected.
Marijuana:	Excessive sedation. Avoid.
Tobacco:	None expected.

METHENAMINE

BRAND NAMES

Azo-Mandelamine	Renalgin
Hexamine	Sterine
Hip-Rex	Trac 2X
Hiprex	Urex
Mandelamine	Urised
Mandelets	Uroblue
Methandine	Uro-phosphate
Prov-U-Sep	Uroquid-Acid

BASIC INFORMATION

Habit forming? No
Prescription needed? Yes
Available as generic? Yes
Drug class: Anti-infective (urinary)

 USES

Suppresses chronic urinary-tract infections.

 DOSAGE & USAGE INFORMATION

How to take:
- Tablet—Swallow with liquid or food to lessen stomach irritation. If you can't swallow whole, crumble tablet and take with liquid or food.
- Liquid form—Use a measuring spoon to ensure correct dose.
- Granules—Dissolve dose in 4 oz. of water. Drink all the liquid.

When to take:
At the same times each day.

If you forget a dose:
Take as soon as you remember up to 8 hours late. If more than 8 hours, wait for next scheduled dose (don't double this dose).

What drug does:
A chemical reaction in the urine changes methenamine into formaldehyde, which destroys certain bacteria.

Continued next column

 OVERDOSE

SYMPTOMS:
Bloody urine, weakness, deep breathing, stupor, coma.
WHAT TO DO:
- Dial 0 (operator) or 911 (emergency) for an ambulance or medical help. Then give first aid immediately.
- See emergency information on inside covers.

Time lapse before drug works:
Continual use for 3 to 6 months.

Don't take with:
See Interaction column and consult doctor.

 POSSIBLE ADVERSE REACTIONS OR SIDE EFFECTS

SYMPTOMS	WHAT TO DO
Life-threatening:	
None expected.	
Common:	
• Rash.	Discontinue. Call doctor right away.
• Nausea, difficult urination.	Continue. Call doctor when convenient.
Infrequent:	
• Blood in urine.	Discontinue. Call doctor right away.
• Burning on urination, lower back pain.	Continue. Call doctor when convenient.
Rare:	
None expected.	

WARNINGS & PRECAUTIONS

Don't take if:
- You are allergic to methenamine.
- You have a severe impairment of kidney or liver function.
- The urine cannot or should not be acidified (check with your doctor).

Before you start, consult your doctor:
- If you have had kidney or liver disease.
- If you plan to become pregnant within medication period.
- If you have had gout.

Over age 60:
Don't exceed recommended dose.

Pregnancy:
Studies inconclusive on harm to unborn child. Avoid if possible, especially first 3 months.

Breast-feeding:
Drug passes into milk in small amounts. Consult doctor.

Infants & children:
Use only under medical supervision.

Prolonged use:
No problems expected.

Skin & sunlight:
No problems expected.

Driving, piloting or hazardous work:
No problems expected.

Discontinuing:
Don't discontinue without doctor's advice until you complete prescribed dose, even though symptoms diminish or disappear.

Others:
Requires an acid urine to be effective. Eat more protein foods, cranberries, cranberry juice with vitamin C, plums, prunes.

POSSIBLE INTERACTION WITH OTHER DRUGS

GENERIC NAME OR DRUG CLASS	COMBINED EFFECT
Antacids	Decreased methenamine effect.
Carbonic anhydrase inhibitors	Decreased methenamine effect.
Citrates	Decreases effects of methenamine.
Diuretics (thiazide)	Decreased urine acidity.
Sodium bicarbonate	Decreased methenamine effect.
Sulfa drugs	Possible kidney damage.
Vitamin C (1 to 4 grams per day)	Increased effect of methenamine, contributing to urine's acidity.

POSSIBLE INTERACTION WITH OTHER SUBSTANCES

INTERACTS WITH	COMBINED EFFECT
Alcohol:	Possible brain depression. Avoid or use with caution.
Beverages: Milk.	Decreased methenamine effect.
Cocaine:	None expected.
Foods:	None expected.
Marijuana:	Drowsiness, muscle weakness or blood-pressure drop.
Tobacco:	None expected.

METHICILLIN

BRAND NAMES

Azapen   Staphcillin
Celbenin

BASIC INFORMATION

Habit forming? No
Prescription needed? Yes
Available as generic? Yes
Drug class: Antibiotic (penicillin)

 USES

Treatment of bacterial infections that are
susceptible to methicillin.

 **DOSAGE & USAGE
INFORMATION**

How to take:
By injection only.

When to take:
Follow doctor's instructions.

If you forget a dose:
Consult doctor.

What drug does:
Destroys susceptible bacteria. Does not kill
viruses.

Time lapse before drug works:
May be several days before medicine affects
infection.

Don't take with:
See Interaction column and consult doctor.

 OVERDOSE

SYMPTOMS:
Severe diarrhea, nausea or vomiting.
WHAT TO DO:
**Overdose unlikely to threaten life. If person
takes much larger amount than prescribed,
call doctor, poison-control center or hospital
emergency room for instructions.**

 **POSSIBLE
ADVERSE REACTIONS
OR SIDE EFFECTS**

SYMPTOMS	WHAT TO DO
Life-threatening:	
Hives, rash, intense itching, faintness soon after a dose (anaphylaxis).	Seek emergency treatment immediately.
Common:	
Dark or discolored tongue.	Continue. Tell doctor at next visit.
Infrequent:	
Mild nausea, vomiting, diarrhea.	Continue. Call doctor when convenient.
Rare:	
Unexplained bleeding.	Discontinue. Call doctor right away.

WARNINGS & PRECAUTIONS

Don't take if:
You are allergic to methicillin, cephalosporin antibiotics, other penicillins or penicillamine. Life-threatening reaction may occur.

Before you start, consult your doctor:
If you are allergic to any substance or drug.

Over age 60:
You may have skin reactions, particularly around genitals and anus.

Pregnancy:
Studies inconclusive on harm to unborn child. Animal studies show fetal abnormalities. Decide with your doctor whether drug benefits justify risk to unborn child.

Breast-feeding:
Drug passes into milk. Child may become sensitive to penicillins and have allergic reactions to penicillin drugs. Avoid methicillin or discontinue nursing until you finish medicine. Consult doctor for advice on maintaining milk supply.

Infants & children:
No problems expected.

Prolonged use:
- You may become more susceptible to infections caused by germs not responsive to methicillin.
- May cause kidney damage. Laboratory studies to detect damage recommended if you take for a long time.

Skin & sunlight:
No problems expected.

Driving, piloting or hazardous work:
Usually not dangerous. Most hazardous reactions likely to occur a few minutes after taking methicillin.

Discontinuing:
Don't discontinue without doctor's advice until you complete prescribed dose, even though symptoms diminish or disappear.

Others:
No problems expected.

POSSIBLE INTERACTION WITH OTHER DRUGS

GENERIC NAME OR DRUG CLASS	COMBINED EFFECT
Beta-adrenergic blockers	Increased chance of anaphylaxis (see emergency information on inside front cover).
Chloramphenicol	Decreased effect of both drugs.
Erythromycins	Decreased effect of both drugs.
Loperamide	Decreased methicillin effect.
Paromomycin	Decreased effect of both drugs.
Tetracyclines	Decreased effect of both drugs.
Troleandomycin	Decreased effect of both drugs.

POSSIBLE INTERACTION WITH OTHER SUBSTANCES

INTERACTS WITH	COMBINED EFFECT
Alcohol:	Occasional stomach irritation.
Beverages:	None expected.
Cocaine:	No proven problems.
Foods:	None expected.
Marijuana:	No proven problems.
Tobacco:	None expected.

METHOCARBAMOL

BRAND NAMES

Delaxin
Forbaxin
Marbaxin
Marbaxin-750
Metho-500

Robamol
Robaxin
Robaxisal
Spinaxin
Tumol

BASIC INFORMATION

Habit forming? No
Prescription needed? Yes
Available as generic? Yes
Drug class: Muscle relaxant (skeletal)

 USES

Pain reliever for skeletal-muscle spasms.

 DOSAGE & USAGE INFORMATION

How to take:
Tablet—Swallow with liquid. If you can't swallow whole, crumble tablet and take with liquid or food.

When to take:
As directed on label.

If you forget a dose:
Take as soon as you remember up to 2 hours late. If more than 2 hours, wait for next scheduled dose (don't double this dose).

What drug does:
Blocks reflex nerve impulses in brain and spinal cord.

Continued next column

 OVERDOSE

SYMPTOMS:
Unsteadiness, lack of coordination, extreme weakness, paralysis, weak and rapid pulse, shallow breathing, cold and sweaty skin.
WHAT TO DO:
- Dial 0 (operator) or 911 (emergency) for an ambulance or medical help. Then give first aid immediately.
- If patient is unconscious and not breathing, give mouth-to-mouth breathing. If there is no heartbeat, use cardiac massage and mouth-to-mouth breathing (CPR). Don't try to make patient vomit. If you can't get help quickly, take patient to nearest emergency facility.
- See emergency information on inside covers.

Time lapse before drug works:
30 to 45 minutes.

Don't take with:
- Non-prescription drugs containing alcohol without consulting doctor.
- See Interaction column and consult doctor.

 POSSIBLE ADVERSE REACTIONS OR SIDE EFFECTS

SYMPTOMS	WHAT TO DO
Life-threatening: None expected.	
Common:	
• Blurred or double vision.	Discontinue. Call doctor right away.
• Dizziness, drowsiness, lightheadedness.	Continue. Call doctor when convenient.
Infrequent:	
• Rash, itchy skin.	Discontinue. Call doctor right away.
• Headache, bloodshot eyes, metallic taste, fever.	Continue. Call doctor when convenient.
• Stuffy nose, nausea.	Continue. Tell doctor at next visit.
Rare: None expected.	

WARNINGS & PRECAUTIONS

Don't take if:
You are allergic to any muscle relaxant.

Before you start, consult your doctor:
- If you have epilepsy.
- If you have myasthenia gravis.
- If you have impaired kidney function.

Over age 60:
Adverse reactions and side effects may be more frequent and severe than in younger persons.

Pregnancy:
No proven harm to unborn child. Avoid if possible.

Breast-feeding:
Drug filters into milk. May harm child. Avoid.

Infants & children:
Not recommended.

Prolonged use:
No problems expected.

Skin & sunlight:
No problems expected.

Driving, piloting or hazardous work:
Don't drive or pilot aircraft until you learn how medicine affects you. Don't work around dangerous machinery. Don't climb ladders or work in high places. Danger increases if you drink alcohol or take medicine affecting alertness and reflexes, such as antihistamines, tranquilizers, sedatives, pain medicine, narcotics and mind-altering drugs.

Discontinuing:
May be unnecessary to finish medicine. Follow doctor's instructions.

Others:
No problems expected.

POSSIBLE INTERACTION WITH OTHER DRUGS

GENERIC NAME OR DRUG CLASS	COMBINED EFFECT
Antidepressants (tricyclic)	Increased effect of both drugs.
Antimyasthenics	Decreased antimyasthenic effect.
Dronabinol	Increased effect of dronabinol on central nervous system. Avoid combination.
Narcotics	Increased sedative effect.
Sedatives	Increased sedative effect.
Sleep inducers	Increased effect of sleep inducer.
Tranquilizers	Increased tranquilizer effect.

POSSIBLE INTERACTION WITH OTHER SUBSTANCES

INTERACTS WITH	COMBINED EFFECT
Alcohol:	Depressed brain function. Avoid.
Beverages:	None expected.
Cocaine:	May increase muscle spasms.
Foods:	None expected.
Marijuana:	Drowsiness, muscle weakness, lack of coordination, fainting.
Tobacco:	None expected.

545

METHOTREXATE

BRAND NAMES

Folex
Folex PFS

Mexate
Mexate AQ

BASIC INFORMATION

Habit forming? No
Prescription needed? Yes
Available as generic? Yes
Drug class: Antimetabolite, antipsoriatic

 ## USES

- Treatment for some kinds of cancer.
- Treatment for psoriasis in patients with severe problems.

 ## DOSAGE & USAGE INFORMATION

How to take:
Tablet—Swallow with liquid.

When to take:
At the same time each day.

If you forget a dose:
Skip the missed dose. Don't double the next dose.

What drug does:
Inhibits abnormal-cell reproduction.

Time lapse before drug works:
May require 6 weeks for maximum effect.

Don't take with:
See Interaction column and consult doctor.

 ## OVERDOSE

SYMPTOMS:
Headache, stupor, seizures.
WHAT TO DO:

- Dial 0 (operator) or 911 (emergency) for an ambulance or medical help. Then give first aid immediately.
- If patient is unconscious and not breathing, give mouth-to-mouth breathing. If there is no heartbeat, use cardiac massage and mouth-to-mouth breathing (CPR). Don't try to make patient vomit. If you can't get help quickly, take patient to nearest emergency facility.
- See emergency information on inside covers.

 ## POSSIBLE ADVERSE REACTIONS OR SIDE EFFECTS

SYMPTOMS	WHAT TO DO
Life-threatening:	
None expected.	
Common:	
• Black stools or bloody vomit.	Discontinue. Seek emergency treatment.
• Sore throat, fever, mouth sores; chills; unusual bleeding or bruising.	Discontinue. Call doctor right away.
• Stomach pain, nausea, vomiting.	Continue. Call doctor when convenient.
Infrequent:	
• Seizures.	Discontinue. Seek emergency treatment.
• Dizziness when standing after sitting or lying, drowsiness, headache, confusion, blurred vision, shortness of breath, joint pain, blood in urine, jaundice.	Discontinue. Call doctor right away.
• Cough.	Continue. Call doctor when convenient.
• Acne, boils, hair loss, itchy skin.	Continue. Tell doctor at next visit.
Rare:	
None expected.	

WARNINGS & PRECAUTIONS

Don't take if:
You are allergic to any antimetabolite.

Before you start, consult your doctor:
- If you are alcoholic.
- If you have blood, liver or kidney disease.
- If you have colitis or peptic ulcer.
- If you have gout.
- If you have an infection.
- If you plan to become pregnant within 3 months.

Over age 60:
Adverse reactions and side effects may be more frequent and severe than in younger persons.

Pregnancy:
- Psoriasis—Risk to unborn child outweighs drug benefits. Don't use.
- Cancer—Consult doctor.

Breast-feeding:
Drug passes into milk. Avoid drug or discontinue nursing.

Infants & children:
Use only under special medical supervision.

Prolonged use:
Adverse reactions more likely the longer drug is required.

Skin & sunlight:
No problems expected.

Driving, piloting or hazardous work:
Avoid if you feel dizzy, drowsy or confused. Otherwise, no problems expected.

Discontinuing:
Don't discontinue without doctor's advice until you complete prescribed dose, even though symptoms diminish or disappear. Some side effects may follow discontinuing. Report to doctor blurred vision, convulsions, confusion, persistent headache.

Others:
- Drink more water than usual to cause frequent urination.
- Don't give this medicine to anyone else for any purpose. It is a strong drug that requires close medical supervision.
- Report for frequent medical follow-up and laboratory studies.

POSSIBLE INTERACTION WITH OTHER DRUGS

GENERIC NAME OR DRUG CLASS	COMBINED EFFECT
Anticoagulants (oral)	Increased anticoagulant effect.
Anticonvulsants (hydantoin)	Possible methotrexate toxicity.
Antigout drugs	Decreased antigout effect.
Asparaginase	Decreased methotrexate effect.
Flurouracil	Decreased methotrexate effect.
Oxyphenbutazone	Possible methotrexate toxicity.
Phenylbutazone	Possible methotrexate toxicity.
Probenecid	Possible methotrexate toxicity.
Pyrimethamine	Increased toxic effect of methotrexate.
Salicylates (including aspirin)	Possible methotrexate toxicity.
Sulfa drugs	Possible methotrexate toxicity.
Tetracyclines	Possible methotrexate toxicity.

POSSIBLE INTERACTION WITH OTHER SUBSTANCES

INTERACTS WITH	COMBINED EFFECT
Alcohol:	Likely liver damage. Avoid.
Beverages:	Extra fluid intake decreases chance of methotrexate toxicity.
Cocaine:	Increased chance of methotrexate adverse reactions. Avoid.
Foods:	None expected.
Marijuana:	None expected.
Tobacco:	None expected.

METHSUXIMIDE

BRAND NAMES

Celontin

BASIC INFORMATION

Habit forming? No
Prescription needed? Yes
Available as generic? No
Drug class: Anticonvulsant (succinimide)

 USES

Controls seizures in treatment of epilepsy.

 DOSAGE & USAGE INFORMATION

How to take:
Capsule—Swallow with liquid or food to lessen stomach irritation.

When to take:
Every day in regularly spaced doses, according to prescription.

If you forget a dose:
Take as soon as you remember up to 2 hours late. If more than 2 hours, wait for next scheduled dose (don't double this dose).

What drug does:
Depresses nerve transmissions in part of brain that controls muscles.

Time lapse before drug works:
3 hours.

Don't take with:
See Interaction column and consult doctor.

 OVERDOSE

SYMPTOMS:
Coma
WHAT TO DO:
- Dial 0 (operator) or 911 (emergency) for an ambulance or medical help. Then give first aid immediately.
- If patient is unconscious and not breathing, give mouth-to-mouth breathing. If there is no heartbeat, use cardiac massage and mouth-to-mouth breathing (CPR). Don't try to make patient vomit. If you can't get help quickly, take patient to nearest emergency facility.
- See emergency information on inside covers.

 POSSIBLE ADVERSE REACTIONS OR SIDE EFFECTS

SYMPTOMS	WHAT TO DO
Life-threatening: None expected.	
Common: Nausea, vomiting, stomach cramps, appetite loss.	Continue. Call doctor when convenient.
Infrequent: Dizziness, drowsiness, headache, irritability, mood change.	Continue. Call doctor when convenient.
Rare: • Rash, sore throat, fever, unusual bleeding or bruising.	Discontinue. Call doctor right away.
• Swollen lymph glands.	Continue. Call doctor when convenient.

WARNINGS & PRECAUTIONS

Don't take if:
You are allergic to any succinimide anticonvulsant.

Before you start, consult your doctor:
- If you plan to become pregnant within medication period.
- If you take other anticonvulsants.
- If you have blood disease.
- If you have kidney or liver disease.

Over age 60:
Adverse reactions and side effects may be more frequent and severe than in younger persons.

Pregnancy:
Risk to unborn child outweighs drug benefits. Don't use.

Breast-feeding:
Drug passes into milk. Avoid drug or discontinue nursing.

Infants & children:
Use only under medical supervision.

Prolonged use:
No problems expected.

Skin & sunlight:
No problems expected.

Driving, piloting or hazardous work:
Don't drive or pilot aircraft until you learn how medicine affects you. Don't work around dangerous machinery. Don't climb ladders or work in high places. Danger increases if you drink alcohol or take medicine affecting alertness and reflexes, such as antihistamines, tranquilizers, sedatives, pain medicine, narcotics and mind-altering drugs.

Discontinuing:
Don't discontinue without doctor's advice until you complete prescribed dose, even though symptoms diminish or disappear.

Others:
- Your response to medicine should be checked regularly by your doctor. Dose and schedule may have to be altered frequently to fit individual needs.
- Periodic blood-cell counts, kidney- and liver-function studies recommended.

POSSIBLE INTERACTION WITH OTHER DRUGS

GENERIC NAME OR DRUG CLASS	COMBINED EFFECT
Anticonvulsants (other)	Increased effect of both drugs.
Antidepressants (tricyclic)	May provoke seizures.
Antipsychotics	May provoke seizures.

POSSIBLE INTERACTION WITH OTHER SUBSTANCES

INTERACTS WITH	COMBINED EFFECT
Alcohol:	May provoke seizures.
Beverages:	None expected.
Cocaine:	May provoke seizures.
Foods:	None expected.
Marijuana:	May provoke seizures.
Tobacco:	None expected.

METHYCLOTHIAZIDE

BRAND NAMES

Aquatensen   Enduron
Diutensen   Enduronyl
Duretic

BASIC INFORMATION

Habit forming? No
Prescription needed? Yes
Available as generic? Yes
Drug class: Antihypertensive, diuretic
    (thiazide)

USES

- Controls, but doesn't cure, high blood pressure.
- Reduces fluid retention (edema) caused by conditions such as heart disorders and liver disease.

DOSAGE & USAGE INFORMATION

How to take:
Tablet or capsule—Swallow with liquid. If you can't swallow whole, crumble tablet or open capsule and take with liquid or food. Don't exceed dose.

When to take:
At the same time each day.

If you forget a dose:
Take as soon as you remember up to 2 hours late. If more than 2 hours, wait for next scheduled dose (don't double this dose).

What drug does:
- Forces sodium and water excretion, reducing body fluid.
- Relaxes muscle cells of small arteries.
- Reduced body fluid and relaxed arteries lower blood pressure.

Continued next column

OVERDOSE

SYMPTOMS:
Cramps, weakness, drowsiness, weak pulse, coma.
WHAT TO DO:
- Dial 0 (operator) or 911 (emergency) for an ambulance or medical help. Then give first aid immediately.
- See emergency information on inside covers.

Time lapse before drug works:
4 to 6 hours. May require several weeks to lower blood pressure.

Don't take with:
- See Interaction column and consult doctor.
- Non-prescription drugs without consulting doctor.

POSSIBLE ADVERSE REACTIONS OR SIDE EFFECTS

SYMPTOMS	WHAT TO DO
Life-threatening: None expected.	
Common: None expected.	
Infrequent: • Blurred vision, severe abdominal pain, nausea, vomiting, irregular heartbeat, weak pulse.	Discontinue. Call doctor right away.
• Dizziness, mood change, headache, weakness, tiredness, weight changes.	Continue. Call doctor when convenient.
• Dry mouth, thirst.	Continue. Tell doctor at next visit.
Rare: • Rash or hives.	Discontinue. Seek emergency treatment.
• Jaundice, sore throat, fever.	Discontinue. Call doctor right away.

WARNINGS & PRECAUTIONS

Don't take if:
You are allergic to any thiazide diuretic drug.

Before you start, consult your doctor:
- If you are allergic to any sulfa drug.
- If you have gout.
- If you have liver, pancreas or kidney disorder.

Over age 60:
Adverse reactions and side effects may be more frequent and severe than in younger persons, especially dizziness and excessive potassium loss.

Pregnancy:
Risk to unborn child outweighs drug benefits. Don't use.

Breast-feeding:
Drug passes into milk. Avoid drug or discontinue nursing.

Infants & children:
No problems expected.

Prolonged use:
You may need medicine to treat high blood pressure for the rest of your life.

Skin & sunlight:
May cause rash or intensify sunburn in areas exposed to sun or sunlamp.

Driving, piloting or hazardous work:
Don't drive or pilot aircraft until you learn how medicine affects you. Don't work around dangerous machinery. Don't climb ladders or work in high places. Danger increases if you drink alcohol or take medicine affecting alertness and reflexes, such as antihistamines, tranquilizers, sedatives, pain medicine, narcotics and mind-altering drugs.

Discontinuing:
Don't discontinue without medical advice.

Others:
- Hot weather and fever may cause dehydration and drop in blood pressure. Dose may require temporary adjustment. Weigh daily and report any unexpected weight decreases to your doctor.
- May cause rise in uric acid, leading to gout.
- May cause blood-sugar rise in diabetics.

POSSIBLE INTERACTION WITH OTHER DRUGS

GENERIC NAME OR DRUG CLASS	COMBINED EFFECT
Acebutolol	Increased antihypertensive effect. Dosages of both drugs may require adjustments.
Allopurinol	Decreased allopurinol effect.
Amiodarone	Increased risk of heartbeat irregularity due to low potassium.
Antidepressants (tricyclic)	Dangerous drop in blood pressure. Avoid combination unless under medical supervision.
Barbiturates	Increased methyclothiazide effect.
Calcium supplements	Increased calcium in blood.
Cholestyramine	Decreased methyclothiazide effect.
Cortisone drugs	Excessive potassium loss that causes dangerous heart rhythms.

Digitalis preparations	Excessive potassium loss that causes dangerous heart rhythms.
Diuretics (thiazide)	Increased effect of other thiazide diuretics.
Indapamide	Increased diuretic effect.
Labetolol	Increased antihypertensive effects.
Lithium	Increased effect of lithium.
MAO inhibitors	Increased metolazone effect.
Nitrates	Excessive blood-pressure drop.
Oxprenolol	Increased antihypertensive effect. Dosages of both drugs may require adjustments.
Potassium supplements	Decreased potassium effect.
Probenecid	Decreased probenecid effect.

POSSIBLE INTERACTION WITH OTHER SUBSTANCES

INTERACTS WITH	COMBINED EFFECT
Alcohol:	Dangerous blood-pressure drop.
Beverages:	None expected.
Cocaine:	None expected.
Foods: Licorice.	Excessive potassium loss that causes dangerous heart rhythms.
Marijuana:	May increase blood pressure.
Tobacco:	None expected.

METHYLCELLULOSE

BRAND NAMES

Anorex-CCK
Cellothyl
Citrucel
Cologel

Gonio-Gel
Hydrolose
Lacril
Murocel

BASIC INFORMATION

Habit forming? No
Prescription needed? No
Available as generic? Yes
Drug class: Laxative (bulk-forming)

 ## USES

Relieves constipation and prevents straining for bowel movement.

 ## DOSAGE & USAGE INFORMATION

How to take:
- Liquid, powder, flakes, granules—Dilute dose in 8 oz. cold water or fruit juice.
- Capsules—Swallow with 8 oz. cold liquid. Drink 6 to 8 glasses of water each day in addition to the one with each dose.

When to take:
At the same time each day, preferably morning.

If you forget a dose:
Take as soon as you remember. Resume regular schedule.

What drug does:
Absorbs water, stimulating the bowel to form a soft, bulky stool.

Time lapse before drug works:
May require 2 or 3 days to begin, then works in 12 to 24 hours.

Don't take with:
- See Interaction column and consult doctor.
- Don't take within 2 hours of taking another medicine. Laxative interferes with medicine absorption.

 ## OVERDOSE

SYMPTOMS:
None expected.
WHAT TO DO:
Overdose unlikely to threaten life. If person takes much larger amount than prescribed, call doctor, poison-control center or hospital emergency room for instructions.

 ## POSSIBLE ADVERSE REACTIONS OR SIDE EFFECTS

SYMPTOMS	WHAT TO DO
Life-threatening:	
None expected.	
Common:	
None expected.	
Infrequent:	
Swallowing difficulty, "lump in throat" sensation, nausea, vomiting, diarrhea.	Continue. Call doctor when convenient.
Rare:	
Itchy skin, rash, intestinal blockage, asthma.	Discontinue. Call doctor right away.

WARNINGS & PRECAUTIONS

Don't take if:
- You are allergic to any bulk-forming laxative.
- You have symptoms of appendicitis, inflamed bowel or intestinal blockage.
- You have missed a bowel movement for only 1 or 2 days.

Before you start, consult your doctor:
- If you have diabetes.
- If you have a laxative habit.
- If you have rectal bleeding.
- If you have difficulty swallowing.
- If you take other laxatives.

Over age 60:
Adverse reactions and side effects may be more frequent and severe than in younger persons.

Pregnancy:
Most bulk-forming laxatives contain sodium or sugars which may cause fluid retention. Avoid if possible.

Breast-feeding:
No problems expected.

Infants & children:
Use only under medical supervision.

Prolonged use:
Don't take for more than 1 week unless under a doctor's supervision. May cause laxative dependence.

Skin & sunlight:
No problems expected.

Driving, piloting or hazardous work:
No problems expected.

Discontinuing:
May be unnecessary to finish medicine. Follow doctor's instructions.

Others:
Don't take to "flush out" your system or as a "tonic."

 ## POSSIBLE INTERACTION WITH OTHER DRUGS

GENERIC NAME OR DRUG CLASS	COMBINED EFFECT
Antibiotics	Decreased antibiotic effect.
Anticoagulants	Decreased anticoagulant effect.
Digitalis preparations	Decreased digitalis effect.
Salicylates (including aspirin)	Decreased salicylate effect.

 ## POSSIBLE INTERACTION WITH OTHER SUBSTANCES

INTERACTS WITH	COMBINED EFFECT
Alcohol:	None expected.
Beverages:	None expected.
Cocaine:	None expected.
Foods:	None expected.
Marijuana:	None expected.
Tobacco:	None expected.

METHYLDOPA

BRAND NAMES

Aldoclor
Aldoril D30
Aldoril D50
Aldoril-15

Aldoril-25
Apo-Methyldopa
Medimet
PMS Dopazide

BASIC INFORMATION

Habit forming? No
Prescription needed? Yes
Available as generic? Yes
Drug class: Antihypertensive

 USES

Reduces high blood pressure.

 DOSAGE & USAGE INFORMATION

How to take:
Liquid or tablet—Swallow with liquid. If you can't swallow whole, crumble tablet and take with liquid or food.

When to take:
At the same times each day.

If you forget a dose:
Take as soon as you remember up to 2 hours late. If more than 2 hours, wait for next scheduled dose (don't double this dose).

What drug does:
Relaxes walls of small arteries to decrease blood pressure.

Continued next column

 OVERDOSE

SYMPTOMS:
Drowsiness; exhaustion; stupor; confusion; slow, weak pulse.
WHAT TO DO:
- **Dial 0 (operator) or 911 (emergency) for an ambulance or medical help. Then give first aid immediately.**
- **If patient is unconscious and not breathing, give mouth-to-mouth breathing. If there is no heartbeat, use cardiac massage and mouth-to-mouth breathing (CPR). Don't try to make patient vomit. If you can't get help quickly, take patient to nearest emergency facility.**
- **See emergency information on inside covers.**

Time lapse before drug works:
Continual use for 2 to 4 weeks may be necessary to determine effectiveness.

Don't take with:
See Interaction column and consult doctor.

 POSSIBLE ADVERSE REACTIONS OR SIDE EFFECTS

SYMPTOMS	WHAT TO DO
Life-threatening: None expected.	
Common: Depression, nightmares, drowsiness, weakness, stuffy nose, dry mouth, fluid retention, swollen feet or legs.	Continue. Call doctor when convenient.
Infrequent: ● Fast heartbeat.	Discontinue. Call doctor right away.
● Insomnia, nausea, vomiting, diarrhea.	Continue. Call doctor when convenient.
● Swollen breasts, diminished sex drive.	Continue. Tell doctor at next visit.
Rare: Rash, jaundice, unexplained fever.	Discontinue. Call doctor right away.

WARNINGS & PRECAUTIONS

Don't take if:
You will have surgery within 2 months, including dental surgery, requiring general or spinal anesthesia.

Before you start, consult your doctor:
If you have liver disease.

Over age 60:
- Increased susceptibility to dizziness, unsteadiness, fainting, falling.
- Drug can produce or intensify Parkinson's disease.

Pregnancy:
No proven problems. Consult doctor.

Breast-feeding:
No proven problems. Consult doctor.

Infants & children:
Not used.

Prolonged use:
- May cause anemia.
- Severe edema (fluid retention).

Skin & sunlight:
No problems expected.

Driving, piloting or hazardous work:
Don't drive or pilot aircraft until you learn how medicine affects you. Don't work around dangerous machinery. Don't climb ladders or work in high places. Danger increases if you drink alcohol or take medicine affecting alertness and reflexes, such as antihistamines, tranquilizers, sedatives, pain medicine, narcotics and mind-altering drugs.

Discontinuing:
Don't discontinue without consulting doctor. Dose may require gradual reduction if you have taken drug for a long time. Doses of other drugs may also require adjustment.

Others:
Avoid heavy exercise, exertion, sweating.

POSSIBLE INTERACTION WITH OTHER DRUGS

GENERIC NAME OR DRUG CLASS	COMBINED EFFECT
Amphetamines	Decreased methyldopa effect.
Anticoagulants (oral)	Increased anticoagulant effect.
Antidepressants (tricyclic)	Dangerous blood-pressure rise. Decreased methyldopa effect.
Antihypertensives	Increased antihypertensive effect.
Digitalis preparations	Excessively slow heartbeat.
Diuretics (thiazide)	Increased methyldopa effect.
Enalapril	Possible excessive potassium in blood.
Levodopa	Decreased levodopa effect.
MAO inhibitors	Dangerous blood-pressure rise.
Pentoxifylline	Increased antihypertensive effect.

POSSIBLE INTERACTION WITH OTHER SUBSTANCES

INTERACTS WITH	COMBINED EFFECT
Alcohol:	Increased sedation. Excessive blood-pressure drop. Avoid.
Beverages:	None expected.
Cocaine:	Decreased methyldopa effect.
Foods:	None expected.
Marijuana:	Possible fainting.
Tobacco:	Possible increased blood pressure.

METHYLDOPA & THIAZIDE DIURETICS

BRAND NAMES

Aldomet   Medimet-250
Dopamet   Novomedopa

BASIC INFORMATION

Habit forming? No
Prescription needed? Yes
Available as generic? Yes
**Drug class: Antihypertensive, diuretic
(thiazide)**

 USES

- Controls, but doesn't cure, high blood pressure.
- Reduces fluid retention (edema).

 DOSAGE & USAGE INFORMATION

How to take:
Tablet or capsule—Swallow with liquid. If you can't swallow whole, crumble tablet or open capsule and take with liquid or food.

When to take:
At the same times each day.

If you forget a dose:
Take as soon as you remember up to 2 hours late. If more than 2 hours, wait for next scheduled dose (don't double this dose).

Continued next column

 OVERDOSE

SYMPTOMS:
Drowsiness; exhaustion; cramps; weakness; stupor; confusion; slow, weak pulse; coma.
WHAT TO DO:

- **Dial 0 (operator) or 911 (emergency) for an ambulance or medical help. Then give first aid immediately.**
- **If patient is unconscious and not breathing, give mouth-to-mouth breathing. If there is no heartbeat, use cardiac massage and mouth-to-mouth breathing (CPR). Don't try to make patient vomit. If you can't get help quickly, take patient to nearest emergency facility.**
- **See emergency information on inside covers.**

What drug does:

- Relaxes walls of small arteries to decrease blood pressure.
- Forces sodium and water excretion, reducing body fluid.
- Reduced body fluid and relaxed arteries lower blood pressure.

Time lapse before drug works:
Continual use for 2 to 4 weeks may be necessary to determine effectiveness.

Don't take with:

- Non-prescription drugs without consulting doctor.
- See Interaction column and consult doctor.

 POSSIBLE ADVERSE REACTIONS OR SIDE EFFECTS

SYMPTOMS	WHAT TO DO
Life-threatening:	
Irregular heartbeat, weak pulse.	Discontinue. Seek emergency treatment.
Common:	
Depression, nightmares, drowsiness, weakness, stuffy nose, dry mouth, swollen feet and ankles, dizziness.	Continue. Call doctor when convenient.
Infrequent:	
• Fast heartbeat, change in vision, abdominal pain, nervousness.	Discontinue. Call doctor right away.
• Insomnia, nausea, vomiting, diarrhea, headache.	Continue. Call doctor when convenient.
Rare:	
• Rash; jaundice; hives; sore throat, fever, mouth sores.	Discontinue. Call doctor right away.
• Weight gain or loss.	Continue. Call doctor when convenient.

 WARNINGS & PRECAUTIONS

Don't take if:

- You are allergic to any thiazide diuretic drug.
- If you will have surgery within 2 months, including dental surgery, requiring general or spinal anesthesia.

Before you start, consult your doctor:

- If you are allergic to any sulfa drug.
- If you have gout, liver, pancreas or kidney disorder.

Over age 60:

- Increased susceptibility to dizziness, unsteadiness, fainting, falling.

- Drug can produce or intensify Parkinson's disease.

Pregnancy:
Risk to unborn child outweighs drug benefits. Don't use.

Breast-feeding:
Drug passes into milk. Avoid drug or discontinue nursing until you finish medicine. Consult doctor for advice on maintaining milk supply.

Infants & children:
Not recommended.

Prolonged use:
- May cause anemia.
- Severe edema (fluid retention).

Skin & sunlight:
May cause rash or intensify sunburn in areas exposed to sun or sunlamp.

Driving, piloting or hazardous work:
Don't drive or pilot aircraft until you learn how medicine affects you. Don't work around dangerous machinery. Don't climb ladders or work in high places. Danger increases if you drink alcohol or take medicine affecting alertness and reflexes, such as antihistamines, tranquilizers, sedatives, pain medicine, narcotics and mind-altering drugs.

Discontinuing:
Don't discontinue without consulting doctor. Dose may require gradual reduction if you have taken drug for a long time. Doses of other drugs may also require adjustment.

Others:
- Hot weather and fever may cause dehydration and drop in blood pressure. Dose may require temporary adjustment. Weigh daily and report any unexpected weight decreases to your doctor.
- May cause rise in uric acid, leading to gout.
- May cause blood-sugar rise in diabetics.
- Avoid heavy exercise, exertion, sweating.

POSSIBLE INTERACTION WITH OTHER DRUGS

GENERIC NAME OR DRUG CLASS	COMBINED EFFECT
Acebutolol	Increased antihypertensive effect. Dosages of both drugs may require adjustments.
Allopurinol	Decreased allopurinol effect.
Amphetamines	Decreased methyldopa effect.
Anticoagulants (oral)	Increased anticoagulant effect.
Antidepressants (tricyclic)	Dangerous changes in blood pressure. Avoid combination unless under medical supervision.
Antihypertensives	Increased antihypertensive effect.
Barbiturates	Increased hydrochlorothiazide effect.
Cholestyamine	Decreased hydrochlorothiazide effect.
Cortisone drugs	Excessive potassium loss that causes dangerous heart rhythms.
Digitalis preparations	Excessive potassium loss that causes dangerous heart rhythms.
Diuretics (thiazide)	Increased effect of both drugs.
Indapamide	Increased diuretic effect.
Levodopa	Decreased levodopa effect.
Lithium	Increased lithium effect.

Continued page 968

POSSIBLE INTERACTION WITH OTHER SUBSTANCES

INTERACTS WITH	COMBINED EFFECT
Alcohol:	Increased sedation. Excessive blood-pressure drop. Avoid.
Beverages:	None expected.
Cocaine:	Decreased methyldopa effect.
Foods: Licorice.	Excessive potassium loss that causes dangerous heart rhythms.
Marijuana:	May increase blood pressure.
Tobacco:	Possible increased blood pressure.

METHYLERGONOVINE

BRAND NAMES

Methergine   Methylergometrine
Methylergobasine-
  Sandoz

BASIC INFORMATION

Habit forming? No
Prescription needed? Yes
Available as generic? Yes
Drug class: Ergot preparation (uterine
              stimulant)

 ## USES

Retards excessive post-delivery bleeding.

 ## DOSAGE & USAGE INFORMATION

How to take:
Tablet—Swallow with liquid or food to lessen stomach irritation.

When to take:
At the same times each day.

If you forget a dose:
Don't take missed dose and don't double next one. Wait for next scheduled dose.

What drug does:
Causes smooth-muscle cells of uterine wall to contract and surround bleeding blood vessels of relaxed uterus.

Time lapse before drug works:
Tablets—20 to 30 minutes.

Don't take with:
See Interaction column and consult doctor.

 ## OVERDOSE

SYMPTOMS:
Vomiting, diarrhea, weak pulse, low blood pressure, convulsions.
WHAT TO DO:
- **Dial 0 (operator) or 911 (emergency) for an ambulance or medical help. Then give first aid immediately.**
- **If patient is unconscious and not breathing, give mouth-to-mouth breathing. If there is no heartbeat, use cardiac massage and mouth-to-mouth breathing (CPR). Don't try to make patient vomit. If you can't get help quickly, take patient to nearest emergency facility.**
- **See emergency information on inside covers.**

 ## POSSIBLE ADVERSE REACTIONS OR SIDE EFFECTS

SYMPTOMS	WHAT TO DO
Life-threatening:	
None expected.	
Common:	
Nausea, vomiting.	Discontinue. Call doctor right away.
Infrequent:	
• Confusion, ringing in ears, diarrhea, muscle cramps.	Discontinue. Call doctor right away.
• Unusual sweating.	Continue. Call doctor when convenient.
Rare:	
Sudden, severe headache; shortness of breath; chest pain; numb, cold hands and feet.	Discontinue. Seek emergency treatment.

WARNINGS & PRECAUTIONS

Don't take if:
You are allergic to any ergot preparation.

Before you start, consult your doctor:
- If you have coronary-artery or blood-vessel disease.
- If you have liver or kidney disease.
- If you have high blood pressure.
- If you have postpartum infection.

Over age 60:
Not recommended.

Pregnancy:
Risk to unborn child outweighs drug benefits. Don't use.

Breast-feeding:
Drug passes into milk. Avoid drug or discontinue nursing until you finish medicine. Consult doctor for advice on maintaining milk supply.

Infants & children:
Not recommended.

Prolonged use:
Not recommended.

Skin & sunlight:
No problems expected.

Driving, piloting or hazardous work:
No problems expected.

Discontinuing:
May be unnecessary to finish medicine. Follow doctor's instructions.

Others:
Drug should be used for short time only following childbirth or miscarriage.

POSSIBLE INTERACTION WITH OTHER DRUGS

GENERIC NAME OR DRUG CLASS	COMBINED EFFECT
Ergot preparations (other)	Increased methylergonovine effect.

POSSIBLE INTERACTION WITH OTHER SUBSTANCES

INTERACTS WITH	COMBINED EFFECT
Alcohol:	None expected.
Beverages:	None expected.
Cocaine:	None expected.
Foods:	None expected.
Marijuana:	None expected.
Tobacco:	None expected.

METHYLPHENIDATE

BRAND NAMES

Methidate   Ritalin SR
Ritalin

BASIC INFORMATION

Habit forming? Yes
Available as generic? Yes
Prescription needed? Yes
Drug class: Sympathomimetic

 USES

- Treatment for hyperactive children.
- Treatment for drowsiness and fatigue in adults.
- Treatment for narcolepsy (uncontrollable attacks of sleepiness).

 DOSAGE & USAGE INFORMATION

How to take:
Tablet or capsule—Swallow with liquid or food to lessen stomach irritation. If you can't swallow whole, crumble tablet or open capsule and take with liquid or food.

When to take:
At the same times each day.

If you forget a dose:
Take as soon as you remember up to 2 hours late. If more than 2 hours, wait for next scheduled dose (don't double this dose).

Continued next column

 OVERDOSE

SYMPTOMS:
Rapid heartbeat, fever, confusion,
hallucinations, convulsions, coma.
WHAT TO DO:
- **Dial 0 (operator) or 911 (emergency) for an ambulance or medical help. Then give first aid immediately.**
- **If patient is unconscious and not breathing, give mouth-to-mouth breathing. If there is no heartbeat, use cardiac massage and mouth-to-mouth breathing (CPR). Don't try to make patient vomit. If you can't get help quickly, take patient to nearest emergency facility.**
- **See emergency information on inside covers.**

What drug does:
Stimulates brain to improve alertness, concentration and attention span. Calms the hyperactive child.

Time lapse before drug works:
- 1 month or more for maximum effect on child.
- 30 minutes to stimulate adults.

Don't take with:
See Interaction column and consult doctor.

 POSSIBLE ADVERSE REACTIONS OR SIDE EFFECTS

SYMPTOMS	WHAT TO DO
Life-threatening:	
None expected.	
Common:	
• Mood change.	Continue. Call doctor when convenient.
• Nervousness, insomnia, dizziness, headache, appetite loss.	Continue. Tell doctor at next visit.
Infrequent:	
• Rash or hives; chest pain; fast, irregular heartbeat; unusual bruising; joint pain; uncontrollable movements; unexplained fever.	Discontinue. Call doctor right away.
• Nausea, abdominal pain.	Continue. Call doctor when convenient.
Rare:	
• Blurred vision, sore throat, fever.	Discontinue. Call doctor right away.
• Unusual tiredness.	Continue. Call doctor when convenient.

WARNINGS & PRECAUTIONS

Don't take if:
- You are allergic to methylphenidate.
- You have glaucoma.
- Patient is younger than 6.

Before you start, consult your doctor:
- If you have epilepsy.
- If you have high blood pressure.
- If you take MAO inhibitors.

Over age 60:
Adverse reactions and side effects may be more frequent and severe than in younger persons.

Pregnancy:
No proven harm to unborn child. Avoid if possible.

Breast-feeding:
No proven problems. Consult doctor.

Infants & children:
Use only under medical supervision for children 6 or older.

Prolonged use:
Rare possibility of physical growth retardation.

Skin & sunlight:
No problems expected.

Driving, piloting or hazardous work:
No problems expected.

Discontinuing:
Don't discontinue abruptly. Don't discontinue without doctor's advice until you complete prescribed dose, even though symptoms diminish or disappear.

Others:
Dose must be carefully adjusted by doctor.

POSSIBLE INTERACTION WITH OTHER DRUGS

GENERIC NAME OR DRUG CLASS	COMBINED EFFECT
Acebutolol	Decreased effects of both drugs.
Anticholinergics	Increased anticholinergic effect.
Anticoagulants (oral)	Increased anticoagulant effect.
Anticonvulsants	Increased anticonvulsant effect.
Antidepressants (tricyclic)	Increased antidepressant effect. Decreased methylphenidate effect.
Guanethidine	Decreased guanethidine effect.
MAO inhibitors	Dangerous rise in blood pressure.
Minoxidil	Decreased minoxidil effect.
Nitrates	Possible decreased effects of both drugs.
Oxprenolol	Decreased effects of both drugs.
Oxyphenbutazone	Increased oxyphenbutazone effect.
Phenylbutazone	Increased phenylbutazone effect.

POSSIBLE INTERACTION WITH OTHER SUBSTANCES

INTERACTS WITH	COMBINED EFFECT
Alcohol:	None expected.
Beverages: Caffeine drinks.	May raise blood pressure.
Cocaine:	Overstimulation. Avoid.
Foods: Foods containing tyramine (see Glossary).	May raise blood pressure.
Marijuana:	None expected.
Tobacco:	None expected.

METHYLPREDNISOLONE

BRAND NAMES

See complete list of brand names in the *Brand Name Directory,* page 951.

BASIC INFORMATION

Habit forming? No
Prescription needed? Yes
Available as generic? Yes
Drug class: Cortisone drug (adrenal corticosteroid)

 USES

- Reduces inflammation caused by many different medical problems.
- Treatment for some allergic diseases, blood disorders, kidney diseases, asthma and emphysema.
- Replaces corticosteroid deficiencies.

 DOSAGE & USAGE INFORMATION

How to take:
Tablet—Swallow with liquid or food to lessen stomach irritation. If you can't swallow whole, crumble tablet and take with liquid or food.

When to take:
At the same times each day. Take once-a-day or once-every-other-day doses in mornings.

If you forget a dose:
- Several-doses-per-day prescription—Take as soon as you remember up to 2 hours late. If more than 2 hours, wait for next scheduled dose (don't double this dose).
- Once-a-day dose or less—Wait for next dose. Double this dose.

What drug does:
Decreases inflammatory responses.

Time lapse before drug works:
2 to 4 days.

Don't take with:
See Interaction column and consult doctor.

 OVERDOSE

SYMPTOMS:
Headache, convulsions, heart failure.
WHAT TO DO:
- **Dial 0 (operator) or 911 (emergency) for an ambulance or medical help. Then give first aid immediately.**
- **See emergency information on inside covers.**

 POSSIBLE ADVERSE REACTIONS OR SIDE EFFECTS

SYMPTOMS	WHAT TO DO
Life-threatening: None expected.	
Common: Acne, poor wound healing, thirst, indigestion, nausea, vomiting.	Continue. Call doctor when convenient.
Infrequent:	
• Black, bloody or tarry stools.	Discontinue. Seek emergency treatment.
• Blurred vision, halos around lights, sore throat, fever, muscle cramps, swollen legs or feet.	Discontinue. Call doctor right away.
• Mood change, insomnia, restlessness, frequent urination, weight gain, round face, fatigue, weakness, TB recurrence, irregular menstrual periods.	Continue. Call doctor when convenient.
Rare:	
• Irregular heartbeat.	Discontinue. Seek emergency treatment.
• Rash.	Discontinue. Call doctor right away.

 WARNINGS & PRECAUTIONS

Don't take if:
- You are allergic to any cortisone drug.
- You have tuberculosis or fungus infection.
- You have herpes infection of eyes, lips or genitals.

Before you start, consult your doctor:
- If you have had tuberculosis.
- If you have congestive heart failure.
- If you have diabetes.
- If you have peptic ulcer.
- If you have glaucoma.
- If you have underactive thyroid.
- If you have high blood pressure.
- If you have myasthenia gravis.
- If you have blood clots in legs or lungs.

Over age 60:
Adverse reactions and side effects may be more frequent and severe than in younger persons. Likely to aggravate edema, diabetes or ulcers. Likely to cause cataracts and osteoporosis (softening of the bones).

Pregnancy:
Risk to unborn child outweighs drug benefits.
Don't use.

Breast-feeding:
Drug passes into milk. Avoid drug or
discontinue nursing until you finish medicine.
Consult doctor for advice on maintaining milk
supply.

Infants & children:
Use only under medical supervision.

Prolonged use:
- Retards growth in children.
- Possible glaucoma, cataracts, diabetes,
  fragile bones and thin skin.
- Functional dependence.

Skin & sunlight:
No problems expected.

Driving, piloting or hazardous work:
No problems expected.

Discontinuing:
- Don't discontinue without doctor's advice until
  you complete prescribed dose, even though
  symptoms diminish or disappear.
- Drug affects your response to surgery, illness,
  injury or stress for 2 years after discontinuing.
  Tell anyone who takes medical care of you
  within 2 years about drug.

Others:
Avoid immunizations if possible.

POSSIBLE INTERACTION WITH OTHER DRUGS

GENERIC NAME OR DRUG CLASS	COMBINED EFFECT
Amphoterecin B	Potassium depletion.
Anticholinergics	Possible glaucoma.
Anticoagulants (oral)	Decreased anticoagulant effect.
Anticonvulsants (hydantoin)	Decreased methylprednisolone effect.
Antidiabetics (oral)	Decreased antidiabetic effect.
Antihistamines	Decreased methylprednisolone effect.
Aspirin	Increased methylprednisolone effect.
Barbiturates	Decreased methylprednisolone effect. Oversedation.
Beta-adrenergic blockers	Decreased methylprednisolone effect.
Chloral hydrate	Decreased methylprednisolone effect.
Chlorthalidone	Potassium depletion.
Cholinergics	Decreased cholinergic effect.
Contraceptives (oral)	Increased methylprednisolone effect.
Digitalis preparations	Dangerous potassium depletion. Possible digitalis toxicity.
Diuretics (thiazide)	Potassium depletion.
Ephedrine	Decreased methylprednisolone effect.
Estrogens	Increased methylprednisolone effect.
Ethacrynic acid	Potassium depletion.
Furosemide	Potassium depletion.
Glutethimide	Decreased methylprednisolone effect.
Indapamide	Possible excessive potassium loss, causing dangerous heartbeat irregularity.
Indomethacin	Increased methylprednisolone effect.
Insulin	Decreased insulin effect.
Isoniazid	Decreased isoniazid effect.
Oxyphenbutazone	Possible ulcers.
Phenylbutazone	Possible ulcers.

Continued page 969

POSSIBLE INTERACTION WITH OTHER SUBSTANCES

INTERACTS WITH	COMBINED EFFECT
Alcohol:	Risk of stomach ulcers.
Beverages:	No proven problems.
Cocaine:	Overstimulation. Avoid.
Foods:	No proven problems.
Marijuana:	Decreased immunity.
Tobacco:	Increased methylprednisolone effect. Possible toxicity.

METHYSERGIDE

BRAND NAMES

Sansert

BASIC INFORMATION

Habit forming? Yes
Prescription needed? Yes
Available as generic? No
Drug class: Vasoconstrictor (antiserotonin)

 ## USES

Prevents migraine and other recurring vascular headaches.

 ## DOSAGE & USAGE INFORMATION

How to take:
Tablet—Swallow with liquid or with food to lessen stomach irritation. If you can't swallow whole, crumble tablet and take with liquid or food.

When to take:
At the same times each day.

If you forget a dose:
Don't take missed dose. Wait for next scheduled dose (don't double this dose).

What drug does:
Blocks the action of serotonin, a chemical that constricts blood vessels.

Time lapse before drug works:
About 3 weeks.

Don't take with:
See Interaction column and consult doctor.

 ## OVERDOSE

SYMPTOMS:
Nausea, vomiting, abdominal pain, severe diarrhea, lack of coordination, extreme thirst.
WHAT TO DO:
Overdose unlikely to threaten life. If person takes much larger amount than prescribed, call doctor, poison-control center or hospital emergency room for instructions.

 ## POSSIBLE ADVERSE REACTIONS OR SIDE EFFECTS

SYMPTOMS	WHAT TO DO
Life-threatening:	
None expected.	
Common:	
● Itchy skin.	Discontinue. Call doctor right away.
● Nausea, vomiting, diarrhea, numbness or tingling of extremities, leg weakness.	Continue. Call doctor when convenient.
● Drowsiness.	Continue. Tell doctor at next visit.
Infrequent:	
● Anxiety, agitation, hallucinations, unusually fast or slow heartbeat.	Discontinue. Call doctor right away.
● Change in vision.	Continue. Call doctor when convenient.
Rare:	
● Extreme thirst, chest pain, shortness of breath, fever, pale or swollen extremities, leg cramps, lower back pain, side or groin pain, appetite loss.	Discontinue. Call doctor right away.
● Painful or difficult urination.	Continue. Call doctor when convenient.
● Weight change, hair loss.	Continue. Tell doctor at next visit.

WARNINGS & PRECAUTIONS

Don't take if:
- You are allergic to any antiserotonin.
- You plan to become pregnant within medication period.
- You have an infection.
- You have a heart or blood-vessel disease.
- You have a chronic lung disease.
- You have a collagen (connective tissue) disorder.
- You have impaired liver or kidney function.

Before you start, consult your doctor:
- If you have been allergic to any ergot preparation.
- If you have had a peptic ulcer.

Over age 60:
Adverse reactions and side effects may be more frequent and severe than in younger persons.

Pregnancy:
Manufacturer suggests risk to unborn child outweighs drug benefits, even though studies are inconclusive.

Breast-feeding:
Drug probably passes into milk. Avoid drug or discontinue nursing until you finish medicine. Consult doctor for advice on maintaining milk supply.

Infants & children:
Not recommended.

Prolonged use:
Possible fibrosis, a condition in which scar tissue is deposited on heart valves, in lung tissue, blood vessels and internal organs. After 6 months, decrease dose over 2 to 3 weeks. Then discontinue for at least 2 months for re-evaluation.

Skin & sunlight:
No problems expected.

Driving, piloting or hazardous work:
Avoid if you feel drowsy or dizzy. Otherwise, no problems expected.

Discontinuing:
- Don't discontinue without consulting doctor. Dose may require gradual reduction if you have taken drug for a long time. Doses of other drugs may also require adjustment.
- Probably should discontinue drug if you don't improve after 3 weeks' use.

Others:
- Periodic laboratory tests for liver function and blood counts recommended.
- Potential for abuse.

POSSIBLE INTERACTION WITH OTHER DRUGS

GENERIC NAME OR DRUG CLASS	COMBINED EFFECT
Ergot preparations	Unpredictable increased or decreased effect of either drug.
Narcotics	Decreased narcotic effect.

POSSIBLE INTERACTION WITH OTHER SUBSTANCES

INTERACTS WITH	COMBINED EFFECT
Alcohol:	None expected. However, alcohol may trigger a migraine headache.
Beverages: Caffeine drinks.	Decreased methysergide effect.
Cocaine:	May make headache worse.
Foods:	None expected. Avoid foods to which you are allergic.
Marijuana:	No proven problems.
Tobacco:	Blood-vessel constriction. Makes headache worse.

METOCLOPRAMIDE

BRAND NAMES

Emex	Maxolon
Maxeran	Reglan

BASIC INFORMATION

Habit forming? No
Prescription needed? Yes
Available as generic? Yes
Drug class: Antiemetic; dopaminergic
    blocker

 USES

- Relieves nausea and vomiting caused by chemotherapy and drug related postoperative factors.
- Relieves symptoms of esophagitis.

 DOSAGE & USAGE INFORMATION

How to take:
Tablet or capsule—Swallow with liquid or food to lessen stomach irritation.

When to take:
30 minutes before symptoms expected, up to 4 times a day.

If you forget a dose:
Take as soon as you remember up to 2 hours late. If more than 2 hours, wait for next scheduled dose (don't double this dose).

What drug does:
- Prevents smooth muscle in stomach from relaxing.
- Affects vomiting center in brain.

Continued next column

 OVERDOSE

SYMPTOMS:
Severe drowsiness, mental confusion, trembling, seizure, coma.
WHAT TO DO:
- Dial 0 (operator) or 911 (emergency) for an ambulance or medical help. Then give first aid immediately.
- If patient is unconscious and not breathing, give mouth-to-mouth breathing. If there is no heartbeat, use cardiac massage and mouth-to-mouth breathing (CPR). Don't try to make patient vomit. If you can't get help quickly, take patient to nearest emergency facility.
- See emergency information on inside covers.

Time lapse before drug works:
30 to 60 minutes.

Don't take with:
See Interaction column and consult doctor.

 POSSIBLE ADVERSE REACTIONS OR SIDE EFFECTS

SYMPTOMS	WHAT TO DO
Life-threatening: None expected.	
Common: Drowsiness, restlessness.	Continue. Call doctor when convenient.
Frequent Rash.	Continue. Call doctor when convenient.
Infrequent: ● Wheezing, shortness of breath.	Discontinue. Call doctor right away.
● Dizziness; headache; insomnia; tender, swollen breasts; increased milk flow.	Continue. Call doctor when convenient.
Rare: Constipation, diarrhea, nausea.	Continue. Call doctor when convenient.

WARNINGS & PRECAUTIONS

Don't take if:
You are allergic to procaine, procainamide or metoclopramide.

Before you start, consult your doctor:
- If you have Parkinson's disease.
- If you have liver or kidney disease.
- If you have epilepsy.
- If you have bleeding from gastrointestinal tract or intestinal obstruction.
- If you will have surgery within 2 months, including dental surgery, requiring general or spinal anesthesia.

Over age 60:
Adverse reactions and side effects may be more frequent and severe than in younger persons.

Pregnancy:
No proven harm to unborn child. Avoid if possible.

Breast-feeding:
Unknown effect.

Infants & children:
Adverse reactions more likely to occur than in adults.

Prolonged use:
Adverse reactions including muscle spasms and trembling hands more likely to occur.

Skin & sunlight:
No problems expected.

Driving, piloting or hazardous work:
Don't drive or pilot aircraft until you learn how medicine affects you. Don't work around dangerous machinery. Don't climb ladders or work in high places. Danger increases if you drink alcohol or take medicine affecting alertness and reflexes, such as antihistamines, tranquilizers, sedatives, pain medicine, narcotics and mind-altering drugs.

Discontinuing:
May be unnecessary to finish medicine. Follow doctor's instructions.

Others:
No problems expected.

POSSIBLE INTERACTION WITH OTHER DRUGS

GENERIC NAME OR DRUG CLASS	COMBINED EFFECT
Acetaminophen	Slow stomach emptying.
Bromocriptine	Decreased bromocriptine effect.
Central nervous system depressants: antidepressants, antihistamines, muscle relaxants, narcotics, sedatives, sleeping pills, tranquilizers.	Excess sedation.
Digitalis preparations	Decreased absorption of digitalis.
Levodopa	Slow stomach emptying.
Phenothiazines	Increased chance of muscle spasm and trembling.
Tetracycline	Slow stomach emptying.

POSSIBLE INTERACTION WITH OTHER SUBSTANCES

INTERACTS WITH	COMBINED EFFECT
Alcohol:	Excess sedation. Avoid.
Beverages: Coffee.	Decreased metoclopramide effect.
Cocaine:	Decreased metoclopramide effect.
Foods:	No problems expected.
Marijuana:	Decreased metoclopramide effect.
Tobacco:	Decreased metoclopramide effect.

METOLAZONE

BRAND NAMES

Diulo   Zaroxolyn

BASIC INFORMATION

Habit forming? No
Prescription needed? Yes
Available as generic? Yes
Drug class: Antihypertensive, diuretic
          (thiazide)

 ## USES

- Controls, but doesn't cure, high blood pressure.
- Reduces fluid retention (edema) caused by conditions such as heart disorders and liver disease.

 ## DOSAGE & USAGE INFORMATION

How to take:
Tablet or capsule—Swallow with 8 oz. of liquid. If you can't swallow whole, crumble tablet or open capsule and take with liquid or food. Don't exceed dose.

When to take:
At the same time each day.

If you forget a dose:
Take as soon as you remember up to 2 hours late. If more than 2 hours, wait for next scheduled dose (don't double this dose).

What drug does:
- Forces sodium and water excretion, reducing body fluid.
- Relaxes muscle cells of small arteries.
- Reduced body fluid and relaxed arteries lower blood pressure.

Time lapse before drug works:
4 to 6 hours. May require several weeks to lower blood pressure.

Continued next column

 ## OVERDOSE

SYMPTOMS:
Cramps, weakness, drowsiness, weak pulse, coma.
WHAT TO DO:
- **Dial 0 (operator) or 911 (emergency) for an ambulance or medical help. Then give first aid immediately.**
- **See emergency information on inside covers.**

Don't take with:
- See Interaction column and consult doctor.
- Non-prescription drugs without consulting doctor.

 ## POSSIBLE ADVERSE REACTIONS OR SIDE EFFECTS

SYMPTOMS	WHAT TO DO
Life-threatening: None expected.	
Common: None expected.	
Infrequent:	
• Blurred vision, severe abdominal pain, nausea, vomiting, irregular heartbeat, weak pulse.	Discontinue. Call doctor right away.
• Dizziness, mood change, headache, weakness, tiredness, weight changes.	Continue. Call doctor when convenient.
• Dry mouth, thirst.	Continue. Tell doctor at next visit.
Rare:	
• Rash or hives.	Discontinue. Seek emergency treatment.
• Jaundice, sore throat, fever.	Discontinue. Call doctor right away.

 ## WARNINGS & PRECAUTIONS

Don't take if:
You are allergic to any thiazide diuretic drug.

Before you start, consult your doctor:
- If you are allergic to any sulfa drug.
- If you have gout.
- If you have liver, pancreas or kidney disorder.

Over age 60:
Adverse reactions and side effects may be more frequent and severe than in younger persons, especially dizziness and excessive potassium loss.

Pregnancy:
Risk to unborn child outweighs drug benefits. Don't use.

Breast-feeding:
Drug passes into milk. Avoid this medicine or discontinue nursing.

Infants & children:
No problems expected.

Prolonged use:
You may need medicine to treat high blood pressure for the rest of your life.

Skin & sunlight:
May cause rash or intensify sunburn in areas exposed to sun or sunlamp.

Driving, piloting or hazardous work:
Don't drive or pilot aircraft until you learn how medicine affects you. Don't work around dangerous machinery. Don't climb ladders or work in high places. Danger increases if you drink alcohol or take medicine affecting alertness and reflexes, such as antihistamines, tranquilizers, sedatives, pain medicine, narcotics and mind-altering drugs.

Discontinuing:
Don't discontinue without medical advice.

Others:
- Hot weather and fever may cause dehydration and drop in blood pressure. Dose may require temporary adjustment. Weigh daily and report any unexpected weight decreases to your doctor.
- May cause rise in uric acid, leading to gout.
- May cause blood-sugar rise in diabetics.

POSSIBLE INTERACTION WITH OTHER DRUGS

GENERIC NAME OR DRUG CLASS	COMBINED EFFECT
Acebutolol	Increased antihypertensive effect. Dosages of both drugs may require adjustments.
Allopurinol	Decreased allopurinol effect.
Amiodarone	Increased risk of heartbeat irregularity due to low potassium.
Antidepressants (tricyclic)	Dangerous drop in blood pressure. Avoid combination unless under medical supervision.
Barbiturates	Increased metolazone effect.
Calcium supplements	Increased calcium in blood.
Cholestyramine	Decreased metolazone effect.
Cortisone drugs	Excessive potassium loss that causes dangerous heart rhythms.

Digitalis preparations	Excessive potassium loss that causes dangerous heart rhythms.
Diuretics (thiazide)	Increased effect of other thiazide diuretics.
Enalapril	Possible excessive potassium in blood.
Indapamide	Increased diuretic effect.
Labetolol	Increased antihypertensive effects.
Lithium	Increased effect of lithium.
MAO inhibitors	Increased metolazone effect.
Nitrates	Excessive blood-pressure drop.
Oxprenolol	Increased antihypertensive effect. Dosages of both drugs may require adjustments.
Potassium supplements	Decreased potassium effect.
Probenecid	Decreased probenecid effect.

POSSIBLE INTERACTION WITH OTHER SUBSTANCES

INTERACTS WITH	COMBINED EFFECT
Alcohol:	Dangerous blood-pressure drop.
Beverages:	None expected.
Cocaine:	None expected.
Foods: Licorice.	Excessive potassium loss that causes dangerous heart rhythms.
Marijuana:	May increase blood pressure.
Tobacco:	None expected.

METOPROLOL

BRAND NAMES

Apo-metoprolol	Lopressor
Betaloc	Lopressor SR
Betaloc Durules	Novometoprol

BASIC INFORMATION

Habit forming? No
Prescription needed? Yes
Available as generic? No
Drug class: Beta-adrenergic blocker

 USES

- Reduces angina attacks.
- Stabilizes irregular heartbeat.
- Lowers blood pressure.
- Reduces frequency of migraine headaches. (Does not relieve headache pain.)
- Other uses prescribed by your doctor.

 DOSAGE & USAGE INFORMATION

How to take:
Tablet or capsule—Swallow with liquid. If you can't swallow whole, crumble tablet or open capsule and take with liquid or food.

When to take:
With meals or immediately after.

If you forget a dose:
Take as soon as you remember. Return to regular schedule, but allow 3 hours between doses.

What drug does:
- Blocks certain actions of sympathetic nervous system.
- Lowers heart's oxygen requirements.
- Slows nerve impulses through heart.
- Reduces blood vessel contraction in heart, scalp and other body parts.

Continued next column

 OVERDOSE

SYMPTOMS:
Weakness, slow or weak pulse, blood-pressure drop, fainting, convulsions, cold and sweaty skin.
WHAT TO DO:
- Dial 0 (operator) or 911 (emergency) for an ambulance or medical help. Then give first aid immediately.
- See emergency information on inside covers.

Time lapse before drug works:
1 to 4 hours.

Don't take with:
Non-prescription drugs or drugs in Interaction column without consulting doctor.

 POSSIBLE ADVERSE REACTIONS OR SIDE EFFECTS

SYMPTOMS	WHAT TO DO
Life-threatening:	
None expected.	
Common:	
• Pulse slower than 50 beats per minute.	Discontinue. Call doctor right away.
• Drowsiness, numbness or tingling of fingers or toes, dizziness, diarrhea, nausea, fatigue, weakness.	Continue. Call doctor when convenient.
• Cold hands, feet; dry mouth, eyes, skin.	Continue. Tell doctor at next visit.
Infrequent:	
• Hallucinations, nightmares, insomnia, headache, difficult breathing, joint pain.	Discontinue. Call doctor right away.
• Confusion, depression, reduced alertness.	Continue. Call doctor when convenient.
• Constipation.	Continue. Tell doctor at next visit.
Rare:	
• Rash, sore throat, fever.	Discontinue. Call doctor right away.
• Unusual bleeding or bruising.	Continue. Call doctor when convenient.

 WARNINGS & PRECAUTIONS

Don't take if:
- You are allergic to any beta-adrenergic blocker.
- You have asthma or hay fever symptoms.
- You have taken MAO inhibitors in past 2 weeks.

Before you start, consult your doctor:
- If you have heart disease or poor circulation to the extremities.
- If you have hay fever, asthma, chronic bronchitis, emphysema.
- If you have overactive thyroid function.
- If you have impaired liver or kidney function.
- If you will have surgery within 2 months, including dental surgery, requiring general or spinal anesthesia.
- If you have diabetes or hypoglycemia.

Over age 60:
Adverse reactions and side effects may be more frequent and severe than in younger persons.

Pregnancy:
Risk to unborn child outweighs drug benefits. Don't use.

Breast-feeding:
Drug passes into milk. Avoid drug or discontinue nursing until you finish medicine. Consult doctor for advice on maintaining milk supply.

Infants & children:
Not recommended.

Prolonged use:
Weakens heart muscle contractions.

Skin & sunlight:
No problems expected.

Driving, piloting or hazardous work:
Don't drive or pilot aircraft until you learn how medicine affects you. Don't work around dangerous machinery. Don't climb ladders or work in high places. Danger increases if you drink alcohol or take medicine affecting alertness and reflexes.

Discontinuing:
Don't discontinue without consulting doctor. Dose may require gradual reduction if you have taken drug for a long time. Doses of other drugs may also require adjustment.

Others:
May mask hypoglycemia.

POSSIBLE INTERACTION WITH OTHER DRUGS

GENERIC NAME OR DRUG CLASS	COMBINED EFFECT
Acebutolol	Increased antihypertensive effects of both drugs. Dosages may require adjustment.
Albuterol	Decreased albuterol effect and beta-adrenergic blocking effect.
Antidiabetics	Increased antidiabetic effect.
Antihistamines	Decreased antihistamine effect.
Antihypertensives	Increased antihypertensive effect.
Anti-inflammatory drugs	Decreased anti-inflammatory effect.
Barbiturates	Increased barbiturate effect. Dangerous sedation.
Digitalis preparations	Can either increase or decrease heart rate. Improves irregular heartbeat.
Indapamide	Increased effects of both drugs. Can help control high blood pressure.
Molindone	Increased tranquilizer effect.
Narcotics	Increased narcotic effect. Dangerous sedation.
Nitrates	Possible excessive blood-pressure drop.
Pentoxifylline	Increased antihypertensive effect.
Phenytoin	Increased metoprolol effect.
Quinidine	Slows heart excessively.
Reserpine	Possible increased effects of both drugs. Slow heartbeat and low blood pressure may result.
Tocainide	May worsen congestive heart failure.

POSSIBLE INTERACTION WITH OTHER SUBSTANCES

INTERACTS WITH	COMBINED EFFECT
Alcohol:	Excessive blood pressure drop. Avoid.
Beverages:	None expected.
Cocaine:	Irregular heartbeat. Avoid.
Foods:	None expected.
Marijuana:	Daily use—Impaired circulation to hands and feet.
Tobacco:	Possible irregular heartbeat.

METRONIDAZOLE

BRAND NAMES

Apo-Metronidazole	Metryl IV
Flagyl	Neo-Tric
Flagyl I.V.	Novonidazol
Flagyl I.V. RTU	PMS Metronidazole
Metric 21	Protostat
Metro I.V.	Satric
Metronid	SK-Metronidazole
Metryl	Trikacide

BASIC INFORMATION

Habit forming? No
Prescription needed? Yes
Available as generic? Yes
Drug class: Antiprotozoal

USES

Treatment for infections susceptible to metronidazole, such as trichomoniasis and amebiasis.

DOSAGE & USAGE INFORMATION

How to take:
- Tablet or capsule—Swallow with liquid or food to lessen stomach irritation. If you can't swallow whole, crumble tablet or open capsule and take with liquid or food.
- Suppositories—Remove wrapper and moisten suppository with water. Gently insert larger end into vagina. Push well into vagina with finger or applicator.

When to take:
At the same times each day.

If you forget a dose:
Take as soon as you remember up to 2 hours late. If more than 2 hours, wait for next scheduled dose (don't double this dose).

What drug does:
Kills organisms causing the infection.

Continued next column

OVERDOSE

SYMPTOMS:
Weakness, nausea, vomiting, diarrhea, confusion, seizures.
WHAT TO DO:
Overdose unlikely to threaten life. If person takes much larger amount than prescribed, call doctor, poison-control center or hospital emergency room for instructions.

Time lapse before drug works:
Begins in 1 hour. May require regular use for 10 days to cure infection.

Don't take with:
- See Interaction column and consult doctor.
- Non-prescription medicines containing alcohol.

POSSIBLE ADVERSE REACTIONS OR SIDE EFFECTS

SYMPTOMS	WHAT TO DO
Life-threatening: None expected.	
Common:	
• Appetite loss, nausea, stomach pain, diarrhea, vomiting.	Discontinue. Call doctor right away.
• Unpleasant taste.	Continue. Tell doctor at next visit.
Infrequent:	
• Dizziness; headache; rash; hives; skin redness; itchy skin; mouth irritation, soreness or infection; sore throat; fever.	Discontinue. Call doctor right away.
• Vaginal irritation, discharge, dryness; fatigue; weakness.	Continue. Call doctor when convenient.
• Constipation.	Continue. Tell doctor at next visit.
Rare: Mood change; unsteadiness; numbness, tingling, weakness or pain in hands or feet.	Discontinue. Call doctor right away.

WARNINGS & PRECAUTIONS

Don't take if:
- You are allergic to metronidazole.
- You have had a blood-cell or bone-marrow disorder.

Before you start, consult your doctor:
- If you plan to become pregnant within medication period.
- If you have a brain or nervous-system disorder.
- If you have liver or heart disease.
- If you drink alcohol.

Over age 60:
Adverse reactions and side effects may be more frequent and severe than in younger persons.

Pregnancy:
Risk to unborn child outweighs drug benefits. Manufacturer advises against use during first 3 months and only limited use after that. Don't use.

Breast-feeding:
Drug passes into milk. Avoid drug or discontinue nursing until you finish medicine. Consult doctor for advice on maintaining milk supply.

Infants & children:
Use in children for amoeba infection only under close medical supervision.

Prolonged use:
No problems expected.

Skin & sunlight:
No problems expected.

Driving, piloting or hazardous work:
Avoid if you feel dizzy or unsteady. Otherwise, no problems expected.

Discontinuing:
Don't discontinue without doctor's advice until you complete prescribed dose, even though symptoms diminish or disappear.

Others:
No problems expected.

POSSIBLE INTERACTION WITH OTHER DRUGS

GENERIC NAME OR DRUG CLASS	COMBINED EFFECT
Anticoagulants (oral)	Decreased anticoagulant effect. Possible bleeding or bruising.
Disulfiram	Disulfiram reaction (see Glossary). Avoid.
Oxytetracycline	Decreased metronidazole effect.

POSSIBLE INTERACTION WITH OTHER SUBSTANCES

INTERACTS WITH	COMBINED EFFECT
Alcohol:	Possible disulfiram reaction (see Glossary). Avoid alcohol in *any* form or amount.
Beverages:	None expected.
Cocaine:	Decreased metronidazole effect. Avoid.
Foods:	None expected.
Marijuana:	None expected.
Tobacco:	None expected.

MEXILETINE

BRAND NAMES

Mexitil

BASIC INFORMATION

Habit forming? No
Prescription needed? Yes
Available as generic? No
Drug class: Antiarrhythmic

 USES

Stabilizes irregular heartbeat.

 DOSAGE & USAGE INFORMATION

How to take:
Swallow whole with food, milk or antacid to lessen stomach irritation.

When to take:
At the same times each day as directed by your doctor.

If you forget a dose:
Take as soon as you remember up to 4 hours late. If more than 4 hours, wait for next scheduled dose (don't double this dose).

What drug does:
Blocks the fast sodium channel in heart tissue.

Time lapse before drug works:
30 minutes to 2 hours.

Don't take with:
See Interaction column and consult doctor.

 OVERDOSE

SYMPTOMS:
Nausea, vomiting, seizures, cardiac arrest.
WHAT TO DO:
- **Dial 0 (operator) or 911 (emergency) for an ambulance or medical help. Then give first aid immediately.**
- **See emergency information on inside covers.**

 POSSIBLE ADVERSE REACTIONS OR SIDE EFFECTS

SYMPTOMS	WHAT TO DO
Life-threatening:	
Chest pain, shortness of breath, irregular or fast heartbeat.	Discontinue. Seek emergency treatment.
Common:	
Dizziness, anxiety, shakiness, unsteadiness when walking, heartburn, nausea, vomiting.	Discontinue. Call doctor right away.
Infrequent:	
Sore throat, fever, mouth sores; blurred vision; confusion; constipation; diarrhea; headache; numbness or tingling in hands or feet; ringing in ears; unexplained bleeding or bruising; rash; slurred speech; insomnia; weakness.	Discontinue. Call doctor right away.
Rare:	
Jaundice.	Discontinue. Call doctor right away.

WARNINGS & PRECAUTIONS

Don't take if:
- If you are allergic to mexiletine, lidocaine or tocainide.
- If you take other heart medicine such as digitalis.

Before you start, consult your doctor:
- If you have had liver or kidney disease or impaired kidney function.
- If you have had lupus.
- If you have a history of seizures.
- If you will have surgery within 2 months, including dental surgery, requiring general or spinal anesthesia.

Over age 60:
Adverse reactions and side effects may be more frequent and severe than in younger persons. Ask doctor about smaller doses.

Pregnancy:
Risk to unborn child outweighs drug benefits. Don't use.

Breast-feeding:
Drug passes into milk. Avoid drug or discontinue nursing until you finish medicine. Consult doctor for advice on maintaining milk supply.

Infants & children:
Use only under close medical supervision.

Prolonged use:
May possibly cause lupus-like illness.

Skin & sunlight:
No problems expected.

Driving, piloting or hazardous work:
Use caution if you feel dizzy or weak. Otherwise, no problems expected.

Discontinuing:
Don't discontinue without consulting doctor. Dose may require gradual reduction if you have taken drug for a long time. Doses of other drugs may also require adjustment.

Others:
No problems expected.

POSSIBLE INTERACTION WITH OTHER DRUGS

GENERIC NAME OR DRUG CLASS	COMBINED EFFECT
Urinary acidifiers (ammonium chloride, ascorbic acid, potassium or sodium phosphate)	May decrease effectiveness of medicine.
Urinary alkalizers (acetazolamide, antacids with calcium or magnesium, methazolamide, dichlorphenamide, sodium bicarbonate, citric acid, potassium citrate, sodium citrate)	May slow elimination of mexiletine and cause need to adjust dosage.

POSSIBLE INTERACTION WITH OTHER SUBSTANCES

INTERACTS WITH	COMBINED EFFECT
Alcohol:	Causes irregular effectiveness of mexiletine. Avoid.
Beverages: Caffeine drinks, iced drinks.	Irregular heartbeat.
Cocaine:	Decreased mexiletine effect.
Foods:	None expected.
Marijuana:	Irregular heartbeat. Avoid.
Tobacco:	Dangerous combination. May lead to liver problems and reduce effectiveness of mexiletine.

MINOXIDIL

BRAND NAMES

Loniten

BASIC INFORMATION

Habit forming? No
Prescription needed? Yes
Available as generic? No
Drug class: Antihypertensive

 ## USES

- Treatment for high blood pressure in conjunction with other drugs, such as beta-adrenergic blockers and diuretics.
- Treatment for congestive heart failure.
- Can stimulate hair growth.

 ## DOSAGE & USAGE INFORMATION

How to take:
Tablet or capsule—Swallow with liquid. If you can't swallow whole, crumble tablet or open capsule and take with liquid or food.

When to take:
At the same time each day, according to instructions on prescription label.

If you forget a dose:
Take as soon as you remember up to 2 hours late. If more than 2 hours, wait for next scheduled dose (don't double this dose).

What drug does:
Relaxes small blood vessels (arterioles) so blood can pass through more easily.

Time lapse before drug works:
2 to 3 hours for effect to begin; 3 to 7 days of continuous use may be necessary for maximum blood-pressure response.

Don't take with:
See Interaction column and consult doctor.

 ## OVERDOSE

SYMPTOMS:
Low blood pressure, fainting, coma.
WHAT TO DO:
- Dial 0 (operator) or 911 (emergency) for an ambulance or medical help. Then give first aid immediately.
- See emergency information on inside covers.

 ## POSSIBLE ADVERSE REACTIONS OR SIDE EFFECTS

SYMPTOMS	WHAT TO DO
Life-threatening: None expected.	
Common: Excessive hair growth.	Continue. Call doctor when convenient.
Frequent: Flushed skin or redness.	Continue. Call doctor when convenient.
Infrequent: • Chest pain, irregular or slow heartbeat, shortness of breath, swollen feet or legs, rapid weight gain.	Discontinue. Call doctor right away.
• Numbness of hands, feet, or face; headache; tender breasts.	Continue. Call doctor when convenient.
Rare: Rash.	Discontinue. Call doctor right away.

WARNINGS & PRECAUTIONS

Don't take if:
You are allergic to minoxidil.

Before you start, consult your doctor:
- If you have had recent stroke, heart attack or angina pectoris in past 3 weeks.
- If you have impaired kidney function.

Over age 60:
Adverse reactions and side effects may be more frequent and severe than in younger persons.

Pregnancy:
Human studies not available. Avoid if possible.

Breast-feeding:
Human studies not available. Avoid if possible.

Infants & children:
Not recommended. Safety and dosage have not been established.

Prolonged use:
Request periodic blood examinations that include potassium levels.

Skin & sunlight:
No problems expected.

Driving, piloting or hazardous work:
Avoid if you become dizzy or faint. Otherwise, no problems expected.

Discontinuing:
Don't discontinue without consulting doctor. Dose may require gradual reduction if you have taken drug for a long time. Doses of other drugs may also require adjustment.

Others:
- Check pulse regularly. If it exceeds 20 or more beats per minute over your normal rate, consult doctor immediately.
- Check blood pressure frequently.

POSSIBLE INTERACTION WITH OTHER DRUGS

GENERIC NAME OR DRUG CLASS	COMBINED EFFECT
Anesthesia	Drastic drop in blood pressure.
Antihypertensives (other)	Dosage adjustments may be necessary to keep blood pressure at desired level.
Anti-inflammatory drugs (non-steroidal)	Decreased minoxidil effect.
Diuretics	Dosage adjustments may be necessary to keep blood pressure at desired level.
Enalapril	Possible excessive potassium in blood.
Ketoprofen	Decreased minoxidil effect.
Nitrates	Drastic drop in blood pressure.
Suprofen	Decreased minoxidil effect.
Sympathomimetics	Decreased minoxidil effect.

POSSIBLE INTERACTION WITH OTHER SUBSTANCES

INTERACTS WITH	COMBINED EFFECT
Alcohol:	Possible excessive blood-pressure drop.
Beverages:	None expected.
Cocaine:	Increased dizziness. Avoid.
Foods: Salt substitutes.	Possible excessive potassium levels in blood.
Marijuana:	Increased dizziness.
Tobacco:	May decrease minoxidil effect. Avoid.

MITOTANE

BRAND NAMES

Lysodren

BASIC INFORMATION

Habit forming? No
Prescription needed? Yes
Available as generic? No
Drug class: Antineoplastic

 USES

- Treatment for some kinds of cancer.
- Treatment of Cushing's disease.

 DOSAGE & USAGE INFORMATION

How to take:
Tablet or capsule—Take with liquid after light meal. Don't drink fluid with meals. Drink extra fluids between meals. Avoid sweet and fatty foods.

When to take:
At the same time each day.

If you forget a dose:
Take as soon as you remember. Don't ever double dose.

What drug does:
Suppresses adrenal cortex to prevent manufacture of excess cortisone.

Time lapse before drug works:
2 to 3 weeks for full effect.

Don't take with:
See Interaction column and consult doctor.

 OVERDOSE

SYMPTOMS:
Headache, vomiting blood, stupor, seizure.
WHAT TO DO:
- Dial 0 (operator) or 911 (emergency) for an ambulance or medical help. Then give first aid immediately.
- If patient is unconscious and not breathing, give mouth-to-mouth breathing. If there is no heartbeat, use cardiac massage and mouth-to-mouth breathing (CPR). Don't try to make patient vomit. If you can't get help quickly, take patient to nearest emergency facility.
- See emergency information on inside covers.

 POSSIBLE ADVERSE REACTIONS OR SIDE EFFECTS

SYMPTOMS	WHAT TO DO
Life-threatening: None expected.	
Common:	
• Darkened skin, appetite loss, nausea, vomiting.	Continue. Call doctor when convenient.
• Mental depression.	Continue. Tell doctor at next visit.
Infrequent:	
• Fever, chills, sore throat.	Discontinue. Seek emergency treatment.
• Unusual bleeding or bruising.	Discontinue. Call doctor right away.
• Rash, hair loss, purple bands on nails, blurred vision, seeing double, cough, difficult breathing, numbness or tingling in feet and toes, tiredness, weakness, dizziness when standing after sitting or lying.	Continue. Call doctor when convenient.
Rare:	
Blood in urine.	Continue. Call doctor when convenient.

WARNINGS & PRECAUTIONS

Don't take if:
You are allergic to adrenocorticosteroids or any antineoplastic drug.

Before you start, consult your doctor:
- If you have liver disease.
- If you have infection.

Over age 60:
Adverse reactions and side effects may be more frequent and severe than in younger persons.

Pregnancy:
Consult doctor. Risk to child is significant.

Breast-feeding:
Drug passes into milk. Don't nurse.

Infants & children:
Use only under care of medical supervisors who are experienced in anticancer drugs.

Prolonged use:
Adverse reactions more likely the longer drug is required.

Skin & sunlight:
No problems expected.

Driving, piloting or hazardous work:
No problems expected.

Discontinuing:
- Don't discontinue without consulting doctor. Dose may require gradual reduction if you have taken drug for a long time. Doses of other drugs may also require adjustment.
- Some side effects may follow discontinuing. Report any new symptoms.

Others:
No problems expected.

POSSIBLE INTERACTION WITH OTHER DRUGS

GENERIC NAME OR DRUG CLASS	COMBINED EFFECT
Antidepressants	Increased central nervous system depression.
Antihistamines	Increased central nervous system depression.
Corticosteroids	Decreased effect of corticosteroid.
Mind-altering drugs (LSD, etc.)	Increased central nervous system depression.
Narcotics	Increased central nervous system depression.
Sedatives	Increased central nervous system depression.
Sleeping pills	Increased central nervous system depression.
Tranquilizers	Increased central nervous system depression.

POSSIBLE INTERACTION WITH OTHER SUBSTANCES

INTERACTS WITH	COMBINED EFFECT
Alcohol:	Increased depression. Avoid.
Beverages:	No problems expected.
Cocaine:	Increased toxicity. Avoid.
Foods:	Reduced irritation in stomach.
Marijuana:	No problems expected.
Tobacco:	Increased possibility of lung toxicity.

MOLINDONE

BRAND NAMES

Moban

BASIC INFORMATION

Habit forming? No
Prescription needed? Yes
Available as generic? No
Drug class: Antipsychotic

 USES

Treats severe emotional, mental or nervous problems.

 DOSAGE & USAGE INFORMATION

How to take:
Tablet or capsule—Swallow with liquid or food to lessen stomach irritation. If you can't swallow whole, crumble tablet and take with food or liquid.

When to take:
Follow instructions on prescription label or side of package. Doses should be evenly spaced. For example, 4 times a day means every 6 hours.

If you forget a dose:
Take as soon as you remember up to 2 hours late. If more than 2 hours, wait for next scheduled dose (don't double this dose).

What drug does:
Corrects an imbalance in nerve impulses from the brain.

Time lapse before drug works:
- Nausea and vomiting—1 hour or less.
- Nervous and mental disorders—4-6 weeks.

Don't take with:
- Antacid or medicine for diarrhea.
- Non-prescription drug for cough, cold or allergy.
- See Interaction column and consult doctor.

 OVERDOSE

SYMPTOMS:
Stupor, convulsions, coma.
WHAT TO DO:
- Dial 0 (operator) or 911 (emergency) for an ambulance or medical help. Then give first aid immediately.
- See emergency information on inside covers.

 POSSIBLE ADVERSE REACTIONS OR SIDE EFFECTS

SYMPTOMS	WHAT TO DO
Life-threatening:	
None expected.	
Common:	
• Muscle spasms of face and neck, unsteady gait.	Discontinue. Seek emergency treatment.
• Restlessness, tremor, drowsiness.	Discontinue. Call doctor right away.
• Decreased sweating, dry mouth, runny nose, constipation.	Continue. Call doctor when convenient.
Infrequent:	
• Fainting.	Discontinue. Seek emergency treatment.
• Rash.	Discontinue. Call doctor right away.
• Frequent urination, diminished sex drive, swollen breasts, menstrual irregularities.	Continue. Call doctor when convenient.
Rare:	
Change in vision, sore throat, fever, jaundice.	Discontinue. Call doctor right away.

WARNINGS & PRECAUTIONS

Don't take if:
- You are allergic to any phenothiazine.
- You have a blood or bone-marrow disease.

Before you start, consult your doctor:
- If you will have surgery within 2 months, including dental surgery, requiring general or spinal anesthesia.
- If you have asthma, emphysema or other lung disorder.
- If you take non-prescription ulcer medicine, asthma medicine or amphetamines.

Over age 60:
Adverse reactions and side effects may be more frequent and severe than in younger persons. More likely to develop involuntary movement of jaws, lips, tongue, chewing. Report this to your doctor immediately. Early treatment can help.

Pregnancy:
Risk to unborn child outweighs drug benefits. Don't use.

Breast-feeding:
Drug passes into milk. Avoid drug or discontinue nursing until you finish medicine. Consult doctor for advice on maintaining milk supply.

Infants & children:
Don't give to children younger than 2.

Prolonged use:
May lead to tardive dyskinesia (involuntary movement of jaws, lips, tongue, chewing).

Skin & sunlight:
May cause rash or intensify sunburn in areas exposed to sun or sunlamp. Skin may remain sensitive for 3 months after discontinuing.

Driving, piloting or hazardous work:
Don't drive or pilot aircraft until you learn how medicine affects you. Don't work around dangerous machinery. Don't climb ladders or work in high places. Danger increases if you drink alcohol or take medicine affecting alertness and reflexes.

Discontinuing:
- Nervous and mental disorders—Don't discontinue without doctor's advice until you complete prescribed dose, even though symptoms diminish or disappear.
- Nausea and vomiting—May be unnecessary to finish medicine. Follow doctor's instructions.

Others:
No problems expected.

POSSIBLE INTERACTION WITH OTHER DRUGS

GENERIC NAME OR DRUG CLASS	COMBINED EFFECT
Anticholinergics	Increased anticholinergic effect.
Antidepressants (tricyclic)	Increased fluphenazine effect.
Antihistamines	Increased antihistamine effect.
Appetite suppressants	Decreased suppressant effect.
Dronabinol	Increased effects of both drugs. Avoid.
Levodopa	Decreased levodopa effect.
Mind-altering drugs	Increased effect of mind-altering drugs.
Narcotics	Increased narcotic effect.
Phenytoin	Increased phenytoin effect.
Quinidine	Impaired heart function. Dangerous mixture.
Sedatives	Increased sedative effect.
Tranquilizers (other)	Increased tranquilizer effect.

POSSIBLE INTERACTION WITH OTHER SUBSTANCES

INTERACTS WITH	COMBINED EFFECT
Alcohol:	Dangerous oversedation.
Beverages:	None expected.
Cocaine:	Decreased fluphenazine effect. Avoid.
Foods:	None expected.
Marijuana:	Drowsiness. May increase antinausea effect.
Tobacco:	None expected.

BRAND AND GENERIC NAMES

Eutonyl	PARGYLINE
ISOCARBOXAZID	Parnate
Marplan	PHENELZINE
Nardil	TRANYLCYPROMINE

BASIC INFORMATION

Habit forming? No
Prescription needed? Yes
Available as generic? No
Drug class: MAO (monamine oxidase)
inhibitor, antidepressant

USES

- Treatment for depression.
- Pargyline sometimes used to lower blood pressure.

DOSAGE & USAGE INFORMATION

How to take:
Tablet—Swallow with liquid. If you can't swallow whole, crumble tablet and take with liquid or food.

When to take:
At the same times each day.

If you forget a dose:
Take as soon as you remember up to 2 hours late. If more than 2 hours, wait for next scheduled dose (don't double this dose).

What drug does:
Inhibits nerve transmissions in brain that may cause depression.

Time lapse before drug works:
4 to 6 weeks for maximum effect.

Continued next column

OVERDOSE

SYMPTOMS:
Restlessness, agitation, fever, convulsions, coma.
WHAT TO DO:
- Dial 0 (operator) or 911 (emergency) for an ambulance or medical help. Then give first aid immediately.
- See emergency information on inside covers.

Don't take with:
- Non-prescription diet pills, nose drops, medicine for asthma, cough, cold or allergy, or medicine containing caffeine or alcohol.
- See Interaction column and consult doctor.

POSSIBLE ADVERSE REACTIONS OR SIDE EFFECTS

SYMPTOMS	WHAT TO DO
Life-threatening: None expected.	
Common:	
• Fatigue, weakness.	Continue. Call doctor when convenient.
• Dizziness when changing position, dry mouth, constipation, difficult urination.	Continue. Tell doctor at next visit.
Infrequent:	
• Fainting.	Discontinue. Seek emergency treatment.
• Severe headache, chest pain.	Discontinue. Call doctor right away.
• Hallucinations, insomnia, nightmares, diarrhea, rapid or pounding heartbeat, swollen feet or legs.	Continue. Call doctor when convenient.
• Diminished sex drive.	Continue. Tell doctor at next visit.
Rare: Rash, nausea, vomiting, stiff neck, jaundice, fever.	Discontinue. Call doctor right away.

WARNINGS & PRECAUTIONS

Don't take if:
- You are allergic to any MAO inhibitor.
- You have heart disease, congestive heart failure, heart-rhythm irregularities or high blood pressure.
- You have liver or kidney disease.

Before you start, consult your doctor:
- If you are alcoholic.
- If you have asthma.
- If you have had a stroke.
- If you have diabetes or epilepsy.
- If you have overactive thyroid.
- If you have schizophrenia.
- If you have Parkinson's disease.
- If you have adrenal-gland tumor.
- If you will have surgery within 2 months, including dental surgery, requiring general or spinal anesthesia.

MONAMINE OXIDASE (MAO) INHIBITORS

Over age 60:
Not recommended.

Pregnancy:
No proven harm to unborn child. Avoid if possible.

Breast-feeding:
Safety not established. Consult doctor.

Infants & children:
Not recommended.

Prolonged use:
May be toxic to liver.

Skin & sunlight:
May cause rash or intensify sunburn in areas exposed to sun or sunlamp.

Driving, piloting or hazardous work:
Don't drive or pilot aircraft until you learn how medicine affects you. Don't work around dangerous machinery. Don't climb ladders or work in high places. Danger increases if you drink alcohol or take medicine affecting alertness and reflexes.

Discontinuing:
- Don't discontinue without doctor's advice until you complete prescribed dose, even though symptoms diminish or disappear.
- Follow precautions regarding foods, drinks and other medicines for 2 weeks after discontinuing.

Others:
- May affect blood-sugar levels in patients with diabetes.
- Fever may indicate that MAO inhibitor dose requires adjustment.

 POSSIBLE INTERACTION WITH OTHER DRUGS

GENERIC NAME OR DRUG CLASS	COMBINED EFFECT
Acebutolol	Possible blood-pressure rise if MAO inhibitor is discontinued after simultaneous use with acebutolol.
Amphetamines	Blood-pressure rise to life-threatening level.
Anticholinergics	Increased anticholinergic effect.
Anticonvulsants	Changed seizure pattern.
Antidepressants (tricyclic)	Blood-pressure rise to life-threatening level. Possible fever, convulsions, delirium.
Antidiabetics (oral and insulin)	Excessively low blood sugar.
Antihypertensives	Excessively low blood pressure.
Caffeine	Irregular heartbeat or high blood pressure.
Carbamazepine	Fever, seizures. Avoid.
Cyclobenzaprine	Fever, seizures. Avoid.
Diuretics	Excessively low blood pressure.
Guanethidine	Blood-pressure rise to life-threatening level.
Indapamide	Increased indapamide effect.
Levodopa	Sudden, severe blood-pressure rise.
MAO inhibitors (others, when taken together)	High fever, convulsions, death.
Oxprenolol	Possible blood-pressure rise if MAO inhibitor is discontinued after simultaneous use with oxprenolol.
Terfenadine	Increased side effects of MAO inhibitors.

 POSSIBLE INTERACTION WITH OTHER SUBSTANCES

INTERACTS WITH	COMBINED EFFECT
Alcohol:	Increased sedation to dangerous level.
Beverages: Caffeine drinks.	Irregular heartbeat or high blood pressure.
Drinks containing tyramine (see Glossary).	Blood-pressure rise to life-threatening level.
Cocaine:	Overstimulation. Possibly fatal.
Foods: Foods containing tyramine (see Glossary).	Blood-pressure rise to life-threatening level.
Marijuana:	Overstimulation. Avoid.
Tobacco:	No proven problems.

NADOLOL

BRAND NAMES

Corgard   Corzide

BASIC INFORMATION

Habit forming? No
Prescription needed? Yes
Available as generic? No
Drug class: Beta-adrenergic blocker

 USES

- Reduces angina attacks.
- Stabilizes irregular heartbeat.
- Lowers blood pressure.
- Reduces frequency of migraine headaches. (Does not relieve headache pain.)
- Other uses prescribed by your doctor.

 DOSAGE & USAGE INFORMATION

How to take:
Tablet or capsule—Swallow with liquid. If you can't swallow whole, crumble tablet or open capsule and take with liquid or food.

When to take:
With meals or immediately after.

If you forget a dose:
Take as soon as you remember. Return to regular schedule, but allow 3 hours between doses.

What drug does:
- Blocks certain actions of sympathetic nervous system.
- Lowers heart's oxygen requirements.
- Slows nerve impulses through heart.
- Reduces blood vessel contraction in heart, scalp and other body parts.

Time lapse before drug works:
1 to 4 hours.

Continued next column

 OVERDOSE

SYMPTOMS:
Weakness, slow or weak pulse, blood-pressure drop, fainting, convulsions, cold and sweaty skin.
WHAT TO DO:
- **Dial 0 (operator) or 911 (emergency) for an ambulance or medical help. Then give first aid immediately.**
- **See emergency information on inside covers.**

Don't take with:
Non-prescription drugs or drugs in Interaction column without consulting doctor.

 POSSIBLE ADVERSE REACTIONS OR SIDE EFFECTS

SYMPTOMS	WHAT TO DO
Life-threatening:	
None expected.	
Common:	
• Pulse lower than 50 beats per minute.	Discontinue. Call doctor right away.
• Drowsiness, numbness or tingling in fingers or toes, dizziness, nausea, diarrhea, fatigue, weakness.	Continue. Call doctor when convenient.
• Cold hands, feet; dry mouth, eyes, skin.	Continue. Tell doctor at next visit.
Infrequent:	
• Hallucinations, nightmares, insomnia, headache, difficult breathing, joint pain.	Discontinue. Call doctor right away.
• Confusion, depression, reduced alertness.	Continue. Call doctor when convenient.
• Constipation.	Continue. Tell doctor at next visit.
Rare:	
• Rash, sore throat, fever.	Discontinue. Call doctor right away.
• Unusual bleeding or bruising.	Continue. Call doctor when convenient.

 WARNINGS & PRECAUTIONS

Don't take if:
- You are allergic to any beta-adrenergic blocker.
- You have asthma.
- You have hay fever symptoms.
- You have taken MAO inhibitors in past 2 weeks.

Before you start, consult your doctor:
- If you have heart disease or poor circulation to the extremities.
- If you have hay fever, asthma, chronic bronchitis, emphysema.
- If you have overactive thyroid function.
- If you have impaired liver or kidney function.
- If you will have surgery within 2 months, including dental surgery, requiring general or spinal anesthesia.
- If you have diabetes or hypoglycemia.

Over age 60:
Adverse reactions and side effects may be more frequent and severe than in younger persons.

Pregnancy:
Risk to unborn child outweighs drug benefits. Don't use.

Breast-feeding:
Drug passes into milk. Avoid drug or discontinue nursing until you finish medicine. Consult doctor for advice on maintaining milk supply.

Infants & children:
Not recommended.

Prolonged use:
Weakens heart muscle contractions.

Skin & sunlight:
No problems expected.

Driving, piloting or hazardous work:
Don't drive or pilot aircraft until you learn how medicine affects you. Don't work around dangerous machinery. Don't climb ladders or work in high places. Danger increases if you drink alcohol or take medicine affecting alertness and reflexes.

Discontinuing:
Don't discontinue without consulting doctor. Dose may require gradual reduction if you have taken drug for a long time. Doses of other drugs may also require adjustment.

Others:
May mask hypoglycemia.

POSSIBLE INTERACTION WITH OTHER DRUGS

GENERIC NAME OR DRUG CLASS	COMBINED EFFECT
Acebutolol	Increased antihypertensive effects of both drugs. Dosages may require adjustment.
Albuterol	Decreased albuterol effect and beta-adrenergic blocking effect
Antidiabetics	Increased antidiabetic effect.
Antihistamines	Decreased antihistamine effect.
Antihypertensives	Increased antihypertensive effect.
Anti-inflammatory drugs	Decreased effect of anti-inflammatory.

Barbiturates	Increased barbiturate effect. Dangerous sedation.
Digitalis preparations	Increased or decreased heart rate. Improves irregular heartbeat.
Narcotics	Increased narcotic effect. Dangerous sedation.
Nitrates	Possible excessive blood-pressure drop.
Pentoxifylline	Increased antihypertensive effect.
Phenytoin	Increased nadolol effect.
Quinidine	Slows heart excessively.
Reserpine	Increased reserpine effect. Oversedation, depression.
Tocainide	May worsen congestive heart failure.

POSSIBLE INTERACTION WITH OTHER SUBSTANCES

INTERACTS WITH	COMBINED EFFECT
Alcohol:	Excessive blood-pressure drop. Avoid.
Beverages:	None expected.
Cocaine:	Irregular heartbeat. Avoid.
Foods:	None expected.
Marijuana:	Daily use—Impaired circulation to hands and feet.
Tobacco:	Possible irregular heartbeat.

NAFCILLIN

BRAND NAMES

Nafcil   Unipen
Nallpen

BASIC INFORMATION

Habit forming? No
Prescription needed? Yes
Available as generic? Yes
Drug class: Antibiotic (penicillin)

 USES

Treatment of bacterial infections that are
susceptible to nafcillin.

 DOSAGE & USAGE INFORMATION

How to take:
- Tablets or capsules—Swallow with liquid on
  an empty stomach 1 hour before or 2 hours
  after eating.
- Liquid—Take with cold beverage. Liquid form
  is perishable and effective for only 7 days at
  room temperature. Effective for 14 days if
  stored in refrigerator. Don't freeze.

When to take:
Follow instructions on prescription label or side
of package. Doses should be evenly spaced.
For example, 4 times a day means every 6
hours.

If you forget a dose:
Take as soon as you remember. Continue
regular schedule.

What drug does:
Destroys susceptible bacteria. Does not kill
viruses.

Time lapse before drug works:
May be several days before medicine affects
infection.

Don't take with:
See Interaction column and consult doctor.

 OVERDOSE

SYMPTOMS:
Severe diarrhea, nausea or vomiting.
WHAT TO DO:
**Overdose unlikely to threaten life. If person
takes much larger amount than prescribed,
call doctor, poison-control center or hospital
emergency room for instructions.**

 POSSIBLE ADVERSE REACTIONS OR SIDE EFFECTS

SYMPTOMS	WHAT TO DO
Life-threatening:	
Hives, rash, intense itching, faintness soon after a dose (anaphylaxis).	Seek emergency treatment immediately.
Common:	
Dark or discolored tongue.	Continue. Tell doctor at next visit.
Infrequent:	
Mild nausea, vomiting, diarrhea.	Continue. Call doctor when convenient.
Rare:	
Unexplained bleeding.	Discontinue. Call doctor right away.

WARNINGS & PRECAUTIONS

Don't take if:
You are allergic to nafcillin, cephalosporin antibiotics, other penicillins or penicillamine. Life-threatening reaction may occur.

Before you start, consult your doctor:
If you are allergic to any substance or drug.

Over age 60:
You may have skin reactions, particularly around genitals and anus.

Pregnancy:
Studies inconclusive on harm to unborn child. Animal studies show fetal abnormalities. Decide with your doctor whether drug benefits justify risk to unborn child.

Breast-feeding:
Drug passes into milk. Child may become sensitive to penicillins and have allergic reactions to penicillin drugs. Avoid nafcillin or discontinue nursing until you finish medicine. Consult doctor for advice on maintaining milk supply.

Infants & children:
No problems expected.

Prolonged use:
You may become more susceptible to infections caused by germs not responsive to nafcillin.

Skin & sunlight:
No problems expected.

Driving, piloting or hazardous work:
Usually not dangerous. Most hazardous reactions likely to occur a few minutes after taking nafcillin.

Discontinuing:
Don't discontinue without doctor's advice until you complete prescribed dose, even though symptoms diminish or disappear.

Others:
Absorption of this drug in oral form is unpredictable. Injections are more reliable.

POSSIBLE INTERACTION WITH OTHER DRUGS

GENERIC NAME OR DRUG CLASS	COMBINED EFFECT
Beta-adrenergic blockers	Increased chance of anaphylaxis (see emergency information on inside front cover).
Chloramphenicol	Decreased effect of both drugs.
Erythromycins	Decreased effect of both drugs.
Loperamide	Decreased nafcillin effect.
Paromomycin	Decreased effect of both drugs.
Tetracyclines	Decreased effect of both drugs.
Troleandomycin	Decreased effect of both drugs.

POSSIBLE INTERACTION WITH OTHER SUBSTANCES

INTERACTS WITH	COMBINED EFFECT
Alcohol:	Occasional stomach irritation.
Beverages:	None expected.
Cocaine:	No proven problems.
Foods:	None expected.
Marijuana:	No proven problems.
Tobacco:	None expected.

NALIDIXIC ACID

BRAND NAMES

NegGram

BASIC INFORMATION

Habit forming? No
Prescription needed? Yes
Available as generic? No
Drug class: Antimicrobial

 USES

Treatment for urinary-tract infections.

 DOSAGE & USAGE INFORMATION

How to take:
- Tablet—Swallow with food or milk to lessen stomach irritation. If you can't swallow whole, crumble tablet and take with liquid or food.
- Liquid—Take with liquid or food.

When to take:
At the same times each day.

If you forget a dose:
Take as soon as you remember up to 2 hours late. If more than 2 hours, wait for next scheduled dose (don't double this dose).

What drug does:
Destroys bacteria susceptible to nalidixic acid.

Time lapse before drug works:
1 to 2 weeks.

Don't take with:
See Interaction column and consult doctor.

 OVERDOSE

SYMPTOMS:
Lethargy, stomach upset, behavioral changes, convulsions and stupor.
WHAT TO DO:
- **Dial 0 (operator) or 911 (emergency) for an ambulance or medical help. Then give first aid immediately.**
- **If patient is unconscious and not breathing, give mouth-to-mouth breathing. If there is no heartbeat, use cardiac massage and mouth-to-mouth breathing (CPR). Don't try to make patient vomit. If you can't get help quickly, take patient to nearest emergency facility.**
- **See emergency information on inside covers.**

 POSSIBLE ADVERSE REACTIONS OR SIDE EFFECTS

SYMPTOMS	WHAT TO DO
Life-threatening: None expected.	
Common: Rash; itchy skin; decreased, blurred or double vision; halos around lights or excess brightness; changes in color vision; nausea; vomiting; diarrhea.	Discontinue. Call doctor right away.
Infrequent: Dizziness, drowsiness.	Continue. Call doctor when convenient.
Rare: Paleness, sore throat or fever, severe stomach pain, pale stool, unusual bleeding or bruising, jaundice, fatigue, weakness.	Discontinue. Call doctor right away.

WARNINGS & PRECAUTIONS

Don't take if:
- You are allergic to nalidixic acid.
- You have a seizure disorder (epilepsy, convulsions).

Before you start, consult your doctor:
- If you plan to become pregnant within medication period.
- If you have or have had kidney or liver disease.
- If you have impaired circulation of the brain (hardened arteries).
- If you have Parkinson's disease.
- If you have diabetes (it may affect urine-sugar tests).

Over age 60:
Adverse reactions and side effects may be more frequent and severe than in younger persons.

Pregnancy:
Risk to unborn child outweighs drug benefits. Don't use, especially during first 3 months.

Breast-feeding:
No problems expected, unless you have impaired kidney function. Consult doctor.

Infants & children:
Don't give to infants younger than 3 months.

Prolonged use:
No problems expected.

Skin & sunlight:
May cause rash or intensify sunburn in areas exposed to sun or sunlamp.

Driving, piloting or hazardous work:
Avoid if you feel drowsy, dizzy or have vision problems. Otherwise, no problems expected.

Discontinuing:
Don't discontinue without consulting doctor. Dose may require gradual reduction if you have taken drug for a long time. Doses of other drugs may also require adjustment.

Others:
Periodic blood counts and liver- and kidney-function tests recommended.

POSSIBLE INTERACTION WITH OTHER DRUGS

GENERIC NAME OR DRUG CLASS	COMBINED EFFECT
Antacids	Decreased absorption of nalidixic acid.
Anticoagulants (oral)	Increased anticoagulant effect.
Calcium supplements	Decreased effect of nalidixic acid.
Nitrofurantoin	Decreased effect of nalidixic acid.
Probenecid	Decreased effect of nalidixic acid.
Vitamin C (in large doses)	Increased effect of nalidixic acid.

POSSIBLE INTERACTION WITH OTHER SUBSTANCES

INTERACTS WITH	COMBINED EFFECT
Alcohol:	Impaired alertness, judgment and coordination.
Beverages:	None expected.
Cocaine:	Impaired judgment and coordination.
Foods:	None expected.
Marijuana:	Impaired alertness, judgment and coordination.
Tobacco:	None expected.

NAPROXEN

BRAND NAMES

Anaprox
Apo-Naproxen
Naprosyn

Naxen
Novonaprox
Synflex

BASIC INFORMATION

Habit forming? No
Prescription needed? Yes
Available as generic? No
Drug class: Anti-inflammatory (non-steroid)

 USES

- Treatment for joint pain, stiffness, inflammation and swelling of arthritis and gout.
- Pain reliever.
- Treatment for dysmenorrhea (painful or difficult menstruation).

 DOSAGE & USAGE INFORMATION

How to take:
Tablet—Swallow with liquid or food to lessen stomach irritation. If you can't swallow whole, crumble tablet and take with liquid or food.

When to take:
At the same times each day.

If you forget a dose:
Take as soon as you remember up to 2 hours late. If more than 2 hours, wait for next scheduled dose (don't double this dose).

What drug does:
Reduces tissue concentration of prostaglandins (hormones which produce inflammation and pain).

Time lapse before drug works:
Begins in 4 to 24 hours. May require 3 weeks regular use for maximum benefit.

Continued next column

 OVERDOSE

SYMPTOMS:
Confusion, agitation, incoherence, convulsions, possible hemorrhage from stomach or intestine, coma.
WHAT TO DO:
- **Dial 0 (operator) or 911 (emergency) for an ambulance or medical help. Then give first aid immediately.**
- **See emergency information on inside covers.**

Don't take with:
See Interaction column and consult doctor.

 POSSIBLE ADVERSE REACTIONS OR SIDE EFFECTS

SYMPTOMS	WHAT TO DO
Life-threatening: None expected.	
Common:	
• Dizziness, nausea, pain.	Continue. Call doctor when convenient.
• Headache.	Continue. Tell doctor at next visit.
Infrequent: Depression, drowsiness, ringing in ears, constipation or diarrhea, vomiting, swollen feet or legs.	Continue. Call doctor when convenient.
Rare:	
• Convulsions; confusion; rash, hives or itchy skin; blurred vision; black, bloody or tarry stool; difficult breathing; tightness in chest; rapid heartbeat; unusual bleeding or bruising; blood in urine; jaundice.	Discontinue. Call doctor right away.
• Urgent, frequent, painful or difficult urination; fatigue; weakness.	Continue. Call doctor when convenient.

WARNINGS & PRECAUTIONS

Don't take if:
- You are allergic to aspirin or any non-steroid, anti-inflammatory drug.
- You have gastritis, peptic ulcer, enteritis, ileitis, ulcerative colitis, asthma, heart failure, high blood pressure or bleeding problems.
- You have had recent rectal bleeding and suppository form has been prescribed.
- Patient is younger than 15.

Before you start, consult your doctor:
- If you have epilepsy.
- If you have Parkinson's disease.
- If you have been mentally ill.
- If you have had kidney disease or impaired kidney function.

Over age 60:
Adverse reactions and side effects may be more frequent and severe than in younger persons.

Pregnancy:
Studies inconclusive on harm to unborn child. Decide with your doctor whether drug benefits justify risk to unborn child.

Breast-feeding:
May harm child. Avoid.

Infants & children:
Not recommended for anyone younger than 15. Use only under medical supervision.

Prolonged use:
- Eye damage.
- Reduced hearing.
- Sore throat, fever.
- Weight gain.

Skin & sunlight:
No problems expected.

Driving, piloting or hazardous work:
Don't drive or pilot aircraft until you learn how medicine affects you. Don't work around dangerous machinery. Don't climb ladders or work in high places. Danger increases if you drink alcohol or take medicine affecting alertness and reflexes, such as antihistamines, tranquilizers, sedatives, pain medicine, narcotics and mind-altering drugs.

Discontinuing:
Don't discontinue without consulting doctor. Dose may require gradual reduction if you have taken drug for a long time. Doses of other drugs may also require adjustment.

Others:
No problems expected.

POSSIBLE INTERACTION WITH OTHER DRUGS

GENERIC NAME OR DRUG CLASS	COMBINED EFFECT
Acebutolol	Decreased antihypertensive effect of acebutolol.
Anticoagulants, (oral)	Increased risk of bleeding.
Aspirin	Increased risk of stomach ulcer.
Cortisone drugs	Increased risk of stomach ulcer.
Furosemide	Decreased diuretic effect of furosemide.
Gold compounds	Possible increased likelihood of kidney damage.
Ketoprofen	Increased possibility of internal bleeding.
Minoxidil	Decreased minoxidil effect.
Oxprenolol	Decreased antihypertensive effect of oxprenolol.
Oxyphenbutazone	Possible stomach ulcer.
Phenylbutazone	Possible stomach ulcer.
Probenecid	Increased naproxen effect.
Thyroid hormones	Rapid heartbeat, blood-pressure rise.

POSSIBLE INTERACTION WITH OTHER SUBSTANCES

INTERACTS WITH	COMBINED EFFECT
Alcohol:	Possible stomach ulcer or bleeding.
Beverages:	None expected.
Cocaine:	None expected.
Foods:	None expected.
Marijuana:	Increased pain relief from naproxen.
Tobacco:	None expected.

NARCOTIC & ACETAMINOPHEN

BRAND NAMES

See complete list of brand names in the *Brand Name Directory,* page 951.

BASIC INFORMATION

Habit forming? Yes
Prescription needed? Yes
Available as generic? Yes
Drug class: Narcotic, analgesic,
           fever-reducer

 ## USES

- Relieves pain.
- Suppresses cough.

 ## DOSAGE & USAGE INFORMATION

How to take:
- Tablet or capsule—Swallow with liquid. If you can't swallow whole, crumble tablet or open capsule and take with liquid or food.
- Drops or liquid—Dilute dose in beverage before swallowing.

When to take:
When needed. No more often than every 4 hours.

If you forget a dose:
Take as soon as you remember. Wait 4 hours for next dose.

Continued next column

 ## OVERDOSE

SYMPTOMS:
Stomach upset; irritability; convulsions; deep sleep; slow breathing; slow pulse; flushed, warm skin; constricted pupils; coma.
WHAT TO DO:
- **Dial 0 (operator) or 911 (emergency) for an ambulance or medical help. Then give first aid immediately.**
- **If patient is unconscious and not breathing, give mouth-to-mouth breathing. If there is no heartbeat, use cardiac massage and mouth-to-mouth breathing (CPR). Don't try to make patient vomit. If you can't get help quickly, take patient to nearest emergency facility.**
- **See emergency information on inside covers.**

What drug does:
- May affect hypothalamus—the part of the brain that helps regulate body heat and receives body's pain messages.
- Blocks pain messages to brain and spinal cord.
- Reduces sensitivity of brain's cough-control center.

Time lapse before drug works:
15 to 30 minutes. May last 4 hours.

Don't take with:
- Other drugs with acetaminophen. Too much acetaminophen can damage liver and kidneys.
- See Interaction column and consult doctor.

 ## POSSIBLE ADVERSE REACTIONS OR SIDE EFFECTS

SYMPTOMS	WHAT TO DO
Life-threatening: Irregular or slow heartbeat, difficult breathing.	Discontinue. Seek emergency treatment.
Common: Dizziness, agitation, tiredness.	Continue. Call doctor when convenient.
Infrequent: Abdominal pain, constipation, vomiting.	Discontinue. Call doctor right away.
Rare: • Fatigue; itchy skin; rash; sore throat, fever, mouth sores; bruising and bleeding increased; painful or difficult urination; blood in urine; anemia; blurred vision.	Discontinue. Call doctor right away.
• Depression.	Continue. Call doctor when convenient.

 ## WARNINGS & PRECAUTIONS

Don't take if:
- You are allergic to any narcotic or acetaminophen.
- Your symptoms don't improve after 2 days use. Call your doctor.

Before you start, consult your doctor:
- If you have bronchial asthma, kidney disease or liver damage.
- If you will have surgery within 2 months, including dental surgery, requiring general or spinal anesthesia.

NARCOTIC & ACETAMINOPHEN

Over age 60:
More likely to be drowsy, dizzy, unsteady or constipated. Don't exceed recommended dose. You can't eliminate drug as efficiently as younger persons. Use only if absolutely necessary.

Pregnancy:
Decide with your doctor whether drug benefits justify risk to unborn child. Abuse by pregnant woman will result in addicted newborn. Withdrawal of newborn can be life-threatening.

Breast-feeding:
Drug filters into milk. May harm child. Avoid.

Infants & children:
Not recommended.

Prolonged use:
- Causes psychological and physical dependence (addiction).
- May affect blood stream and cause anemia. Limit use to 5 days for children 12 and under, and 10 days for adults.

Skin & sunlight:
May cause rash or intensify sunburn in areas exposed to sun or sunlamp.

Driving, piloting or hazardous work:
Don't drive or pilot aircraft until you learn how medicine affects you. Don't work around dangerous machinery. Don't climb ladders or work in high places. Danger increases if you drink alcohol or take medicine affecting alertness and reflexes, such as antihistamines, tranquilizers, sedatives, pain medicine, narcotics and mind-altering drugs.

Discontinuing:
Discontinue in 2 days if symptoms don't improve.

Others:
No problems expected.

POSSIBLE INTERACTION WITH OTHER DRUGS

GENERIC NAME OR DRUG CLASS	COMBINED EFFECT
Analgesics (other)	Increased analgesic effect.
Anticoagulants (other)	May increase anticoagulant effect. Prothrombin times should be monitored.
Anticholinergics	Increased anticholinergic effect.
Antidepressants	Increased sedative effect.
Antihistamines	Increased sedative effect.
Mind-altering drugs	Increased sedative effect.
Narcotics (other)	Increased narcotic effect.
Nitrates	Excessive blood-pressure drop.
Phenobarbital and other barbiturates	Quicker elimination and decreased effect of acetaminophen.
Phenothiazines	Increased phenothiazine effect.
Sedatives	Increased sedative effect.
Sleep inducers	Increased sedative effect.
Terfenadine	Possible oversedation.
Tetracyclines	May slow tetracycline absorption. Space doses 2 hours apart.
Tranquilizers	Increased sedative effect.

POSSIBLE INTERACTION WITH OTHER SUBSTANCES

INTERACTS WITH	COMBINED EFFECT
Alcohol:	Increases alcohol's intoxicating effect. Avoid.
Beverages:	None expected.
Cocaine:	Increased cocaine toxic effects. Avoid.
Foods:	None expected.
Marijuana:	Impairs physical and mental performance. Avoid.
Tobacco:	None expected.

BRAND AND GENERIC NAMES

See complete list of brand names in the *Brand Name Directory,* page 952.

BASIC INFORMATION

Habit forming? Yes
Prescription needed? Yes
Available as generic? Yes
Drug class: Narcotic

 ## USES

- Relieves pain.
- Suppresses cough.

 ## DOSAGE & USAGE INFORMATION

How to take:
- Tablet or capsule—Swallow with liquid. If you can't swallow whole, crumble tablet or open capsule and take with liquid or food.
- Drops or liquid—Dilute dose in beverage before swallowing.

When to take:
When needed. No more often than every 4 hours.

If you forget a dose:
Take as soon as you remember. Wait 4 hours for next dose.

What drug does:
- Blocks pain messages to brain and spinal cord.
- Reduces sensitivity of brain's cough-control center.

Continued next column

 ## OVERDOSE

SYMPTOMS:
Deep sleep, slow breathing; slow pulse; flushed, warm skin; constricted pupils.
WHAT TO DO:
- **Dial 0 (operator) or 911 (emergency) for an ambulance or medical help. Then give first aid immediately.**
- **If patient is unconscious and not breathing, give mouth-to-mouth breathing. If there is no heartbeat, use cardiac massage and mouth-to-mouth breathing (CPR). Don't try to make patient vomit. If you can't get help quickly, take patient to nearest emergency facility.**
- **See emergency information on inside covers.**

Time lapse before drug works:
30 minutes.

Don't take with:
See Interaction column and consult doctor.

 ## POSSIBLE ADVERSE REACTIONS OR SIDE EFFECTS

SYMPTOMS	WHAT TO DO
Life-threatening: None expected.	
Common: Dizziness, flushed face, difficult urination, unusual tiredness.	Continue. Call doctor when convenient.
Infrequent: Severe constipation, abdominal pain, vomiting.	Discontinue. Call doctor right away.
Rare: • Hives, rash, itchy skin, face swelling, slow heartbeat, irregular breathing.	Discontinue. Call doctor right away.
• Depression, blurred vision.	Continue. Call doctor when convenient.

WARNINGS & PRECAUTIONS

Don't take if:
You are allergic to any narcotic.

Before you start, consult your doctor:
- If you have impaired liver or kidney function.
- If you will have surgery within 2 months, including dental surgery, requiring general or spinal anesthesia.

Over age 60:
More likely to be drowsy, dizzy, unsteady or constipated. Use only if absolutely necessary.

Pregnancy:
Decide with your doctor whether drug benefits justify risk to unborn child. Abuse by pregnant woman will result in addicted newborn. Withdrawal of newborn can be life-threatening.

Breast-feeding:
Drug filters into milk. May harm child. Avoid.

Infants & children:
Not recommended.

Prolonged use:
Causes psychological and physical dependence (addiction).

Skin & sunlight:
May cause rash or intensify sunburn in areas exposed to sun or sunlamp.

Driving, piloting or hazardous work:
Don't drive or pilot aircraft until you learn how medicine affects you. Don't work around dangerous machinery. Don't climb ladders or work in high places. Danger increases if you drink alcohol or take medicine affecting alertness and reflexes, such as antihistamines, tranquilizers, sedatives, pain medicine, narcotics and mind-altering drugs.

Discontinuing:
May be unnecessary to finish medicine. Follow doctor's instructions.

Others:
No problems expected.

POSSIBLE INTERACTION WITH OTHER DRUGS

GENERIC NAME OR DRUG CLASS	COMBINED EFFECT
Analgesics (other)	Increased analgesic effect.
Anticholinergics	Increased anticholinergic effect.
Antidepressants	Increased sedative effect.
Antihistamines	Increased sedative effect.
Mind-altering drugs	Increased sedative effect.
Molindone	Increased narcotic effect.
Narcotics (other)	Increased narcotic effect.
Nitrates	Excessive blood-pressure drop.
Phenothiazines	Increased phenothiazine effect.
Sedatives	Increased sedative effect.
Sleep inducers	Increased sedative effect.
Terfenadine	Possible oversedation.
Tranquilizers	Increased sedative effect.

POSSIBLE INTERACTION WITH OTHER SUBSTANCES

INTERACTS WITH	COMBINED EFFECT
Alcohol:	Increases alcohol's intoxicating effect. Avoid.
Beverages:	None expected.
Cocaine:	Increased cocaine toxic effects. Avoid.
Foods:	None expected.
Marijuana:	Impairs physical and mental performance. Avoid.
Tobacco:	None expected.

BRAND NAMES

See complete list of brand names in the *Brand Name Directory,* page 952.

BASIC INFORMATION

Habit forming? Yes
Prescription needed? Yes
Available as generic? Yes
Drug class: Narcotic, analgesic, anti-inflammatory

 USES

- Reduces pain, fever, inflammation.
- Suppresses cough.

 DOSAGE & USAGE INFORMATION

How to take:
Tablet or capsule—Swallow with liquid. If you can't swallow whole, crumble tablet or open capsule and take with liquid or food.

When to take:
When needed. No more often than every 4 hours.

If you forget a dose:
Take as soon as you remember. Wait 4 hours for next dose.

What drug does:
- Affects hypothalamus, the part of the brain which regulates temperature by dilating small blood vessels in skin.

Continued next column

 OVERDOSE

SYMPTOMS:
Ringing in ears; nausea; vomiting; dizziness; fever; deep sleep; slow breathing; slow pulse; flushed, warm skin; constricted pupils; hallucinations; convulsions; coma.
WHAT TO DO:
- **Dial 0 (operator) or 911 (emergency) for an ambulance or medical help. Then give first aid immediately.**
- **If patient is unconscious and not breathing, give mouth-to-mouth breathing. If there is no heartbeat, use cardiac massage and mouth-to-mouth breathing (CPR). Don't try to make patient vomit. If you can't get help quickly, take patient to nearest emergency facility.**
- **See emergency information on inside covers.**

- Prevents clumping of platelets (small blood cells) so blood vessels remain open.
- Decreases prostaglandin effect.
- Suppresses body's pain messages.
- Reduces sensitivity of brain's cough-control center.

Time lapse before drug works:
30 minutes.

Don't take with:
- Tetracyclines. Space doses 1 hour apart.
- See Interaction column and consult doctor.

 POSSIBLE ADVERSE REACTIONS OR SIDE EFFECTS

SYMPTOMS	WHAT TO DO
Life-threatening:	
• Hives, rash, intense itching, faintness soon after a dose (anaphylaxis).	Seek emergency treatment immediately.
• Clot or pain over blood vessel, cold hands, feet.	Discontinue. Seek emergency treatment.
Common:	
• Nausea, abdominal cramps or pain.	Discontinue. Call doctor right away.
• Dizziness, red or flushed face, frequent urination, unusual tiredness, ringing in ears, heartburn, indigestion.	Continue. Call doctor when convenient.
Infrequent:	
Constipation, abdominal pain or cramps, vomiting.	Discontinue. Call doctor right away.
Rare:	
• Slow heartbeat; change in vision; black, bloody or tarry stool; blood in urine; jaundice.	Discontinue. Call doctor right away.
• Depression, blurred vision.	Continue. Call doctor when convenient.

 WARNINGS & PRECAUTIONS

Don't take if:
- You are allergic to any narcotic or subject to any substance abuse.
- You have a peptic ulcer of stomach or duodenum or a bleeding disorder.

Before you start, consult your doctor:
- If you have impaired liver or kidney function, asthma or nasal polyps.
- If you have had stomach or duodenal ulcers, gout.

- If you will have surgery within 2 months, including dental surgery, requiring general or spinal anesthesia.

Over age 60:
- More likely to be drowsy, dizzy, unsteady or constipated. Use only if absolutely necessary.
- More likely to cause hidden bleeding in stomach or intestines. Watch for dark stools.

Pregnancy:
Risk to unborn child outweighs drug benefits. Don't use.

Breast-feeding:
Drug passes into milk and may harm child. Avoid drug or discontinue nursing until you finish medicine. Consult doctor for advice on maintaining milk supply.

Infants & children:
Not recommended.

Prolonged use:
- Causes psychological and physical dependence (addiction).
- Kidney damage. Periodic kidney-function test recommended.

Skin & sunlight:
May cause rash or intensify sunburn in areas exposed to sun or sunlamp.

Driving, piloting or hazardous work:
Don't drive or pilot aircraft until you learn how medicine affects you. Don't work around dangerous machinery. Don't climb ladders or work in high places. Danger increases if you drink alcohol or take medicine affecting alertness and reflexes, such as antihistamines, tranquilizers, sedatives, pain medicine, narcotics and mind-altering drugs.

Discontinuing:
May be unnecessary to finish medicine. Follow doctor's instructions.

Others:
- Aspirin can complicate surgery, pregnancy, labor and delivery, and illness.
- Urine tests for blood sugar may be inaccurate.

POSSIBLE INTERACTION WITH OTHER DRUGS

GENERIC NAME OR DRUG CLASS	COMBINED EFFECT
Acebutolol	Decreased antihypertensive effect of acebutolol.
Allopurinol	Decreased allopurinol effect.
Antacids	Decreased aspirin effect.

Anticoagulants	Increased anticoagulant effect. Abnormal bleeding.
Antidepressants	Increased sedative effect.
Antidiabetics (oral)	Low blood sugar.
Anti-inflammatory drugs (non-steroid)	Risk of stomach bleeding and ulcers.
Aspirin (other)	Likely aspirin toxicity.
Cortisone drugs	Increased cortisone effect. Risk of ulcers and stomach bleeding.
Furosemide	Possible aspirin toxicity.
Gold compounds	Increased likelihood of kidney damage.
Indomethacin	Risk of stomach bleeding and ulcers.
Methotrexate	Increased methotrexate effect.
Minoxidil	Decreased minoxidil effect.
Narcotics (other)	Increased narcotic effect.
Nitrates	Excessive blood-pressure drop.
Oxprenolol	Decreased antihypertensive effect of oxprenolol.
Para-aminosalicylic acid (PAS)	Possible aspirin toxicity.
Penicillins	Increased effect of both drugs.

Continued page 969

POSSIBLE INTERACTION WITH OTHER SUBSTANCES

INTERACTS WITH	COMBINED EFFECT
Alcohol:	Possible stomach irritation and bleeding. Increases alcohol's intoxicating effect. Avoid.
Beverages:	None expected.
Cocaine:	Decreased cocaine toxic effects. Avoid.
Foods:	None expected.
Marijuana:	Impairs physical and mental performance. Avoid.
Tobacco:	None expected.

NEOMYCIN (ORAL)

BRAND NAMES

Mycifradin   Neobiotic

BASIC INFORMATION

Habit forming? No
Prescription needed? Yes
Available as generic? Yes
Drug class: Antibiotic

USES

- Clears intestinal tract of germs prior to surgery.
- Treats some causes of diarrhea.
- Lowers blood cholesterol.
- Lessens symptoms of hepatic coma.

DOSAGE & USAGE INFORMATION

How to take:
Tablet or capsule—Swallow with liquid or food to lessen stomach irritation. If you can't swallow whole, crumble tablet or open capsule and take with liquid or food.

When to take:
According to directions on prescription.

If you forget a dose:
Take as soon as you remember up to 2 hours late. If more than 2 hours, wait for next scheduled dose (don't double this dose).

What drug does:
Kills germs susceptible to neomycin.

Time lapse before drug works:
2 to 3 days.

Continued next column

OVERDOSE

SYMPTOMS:
Loss of hearing, difficulty breathing, respiratory paralysis.
WHAT TO DO:
- Dial 0 (operator) or 911 (emergency) for an ambulance or medical help. Then give first aid immediately.
- If patient is unconscious and not breathing, give mouth-to-mouth breathing. If there is no heartbeat, use cardiac massage and mouth-to-mouth breathing (CPR). Don't try to make patient vomit. If you can't get help quickly, take patient to nearest emergency facility.
- See emergency information on inside covers.

Don't take with:
See Interaction column and consult doctor.

POSSIBLE ADVERSE REACTIONS OR SIDE EFFECTS

SYMPTOMS	WHAT TO DO
Life-threatening: None expected.	
Common: Sore mouth, nausea, vomiting.	Continue. Call doctor when convenient.
Infrequent: None expected.	
Rare: Clumsiness, dizziness, rash, hearing loss, ringing or noises in ear, frothy stools, gaseousness, decreased frequency of urination.	Discontinue. Call doctor right away.

WARNINGS & PRECAUTIONS

Don't take if:
You are allergic to neomycin or any aminoglycoside. (See Interactions column.)

Before you start, consult your doctor:
- If you will have surgery within 2 months, including dental surgery, requiring general or spinal anesthesia.
- If you have hearing loss or loss of balance secondary to 8th cranial nerve disease.
- If you have intestinal obstruction.
- If you have myasthenia gravis, Parkinson's disease, kidney disease, ulcers in intestines.

Over age 60:
Adverse reactions and side effects may be more frequent and severe than in younger persons.

Pregnancy:
No proven harm to unborn child. Avoid if possible.

Breast-feeding:
Avoid if possible.

Infants & children:
Only under close medical supervision.

Prolonged use:
Adverse effects more likely.

Skin & sunlight:
No problems expected.

Driving, piloting or hazardous work:
No problems expected.

Discontinuing:
May be unnecessary to finish medicine. Follow doctor's instructions.

Others:
No problems expected.

POSSIBLE INTERACTION WITH OTHER DRUGS

GENERIC NAME OR DRUG CLASS	COMBINED EFFECT
Aminoglycosides: Amikacin, Gentamicin, Kanamycin, Streptomycin, Tobramycin	Increases chance of toxic effect on hearing, kidney, muscles.
Capreomycin Cisplatin Ethacrynic acid Furosemide Mercaptomerin Vancomycin	Increases chance of toxic effects on hearing, kidneys.
Cephalothin	Increased chance of toxic effect on kidneys.

POSSIBLE INTERACTION WITH OTHER SUBSTANCES

INTERACTS WITH	COMBINED EFFECT
Alcohol:	Increased chance of toxicity. Avoid.
Beverages:	No problems expected.
Cocaine:	Increased chance of toxicity. Avoid.
Foods:	No problems expected.
Marijuana:	Increased chance of toxicity. Avoid.
Tobacco:	No problems expected.

NEOSTIGMINE

BRAND NAMES

Prostigmin

BASIC INFORMATION

Habit forming? No
Prescription needed? Yes
Available as generic? Yes
Drug class: Cholinergic (anticholinesterase)

 USES

- Treatment of myasthenia gravis.
- Treatment of urinary retention and abdominal distention.
- Antidote to adverse effects of muscle relaxants used in surgery.

 DOSAGE & USAGE INFORMATION

How to take:
Tablet—Swallow with liquid or food to lessen stomach irritation.

When to take:
As directed, usually 3 or 4 times a day.

If you forget a dose:
Take as soon as you remember up to 2 hours late. If more than 2 hours, wait for next scheduled dose (don't double this dose).

What drug does:
Inhibits the chemical activity of an enzyme (cholinesterase) so nerve impulses can cross the junction of nerves and muscles.

Time lapse before drug works:
3 hours.

Don't take with:
See Interaction column and consult doctor.

 OVERDOSE

SYMPTOMS:
Muscle weakness, cramps, twitching or clumsiness; severe diarrhea, nausea, vomiting, stomach cramps or pain; breathing difficulty; confusion, irritability, nervousness, restlessness, fear; unusually slow heartbeat; seizures.
WHAT TO DO:
- **Dial 0 (operator) or 911 (emergency) for an ambulance or medical help. Then give first aid immediately.**
- **See emergency information on inside covers.**

 POSSIBLE ADVERSE REACTIONS OR SIDE EFFECTS

SYMPTOMS	WHAT TO DO
Life-threatening: None expected.	
Common:	
• Mild diarrhea, nausea, vomiting, stomach cramps or pain.	Discontinue. Call doctor right away.
• Excess saliva, unusual sweating.	Continue. Call doctor when convenient.
Infrequent:	
• Confusion, irritability.	Discontinue. Seek emergency treatment.
• Constricted pupils, watery eyes, lung congestion, frequent urge to urinate.	Continue. Call doctor when convenient.
Rare: None expected.	

WARNINGS & PRECAUTIONS

Don't take if:
- You are allergic to any cholinergic or bromide.
- You take mecamylamine.

Before you start, consult your doctor:
- If you plan to become pregnant within medication period.
- If you have bronchial asthma.
- If you have heartbeat irregularities.
- If you have urinary obstruction or urinary-tract infection.

Over age 60:
Adverse reactions and side effects may be more frequent and severe than in younger persons.

Pregnancy:
No proven harm to unborn child. Avoid if possible. May increase uterus contractions close to delivery.

Breast-feeding:
No problems expected, but consult doctor.

Infants & children:
Not recommended.

Prolonged use:
Medication may lose effectiveness. Discontinuing for a few days may restore effect.

Skin & sunlight:
No problems expected.

Driving, piloting or hazardous work:
Don't drive or pilot aircraft until you learn how medicine affects you. Don't work around dangerous machinery. Don't climb ladders or work in high places. Danger increases if you drink alcohol or take medicine affecting alertness and reflexes, such as antihistamines, tranquilizers, sedatives, pain medicine, narcotics and mind-altering drugs.

Discontinuing:
Don't discontinue without doctor's advice until you complete prescribed dose, even though symptoms diminish or disappear.

Others:
No problems expected.

POSSIBLE INTERACTION WITH OTHER DRUGS

GENERIC NAME OR DRUG CLASS	COMBINED EFFECT
Anesthetics (local or general)	Decreased neostigmine effect.
Antiarrhythmics	Decreased neostigmine effect.
Antibiotics	Decreased neostigmine effect.
Anticholinergics	Decreased neostigmine effect. May mask severe side effects.
Cholinergics (other)	Reduced intestinal-tract function. Possible brain and nervous-system toxicity.
Mecamylamine	Decreased neostigmine effect.
Nitrates	Decreased neostigmine effect.
Quinidine	Decreased neostigmine effect.

POSSIBLE INTERACTION WITH OTHER SUBSTANCES

INTERACTS WITH	COMBINED EFFECT
Alcohol:	No proven problems with small doses.
Beverages:	None expected.
Cocaine:	Decreased neostigmine effect. Avoid.
Foods:	None expected.
Marijuana:	No proven problems.
Tobacco:	No proven problems.

BRAND NAMES

See complete list of brand names in the
Brand Name Directory, page 953.

**There are numerous other multiple
vitamin-mineral supplements available.**

BASIC INFORMATION

Habit forming? No
Prescription needed?
  Tablets: No
  Liquid, capsules: Yes
Available as generic? Yes
**Drug class: Vitamin supplement, vasodilator,
        antihyperlipidemic**

 ## USES

- Replacement for niacin deficiency caused by
  inadequate diet.
- Treatment for vertigo (dizziness) and ringing
  in ears.
- Prevention of premenstrual headache.
- Reduction of blood levels of cholesterol and
  triglycerides.
- Treatment for pellagra.

 ## DOSAGE & USAGE
INFORMATION

How to take:
- Tablet, capsule or liquid—Swallow with liquid
  or food to lessen stomach irritation.
- Extended-release tablets or
  capsules—Swallow each dose whole.

When to take:
At the same times each day.

If you forget a dose:
Take as soon as you remember. Wait 4 hours
for next dose.

What drug does:
- Corrects niacin deficiency.
- Dilates blood vessels.
- In large doses, decreases cholesterol
  production.

Continued next column

 ## OVERDOSE

SYMPTOMS:
**Body flush, nausea, vomiting, abdominal
cramps, diarrhea, weakness,
lightheadedness, fainting, sweating.**
WHAT TO DO:
**Overdose unlikely to threaten life. If person
takes much larger amount than prescribed,
call doctor, poison-control center or hospital
emergency room for instructions.**

Time lapse before drug works:
15 to 20 minutes.

Don't take with:
See Interaction column and consult doctor.

 ## POSSIBLE
ADVERSE REACTIONS
OR SIDE EFFECTS

SYMPTOMS	WHAT TO DO
Life-threatening:	
None expected.	
Common:	
None expected.	
Infrequent:	
• Headache, dizziness, faintness, temporary numbness and tingling in hands and feet.	Continue. Call doctor when convenient.
• "Hot" feeling, flush.	No action necessary.
Rare:	
Jaundice.	Discontinue. Call doctor right away.

NIACIN (NICOTINIC ACID)

 WARNINGS & PRECAUTIONS

Don't take if:
- You are allergic to niacin or any niacin-containing vitamin mixtures.
- You have impaired liver function.
- You have active peptic ulcer.

Before you start, consult your doctor:
- If you have diabetes.
- If you have gout.
- If you have gallbladder or liver disease.

Over age 60:
Response to drug cannot be predicted. Dose must be individualized.

Pregnancy:
Risk to unborn child outweighs drug benefits. Don't use.

Breast-feeding:
Studies inconclusive. Consult doctor.

Infants & children:
- Use only under supervision.
- Keep vitamin-mineral supplements out of children's reach.

Prolonged use:
Possible impaired liver function.

Skin & sunlight:
No problems expected.

Driving, piloting or hazardous work:
Avoid if you feel dizzy or faint. Otherwise, no problems expected.

Discontinuing:
May be unnecessary to finish medicine. Follow doctor's instructions.

Others:
- A balanced diet should provide all the niacin a healthy person needs and make supplements unnecessary. Best sources are meat, eggs and dairy products.
- Store in original container in cool, dry, dark place. Bathroom medicine chest too moist.
- Obesity reduces effectiveness.

 POSSIBLE INTERACTION WITH OTHER DRUGS

GENERIC NAME OR DRUG CLASS	COMBINED EFFECT
Antidiabetics	Decreased antidiabetic effect.
Beta-adrenergic blockers	Excessively low blood pressure.
Guanethidine	Increased guanethidine effect.
Isoniazid	Decreased niacin effect.
Mecamylamine	Excessively low blood pressure.
Methyldopa	Excessively low blood pressure.
Pargyline	Excessively low blood pressure.

 POSSIBLE INTERACTION WITH OTHER SUBSTANCES

INTERACTS WITH	COMBINED EFFECT
Alcohol:	Excessively low blood pressure. Use caution.
Beverages:	None expected.
Cocaine:	Increased flushing.
Foods:	None expected.
Marijuana:	None expected.
Tobacco:	Decreased niacin effect.

NICOTINE RESIN COMPLEX

BRAND NAMES

Nicorette

BASIC INFORMATION

Habit forming? Yes
Prescription needed? Yes
Available as generic? No
Drug class: Antismoking agent

 ## USES

Treats smoking addiction.

 ## DOSAGE & USAGE INFORMATION

How to take:
Follow detailed instructions on patient instruction sheet provided with prescription.

When to take:
Follow detailed instructions on patient instruction sheet provided with prescription.

If you forget a dose:
Follow detailed instructions on patient instruction sheet provided with prescription.

What drug does:
Satisfies physical craving for nicotine in addicted persons and avoids peaks in blood nicotine level resulting from smoking.

Time lapse before drug works:
30 minutes.

Don't take with:
See Interaction column and consult doctor.

 ## OVERDOSE

SYMPTOMS:
Vomiting, irregular heartbeat.
WHAT TO DO:
Overdose unlikely to threaten life. If person takes much larger amount than prescribed, call doctor, poison-control center or hospital emergency room for instructions.

 ## POSSIBLE ADVERSE REACTIONS OR SIDE EFFECTS

SYMPTOMS	WHAT TO DO
Life-threatening: None expected.	
Frequent: Increased irritability causing heartbeat irregularity.	Continue. Call doctor when convenient.
Common:	
● Injury to loose teeth, jaw muscle ache.	Continue. Call doctor when convenient.
● Belching, mouth irritation or tingling, excessive salivation.	Continue. Tell doctor at next visit.
Infrequent:	
● Nausea and vomiting, abdominal pain.	Discontinue. Call doctor right away.
● Lightheadedness, headache, hiccups.	Continue. Call doctor when convenient.
Rare: None expected.	

WARNINGS & PRECAUTIONS

Don't take if:
- You are a non-smoker.
- You are pregnant or intend to become pregnant.
- You recently suffered a heart attack.

Before you start, consult your doctor:
- If you have coronary artery disease.
- If you have active temperomandibular joint disease.
- If you have severe angina.
- If you have peptic ulcer.

Over age 60:
Adverse reactions and side effects may be more frequent and severe than in younger persons.

Pregnancy:
Risk to unborn child outweighs drug benefits. Don't use.

Breast-feeding:
Drug passes into milk. Avoid drug or discontinue nursing until you finish medicine. Consult doctor for advice on maintaining milk supply.

Infants & children:
Don't use.

Prolonged use:
May cause addiction and greater likelihood of toxicity.

Skin & sunlight:
No problems expected.

Driving, piloting or hazardous work:
No problems expected.

Discontinuing:
May be unnecessary to finish medicine. Follow doctor's instructions.

Others:
No problems expected.

POSSIBLE INTERACTION WITH OTHER DRUGS

GENERIC NAME OR DRUG CLASS	COMBINED EFFECT
Beta-adrenergic blockers	Decreased blood pressure (slight).
Caffeine	Increased effect of caffeine.
Cortisone drugs	Increased cortisone circulating in blood.
Furosemide	Increased effect of furosemide.
Glutethimide	Increased absorption of glutethimide.
Imipramine	Increased effect of imipramine.
Pentazocine	Increased effect of pentazocine.
Phenacetin	Increased effect of phenacetin.
Propoxyphene	Decreased blood level of propoxyphene.
Theophylline	Increased effect of theophylline.

POSSIBLE INTERACTION WITH OTHER SUBSTANCES

INTERACTS WITH	COMBINED EFFECT
Alcohol:	Increased cardiac irritability. Avoid.
Beverages: Caffeine.	Increased cardiac irritability. Avoid any beverage with caffeine.
Cocaine:	Increased cardiac irritability. Avoid.
Foods:	No problems expected.
Marijuana:	Increased toxic effects. Avoid.
Tobacco:	Increased toxic effects. Avoid.

NIFEDIPINE

BRAND NAMES

Adalat   **Procardia**

BASIC INFORMATION

Habit forming? No
Prescription needed? Yes
Available as generic? No
Drug class: Calcium-channel blocker,
              antiarrhythmic, antianginal

 USES

Prevents angina attacks.

 DOSAGE & USAGE INFORMATION

How to take:
Capsule—Swallow with liquid.

When to take:
At the same times each day 1 hour before or 2 hours after eating.

If you forget a dose:
Take as soon as you remember up to 2 hours late. If more than 2 hours, wait for next scheduled dose (don't double this dose).

What drug does:
- Reduces work that heart must perform.
- Reduces normal artery pressure.
- Increases oxygen to heart muscle.

Time lapse before drug works:
1 to 2 hours.

Don't take with:
See Interaction column and consult doctor.

 OVERDOSE

SYMPTOMS:
Unusually fast or unusually slow heartbeat, loss of consciousness, cardiac arrest.
WHAT TO DO:
- **Dial 0 (operator) or 911 (emergency) for an ambulance or medical help. Then give first aid immediately.**
- **If patient is unconscious and not breathing, give mouth-to-mouth breathing. If there is no heartbeat, use cardiac massage and mouth-to-mouth breathing (CPR). Don't try to make patient vomit. If you can't get help quickly, take patient to nearest emergency facility.**
- **See emergency information on inside covers.**

 POSSIBLE ADVERSE REACTIONS OR SIDE EFFECTS

SYMPTOMS	WHAT TO DO
Life-threatening: None expected.	
Common: Tiredness.	Continue. Tell doctor at next visit.
Infrequent: • Unusually fast or unusually slow heartbeat, wheezing, cough, shortness of breath.	Discontinue. Call doctor right away.
• Dizziness; numbness or tingling in hands or feet; swelling of ankles, feet, legs; difficult urination.	Continue. Call doctor when convenient.
• Nausea, constipation.	Continue. Tell doctor at next visit.
Rare: • Fainting, chest pain.	Discontinue. Call doctor right away.
• Headache.	Continue. Tell doctor at next visit.

 WARNINGS & PRECAUTIONS

Don't take if:
- You are allergic to nifedipine.
- You have very low blood pressure.

Before you start, consult your doctor:
- If you have kidney or liver disease.
- If you have high blood pressure.
- If you have heart disease other than coronary-artery disease.

Over age 60:
Adverse reactions and side effects may be more frequent and severe than in younger persons.

Pregnancy:
No proven harm to unborn child: Avoid if possible.

Breast-feeding:
Safety not established. Avoid if possible.

Infants & children:
Not recommended.

Prolonged use:
No problems expected.

Skin & sunlight:
No problems expected.

Driving, piloting or hazardous work:
Avoid if you feel dizzy. Otherwise, no problems expected.

Discontinuing:
Don't discontinue without doctor's advice until you complete prescribed dose, even though symptoms diminish or disappear.

Others:
- Learn to check your own pulse rate. If it drops to 50 beats per minute or lower, don't take nifedipine until you consult your doctor.
- Drug may lower blood-sugar level if daily dose is more than 60 mg.

POSSIBLE INTERACTION WITH OTHER DRUGS

GENERIC NAME OR DRUG CLASS	COMBINED EFFECT
Amiodarone	Increased likelihood of slow heartbeat.
Anticoagulants (oral)	Increased anticoagulant effect.
Anticonvulsants (hydantoin)	Increased anticonvulsant effect.
Antihypertensives	Dangerous blood-pressure drop.
Beta-adrenergic blockers	Possible irregular heartbeat. May worsen congestive heart failure.
Calcium (large doses)	Decreased nifedipine effect.
Digitalis preparations	Increased digitalis effect. May need to reduce dose.
Disopyramide	May cause dangerously slow, fast or irregular heartbeat.
Diuretics	Dangerous blood-pressure drop.
Enalapril	Possible excessive potassium in blood.
Flecainide	Possible irregular heartbeat.
Ketoprofen	Increases chance of toxicity of nifedipine.
Nitrates	Reduced angina attacks.
Quinidine	Increased quinidine effect.
Suprofen	Increases chances of toxicity of nifedipine.

Tocainide	Increased likelihood of adverse reactions from either drug.
Vitamin D (large doses)	Decreased nifedipine effect.

POSSIBLE INTERACTION WITH OTHER SUBSTANCES

INTERACTS WITH	COMBINED EFFECT
Alcohol:	Dangerously low blood pressure. Avoid.
Beverages:	None expected.
Cocaine:	Possible irregular heartbeat. Avoid.
Foods:	None expected.
Marijuana:	Possible irregular heartbeat. Avoid.
Tobacco:	Possible rapid heartbeat. Avoid.

NITRATES

BRAND NAMES

See complete list of brand names in the *Brand Name Directory,* page 953.

BASIC INFORMATION

Habit forming? No
Prescription needed? Yes
Available as generic? Yes
Drug class: Antianginal (nitrate)

 USES

Reduces frequency and severity of angina attacks.

 DOSAGE & USAGE INFORMATION

How to take:
- Extended-release tablets or capsules—Swallow each dose whole with liquid.
- Chewable tablet—Chew tablet at earliest sign of angina, and hold in mouth for 2 minutes.
- Regular tablet or capsule—Swallow whole with liquid. Don't crush, chew or open.
- Ointment—Apply as directed.
- Sublingual tablets—Place under tongue every 3 to 5 minutes at earliest sign of angina. If you don't have complete relief with 3 or 4 tablets, call doctor.

When to take:
- Swallowed tablets—Take at the same times each day, 1 or 2 hours after meals.
- Ointment—Follow prescription directions.

If you forget a dose:
Take as soon as you remember up to 2 hours late. If more than 2 hours, wait for next scheduled dose (don't double this dose).

Continued next column

 OVERDOSE

SYMPTOMS:
Dizziness; blue fingernails and lips; fainting; shortness of breath; weak, fast heartbeat; convulsions.
WHAT TO DO:
- **Dial 0 (operator) or 911 (emergency) for an ambulance or medical help. Then give first aid immediately.**
- **See emergency information on inside covers.**

What drug does:
Relaxes blood vessels, increasing blood flow to heart muscle.

Time lapse before drug works:
- Sublingual tablets—1 to 3 minutes.
- Other forms—15 to 30 minutes. Will not stop an attack, but may prevent attacks.

Don't take with:
See Interaction column and consult doctor.

 POSSIBLE ADVERSE REACTIONS OR SIDE EFFECTS

SYMPTOMS	WHAT TO DO
Life-threatening:	
None expected.	
Common:	
Headache, flushed face and neck, dry mouth, nausea, vomiting, rapid heartbeat.	Continue. Tell doctor at next visit.
Infrequent:	
• Fainting.	Discontinue. Call doctor right away.
• Restlessness, blurred vision.	Continue. Call doctor when convenient.
Rare:	
• Rash.	Discontinue. Call doctor right away.
• Severe irritation, peeling.	Continue. Call doctor when convenient.

WARNINGS & PRECAUTIONS

Don't take if:
You are allergic to nitrates, including nitroglycerin.

Before you start, consult your doctor:
- If you are taking non-prescription drugs.
- If you plan to become pregnant within medication period.
- If you have glaucoma.
- If you have reacted badly to any vasodilator drug.
- If you drink alcoholic beverages or smoke marijuana.

Over age 60:
Adverse reactions and side effects may be more frequent and severe than in younger persons.

Pregnancy:
No proven harm to unborn child. Avoid if possible.

Breast-feeding:
No problems expected. Consult your doctor.

Infants & children:
Not recommended.

Prolonged use:
Drug may become less effective and require higher doses.

Skin & sunlight:
No problems expected.

Driving, piloting or hazardous work:
Don't drive or pilot aircraft until you learn how medicine affects you. Don't work around dangerous machinery. Don't climb ladders or work in high places. Danger increases if you drink alcohol or take medicine affecting alertness and reflexes.

Discontinuing:
Except for sublingual tablets, don't discontinue without doctor's advice until you complete prescribed dose, even though symptoms diminish or disappear.

Others:
- If discomfort is not caused by angina, nitrate medication will not bring relief. Call doctor if discomfort persists.
- Periodic urine and laboratory blood studies of white cell counts recommended if you take nitrates.
- Keep sublingual tablets in original container. Always carry them with you, but keep from body heat if possible.

POSSIBLE INTERACTION WITH OTHER DRUGS

GENERIC NAME OR DRUG CLASS	COMBINED EFFECT
Anticholinergics	Increased internal-eye pressure.
Antidepressants (tricyclic)	Excessive blood-pressure drop.
Antihypertensives	Excessive blood-pressure drop.
Beta-adrenergic blockers	Excessive blood-pressure drop.
Cholinergics	Decreased cholinergic effect.
Ephedrine	Decreased nitrate effect.
Labetolol	Increased antihypertensive effects.
Narcotics	Excessive blood-pressure drop.
Sympathomimetics	Possible reduced effects of both medicines.

POSSIBLE INTERACTION WITH OTHER SUBSTANCES

INTERACTS WITH	COMBINED EFFECT
Alcohol:	Excessive blood-pressure drop.
Beverages:	None expected.
Cocaine:	Flushed face and headache. Avoid.
Foods:	None expected.
Marijuana:	Decreased nitrate effect.
Tobacco:	Decreased nitrate effect.

NITROFURANTOIN

BRAND NAMES

Apo-Nitrofurantoin	Nephronex
Cyantin	Nifuran
Furadantin	Nitrex
Furalan	Nitrodan
Furaloid	Novofuran
Furantoin	Sarodant
Furatine	Trantoin
Macrodantin	Urotoin

BASIC INFORMATION

Habit forming? No
Prescription needed? Yes
Available as generic? Yes
Drug class: Antimicrobial

USES

Treatment for urinary-tract infections.

DOSAGE & USAGE INFORMATION

How to take:
- Tablet or capsule—Swallow with food or milk to lessen stomach irritation. If you can't swallow whole, crumble tablet or open capsule and take with liquid or food.
- Liquid—Shake well and take with food. Use a measuring spoon to ensure accuracy.

When to take:
At the same times each day.

If you forget a dose:
Take as soon as you remember up to 2 hours late. If more than 2 hours, wait for next scheduled dose (don't double this dose).

What drug does:
Prevents susceptible bacteria in the urinary tract from growing and multiplying.

Time lapse before drug works:
1 to 2 weeks.

Don't take with:
See Interaction column and consult doctor.

OVERDOSE

SYMPTOMS:
Nausea, vomiting, abdominal pain, diarrhea.
WHAT TO DO:
Overdose unlikely to threaten life. If person takes much larger amount than prescribed, call doctor, poison-control center or hospital emergency room for instructions.

POSSIBLE ADVERSE REACTIONS OR SIDE EFFECTS

SYMPTOMS	WHAT TO DO
Life-threatening:	
Hives, rash, intense itching, faintness soon after a dose (anaphylaxis).	Seek emergency treatment immediately.
Common:	
• Diarrhea, appetite loss, nausea, vomiting, chest pain, cough, difficult breathing, chills or unexplained fever.	Discontinue. Call doctor right away.
• Rusty colored or brown urine.	No action necessary.
Infrequent:	
• Rash, itchy skin, numbness, tingling or burning of face or mouth, fatigue, weakness.	Discontinue. Call doctor right away.
• Dizziness, drowsiness, headache, paleness (in children), discolored teeth (from liquid form).	Continue. Call doctor when convenient.
Rare:	
Jaundice.	Discontinue. Call doctor right away.

WARNINGS & PRECAUTIONS

Don't take if:
- You are allergic to nitrofurantoin.
- You have impaired kidney function.
- You drink alcohol.

Before you start, consult your doctor:
- If you are prone to allergic reactions.
- If you are pregnant and within 2 weeks of delivery.
- If you have had kidney disease, lung disease, anemia, nerve damage, or G6PD deficiency (a metabolic deficiency).
- If you have diabetes. Drug may affect urine sugar tests.

Over age 60:
Adverse reactions and side effects may be more frequent and severe than in younger persons.

Pregnancy:
Risk to unborn child outweighs drug benefits, especially in last month of pregnancy. Don't use.

Breast-feeding:
Drug passes into milk. Avoid drug or discontinue nursing until you finish medicine. Consult doctor for advice on maintaining milk supply.

Infants & children:
Don't give to infants younger than 1 month. Use only under medical supervision for older children.

Prolonged use:
Chest pain, cough, shortness of breath.

Skin & sunlight:
No problems expected.

Driving, piloting or hazardous work:
Avoid if you feel dizzy or drowsy. Otherwise, no problems expected.

Discontinuing:
Don't discontinue without consulting doctor. Dose may require gradual reduction if you have taken drug for a long time. Doses of other drugs may also require adjustment.

Others:
Periodic blood counts, liver-function tests, and chest X-rays recommended.

POSSIBLE INTERACTION WITH OTHER DRUGS

GENERIC NAME OR DRUG CLASS	COMBINED EFFECT
Nalidixic acid	Decreased nitrofurantoin effect.
Phenobarbital	Decreased nitrofurantoin effect.
Probenecid	Increased nitrofurantoin effect.
Sulfinpyrazone	Possible nitrofurantoin toxicity.

POSSIBLE INTERACTION WITH OTHER SUBSTANCES

INTERACTS WITH	COMBINED EFFECT
Alcohol:	Possible disulfiram reaction (see Glossary). Avoid.
Beverages:	None expected.
Cocaine:	No proven problems.
Foods:	None expected.
Marijuana:	None expected.
Tobacco:	None expected.

NORETHINDRONE

BRAND NAMES

Micronor	Norlutin
Modicon 21	Nor-Q.D.
Norinyl 1 + 35	Ortho-Novum 1/35
21-Day Tablets	Ovcon
Norlestrin	Tri-Norinyl
Norlutate	

BASIC INFORMATION

Habit forming? No
Prescription needed? Yes
Available as generic? No
Drug class: Female sex hormone (progestin)

USES

- Treatment for menstrual or uterine disorders caused by progestin imbalance.
- Contraceptive.

DOSAGE & USAGE INFORMATION

How to take:
Tablet or capsule—Swallow with liquid or food to lessen stomach irritation. You may crumble tablet or open capsule.

When to take:
At the same time each day.

If you forget a dose:
- Menstrual disorders—Take up to 2 hours late. If more than 2 hours, wait for next dose (don't double this dose).
- Contraceptive—Consult your doctor. You may need to use another birth-control method until next period.

What drug does:
- Creates a uterine lining similar to pregnancy that prevents bleeding.
- Suppresses a pituitary gland hormone responsible for ovulation.
- Stimulates cervical mucus, which stops sperm penetration and prevents pregnancy.

Continued next column

OVERDOSE

SYMPTOMS:
Nausea, vomiting, fluid retention, breast discomfort or enlargement, vaginal bleeding.
WHAT TO DO:
Overdose unlikely to threaten life. If person takes much larger amount than prescribed, call doctor, poison-control center or hospital emergency room for instructions.

Time lapse before drug works:
- Menstrual disorders—24 to 48 hours.
- Contraception—3 weeks.

Don't take with:
See Interaction column and consult doctor.

POSSIBLE ADVERSE REACTIONS OR SIDE EFFECTS

SYMPTOMS	WHAT TO DO
Life-threatening: Blood clot in leg, brain or lung.	Seek emergency treatment immediately.
Common: Appetite or weight changes, swollen ankles or feet, unusual tiredness or weakness.	Continue. Tell doctor at next visit.
Infrequent: • Prolonged vaginal bleeding.	Discontinue. Call doctor right away.
• Depression.	Continue. Call doctor when convenient.
• Acne, increased facial or body hair, nausea, breast tenderness.	Continue. Tell doctor at next visit.
Rare: Rash, stomach or side pain, jaundice.	Discontinue. Call doctor right away.

WARNINGS & PRECAUTIONS

Don't take if:
- You are allergic to any progestin hormone.
- You may be pregnant.
- You have liver or gallbladder disease.
- You have had thrombophlebitis, embolism or stroke.
- You have unexplained vaginal bleeding.
- You have had breast or uterine cancer.

Before you start, consult your doctor:
- If you have heart or kidney disease.
- If you have diabetes.
- If you have a seizure disorder.
- If you suffer migraines.
- If you are easily depressed.

Over age 60:
Not recommended.

Pregnancy:
May harm child. Discontinue at first sign of pregnancy.

Breast-feeding:
Drug passes into milk. Avoid drug or discontinue nursing until you finish medicine. Consult doctor for advice on maintaining milk supply.

Infants & children:
Use only for female children under medical supervision.

Prolonged use:
No problems expected.

Skin & sunlight:
No problems expected.

Driving, piloting or hazardous work:
No problems expected.

Discontinuing:
Consult doctor. This medicine stays in the body and causes fetal abnormalities. Wait at least 3 months before becoming pregnant.

Others:
- Patients with diabetes must be monitored closely.
- Symptoms of blood clot in leg, brain or lung are: chest, groin, leg pain; sudden, severe headache; loss of coordination; vision change; shortness of breath; slurred speech.

POSSIBLE INTERACTION WITH OTHER DRUGS

GENERIC NAME OR DRUG CLASS	COMBINED EFFECT
Antihistamines	Decreased norethindrone effect.
Oxyphenbutazone	Decreased norethindrone effect.
Phenobarbital	Decreased norethindrone effect.
Phenothiazines	Increased phenothiazine effect.
Phenylbutazone	Decreased norethindrone effect.

POSSIBLE INTERACTION WITH OTHER SUBSTANCES

INTERACTS WITH	COMBINED EFFECT
Alcohol:	None expected.
Beverages:	None expected.
Cocaine:	Decreased norethindrone effect.
Foods: Salt.	Fluid retention.
Marijuana:	Possible menstrual irregularities or bleeding between periods.
Tobacco:	Possible blood clots in lung, brain, legs. Avoid.

NORETHINDRONE ACETATE

BRAND NAMES

Aygestin	Norlutate Acetate
Micronor	Norlutin
Norlutate	Nor-O.-D.

BASIC INFORMATION

Habit forming? No
Prescription needed? Yes
Available as generic? No
Drug class: Female sex hormone (progestin)

USES

- Treatment for menstrual or uterine disorders caused by progestin imbalance.
- Contraceptive.
- Treatment for cancer of breast and uterus.

DOSAGE & USAGE INFORMATION

How to take:
Tablet or capsule—Swallow with liquid or food to lessen stomach irritation. You may crumble tablet or open capsule.

When to take:
At the same time each day.

If you forget a dose:
- Menstrual disorders—Take up to 2 hours late. If more than 2 hours, wait for next dose (don't double this dose).
- Contraceptive—Consult your doctor. You may need to use another birth-control method until next period.

What drug does:
- Creates a uterine lining similar to pregnancy that prevents bleeding.
- Suppresses a pituitary gland hormone responsible for ovulation.
- Stimulates cervical mucus, which stops sperm penetration and prevents pregnancy.

Continued next column

OVERDOSE

SYMPTOMS:
Nausea, vomiting, fluid retention, breast discomfort or enlargement, vaginal bleeding.
WHAT TO DO:
Overdose unlikely to threaten life. If person takes much larger amount than prescribed, call doctor, poison-control center or hospital emergency room for instructions.

Time lapse before drug works:
- Menstrual disorders—24 to 48 hours.
- Contraception—3 weeks.
- Cancer—May require 2 to 3 months.

Don't take with:
See Interaction column and consult doctor.

POSSIBLE ADVERSE REACTIONS OR SIDE EFFECTS

SYMPTOMS	WHAT TO DO
Life-threatening:	
Blood clot in leg, brain or lung.	Seek emergency treatment immediately.
Common:	
Appetite or weight changes, swollen ankles or feet, unusual tiredness or weakness.	Continue. Tell doctor at next visit.
Infrequent:	
• Prolonged vaginal bleeding.	Discontinue. Call doctor right away.
• Depression.	Continue. Call doctor when convenient.
• Acne, increased facial or body hair, nausea, breast tenderness.	Continue. Tell doctor at next visit.
Rare:	
Rash, stomach or side pain, jaundice.	Discontinue. Call doctor right away.

WARNINGS & PRECAUTIONS

Don't take if:
- You are allergic to any progestin hormone.
- You may be pregnant.
- You have liver or gallbladder disease.
- You have had thrombophlebitis, embolism or stroke.
- You have unexplained vaginal bleeding.
- You have had breast or uterine cancer.

Before you start, consult your doctor:
- If you have heart or kidney disease.
- If you have diabetes.
- If you have a seizure disorder.
- If you suffer migraines.
- If you are easily depressed.

Over age 60:
Not recommended.

Pregnancy:
May harm child. Discontinue at first sign of pregnancy.

Breast-feeding:
Drug passes into milk. Avoid drug or discontinue nursing until you finish medicine. Consult doctor for advice on maintaining milk supply.

Infants & children:
Use only for female children under medical supervision.

Prolonged use:
No problems expected.

Skin & sunlight:
No problems expected.

Driving, piloting or hazardous work:
No problems expected.

Discontinuing:
Consult doctor. This medicine stays in the body and causes fetal abnormalities. Wait at least 3 months before becoming pregnant.

Others:
- Patients with diabetes must be monitored closely.
- Symptoms of blood clot in leg, brain or lung are: chest, groin, leg pain; sudden, severe headache; loss of coordination; vision change; shortness of breath; slurred speech.

POSSIBLE INTERACTION WITH OTHER DRUGS

GENERIC NAME OR DRUG CLASS	COMBINED EFFECT
Antihistamines	Decreased norethindrone acetate effect.
Oxyphenbutazone	Decreased norethindrone acetate effect.
Phenobarbital	Decreased norethindrone acetate effect.
Phenothiazines	Increased phenothiazine effect.
Phenylbutazone	Decreased norethindrone acetate effect.

POSSIBLE INTERACTION WITH OTHER SUBSTANCES

INTERACTS WITH	COMBINED EFFECT
Alcohol:	None expected.
Beverages:	None expected.
Cocaine:	Decreased norethindrone acetate effect.
Foods: Salt.	Fluid retention.
Marijuana:	Possible menstrual irregularities or bleeding between periods.
Tobacco:	Possible blood clots in lung, brain, legs. Avoid.

NORFLOXACIN

BRAND NAMES

Noroxin

BASIC INFORMATION

Habit forming? No
Prescription needed? Yes
Available as generic? No
Drug class: Antibacterial, fluoroquinolones

 USES

- Treats infections of the kidney, ureter, bladder and urethra. Cure rate reported to be about 95%.
- Treats traveler's diarrhea, gonorrhea, bacterial gastroenteritis.

 DOSAGE & USAGE INFORMATION

How to take:
Tablets or capsules—On an empty stomach 1 hour before or 2 hours after meals. Take with lots of water.

When to take:
As directed. Usually every 12 hours on empty stomach.

If you forget a dose:
Take as soon as you remember up to 6 hours late. If more than 6 hours, wait for next scheduled dose (don't double this dose).

What drug does:
Interferes with nutrient necessary for growth and reproduction of bacteria. Will not kill viruses.

Time lapse before drug works:
2 hours to peak level in blood. May require 7 to 21 days of treatment to cure infections.

Don't take with:
- Food, antacids.
- See Interaction column and consult doctor.

 OVERDOSE

SYMPTOMS:
Seizures
WHAT TO DO:
- Dial 0 (operator) or 911 (emergency) for an ambulance or medical help. Then give first aid immediately.
- See emergency information on inside covers.

 POSSIBLE ADVERSE REACTIONS OR SIDE EFFECTS

SYMPTOMS	WHAT TO DO
Life-threatening: None expected.	
Common: None expected.	
Infrequent: Nausea, abdominal pain, heartburn, insomnia, diarrhea, dizziness, fatigue, rash, vulvar irritation, crystals in urine.	Discontinue. Call doctor right away.
Rare: Anemia, joint pain, joint swelling.	Discontinue. Call doctor right away.

WARNINGS & PRECAUTIONS

Don't take if:
You are allergic to any fluoroquinolone.

Before you start, consult your doctor:
If you have chronic kidney disease with loss of kidney function.

Over age 60:
Adverse reactions and side effects may be more frequent and severe than in younger persons. Ask doctor about smaller doses.

Pregnancy:
Safety to unborn child unestablished. Avoid if possible.

Breast-feeding:
Drug passes into milk. Avoid drug or discontinue nursing until you finish medicine. Consult doctor for advice on maintaining milk supply.

Infants & children:
Use only under close medical supervision.

Prolonged use:
No problems expected.

Skin & sunlight:
No problems expected.

Driving, piloting or hazardous work:
Avoid if you feel drowsy or dizzy.

Discontinuing:
No problems expected.

Others:
No problems expected.

POSSIBLE INTERACTION WITH OTHER DRUGS

GENERIC NAME OR DRUG CLASS	COMBINED EFFECT
Antacids	Decreased absorption of norfloxacin.
Probenecid	Enhances effect of norfloxacin.

POSSIBLE INTERACTION WITH OTHER SUBSTANCES

INTERACTS WITH	COMBINED EFFECT
Alcohol:	Decreased effect of norfloxacin.
Beverages:	None expected.
Cocaine:	Decreased effect of norfloxacin.
Foods:	None expected.
Marijuana:	Decreased effect of norfloxacin.
Tobacco:	May stimulate irritated gastrointestinal tract. Avoid.

NORGESTREL

BRAND NAMES

Lo-Ovral   Ovrette
Ovral

BASIC INFORMATION

Habit forming? No
Prescription needed? Yes
Available as generic? No
Drug class: Female sex hormone (progestin)

 ## USES

Contraceptive.

 ## DOSAGE & USAGE INFORMATION

How to take:
Tablet or capsule—Swallow with liquid or food to lessen stomach irritation. You may crumble tablet or open capsule.

When to take:
At the same time each day.

If you forget a dose:
Consult your doctor. You may need to use another birth-control method until next period, then resume norgestrel.

What drug does:
- Creates a uterine lining similar to pregnancy that prevents bleeding.
- Suppresses a pituitary gland hormone responsible for ovulation.
- Stimulates cervical mucus, which stops sperm penetration and prevents pregnancy.

Time lapse before drug works:
3 weeks. Use another method of birth control until then.

Don't take with:
See Interaction column and consult doctor.

 ## OVERDOSE

SYMPTOMS:
Nausea, vomiting, fluid retention, breast discomfort or enlargement, vaginal bleeding.
WHAT TO DO:
Overdose unlikely to threaten life. If person takes much larger amount than prescribed, call doctor, poison-control center or hospital emergency room for instructions.

 ## POSSIBLE ADVERSE REACTIONS OR SIDE EFFECTS

SYMPTOMS	WHAT TO DO
Life-threatening: Blood clot in leg, brain or lung.	Seek emergency treatment immediately.
Common: Appetite or weight changes, swollen ankles or feet, unusual tiredness or weakness.	Continue. Tell doctor at next visit.
Infrequent: • Prolonged vaginal bleeding.	Discontinue. Call doctor right away.
• Depression.	Continue. Call doctor when convenient.
• Acne, increased facial or body hair, nausea, breast tenderness.	Continue. Tell doctor at next visit.
Rare: Rash, stomach or side pain, jaundice.	Discontinue. Call doctor right away.

WARNINGS & PRECAUTIONS

Don't take if:
- You are allergic to any progestin hormone.
- You may be pregnant.
- You have liver or gallbladder disease.
- You have had thrombophlebitis, embolism or stroke.
- You have unexplained vaginal bleeding.
- You have had breast or uterine cancer.

Before you start, consult your doctor:
- If you have heart or kidney disease.
- If you have diabetes.
- If you have a seizure disorder.
- If you suffer migraines.
- If you are easily depressed.

Over age 60:
Not recommended.

Pregnancy:
May harm child. Discontinue at first sign of pregnancy.

Breast-feeding:
Drug passes into milk. Avoid drug or discontinue nursing until you finish medicine. Consult doctor for advice on maintaining milk supply.

Infants & children:
Use only for female children under medical supervision.

Prolonged use:
No problems expected.

Skin & sunlight:
No problems expected.

Driving, piloting or hazardous work:
No problems expected.

Discontinuing:
Consult doctor. This medicine stays in the body and causes fetal abnormalities. Wait at least 3 months before becoming pregnant.

Others:
- Patients with diabetes must be monitored closely.
- Symptoms of blood clot in leg, brain or lung are: chest, groin, leg pain; sudden, severe headache; loss of coordination; vision change; shortness of breath; slurred speech.

POSSIBLE INTERACTION WITH OTHER DRUGS

GENERIC NAME OR DRUG CLASS	COMBINED EFFECT
Antihistamines	Decreased norgestrel effect.
Oxyphenbutazone	Decreased norgestrel effect.
Phenobarbital	Decreased norgestrel effect.
Phenothiazines	Increased phenothiazine effect.
Phenylbutazone	Decreased norgestrel effect.

POSSIBLE INTERACTION WITH OTHER SUBSTANCES

INTERACTS WITH	COMBINED EFFECT
Alcohol:	None expected.
Beverages:	None expected.
Cocaine:	Decreased norgestrel effect.
Foods: Salt.	Fluid retention.
Marijuana:	Possible menstrual irregularities or bleeding between periods.
Tobacco:	Possible blood clots in lung, brain, legs. Avoid.

NYLIDRIN

BRAND NAMES

Arlidin
Arlidin Forte
Circlidrin

Pervadil
PMS Nylidrin
Rolidrin

BASIC INFORMATION

Habit forming? No
Prescription needed? Yes
Available as generic? Yes
Drug class: Vasodilator

USES

- Improves poor circulation in extremities.
- Reduces dizziness caused by poor circulation in inner ear.

DOSAGE & USAGE INFORMATION

How to take:
Tablet—Swallow with liquid or food to lessen stomach irritation. If you can't swallow whole, crumble tablet and take with liquid or food.

When to take:
At the same times each day.

If you forget a dose:
Take as soon as you remember up to 2 hours late. If more than 2 hours, wait for next scheduled dose (don't double this dose).

What drug does:
Stimulates nerves that dilate blood vessels, increasing oxygen and nutrients.

Continued next column

OVERDOSE

SYMPTOMS:
Blood-pressure drop; nausea, vomiting; rapid, irregular heartbeat, chest pain; blurred vision; metallic taste.
WHAT TO DO:
- **Dial 0 (operator) or 911 (emergency) for an ambulance or medical help. Then give first aid immediately.**
- **If patient is unconscious and not breathing, give mouth-to-mouth breathing. If there is no heartbeat, use cardiac massage and mouth-to-mouth breathing (CPR). Don't try to make patient vomit. If you can't get help quickly, take patient to nearest emergency facility.**
- **See emergency information on inside covers.**

Time lapse before drug works:
10 to 30 minutes.

Don't take with:
See Interaction column and consult doctor.

POSSIBLE ADVERSE REACTIONS OR SIDE EFFECTS

SYMPTOMS	WHAT TO DO
Life-threatening: None expected.	
Common: • Chest pain.	Discontinue. Call doctor right away.
• Blurred vision, fever, low blood pressure on standing, decreased or difficult urination.	Continue. Call doctor when convenient.
• Metallic taste.	Continue. Tell doctor at next visit.
Infrequent: • Rapid or irregular heartbeat.	Discontinue. Call doctor right away.
• Dizziness, weakness, tiredness.	Continue. Call doctor when convenient.
Rare: • Shakiness, chills.	Discontinue. Call doctor right away.
• Headache, flushed face, nausea, vomiting, nervousness.	Continue. Call doctor when convenient.

WARNINGS & PRECAUTIONS

Don't take if:
- You are allergic to any vasodilator drugs.
- You have had a heart attack or stroke within 4 weeks.
- You have an active peptic ulcer.

Before you start, consult your doctor:
- If you have had heart disease, heart-rhythm disorders (especially rapid heartbeat), a stroke or poor circulation to the brain.
- If you have glaucoma.
- If you have an overactive thyroid gland.
- If you plan to become pregnant within medication period.
- If you use tobacco.

Over age 60:
Adverse reactions and side effects may be more frequent and severe than in younger persons.

Pregnancy:
No proven harm to unborn child. Avoid if possible.

Breast-feeding:
No proven problems. Consult doctor.

Infants & children:
Not recommended.

Prolonged use:
No problems expected.

Skin & sunlight:
No problems expected.

Driving, piloting or hazardous work:
Don't drive or pilot aircraft until you learn how medicine affects you. Don't work around dangerous machinery. Don't climb ladders or work in high places. Danger increases if you drink alcohol or take medicine affecting alertness and reflexes, such as antihistamines, tranquilizers, sedatives, pain medicine, narcotics and mind-altering drugs.

Discontinuing:
Don't discontinue without consulting doctor. If your condition worsens, contact your doctor immediately. Dose may require gradual reduction if you have taken drug for a long time. Doses of other drugs may also require adjustment.

Others:
No problems expected.

POSSIBLE INTERACTION WITH OTHER DRUGS

GENERIC NAME OR DRUG CLASS	COMBINED EFFECT
Beta-adrenergic blockers	Decreased effect of nylidrin.
Phenothiazines	Increased blood level of phenothiazines.

POSSIBLE INTERACTION WITH OTHER SUBSTANCES

INTERACTS WITH	COMBINED EFFECT
Alcohol:	Possible increased stomach-acid secretion. Use with caution.
Beverages:	None expected.
Cocaine:	Increased adverse effects of nylidrin.
Foods:	None expected.
Marijuana:	None expected.
Tobacco:	Decreased nylidrin effect. Worsens circulation. Avoid.

NYSTATIN

BRAND NAMES

Achrostatin V	Mytrex
Candex	Nadostine
Declostatin	Nilstat
Korostatin	Nyaderm
Mycolog	Nystaform
Mycostatin	Nystex
Myco-Triacet	O-V statin
Mykinac	Terrastatin

BASIC INFORMATION

Habit forming? No
Prescription needed? Yes
Available as generic? Yes
Drug class: Antifungal

 USES

Treatment of fungus infections susceptible to nystatin.

 DOSAGE & USAGE INFORMATION

How to take:
- Tablet or capsule—Swallow with liquid. If you can't swallow whole, crumble tablet or open capsule and take with liquid or food.
- Suppositories—Remove wrapper and moisten suppository with water. Gently insert larger end into vagina. Push well into vagina with finger.
- Ointment, cream or lotion—Use as directed by doctor and label.
- Liquid—Take as directed. Instruction varies by preparation.

When to take:
At the same time each day.

If you forget a dose:
Take as soon as you remember up to 2 hours late. If more than 2 hours, wait for next scheduled dose (don't double this dose).

Continued next column

 OVERDOSE

SYMPTOMS:
Mild overdose may cause nausea, vomiting, diarrhea.
WHAT TO DO:
Overdose unlikely to threaten life. If person takes much larger amount than prescribed, call doctor, poison-control center or hospital emergency room for instructions.

What drug does:
Prevents growth and reproduction of fungus.

Time lapse before drug works:
Begins immediately. May require 3 weeks for maximum benefit, depending on location and severity of infection.

Don't take with:
See Interaction column and consult doctor.

 POSSIBLE ADVERSE REACTIONS OR SIDE EFFECTS

SYMPTOMS	WHAT TO DO
Life-threatening:	
None expected.	
Common:	
(at high doses)	
Nausea, stomach pain, vomiting, diarrhea.	Discontinue. Call doctor right away.
Infrequent:	
Mild irritation, itch at application site.	Discontinue. Call doctor right away.
Rare:	
None expected.	

WARNINGS & PRECAUTIONS

Don't take if:
You are allergic to nystatin.

Before you start, consult your doctor:
If you plan to become pregnant within medication period.

Over age 60:
No problems expected.

Pregnancy:
No proven harm to unborn child. Avoid if possible.

Breast-feeding:
No proven problems. Consult doctor.

Infants & children:
No problems expected.

Prolonged use:
No problems expected.

Skin & sunlight:
No problems expected.

Driving, piloting or hazardous work:
No problems expected.

Discontinuing:
Don't discontinue without doctor's advice until you complete prescribed dose, even though symptoms diminish or disappear.

Others:
No problems expected.

POSSIBLE INTERACTION WITH OTHER DRUGS

GENERIC NAME OR DRUG CLASS	COMBINED EFFECT
None	

POSSIBLE INTERACTION WITH OTHER SUBSTANCES

INTERACTS WITH	COMBINED EFFECT
Alcohol:	None expected.
Beverages:	None expected.
Cocaine:	None expected.
Foods:	None expected.
Marijuana:	None expected.
Tobacco:	None expected.

ORPHENADRINE

BRAND NAMES

Banflex	Neocyten
Disipal	Norflex
Flexoject	O-Flex
Flexon	Orflagen
K-Flex	Orphenate
Marflex	Ro-Orphena
Myolin	Tega-Flex
Myotrol	X-Otag

BASIC INFORMATION

Habit forming? No
Prescription needed?
  U.S.: Yes
  Canada: No
Available as generic? Yes
Drug class: Muscle relaxant, anticholinergic,
      antihistamine, antiparkinsonism

 USES

- Reduces muscle-strain discomfort.
- Relieves symptoms of Parkinson's disease.

 DOSAGE & USAGE INFORMATION

How to take:
Tablet—Swallow with liquid. If you can't swallow whole, crumble tablet and take with liquid or food.

When to take:
At the same times each day.

If you forget a dose:
Take as soon as you remember up to 6 hours late. If more than 6 hours, wait for next scheduled dose (don't double this dose).

What drug does:
Sedative and analgesic effects reduce spasm and pain in skeletal muscles.

Continued next column

 OVERDOSE

SYMPTOMS:
Fainting, confusion, widely dilated pupils, rapid pulse, convulsions, coma.
WHAT TO DO:
- **Dial 0 (operator) or 911 (emergency) for an ambulance or medical help. Then give first aid immediately.**
- **See emergency information on inside covers.**

Time lapse before drug works:
1 to 2 hours.

Don't take with:
See Interaction column and consult doctor.

 POSSIBLE ADVERSE REACTIONS OR SIDE EFFECTS

SYMPTOMS	WHAT TO DO
Life-threatening:	
None expected.	
Common:	
None expected.	
Infrequent:	
• Weakness, headache, dizziness, drowsiness, agitation, tremor, confusion, rapid or pounding heartbeat.	Discontinue. Call doctor right away.
• Dry mouth, nausea, vomiting, constipation, urinary hesitancy or retention.	Continue. Call doctor when convenient.
Rare:	
Rash, itchy skin, blurred vision, dilated pupils.	Discontinue. Call doctor right away.

WARNINGS & PRECAUTIONS

Don't take if:
You are allergic to orphenadrine.

Before you start, consult your doctor:
- If you have glaucoma.
- If you have myasthenia gravis.
- If you have difficulty emptying bladder.
- If you have had heart disease or heart-rhythm disturbance.
- If you have had a peptic ulcer.

Over age 60:
Adverse reactions and side effects may be more frequent and severe than in younger persons.

Pregnancy:
No proven harm to unborn child. Avoid if possible.

Breast-feeding:
No proven problems. Consult doctor.

Infants & children:
Not recommended for children younger than 12.

Prolonged use:
Increased internal-eye pressure.

Skin & sunlight:
No problems expected.

Driving, piloting or hazardous work:
Don't drive or pilot aircraft until you learn how medicine affects you. Don't work around dangerous machinery. Don't climb ladders or work in high places. Danger increases if you drink alcohol or take medicine affecting alertness and reflexes, such as antihistamines, tranquilizers, sedatives, pain medicine, narcotics and mind-altering drugs.

Discontinuing:
May be unnecessary to finish medicine. Follow doctor's instructions.

Others:
No problems expected.

POSSIBLE INTERACTION WITH OTHER DRUGS

GENERIC NAME OR DRUG CLASS	COMBINED EFFECT
Anticholinergics	Increased anticholinergic effect.
Antidepressants (tricyclic)	Increased sedation.
Chlorpromazine	Hypoglycemia (low blood sugar).
Griseofulvin	Decreased griseofulvin effect.
Levodopa	Increased effect of levodopa. (Improves effectiveness in treating Parkinson's disease.)
Nitrates	Increased internal-eye pressure.
Phenylbutazone	Decreased phenylbutazone effect.
Potassium supplements	Increased possibility of intestinal ulcers with oral potassium tablets.
Propoxyphene	Possible confusion, nervousness, tremors.
Terfenadine	Possible increased orphenadrine effect.

POSSIBLE INTERACTION WITH OTHER SUBSTANCES

INTERACTS WITH	COMBINED EFFECT
Alcohol:	Increased drowsiness. Avoid.
Beverages:	None expected.
Cocaine:	Decreased orphenadrine effect. Avoid.
Foods:	None expected.
Marijuana:	Increased drowsiness, mouth dryness, muscle weakness, fainting.
Tobacco:	None expected.

ORPHENADRINE, ASPIRIN & CAFFEINE

BRAND NAMES

Back-Ese   Norgesic Forte
Norgesic

BASIC INFORMATION

Habit forming? Yes
Prescription needed? Yes
Available as generic? No
**Drug class: Stimulant, vasoconstrictor,
      muscle relaxant, analgesic,
      anti-inflammatory**

USES

- Reduces muscle-strain discomfort.
- Reduces pain, fever, inflammation.
- Relieves swelling, stiffness, joint pain.
- Treatment for drowsiness and fatigue.

DOSAGE & USAGE INFORMATION

How to take:
Tablet or capsule—Swallow with liquid. If you
can't swallow whole, crumble tablet or open
capsule and take with liquid or food.

When to take:
At the same times each day.

If you forget a dose:
Take as soon as you remember up to 2 hours
late. If more than 2 hours, wait for next
scheduled dose (don't double this dose).

What drug does:
- Sedative and analgesic effects reduce spasm
  and pain in skeletal muscles.
- Affects hypothalamus, the part of the brain
  which regulates temperature by dilating small
  blood vessels in skin.
- Prevents clumping of platelets (small blood
  cells) so blood vessels remain open.

Continued next column

OVERDOSE

SYMPTOMS:
**Fainting, confusion, widely dilated pupils,
rapid pulse, ringing in ears, nausea,
vomiting, dizziness, fever, deep and rapid
breathing, excitement, rapid heartbeat,
hallucinations, coma.**
WHAT TO DO:
- **Dial 0 (operator) or 911 (emergency) for an
  ambulance or medical help. Then give first
  aid immediately.**
- **See emergency information on inside
  covers.**

- Decreases prostaglandin effect.
- Suppresses body's pain messages.
- Constricts blood-vessel walls.
- Stimulates central nervous system.

Time lapse before drug works:
1 hour.

Don't take with:
- Tetracyclines. Space doses 1 hour apart.
- Non-prescription drugs without consulting
  doctor.
- See Interaction column and consult doctor.

POSSIBLE ADVERSE REACTIONS OR SIDE EFFECTS

SYMPTOMS	WHAT TO DO
Life-threatening:	
Hives, rash, intense itching, faintness soon after a dose (anaphylaxis).	Seek emergency treatment immediately.
Common:	
• Nausea, vomiting, abdominal cramps, nervousness, urgent urination, low blood sugar (hunger, anxiety, cold sweats, rapid pulse).	Discontinue. Call doctor right away.
• Ringing in ears, heartburn, indigestion, insomnia.	Continue. Call doctor when convenient.
Infrequent:	
• Weakness, headache, dizziness, drowsiness, agitation, tremor, confusion, irregular heartbeat.	Discontinue. Call doctor right away.
• Dry mouth, constipation.	Continue. Call doctor when convenient.
Rare:	
• Black or bloody vomit.	Discontinue. Seek emergency treatment.
• Change in vision; blurred vision; black, bloody or tarry stool; bloody urine; jaundice; dilated pupils.	Discontinue. Call doctor right away.
• Drowsiness.	Continue. Call doctor when convenient.

WARNINGS & PRECAUTIONS

Don't take if:
- You need to restrict sodium in your diet.
  Buffered effervescent tablets and sodium
  salicylate are high in sodium.

- Aspirin has a strong vinegar-like odor, which means it has decomposed.
- You have a peptic ulcer of stomach or duodenum, a bleeding disorder, heart disease.
- You are allergic to any stimulant or orphenadrine.

Before you start, consult your doctor:
- If you have had stomach or duodenal ulcers, gout, heart disease or heart-rhythm disturbance, peptic ulcer.
- If you have asthma, nasal polyps, irregular heartbeat, hypoglycemia (low blood sugar), epilepsy, glaucoma, myasthenia gravis, difficulty emptying bladder.

Over age 60:
- More likely to cause hidden bleeding in stomach or intestines. Watch for dark stools.
- Adverse reactions and side effects may be more frequent and severe than in younger persons.

Pregnancy:
Risk to unborn child outweighs drug benefits. Don't use.

Breast-feeding:
Drug passes into milk. Avoid drug or discontinue nursing until you finish medicine. Consult doctor for advice on maintaining milk supply.

Infants & children:
- Overdose frequent and severe. Keep bottles out of children's reach.
- Consult doctor before giving to persons under age 18 who have fever and discomfort of viral illness, especially chicken pox and influenza. Probably increases risk of Reye's syndrome.
- Not recommended for children younger than 12.

Prolonged use:
- Kidney damage. Periodic kidney-function test recommended.
- Stomach ulcers more likely.
- Increased internal-eye pressure.

Skin & sunlight:
Aspirin combined with sunscreen may decrease sunburn.

Driving, piloting or hazardous work:
Don't drive or pilot aircraft until you learn how medicine affects you. Don't work around dangerous machinery. Don't climb ladders or work in high places. Danger increases if you drink alcohol or take medicine affecting alertness and reflexes, such as antihistamines, tranquilizers, sedatives, pain medicine, narcotics and mind-altering drugs.

Discontinuing:
- For chronic illness—Don't discontinue without doctor's advice until you complete prescribed dose, even though symptoms diminish or disappear.
- May be unnecessary to finish medicine if you take it for a short-term illness. Follow doctor's instructions.

Others:
- Aspirin can complicate surgery, pregnancy, labor and delivery, and illness.
- For arthritis—Don't change dose without consulting doctor.
- Urine tests for blood sugar may be inaccurate.
- May produce or aggravate fibrocystic breast disease in women.

 ## POSSIBLE INTERACTION WITH OTHER DRUGS

GENERIC NAME OR DRUG CLASS	COMBINED EFFECT
Acebutolol	Decreased antihypertensive effect of acebutolol.
Allopurinol	Decreased allopurinol effect.
Antacids	Decreased aspirin effect.
Anticholinergics	Increased anticholinergic effect.
Anticoagulants	Increased anticoagulant effect. Abnormal bleeding.

Continued page 969

 ## POSSIBLE INTERACTION WITH OTHER SUBSTANCES

INTERACTS WITH	COMBINED EFFECT
Alcohol:	Possible stomach irritation and bleeding, increased drowsiness. Avoid.
Beverages: Caffeine drinks.	Increased caffeine effect.
Cocaine:	Decreased orphenadrine effect. Overstimulation. Avoid.
Foods:	No proven problems.
Marijuana:	Increased effect of drugs. May lead to dangerous, rapid heartbeat. Increased dry mouth. Avoid.
Tobacco:	Increased heartbeat. Avoid.

OXACILLIN

BRAND NAMES

Bactocill   Prostaphlin

BASIC INFORMATION

Habit forming? No
Prescription needed? Yes
Available as generic? Yes
Drug class: Antibiotic (penicillin)

USES

Treatment of bacterial infections that are susceptible to oxacillin.

DOSAGE & USAGE INFORMATION

How to take:
- Tablets or capsules—Swallow with liquid on an empty stomach 1 hour before or 2 hours after eating.
- Liquid—Take with cold beverage. Liquid form is perishable and effective for only 7 days at room temperature. Effective for 14 days if stored in refrigerator. Don't freeze.

When to take:
Follow instructions on prescription label or side of package. Doses should be evenly spaced. For example, 4 times a day means every 6 hours.

If you forget a dose:
Take as soon as you remember. Continue regular schedule.

What drug does:
Destroys susceptible bacteria. Does not kill viruses.

Time lapse before drug works:
May be several days before medicine affects infection.

Don't take with:
See Interaction column and consult doctor.

OVERDOSE

SYMPTOMS:
Severe diarrhea, nausea or vomiting.
WHAT TO DO:
Overdose unlikely to threaten life. If person takes much larger amount than prescribed, call doctor, poison-control center or hospital emergency room for instructions.

POSSIBLE ADVERSE REACTIONS OR SIDE EFFECTS

SYMPTOMS	WHAT TO DO
Life-threatening:	
Hives, rash, intense itching, faintness soon after a dose (anaphylaxis).	Seek emergency treatment immediately.
Common:	
Dark or discolored tongue.	Continue. Tell doctor at next visit.
Infrequent:	
Mild nausea, vomiting, diarrhea.	Continue. Call doctor when convenient.
Rare:	
Unexplained bleeding.	Discontinue. Call doctor right away.

WARNINGS & PRECAUTIONS

Don't take if:
You are allergic to oxacillin, cephalosporin antibiotics, other penicillins or penicillamine. Life-threatening reaction may occur.

Before you start, consult your doctor:
If you are allergic to any substance or drug.

Over age 60:
You may have skin reactions, particularly around genitals and anus.

Pregnancy:
Studies inconclusive on harm to unborn child. Animal studies show fetal abnormalities. Decide with your doctor whether drug benefits justify risk to unborn child.

Breast-feeding:
Drug passes into milk. Child may become sensitive to penicillins and have allergic reactions to penicillin drugs. Avoid oxacillin or discontinue nursing until you finish medicine. Consult doctor for advice on maintaining milk supply.

Infants & children:
No problems expected.

Prolonged use:
You may become more susceptible to infections caused by germs not responsive to oxacillin.

Skin & sunlight:
No problems expected.

Driving, piloting or hazardous work:
Usually not dangerous. Most hazardous reactions likely to occur a few minutes after taking oxacillin.

Discontinuing:
Don't discontinue without doctor's advice until you complete prescribed dose, even though symptoms diminish or disappear.

Others:
No problems expected.

POSSIBLE INTERACTION WITH OTHER DRUGS

GENERIC NAME OR DRUG CLASS	COMBINED EFFECT
Beta-adrenergic blockers	Increased chance of anaphylaxis (see emergency information on inside front cover).
Chloramphenicol	Decreased effect of both drugs.
Erythromycins	Decreased effect of both drugs.
Loperamide	Decreased oxacillin effect.
Paromomycin	Decreased effect of both drugs.
Tetracyclines	Decreased effect of both drugs.
Troleandomycin	Decreased effect of both drugs.

POSSIBLE INTERACTION WITH OTHER SUBSTANCES

INTERACTS WITH	COMBINED EFFECT
Alcohol:	Occasional stomach irritation.
Beverages:	None expected.
Cocaine:	No proven problems.
Foods:	None expected.
Marijuana:	No proven problems.
Tobacco:	None expected.

OXAZEPAM

BRAND NAMES

Apo-Oxazepam	Serax
Ox-Pam	Zapex

BASIC INFORMATION

Habit forming? Yes
Prescription needed? Yes
Available as generic? No
Drug class: Tranquilizer (benzodiazepine)

 USES

Treatment for nervousness or tension.

 DOSAGE & USAGE INFORMATION

How to take:
Tablet or capsule—Swallow with liquid. If you can't swallow whole, crumble tablet or open capsule and take with liquid or food.

When to take:
At the same time each day, according to instructions on prescription label.

If you forget a dose:
Take as soon as you remember up to 2 hours late. If more than 2 hours, wait for next scheduled dose (don't double this dose).

What drug does:
Affects limbic system of brain—part that controls emotions.

Time lapse before drug works:
2 hours. May take 6 weeks for full benefit.

Don't take with:
See Interaction column and consult doctor.

 OVERDOSE

SYMPTOMS:
Drowsiness, weakness, tremor, stupor, coma.
WHAT TO DO:
- Dial 0 (operator) or 911 (emergency) for an ambulance or medical help. Then give first aid immediately.
- If patient is unconscious and not breathing, give mouth-to-mouth breathing. If there is no heartbeat, use cardiac massage and mouth-to-mouth breathing (CPR). Don't try to make patient vomit. If you can't get help quickly, take patient to nearest emergency facility.
- See emergency information on inside covers.

 POSSIBLE ADVERSE REACTIONS OR SIDE EFFECTS

SYMPTOMS	WHAT TO DO
Life-threatening:	
None expected.	
Common:	
Clumsiness, drowsiness, dizziness.	Continue. Call doctor when convenient.
Infrequent:	
• Hallucinations, confusion, depression, irritability, rash, itchy skin, change in vision.	Discontinue. Call doctor right away.
• Constipation or diarrhea, nausea, vomiting, difficult urination.	Continue. Call doctor when convenient.
Rare:	
• Slow heartbeat, difficult breathing.	Discontinue. Seek emergency treatment.
• Mouth, throat ulcers; jaundice.	Discontinue. Call doctor right away.

WARNINGS & PRECAUTIONS

Don't take if:
- You are allergic to any benzodiazepine.
- You have myasthenia gravis.
- You are active or recovering alcoholic.
- Patient is younger than 6 months.

Before you start, consult your doctor:
- If you have liver, kidney or lung disease.
- If you have diabetes, epilepsy or porphyria.

Over age 60:
Adverse reactions and side effects may be more frequent and severe than in younger persons. You need smaller doses for shorter periods of time. May develop agitation, rage or "hangover" effect.

Pregnancy:
Risk to unborn child outweighs drug benefits. Don't use.

Breast-feeding:
Drug passes into milk. Avoid drug or discontinue nursing until you finish medicine. Consult doctor for advice on maintaining milk supply.

Infants & children:
Use only under medical supervision for children older than 6 months.

Prolonged use:
May impair liver function.

Skin & sunlight:
No problems expected.

Driving, piloting or hazardous work:
Don't drive or pilot aircraft until you learn how medicine affects you. Don't work around dangerous machinery. Don't climb ladders or work in high places. Danger increases if you drink alcohol or take medicine affecting alertness and reflexes.

Discontinuing:
Don't discontinue without consulting doctor. Dose may require gradual reduction if you have taken drug for a long time. Doses of other drugs may also require adjustment.

Others:
- Hot weather, heavy exercise and profuse sweat may reduce excretion and cause overdose.
- Blood sugar may rise in diabetics, requiring insulin adjustment.

POSSIBLE INTERACTION WITH OTHER DRUGS

GENERIC NAME OR DRUG CLASS	COMBINED EFFECT
Anticonvulsants	Change in seizure frequency or severity.
Antidepressants	Increased sedative effect of both drugs.
Antihistamines	Increased sedative effect of both drugs.
Antihypertensives	Excessively low blood pressure.
Cimetidine	Excess sedation.
Disulfiram	Increased oxazepam effect.
Dronabinol	Increased effects of both drugs. Avoid.
MAO inhibitors	Convulsions, deep sedation, rage.
Molindone	Increased tranquilizer effect.
Narcotics	Increased sedative effect of both drugs.
Sedatives	Increased sedative effect of both drugs.
Sleep inducers	Increased sedative effect of both drugs.
Terfenadine	Possible oversedation.
Tranquilizers	Increased sedative effect of both drugs.

POSSIBLE INTERACTION WITH OTHER SUBSTANCES

INTERACTS WITH	COMBINED EFFECT
Alcohol:	Heavy sedation. Avoid.
Beverages:	None expected.
Cocaine:	Decreased oxazepam effect.
Foods:	None expected.
Marijuana:	Heavy sedation. Avoid.
Tobacco:	Decreased oxazepam effect.

OXPRENOLOL

BRAND NAMES

Slow-trasicor   Trasicor

BASIC INFORMATION

Habit forming? No
Prescription needed? Yes
Available as generic? No
Drug class: Beta-adrenergic blocker

 ## USES

- Reduces frequency and severity of angina attacks.
- Stabilizes irregular heartbeat.
- Lowers blood pressure.
- Reduces frequency of migraine headaches. (Does not relieve headache pain.)

 ## DOSAGE & USAGE INFORMATION

How to take:
Tablet or capsule—Swallow with liquid. If you can't swallow whole, crumble tablet or open capsule and take with liquid or food.

When to take:
With meals or immediately after.

If you forget a dose:
Take as soon as you remember. Return to regular schedule, but allow 3 hours between doses.

What drug does:
- Blocks actions of sympathetic nervous system.
- Lowers heart's oxygen requirements.
- Slows nerve impulses through heart.
- Reduces blood-vessel contraction in several major organs and glands.

Time lapse before drug works:
1 to 4 hours.

Continued next column

 ## OVERDOSE

SYMPTOMS:
Weakness, slow or weak pulse, blood-pressure drop, fainting, convulsions, cold and sweaty skin.
WHAT TO DO:
- **Dial 0 (operator) or 911 (emergency) for an ambulance or medical help. Then give first aid immediately.**
- **See emergency information on inside covers.**

Don't take with:
Non-prescription drugs or drugs in interaction column without consulting doctor.

 ## POSSIBLE ADVERSE REACTIONS OR SIDE EFFECTS

SYMPTOMS	WHAT TO DO
Life-threatening:	
None expected.	
Common:	
• Pulse slower than 50 beats per minute.	Discontinue. Call doctor right away.
• Drowsiness, numbness or tingling of fingers or toes, dizziness, diarrhea, nausea, fatigue, weakness.	Continue. Call doctor when convenient.
• Dry skin, eyes or mouth; cold hands, feet.	Continue. Tell doctor at next visit.
Infrequent:	
• Hallucinations, nightmares, insomnia, headache, difficult breathing.	Discontinue. Call doctor right away.
• Confusion, depression, reduced alertness.	Continue. Call doctor when convenient.
• Constipation.	Continue. Tell doctor at next visit.
Rare:	
• Rash, sore throat, fever.	Discontinue. Call doctor right away.
• Unexplained bleeding or bruising.	Continue. Call doctor when convenient.

 ## WARNINGS & PRECAUTIONS

Don't take if:
- You are allergic to any beta-adrenergic blocker.
- You have asthma.
- You have hay-fever symptoms.
- You have taken MAO inhibitors in past 2 weeks.

Before you start, consult your doctor:
- If you have heart disease or poor circulation to extremities.
- If you have hay fever, asthma, chronic bronchitis or emphysema.
- If you have overactive thyroid function.
- If you have impaired liver or kidney function.
- If you will have surgery within 2 months, including dental surgery, requiring general or spinal anesthesia.
- If you have diabetes or hypoglycemia.

Over age 60:
Adverse reactions and side effects may be more frequent and severe than in younger persons.

Pregnancy:
Risk to unborn child outweighs drug benefits. Don't use.

Breast-feeding:
Drug passes into milk. Avoid drug or discontinue nursing until you finish medicine. Consult doctor for advice on maintaining milk supply.

Infants & children:
Not recommended. Safety and dosage have not been established.

Prolonged use:
Weakens heart-muscle contractions.

Skin & sunlight:
No problems expected.

Driving, piloting or hazardous work:
Don't drive or pilot aircraft until you learn how medicine affects you. Don't work around dangerous machinery. Don't climb ladders or work in high places. Danger increases if you drink alcohol or take medicine affecting alertness and reflexes.

Discontinuing:
Don't discontinue without consulting doctor. Dose may require gradual reduction if you have taken drug for a long time. Doses of other drugs may also require adjustment.

Others:
May mask hypoglycemia.

POSSIBLE INTERACTION WITH OTHER DRUGS

GENERIC NAME OR DRUG CLASS	COMBINED EFFECT
Albuterol	Decreased albuterol effect and beta-adrenergic blocking effect.
Anesthetics used in surgery	Increased antihypertensive effect.
Antidiabetics	May make blood-sugar levels difficult to control.
Antihypertensives	Increased antihypertensive effect.
Anti-inflammatory drugs	Decreased antihypertensive effect of oxprenolol.
Calcium-channel blockers	May worsen congestive heart failure.
Clonidine	Possible blood-pressure rise once clonidine is discontinued.
Digitalis preparations	Increased **or** decreased heart rate. Improves irregular heartbeat.
Diuretics	Increased antihypertensive effect.
Ketoprofen	Decreased antihypertensive effect of oxprenolol
MAO inhibitors	Possible excessive blood-pressure rise once MAO inhibitor is discontinued.
Molindone	Increased tranquilizer effect.
Pentoxifylline	Increased antihypertensive effect.
Reserpine	Possible excessively low blood pressure and slow heartbeat.
Suprofen	Decreased antihypertensive effect of oxprenolol.
Sympathomimetics	Decreased effects of both drugs.
Timolol eyedrops	Possible increased oxprenolol effect.
Xanthine bronchodilators	Decreased effects of both drugs.

POSSIBLE INTERACTION WITH OTHER SUBSTANCES

INTERACTS WITH	COMBINED EFFECT
Alcohol:	Excessive blood pressure drop. Avoid.
Beverages:	None expected.
Cocaine:	Irregular heartbeat. Avoid.
Foods:	None expected.
Marijuana:	Daily use—Impaired circulation to hands and feet.
Tobacco:	Possible irregular heartbeat.

OXTRIPHYLLINE & GUAIFENESIN

BRAND NAMES

Brondecon   Brondelate

BASIC INFORMATION

Habit forming? No
Prescription needed? Yes
Available as generic? No
Drug class: Bronchodilator (xanthine), cough/cold preparation

 USES

- Treatment for bronchial asthma symptoms.
- Loosens mucus in respiratory passages from allergies and infections.

 DOSAGE & USAGE INFORMATION

How to take:
Tablet or capsule—Swallow with liquid. If you can't swallow whole, crumble tablet or open capsule and take with liquid or food.

When to take:
Most effective taken on empty stomach 1 hour before or 2 hours after eating. However, may take with food to lessen stomach upset.

If you forget a dose:
Take as soon as you remember up to 2 hours late. If more than 2 hours, wait for next scheduled dose (don't double this dose).

What drug does:
- Relaxes and expands bronchial tubes.
- Increases production of watery fluids to thin mucus so it can be coughed out or absorbed.

Time lapse before drug works:
15 to 30 minutes.

Don't take with:
- Any stimulant.
- See Interaction column and consult doctor.

 OVERDOSE

SYMPTOMS:
Restlessness, irritability, confusion, delirium, convulsions, rapid pulse, nausea, vomiting, coma.
WHAT TO DO:
- **Dial 0 (operator) or 911 (emergency) for an ambulance or medical help. Then give first aid immediately.**
- **See emergency information on inside covers.**

 POSSIBLE ADVERSE REACTIONS OR SIDE EFFECTS

SYMPTOMS	WHAT TO DO
Life-threatening: Difficult breathing, irregular or fast heartbeat.	Discontinue. Seek emergency treatment.
Common: Headache, irritability, nervousness, restlessness, insomnia, nausea, vomiting, abdominal pain, drowsiness.	Continue. Call doctor when convenient.
Infrequent: • Hives, rash, red or flushed face, diarrhea.	Discontinue. Call doctor right away.
• Dizziness, lightheadedness, appetite loss.	Continue. Call doctor when convenient.
Rare: None expected.	

WARNINGS & PRECAUTIONS

Don't take if:
- You are allergic to any cough or cold preparation containing guaifenesin or any bronchodilator.
- You have an active peptic ulcer.

Before you start, consult your doctor:
- If you have had impaired kidney or liver function.
- If you gastritis, peptic ulcer, high blood pressure or heart disease.
- If you take medication for gout.

Over age 60:
Adverse reactions and side effects may be more frequent and severe than in younger persons. For drug to work, you must drink 8 to 10 glasses of fluid per day.

Pregnancy:
Risk to unborn child outweighs drug benefits. Don't use.

Breast-feeding:
Drug passes into milk. Avoid drug or discontinue nursing until you finish medicine. Consult doctor for advice on maintaining milk supply.

Infants & children:
Use only under medical supervision.

Prolonged use:
Stomach irritation.

Skin & sunlight:
No problems expected.

Driving, piloting or hazardous work:
Avoid if lightheaded or dizzy. Otherwise, no problems expected.

Discontinuing:
May be unnecessary to finish medicine. Follow doctor's instructions.

Others:
No problems expected.

POSSIBLE INTERACTION WITH OTHER DRUGS

GENERIC NAME OR DRUG CLASS	COMBINED EFFECT
Allopurinol	Decreased allopurinol effect.
Anticoagulants	Risk of bleeding.
Ephedrine	Increased effect of both drugs.
Epinephrine	Increased effect of both drugs.
Erythromycin	Increased bronchodilator effect.
Furosemide	Increased furosemide effect.
Lincomycins	Increased bronchodilator effect.
Lithium	Decreased lithium effect.
Probenecid	Decreased effect of both drugs.
Propranolol	Decreased bronchodilator effect.
Rauwolfia alkaloids	Rapid heartbeat.
Sulfinpyrazone	Decreased sulfinpyrazone effect.
Troleandomycin	Increased bronchodilator effect.

POSSIBLE INTERACTION WITH OTHER SUBSTANCES

INTERACTS WITH	COMBINED EFFECT
Alcohol:	None expected.
Beverages: Caffeine drinks.	Nervousness and insomnia. You must drink 8 to 10 glasses of fluid per day for drug to work.
Cocaine:	Excess stimulation. Avoid.
Foods:	None expected.
Marijuana:	Slightly increased antiasthmatic effect of bronchodilator.
Tobacco:	Decreased bronchodilator effect and harmful for all conditions requiring bronchodilator treatment. Avoid.

OXYMETAZOLINE

BRAND NAMES

See complete list of brand names in the *Brand Name Directory,* page 953.

BASIC INFORMATION

Habit forming? No
Prescription needed? No
Available as generic? Yes
Drug class: Sympathomimetic

 ## USES

Relieves congestion of nose, sinuses and throat from allergies and infections.

 ## DOSAGE & USAGE INFORMATION

How to take:
Nasal solution, nasal spray—Use as directed on label. Avoid contamination. Don't use same container for more than 1 person.

When to take:
When needed, no more often than every 4 hours.

If you forget a dose:
Take as soon as you remember. Wait 4 hours for next dose.

What drug does:
Constricts walls of small arteries in nose, sinuses and eustachian tubes.

Time lapse before drug works:
5 to 30 minutes.

Continued next column

 ## OVERDOSE

SYMPTOMS:
Headache, sweating, anxiety, agitation, rapid and irregular heartbeat.
WHAT TO DO:
- Dial 0 (operator) or 911 (emergency) for an ambulance or medical help. Then give first aid immediately.
- If patient is unconscious and not breathing, give mouth-to-mouth breathing. If there is no heartbeat, use cardiac massage and mouth-to-mouth breathing (CPR). If you can't get help quickly, take patient to nearest emergency facility.
- See emergency information on inside covers.

Don't take with:
- Non-prescription drugs for allergy, cough or cold without consulting doctor.
- See Interaction column and consult doctor.

 ## POSSIBLE ADVERSE REACTIONS OR SIDE EFFECTS

SYMPTOMS	WHAT TO DO
Life-threatening: None expected.	
Common: Runny, stuffy, burning, dry or stinging nose; sneezing; fast, irregular or pounding heartbeat.	Continue. Call doctor when convenient.
Infrequent: Headache or lightheadedness, insomnia, nervousness.	Continue. Call doctor when convenient.
Rare: None expected.	

WARNINGS & PRECAUTIONS

Don't take if:
You are allergic to any sympathomimetic nasal spray.

Before you start, consult your doctor:
• If you have heart disease or high blood pressure.
• If you have diabetes.
• If you have overactive thyroid.
• If you have taken MAO inhibitors in past 2 weeks.

Over age 60:
Adverse reactions and side effects may be more frequent and severe than in younger persons.

Pregnancy:
No proven harm to unborn child. Avoid if possible.

Breast-feeding:
No proven problems. Consult doctor.

Infants & children:
Don't give to children younger than 2.

Prolonged use:
Drug may lose effectiveness, cause increased congestion ("rebound effect," see Glossary) and irritate nasal membranes.

Skin & sunlight:
No problems expected.

Driving, piloting or hazardous work:
No problems expected.

Discontinuing:
May be unnecessary to finish medicine. Follow doctor's instructions.

Others:
No problems expected.

POSSIBLE INTERACTION WITH OTHER DRUGS

GENERIC NAME OR DRUG CLASS	COMBINED EFFECT
Acebutolol	Decreased effects of both drugs.
Antidepressants (tricyclics)	Increased oxymetazoline effect.
MAO inhibitors	Dangerous blood-pressure rise.
Minoxidil	Decreased minoxidil effect.
Nitrates	Possible decreased effects of both drugs.
Oxprenolol	Decreased effects of both drugs.
Sympathomimetics	Increased effect of both drugs, especially harmful side effects.

POSSIBLE INTERACTION WITH OTHER SUBSTANCES

INTERACTS WITH	COMBINED EFFECT
Alcohol:	None expected.
Beverages: Caffeine drinks.	Nervousness or insomnia.
Cocaine:	Overstimulation. Avoid.
Foods:	None expected.
Marijuana:	Overstimulation. Avoid.
Tobacco:	None expected.

OXYPHENBUTAZONE

BRAND NAMES

Oxalid   Tandearil
Oxybutazone

BASIC INFORMATION

Habit forming? No
Prescription needed? Yes
Available as generic? Yes
Drug class: Anti-inflammatory (non-steroid)

 USES

- Treatment for joint pain, stiffness, inflammation and swelling of arthritis and gout.
- Pain reliever.
- Treatment for dysmenorrhea (painful or difficult menstruation).

 DOSAGE & USAGE INFORMATION

How to take:
Tablet or capsule—Swallow with liquid or food to lessen stomach irritation. If you can't swallow whole, crumble tablet or open capsule and take with liquid or food.

When to take:
At the same times each day.

If you forget a dose:
Take as soon as you remember up to 2 hours late. If more than 2 hours, wait for next scheduled dose (don't double this dose).

What drug does:
Reduces tissue concentration of prostaglandins (hormones which produce inflammation and pain).

Time lapse before drug works:
Begins in 4 to 24 hours. May require 3 weeks regular use for maximum benefit.

Continued next column

 OVERDOSE

SYMPTOMS:
Confusion, agitation, incoherence, convulsions, possible hemorrhage from stomach or intestine, coma.
WHAT TO DO:
- **Dial 0 (operator) or 911 (emergency) for an ambulance or medical help. Then give first aid immediately.**
- **See emergency information on inside covers.**

Don't take with:
See Interaction column and consult doctor.

 POSSIBLE ADVERSE REACTIONS OR SIDE EFFECTS

SYMPTOMS	WHAT TO DO
Life-threatening: None expected.	
Common:	
• Dizziness, stomach upset.	Continue. Call doctor when convenient.
• Headache.	Continue. Tell doctor at next visit.
Infrequent: Depression, drowsiness, ringing in ears, constipation or diarrhea, vomiting, swollen feet or legs.	Continue. Call doctor when convenient.
Rare:	
• Convulsions; confusion; rash, hives or itchy skin; blurred vision; sore throat, fever, mouth ulcers; black stools; vomiting blood; difficult breathing; tightness in chest; unusual bleeding or bruising; blood in urine.	Discontinue. Call doctor right away.
• Urgent, frequent, painful or difficult urination; fatigue, weakness; weight gain.	Continue. Call doctor when convenient.

WARNINGS & PRECAUTIONS

Don't take if:
- You are allergic to aspirin or any non-steroid, anti-inflammatory drug.
- You have gastritis, peptic ulcer, enteritis, ileitis, ulcerative colitis.
- Patient is younger than 15.

Before you start, consult your doctor:
- If you have epilepsy.
- If you have Parkinson's disease.
- If you have been mentally ill.
- If you have had kidney disease or impaired kidney function, asthma, high blood pressure, heart failure, temporal arthritis, or polymyalgia rheumatica.

Over age 60:
Adverse reactions and side effects may be more frequent and severe than in younger persons.

Pregnancy:
Studies inconclusive on harm to unborn child. Animal studies show fetal abnormalities. Decide with your doctor whether drug benefits justify risk to unborn child.

Breast-feeding:
Drug filters into milk. May harm child. Avoid.

Infants & children:
Not recommended for those younger than 15. Use only under medical supervision.

Prolonged use:
- Eye damage.
- May cause rare bone-marrow damage, jaundice, reduced hearing.
- Periodic blood counts recommended if you use a long time.

Skin & sunlight:
No problems expected.

Driving, piloting or hazardous work:
Don't drive or pilot aircraft until you learn how medicine affects you. Don't work around dangerous machinery. Don't climb ladders or work in high places. Danger increases if you drink alcohol or take medicine affecting alertness and reflexes, such as antihistamines, tranquilizers, sedatives, pain medicine, narcotics and mind-altering drugs.

Discontinuing:
Don't discontinue without consulting doctor. Dose may require gradual reduction if you have taken drug for a long time. Doses of other drugs may also require adjustment.

Others:
No problems expected.

POSSIBLE INTERACTION WITH OTHER DRUGS

GENERIC NAME OR DRUG CLASS	COMBINED EFFECT
Acebutolol	Decreased antihypertensive effect of acebutolol.
Anticoagulants (oral)	Increased anticoagulant effect.
Antidiabetics (oral)	Increased antidiabetic effect.
Aspirin	Possible stomach ulcer.
Chloroquine	Possible skin toxicity.
Digitoxin	Decreased digitoxin effect.
Gold compounds	Possible increased likelihood of kidney damage.
Hydroxychloroquine	Possible skin toxicity.
Ketoprofen	Increased possibility of internal bleeding.
Methotrexate	Increased toxicity of both drugs to bone marrow.
Minoxidil	Decreased minoxidil effect.
Oxprenolol	Decreased antihypertensive effect of oxprenolol.
Penicillamine	Possible toxicity.
Phenytoin	Possible toxic phenytoin effect.
Trimethoprim	Possible bone-marrow toxicity.

POSSIBLE INTERACTION WITH OTHER SUBSTANCES

INTERACTS WITH	COMBINED EFFECT
Alcohol:	Possible stomach ulcer or bleeding.
Beverages:	None expected.
Cocaine:	None expected.
Foods:	None expected.
Marijuana:	Increased pain relief from oxyphenbutazone.
Tobacco:	None expected.

PANCREATIN, PEPSIN, BILE SALTS, HYOSCYAMINE, ATROPINE, SCOPOLAMINE & PHENOBARBITAL

BRAND NAMES

Donnazyme

BASIC INFORMATION

Habit forming? Yes
Prescription needed? Yes
Available as generic? No
Drug class: Digestant, sedative, anticholinergic

USES

- Replaces deficient digestive enzymes.
- Sometimes used to relieve indigestion.

DOSAGE & USAGE INFORMATION

How to take:
Tablet—Swallow with liquid or food to lessen stomach irritation. If you can't swallow whole, crumble tablet and take with food or liquid.

When to take:
With or after meals.

If you forget a dose:
Skip it and resume schedule. Don't double-dose.

What drug does:
Blocks nerve impulses at parasympathetic nerve endings, preventing smooth muscle contraction and gland secretions.

Time lapse before drug works:
30 to 60 minutes.

Don't take with:
- Any medicine that will decrease mental alertness or reflexes, such as alcohol, other mind-altering drugs, cough/cold medicines,

Continued next column

OVERDOSE

SYMPTOMS:
Hallucinations, excitement, irregular heartbeat (too fast or too slow), fainting, collapse, coma.
WHAT TO DO:
- **Dial 0 (operator) or 911 (emergency) for an ambulance or medical help. Then give first aid immediately.**
- **See emergency information on inside covers.**

antihistamines, allergy medicine, sedatives, tranquilizers (sleeping pills or "downers") barbiturates, seizure medicine, narcotics, other prescription medicine for pain, muscle relaxants, anesthetics.
- See Interaction column and consult doctor.

POSSIBLE ADVERSE REACTIONS OR SIDE EFFECTS

SYMPTOMS	WHAT TO DO
Life-threatening: None expected.	
Common:	
• Constipation, decreased sweating, headache.	Discontinue. Call doctor right away.
• Drowsiness, dry mouth, frequent urination.	Continue. Call doctor when convenient.
Infrequent:	
• Blurred vision.	Discontinue. Call doctor right away.
• Diminished sex drive, swallowing difficulty, sensitivity to light, insomnia.	Continue. Call doctor when convenient.
Rare:	
• Jaundice; unusual bleeding or bruising; swollen feet and ankles; abdominal pain; sore throat, fever, mouth sores; rash; hives; vomiting; joint pain; eye pain; diarrhea; blood in urine.	Discontinue. Call doctor right away.
• Unusual tiredness.	Continue. Call doctor when convenient.

WARNINGS & PRECAUTIONS

Don't take if:
- You are allergic to any of the drugs in this combination.
- You have trouble with stomach bloating, difficulty emptying your bladder completely, narrow-angle glaucoma, severe ulcerative colitis, porphyria.

Before you start, consult your doctor:
- If you have open-angle glaucoma, angina, chronic bronchitis or asthma, liver disease, hiatal hernia, enlarged prostate, myasthenia gravis, epilepsy, kidney or liver damage, anemia, chronic pain.

- If you will have surgery within 2 months, including dental surgery, requiring general or spinal anesthesia.

Over age 60:
Adverse reactions and side effects may be more frequent and severe than in younger persons

Pregnancy:
Risk to unborn child outweighs drug benefits. Don't use.

Breast-feeding:
Drug passes into milk. Avoid drug or discontinue nursing until you finish medicine. Consult doctor for advice on maintaining milk supply.

Infants & children:
Use only under medical supervision.

Prolonged use:
- Chronic constipation, possible fecal impaction.
- May cause addiction, anemia, chronic intoxication.
- May lower body temperature, making exposure to cold temperatures hazardous.

Skin & sunlight:
May cause rash or intensify sunburn in areas exposed to sun or sunlamp.

Driving, piloting or hazardous work:
Don't drive or pilot aircraft until you learn how medicine affects you. Don't work around dangerous machinery. Don't climb ladders or work in high places. Danger increases if you drink alcohol or take medicine affecting alertness and reflexes, such as antihistamines, tranquilizers, sedatives, pain medicine, narcotics and mind-altering drugs.

Discontinuing:
- May be unnecessary to finish medicine. Follow doctor's instructions.
- If you develop withdrawal symptoms of hallucinations, agitation or sleeplessness after discontinuing, call doctor right away.

Others:
- Potential for abuse.
- Enzyme deficiencies probably better treated with identified separate substances rather than a mixture of components.

 POSSIBLE INTERACTION WITH OTHER DRUGS

GENERIC NAME OR DRUG CLASS	COMBINED EFFECT
Amantadine	Increased atropine effect.
Anticholinergics (other)	Increased anticholinergic effect.
Anticoagulants (oral)	Decreased anticoagulant effect.
Antidepressants (tricyclic)	Decreased antidepressant effect. Possible dangerous oversedation.
Antidiabetics (oral)	Increased phenobartital effect.
Antihistamines	Increased atropine effect.
Anti-inflammatory drugs (non-steroidal)	Decreased anti-inflammatory effect.
Aspirin	Decreased aspirin effect.
Beta-adrenergic blockers	Decreased effect of beta-adrenergic blocker.
Contraceptives (oral)	Decreased contraceptive effect.
Cortisone drugs	Decreased cortisone effect.
Dronabinol	Increased phenobarbital effect.
Griseofulvin	Decreased griseofulvin effect.
Haloperidol	Increased internal-eye pressure.

Continued page 970

 POSSIBLE INTERACTION WITH OTHER SUBSTANCES

INTERACTS WITH	COMBINED EFFECT
Alcohol:	Possible fatal oversedation. Avoid.
Beverages:	None expected.
Cocaine:	Excessively rapid heartbeat. Avoid.
Foods:	None expected.
Marijuana:	Excessive sedation, drowsiness and dry mouth.
Tobacco:	May increase stomach acidity, decreasing the effectiveness of Donnazyme. Avoid.

PANCRELIPASE

BRAND NAMES

Cotazym	Ku-Zyme HP
Cotazym-S	Lipancreatin
Festal II	Pancrease
Ilozyme	Viokase

BASIC INFORMATION

Habit forming? No
Prescription needed? Yes
Available as generic? No
Drug class: Enzyme (pancreatic)

USES

- Replaces pancreatic enzyme deficiency caused by surgery or disease.
- Treats fatty stools (steatorrhea).

DOSAGE & USAGE INFORMATION

How to take:
- Capsules—Swallow whole. Do not take with milk or milk products.
- Powder—Sprinkle on liquid or soft food.

When to take:
Before meals.

If you forget a dose:
Take as soon as you remember up to 2 hours late. If more than 2 hours, wait for next scheduled dose (don't double this dose).

What drug does:
Enhances digestion of proteins, carbohydrates and fats.

Time lapse before drug works:
30 minutes.

Don't take with:
See Interaction column and consult doctor.

OVERDOSE

SYMPTOMS:
Shortness of breath, wheezing, diarrhea.
WHAT TO DO:
Overdose unlikely to threaten life. If person takes much larger amount than prescribed, call doctor, poison-control center or hospital emergency room for instructions.

POSSIBLE ADVERSE REACTIONS OR SIDE EFFECTS

SYMPTOMS	WHAT TO DO
Life-threatening:	
None expected.	
Common:	
None expected.	
Infrequent:	
None expected.	
Rare:	
• Rash, hives, blood in urine, swollen feet or legs.	Discontinue. Call doctor right away.
• Nausea, joint pain.	Continue. Call doctor when convenient.

WARNINGS & PRECAUTIONS

Don't take if:
You are allergic to pancreatin, pancrelipase, or pork.

Before you start, consult your doctor:
If you take any other medicines.

Over age 60:
Adverse reactions and side effects may be more frequent and severe than in younger persons.

Pregnancy:
Risk to unborn child outweighs drug benefits. Don't use.

Breast-feeding:
Drug passes into milk. Avoid drug or discontinue nursing until you finish medicine. Consult doctor for advice on maintaining milk supply.

Infants & children:
Under close medical supervision only.

Prolonged use:
No additional problems expected.

Skin & sunlight:
No problems expected.

Driving, piloting or hazardous work:
No problems expected.

Discontinuing:
Don't discontinue without consulting doctor. Dose may require gradual reduction if you have taken drug for a long time. Doses of other drugs may also require adjustment.

Others:
If you take powder form, avoid inhaling.

POSSIBLE INTERACTION WITH OTHER DRUGS

GENERIC NAME OR DRUG CLASS	COMBINED EFFECT
Calcium carbonate antacids.	Decreased effect of pancrelipase.
Iron preparations	Decreased iron absorption.
Magnesium hydroxide antacids	Decreased effect of pancrelipase.

POSSIBLE INTERACTION WITH OTHER SUBSTANCES

INTERACTS WITH	COMBINED EFFECT
Alcohol:	Unknown.
Beverages: Milk.	Decreased effect of pancrelipase.
Cocaine:	Unknown.
Foods: Ice cream, milk products.	Decreased effect of pancrelipase.
Marijuana:	Decreased absorption of pancrelipase.
Tobacco:	Decreased absorption of pancrelipase.

PANTOTHENIC ACID (VITAMIN B-5)

BRAND AND GENERIC NAMES

CALCIUM
  PATOTHENATE
Dexol T.D.
Durasil

Pantholin
PANTOTHENIC ACID

Ingredients in numerous multiple
vitamin-mineral supplements.

BASIC INFORMATION

Habit forming? No
Prescription needed? No
Available as generic? Yes
Drug class: Vitamin supplement

 USES

Prevents and treats vitamin B-5 deficiency.

 DOSAGE & USAGE INFORMATION

How to take:
- Tablet or capsule—Swallow with liquid.
- Extended-release tablets—Swallow each dose whole with liquid.

When to take:
At the same times each day.

If you forget a dose:
Take as soon as you remember, then resume regular schedule.

What drug does:
Acts as co-enzyme in carbohydrate, protein and fat metabolism.

Time lapse before drug works:
15 to 20 minutes.

Don't take with:
- Levodopa—Small amounts of pantothenic acid will nullify levodopa effect. Carbidopa-levodopa combination not affected by this interaction.
- See Interaction column and consult doctor.

 OVERDOSE

SYMPTOMS:
None expected.
WHAT TO DO:
Overdose unlikely to threaten life.

 POSSIBLE ADVERSE REACTIONS OR SIDE EFFECTS

SYMPTOMS	WHAT TO DO
Life-threatening: None expected.	
Common: None expected.	
Infrequent: None expected.	
Rare: None expected.	

WARNINGS & PRECAUTIONS

Don't take if:
You are allergic to pantothenic acid.

Before you start, consult your doctor:
If you have hemophilia.

Over age 60:
No problems expected.

Pregnancy:
Don't exceed recommended dose.

Breast-feeding:
Don't exceed recommended dose.

Infants & children:
Don't exceed recommended dose.

Prolonged use:
Large doses for more than 1 month may cause toxicity.

Skin & sunlight:
No problems expected.

Driving, piloting or hazardous work:
No problems expected.

Discontinuing:
No problems expected.

Others:
Regular pantothenic acid supplements are recommended if you take chloramphenicol, cycloserine, ethionamide, hydralazine, immunosuppressants, isoniazid or penicillamine. These decrease pantothenic acid absorption and can cause anemia or tingling and numbness in hands and feet.

POSSIBLE INTERACTION WITH OTHER DRUGS

GENERIC NAME OR DRUG CLASS	COMBINED EFFECT
None expected.	

POSSIBLE INTERACTION WITH OTHER SUBSTANCES

INTERACTS WITH	COMBINED EFFECT
Alcohol:	None expected.
Beverages:	None expected.
Cocaine:	None expected.
Foods:	None expected.
Marijuana:	None expected.
Tobacco:	May decrease pantothenic acid absorption. Decreased pantothenic acid effect.

PAPAVERINE

BRAND NAMES

See complete list of brand names in the *Brand Name Directory,* page 954.

BASIC INFORMATION

Habit forming? No
Prescription needed? Yes
Available as generic? Yes
Drug class: Vasodilator

 ## USES

Improves poor circulation in the extremities or brain.

 ## DOSAGE & USAGE INFORMATION

How to take:
- Tablet or capsule—Swallow with liquid or food to lessen stomach irritation. If you can't swallow whole, crumble tablet or open capsule and take with liquid or food.
- Extended-release tablets or capsules—Swallow whole with liquid.
- Liquid—Follow label instructions.

When to take:
At the same times each day.

If you forget a dose:
Take as soon as you remember up to 2 hours late. If more than 2 hours, wait for next scheduled dose (don't double this dose).

What drug does:
Relaxes and expands blood-vessel walls, allowing better distribution of oxygen and nutrients.

Time lapse before drug works:
30 to 60 minutes.

Don't take with:
- Non-prescription drugs without consulting doctor.
- See Interaction column and consult doctor.

 ## OVERDOSE

SYMPTOMS:
Weakness, fainting, flush, sweating, stupor, irregular heartbeat.
WHAT TO DO:
- **Dial 0 (operator) or 911 (emergency) for an ambulance or medical help. Then give first aid immediately.**
- **See emergency information on inside covers.**

 ## POSSIBLE ADVERSE REACTIONS OR SIDE EFFECTS

SYMPTOMS	WHAT TO DO
Life-threatening:	
None expected.	
Common:	
• Drowsiness, dizziness, headache, flushed face, stomach irritation, indigestion, nausea, mild constipation, low blood pressure causing lethargy or dizziness (especially on change of position).	Continue. Call doctor when convenient.
• Dry mouth, throat.	Continue. Tell doctor at next visit.
Infrequent:	
• Rash, itchy skin, blurred or double vision, weakness.	Discontinue. Call doctor right away.
• Deep breathing, rapid heartbeat.	Continue. Call doctor when convenient.
Rare:	
Jaundice.	Discontinue. Call doctor right away.

WARNINGS & PRECAUTIONS

Don't take if:
You are allergic to any narcotic.

Before you start, consult your doctor:
- If you plan to become pregnant within medication period.
- If you have had a heart attack, heart disease, angina or stroke.
- If you have Parkinson's disease.

Over age 60:
Adverse reactions and side effects may be more frequent and severe than in younger persons.

Pregnancy:
No proven harm to unborn child. Avoid if possible.

Breast-feeding:
Drug filters into milk. May harm child. Avoid.

Infants & children:
Not recommended.

Prolonged use:
No problems expected.

Skin & sunlight:
No problems expected.

Driving, piloting or hazardous work:
Don't drive or pilot aircraft until you learn how medicine affects you. Don't work around dangerous machinery. Don't climb ladders or work in high places. Danger increases if you drink alcohol or take medicine affecting alertness and reflexes, such as antihistamines, tranquilizers, sedatives, pain medicine, narcotics and mind-altering drugs.

Discontinuing:
May be unnecessary to finish medicine. If drug does not help in 1 to 2 weeks, consult doctor about discontinuing.

Others:
- Periodic liver-function tests recommended.
- Internal eye-pressure measurements recommended if you have glaucoma.

POSSIBLE INTERACTION WITH OTHER DRUGS

GENERIC NAME OR DRUG CLASS	COMBINED EFFECT
Levodopa	Decreased levodopa effect.
Narcotics	Increased papaverine effect.
Pain relievers	Increased papaverine effect.
Sedatives	Increased papaverine effect.
Tranquilizers	Increased papaverine effect.

POSSIBLE INTERACTION WITH OTHER SUBSTANCES

INTERACTS WITH	COMBINED EFFECT
Alcohol:	None expected.
Beverages:	None expected.
Cocaine:	Decreased papaverine effect.
Foods:	None expected.
Marijuana:	None expected.
Tobacco:	Decrease in papaverine's dilation of blood vessels.

PARA-AMINOSALICYLIC ACID (PAS)

BRAND NAMES

Nemasol

Parasal

P.A.S.

P.A.S. Acid

Pasna

Teebacin

BASIC INFORMATION

Habit forming? No
Prescription needed? Yes
Available as generic? Yes
Drug class: Antitubercular

USES

Treatment for tuberculosis.

DOSAGE & USAGE INFORMATION

How to take:
- Tablet—Swallow with liquid or food to lessen stomach irritation.
- Powder—Dissolve dose in water. Stir well and drink all liquid.

When to take:
At the same times each day.

If you forget a dose:
Take as soon as you remember up to 2 hours late. If more than 2 hours, wait for next scheduled dose (don't double this dose).

What drug does:
- Prevents growth of TB germs.
- Makes TB germs more susceptible to other antituberculosis drugs.

Time lapse before drug works:
6 months.

Don't take with:
See Interaction column and consult doctor.

OVERDOSE

SYMPTOMS:
Nausea, vomiting, diarrhea; rapid breathing; convulsions.
WHAT TO DO:
- **Dial 0 (operator) or 911 (emergency) for an ambulance or medical help. Then give first aid immediately.**
- **See emergency information on inside covers.**

POSSIBLE ADVERSE REACTIONS OR SIDE EFFECTS

SYMPTOMS	WHAT TO DO
Life-threatening: None expected.	
Common:	
● Painful urination, chills, low back pain.	Discontinue. Call doctor right away.
● Diarrhea or stomach pain.	Continue. Call doctor when convenient.
Infrequent:	
● Confusion, blood in urine.	Discontinue. Call doctor right away.
● Headache; itchy, dry, puffy skin; light sensitivity; sore throat; fever; constipation or vomiting; swelling in front of neck; decreased sex drive in men; fatigue; weakness.	Continue. Call doctor when convenient.
● Menstrual irregularities.	Continue. Tell doctor at next visit.
Rare: Jaundice.	Discontinue. Call doctor right away.

648

WARNINGS & PRECAUTIONS

Don't take if:
- You are allergic to PAS, aspirin or other salicylates.
- Tablets have turned brownish or purplish.

Before you start, consult your doctor:
- If you have ulcers in stomach or duodenum.
- If you have liver or kidney disease.
- If you have epilepsy.
- If you have adrenal insufficiency.
- If you have heart disease or congestive heart failure.
- If you have cancer.
- If you have overactive thyroid.

Over age 60:
Adverse reactions and side effects may be more frequent and severe than in younger persons.

Pregnancy:
Risk to unborn child outweighs drug benefits. Don't use.

Breast-feeding:
No proven problems. Consult doctor.

Infants & children:
Use only under medical supervision.

Prolonged use:
Enlarged thyroid gland and decreased function.

Skin & sunlight:
No problems expected.

Driving, piloting or hazardous work:
No problems expected.

Discontinuing:
No problems expected.

Others:
- Treatment may need to continue for several years or indefinitely.
- Periodic blood tests and liver- and kidney-function studies recommended.

POSSIBLE INTERACTION WITH OTHER DRUGS

GENERIC NAME OR DRUG CLASS	COMBINED EFFECT
Aminobenzoic acid (PABA)	Decreased effect of PAS.
Anticoagulants (oral)	Increased anticoagulant effect.
Anticonvulsants (hydantoin)	Increased anticonvulsant effect.
Aspirin	Stomach irritation.
Barbiturates	Oversedation.
Folic acid	Decreased effect of folic acid.
Probenecid	Increased PAS effect. Possible toxicity.
Rifampin	Decreased rifampin effect.
Sulfa drugs	Decreased effect of sulfa drugs.
Sulfinpyrazone	Increased PAS effect. Possible toxicity.
Tetracyclines	Reduced absorption of PAS. Space doses 3 hours apart.

POSSIBLE INTERACTION WITH OTHER SUBSTANCES

INTERACTS WITH	COMBINED EFFECT
Alcohol:	Possible liver disease.
Beverages:	None expected
Cocaine:	None expected.
Foods:	None expected.
Marijuana:	None expected.
Tobacco:	None expected, but tobacco smoking may slow recovery. Avoid.

PARAMETHASONE

BRAND NAMES

Haldrone

BASIC INFORMATION

Habit forming? No
Prescription needed? Yes
Available as generic? No
Drug class: Cortisone drug (adrenal corticosteroid)

 USES

- Reduces inflammation caused by many different medical problems.
- Treatment for some allergic diseases, blood disorders, kidney diseases, asthma and emphysema.
- Replaces corticosteroid deficiencies.

 DOSAGE & USAGE INFORMATION

How to take:
Tablet—Swallow with liquid or food to lessen stomach irritation. If you can't swallow whole, crumble tablet and take with liquid or food.

When to take:
At the same times each day. Take once-a-day or once-every-other-day doses in mornings.

If you forget a dose:
- Several-doses-per-day prescription—Take as soon as you remember up to 2 hours late. If more than 2 hours, wait for next scheduled dose (don't double this dose).
- Once-a-day dose or less—Wait for next dose. Double this dose.

What drug does:
Decreases inflammatory responses.

Time lapse before drug works:
2 to 4 days.

Don't take with:
See Interaction column and consult doctor.

 OVERDOSE

SYMPTOMS:
Headache, convulsions, heart failure.

WHAT TO DO:
- Dial 0 (operator) or 911 (emergency) for an ambulance or medical help. Then give first aid immediately.
- Additional emergency information on inside covers.

 POSSIBLE ADVERSE REACTIONS OR SIDE EFFECTS

SYMPTOMS	WHAT TO DO
Life-threatening:	
None expected.	
Common:	
• Acne, poor wound healing, indigestion, nausea, vomiting, thirst.	Continue. Call doctor when convenient.
Infrequent:	
• Black, bloody or tarry stool.	Discontinue. Seek emergency treatment.
• Blurred vision, halos around lights, sore throat, fever, muscle cramps.	Discontinue. Call doctor right away.
• Mood change, insomnia, restlessness, frequent urination, weight gain, round face, fatigue, weakness, TB recurrence, irregular menstrual periods.	Continue. Call doctor when convenient.
Rare:	
• Irregular heartbeat.	Discontinue. Seek emergency treatment.
• Rash.	Discontinue. Call doctor right away.

 WARNINGS & PRECAUTIONS

Don't take if:
- You are allergic to any cortisone drug.
- You have tuberculosis or fungus infection.
- You have herpes infection of eyes, lips or genitals.

Before you start, consult your doctor:
- If you have had tuberculosis.
- If you have congestive heart failure.
- If you have diabetes.
- If you have peptic ulcer.
- If you have glaucoma.
- If you have underactive thyroid.
- If you have high blood pressure.
- If you have myasthenia gravis.
- If you have blood clots in legs or lungs.

Over age 60:
Adverse reactions and side effects may be more frequent and severe than in younger persons. Likely to aggravate edema, diabetes or ulcers. Likely to cause cataracts and osteoporosis (softening of the bones).

Pregnancy:
Risk to unborn child outweighs drug benefits. Don't use.

Breast-feeding:
Drug passes into milk. Avoid drug or discontinue nursing until you finish medicine. Consult doctor for advice on maintaining milk supply.

Infants & children:
Use only under medical supervision.

Prolonged use:
- Retards growth in children.
- Possible glaucoma, cataracts, diabetes, fragile bones and thin skin.
- Functional dependence.

Skin & sunlight:
No problems expected.

Driving, piloting or hazardous work:
No problems expected.

Discontinuing:
- Don't discontinue without doctor's advice until you complete prescribed dose, even though symptoms diminish or disappear.
- Drug affects your response to surgery, illness, injury or stress for 2 years after discontinuing. Tell anyone who takes medical care of you within 2 years about drug.

Others:
Avoid immunizations if possible.

POSSIBLE INTERACTION WITH OTHER DRUGS

GENERIC NAME OR DRUG CLASS	COMBINED EFFECT
Amphoterecin B	Potassium depletion.
Anticholinergics	Possible glaucoma.
Anticoagulants (oral)	Decreased anticoagulant effect.
Anticonvulsants (hydantoin)	Decreased paramethasone effect.
Antidiabetics (oral)	Decreased antidiabetic effect.
Antihistamines	Decreased paramethasone effect.
Aspirin	Increased paramethasone effect.
Barbiturates	Decreased paramethasone effect. Oversedation.
Beta-adrenergic blockers	Decreased paramethasone effect.
Chloral hydrate	Decreased paramethasone effect.

Chlorthalidone	Potassium depletion.
Cholinergics	Decreased cholinergic effect.
Contraceptives (oral)	Increased paramethasone effect.
Digitalis preparations	Dangerous potassium depletion. Possible digitalis toxicity.
Diuretics (thiazide)	Potassium depletion.
Ephedrine	Decreased paramethasone effect.
Estrogens	Increased paramethasone effect.
Ethacrynic acid	Potassium depletion.
Furosemide	Potassium depletion.
Glutethimide	Decreased paramethasone effect.
Indapamide	Possible excessive potassium loss, causing dangerous heartbeat irregularity.
Indomethacin	Increased paramethasone effect.
Insulin	Decreased insulin effect.
Isoniazid	Decreased isoniazid effect.
Oxyphenbutazone	Possible ulcers.
Phenylbutazone	Possible ulcers.
Potassium supplements	Decreased potassium effect.
Rifampin	Decreased paramethasone effect.
Sympathomimetics	Possible glaucoma.

POSSIBLE INTERACTION WITH OTHER SUBSTANCES

INTERACTS WITH	COMBINED EFFECT
Alcohol:	Risk of stomach ulcers.
Beverages:	No proven problems.
Cocaine:	Overstimulation. Avoid.
Foods:	No proven problems.
Marijuana:	Decreased immunity.
Tobacco:	Increased paramethasone effect. Possible toxicity.

PAREGORIC

BRAND NAMES

Brown Mixture	Kaoparin
CM with Paregoric	Opium Tincture
Diban	Parepectolin
Donnagel-PG	Pomalin

BASIC INFORMATION

Habit forming? Yes
Prescription needed? Yes
Available as generic? Yes
Drug class: Narcotic, antidiarrheal

 USES

Reduces intestinal cramps and diarrhea.

 DOSAGE & USAGE INFORMATION

How to take:
Drops or liquid—Dilute dose in beverage before swallowing.

When to take:
As needed for diarrhea, no more often than every 4 hours.

If you forget a dose:
Take as soon as you remember. Wait 4 hours for next dose.

What drug does:
Anesthetizes surface membranes of intestines and blocks nerve impulses.

Time lapse before drug works:
2 to 6 hours.

Don't take with:
See Interaction column and consult doctor.

 OVERDOSE

SYMPTOMS:
Deep sleep; slow breathing; slow pulse; flushed, warm skin; constricted pupils.
WHAT TO DO:
- **Dial 0 (operator) or 911 (emergency) for an ambulance or medical help. Then give first aid immediately.**
- **If patient is unconscious and not breathing, give mouth-to-mouth breathing. If there is no heartbeat, use cardiac massage and mouth-to-mouth breathing (CPR). Don't try to make patient vomit. If you can't get help quickly, take patient to nearest emergency facility.**
- **See emergency information on inside covers.**

 POSSIBLE ADVERSE REACTIONS OR SIDE EFFECTS

SYMPTOMS	WHAT TO DO
Life-threatening: None expected.	
Common: Dizziness, flushed face, unusual tiredness, difficult urination.	Continue. Call doctor when convenient.
Infrequent: Severe constipation, abdominal pain, vomiting.	Discontinue. Call doctor right away.
Rare:	
• Hives, rash, itchy skin, slow heartbeat, irregular breathing.	Discontinue. Call doctor right away.
• Depression.	Continue. Call doctor when convenient.

WARNINGS & PRECAUTIONS

Don't take if:
You are allergic to any narcotic.

Before you start, consult your doctor:
If you have impaired liver or kidney function.

Over age 60:
More likely to be drowsy, dizzy, unsteady or constipated.

Pregnancy:
No proven harm to unborn child. Avoid if possible.

Breast-feeding:
Drug filters into milk. May depress infant. Avoid.

Infants & children:
Use only under medical supervision.

Prolonged use:
Causes psychological and physical dependence.

Skin & sunlight:
No problems expected.

Driving, piloting or hazardous work:
Don't drive or pilot aircraft until you learn how medicine affects you. Don't work around dangerous machinery. Don't climb ladders or work in high places. Danger increases if you drink alcohol or take medicine affecting alertness and reflexes, such as antihistamines, tranquilizers, sedatives, pain medicine, narcotics and mind-altering drugs.

Discontinuing:
May be unnecessary to finish medicine. Follow doctor's instructions.

Others:
Great potential for abuse.

POSSIBLE INTERACTION WITH OTHER DRUGS

GENERIC NAME OR DRUG CLASS	COMBINED EFFECT
Analgesics	Increased analgesic effect.
Antidepressants	Increased sedative effect.
Antihistamines	Increased sedative effect.
Mind-altering drugs	Increased sedative effect.
Narcotics (other)	Increased narcotic effect.
Phenothiazines	Increased sedative effect of paregoric.
Sedatives	Excessive sedation.
Sleep inducers	Increased effect of sleep inducers.
Tranquilizers	Increased tranquilizer effect.

POSSIBLE INTERACTION WITH OTHER SUBSTANCES

INTERACTS WITH	COMBINED EFFECT
Alcohol:	Increases alcohol's intoxicating effect. Avoid.
Beverages:	None expected.
Cocaine:	None expected.
Foods:	None expected.
Marijuana:	Impairs physical and mental performance.
Tobacco:	None expected.

PARGYLINE & METHYCLOTHIAZIDE

BRAND NAMES

Eutron

BASIC INFORMATION

Habit forming? No
Prescription needed? Yes
Available as generic? No
Drug class: Antihypertensive, MAO inhibitor

 ## USES

- Controls, but doesn't cure, high blood pressure.
- Reduces fluid retention (edema) caused by conditions such as heart disorders and liver disease.

 ## DOSAGE & USAGE INFORMATION

How to take:
Tablet or capsule—Swallow with liquid. If you can't swallow whole, crumble tablet or open capsule and take with liquid or food. Don't exceed dose.

When to take:
At the same times each day.

If you forget a dose:
Take as soon as you remember up to 2 hours late. If more than 2 hours, wait for next scheduled dose (don't double this dose).

What drug does:
- Forces sodium and water excretion, reducing body fluid.
- Relaxes muscle cells of small arteries.
- Reduced body fluid and relaxed arteries lower blood pressure.
- Inhibits nerve transmissions in brain that may cause hypertension.

Time lapse before drug works:
4 to 6 weeks for maximum effect.

Continued next column

 ## OVERDOSE

SYMPTOMS:
Cramps, weakness, drowsiness, weak pulse, restlessness, agitation, fever, convulsions, coma.
WHAT TO DO:
- **Dial 0 (operator) or 911 (emergency) for an ambulance or medical help. Then give first aid immediately.**
- **See emergency information on inside covers.**

Don't take with:

- Non-prescription drugs without consulting doctor.
- Non-prescription diet pills, nose drops, medicine for asthma, cough, cold or allergy, or medicine containing caffeine or alcohol.
- See Interaction column and consult doctor.

 ## POSSIBLE ADVERSE REACTIONS OR SIDE EFFECTS

SYMPTOMS	WHAT TO DO
Life-threatening:	
Irregular heartbeat, weak pulse, chest pain, fast heartbeat.	Discontinue. Seek emergency treatment.
Common:	
• Constipation, frequent urination.	Discontinue. Call doctor right away.
• Dry mouth, increased thirst, muscle cramps, muscle pain.	Continue. Call doctor when convenient.
Infrequent:	
• Fainting.	Discontinue. Seek emergency treatment.
• Blurred vision, abdominal pain, nausea, vomiting, swollen feet and ankles, chills.	Discontinue. Call doctor right away.
• Dizziness, mood change, headache, muscle cramps, weakness, tiredness, weight gain or loss, nightmares, restlessness, shakiness.	Continue. Call doctor when convenient.
Rare:	
Sore throat; jaundice; headache; nausea; vomiting; fever; hallucinations; joint pain; rash; hives; sore throat, fever, mouth sores; unusual bruising; stiff or sore neck.	Discontinue. Call doctor right away.

 ## WARNINGS & PRECAUTIONS

Don't take if:
- You are allergic to any MAO inhibitor.
- You are allergic to any thiazide diuretic drug.

Before you start, consult your doctor:
- If you are alcoholic or allergic to any sulfa drug.

- If you have asthma, diabetes, epilepsy, overactive thyroid, schizophrenia, Parkinson's disease, adrenal-gland tumor, gout, liver, pancreas or kidney disorder.
- If you have had a stroke.
- If you will have surgery within 2 months, including dental surgery, requiring general or spinal anesthesia.

Over age 60:
Not recommended.

Pregnancy:
Risk to unborn child outweighs drug benefits. Don't use.

Breast-feeding:
Drug passes into milk. Avoid drug or discontinue nursing until you finish medicine. Consult doctor for advice on maintaining milk supply.

Infants & children:
Not recommended.

Prolonged use:
May be toxic to liver.

Skin & sunlight:
May cause rash or intensify sunburn in areas exposed to sun or sunlamp.

Driving, piloting or hazardous work:
Don't drive or pilot aircraft until you learn how medicine affects you. Don't work around dangerous machinery. Don't climb ladders or work in high places. Danger increases if you drink alcohol or take medicine affecting alertness and reflexes, such as antihistamines, tranquilizers, sedatives, pain medicine, narcotics and mind-altering drugs.

Discontinuing:
- Don't discontinue without doctor's advice until you complete prescribed dose, even though symptoms diminish or disappear.
- Follow precautions regarding foods, drinks and other medicines for 2 weeks after discontinuing.

Others:
- May affect blood-sugar levels in patients with diabetes.
- Hot weather and fever may cause dehydration and drop in blood pressure. Dose may require temporary adjustment. Weigh daily and report any unexpected weight decreases to your doctor.
- May cause rise in uric acid, leading to gout.

POSSIBLE INTERACTION WITH OTHER DRUGS

GENERIC NAME OR DRUG CLASS	COMBINED EFFECT
Acebutolol	Increased antihypertensive effect. Dosages of both drugs may require adjustments.
Allopurinol	Decreased allopurinol effect.
Amphetamines	Blood-pressure rise to life-threatening level.
Anticholinergics	Increased anticholinergic effect.
Anticonvulsants	Changed seizure pattern.
Antidepressants (tricyclic)	Blood-pressure rise to life-threatening level. Possible fever, convulsions, delirium.
Antidiabetics (oral and insulin)	Excessively low blood sugar.

Continued page 970

POSSIBLE INTERACTION WITH OTHER SUBSTANCES

INTERACTS WITH	COMBINED EFFECT
Alcohol:	Dangerous blood-pressure drop, increased sedation to dangerous level.
Beverages: Caffeine drinks.	Irregular heartbeat or high blood pressure.
Drinks containing tyramine (see Glossary).	Blood-pressure rise to life-threatening level.
Cocaine:	Overstimulation. Possibly fatal.
Foods: Foods containing tyramine (see Glossary).	Blood-pressure rise to life-threatening level.
Licorice.	Excessive potassium loss that causes dangerous heart rhythms.
Marijuana:	Overstimulation. May increase blood pressure. Avoid.
Tobacco:	No proven problems.

PEMOLINE

BRAND NAMES

Cylert

BASIC INFORMATION

Habit forming? Yes
Prescription needed? Yes
Available as generic? No
Drug class: Central nervous system stimulant

 USES

- Decreases overactivity and lengthens attention span in hyperactive children.
- Treatment of minimal brain dysfunction.

 DOSAGE & USAGE INFORMATION

How to take:
Tablet or capsule—Swallow with liquid or food to lessen stomach irritation. If you can't swallow whole, crumble tablet or open capsule and take with liquid or food.

When to take:
At the same times each day.

If you forget a dose:
Take as soon as you remember up to 2 hours late. If more than 2 hours, wait for next scheduled dose (don't double this dose).

What drug does:
Stimulates brain to improve alertness, concentration and attention span. Calms the hyperactive child.

Continued next column

 OVERDOSE

SYMPTOMS:
Rapid heartbeat, hallucinations, fever, confusion, convulsions, coma.
WHAT TO DO:
- **Dial 0 (operator) or 911 (emergency) for an ambulance or medical help. Then give first aid immediately.**
- **If patient is unconscious and not breathing, give mouth-to-mouth breathing. If there is no heartbeat, use cardiac massage and mouth-to-mouth breathing (CPR). Don't try to make patient vomit. If you can't get help quickly, take patient to nearest emergency facility.**
- **See emergency information on inside covers.**

Time lapse before drug works:
- 1 month or more for maximum effect on child.
- 30 minutes to stimulate adults.

Don't take with:
See Interaction column and consult doctor.

 POSSIBLE ADVERSE REACTIONS OR SIDE EFFECTS

SYMPTOMS	WHAT TO DO
Life-threatening: None expected.	
Common: Insomnia.	Continue. Call doctor when convenient.
Infrequent: • Irritability, depression dizziness, headache, drowsiness, unusual movement of eyes, rapid heartbeat.	Discontinue. Call doctor right away.
• Rash, unusual movements of tongue, appetite loss, abdominal pain, nausea, weight loss.	Continue. Call doctor when convenient.
Rare: Jaundice.	Discontinue. Call doctor right away.

656

WARNINGS & PRECAUTIONS

Don't take if:
You are allergic to pemoline.

Before you start, consult your doctor:
- If you have liver disease.
- If you have kidney disease.
- If patient younger than 6 years.
- If there is marked emotional instability.

Over age 60:
Adverse reactions and side effects may be more frequent and severe than in younger persons.

Pregnancy:
No proven harm to unborn child. Avoid if possible.

Breast-feeding:
No problems expected. Consult doctor.

Infants & children:
Use only under close medical supervision for children 6 or older.

Prolonged use:
Rare possibility of physical growth retardation.

Skin & sunlight:
No problems expected.

Driving, piloting or hazardous work:
Don't drive or pilot aircraft until you learn how medicine affects you. Don't work around dangerous machinery. Don't climb ladders or work in high places. Danger increases if you drink alcohol or take medicine affecting alertness and reflexes, such as antihistamines, tranquilizers, sedatives, pain medicine, narcotics and mind-altering drugs.

Discontinuing:
Don't discontinue without consulting doctor. Dose may require gradual reduction if you have taken drug for a long time. Doses of other drugs may also require adjustment.

Others:
Dose must be carefully adjusted by doctor.

 ## POSSIBLE INTERACTION WITH OTHER DRUGS

GENERIC NAME OR DRUG CLASS	COMBINED EFFECT
None identified.	

POSSIBLE INTERACTION WITH OTHER SUBSTANCES

INTERACTS WITH	COMBINED EFFECT
Alcohol:	More chance of depression. Avoid.
Beverages: Caffeine drinks.	May raise blood pressure. Avoid.
Cocaine:	Overstimulation. Avoid.
Foods:	No problems expected.
Marijuana:	Unknown.
Tobacco:	Unknown.

PENICILLAMINE

BRAND NAMES

Cuprimine   Distamine
Depen   Pendramine

BASIC INFORMATION

Habit forming? No
Prescription needed? Yes
Available as generic? Yes
Drug class: Chelating agent, antirheumatic, antidote (heavy-metal)

USES

- Treatment for rheumatoid arthritis.
- Prevention of kidney stones.
- Treatment for heavy-metal poisoning.

DOSAGE & USAGE INFORMATION

How to take:
Tablets or capsules—With liquid on an empty stomach 1 hour before or 2 hours after eating.

When to take:
At the same times each day.

If you forget a dose:
- 1 dose a day—Take as soon as you remember up to 12 hours late. If more than 12 hours, wait for next scheduled dose (don't double this dose).
- More than 1 dose a day—Take as soon as you remember up to 2 hours late. If more than 2 hours, wait for next scheduled dose (don't double this dose).

What drug does:
- Combines with heavy metals so kidney can excrete them.
- Combines with cysteine (amino acid found in many foods) to prevent cysteine kidney stones.
- May improve protective function of some white-blood cells against rheumatoid arthritis.

Continued next column

OVERDOSE

SYMPTOMS:
Ulcers, sores, convulsions, coughing up blood, coma.
WHAT TO DO:
- **Dial 0 (operator) or 911 (emergency) for an ambulance or medical help. Then give first aid immediately.**
- **See emergency information on inside covers.**

Time lapse before drug works:
2 to 3 months.

Don't take with:
See Interaction column and consult doctor.

POSSIBLE ADVERSE REACTIONS OR SIDE EFFECTS

SYMPTOMS	WHAT TO DO
Life-threatening: None expected.	
Common: Rash, itchy skin, joint pain, fever, swollen lymph glands.	Discontinue. Call doctor right away.
Infrequent: • Sore throat, fever, unusual bruising, swollen feet or legs, bloody or cloudy urine, weight gain, fatigue, weakness.	Discontinue. Call doctor right away.
• Appetite loss, nausea, diarrhea, vomiting.	Continue. Call doctor when convenient.
Rare: Double or blurred vision, pain, ringing in ears, ulcers, sores, white spots in mouth, difficult breathing, coughing up blood, jaundice.	Discontinue. Call doctor right away.

WARNINGS & PRECAUTIONS

Don't take if:
- You are allergic to penicillamine.
- You have severe anemia.

Before you start, consult your doctor:
- If you have kidney disease.
- If you are allergic to any pencillin antibiotic.

Over age 60:
More likely to damage blood cells and kidneys.

Pregnancy:
Risk to unborn child outweighs drug benefits. Don't use.

Breast-feeding:
Drug filters into milk. May harm child. Avoid.

Infants & children:
Use only under medical supervision.

Prolonged use:
May damage blood cells, kidney, liver.

Skin & sunlight:
No problems expected.

Driving, piloting or hazardous work:
No problems expected.

Discontinuing:
No problems expected.

Others:
Request laboratory studies on blood and urine every 2 weeks. Kidney- and liver-function studies recommended every 6 months.

POSSIBLE INTERACTION WITH OTHER DRUGS

GENERIC NAME OR DRUG CLASS	COMBINED EFFECT
Flecainide	Possible decreased blood-cell production in bone marrow.
Gold compounds	Damage to blood cells and kidney.
Immunosuppressants	Damage to blood cells and kidney.
Iron supplements	Decreased effect of penicillamine. Wait 2 hours between doses.
Oxyphenbutazone	Damage to blood cells and kidney.
Phenylbutazone	Damage to blood cells and kidney.
Quinine	Damage to blood cells and kidney.
Tocainide	Possible decreased blood-cell production in bone marrow.

POSSIBLE INTERACTION WITH OTHER SUBSTANCES

INTERACTS WITH	COMBINED EFFECT
Alcohol:	Increased side effects of penicillamine.
Beverages:	None expected.
Cocaine:	Increased side effects of penicillamine.
Foods:	None expected.
Marijuana:	Increased side effects of penicillamine.
Tobacco:	None expected.

PENICILLIN G

BRAND NAMES

Ayercillin	Penioral
Bicillin	Pentids
Bicillin L.A.	Permapen
Crystapen	Pfizerpen
Crysticillin	Pfizerpen-AS
Duracillin	Pfizerpen G
Duracillin A.S.	SK-Penicillin G
Megacillin	Wycillin
Novopen-G	

BASIC INFORMATION

Habit forming? No
Prescription needed? Yes
Available as generic? Yes
Drug class: Antibiotic (penicillin)

 USES

Treatment of bacterial infections that are susceptible to penicillin G.

 DOSAGE & USAGE INFORMATION

How to take:
- Tablets or capsules—Swallow with liquid on an empty stomach 1 hour before or 2 hours after eating.
- Liquid—Take with cold beverage. Liquid form is perishable and effective for only 7 days at room temperature. Effective for 14 days if stored in refrigerator. Don't freeze.

When to take:
Follow instructions on prescription label or side of package. Doses should be evenly spaced. For example, 4 times a day means every 6 hours.

If you forget a dose:
Take as soon as you remember. Continue regular schedule.

What drug does:
Destroys susceptible bacteria. Does not kill viruses.

Continued next column

 OVERDOSE

SYMPTOMS:
Severe diarrhea, nausea or vomiting.
WHAT TO DO:
Overdose unlikely to threaten life. If person takes much larger amount than prescribed, call doctor, poison-control center or hospital emergency room for instructions.

Time lapse before drug works:
May be several days before medicine affects infection.

Don't take with:
See Interaction column and consult doctor.

 POSSIBLE ADVERSE REACTIONS OR SIDE EFFECTS

SYMPTOMS	WHAT TO DO
Life-threatening:	
Hives, rash, intense itching, faintness soon after a dose (anaphylaxis).	Seek emergency treatment immediately.
Common:	
Dark or discolored tongue.	Continue. Tell doctor at next visit.
Infrequent:	
Mild nausea, vomiting, diarrhea.	Continue. Call doctor when convenient.
Rare:	
Unexplained bleeding.	Discontinue. Call doctor right away.

WARNINGS &
PRECAUTIONS

Don't take if:
You are allergic to penicillin G, cephalosporin antibiotics, other penicillins or penicillamine. Life-threatening reaction may occur.

Before you start, consult your doctor:
If you are allergic to any substance or drug.

Over age 60:
You may have skin reactions, particularly around genitals and anus.

Pregnancy:
Studies inconclusive on harm to unborn child. Animal studies show fetal abnormalities. Decide with your doctor whether drug benefits justify risk to unborn child.

Breast-feeding:
Drug passes into milk. Child may become sensitive to penicillins and have allergic reactions to penicillin drugs. Avoid penicillin G or discontinue nursing until you finish medicine. Consult doctor for advice on maintaining milk supply.

Infants & children:
No problems expected.

Prolonged use:
You may become more susceptible to infections caused by germs not responsive to penicillin G.

Skin & sunlight:
No problems expected.

Driving, piloting or hazardous work:
Usually not dangerous. Most hazardous reactions likely to occur a few minutes after taking penicillin G.

Discontinuing:
Don't discontinue without doctor's advice until you complete prescribed dose, even though symptoms diminish or disappear.

Others:
Urine sugar test for diabetes may show false positive result.

 ## POSSIBLE INTERACTION
WITH OTHER DRUGS

GENERIC NAME OR DRUG CLASS	COMBINED EFFECT
Beta-adrenergic blockers	Increased chance of anaphylaxis (see emergency information on inside front cover).
Calcium supplements	Decreased penicillin effect.
Chloramphenicol	Decreased effect of both drugs.
Erythromycins	Decreased effect of both drugs.
Loperamide	Decreased penicillin effect.
Paromomycin	Decreased effect of both drugs.
Tetracyclines	Decreased effect of both drugs.
Troleandomycin	Decreased effect of both drugs.

 ## POSSIBLE INTERACTION
WITH OTHER SUBSTANCES

INTERACTS WITH	COMBINED EFFECT
Alcohol:	Occasional stomach irritation.
Beverages:	None expected.
Cocaine:	No proven problems.
Foods:	Decreased effect of penicillin G.
Marijuana:	No proven problems.
Tobacco:	None expected.

PENICILLIN V

BRAND NAMES

Beepen-VK	Penapar VK
Betapen-VK	Pfizerpen VK
Compocillin VK	Robicillin VK
Ledercillin VK	SK-Penicillin VK
Nadopen-V	Uticillin VK
Novapen V	V-Cillin
Novopen-VK	V-Cillin K
Pen-Vee K	Veetids

BASIC INFORMATION

Habit forming? No
Prescription needed? Yes
Available as generic? Yes
Drug class: Antibiotic (penicillin)

 USES

- Treatment of bacterial infections that are susceptible to penicillin V.
- Prevention of streptococcal infections in susceptible persons such as those with heart valves damaged by rheumatic fever.

 DOSAGE & USAGE INFORMATION

How to take:
- Tablets or capsules—Swallow with liquid on an empty stomach 1 hour before meals or 2 hours after eating.
- Liquid—Take with cold beverage. Liquid form is perishable and effective for only 7 days at room temperature. Effective for 14 days if stored in refrigerator. Don't freeze.

When to take:
Follow instructions on prescription label or side of package. Doses should be evenly spaced. For example, 4 times a day means every 6 hours.

If you forget a dose:
Take as soon as you remember. Continue regular schedule.

Continued next column

 OVERDOSE

SYMPTOMS:
Severe diarrhea, nausea or vomiting.
WHAT TO DO:
Overdose unlikely to threaten life. If person takes much larger amount than prescribed, call doctor, poison-control center or hospital emergency room for instructions.

What drug does:
Destroys susceptible bacteria. Does not kill viruses.

Time lapse before drug works:
May be several days before penicillin V affects infection.

Don't take with:
See Interaction column and consult doctor.

 POSSIBLE ADVERSE REACTIONS OR SIDE EFFECTS

SYMPTOMS	WHAT TO DO
Life-threatening:	
Hives, rash, intense itching, faintness soon after a dose (anaphylaxis).	Seek emergency treatment immediately.
Common:	
Dark or discolored tongue.	Continue. Tell doctor at next visit.
Infrequent:	
Mild nausea, vomiting, diarrhea.	Continue. Call doctor when convenient.
Rare:	
Unexplained bleeding.	Discontinue. Call doctor right away.

WARNINGS & PRECAUTIONS

Don't take if:
You are allergic to penicillin V, cephalosporin antibiotics, other penicillins or penicillamine. Life-threatening reaction may occur.

Before you start, consult your doctor:
If you are allergic to any substance or drug.

Over age 60:
You may have skin reactions, particularly around genitals and anus.

Pregnancy:
Studies inconclusive on danger to unborn child. Decide with your doctor whether drug benefits justify risk to unborn child.

Breast-feeding:
Drug passes into milk. Child may become sensitive to penicillin. Child more likely to have future allergic reactions to penicillin. Avoid penicillin V or discontinue nursing until you finish medicine. Consult doctor for advice on maintaining milk supply.

Infants & children:
No problems expected.

Prolonged use:
You may become more susceptible to infections caused by germs not responsive to penicillin V.

Skin & sunlight:
No problems expected.

Driving, piloting or hazardous work:
Usually not dangerous. Most hazardous reactions likely to occur a few minutes after taking penicillin V.

Discontinuing:
Don't discontinue without doctor's advice until you have finished prescribed dose, even if symptoms diminish or disappear.

Others:
No problems expected.

POSSIBLE INTERACTION WITH OTHER DRUGS

GENERIC NAME OR DRUG CLASS	COMBINED EFFECT
Beta-adrenergic blockers	Increased chance of anaphylaxis (see emergency information on inside front cover).
Calcium supplements	Decreased penicillin effect.
Chloramphenicol	Decreased effect of both drugs.
Erythromycins	Decreased effect of both drugs.
Loperamide	Decreased penicillin effect.
Paromomycin	Decreased effect of both drugs.
Tetracyclines	Decreased effect of both drugs.
Troleandomycin	Decreased effect of both drugs.

POSSIBLE INTERACTION WITH OTHER SUBSTANCES

INTERACTS WITH	COMBINED EFFECT
Alcohol:	Occasional stomach irritation.
Beverages:	None expected.
Cocaine:	No proven problems.
Foods:	Decreased effect of penicillin V.
Marijuana:	No proven problems.
Tobacco:	None expected.

PENTOBARBITAL

BRAND NAMES

Carbrital	Pentogen
Nembutal	Quless
Nova-Rectal	Wigraine-PB
Novopentobarb	

BASIC INFORMATION

Habit forming? Yes
Prescription needed? Yes
Available as generic? Yes
Drug class: Sedative, hypnotic (barbiturate)

USES

- Reduces anxiety or nervous tension (low dose).
- Relieves insomnia (higher bedtime dose).

DOSAGE & USAGE INFORMATION

How to take:
- Tablet, capsule or liquid—Swallow with food or liquid to lessen stomach irritation. If you can't swallow whole, crumble tablet or open capsule and take with liquid or food.
- Suppositories—Remove wrapper and moisten suppository with water. Gently insert larger end into rectum. Push well into rectum with finger.

When to take:
At the same times each day.

If you forget a dose:
Take as soon as you remember up to 2 hours late. If more than 2 hours, wait for next scheduled dose (don't double this dose).

What drug does:
May partially block nerve impulses at nerve-cell connections.

Time lapse before drug works:
60 minutes.

Continued next column

OVERDOSE

SYMPTOMS:
Deep sleep, weak pulse, coma.
WHAT TO DO:
- **Dial 0 (operator) or 911 (emergency) for an ambulance or medical help. Then give first aid immediately.**
- **See emergency information on inside covers.**

Don't take with:
- Non-prescription drugs without consulting doctor.
- See Interaction column and consult doctor.

POSSIBLE ADVERSE REACTIONS OR SIDE EFFECTS

SYMPTOMS	WHAT TO DO
Life-threatening: None expected.	
Common: Dizziness, drowsiness, "hangover" effect.	Continue. Call doctor when convenient.
Infrequent:	
• Rash or hives; face, lip swelling; swollen eyelids; sore throat, fever.	Discontinue. Call doctor right away.
• Depression, confusion, slurred speech, diarrhea, nausea, vomiting, joint or muscle pain.	Continue. Call doctor when convenient.
Rare:	
• Agitation, slow heartbeat, difficult breathing, jaundice.	Discontinue. Call doctor right away.
• Unexplained bleeding or bruising.	Continue. Call doctor when convenient.

WARNINGS & PRECAUTIONS

Don't take if:
- You are allergic to any barbiturate.
- You have porphyria.

Before you start, consult your doctor:
- If you have epilepsy.
- If you have kidney or liver damage.
- If you have asthma.
- If you have anemia.
- If you have chronic pain.
- If you will have surgery within 2 months, including dental surgery, requiring general or spinal anesthesia.

Over age 60:
Adverse reactions and side effects may be more frequent and severe than in younger persons. Use small doses.

Pregnancy:
Risk to unborn child outweighs drug benefits. Don't use.

Breast-feeding:
Drug passes into milk. Avoid drug or discontinue nursing until you finish medicine. Consult doctor for advice on maintaining milk supply.

Infants & children:
Use only under doctor's supervision.

Prolonged use:
- May cause addiction, anemia, chronic intoxication.
- May lower body temperature, making exposure to cold temperatures hazardous.

Skin & sunlight:
May cause rash or intensify sunburn in areas exposed to sun or sunlamp.

Driving, piloting or hazardous work:
Don't drive or pilot aircraft until you learn how medicine affects you. Don't work around dangerous machinery. Don't climb ladders or work in high places. Danger increases if you drink alcohol or take medicine affecting alertness and reflexes.

Discontinuing:
May be unnecessary to finish medicine. Follow doctor's instructions. If you develop withdrawal symptoms of hallucinations, agitation or sleeplessness after discontinuing, call doctor right away.

Others:
Great potential for abuse.

 POSSIBLE INTERACTION WITH OTHER DRUGS

GENERIC NAME OR DRUG CLASS	COMBINED EFFECT
Anticoagulants (oral)	Decreased anticoagulant effect.
Anticonvulsants	Changed seizure patterns.
Antidepressants (tricyclics)	Decreased antidepressant effect. Possible dangerous oversedation.
Antidiabetics (oral)	Increased pentobarbital effect.
Antihistamines	Dangerous sedation. Avoid.
Anti-inflammatory drugs (non-steroidal)	Decreased anti-inflammatory effect.
Aspirin	Decreased aspirin effect.
Beta-adrenergic blockers	Decreased effect of beta-adrenergic blocker.
Contraceptives (oral)	Decreased contraceptive effect.
Cortisone drugs	Decreased cortisone effect.

Digitoxin	Decreased digitoxin effect.
Doxycycline	Decreased doxycycline effect.
Dronabinol	Increased effects of both drugs. Avoid.
Griseofulvin	Decreased griseofulvin effect.
Indapamide	Increased indapamide effect.
MAO inhibitors	Increased pentobarbital effect.
Mind-altering drugs	Dangerous sedation. Avoid.
Molindone	Increased sedative effect.
Narcotics	Dangerous sedation. Avoid.
Pain relievers	Dangerous sedation. Avoid.
Sedatives	Dangerous sedation. Avoid.
Sleep inducers	Dangerous sedation. Avoid.
Tranquilizers	Dangerous sedation. Avoid.
Valproic acid	Increased pentobarbital effect.

 POSSIBLE INTERACTION WITH OTHER SUBSTANCES

INTERACTS WITH	COMBINED EFFECT
Alcohol:	Possible fatal oversedation. Avoid.
Beverages:	None expected.
Cocaine:	Decreased pentobarbital effect.
Foods:	None expected.
Marijuana:	Excessive sedation. Avoid.
Tobacco:	None expected.

PENTOXIFYLLINE

BRAND NAMES

Trental

BASIC INFORMATION

Habit forming? No
Prescription needed? Yes
Available as generic? No
Drug class: Hemorrheologic agent

 USES

Reduces pain in legs caused by poor circulation.

 DOSAGE & USAGE INFORMATION

How to take:
Extended-release tablets—Swallow whole with water and food.

When to take:
At mealtimes. Taking with food decreases the likelihood of irritating the stomach to cause nausea.

If you forget a dose:
Take as soon as you remember up to 3 hours late. If more than 3 hours, wait for next scheduled dose (don't double this dose).

What drug does:
- Reduces "stickiness" of red blood cells and improves flexibility of the red cells.
- Improves blood flow through blood vessels.

Time lapse before drug works:
1 hour. Several weeks for full effect on circulation.

Don't take with:
- Tobacco or medicines to treat hypertension.
- See Interaction column and consult doctor.

 OVERDOSE

SYMPTOMS:
Drowsiness, flushed face, fainting, nervousness, convulsions, coma.
WHAT TO DO:
- **Dial 0 (operator) or 911 (emergency) for an ambulance or medical help. Then give first aid immediately.**
- **See emergency information on inside covers.**

 POSSIBLE ADVERSE REACTIONS OR SIDE EFFECTS

SYMPTOMS	WHAT TO DO
Life-threatening:	
Chest pain, irregular heartbeat.	Discontinue. Seek emergency treatment.
Common:	
None expected.	
Infrequent:	
Dizziness, headache, nausea, vomiting.	Discontinue. Call doctor right away.
Rare:	
None expected.	

WARNINGS & PRECAUTIONS

Don't take if:
You are allergic to pentoxifylline.

Before you start, consult your doctor:
If you are allergic to caffeine, theophylline, theobromine, aminophyllin, dyphyllin, oxtriphylline, theobromine.

Over age 60:
Adverse reactions and side effects may be more frequent and severe than in younger persons. Ask doctor about smaller doses.

Pregnancy:
Safety to unborn child unestablished. Avoid if possible.

Breast-feeding:
No problems expected, but ask doctor.

Infants & children:
Not recommended.

Prolonged use:
No problems expected.

Skin & sunlight:
No problems expected.

Driving, piloting or hazardous work:
Wait to see if drug causes drowsiness or dizziness. If none, no problems expected.

Discontinuing:
No problems expected.

Others:
Don't smoke.

POSSIBLE INTERACTION WITH OTHER DRUGS

GENERIC NAME OR DRUG CLASS	COMBINED EFFECT
Anithypertensives (high blood pressure medicine such as Acebutolol, Alseroxylen, Amiloride, Atenolol, Butmetanide, Captopril, Chlorothiazide, Chlorthalidone, Clonidine, Cyclothiazide, Guanethidine, Hydralazine, Methyldopa, Metoprolol, Spironolactone, Verapamil, Nadolol, Oxprenolol, Pindolol, Propranolol, Timolol)	Increased effect of hypertensive medication.

POSSIBLE INTERACTION WITH OTHER SUBSTANCES

INTERACTS WITH	COMBINED EFFECT
Alcohol:	Unknown. Best to avoid.
Beverages: Coffee, tea or other caffeine-containing beverages.	May decrease effectiveness of pentoxifylline.
Cocaine:	Reduces pentoxifylline effect.
Foods:	None expected.
Marijuana:	Decreased effect of pentoxifylline.
Tobacco:	Decreased effect of pentoxifylline.

PERPHENAZINE

BRAND NAMES

Apo-Perphenazine	Phenazine
Etrafon	Triavil
PMS Levazine	Trilafon

BASIC INFORMATION

Habit forming? No
Prescription needed? Yes
Available as generic? Yes
**Drug class: Tranquilizer, antiemetic
(phenothiazine)**

 USES

- Stops nausea, vomiting.
- Reduces anxiety, agitation.

 DOSAGE & USAGE INFORMATION

How to take:
- Tablet or capsule—Swallow with liquid or food to lessen stomach irritation.
- Suppositories—Remove wrapper and moisten suppository with water. Gently insert into rectum, large end first.
- Drops or liquid—Dilute dose in beverage.

When to take:
- Nervous and mental disorders—Take at the same times each day.
- Nausea and vomiting—Take as needed, no more often than every 4 hours.

If you forget a dose:
- Nervous and mental disorders—Take up to 2 hours late. If more than 2 hours, wait for next scheduled dose (don't double this dose).
- Nausea and vomiting—Take as soon as you remember. Wait 4 hours for next dose.

What drug does:
- Suppresses brain's vomiting center.
- Suppresses brain centers that control abnormal emotions and behavior.

Continued next column

 OVERDOSE

SYMPTOMS:
Stupor, convulsions, coma.
WHAT TO DO:
- **Dial 0 (operator) or 911 (emergency) for an ambulance or medical help. Then give first aid immediately.**
- **See emergency information on inside covers.**

Time lapse before drug works:
- Nausea and vomiting—1 hour or less.
- Nervous and mental disorders—4-6 weeks.

Don't take with:
- Antacid or medicine for diarrhea.
- Non-prescription drug for cough, cold or allergy.
- See Interaction column and consult doctor.

 POSSIBLE ADVERSE REACTIONS OR SIDE EFFECTS

SYMPTOMS	WHAT TO DO
Life-threatening: None expected.	
Common:	
• Muscle spasms of face and neck, unsteady gait.	Discontinue. Seek emergency treatment.
• Restlessness, tremor, drowsiness.	Discontinue. Call doctor right away.
• Decreased sweating, dry mouth, runny nose, constipation.	Continue. Call doctor when convenient.
Infrequent:	
• Fainting.	Discontinue. Seek emergency treatment.
• Rash.	Discontinue. Call doctor right away.
• Difficult urination, diminished sex drive, swollen breasts, menstrual irregularities.	Continue. Call doctor when convenient.
Rare: Change in vision, jaundice, sore throat, fever.	Discontinue. Call doctor right away.

WARNINGS & PRECAUTIONS

Don't take if:
- You are allergic to any phenothiazine.
- You have a blood or bone-marrow disease.

Before you start, consult your doctor:
- If you will have surgery within 2 months, including dental surgery, requiring general or spinal anesthesia.
- If you have asthma, emphysema or other lung disorder.
- If you take non-prescription ulcer medicine, asthma medicine or amphetamines.

Over age 60:
Adverse reactions and side effects may be more frequent and severe than in younger persons. More likely to develop involuntary movement of jaws, lips, tongue, chewing. Report this to your doctor immediately. Early treatment can help.

Pregnancy:
Risk to unborn child outweighs drug benefits. Don't use.

Breast-feeding:
Drug passes into milk. Avoid drug or discontinue nursing until you finish medicine. Consult doctor for advice on maintaining milk supply.

Infants & children:
Don't give to children younger than 2.

Prolonged use:
May lead to tardive dyskinesia (involuntary movement of jaws, lips, tongue, chewing).

Skin & sunlight:
May cause rash or intensify sunburn in areas exposed to sun or sunlamp. Skin may remain sensitive for 3 months after discontinuing.

Driving, piloting or hazardous work:
Don't drive or pilot aircraft until you learn how medicine affects you. Don't work around dangerous machinery. Don't climb ladders or work in high places. Danger increases if you drink alcohol or take medicine affecting alertness and reflexes.

Discontinuing:
- Nervous and mental disorders—Don't discontinue without doctor's advice until you complete prescribed dose, even though symptoms diminish or disappear.
- Nausea and vomiting—May be unnecessary to finish medicine. Follow doctor's instructions.

Others:
No problems expected.

POSSIBLE INTERACTION WITH OTHER DRUGS

GENERIC NAME OR DRUG CLASS	COMBINED EFFECT
Anticholinergics	Increased anticholinergic effect.
Antidepressants (tricyclic)	Increased perphenazine effect.
Antihistamines	Increased antihistamine effect.
Appetite suppressants	Decreased suppressant effect.
Dronabinol	Increased effects of both drugs. Avoid.
Levodopa	Decreased levodopa effect.
Mind-altering drugs	Increased effect of mind-altering drugs.
Molindone	Increased tranquilizer effect.
Narcotics	Increased narcotic effect.
Phenytoin	Increased phenytoin effect.
Quinidine	Impaired heart function. Dangerous mixture.
Sedatives	Increased sedative effect.
Tranquilizers (other)	Increased tranquilizer effect.

POSSIBLE INTERACTION WITH OTHER SUBSTANCES

INTERACTS WITH	COMBINED EFFECT
Alcohol:	Dangerous oversedation.
Beverages:	None expected.
Cocaine:	Decreased perphenazine effect. Avoid.
Foods:	None expected.
Marijuana:	Drowsiness. May increase antinausea effect.
Tobacco:	None expected.

PERPHENAZINE & AMITRIPTYLINE

BRAND NAMES

Etrafon   Triavil

BASIC INFORMATION

Habit forming? No
Prescription needed? Yes
Available as generic? Yes
Drug class: Tranquilizer (phenothiazine),
antidepressant

 ## USES

- Decreases nausea, vomiting.
- Gradually relieves, but doesn't cure, symptoms of depression, anxiety, agitation.

 ## DOSAGE & USAGE INFORMATION

How to take:
Tablet or capsule—Swallow with liquid.

When to take:
At the same time each day.

If you forget a dose:
Bedtime dose—If you forget your once-a-day bedtime dose, don't take it more than 3 hours late. If more than 3 hours, wait for next scheduled dose (don't double this dose).

What drug does:
- Suppresses brain's vomiting center.
- Suppresses brain centers that control abnormal emotions and behavior.
- Probably affects part of brain that controls messages between nerve cells.

Continued next column

 ## OVERDOSE

SYMPTOMS:
Stupor, convulsions, hallucinations, coma.
WHAT TO DO:
- **Dial 0 (operator) or 911 (emergency) for an ambulance or medical help. Then give first aid immediately.**
- **If patient is unconscious and not breathing, give mouth-to-mouth breathing. If there is no heartbeat, use cardiac massage and mouth-to-mouth breathing (CPR). Don't try to make patient vomit. If you can't get help quickly, take patient to nearest emergency facility.**
- **See emergency information on inside covers.**

Time lapse before drug works:
- Nausea and vomiting—1 hour or less.
- Nervous and mental disorders—4-6 weeks.
- Begins in 1 to 2 weeks. May require 4 to 6 weeks for maximum benefit.

Don't take with:
- Antacid or medicine for diarrhea.
- Non-prescription drug for cough, cold or allergy.
- Non-prescription drugs without consulting doctor.
- See Interaction column and consult doctor.

 ## POSSIBLE ADVERSE REACTIONS OR SIDE EFFECTS

SYMPTOMS	WHAT TO DO
Life-threatening:	
Seizures, irregular heartbeat, weak pulse, fainting, muscle spasms.	Discontinue. Seek emergency treatment.
Common:	
• Headache, constipation, nausea, vomiting, irregular heartbeat, drowsiness.	Discontinue. Call doctor right away.
• Insomnia, dry mouth, "sweet tooth," decreased sweating, runny nose, constipation.	Continue. Call doctor when convenient.
Infrequent:	
• Hallucinations, dizziness, tremor, blurred vision, eye pain, vomiting.	Discontinue. Call doctor right away.
• Frequent urination, diminished sex drive, breast swelling, menstrual irregularities.	Continue. Call doctor when convenient.
Rare:	
• Rash; itchy skin; sore throat; jaundice; fever; change in vision; sore throat, fever, mouth sores.	Discontinue. Call doctor right away.
• Fatigue, weakness.	Continue. Call doctor when convenient.

WARNINGS & PRECAUTIONS

Don't take if:
- You are allergic to any phenothiazine, tricyclic antidepressant.
- You have a blood or bone-marrow disease or glaucoma.
- You drink alcohol.
- You have had a heart attack within 6 weeks.
- You have taken MAO inhibitors within 2 weeks.
- Patient is younger than 12.

Before you start, consult your doctor:
- If you have asthma, emphysema or other lung disorder.
- If you have an enlarged prostate, heart disease, high blood pressure, stomach or intestinal problems, overactive thyroid, liver disease.
- If you take non-prescription ulcer medicine, asthma medicine or amphetamines.
- If you will have surgery within 2 months, including dental surgery, requiring general or spinal anesthesia.

Over age 60:
Adverse reactions and side effects may be more frequent and severe than in younger persons. More likely to develop involuntary movement of jaws, lips, tongue, chewing, difficult urination. Report this to your doctor immediately. Early treatment can help.

Pregnancy:
Risk to unborn child outweighs drug benefits. Don't use.

Breast-feeding:
Drug passes into milk. Avoid drug or discontinue nursing until you finish medicine. Consult doctor for advice on maintaining milk supply.

Infants & children:
Don't give to children younger than 12.

Prolonged use:
May lead to tardive dyskinesia (involuntary movement of jaws, lips, tongue, chewing).

Skin & sunlight:
May cause rash or intensify sunburn in areas exposed to sun or sunlamp. Skin may remain sensitive for 3 months after discontinuing.

Driving, piloting or hazardous work:
Don't drive or pilot aircraft until you learn how medicine affects you. Don't work around dangerous machinery. Don't climb ladders or work in high places. Danger increases if you drink alcohol or take medicine affecting alertness and reflexes, such as antihistamines, tranquilizers, sedatives, pain medicine, narcotics and mind-altering drugs.

Discontinuing:
- Nervous and mental disorders—Don't discontinue without doctor's advice until you complete prescribed dose, even though symptoms diminish or disappear.
- Dose may require gradual reduction if you have taken drug for a long time. Doses of other drugs may also require adjustment.

Others:
No problems expected.

POSSIBLE INTERACTION WITH OTHER DRUGS

GENERIC NAME OR DRUG CLASS	COMBINED EFFECT
Anticholinergics	Increased anticholinergic effect, increased sedation.
Anticoagulants (oral)	Increased anticoagulant effect.
Antihistamines	Increased antihistamine effect.
Appetite suppressants	Decreased suppressant effect.
Barbiturates	Decreased antidepressant effect.
Clonidine	Decreased clonidine effect.
Diuretics (thiazide)	Increased antidepressant effect.
Dronabinol	Increased effect of both drugs.
Ethchlorvynol	Delirium.

Continued page 971

POSSIBLE INTERACTION WITH OTHER SUBSTANCES

INTERACTS WITH	COMBINED EFFECT
Alcohol: Beverages or medicines with alcohol.	Excessive intoxication. Avoid.
Beverages: Coffee.	Reduces effectiveness.
Cocaine:	Excessive intoxication. Avoid.
Foods:	None expected.
Marijuana:	Excessive drowsiness. Avoid.
Tobacco:	None expected.

PHENACETIN

BRAND NAMES

A.P.C. Tablets
Aspirin Compound
  with Codeine
Emprazil
Fiorinal
P.A.C. Compound
Percodan

Propoxyphene
  Compound 65
Sinubid
SK-65 Compound
Soma Compound
Tabloid APC with
  Codeine

BASIC INFORMATION

Habit forming? No
Prescription needed? Yes
Available as generic? Yes
Drug class: Analgesic, fever reducer

USES

- Relieves pain.
- Reduces fever.

DOSAGE & USAGE INFORMATION

How to take:
- Tablet or capsule—Swallow with liquid or food to lessen stomach irritation. You may chew or crush tablets.
- Extended-release tablets or capsules—Swallow each dose whole with liquid.

When to take:
At the same times each day.

If you forget a dose:
Take as soon as you remember up to 2 hours late. If more than 2 hours, wait for next scheduled dose (don't double this dose).

What drug does:
Reduces level of prostaglandins, a chemical involved in producing inflammation, fever, pain.

Time lapse before drug works:
15 minutes.

Don't take with:
See Interaction column and consult doctor.

OVERDOSE

SYMPTOMS:
Sweating, bloody urine, convulsions, coma.
WHAT TO DO:
- Dial 0 (operator) or 911 (emergency) for an ambulance or medical help. Then give first aid immediately.
- See emergency information on inside covers.

POSSIBLE ADVERSE REACTIONS OR SIDE EFFECTS

SYMPTOMS	WHAT TO DO
Life-threatening: None expected.	
Common: None expected.	
Infrequent:	
• Rash; itchy skin; hives; sore throat, fever, mouth sores.	Discontinue. Call doctor right away.
• Confusion, drowsiness, nausea.	Continue. Call doctor when convenient.
Rare:	
• Black, bloody or tarry stools.	Discontinue. Seek emergency treatment.
• Easy bruising, swollen feet or legs, blood in urine, anemia, blue fingernails, fatigue, weakness.	Discontinue. Call doctor right away.

WARNINGS & PRECAUTIONS

Don't take if:
You are allergic to phenacetin, aspirin or any of the many mixtures which contain either.

Before you start, consult your doctor:
- If you have kidney or liver disease.
- If you have G6PD deficiency.

Over age 60:
Adverse reactions and side effects may be more frequent and severe than in younger persons.

Pregnancy:
May cause anemia in newborn. Avoid if possible.

Breast-feeding:
Drug passes into milk. Avoid drug or discontinue nursing until you finish medicine. Consult doctor for advice on maintaining milk supply.

Infants & children:
Not recommended.

Prolonged use:
Kidney damage. Don't take regularly without medical advice.

Skin & sunlight:
No problems expected.

Driving, piloting or hazardous work:
No problems expected.

Discontinuing:
May be unnecessary to finish medicine. Follow doctor's instructions.

Others:
No problems expected.

POSSIBLE INTERACTION WITH OTHER DRUGS

GENERIC NAME OR DRUG CLASS	COMBINED EFFECT
Phenobarbital	Decreased phenacetin effect.

POSSIBLE INTERACTION WITH OTHER SUBSTANCES

INTERACTS WITH	COMBINED EFFECT
Alcohol:	None expected.
Beverages:	None expected.
Cocaine:	None expected.
Foods:	None expected.
Marijuana:	Increased pain relief.
Tobacco:	None expected.

PHENAZOPYRIDINE

BRAND NAMES

Azo-100	Phen-Azo
Azodine	Phenazodine
Azo-Gantanol	Pyridiate
Azo-Gantrisin	Pyridium
Azo-Mandelamine	Pyridium Plus
Azo-Standard	Pyrodine
Azotrex	Pyronium
Baridium	Thiosulfil-A
Di-Azo	Urobiotic

BASIC INFORMATION

Habit forming? No
Prescription needed? Yes
Available as generic? Yes
Drug class: Analgesic (urinary)

 ## USES

Relieves pain of lower urinary-tract irritation, as in cystitis, urethritis or prostatitis. Relieves symptoms only. Phenazopyridine alone does not cure infections.

 ## DOSAGE & USAGE INFORMATION

How to take:
Tablet or capsule—Swallow with liquid or food to lessen stomach irritation.

When to take:
At the same times each day.

If you forget a dose:
Take as soon as you remember up to 2 hours late. If more than 2 hours, wait for next scheduled dose (don't double this dose).

What drug does:
Anesthetizes lower urinary tract. Relieves pain, burning, pressure and urgency to urinate.

Time lapse before drug works:
1 to 2 hours.

Don't take with:
No restrictions.

 ## OVERDOSE

SYMPTOMS:
Shortness of breath, weakness.
WHAT TO DO:
Overdose unlikely to threaten life. If person takes much larger amount than prescribed, call doctor, poison-control center or hospital emergency room for instructions.

 ## POSSIBLE ADVERSE REACTIONS OR SIDE EFFECTS

SYMPTOMS	WHAT TO DO
Life-threatening:	
None expected.	
Common:	
Red-orange urine.	No action necessary.
Infrequent:	
Indigestion, fatigue, weakness.	Continue. Call doctor when convenient.
Rare:	
• Rash, jaundice.	Discontinue. Call doctor right away.
• Headache, anemia.	Continue. Call doctor when convenient.

WARNINGS & PRECAUTIONS

Don't take if:
- You have hepatitis.
- You are allergic to any urinary analgesic.

Before you start, consult your doctor:
If you have kidney or liver disease.

Over age 60:
Adverse reactions and side effects may be more frequent and severe than in younger persons.

Pregnancy:
No proven harm to unborn child. Avoid if possible.

Breast-feeding:
No problems expected.

Infants & children:
Not recommended.

Prolonged use:
- Orange or yellow skin.
- Anemia. Occasional blood studies recommended.

Skin & sunlight:
No problems expected.

Driving, piloting or hazardous work:
No problems expected.

Discontinuing:
May be unnecessary to finish medicine. Follow doctor's instructions.

Others:
No problems expected.

POSSIBLE INTERACTION WITH OTHER DRUGS

GENERIC NAME OR DRUG CLASS	COMBINED EFFECT
None	

POSSIBLE INTERACTION WITH OTHER SUBSTANCES

INTERACTS WITH	COMBINED EFFECT
Alcohol:	None expected.
Beverages:	None expected.
Cocaine:	None expected.
Foods:	None expected.
Marijuana:	None expected.
Tobacco:	None expected.

PHENIRAMINE

BRAND NAMES

Citra Capsules
Citra Forte
Dri-Hist No. 2 Meta
  Caps
Dristan Nasal Spray
Fiogesic
Inhistor
Poly-Histine D
Robitussin-AC
Ru-Tuss

S-T Forte
Symptrol
Triaminic
Triaminicin
Triaminicol
Tussagesic
Tussaminic
Tussirex Sugar-Free
Ursinus

BASIC INFORMATION

Habit forming? No
Prescription needed?
  High strength: Yes
  Low strength: No
Available as generic? Yes
Drug class: Antihistamine

 USES

Reduces allergic symptoms such as hay fever,
hives, rash or itching.

 DOSAGE & USAGE INFORMATION

How to take:
- Tablet, syrup or capsule—Swallow with liquid
  or food to lessen stomach irritation.
- Extended-release tablets or
  capsules—Swallow each dose whole.

When to take:
Varies with form. Follow label directions.

If you forget a dose:
Take as soon as you remember up to 2 hours
late. If more than 2 hours, wait for next
scheduled dose (don't double this dose).

Continued next column

 OVERDOSE

SYMPTOMS:
Convulsions, red face, hallucinations, coma.
WHAT TO DO:
- Dial 0 (operator) or 911 (emergency) for an
  ambulance or medical help. Then give first
  aid immediately.
- See emergency information on inside
  covers.

What drug does:
Blocks action of histamine after an allergic
response triggers histamine release in sensitive
cells.

Time lapse before drug works:
30 minutes.

Don't take with:
See Interaction column and consult doctor.

 POSSIBLE ADVERSE REACTIONS OR SIDE EFFECTS

SYMPTOMS	WHAT TO DO
Life-threatening: None expected.	
Common: Drowsiness, dizziness, dry mouth, nose, throat, nausea.	Continue. Tell doctor at next visit.
Infrequent:	
• Change in vision.	Discontinue. Call doctor right away.
• Less tolerance for contact lenses, difficult urination.	Continue. Call doctor when convenient.
• Appetite loss.	Continue. Tell doctor at next visit.
Rare: Nightmares, agitation, irritability, sore throat, fever, rapid heartbeat, unusual bleeding or bruising, fatigue, weakness.	Discontinue. Call doctor right away.

WARNINGS & PRECAUTIONS

Don't take if:
You are allergic to any antihistamine.

Before you start, consult your doctor:
- If you have glaucoma.
- If you have enlarged prostate.
- If you have asthma.
- If you have kidney disease.
- If you have peptic ulcer.
- If you will have surgery within 2 months, including dental surgery, requiring general or spinal anesthesia.

Over age 60:
Don't exceed recommended dose. Adverse reactions and side effects may be more frequent and severe than in younger persons, especially urination difficulty, diminished alertness and other brain and nervous-system symptoms.

Pregnancy:
No proven harm to unborn child. Avoid if possible.

Breast-feeding:
Drug passes into milk. Avoid drug or discontinue nursing until you finish medicine. Consult doctor for advice on maintaining milk supply.

Infants & children:
Not recommended for premature or newborn infants. Otherwise, no problems expected.

Prolonged use:
Avoid. May damage bone-marrow and nerve cells.

Skin & sunlight:
May cause rash or intensify sunburn in areas exposed to sun or sunlamp.

Driving, piloting or hazardous work:
Don't drive or pilot aircraft until you learn how medicine affects you. Don't work around dangerous machinery. Don't climb ladders or work in high places. Danger increases if you drink alcohol or take medicine affecting alertness and reflexes, such as antihistamines, tranquilizers, sedatives, pain medicine, narcotics and mind-altering drugs.

Discontinuing:
No problems expected.

Others:
May mask symptoms of hearing damage from aspirin, other salicylates, cisplatin, paromomycin, vancomycin or anticonvulsants. Consult doctor if you use these.

POSSIBLE INTERACTION WITH OTHER DRUGS

GENERIC NAME OR DRUG CLASS	COMBINED EFFECT
Anticholinergics	Increased anticholinergic effect.
Antidepressants (tricyclic)	Increased pheniramine effect.
Antihistamines (other)	Excess sedation. Avoid.
Dronabinol	Increased effects of both drugs. Avoid.
Hypnotics	Excess sedation. Avoid.
MAO inhibitors	Increased pheniramine effect.
Mind-altering drugs	Excess sedation. Avoid.
Narcotics	Excess sedation. Avoid.
Sedatives	Excess sedation. Avoid.
Sleep inducers	Excess sedation. Avoid.
Tranquilizers	Excess sedation. Avoid.

POSSIBLE INTERACTION WITH OTHER SUBSTANCES

INTERACTS WITH	COMBINED EFFECT
Alcohol:	Excess sedation. Avoid.
Beverages: Caffeine drinks.	Less pheniramine sedation.
Cocaine:	Decreased pheniramine effect. Avoid.
Foods:	None expected.
Marijuana:	Excess sedation. Avoid.
Tobacco:	None expected.

PHENOBARBITAL

BRAND NAMES

See complete list of brand names in the *Brand Name Directory,* page 953.

BASIC INFORMATION

Habit forming? Yes
Prescription needed? Yes
Available as generic? Yes
Drug class: Sedative, hypnotic (barbiturate), anticonvulsant

USES

- Reduces anxiety or nervous tension (low dose).
- Relieves insomnia (higher bedtime dose).
- Prevents convulsions or seizures, such as epilepsy.

DOSAGE & USAGE INFORMATION

How to take:
- Tablet, liquid or capsule—Swallow with liquid or food to lessen stomach irritation. If you can't swallow whole, crumble tablet or open capsule and take with liquid or food.
- Extended-release tablets or capsules—Swallow each dose whole.
- Drops—Dilute dose in beverage before swallowing.

When to take:
At the same times each day.

If you forget a dose:
Take as soon as you remember up to 2 hours late. If more than 2 hours, wait for next scheduled dose (don't double this dose).

What drug does:
May partially block nerve impulses at nerve-cell connections.

Continued next column

OVERDOSE

SYMPTOMS:
Deep sleep, weak pulse, coma.
WHAT TO DO:
- **Dial 0 (operator) or 911 (emergency) for an ambulance or medical help. Then give first aid immediately.**
- **See emergency information on inside covers.**

Time lapse before drug works:
60 minutes.

Don't take with:
- Non-prescription drugs without consulting doctor.
- See Interaction column and consult doctor.

POSSIBLE ADVERSE REACTIONS OR SIDE EFFECTS

SYMPTOMS	WHAT TO DO
Life-threatening: None expected.	
Common: Dizziness, drowsiness, "hangover" effect.	Continue. Call doctor when convenient.
Infrequent:	
• Rash or hives, face or lip swelling, swollen eyelids, sore throat, fever.	Discontinue. Call doctor right away.
• Depression, confusion, slurred speech, diarrhea, nausea, vomiting, joint or muscle pain.	Continue. Call doctor when convenient.
Rare:	
• Agitation, slow heartbeat, difficult breathing, jaundice.	Discontinue. Call doctor right away.
• Unexplained bleeding or bruising.	Continue. Call doctor when convenient.

WARNINGS & PRECAUTIONS

Don't take if:
- You are allergic to any barbiturate.
- You have porphyria.

Before you start, consult your doctor:
- If you have epilepsy.
- If you have kidney or liver damage.
- If you have asthma.
- If you have anemia.
- If you have chronic pain.
- If you will have surgery within 2 months, including dental surgery, requiring general or spinal anesthesia.

Over age 60:
Adverse reactions and side effects may be more frequent and severe than in younger persons. Use small doses.

Pregnancy:
Risk to unborn child outweighs drug benefits. Don't use.

Breast-feeding:
Drug passes into milk. Avoid drug or discontinue nursing until you finish medicine. Consult doctor for advice on maintaining milk supply.

Infants & children:
Use only under doctor's supervision.

Prolonged use:
- May cause addiction, anemia, chronic intoxication.
- May lower body temperature, making exposure to cold temperatures hazardous.

Skin & sunlight:
May cause rash or intensify sunburn in areas exposed to sun or sunlamp.

Driving, piloting or hazardous work:
Don't drive or pilot aircraft until you learn how medicine affects you. Don't work around dangerous machinery. Don't climb ladders or work in high places. Danger increases if you drink alcohol or take medicine affecting alertness and reflexes.

Discontinuing:
May be unnecessary to finish medicine. Follow doctor's instructions. If you develop withdrawal symptoms of hallucinations, agitation or sleeplessness after discontinuing, call doctor right away.

Others:
Great potential for abuse.

 ## POSSIBLE INTERACTION WITH OTHER DRUGS

GENERIC NAME OR DRUG CLASS	COMBINED EFFECT
Anticoagulants (oral)	Decreased anticoagulant effect.
Anticonvulsants	Changed seizure patterns.
Antidepressants (tricyclics)	Decreased antidepressant effect. Possible dangerous oversedation.
Antidiabetics (oral)	Increased phenobarbital effect.
Antihistamines	Dangerous sedation. Avoid.
Anti-inflammatory drugs (non-steroidal)	Decreased anti-inflammatory effect.
Aspirin	Decreased aspirin effect.
Beta-adrenergic blockers	Decreased effect of beta-adrenergic blocker.

Contraceptives (oral)	Decreased contraceptive effect.
Cortisone drugs	Decreased cortisone effect.
Digitoxin	Decreased digitoxin effect.
Doxycycline	Decreased doxycycline effect.
Dronabinol	Increased effects of both drugs. Avoid.
Griseofulvin	Decreased griseofulvin effect.
Indapamide	Increased indapamide effect.
MAO inhibitors	Increased phenobarbital effect.
Mind-altering drugs	Dangerous sedation. Avoid.
Molindone	Increased sedative effect.
Narcotics	Dangerous sedation. Avoid.
Pain relievers	Dangerous sedation. Avoid.
Sedatives	Dangerous sedation. Avoid.
Sleep inducers	Dangerous sedation. Avoid.
Tranquilizers	Dangerous sedation. Avoid.
Valproic acid	Increased phenobarbital effect.

 ## POSSIBLE INTERACTION WITH OTHER SUBSTANCES

INTERACTS WITH	COMBINED EFFECT
Alcohol:	Possible fatal oversedation. Avoid.
Beverages:	None expected.
Cocaine:	Decreased phenobarbital effect.
Foods:	None expected.
Marijuana:	Excessive sedation. Avoid.
Tobacco:	None expected.

PHENOLPHTHALEIN

BRAND NAMES

Agoral	Evac-U-Lax
Alophen	Ex-Lax
Correctol	Feen-A-Mint
Espotabs	Fructines-Vichy
Evac-Q-Kit	Phenolax
Evac-Q-Kwik	Prulet
Evac-U-Gen	Trilax

BASIC INFORMATION

Habit forming? No
Prescription needed? No
Available as generic? Yes
Drug class: Laxative (stimulant)

 USES

Constipation relief.

 DOSAGE & USAGE INFORMATION

How to take:
- Tablet or wafer—Swallow with liquid. If you can't swallow whole, chew or crumble and take with liquid or food.
- Liquid—Drink 6 to 8 glasses of water each day, in addition to one taken with each dose.
- Chewable tablets—Chew thoroughly before swallowing.

When to take:
Usually at bedtime with a snack, unless directed otherwise.

If you forget a dose:
Take as soon as you remember.

What drug does:
Acts on smooth muscles of intestine wall to cause vigorous bowel movement.

Time lapse before drug works:
6 to 10 hours.

Continued next column

 OVERDOSE

SYMPTOMS:
Vomiting, electrolyte depletion.
WHAT TO DO:
Overdose unlikely to threaten life. If person takes much larger amount than prescribed, call doctor, poison-control center or hospital emergency room for instructions.

Don't take with:
- See Interaction column and consult doctor.
- Don't take within 2 hours of taking another medicine. Laxative interferes with medicine absorption.

 POSSIBLE ADVERSE REACTIONS OR SIDE EFFECTS

SYMPTOMS	WHAT TO DO
Life-threatening: None expected.	
Common:	
• Rectal irritation.	Continue. Call doctor when convenient.
• Pink to orange urine.	No action necessary.
Infrequent:	
• Dangerous potassium loss.	Discontinue. Call doctor right away.
• Belching, cramps, nausea.	Continue. Call doctor when convenient.
Rare: Irritability, confusion, headache, rash, difficult breathing, irregular heartbeat, muscle cramps, unusual tiredness or weakness, burning on urination.	Discontinue. Call doctor right away.

WARNINGS & PRECAUTIONS

Don't take if:
- You have symptoms of appendicitis, inflamed bowel or intestinal blockage.
- You are allergic to a stimulant laxative.
- You have missed a bowel movement for only 1 or 2 days.

Before you start, consult your doctor:
- If you have a colostomy or ileostomy.
- If you have congestive heart disease.
- If you have diabetes.
- If you have high blood pressure.
- If you have a laxative habit.
- If you have rectal bleeding.
- If you take other laxatives.

Over age 60:
Adverse reactions and side effects may be more frequent and severe than in younger persons.

Pregnancy:
Risk to mother and unborn child outweighs drug benefits. Don't use.

Breast-feeding:
Drug passes into milk. Avoid drug or discontinue nursing until you finish medicine. Consult doctor for advice on maintaining milk supply.

Infants & children:
Use only under medical supervision.

Prolonged use:
Don't take for more than 1 week unless under a doctor's supervision. May cause laxative dependence.

Skin & sunlight:
No problems expected.

Driving, piloting or hazardous work:
No problems expected.

Discontinuing:
May be unnecessary to finish medicine. Follow doctor's instructions.

Others:
Don't take to "flush out" your system or as a "tonic."

POSSIBLE INTERACTION WITH OTHER DRUGS

GENERIC NAME OR DRUG CLASS	COMBINED EFFECT
Antacids	Tablet coating may dissolve too rapidly, irritating stomach or bowel.
Antihypertensives	May cause dangerous low potassium level.
Diuretics	May cause dangerous low potassium level.

POSSIBLE INTERACTION WITH OTHER SUBSTANCES

INTERACTS WITH	COMBINED EFFECT
Alcohol:	None expected.
Beverages: Milk.	Tablet coating may dissolve too rapidly, irritating stomach or bowel.
Cocaine:	None expected.
Foods:	None expected.
Marijuana:	None expected.
Tobacco:	None expected.

PHENPROCOUMON

BRAND NAMES

Liquamar   Marcumar

BASIC INFORMATION

Habit forming? No
Prescription needed? Yes
Available as generic? Yes
Drug class: Anticoagulant

 ## USES

Reduces blood clots. Used for abnormal clotting inside blood vessels.

 ## DOSAGE & USAGE INFORMATION

How to take:
Tablet—Swallow with liquid. If you can't swallow whole, crumble tablet and take with liquid or food.

When to take:
At the same time each day.

If you forget a dose:
Take as soon as you remember up to 12 hours late. If more than 12 hours, wait for next scheduled dose (don't double this dose). Inform your doctor of any missed doses.

What drug does:
Blocks action of vitamin K necessary for blood clotting.

Time lapse before drug works:
36 to 48 hours.

Don't take with:
See Interaction column and consult doctor.

 ## OVERDOSE

SYMPTOMS:
Bloody vomit and bloody or black stools, red urine.
WHAT TO DO:
- **Dial 0 (operator) or 911 (emergency) for an ambulance or medical help. Then give first aid immediately.**
- **See emergency information on inside covers.**

 ## POSSIBLE ADVERSE REACTIONS OR SIDE EFFECTS

SYMPTOMS	WHAT TO DO
Life-threatening:	
None expected.	
Common:	
Bloating, gaseousness.	Continue. Tell doctor at next visit.
Infrequent:	
• Black stools or bloody vomit, coughing up blood.	Discontinue. Seek emergency treatment.
• Rash, hives, itchy skin, blurred vision, sore throat, easy bruising or bleeding, cloudy or red urine, back pain, jaundice, fever, chills, fatigue, weakness.	Discontinue. Call doctor right away.
• Diarrhea, cramps, nausea, vomiting, swollen feet or legs, hair loss.	Continue. Call doctor when convenient.
Rare:	
Dizziness, headache, mouth sores.	Discontinue. Call doctor right away.

PHENPROCOUMON

WARNINGS & PRECAUTIONS

Don't take if:
- You have been allergic to any oral anticoagulant.
- You have a bleeding disorder.
- You have an active peptic ulcer.
- You have ulcerative colitis.

Before you start, consult your doctor:
- If you take any other drugs, including non-prescription drugs.
- If you have high blood pressure.
- If you have heavy or prolonged menstrual periods.
- If you have diabetes.
- If you have a bladder catheter.
- If you have serious liver or kidney disease.
- If you will have surgery within 2 months, including dental surgery, requiring general or spinal anesthesia.

Over age 60:
Adverse reactions and side effects may be more frequent and severe than in younger persons.

Pregnancy:
Risk to unborn child outweighs drug benefits. Don't use.

Breast-feeding:
Drug filters into milk. May harm child. Avoid.

Infants & children:
Use only under doctor's supervision.

Prolonged use:
No problems expected.

Skin & sunlight:
No problems expected.

Driving, piloting or hazardous work:
- Avoid hazardous activities that could cause injury.
- Don't drive if you feel dizzy or have blurred vision.

Discontinuing:
Don't discontinue without consulting doctor. Dose may require gradual reduction if you have taken drug for a long time. Doses of other drugs may also require adjustment.

Others:
Carry identification to state you take anticoagulants.

POSSIBLE INTERACTION WITH OTHER DRUGS

GENERIC NAME OR DRUG CLASS	COMBINED EFFECT
Acetaminophen	Increased phenprocoumon effect.
Allopurinol	Increased phenprocoumon effect.
Androgens	Increased phenprocoumon effect.
Antacids (large doses)	Decreased phenprocoumon effect.
Antibiotics	Increased phenprocoumon effect.
Anticonvulsants (hydantoin)	Increased effect of both drugs.
Antidepressants (tricyclic)	Increased phenprocoumon effect.
Antidiabetics (oral)	Increased phenprocoumon effect.
Antihistamines	Unpredictable increased or decreased anticoagulant effect.
Barbiturates	Decreased phenprocoumon effect.
Benzodiazepines	Unpredictable increased or decreased anticoagulant effect.
Carbamazepine	Decreased phenprocoumon effect.
Chloral hydrate	Unpredictable increased or decreased anticoagulant effect.

Continued page 971

POSSIBLE INTERACTION WITH OTHER SUBSTANCES

INTERACTS WITH	COMBINED EFFECT
Alcohol:	Can increase or decrease effect of anticoagulant. Use with caution.
Beverages:	None expected.
Cocaine:	None expected.
Foods: High in vitamin K such as fish, liver, spinach, cabbage.	May decrease anticoagulant effect.
Marijuana:	None expected.
Tobacco:	None expected.

PHENSUXIMIDE

BRAND NAMES

Milontin

BASIC INFORMATION

Habit forming? No
Prescription needed? Yes
Available as generic? No
Drug class: Anticonvulsant (succinimide)

 USES

Controls seizures in treatment of epilepsy.

 DOSAGE & USAGE INFORMATION

How to take:
Capsule or syrup—Swallow with liquid or food to lessen stomach irritation.

When to take:
Every day in regularly-spaced doses, according to prescription.

If you forget a dose:
Take as soon as you remember up to 2 hours late. If more than 2 hours, wait for next scheduled dose (don't double this dose).

What drug does:
Depresses nerve transmissions in part of brain that controls muscles.

Time lapse before drug works:
3 hours.

Don't take with:
See Interaction column and consult doctor.

 OVERDOSE

SYMPTOMS:
Coma
WHAT TO DO:
- Dial 0 (operator) or 911 (emergency) for an ambulance or medical help. Then give first aid immediately.
- If patient is unconscious and not breathing, give mouth-to-mouth breathing. If there is no heartbeat, use cardiac massage and mouth-to-mouth breathing (CPR). Don't try to make patient vomit. If you can't get help quickly, take patient to nearest emergency facility.
- See emergency information on inside covers.

 POSSIBLE ADVERSE REACTIONS OR SIDE EFFECTS

SYMPTOMS	WHAT TO DO
Life-threatening: None expected.	
Common: Nausea, vomiting, stomach cramps, appetite loss.	Continue. Call doctor when convenient.
Infrequent: Dizziness, drowsiness, headache, irritability, mood change.	Continue. Call doctor when convenient.
Rare: • Rash, sore throat, fever, unusual bleeding or bruising.	Discontinue. Call doctor right away.
• Swollen lymph glands.	Continue. Call doctor when convenient.

WARNINGS & PRECAUTIONS

Don't take if:
You are allergic to any succinimide anticonvulsant.

Before you start, consult your doctor:
- If you plan to become pregnant within medication period.
- If you take other anticonvulsants.
- If you have blood disease.
- If you have kidney or liver disease.

Over age 60:
Adverse reactions and side effects may be more frequent and severe than in younger persons.

Pregnancy:
Risk to unborn child outweighs drug benefits. Don't use.

Breast-feeding:
Drug passes into milk. Avoid drug or discontinue nursing.

Infants & children:
Use only under medical supervision.

Prolonged use:
No problems expected.

Skin & sunlight:
No problems expected.

Driving, piloting or hazardous work:
Don't drive or pilot aircraft until you learn how medicine affects you. Don't work around dangerous machinery. Don't climb ladders or work in high places. Danger increases if you drink alcohol or take medicine affecting alertness and reflexes, such as antihistamines, tranquilizers, sedatives, pain medicine, narcotics and mind-altering drugs.

Discontinuing:
Don't discontinue without doctor's advice until you complete prescribed dose, even though symptoms diminish or disappear.

Others:
- Your response to medicine should be checked regularly by your doctor. Dose and schedule may have to be altered frequently to fit individual needs.
- Periodic blood-cell counts, kidney- and liver-function studies recommended.

POSSIBLE INTERACTION WITH OTHER DRUGS

GENERIC NAME OR DRUG CLASS	COMBINED EFFECT
Anticonvulsants (other)	Increased effect of both drugs.
Antidepressants (tricyclic)	May provoke seizures.
Antipsychotics	May provoke seizures.

POSSIBLE INTERACTION WITH OTHER SUBSTANCES

INTERACTS WITH	COMBINED EFFECT
Alcohol:	May provoke seizures.
Beverages:	None expected.
Cocaine:	May provoke seizures.
Foods:	None expected.
Marijuana:	May provoke seizures.
Tobacco:	None expected.

PHENYLBUTAZONE

BRAND NAMES

Algoverine
Apo-Phenylbutazone
Azolid
Buffazone
Butagesic
Butazolidin
Intrabutazone

Malgesic
Nadozone
Neo-Zoline
Novobutazone
Phenbuff
Phenbutazone
Sterazolidin

BASIC INFORMATION

Habit forming? No
Available as generic? Yes
Prescription needed? Yes
Drug class: Anti-inflammatory (non-steroid)

 USES

- Treatment for joint pain, stiffness, inflammation and swelling of arthritis and gout.
- Pain reliever.
- Treatment for dysmenorrhea (painful or difficult menstruation).

 DOSAGE & USAGE INFORMATION

How to take:
Tablet or capsule—Swallow with liquid or food to lessen stomach irritation. If you can't swallow whole, crumble tablet or open capsule and take with liquid or food.

When to take:
At the same times each day.

If you forget a dose:
Take as soon as you remember up to 2 hours late. If more than 2 hours, wait for next scheduled dose (don't double this dose).

Continued next column

 OVERDOSE

SYMPTOMS:
Confusion, agitation, incoherence, convulsions, possible hemorrhage from stomach or intestine, coma.
WHAT TO DO:
- **Dial 0 (operator) or 911 (emergency) for an ambulance or medical help. Then give first aid immediately.**
- **See emergency information on inside covers.**

What drug does:
Reduces tissue concentration of prostaglandins (hormones which produce inflammation and pain).

Time lapse before drug works:
Begins in 4 to 24 hours. May require 3 weeks regular use for maximum benefit.

Don't take with:
See Interaction column and consult doctor.

 POSSIBLE ADVERSE REACTIONS OR SIDE EFFECTS

SYMPTOMS	WHAT TO DO
Life-threatening: None expected.	
Common: • Dizziness, stomach upset.	Continue. Call doctor when convenient.
• Headache.	Continue. Tell doctor at next visit.
Infrequent: Depression, drowsiness, ringing in ears, constipation or diarrhea, vomiting, swollen feet or legs.	Continue. Call doctor when convenient.
Rare: • Convulsions; confusion; rash, hives or itchy skin; blurred vision; sore throat, fever, mouth ulcers; black stools; vomiting blood; difficult breathing; tightness in chest; unusual bleeding or bruising; blood in urine.	Discontinue. Call doctor right away.
• Frequent, painful or difficult urination; fatigue; weakness; weight gain.	Continue. Call doctor when convenient.

 WARNINGS & PRECAUTIONS

Don't take if:
- You are allergic to aspirin or any non-steroid, anti-inflammatory drug.
- You have gastritis, peptic ulcer, enteritis, ileitis, ulcerative colitis.
- Patient is younger than 15.

Before you start, consult your doctor:
- If you have epilepsy.
- If you have Parkinson's disease.
- If you have been mentally ill.
- If you have had kidney disease or impaired kidney function, asthma, high blood pressure, heart failure, temporal arthritis, or polymyalgia rheumatica.

Over age 60:
Adverse reactions and side effects may be more frequent and severe than in younger persons.

Pregnancy:
Studies inconclusive on harm to unborn child. Animal studies show fetal abnormalities. Decide with your doctor whether drug benefits justify risk to unborn child.

Breast-feeding:
Drug filters into milk. May harm child. Avoid.

Infants & children:
Not recommended for those younger than 15. Use only under medical supervision.

Prolonged use:
- Eye damage.
- May cause rare bone-marrow damage, jaundice (yellow skin and eyes), reduced hearing.
- Periodic blood counts recommended if you use a long time.

Skin & sunlight:
No problems expected.

Driving, piloting or hazardous work:
Don't drive or pilot aircraft until you learn how medicine affects you. Don't work around dangerous machinery. Don't climb ladders or work in high places. Danger increases if you drink alcohol or take medicine affecting alertness and reflexes, such as antihistamines, tranquilizers, sedatives, pain medicine, narcotics and mind-altering drugs.

Discontinuing:
Don't discontinue without consulting doctor. Dose may require gradual reduction if you have taken drug for a long time. Doses of other drugs may also require adjustment.

Others:
No problems expected.

 ## POSSIBLE INTERACTION WITH OTHER DRUGS

GENERIC NAME OR DRUG CLASS	COMBINED EFFECT
Acebutolol	Decreased acebutolol effect.
Anticoagulants (oral)	Increased anticoagulant effect.
Aspirin	Possible stomach ulcer.
Antidiabetics (oral)	Increased antidiabetic effect.
Chloroquine	Possible skin toxicity.
Digitoxin	Decreased digitoxin effect.
Flecainide	Possible decreased blood-cell production in bone marrow.
Gold compounds	Possible increased likelihood of kidney damage.
Hydroxychloroquine	Possible skin toxicity.
Ketoprofen	Increased possibility of internal bleeding.
Methotrexate	Increased toxicity of both drugs to bone marrow.
Minoxidil	Decreased minoxidil effect.
Oxprenolol	Decreased antihypertensive effect of oxprenolol.
Penicillamine	Possible toxicity.
Phenytoin	Possible toxic phenytoin effect.
Tocainide	Possible decreased blood-cell production in bone marrow.
Trimethoprim	Possible bone-marrow toxicity.

 ## POSSIBLE INTERACTION WITH OTHER SUBSTANCES

INTERACTS WITH	COMBINED EFFECT
Alcohol:	Possible stomach ulcer or bleeding.
Beverages:	None expected.
Cocaine:	None expected.
Foods:	None expected.
Marijuana:	Increased pain relief from phenylbutazone.
Tobacco:	None expected.

PHENYLEPHRINE

BRAND NAMES

See complete list of brand names in the *Brand Name Directory,* page 954.

BASIC INFORMATION

Habit forming? No
Prescription needed? No
Available as generic? Yes
Drug class: Sympathomimetic

 ## USES

Temporary relief of congestion of nose, sinuses and throat caused by allergies, colds or sinusitis.

 ## DOSAGE & USAGE INFORMATION

How to take:
- Syrup, tablet or capsule—Swallow with liquid or food to lessen stomach irritation.
- Extended-release tablets or capsules—Swallow each dose whole.
- Nasal solution, nasal spray, nasal jelly—Take as directed on package.

When to take:
As needed, no more often than every 4 hours.

If you forget a dose:
Take when you remember. Wait 4 hours for next dose. Never double a dose.

What drug does:
Contracts blood-vessel walls of nose, sinus and throat tissues, enlarging airways.

Time lapse before drug works:
5 to 30 minutes.

Don't take with:
- Non-prescription drugs for asthma, cough, cold, allergy, appetite suppressants, sleeping pills or drugs containing caffeine without consulting doctor.
- See Interaction column and consult doctor.

 ## OVERDOSE

SYMPTOMS:
Headache, heart palpitations, vomiting, blood-pressure rise, slow and forceful pulse.
WHAT TO DO:
- **Dial 0 (operator) or 911 (emergency) for an ambulance or medical help. Then give first aid immediately.**
- **See emergency information on inside covers.**

 ## POSSIBLE ADVERSE REACTIONS OR SIDE EFFECTS

SYMPTOMS	WHAT TO DO
Life-threatening:	
None expected.	
Common:	
• Fast or pounding heartbeat.	Discontinue. Call doctor right away.
• Headache or dizziness; shakiness; insomnia; nervousness; burning, dryness, stinging inside nose.	Continue. Call doctor when convenient.
Infrequent:	
Paleness.	Continue. Call doctor when convenient.
Rare:	
Unusual sweating.	Discontinue. Call doctor right away.

WARNINGS & PRECAUTIONS

Don't take if:
You are allergic to any sympathomimetic.

Before you start, consult your doctor:
- If you have high blood pressure.
- If you have heart disease.
- If you have diabetes.
- If you have overactive thyroid.
- If you have taken MAO inhibitors in past 2 weeks.

Over age 60:
Adverse reactions and side effects may be more frequent and severe than in younger persons.

Pregnancy:
Risk to unborn child outweighs drug benefits. Don't use.

Breast-feeding:
Drug passes into milk. Avoid drug or discontinue nursing until you finish medicine. Consult doctor for advice on maintaining milk supply.

Infants & children:
Use only under close supervision.

Prolonged use:
- "Rebound" congestion (see Glossary) and chemical irritation of nasal membranes.
- May cause functional dependence.

Skin & sunlight:
No problems expected.

Driving, piloting or hazardous work:
No problems expected.

Discontinuing:
May be unnecessary to finish medicine. Follow doctor's instructions.

Others:
No problems expected.

POSSIBLE INTERACTION WITH OTHER DRUGS

GENERIC NAME OR DRUG CLASS	COMBINED EFFECT
Acebutolol	Decreased effects of both drugs.
Amphetamines	Increased nervousness.
Antiasthmatics	Nervous stimulation.
Antidepressants (tricyclic)	Increased phenylephrine effect.
Antihypertensives	Decreased antihypertensive effect.
MAO inhibitors	Dangerous blood-pressure rise.
Nitrates	Possible decreased effects of both drugs.
Oxprenolol	Decreased effects of both drugs.
Sedatives	Decreased sedative effect.
Sympathomimetics (other)	Increased stimulant effect.
Tranquilizers	Decreased tranquilizer effect.

POSSIBLE INTERACTION WITH OTHER SUBSTANCES

INTERACTS WITH	COMBINED EFFECT
Alcohol:	None expected.
Beverages: Caffeine drinks.	Excess brain stimulation.
Cocaine:	Excess brain stimulation.
Foods:	None expected.
Marijuana:	None expected.
Tobacco:	None expected.

PHENYLPROPANOLAMINE

BRAND NAMES

See complete list of brand names in the *Brand Name Directory,* page 954.

BASIC INFORMATION

Habit forming? No
Prescription needed?
  High strength: Yes
  Low strength: No
Available as generic? Yes
Drug class: Sympathomimetic

USES

- Relieves bronchial asthma.
- Decreases congestion of breathing passages.
- Suppresses allergic reactions.
- Decreases appetite.

DOSAGE & USAGE INFORMATION

How to take:
- Tablet or capsule—Swallow with liquid. You may chew or crush tablet.
- Extended-release tablets or capsules—Swallow each dose whole.
- Syrup—Take as directed on bottle.

When to take:
As needed, no more often than every 4 hours.

If you forget a dose:
Take up to 2 hours late. If more than 2 hours, wait for next dose (don't double this dose).

What drug does:
- Prevents cells from releasing allergy-causing chemicals (histamines).
- Relaxes muscles of bronchial tubes.
- Decreases blood-vessel size and blood flow, thus causing decongestion.

Time lapse before drug works:
30 to 60 minutes.

Continued next column

OVERDOSE

SYMPTOMS:
Severe anxiety, confusion, delirium, muscle tremors, rapid and irregular pulse.
WHAT TO DO:
- **Dial 0 (operator) or 911 (emergency) for an ambulance or medical help. Then give first aid immediately.**
- **See emergency information on inside covers.**

Don't take with:
- Non-prescription drugs for cough, cold, allergy or asthma without consulting doctor.
- See Interaction column and consult doctor.

POSSIBLE ADVERSE REACTIONS OR SIDE EFFECTS

SYMPTOMS	WHAT TO DO
Life-threatening:	
None expected.	
Common:	
• Rapid heartbeat.	Discontinue. Call doctor right away.
• Nervousness, headache, paleness.	Continue. Call doctor when convenient.
• Insomnia.	Continue. Tell doctor at next visit.
Infrequent:	
• Irregular heartbeat.	Discontinue. Call doctor right away.
• Dizziness, appetite loss, nausea, vomiting, difficult urination.	Continue. Call doctor when convenient.
Rare:	
Tightness in chest.	Discontinue. Call doctor right away.

WARNINGS & PRECAUTIONS

Don't take if:
You are allergic to any sympathomimetic drug.

Before you start, consult your doctor:
- If you have high blood pressure.
- If you have diabetes.
- If you have overactive thyroid gland.
- If you have difficulty urinating.
- If you have taken any MAO inhibitors in past 2 weeks.
- If you have taken digitalis preparations in the last 7 days.
- If you will have surgery within 2 months, including dental surgery, requiring general or spinal anesthesia.

Over age 60:
More likely to develop high blood pressure, heart-rhythm disturbances, angina and to feel drug's stimulant effects.

Pregnancy:
No proven harm to unborn child. Avoid if possible.

Breast-feeding:
Drug passes into milk. Avoid drug or discontinue nursing until you finish medicine. Consult doctor for advice on maintaining milk supply.

Infants & children:
No special problems expected.

Prolonged use:
- Excessive doses—Rare toxic psychosis.
- Men with enlarged prostate gland may have more urination difficulty.

Skin & sunlight:
No known problems.

Driving, piloting or hazardous work:
No restrictions unless you feel dizzy.

Discontinuing:
May be unnecessary to finish medicine. Follow doctor's instructions.

Others:
No problems expected.

 ## POSSIBLE INTERACTION WITH OTHER DRUGS

GENERIC NAME OR DRUG CLASS	COMBINED EFFECT
Acebutolol	Decreased effects of both drugs.
Anesthetics (general)	Increased phenylpropanolamine effect.
Antidepressants (tricyclic)	Increased effect of phenylpropanolamine. Excessive stimulation of heart and blood pressure.
Antihypertensives	Decreased antihypertensive effect.
Digitalis preparations	Serious heart-rhythm disturbances.
Epinephrine	Increased epinephrine effect.
Ergot preparations	Serious blood-pressure rise.
Guanethidine	Decreased effect of both drugs.
MAO inhibitors	Increased phenylpropanolamine effect. Dangerous blood-pressure rise.
Nitrates	Possible decreased effects of both drugs.
Oxprenolol	Decreased effects of both drugs.

 ## POSSIBLE INTERACTION WITH OTHER SUBSTANCES

INTERACTS WITH	COMBINED EFFECT
Alcohol:	None expected.
Beverages: Caffeine drinks.	Nervousness or insomnia.
Cocaine:	Rapid heartbeat. Avoid.
Foods:	None expected.
Marijuana:	Rapid heartbeat, possible heart-rhythm disturbance. Avoid.
Tobacco:	None expected.

PHENYLTOLOXAMINE

BRAND NAMES

See complete list of brand names in the *Brand Name Directory,* page 955.

BASIC INFORMATION

Habit forming? No
Prescription needed? No
Available as generic? No
Drug class: Antihistamine

 ## USES

Relieves symptoms of hay fever, allergic reactions and infections of nose and throat.

 ## DOSAGE & USAGE INFORMATION

How to take:
- Extended-release tablets or capsules—Swallow each dose whole with liquid.
- Syrup—Take as directed on label.
- Pediatric drops—Dilute dose in beverage before swallowing.

When to take:
As needed, no more often than every 3 hours.

If you forget a dose:
Take as soon as you remember. Wait 3 hours for next dose (don't double this dose).

What drug does:
Blocks histamine action in sensitized tissues.

Time lapse before drug works:
30 minutes.

Don't take with:
- Non-prescription drugs containing alcohol without consulting doctor.
- See Interaction column and consult doctor.

 ## OVERDOSE

SYMPTOMS:
- Adults—Drowsiness, confusion, incoordination, unsteadiness, muscle tremors, stupor, coma.
- Children—Excitement, hallucinations, overactivity, convulsions.

WHAT TO DO:
- Dial 0 (operator) or 911 (emergency) for an ambulance or medical help. Then give first aid immediately.
- See emergency information on inside covers.

 ## POSSIBLE ADVERSE REACTIONS OR SIDE EFFECTS

SYMPTOMS	WHAT TO DO
Life-threatening: None expected.	
Common: Drowsiness, thick bronchial secretions.	Continue. Tell doctor at next visit.
Infrequent:	
• Stomach upset or pain, rapid heartbeat.	Discontinue. Call doctor right away.
• Confusion; dry mouth, nose, throat; ringing or buzzing in ears; painful or difficult urination, appetite loss.	Continue. Call doctor when convenient.
Rare:	
• Nightmares, agitation, irritability (especially children), change in vision, sore throat, fever, unusual bleeding or bruising, fatigue, weakness.	Discontinue. Call doctor right away.
• Unusual sweating.	Continue. Call doctor when convenient.

WARNINGS & PRECAUTIONS

Don't take if:
- You are allergic to any antihistamine.
- You have asthma attacks.
- You have glaucoma.
- You have urination difficulty.

Before you start, consult your doctor:
- If you have reacted badly to any antihistamine.
- If you have had peptic ulcer disease.
- If you will have surgery within 2 months, including dental surgery, requiring general or spinal anesthesia.

Over age 60:
Likely to be drowsy, dizzy or lethargic and have impaired thinking, judgment and memory. Increases urination problems from enlarged prostate gland.

Pregnancy:
No proven problems. Consult doctor.

Breast-feeding:
Drug passes into milk. Avoid drug or discontinue nursing until you finish medicine. Consult doctor for advice on maintaining milk supply.

Infants & children:
Use only under medical supervision.

Prolonged use:
No problems expected.

Skin & sunlight:
May cause rash or intensify sunburn in areas exposed to sun or sunlamp.

Driving, piloting or hazardous work:
Don't drive or pilot aircraft until you learn how medicine affects you. Don't work around dangerous machinery. Don't climb ladders or work in high places. Danger increases if you drink alcohol or take medicine affecting alertness and reflexes.

Discontinuing:
May be unnecessary to finish medicine. Follow doctor's instructions.

Others:
No problems expected.

POSSIBLE INTERACTION WITH OTHER DRUGS

GENERIC NAME OR DRUG CLASS	COMBINED EFFECT
Amphetamines	Decreased effect of phenyltoloxamine, especially drowsiness.
Anticholinergics	Increased anticholinergic effect.
Anticonvulsants (hydantoin)	Changed pattern of epileptic seizures.
Antidepressants (tricyclic)	Increased phenyltoloxamine effect.
Dronabinol	Increased effects of both drugs. Avoid.
Narcotics	Increased sedation.
Pain relievers	Increased sedation.
Sedatives	Increased sedation.
Sleep inducers	Increased sedation.
Tranquilizers	Increased sedation.

POSSIBLE INTERACTION WITH OTHER SUBSTANCES

INTERACTS WITH	COMBINED EFFECT
Alcohol:	Rapid, excessive sedation. Use caution.
Beverages:	None expected.
Cocaine:	Decreased phenyltoloxamine effect.
Foods:	None expected.
Marijuana:	Excessive sedation.
Tobacco:	None expected.

PHENYTOIN

BRAND NAMES

Dantoin
Dilantin
Dilantin Infatabs
Dilantin Kapseals
Dilantin-125
Dilantin-30-Pediatric
Di-Phen
Diphenylan
Diphenylhydantoin
Novophenytoin

BASIC INFORMATION

Habit forming? No
Prescription needed? Yes
Available as generic? Yes
Drug class: Anticonvulsant (hydantoin)

 USES

- Prevents epileptic seizures.
- Stabilizes irregular heartbeat.

 DOSAGE & USAGE INFORMATION

How to take:
- Tablet or capsule—Swallow with liquid.
- Extended-release tablets or capsules—Swallow each dose whole. If you take regular tablets, you may chew or crush them.

When to take:
At the same time each day.

If you forget a dose:
- If drug taken 1 time per day—Take as soon as you remember up to 12 hours late. If more than 12 hours, wait for next scheduled dose (don't double this dose).
- If taken several times per day—Take as soon as possible, then return to regular schedule.

What drug does:
Promotes sodium loss from nerve fibers. This lessens excitability and inhibits spread of nerve impulses.

Continued next column

 OVERDOSE

SYMPTOMS:
Jerky eye movements; stagger; slurred speech; imbalance; drowsiness; blood-pressure drop; slow, shallow breathing; coma.
WHAT TO DO:
- Dial 0 (operator) or 911 (emergency) for an ambulance or medical help. Then give first aid immediately.
- See emergency information on inside covers.

Time lapse before drug works:
7 to 10 days continual use.

Don't take with:
See Interaction column and consult doctor.

 POSSIBLE ADVERSE REACTIONS OR SIDE EFFECTS

SYMPTOMS	WHAT TO DO
Life-threatening: None expected.	
Common: Enlarged, tender, receding gums with increased likelihood of bleeding; mild dizziness; sleeplessness; constipation; nausea, vomiting.	Continue. Call doctor when convenient.
Infrequent: • Hallucinations, confusion, slurred speech, stagger, rash, change in vision.	Discontinue. Call doctor right away.
• Headache, drowsiness, diarrhea, muscle twitching.	Continue. Call doctor when convenient.
• Increased body and facial hair.	Continue. Tell doctor at next visit.
Rare: Sore throat, fever, stomach pain, unusual bleeding or bruising, jaundice.	Discontinue. Call doctor right away.

WARNINGS & PRECAUTIONS

Don't take if:
You are allergic to any hydantoin anticonvulsant.

Before you start, consult your doctor:
- If you have had impaired liver function or disease.
- If you will have surgery within 2 months, including dental surgery, requiring general or spinal anesthesia.

Over age 60:
Adverse reactions and side effects may be more frequent and severe than in younger persons.

Pregnancy:
Risk to unborn child outweighs drug benefits. Don't use.

Breast-feeding:
Drug passes into milk. Avoid drug or discontinue nursing until you finish medicine. Consult doctor for advice on maintaining milk supply.

Infants & children:
Use only under medical supervision.

Prolonged use:
- Weakened bones.
- Lymph gland enlargement.
- Possible liver damage.
- Numbness and tingling of hands and feet.
- Continual back-and-forth eye movements.
- Bleeding, swollen or tender gums.

Skin & sunlight:
May cause rash or intensify sunburn in areas exposed to sun or sunlamp.

Driving, piloting or hazardous work:
Don't drive or pilot aircraft until you learn how medicine affects you. Don't work around dangerous machinery. Don't climb ladders or work in high places. Danger increases if you drink alcohol or take medicine affecting alertness and reflexes.

Discontinuing:
Don't discontinue without consulting doctor. Dose may require gradual reduction if you have taken drug for a long time. Doses of other drugs may also require adjustment.

Others:
No problems expected.

POSSIBLE INTERACTION WITH OTHER DRUGS

GENERIC NAME OR DRUG CLASS	COMBINED EFFECT
Amiodarone	Increased effect of phenytoin.
Anticoagulants	Increased effect of both drugs.
Antidepressants (tricyclic)	Decreased phenytoin effect. Phenytoin dose requires adjustment.
Antihypertensives	Increased effect of antihypertensive.
Aspirin	Increased phenytoin effect.
Barbiturates	Changed seizure pattern.
Carbonic anhydrase inhibitors	Increased chance of bone disease.
Chloramphenicol	Increased phenytoin effect.
Contraceptives (oral)	Increased seizures. Menstrual irregularities.
Cortisone drugs	Decreased cortisone effect.
Digitalis preparations	Decreased digitalis effect.
Disulfiram	Increased phenytoin effect.
Estrogens	Increased phenytoin effect.
Furosemide	Decreased furosemide effect.

Continued page 972

POSSIBLE INTERACTION WITH OTHER SUBSTANCES

INTERACTS WITH	COMBINED EFFECT
Alcohol:	Possible decreased anticonvulsant effect. Use with caution.
Beverages:	None expected.
Cocaine:	Possible seizures.
Foods:	None expected.
Marijuana:	Drowsiness, unsteadiness, decreased anticonvulsant effect.
Tobacco:	None expected.

PILOCARPINE

BRAND NAMES

Adsorbocarpine
Akarpine
Almocarpine
Isopto Carpine
Minims
Minims Pilocarpine
Miocarpine
Nova-Carpine
Ocusert Pilo

Pilocar
Pilocel
Pilokair
Pilomiotin
Pilopine HS
Piloptic
P.V. Carpine
P.V. Carpine Liquifilm

BASIC INFORMATION

Habit forming? No
Prescription needed?
  U.S.: Yes
  Canada: No
Available as generic? Yes
Drug class: Antiglaucoma

 USES

Treatment for glaucoma.

 DOSAGE & USAGE INFORMATION

How to take:
- Drops—Apply to eyes. Close eyes for 1 or 2 minutes to absorb medicine.
- Eye system—Follow label directions.

When to take:
As directed on label.

Continued next column

 OVERDOSE

SYMPTOMS:
If swallowed—Nausea, vomiting, diarrhea, forceful urination, profuse sweating, rapid pulse, breathing difficulty, loss of consciousness.
WHAT TO DO:
- **Dial 0 (operator) or 911 (emergency) for an ambulance or medical help. Then give first aid immediately.**
- **If patient is unconscious and not breathing, give mouth-to-mouth breathing. If there is no heartbeat, use cardiac massage and mouth-to-mouth breathing (CPR). Don't try to make patient vomit. If you can't get help quickly, take patient to nearest emergency facility.**
- **See emergency information on inside covers.**

If you forget a dose:
Apply as soon as possible and return to prescribed schedule. Don't double dose.

What drug does:
Reduces internal-eye pressure.

Time lapse before drug works:
15 to 30 minutes.

Don't take with:
See Interaction column and consult doctor.

 POSSIBLE ADVERSE REACTIONS OR SIDE EFFECTS

SYMPTOMS	WHAT TO DO
Life-threatening: None expected.	
Common: Pain, blurred or altered vision.	Continue. Call doctor when convenient.
Infrequent: • Headache, eye irritation or twitching, nausea, vomiting, diarrhea, difficult breathing, muscle tremors.	Discontinue. Call doctor right away.
• Profuse sweating, unusual saliva flow.	Continue. Call doctor when convenient.
Rare: None expected.	

WARNINGS & PRECAUTIONS

Don't take if:
You are allergic to pilocarpine.

Before you start, consult your doctor:
- If you take sedatives, sleeping pills, tranquilizers, antidepressants, antihistamines, narcotics or mind-altering drugs.
- If you have asthma.
- If you have conjunctivitis (pink eye).

Over age 60:
Adverse reactions and side effects may be more frequent and severe than in younger persons.

Pregnancy:
No proven harm to unborn child. Avoid if possible.

Breast-feeding:
No proven problems. Consult doctor.

Infants & children:
Not recommended.

Prolonged use:
You may develop tolerance for drug, making it ineffective.

Skin & sunlight:
No problems expected.

Driving, piloting or hazardous work:
Don't drive or pilot aircraft until you learn how medicine affects you. Don't work around dangerous machinery. Don't climb ladders or work in high places. Danger increases if you drink alcohol or take medicine affecting alertness and reflexes, such as antihistamines, tranquilizers, sedatives, pain medicine, narcotics and mind-altering drugs.

Discontinuing:
Doctor may discontinue and substitute another drug to keep treatment effective.

Others:
- Can provoke asthma attack in susceptible individuals.
- Drops may impair vision for 2 to 3 hours.

POSSIBLE INTERACTION WITH OTHER DRUGS

GENERIC NAME OR DRUG CLASS	COMBINED EFFECT
Amphetamines	Decreased pilocarpine effect.
Anticholinergics	Decreased pilocarpine effect.
Appetite suppressants	Decreased pilocarpine effect.
Cortisone drugs	Decreased pilocarpine effect.
Glycopyrrolate	Increased glycopyrrolate effect.
Phenothiazines	Decreased pilocarpine effect.

POSSIBLE INTERACTION WITH OTHER SUBSTANCES

INTERACTS WITH	COMBINED EFFECT
Alcohol:	May prolong alcohol's effect on brain.
Beverages:	None expected.
Cocaine:	Decreased pilocarpine effect. Avoid.
Foods:	None expected.
Marijuana:	Used once or twice weekly—May help lower internal eye pressure.
Tobacco:	None expected.

PINDOLOL

BRAND NAMES

Pindolol   Visken

BASIC INFORMATION

Habit forming? No
Prescription needed? Yes
Available as generic? No
Drug class: Beta-adrenergic blocker

 USES

- Reduces angina attacks.
- Stabilizes irregular heartbeat.
- Lowers blood pressure.
- Reduces frequency of migraine headaches. (Does not relieve headache pain.)
- Other uses prescribed by your doctor.

 DOSAGE & USAGE INFORMATION

How to take:
Tablet or capsule—Swallow with liquid. If you can't swallow whole, crumble tablet or open capsule and take with liquid or food.

When to take:
With meals or immediately after.

If you forget a dose:
Take as soon as you remember. Return to regular schedule, but allow 3 hours between doses.

What drug does:
- Blocks certain actions of sympathetic nervous system.
- Lowers heart's oxygen requirements.
- Slows nerve impulses through heart.
- Reduces blood vessel contraction in heart, scalp and other body parts.

Continued next column

 OVERDOSE

SYMPTOMS:
Weakness, slow or weak pulse, blood-pressure drop, fainting, convulsions, cold and sweaty skin.
WHAT TO DO:
- **Dial 0 (operator) or 911 (emergency) for an ambulance or medical help. Then give first aid immediately.**
- **See emergency information on inside covers.**

Time lapse before drug works:
1 to 4 hours.

Don't take with:
Non-prescription drugs or drugs in Interaction column without consulting doctor.

 POSSIBLE ADVERSE REACTIONS OR SIDE EFFECTS

SYMPTOMS	WHAT TO DO
Life-threatening:	
None expected.	
Common:	
Pulse slower than 50 beats per minute.	Discontinue. Call doctor right away.
Drowsiness, numbness or tingling of fingers or toes, dizziness, diarrhea, nausea, fatigue, weakness.	Continue. Call doctor when convenient.
Cold hands, feet; dry mouth, eyes, skin.	Continue. Tell doctor at next visit.
Infrequent:	
Hallucinations, nightmares, insomnia, headache, difficult breathing, joint pain.	Discontinue. Call doctor right away.
Confusion, depression, reduced alertness.	Continue. Call doctor when convenient.
Constipation.	Continue. Tell doctor at next visit.
Rare:	
Rash, sore throat, fever.	Discontinue. Call doctor right away.
Unusual bleeding and bruising.	Continue. Call doctor when convenient.

 WARNINGS & PRECAUTIONS

Don't take if:
- You are allergic to any beta-adrenergic blocker.
- You have asthma.
- You have hay fever symptoms.
- You have taken MAO inhibitors in past 2 weeks.

Before you start, consult your doctor:
- If you have heart disease or poor circulation to the extremities.
- If you have hay fever, asthma, chronic bronchitis, emphysema.
- If you have overactive thyroid function.
- If you have impaired liver or kidney function.
- If you will have surgery within 2 months, including dental surgery, requiring general or spinal anesthesia.
- If you have diabetes or hypoglycemia.

Over age 60:
Adverse reactions and side effects may be more frequent and severe than in younger persons.

Pregnancy:
Risk to unborn child outweighs drug benefits. Don't use.

Breast-feeding:
Drug passes into milk. Avoid drug or discontinue nursing until you finish medicine. Consult doctor for advice on maintaining milk supply.

Infants & children:
Not recommended.

Prolonged use:
Weakens heart muscle contractions.

Skin & sunlight:
No problems expected.

Driving, piloting or hazardous work:
Don't drive or pilot aircraft until you learn how medicine affects you. Don't work around dangerous machinery. Don't climb ladders or work in high places. Danger increases if you drink alcohol or take medicine affecting alertness and reflexes.

Discontinuing:
Don't discontinue without consulting doctor. Dose may require gradual reduction if you have taken drug for a long time. Doses of other drugs may also require adjustment.

Others:
May mask hypoglycemia.

POSSIBLE INTERACTION WITH OTHER DRUGS

GENERIC NAME OR DRUG CLASS	COMBINED EFFECT
Acebutolol	Increased antihypertensive effects of both drugs. Dosages may require adjustment.
Albuterol	Decreased albuterol effect and beta-adrenergic blocking effect
Antidiabetics	Increased antidiabetic effect.
Antihistamines	Decreased antihistamine effect.
Antihypertensives	Increased antihypertensive effect.
Anti-inflammatory drugs	Decreased anti-inflammatory effect.
Barbiturates	Increased barbiturate effect. Dangerous sedation.
Digitalis preparations	Can either increase or decrease heart rate. Improves irregular heartbeat.
Narcotics	Increased narcotic effect. Dangerous sedation.
Nitrates	Possible excessive blood-pressure drop.
Pentoxifylline	Increased antihypertensive effect.
Phenytoin	Increased pindolol effect.
Quinidine	Slows heart excessively.
Reserpine	Increased reserpine effect. Excessive sedation and depression.
Tocainide	May worsen congestive heart failure.

POSSIBLE INTERACTION WITH OTHER SUBSTANCES

INTERACTS WITH	COMBINED EFFECT
Alcohol:	Excessive blood-pressure drop. Avoid.
Beverages:	None expected.
Cocaine:	Irregular heartbeat. Avoid.
Foods:	None expected.
Marijuana:	Daily use—Impaired circulation to hands and feet.
Tobacco:	Possible irregular heartbeat.

PIPERACETAZINE

BRAND NAMES

Quide

BASIC INFORMATION

Habit forming? No
Prescription needed? Yes
Available as generic? Yes
Drug class: Tranquilizer, antiemetic
           (phenothiazine)

 USES

- Stops nausea, vomiting.
- Reduces anxiety, agitation.

 DOSAGE & USAGE INFORMATION

How to take:

- Tablet or capsule—Swallow with liquid or food to lessen stomach irritation.
- Suppositories—Remove wrapper and moisten suppository with water. Gently insert into rectum, large end first.
- Drops or liquid—Dilute dose in beverage.

When to take:

- Nervous and mental disorders—Take at the same times each day.
- Nausea and vomiting—Take as needed, no more often than every 4 hours.

If you forget a dose:

- Nervous and mental disorders—Take up to 2 hours late. If more than 2 hours, wait for next scheduled dose (don't double this dose).
- Nausea and vomiting—Take as soon as you remember. Wait 4 hours for next dose.

What drug does:

- Suppresses brain's vomiting center.
- Suppresses brain centers that control abnormal emotions and behavior.

Time lapse before drug works:

- Nausea and vomiting—1 hour or less.
- Nervous and mental disorders—4-6 weeks.

Continued next column

 OVERDOSE

SYMPTOMS:
Stupor, convulsions, coma.
WHAT TO DO:
- Dial 0 (operator) or 911 (emergency) for an ambulance or medical help. Then give first aid immediately.
- See emergency information on inside covers.

Don't take with:
- Antacid or medicine for diarrhea.
- Non-prescription drug for cough, cold or allergy.
- See Interaction column and consult doctor.

 POSSIBLE ADVERSE REACTIONS OR SIDE EFFECTS

SYMPTOMS	WHAT TO DO
Life-threatening:	
None expected.	
Common:	
• Muscle spasms of face and neck, unsteady gait.	Discontinue. Seek emergency treatment.
• Restlessness, tremor, drowsiness.	Discontinue. Call doctor right away.
• Decreased sweating, dry mouth, runny nose, constipation.	Continue. Call doctor when convenient.
Infrequent:	
• Fainting.	Discontinue. Seek emergency treatment.
• Rash.	Discontinue. Call doctor right away.
• Difficult urination, diminished sex drive, swollen breasts, menstrual irregularities.	Continue. Call doctor when convenient.
Rare:	
Change in vision, sore throat, fever, jaundice.	Discontinue. Call doctor right away.

WARNINGS & PRECAUTIONS

Don't take if:
- You are allergic to any phenothiazine.
- You have a blood or bone-marrow disease.

Before you start, consult your doctor:
- If you will have surgery within 2 months, including dental surgery, requiring general or spinal anesthesia.
- If you have asthma, emphysema or other lung disorder.
- If you take non-prescription ulcer medicine, asthma medicine or amphetamines.

Over age 60:
Adverse reactions and side effects may be more frequent and severe than in younger persons. More likely to develop involuntary movement of jaws, lips, tongue, chewing. Report this to your doctor immediately. Early treatment can help.

Pregnancy:
Risk to unborn child outweighs drug benefits. Don't use.

Breast feeding:
Drug passes into milk. Avoid drug or discontinue nursing until you finish medicine. Consult doctor for advice on maintaining milk supply.

Infants & children:
Don't give to children younger than 2.

Prolonged use:
May lead to tardive dyskinesia (involuntary movement of jaws, lips, tongue, chewing).

Skin & sunlight:
May cause rash or intensify sunburn in areas exposed to sun or sunlamp. Skin may remain sensitive for 3 months after discontinuing.

Driving, piloting or hazardous work:
Don't drive or pilot aircraft until you learn how medicine affects you. Don't work around dangerous machinery. Don't climb ladders or work in high places. Danger increases if you drink alcohol or take medicine affecting alertness and reflexes.

Discontinuing:
- Nervous and mental disorders—Don't discontinue without doctor's advice until you complete prescribed dose, even though symptoms diminish or disappear.
- Nausea and vomiting—May be unnecessary to finish medicine. Follow doctor's instructions.

Others:
No problems expected.

POSSIBLE INTERACTION WITH OTHER DRUGS

GENERIC NAME OR DRUG CLASS	COMBINED EFFECT
Anticholinergics	Increased anticholinergic effect.
Antidepressants (tricyclic)	Increased piperacetazine effect.
Antihistamines	Increased antihistamine effect.
Appetite suppressants	Decreased suppressant effect.
Dronabinol	Increased effects of both drugs. Avoid.
Levodopa	Decreased levodopa effect.
Mind-altering drugs	Increased effect of mind-altering drugs.
Narcotics	Increased narcotic effect.
Phenytoin	Increased phenytoin effect.
Quinidine	Impaired heart function. Dangerous mixture.
Sedatives	Increased sedative effect.
Tranquilizers (other)	Increased tranquilizer effect.

POSSIBLE INTERACTION WITH OTHER SUBSTANCES

INTERACTS WITH	COMBINED EFFECT
Alcohol:	Dangerous oversedation.
Beverages:	None expected.
Cocaine:	Decreased piperacetazine effect. Avoid.
Foods:	None expected.
Marijuana:	Drowsiness. May increase antinausea effect.
Tobacco:	None expected.

PIROXICAM

BRAND NAMES

Feldene

BASIC INFORMATION

Habit forming? No
Prescription needed? Yes
Available as generic? No
Drug class: Anti-inflammatory (non-steroid)

USES

- Relieves symptoms of rheumatoid arthritis, osteoarthritis and gout.
- Relieves symptoms of ankylosing spondylitis.

DOSAGE & USAGE INFORMATION

How to take:
Tablet—Swallow with liquid or food to lessen stomach irritation. If you can't swallow whole, crumble tablet and take with liquid or food.

When to take:
At the same times each day.

If you forget a dose:
Take as soon as you remember up to 2 hours late. If more than 2 hours, wait for next scheduled dose (don't double this dose).

What drug does:
Reduces tissue concentration of prostaglandins (hormones that produce inflammation and pain).

Time lapse before drug works:
Begins in 4 to 24 hours. May require 3 weeks regular use for maximum benefit.

Don't take with:
See Interaction column and consult doctor.

OVERDOSE

SYMPTOMS:
Confusion, agitation, incoherence, convulsions, possible hemorrhage from stomach or intestine, coma.
WHAT TO DO:
- **Dial 0 (operator) or 911 (emergency) for an ambulance or medical help. Then give first aid immediately.**
- **See emergency information on inside covers.**

POSSIBLE ADVERSE REACTIONS OR SIDE EFFECTS

SYMPTOMS	WHAT TO DO
Life-threatening:	
None expected.	
Common:	
• Dizziness, nausea, pain.	Continue. Call doctor when convenient.
• Headache.	Continue. Tell doctor at next visit.
Infrequent:	
Depression, drowsiness, ringing in ears, swollen feet or legs, constipation or diarrhea, vomiting.	Continue. Call doctor when convenient.
Rare:	
• Convulsions; confusion; rash, hives or itchy skin; blurred vision; black, bloody or tarry stool; difficult breathing; tightness in chest; rapid heartbeat; unusual bleeding or bruising; blood in urine; jaundice.	Discontinue. Call doctor right away.
• Painful or difficult urination, fatigue, weakness.	Continue. Call doctor when convenient.

WARNINGS & PRECAUTIONS

Don't take if:
- You are allergic to aspirin or any non-steroid, anti-inflammatory drug.
- You have gastritis, peptic ulcer, enteritis, ileitis, ulcerative colitis, asthma, heart failure, high blood pressure or bleeding problems.
- Patient is younger than 15.

Before you start, consult your doctor:
- If you have epilepsy.
- If you have Parkinson's disease.
- If you have been mentally ill.
- If you have had kidney disease or impaired kidney function.
- If you will have surgery within 2 months, including dental surgery, requiring general or spinal anesthesia.

Over age 60:
Adverse reactions and side effects may be more frequent and severe than in younger persons. Smaller than average doses may reduce unpleasant side effects.

Pregnancy:
Studies inconclusive on harm to unborn child. Animal studies show fetal abnormalities. Decide with your doctor whether drug benefits justify risk to unborn child.

Breast-feeding:
May harm child. Avoid.

Infants & children:
Not recommended for anyone younger than 15. Use only under medical supervision.

Prolonged use:
- Eye damage, reduced hearing, sore throat, fever.
- Weight gain.
- Request liver-function and bleeding time studies.

Skin & sunlight:
No problems expected.

Driving, piloting or hazardous work:
Don't drive or pilot aircraft until you learn how medicine affects you. Don't work around dangerous machinery. Don't climb ladders or work in high places. Danger increases if you drink alcohol or take medicine affecting alertness and reflexes.

Discontinuing:
Don't discontinue without consulting doctor. Dose may require gradual reduction if you have taken drug for a long time. Doses of other drugs may also require adjustment.

Others:
No problems expected.

POSSIBLE INTERACTION WITH OTHER DRUGS

GENERIC NAME OR DRUG CLASS	COMBINED EFFECT
Acebutolol	Decreased antihypertensive effect of acebutolol.
Anticoagulants (oral)	Increased risk of bleeding.
Aspirin	Increased risk of stomach ulcer.
Cortisone drugs	Increased risk of stomach ulcer.
Furosemide	Decreased diuretic effect of furosemide.
Gold compounds	Possible increased likelihood of kidney damage.
Minoxidil	Decreased minoxidil effect.
Oxprenolol	Decreased antihypertensive effect of oxprenolol.
Oxyphenbutazone	Possible stomach ulcer.
Phenylbutazone	Possible stomach ulcer.
Probenecid	Increased piroxicam effect.
Thyroid hormones	Rapid heartbeat, blood-pressure rise.

POSSIBLE INTERACTION WITH OTHER SUBSTANCES

INTERACTS WITH	COMBINED EFFECT
Alcohol:	Possible stomach ulcer or bleeding.
Beverages:	None expected.
Cocaine:	Depression following cocaine use. Avoid.
Foods:	None expected.
Marijuana:	Increased pain relief from piroxicam, but may be depressing.
Tobacco:	Decreased absorption of piroxicam. Avoid tobacco.

POLOXAMER 188

BRAND NAMES

Alaxin   Poloxalkol

BASIC INFORMATION

Habit forming? No
Prescription needed? No
Available as generic? Yes
Drug class: Laxative (emollient)

 USES

Constipation relief.

 DOSAGE & USAGE INFORMATION

How to take:
- Tablet or capsule—Swallow with liquid. Don't open capsules.
- Drops—Dilute dose in beverage before swallowing.
- Syrup—Take as directed on bottle.

When to take:
At the same time each day, preferably bedtime.

If you forget a dose:
Take as soon as you remember. Wait 12 hours for next dose. Return to regular schedule.

What drug does:
Makes stool hold fluid so it is easier to pass.

Time lapse before drug works:
2 to 3 days of continual use.

Don't take with:
- Other medicines at same time. Wait 2 hours.
- See Interaction column and consult doctor.

 OVERDOSE

SYMPTOMS:
Appetite loss, nausea, vomiting, diarrhea.
WHAT TO DO:
Overdose unlikely to threaten life. If person takes much larger amount than prescribed, call doctor, poison-control center or hospital emergency room for instructions.

 POSSIBLE ADVERSE REACTIONS OR SIDE EFFECTS

SYMPTOMS	WHAT TO DO
Life-threatening:	
None expected.	
Common:	
None expected.	
Infrequent:	
Throat irritation (liquid only), intestinal and stomach cramps.	Continue. Call doctor when convenient.
Rare:	
Rash.	Discontinue. Call doctor right away.

WARNINGS & PRECAUTIONS

Don't take if:
- You are allergic to any emollient laxative.
- You have abdominal pain and fever that might be appendicitis.

Before you start, consult your doctor:
- If you are taking other laxatives.
- To be sure constipation isn't a sign of a serious disorder.

Over age 60:
You must drink 6 to 8 glasses of fluid every 24 hours for drug to work.

Pregnancy:
No problems expected. Consult doctor.

Breast-feeding:
No problems expected.

Infants & children:
No problems expected.

Prolonged use:
Avoid. Overuse of laxatives may damage intestine lining.

Skin & sunlight:
No problems expected.

Driving, piloting or hazardous work:
No problems expected.

Discontinuing:
May be unnecessary to finish medicine. Follow doctor's instructions.

Others:
No problems expected.

 POSSIBLE INTERACTION WITH OTHER DRUGS

GENERIC NAME OR DRUG CLASS	COMBINED EFFECT
Danthron	Possible liver damage.
Digitalis preparations	Toxic absorption of digitalis.
Mineral oil	Increased mineral oil absorption into bloodstream. Avoid.
Phenolphthalein	Increased phenolphthalein absorption. Possible toxicity.

 POSSIBLE INTERACTION WITH OTHER SUBSTANCES

INTERACTS WITH	COMBINED EFFECT
Alcohol:	None expected.
Beverages:	None expected.
Cocaine:	None expected.
Foods:	None expected.
Marijuana:	None expected.
Tobacco:	None expected.

POLYCARBOPHIL CALCIUM

BRAND NAMES

Mitrolan

BASIC INFORMATION

Habit forming? No
Prescription needed? No
Available as generic? No
**Drug class: Laxative (bulk-forming),
             antidiarrheal**

USES

- Relieves constipation and prevents straining for bowel movement.
- Stops diarrhea.

DOSAGE & USAGE INFORMATION

How to take:
- Tablets (laxative)—Swallow with 8 oz. cold liquid. Drink 6 to 8 glasses of water each day in addition to the one with each dose.
- Tablets (diarrhea)—Take without water at half-hour intervals.

When to take:
At the same times each day.

If you forget a dose:
Take as soon as you remember. Resume regular schedule.

What drug does:
Absorbs water, stimulating the bowel to form a soft, bulky stool and decreasing watery diarrhea.

Time lapse before drug works:
May require 2 or 3 days to begin, then works in 12 to 24 hours.

Don't take with:
- See Interaction column and consult doctor.
- Don't take within 2 hours of taking another medicine.

OVERDOSE

SYMPTOMS:
None expected.
WHAT TO DO:
Overdose unlikely to threaten life. If person takes much larger amount than prescribed, call doctor, poison-control center or hospital emergency room for instructions.

POSSIBLE ADVERSE REACTIONS OR SIDE EFFECTS

SYMPTOMS	WHAT TO DO
Life-threatening: None expected.	
Common: None expected.	
Infrequent: Swallowing difficulty, "lump in throat" sensation, nausea, vomiting, diarrhea.	Continue. Call doctor when convenient.
Rare: Itchy skin, rash, intestinal blockage, asthma.	Discontinue. Call doctor right away.

WARNINGS & PRECAUTIONS

Don't take if:
- You are allergic to any bulk-forming laxative.
- You have symptoms of appendicitis, inflamed bowel or intestinal blockage.
- You have missed a bowel movement for only 1 or 2 days.

Before you start, consult your doctor:
- If you have diabetes.
- If you have a laxative habit.
- If you have rectal bleeding.
- If you have difficulty swallowing.
- If you take other laxatives.

Over age 60:
Adverse reactions and side effects may be more frequent and severe than in younger persons.

Pregnancy:
Most bulk-forming laxatives contain sodium or sugars which may cause fluid retention. Avoid if possible.

Breast-feeding:
No problems expected.

Infants & children:
Use only under medical supervision.

Prolonged use:
Don't take for more than 1 week unless under a doctor's supervision. May cause laxative dependence.

Skin & sunlight:
No problems expected.

Driving, piloting or hazardous work:
No problems expected.

Discontinuing:
May be unnecessary to finish medicine. Follow doctor's instructions.

Others:
Don't take to "flush out" your system or as a "tonic."

POSSIBLE INTERACTION WITH OTHER DRUGS

GENERIC NAME OR DRUG CLASS	COMBINED EFFECT
Antibiotics	Decreased antibiotic effect.
Anticoagulants	Decreased anticoagulant effect.
Digitalis preparations	Decreased digitalis effect.
Salicylates (including aspirin)	Decreased salicylate effect.

POSSIBLE INTERACTION WITH OTHER SUBSTANCES

INTERACTS WITH	COMBINED EFFECT
Alcohol:	None expected.
Beverages:	None expected.
Cocaine:	None expected.
Foods:	None expected.
Marijuana:	None expected.
Tobacco:	None expected.

POLYTHIAZIDE

BRAND NAMES

Renese

BASIC INFORMATION

Habit forming? No
Prescription needed? Yes
Available as generic? Yes
Drug class: Antihypertensive, diuretic
(thiazide)

 USES

- Controls, but doesn't cure, high blood pressure.
- Reduces fluid retention (edema) caused by conditions such as heart disorders and liver disease.

 DOSAGE & USAGE INFORMATION

How to take:
Tablet or capsule—Swallow with 8 oz. of liquid. If you can't swallow whole, crumble tablet or open capsule and take with liquid or food. Don't exceed dose.

When to take:
At the same time each day.

If you forget a dose:
Take as soon as you remember up to 2 hours late. If more than 2 hours, wait for next scheduled dose (don't double this dose).

What drug does:
- Forces sodium and water excretion, reducing body fluid.
- Relaxes muscle cells of small arteries.
- Reduced body fluid and relaxed arteries lower blood pressure.

Time lapse before drug works:
4 to 6 hours. May require several weeks to lower blood pressure.

Continued next column

 OVERDOSE

SYMPTOMS:
Cramps, weakness, drowsiness, weak pulse, coma.
WHAT TO DO:
- **Dial 0 (operator) or 911 (emergency) for an ambulance or medical help. Then give first aid immediately.**
- **See emergency information on inside covers.**

Don't take with:
- See Interaction column and consult doctor.
- Non-prescription drugs without consulting doctor.

 POSSIBLE ADVERSE REACTIONS OR SIDE EFFECTS

SYMPTOMS	WHAT TO DO
Life-threatening:	
None expected.	
Common:	
None expected.	
Infrequent:	
• Blurred vision, severe abdominal pain, nausea, vomiting, irregular heartbeat, weak pulse.	Discontinue. Call doctor right away.
• Dizziness, mood change, headache, weakness, tiredness, weight changes.	Continue. Call doctor when convenient.
• Dry mouth, thirst.	Continue. Tell doctor at next visit.
Rare:	
• Rash or hives.	Discontinue. Seek emergency treatment.
• Jaundice, sore throat, fever.	Discontinue. Call doctor right away.

 WARNINGS & PRECAUTIONS

Don't take if:
You are allergic to any thiazide diuretic drug.

Before you start, consult your doctor:
- If you are allergic to any sulfa drug.
- If you have gout.
- If you have liver, pancreas or kidney disorder.

Over age 60:
Adverse reactions and side effects may be more frequent and severe than in younger persons, especially dizziness and excessive potassium loss.

Pregnancy:
Risk to unborn child outweighs drug benefits. Don't use.

Breast-feeding:
Drug passes into milk. Avoid drug or discontinue nursing.

Infants & children:
No problems expected.

Prolonged use:
You may need medicine to treat high blood pressure for the rest of your life.

Skin & sunlight:
May cause rash or intensify sunburn in areas exposed to sun or sunlamp.

Driving, piloting or hazardous work:
Don't drive or pilot aircraft until you learn how medicine affects you. Don't work around dangerous machinery. Don't climb ladders or work in high places. Danger increases if you drink alcohol or take medicine affecting alertness and reflexes, such as antihistamines, tranquilizers, sedatives, pain medicine, narcotics and mind-altering drugs.

Discontinuing:
Don't discontinue without medical advice.

Others:
- Hot weather and fever may cause dehydration and drop in blood pressure. Dose may require temporary adjustment. Weigh daily and report any unexpected weight decreases to your doctor.
- May cause rise in uric acid, leading to gout.
- May cause blood-sugar rise in diabetics.

 POSSIBLE INTERACTION WITH OTHER DRUGS

GENERIC NAME OR DRUG CLASS	COMBINED EFFECT
Acebutolol	Increased antihypertensive effect. Dosages of both drugs may require adjustments.
Allopurinol	Decreased allopurinol effect.
Amiodarone	Increased risk of heartbeat irregularity due to low potassium.
Antidepressants (tricyclic)	Dangerous drop in blood pressure. Avoid combination unless under medical supervision.
Barbiturates	Increased polythiazide effect.
Calcium supplements	Increased calcium in blood.

Cholestyramine	Decreased polythiazide effect.
Cortisone drugs	Excessive potassium loss that causes dangerous heart rhythms.
Digitalis preparations	Excessive potassium loss that causes dangerous heart rhythms.
Diuretics (thiazide)	Increased effect of other thiazide diuretics.
Indapamide	Increased diuretic effect.
Labetolol	Increased antihypertensive effects.
Lithium	Increased effect of lithium.
MAO inhibitors	Increased polythiazide effect.
Nitrates	Excessive blood-pressure drop.
Oxprenolol	Increased antihypertensive effect. Dosages of both drugs may require adjustments.
Potassium supplements	Decreased potassium effect.
Probenecid	Decreased probenecid effect.

 POSSIBLE INTERACTION WITH OTHER SUBSTANCES

INTERACTS WITH	COMBINED EFFECT
Alcohol:	Dangerous blood-pressure drop.
Beverages:	None expected.
Cocaine:	None expected.
Foods: Licorice.	Excessive potassium loss that causes dangerous heart rhythms.
Marijuana:	May increase blood pressure.
Tobacco:	None expected.

POTASSIUM PHOSPHATES

BRAND NAMES

K-Phos Original   **Neutra-Phos K**

BASIC INFORMATION

Habit forming? No
Prescription needed? Yes
Available as generic? No
Drug class: Urinary acidifier, antiurolithic
(antikidney stones) electrolyte
replenisher

USES

- Provides supplement of phosphorous for
  people with diseases which decrease
  phosphorous absorption from food.
- Keeps uric acid to treat or prevent urinary
  tract infections and prevent stone formation.

DOSAGE & USAGE INFORMATION

How to take:
- Tablets—Dissolve tablets in 3/4 to 1 glass of
  water. Let tablets soak 2 to 5 minutes, then
  stir to completely dissolve.
- Capsules—Swallow with food.

When to take:
After meals or with food to prevent or lessen
stomach irritation or loose stools.

If you forget a dose:
Take within 1 hour then return to original
schedule. If later than 1 hour, skip dose. Don't
double-dose.

What drug does:
- Provides supplemental phosphates.
- Makes uric acid.

Time lapse before drug works:
30-60 minutes.

Don't take with:
See Interaction column and consult doctor.

OVERDOSE

SYMPTOMS:
Irregular heartbeat, blood-pressure drop with
weakness, coma, cardiac arrest.
WHAT TO DO:
- **Dial 0 (operator) or 911 (emergency) for an**
  ambulance or medical help. Then give first
  aid immediately.
- **See emergency information on inside**
  covers.

POSSIBLE ADVERSE REACTIONS OR SIDE EFFECTS

SYMPTOMS	WHAT TO DO
Life-threatening: Irregular heart-beat, shortness of breath.	Discontinue. Seek emergency treatment.
Common: Muscle cramps.	Discontinue. Call doctor right away.
Infrequent: Bone and joint pain, numbness or tingling in hands or feet, unusual tiredness, weakness, diarrhea, nausea, abdominal pain, vomiting.	Discontinue. Call doctor right away.
Rare: None expected.	

WARNINGS & PRECAUTIONS

Don't take if:
You have had allergic reaction to potassium, sodium or phosphates; severe kidney disease; severe burns.

Before you start, consult your doctor:
If you have heart problems, adrenal insufficiency, liver disease, high blood pressure, pregnancy, hypoparathyroidism, chronic kidney disease, osteomalacia, pancreatitis, rickets.

Over age 60:
Adverse reactions and side effects may be more frequent and severe than in younger persons. Ask doctor about smaller doses.

Pregnancy:
Risk to unborn child outweighs drug benefits. Don't use.

Breast-feeding:
No data available in humans.

Infants & children:
Use only under medical supervision.

Prolonged use:
Monitor ECG, serum calcium, phosphorous and potassium levels.

Skin & sunlight:
No problems expected.

Driving, piloting or hazardous work:
Avoid if medicine causes dizziness or confusion.

Discontinuing:
Don't discontinue without consulting doctor. Dose may require gradual reduction if you have taken drug for a long time. Doses of other drugs may also require adjustment.

Others:
Protect liquid medicine from freezing.

POSSIBLE INTERACTION WITH OTHER DRUGS

GENERIC NAME OR DRUG CLASS	COMBINED EFFECT
Cortisone drugs	Increased fluid retention.
Captopril	Level of potassium in blood too high.
Digitalis preparations	Level of potassium in blood too high.
Diuretics amiloride, triamterene, spironolactone	Level of potassium in blood too high.
Male hormones	Fluid retention.
Mexiletine	May decrease effectiveness of mexiletine.
Potassium supplements	Level of potassium in blood too high.
Quinidine	Increases quinidine effect.
Salicylates (including aspirin)	Level of salicylates in blood too high.
Vitamin D (calcifidiol and and calcitriol)	Level of phosphorous in blood too high.

POSSIBLE INTERACTION WITH OTHER SUBSTANCES

INTERACTS WITH	COMBINED EFFECT
Alcohol:	None expected.
Beverages: Salty drinks such as tomato juice, commercial thirst quenchers, salt substitutes.	Increased fluid retention.
Cocaine:	May cause irregular heartbeat.
Foods: Salty foods such as canned soups, potato chips, TV dinners, hot dogs, pickles.	Increased fluid retention.
Marijuana:	May cause irregular heartbeat.
Tobacco:	May aggravate irregular heartbeat.

POTASSIUM & SODIUM PHOSPHATES

BRAND AND GENERIC NAMES

DIBASIC POTASSIUM
  & SODIUM
  PHOSPHATES
K-Phos M.F.
K-Phos Neutral
K-Phos 2
MONOBASIC
  POTASSIUM &
  SODIUM
  PHOSPHATES

Neutra-Phos
POTASSIUM &
  SODIUM
  PHOSPHATES
Uro-KP-Neutral

BASIC INFORMATION

Habit forming? No
Prescription needed? Yes
Available as generic? Yes
Drug class: Urinary acidifier, antiurolithic
  (antikidney stones) electrolyte
  replenisher

 USES

- Provides supplement of phosphorous for people with diseases which decrease phosphorous absorption from food.
- Keeps uric acid to treat or prevent urinary tract infections and prevent stone formation.

 DOSAGE & USAGE INFORMATION

How to take:
Dissolve tablets in 3/4 to 1 glass of water. Let tablets soak 2 to 5 minutes, then stir to completely dissolve.

When to take:
After meals or with food to prevent or lessen stomach irritation or loose stools.

If you forget a dose:
Take within 1 hour then return to original schedule. If later than 1 hour, skip dose. Don't double-dose.

Continued next column

 OVERDOSE

SYMPTOMS:
Irregular heartbeat, blood-pressure drop with weakness, coma, cardiac arrest.
WHAT TO DO:
- **Dial 0 (operator) or 911 (emergency) for an ambulance or medical help. Then give first aid immediately.**
- **See emergency information on inside covers.**

What drug does:
- Provides supplemental phosphates.
- Makes uric acid.

Time lapse before drug works:
30-60 minutes.

Don't take with:
See Interaction column and consult doctor.

 POSSIBLE ADVERSE REACTIONS OR SIDE EFFECTS

SYMPTOMS	WHAT TO DO
Life-threatening:	
Irregular heart-beat, difficult breathing, anxiety, weak legs.	Discontinue. Seek emergency treatment.
Common:	
None expected.	
Infrequent:	
Numbness or tingling in hands or feet, diarrhea, nausea, abdominal pain, vomiting, headache, dizziness, muscle cramps, swollen feet and ankles, thirst, weakness.	Discontinue. Call doctor right away.
Rare:	
Confusion.	Discontinue. Call doctor right away.

POTASSIUM & SODIUM PHOSPHATES

WARNINGS & PRECAUTIONS

Don't take if:
You have had allergic reaction to potassium, sodium or phosphates; severe kidney disease; severe burns.

Before you start, consult your doctor:
If you have heart problems, adrenal insufficiency, liver disease, high blood pressure, pregnancy, hypoparathyroidism, chronic kidney disease, osteomalacia, pancreatitis, rickets.

Over age 60:
Adverse reactions and side effects may be more frequent and severe than in younger persons. Ask doctor about smaller doses.

Pregnancy:
Risk to unborn child outweighs drug benefits. Don't use.

Breast-feeding:
No data available in humans.

Infants & children:
Use only under medical supervision.

Prolonged use:
Monitor ECG, serum calcium, phosphorous and potassium levels.

Skin & sunlight:
No problems expected.

Driving, piloting or hazardous work:
Avoid if medicine causes dizziness or confusion.

Discontinuing:
Don't discontinue without consulting doctor. Dose may require gradual reduction if you have taken drug for a long time. Doses of other drugs may also require adjustment.

Others:
Protect liquid medicine from freezing.

POSSIBLE INTERACTION WITH OTHER DRUGS

GENERIC NAME OR DRUG CLASS	COMBINED EFFECT
Captopril	Level of potassium in blood too high.
Cortisone drugs	Increased fluid retention.
Digitalis preparations	Level of potassium in blood too high.
Diuretics such as: amiloride, triamterene, spironolactone	Level of potassium in blood too high.
Male hormones	Fluid retention.
Potassium supplements	Level of potassium in blood too high.
Quinidine	Increases quinidine effect.
Salicylates (including aspirin)	Level of salicylates in blood too high.
Vitamin D (calcifidiol and and calcitriol)	Level of phosphorous in blood too high.

POSSIBLE INTERACTION WITH OTHER SUBSTANCES

INTERACTS WITH	COMBINED EFFECT
Alcohol:	None expected.
Beverages: Salty drinks such as tomato juice, commercial thirst quenchers, salt substitutes.	Increased fluid retention.
Cocaine:	May cause irregular heartbeat.
Foods: Salty foods such as canned soups, potato chips, TV dinners, hot dogs, pickles.	Increased fluid retention.
Marijuana:	May cause irregular heartbeat.
Tobacco:	May aggravate irregular heartbeat.

POTASSIUM SUPPLEMENTS

BRAND NAMES

See complete list of brand names in the *Brand Name Directory,* page 955.

BASIC INFORMATION

Habit forming? No
Prescription needed? Yes
Available as generic? Yes
Drug class: Mineral supplement (potassium)

USES

- Treatment for potassium deficiency from diuretics, cortisone or digitalis medicines.
- Treatment for low potassium associated with some illnesses.

DOSAGE & USAGE INFORMATION

How to take:
- Tablet or capsule—Swallow with liquid or food to lessen stomach irritation. You may chew or crush tablet.
- Extended-release tablets or capsules—Swallow each dose whole with liquid.
- Effervescent tablets, granules, powder or liquid—Dilute dose in water.

When to take:
At the same time each day, preferably with food or immediately after meals.

If you forget a dose:
Take as soon as you remember. Don't double next dose.

What drug does:
Preserves or restores normal function of nerve cells, heart and skeletal-muscle cells, kidneys, and stomach-juice secretions.

Continued next column

OVERDOSE

SYMPTOMS:
Paralysis of arms and legs, irregular heartbeat, blood-pressure drop, convulsions, coma, cardiac arrest.
WHAT TO DO:
- **Dial 0 (operator) or 911 (emergency) for an ambulance or medical help. Then give first aid immediately.**
- **See emergency information on inside covers.**

Time lapse before drug works:
1 to 2 hours. Full benefit may require 12 to 24 hours.

Don't take with:
See Interaction column and consult doctor.

POSSIBLE ADVERSE REACTIONS OR SIDE EFFECTS

SYMPTOMS	WHAT TO DO
Life-threatening: None expected.	
Common: None expected.	
Infrequent: Diarrhea, nausea, vomiting, stomach discomfort.	Continue. Call doctor when convenient.
Rare:	
• Confusion, irregular heartbeat, difficult breathing, unusual fatigue, weakness, heaviness of legs.	Discontinue. Call doctor right away.
• Numbness or tingling in hands or feet.	Continue. Call doctor when convenient.

WARNINGS & PRECAUTIONS

Don't take if:
- You are allergic to any potassium supplement.
- You have acute or chronic kidney disease.

Before you start, consult your doctor:
- If you have Addison's disease or familial periodic paralysis.
- If you have heart disease.
- If you have intestinal blockage.
- If you have a stomach ulcer.
- If you use diuretics.
- If you use heart medicine.
- If you use laxatives or have chronic diarrhea.
- If you use salt substitutes or low-salt milk.

Over age 60:
Observe dose schedule strictly. Potassium balance is critical. Deviation above or below normal can have serious results.

Pregnancy:
No problems expected if you adhere strictly to prescribed dose.

Breast-feeding:
Studies inconclusive on harm to infant. Consult doctor.

Infants & children:
Use only under doctor's supervision.

Prolonged use:
- Slows absorption of vitamin B-12. May cause anemia.
- Request frequent lab tests to monitor potassium levels in blood, especially if you take digitalis preparations.

Skin & sunlight:
No problems expected.

Driving, piloting or hazardous work:
No problems expected.

Discontinuing:
Don't discontinue without consulting doctor. Dose may require gradual reduction if you have taken drug for a long time. Doses of other drugs may also require adjustment.

Others:
- Overdose or underdose serious. Frequent EKGs and laboratory blood studies to measure serum electrolytes and kidney function recommended.
- Prolonged diarrhea may call for increased dosage of potassium.
- Serious injury may necessitate temporary *decrease* in potassium.

POSSIBLE INTERACTION WITH OTHER DRUGS

GENERIC NAME OR DRUG CLASS	COMBINED EFFECT
Amiloride	Dangerous rise in blood potassium.
Atropine	Increased possibility of intestinal ulcers, which sometimes occur with oral potassium tablets.
Belladonna	Increased possibility of intestinal ulcers, which sometimes occur with oral potassium tablets.
Captopril	Possible increased potassium effect.
Cortisone medicines	Decreased effect of potassium.
Digitalis preparations	Possible irregular heartbeat.
Diuretics (thiazide)	Decreased potassium effect.
Laxatives	Possible decreased potassium effect.
Spironolactone	Dangerous rise in blood potassium.
Triamterene	Dangerous rise in blood potassium.
Vitamin B-12	Extended-release tablets may decrease vitamin B-12 absorption and increase vitamin B-12 requirements.

POSSIBLE INTERACTION WITH OTHER SUBSTANCES

INTERACTS WITH	COMBINED EFFECT
Alcohol:	None expected.
Beverages: Salty drinks such as tomato juice, commercial thirst quenchers.	Increased fluid retention.
Cocaine:	May cause irregular heartbeat.
Foods: Salty foods.	Increased fluid retention.
Marijuana:	May cause irregular heartbeat.
Tobacco:	None expected.

PRAZEPAM

BRAND NAMES

Centrax

BASIC INFORMATION

Habit forming? Yes
Prescription needed? Yes
Available as generic? No
Drug class: Tranquilizer (benzodiazepine)

 ## USES

Treatment for nervousness or tension.

 ## DOSAGE & USAGE INFORMATION

How to take:
Tablet or capsule—Swallow with liquid. If you can't swallow whole, crumble tablet or open capsule and take with liquid or food.

When to take:
At the same time each day, according to instructions on prescription label.

If you forget a dose:
Take as soon as you remember up to 2 hours late. If more than 2 hours, wait for next scheduled dose (don't double this dose).

What drug does:
Affects limbic system, the part of the brain that controls emotions.

Time lapse before drug works:
2 hours. May take 6 weeks for full benefit.

Don't take with:
See Interaction column and consult doctor.

 ## OVERDOSE

SYMPTOMS:
Drowsiness, weakness, tremor, stupor, coma.
WHAT TO DO:
- Dial 0 (operator) or 911 (emergency) for an ambulance or medical help. Then give first aid immediately.
- If patient is unconscious and not breathing, give mouth-to-mouth breathing. If there is no heartbeat, use cardiac massage and mouth-to-mouth breathing (CPR). Don't try to make patient vomit. If you can't get help quickly, take patient to nearest emergency facility.
- See emergency information on inside covers.

 ## POSSIBLE ADVERSE REACTIONS OR SIDE EFFECTS

SYMPTOMS	WHAT TO DO
Life-threatening:	
None expected.	
Common:	
Clumsiness, drowsiness, dizziness.	Continue. Call doctor when convenient.
Infrequent:	
• Hallucinations, confusion, depression, irritability, rash, itchy skin, change in vision.	Discontinue. Call doctor right away.
• Constipation or diarrhea, nausea, vomiting, difficult urination.	Continue. Call doctor when convenient.
Rare:	
• Slow heartbeat, difficult breathing.	Discontinue. Seek emergency treatment.
• Mouth and throat ulcers, jaundice.	Discontinue. Call doctor right away.

WARNINGS & PRECAUTIONS

Don't take if:
- You are allergic to any benzodiazepine.
- You have myasthenia gravis.
- You have glaucoma.
- You are active or recovering alcoholic.
- Patient is younger than 6 months.

Before you start, consult your doctor:
- If you have liver, kidney or lung disease.
- If you have diabetes, epilepsy or porphyria.

Over age 60:
Adverse reactions and side effects may be more frequent and severe than in younger persons. You need smaller doses for shorter periods of time. May develop agitation, rage or "hangover" effect.

Pregnancy:
Risk to unborn child outweighs drug benefits. Don't use.

Breast-feeding:
Drug passes into milk. Avoid drug or discontinue nursing until you finish medicine. Consult doctor for advice on maintaining milk supply.

Infants & children:
Use only under medical supervision for children older than 6 months.

Prolonged use:
May impair liver function.

Skin & sunlight:
No problems expected.

Driving, piloting or hazardous work:
Don't drive or pilot aircraft until you learn how medicine affects you. Don't work around dangerous machinery. Don't climb ladders or work in high places. Danger increases if you drink alcohol or take medicine affecting alertness and reflexes.

Discontinuing:
Don't discontinue without consulting doctor. Dose may require gradual reduction if you have taken drug for a long time. Doses of other drugs may also require adjustment.

Others:
- Hot weather, heavy exercise and profuse sweat may reduce excretion and cause overdose.
- Blood sugar may rise in diabetics, requiring insulin adjustment.

POSSIBLE INTERACTION WITH OTHER DRUGS

GENERIC NAME OR DRUG CLASS	COMBINED EFFECT
Anticonvulsants	Change in seizure frequency or severity.
Antidepressants	Increased sedative effect of both drugs.
Antihistamines	Increased sedative effect of both drugs.
Antihypertensives	Excessively low blood pressure.
Cimetidine	Excess sedation.
Disulfiram	Increased prazepam effect.
Dronabinol	Increased effects of both drugs. Avoid.
MAO inhibitors	Convulsions, deep sedation, rage.
Molindone	Increased tranquilizer effect.
Narcotics	Increased sedative effect of both drugs.
Sedatives	Increased sedative effect of both drugs.
Sleep inducers	Increased sedative effect of both drugs.
Tranquilizers	Increased sedative effect of both drugs.

POSSIBLE INTERACTION WITH OTHER SUBSTANCES

INTERACTS WITH	COMBINED EFFECT
Alcohol:	Heavy sedation. Avoid.
Beverages:	None expected.
Cocaine:	Decreased prazepam effect.
Foods:	None expected.
Marijuana:	Heavy sedation. Avoid.
Tobacco:	Decreased prazepam effect.

PRAZOSIN

BRAND NAMES

Minipress

BASIC INFORMATION

Habit forming? No
Prescription needed? Yes
Available as generic? No
Drug class: Antihypertensive

 USES

- Treatment for high blood pressure.
- Improves congestive heart failure.

 DOSAGE & USAGE INFORMATION

How to take:
Tablet or capsule—Swallow with liquid. If you can't swallow whole, crumble tablet or open capsule and take with liquid or food.

When to take:
At the same times each day.

If you forget a dose:
Take as soon as you remember up to 2 hours late. If more than 2 hours, wait for next scheduled dose (don't double this dose).

What drug does:
Expands and relaxes blood-vessel walls to lower blood pressure.

Time lapse before drug works:
30 minutes.

Don't take with:
See Interaction column and consult doctor.

 OVERDOSE

SYMPTOMS:
Extreme weakness; loss of consciousness; cold, sweaty skin; weak, rapid pulse; coma.
WHAT TO DO:
- **Dial 0 (operator) or 911 (emergency) for an ambulance or medical help. Then give first aid immediately.**
- **If patient is unconscious and not breathing, give mouth-to-mouth breathing. If there is no heartbeat, use cardiac massage and mouth-to-mouth breathing (CPR). Don't try to make patient vomit. If you can't get help quickly, take patient to nearest emergency facility.**
- **See emergency information on inside covers.**

 POSSIBLE ADVERSE REACTIONS OR SIDE EFFECTS

SYMPTOMS	WHAT TO DO
Life-threatening:	
None expected.	
Common:	
• Rapid heartbeat.	Discontinue. Call doctor right away.
• Vivid dreams, drowsiness, dizziness.	Continue. Call doctor when convenient.
Infrequent:	
• Rash or itchy skin, blurred vision, shortness of breath, chest pain.	Discontinue. Call doctor right away.
• Appetite loss, constipation or diarrhea, stomach pain, nausea, vomiting, fluid retention, joint or muscle aches.	Continue. Call doctor when convenient.
• Headache, irritability, depression, dry mouth, stuffy nose, increased urination.	Continue. Tell doctor at next visit.
Rare:	
Decreased sexual function.	Continue. Call doctor when convenient.

WARNINGS & PRECAUTIONS

Don't take if:
- You are allergic to prazosin.
- You are depressed.
- You will have surgery within 2 months, including dental surgery, requiring general or spinal anesthesia.

Before you start, consult your doctor:
- If you experience lightheadedness or fainting with other antihypertensive drugs.
- If you are easily depressed.
- If you have impaired brain circulation or have had a stroke.
- If you have coronary heart disease (with or without angina).
- If you have kidney disease or impaired liver function.

Over age 60:
Begin with no more than 1 mg. per day for first 3 days. Increases should be gradual and supervised by your doctor. Don't stand while taking. Sudden changes in position may cause falls. Sit or lie down promptly if you feel dizzy. If you have impaired brain circulation or coronary heart disease, excessive lowering of blood pressure should be avoided. Report problems to your doctor immediately.

Pregnancy:
Studies inconclusive on harm to unborn child. Animal studies show fetal abnormalities. Decide with your doctor whether drug benefits justify risk to child.

Breast-feeding:
No proven problems. Consult doctor.

Infants & children:
Not recommended.

Prolonged use:
No problems expected.

Skin & sunlight:
No problems expected.

Driving, piloting or hazardous work:
Don't drive or pilot aircraft until you learn how medicine affects you. Don't work around dangerous machinery. Don't climb ladders or work in high places.

Discontinuing:
Don't discontinue without doctor's advice until you complete prescribed dose, even though symptoms diminish or disappear.

Others:
First dose likely to cause fainting. Take it at night and get out of bed slowly next morning.

POSSIBLE INTERACTION WITH OTHER DRUGS

GENERIC NAME OR DRUG CLASS	COMBINED EFFECT
Acebutolol	Increased antihypertensive effect. Dosages may require adjustments.
Amitriptyline	Acute agitation.
Amphetamines	Decreased prazosin effect.
Antihypertensives (other)	Increased effect of other drugs.
Chlorpromazine	Acute agitation.
Enalapril	Possible excessive potassium in blood.
MAO inhibitors	Blood-pressure drop.
Nitrates	Possible excessive blood-pressure drop.
Nitroglycerin	Prolonged effect of prazosin.
Oxprenolol	Increased antihypertensive effect. Dosages may require adjustments.

POSSIBLE INTERACTION WITH OTHER SUBSTANCES

INTERACTS WITH	COMBINED EFFECT
Alcohol:	Excessive blood-pressure drop.
Beverages:	None expected.
Cocaine:	Decreased prazosin effect. Avoid.
Foods:	None expected.
Marijuana:	Possible fainting. Avoid.
Tobacco:	Possible spasm of coronary arteries. Avoid.

PRAZOSIN & POLYTHIAZIDE

BRAND NAMES

Minizide

BASIC INFORMATION

Habit forming? No
Prescription needed? Yes
Available as generic? No
**Drug class: Antihypertensive, thiazide
diuretic**

 USES

- Controls, but doesn't cure, high blood pressure.
- Reduces fluid retention (edema) caused by conditions such as heart disorders and liver disease.

 DOSAGE & USAGE INFORMATION

How to take:
Tablet or capsule—Swallow with 8 oz. of liquid. If you can't swallow whole, crumble tablet or open capsule and take with liquid or food. Don't exceed dose.

When to take:
At the same times each day.

If you forget a dose:
Take as soon as you remember up to 2 hours late. If more than 2 hours, wait for next scheduled dose (don't double this dose).

Continued next column

 OVERDOSE

SYMPTOMS:
Extreme weakness; loss of consciousness; cold, sweaty skin; weak, rapid pulse; cramps; weakness; drowsiness; coma.
WHAT TO DO:
- **Dial 0 (operator) or 911 (emergency) for an ambulance or medical help. Then give first aid immediately.**
- **If patient is unconscious and not breathing, give mouth-to-mouth breathing. If there is no heartbeat, use cardiac massage and mouth-to-mouth breathing (CPR). Don't try to make patient vomit. If you can't get help quickly, take patient to nearest emergency facility.**
- **See emergency information on inside covers.**

What drug does:
- Expands and relaxes blood-vessel walls to lower blood pressure.
- Forces sodium and water excretion, reducing body fluid.
- Relaxes muscle cells of small arteries.
- Reduced body fluid and relaxed arteries lower blood pressure.

Time lapse before drug works:
4 to 6 hours. May require several weeks to lower blood pressure.

Don't take with:
- Non-prescription drugs without consulting doctor.
- See Interaction column and consult doctor.

 POSSIBLE ADVERSE REACTIONS OR SIDE EFFECTS

SYMPTOMS	WHAT TO DO
Life-threatening:	
Irregular heartbeat, weak pulse, fast heartbeat, difficult breathing, chest pain.	Discontinue. Seek emergency treatment.
Common:	
Nightmares, vivid dreams, drowsiness, dizziness, dry mouth, stuffy nose.	Continue. Call doctor when convenient.
Infrequent:	
• Blurred vision, abdominal pain, nausea, vomiting.	Discontinue. Call doctor right away.
• Dizziness, mood change, headache, dry mouth, muscle pain, urgent urination, weakness, tiredness, weight gain or loss, runny nose, joint or muscle pain, agitation, depression, rash, appetite loss, constipation.	Continue. Call doctor when convenient.
Rare:	
• Sore throat, fever, mouth sores; jaundice.	Discontinue. Call doctor right away.
• Diminished sex drive.	Continue. Call doctor when convenient.

WARNINGS & PRECAUTIONS

Don't take if:
- You are allergic to any thiazide diuretic drug or prazosin.
- You are depressed.
- You will have surgery within 2 months, including dental surgery, requiring general or spinal anesthesia.

Before you start, consult your doctor:
- If you are allergic to any sulfa drug.
- If you have gout, impaired brain circulation or have had a stroke, coronary heart disease (with or without angina), kidney disease or impaired liver function.
- If you experience lightheadedness or fainting with other antihypertensive drugs.
- If you are easily depressed.

Over age 60:
- Adverse reactions and side effects may be more frequent and severe than in younger persons, especially dizziness and excessive potassium loss.
- Don't stand while taking. Sudden changes in position may cause falls. Sit or lie down promptly if you feel dizzy. If you have impaired brain circulation or coronary heart disease, excessive lowering of blood pressure should be avoided. Report problems to your doctor immediately.

Pregnancy:
Risk to unborn child outweighs drug benefits. Don't use.

Breast-feeding:
Drug passes into milk. Avoid drug or discontinue nursing until you finish medicine. Consult doctor for advice on maintaining milk supply.

Infants & children:
Not recommended.

Prolonged use:
You may need medicine to treat high blood pressure for the rest of your life.

Skin & sunlight:
May cause rash or intensify sunburn in areas exposed to sun or sunlamp.

Driving, piloting or hazardous work:
Don't drive or pilot aircraft until you learn how medicine affects you. Don't work around dangerous machinery. Don't climb ladders or work in high places. Danger increases if you drink alcohol or take medicine affecting alertness and reflexes, such as antihistamines, tranquilizers, sedatives, pain medicine, narcotics and mind-altering drugs.

Discontinuing:
Don't discontinue without consulting doctor.

Others:
- First dose likely to cause fainting. Take it at night and get out of bed slowly next morning.
- Hot weather and fever may cause dehydration and drop in blood pressure. Dose may require temporary adjustment. Weigh daily and report any unexpected weight decreases to your doctor.
- May cause rise in uric acid, leading to gout.
- May cause blood-sugar rise in diabetics.

POSSIBLE INTERACTION WITH OTHER DRUGS

GENERIC NAME OR DRUG CLASS	COMBINED EFFECT
Acebutolol	Increased antihypertensive effect. Dosages may require adjustments.
Allopurinol	Decreased allopurinol effect.
Amitriptyline	Acute agitation.
Amphetamines	Decreased prazosin effect.
Antidepressants (tricyclic)	Dangerous drop in blood pressure. Avoid combination unless under medical supervision.
Barbiturates	Increased polythiazide effect.

Continued page 973

POSSIBLE INTERACTION WITH OTHER SUBSTANCES

INTERACTS WITH	COMBINED EFFECT
Alcohol:	Dangerous blood-pressure drop. Avoid.
Beverages:	None expected.
Cocaine:	Decreased prazosin effect. Avoid.
Foods: Licorice.	Excessive potassium loss that causes dangerous heart rhythms.
Marijuana:	Possible fainting, may increase blood pressure. Avoid.
Tobacco:	Possible spasm of coronary arteries. Avoid.

PREDNISOLONE

BRAND NAMES

See complete list of brand names in the *Brand Name Directory,* page 955.

BASIC INFORMATION

Habit forming? No
Prescription needed? Yes
Available as generic? Yes
Drug class: Cortisone drug (adrenal corticosteroid)

 ## USES

- Reduces inflammation caused by many different medical problems.
- Treatment for some allergic diseases, blood disorders, kidney diseases, asthma and emphysema.
- Replaces corticosteroid deficiencies.

 ## DOSAGE & USAGE INFORMATION

How to take:
Tablet—Swallow with liquid or food to lessen stomach irritation. If you can't swallow whole, crumble tablet and take with liquid or food.

When to take:
At the same times each day. Take once-a-day or once-every-other-day doses in mornings.

If you forget a dose:
- Several-doses-per-day prescription—Take as soon as you remember up to 2 hours late. If more than 2 hours, wait for next scheduled dose (don't double this dose).
- Once-a-day dose or less—Wait for next dose. Double this dose.

What drug does:
Decreases inflammatory responses.

Time lapse before drug works:
2 to 4 days.

Don't take with:
See Interaction column and consult doctor.

 ## OVERDOSE

SYMPTOMS:
Headache, convulsions, heart failure.
WHAT TO DO:
- **Dial 0 (operator) or 911 (emergency) for an ambulance or medical help. Then give first aid immediately.**
- **See emergency information on inside covers.**

 ## POSSIBLE ADVERSE REACTIONS OR SIDE EFFECTS

SYMPTOMS	WHAT TO DO
Life-threatening: None expected.	
Common: Acne, poor wound healing, thirst, indigestion, nausea, vomiting.	Continue. Call doctor when convenient.
Infrequent:	
• Black, bloody or tarry stool.	Discontinue. Seek emergency treatment.
• Blurred vision, halos around lights, sore throat, fever, muscle cramps, swollen legs or feet.	Discontinue. Call doctor right away.
• Mood change, insomnia, restlessness, frequent urination, weight gain, round face, fatigue, weakness, TB recurrence, irregular menstrual periods.	Continue. Call doctor when convenient.
Rare:	
• Irregular heartbeat.	Discontinue. Seek emergency treatment.
• Rash.	Discontinue. Call doctor right away.

 ## WARNINGS & PRECAUTIONS

Don't take if:
- You are allergic to any cortisone drug.
- You have tuberculosis or fungus infection.
- You have herpes infection of eyes, lips or genitals.

Before you start, consult your doctor:
- If you have had tuberculosis.
- If you have congestive heart failure.
- If you have diabetes.
- If you have peptic ulcer.
- If you have glaucoma.
- If you have underactive thyroid.
- If you have high blood pressure.
- If you have myasthenia gravis.
- If you have blood clots in legs or lungs.

Over age 60:
Adverse reactions and side effects may be more frequent and severe than in younger persons. Likely to aggravate edema, diabetes or ulcers. Likely to cause cataracts and osteoporosis (softening of the bones).

Prolonged use:
You may need medicine to treat high blood pressure for the rest of your life.

Skin & sunlight:
May cause rash or intensify sunburn in areas exposed to sun or sunlamp.

Driving, piloting or hazardous work:
Don't drive or pilot aircraft until you learn how medicine affects you. Don't work around dangerous machinery. Don't climb ladders or work in high places. Danger increases if you drink alcohol or take medicine affecting alertness and reflexes, such as antihistamines, tranquilizers, sedatives, pain medicine, narcotics and mind-altering drugs.

Discontinuing:
Don't discontinue without medical advice.

Others:
- Hot weather and fever may cause dehydration and drop in blood pressure. Dose may require temporary adjustment. Weigh daily and report any unexpected weight decreases to your doctor.
- May cause rise in uric acid, leading to gout.
- May cause blood-sugar rise in diabetics.

POSSIBLE INTERACTION WITH OTHER DRUGS

GENERIC NAME OR DRUG CLASS	COMBINED EFFECT
Acebutolol	Increased antihypertensive effect. Dosages of both drugs may require adjustments.
Allopurinol	Decreased allopurinol effect.
Amiodarone	Increased risk of heartbeat irregularity due to low potassium.
Antidepressants (tricyclic)	Dangerous drop in blood pressure. Avoid combination unless under medical supervision.
Barbiturates	Increased polythiazide effect.
Calcium supplements	Increased calcium in blood.

Chlorthalidone	Potassium depletion.
Cholinergics	Decreased cholinergic effect.
Contraceptives (oral)	Increased prednisolone effect.
Digitalis preparations	Dangerous potassium depletion. Possible digitalis toxicity.
Diuretics (thiazide)	Potassium depletion.
Ephedrine	Decreased prednisolone effect.
Estrogens	Increased prednisolone effect.
Ethacrynic acid	Potassium depletion.
Furosemide	Potassium depletion.
Glutethimide	Decreased prednisolone effect.
Indapamide	Possible excessive potassium loss, causing dangerous heartbeat irregularity.
Indomethacin	Increased prednisolone effect.
Insulin	Decreased insulin effect.
Isoniazid	Decreased isoniazid effect.
Oxyphenbutazone	Possible ulcers.
Phenylbutazone	Possible ulcers.
Potassium supplements	Decreased potassium effect.
Rifampin	Decreased prednisolone effect.
Sympathomimetics	Possible glaucoma.

POSSIBLE INTERACTION WITH OTHER SUBSTANCES

INTERACTS WITH	COMBINED EFFECT
Alcohol:	Risk of stomach ulcers.
Beverages:	No proven problems.
Cocaine:	Overstimulation. Avoid.
Foods:	No proven problems.
Marijuana:	Decreased immunity.
Tobacco:	Increased prednisolone effect. Possible toxicity.

PREDNISONE

BRAND NAMES

Apo-Prednisone	Panasol
Colisone	Paracort
Cortan	Prednicen-M
Deltasone	SK-Prednisone
Liquid-Pred	Sterapred
Meticorten	Sterazolidin
Novoprednisone	Winpred
Orasone	

BASIC INFORMATION

Habit forming? No
Prescription needed? Yes
Available as generic? Yes
Drug class: Cortisone drug (adrenal corticosteroid)

USES

- Reduces inflammation caused by many different medical problems.
- Treatment for some allergic diseases, blood disorders, kidney diseases, asthma and emphysema.
- Replaces corticosteroid deficiencies.

DOSAGE & USAGE INFORMATION

How to take:
Tablet or syrup—Swallow with liquid or food to lessen stomach irritation. If you can't swallow whole, crumble tablet.

When to take:
At the same times each day. Take once-a-day or once-every-other-day doses in mornings.

If you forget a dose:
- Several-doses-per-day prescription—Take as soon as you remember up to 2 hours late. If more than 2 hours, wait for next scheduled dose (don't double this dose).
- Once-a-day dose or less—Wait for next dose. Double this dose.

Continued next column

OVERDOSE

SYMPTOMS:
Headache, convulsions, heart failure.
WHAT TO DO:
- Dial 0 (operator) or 911 (emergency) for an ambulance or medical help. Then give first aid immediately.
- See emergency information on inside covers.

What drug does:
Decreases inflammatory responses.

Time lapse before drug works:
2 to 4 days.

Don't take with:
See Interaction column and consult doctor.

POSSIBLE ADVERSE REACTIONS OR SIDE EFFECTS

SYMPTOMS	WHAT TO DO
Life-threatening: None expected.	
Common: Acne, poor wound healing, thirst, indigestion, nausea, vomiting.	Continue. Call doctor when convenient.
Infrequent:	
• Black, bloody or tarry stool.	Discontinue. Seek emergency treatment.
• Blurred vision, halos around lights, sore throat, fever, muscle cramps, swollen legs or feet.	Discontinue. Call doctor right away.
• Mood change, insomnia, restlessness, frequent urination, weight gain, round face, fatigue, weakness, TB recurrence, irregular menstrual periods.	Continue. Call doctor when convenient.
Rare:	
• Irregular heartbeat.	Discontinue. Seek emergency treatment.
• Rash.	Discontinue. Call doctor right away.

WARNINGS & PRECAUTIONS

Don't take if:
- You are allergic to any cortisone drug.
- You have tuberculosis or fungus infection.
- You have herpes infection of eyes, lips or genitals.

Before you start, consult your doctor:
- If you have had tuberculosis.
- If you have congestive heart failure.
- If you have diabetes.
- If you have peptic ulcer.
- If you have glaucoma.
- If you have underactive thyroid.
- If you have high blood pressure.
- If you have myasthenia gravis.
- If you have blood clots in legs or lungs.

Over age 60:
Adverse reactions and side effects may be more frequent and severe than in younger persons. Likely to aggravate edema, diabetes or ulcers. Likely to cause cataracts and osteoporosis (softening of the bones).

Pregnancy:
Risk to unborn child outweighs drug benefits. Don't use.

Breast-feeding:
Drug passes into milk. Avoid drug or discontinue nursing until you finish medicine. Consult doctor for advice on maintaining milk supply.

Infants & children:
Use only under medical supervision.

Prolonged use:
- Retards growth in children.
- Possible glaucoma, cataracts, diabetes, fragile bones and thin skin.
- Functional dependence.

Skin & sunlight:
No problems expected.

Driving, piloting or hazardous work:
No problems expected.

Discontinuing:
- Don't discontinue without doctor's advice until you complete prescribed dose, even though symptoms diminish or disappear.
- Drug affects your response to surgery, illness, injury or stress for 2 years after discontinuing. Tell anyone who takes medical care of you within 2 years about drug.

Others:
Avoid immunizations if possible.

POSSIBLE INTERACTION WITH OTHER DRUGS

GENERIC NAME OR DRUG CLASS	COMBINED EFFECT
Amphoterecin B	Potassium depletion.
Anticholinergics	Possible glaucoma.
Anticoagulants (oral)	Decreased anticoagulant effect.
Anticonvulsants (hydantoin)	Decreased prednisone effect.
Antidiabetics (oral)	Decreased antidiabetic effect.
Antihistamines	Decreased prednisone effect.
Aspirin	Increased prednisone effect.
Barbiturates	Decreased prednisone effect. Oversedation.
Beta-adrenergic blockers	Decreased prednisone effect.
Chloral hydrate	Decreased prednisone effect.
Chlorthalidone	Potassium depletion.
Cholinergics	Decreased cholinergic effect.
Contraceptives (oral)	Increased prednisone effect.
Digitalis preparations	Dangerous potassium depletion. Possible digitalis toxicity.
Diuretics (thiazide)	Potassium depletion.
Ephedrine	Decreased prednisone effect.
Estrogens	Increased prednisone effect.

Continued page 973

POSSIBLE INTERACTION WITH OTHER SUBSTANCES

INTERACTS WITH	COMBINED EFFECT
Alcohol:	Risk of stomach ulcers.
Beverages:	No proven problems.
Cocaine:	Overstimulation. Avoid.
Foods:	No proven problems.
Marijuana:	Decreased immunity.
Tobacco:	Increased prednisone effect. Possible toxicity.

PRIMIDONE

BRAND NAMES

Apo-Primidone   Mysoline
Myidone   Sertan

BASIC INFORMATION

Habit forming? No
Prescription needed? Yes
Available as generic? Yes
Drug class: Anticonvulsant

USES

Prevents epileptic seizures.

DOSAGE & USAGE INFORMATION

How to take:
- Tablet or capsule—Swallow with liquid. If you can't swallow whole, crumble tablet or open capsule and take with liquid or food.
- Liquid—If desired, dilute dose in beverage before swallowing.

When to take:
Daily in regularly spaced doses, according to doctor's prescription.

If you forget a dose:
Take as soon as you remember up to 2 hours late. If more than 2 hours, wait for next scheduled dose (don't double this dose).

What drug does:
Probably inhibits repetitious spread of impulses along nerve pathways.

Continued next column

OVERDOSE

SYMPTOMS:
Slow, shallow breathing; weak, rapid pulse; confusion, deep sleep, coma.
WHAT TO DO:
- Dial 0 (operator) or 911 (emergency) for an ambulance or medical help. Then give first aid immediately.
- If patient is unconscious and not breathing, give mouth-to-mouth breathing. If there is no heartbeat, use cardiac massage and mouth-to-mouth breathing (CPR). Don't try to make patient vomit. If you can't get help quickly, take patient to nearest emergency facility.
- See emergency information on inside covers.

Time lapse before drug works:
2 to 3 weeks.

Don't take with:
See Interaction column and consult doctor.

POSSIBLE ADVERSE REACTIONS OR SIDE EFFECTS

SYMPTOMS	WHAT TO DO
Life-threatening:	
None expected.	
Common:	
• Difficult breathing.	Discontinue. Call doctor right away.
• Confusion, change in vision.	Continue. Call doctor when convenient.
• Clumsiness, dizziness, drowsiness.	Continue. Tell doctor at next visit.
Infrequent:	
• Unusual excitement, particularly in children.	Discontinue. Call doctor right away.
• Headache, fatigue, weakness.	Continue. Call doctor when convenient.
Rare:	
• Rash or hives, nausea, vomiting, appetite loss.	Discontinue. Call doctor right away.
• Swollen eyelids.	Continue. Call doctor when convenient.
• Decreased sexual ability.	Continue. Tell doctor at next visit.

WARNINGS & PRECAUTIONS

Don't take if:
- You are allergic to any barbiturate.
- You have had porphyria.

Before you start, consult your doctor:
- If you have had liver, kidney or lung disease or asthma.
- If you have lupus.

Over age 60:
Adverse reactions and side effects may be more frequent and severe than in younger persons.

Pregnancy:
Studies inconclusive on harm to unborn child. Animal studies show fetal abnormalities. Decide with your doctor whether drug benefits justify risk to unborn child.

Breast-feeding:
Drug filters into milk. May harm child. Avoid.

Infants & children:
Use only under medical supervision.

Prolonged use:
- Enlarged lymph and thyroid glands.
- Anemia.
- Rickets in children and osteomalacia (insufficient calcium to bones) in adults.

Skin & sunlight:
None expected.

Driving, piloting or hazardous work:
Don't drive or pilot aircraft until you learn how medicine affects you. Don't work around dangerous machinery. Don't climb ladders or work in high places. Danger increases if you drink alcohol or take medicine affecting alertness and reflexes.

Discontinuing:
Don't discontinue abruptly or without doctor's advice until you complete prescribed dose, even though symptoms diminish or disappear.

Others:
- Tell doctor if you become ill or injured and must interrupt dose schedule.
- Periodic laboratory blood tests of drug level recommended.

 POSSIBLE INTERACTION WITH OTHER DRUGS

GENERIC NAME OR DRUG CLASS	COMBINED EFFECT
Anticoagulants (oral)	Decreased primidone effect.
Anticonvulsants (other)	Changed seizure pattern.
Antidepressants	Increased antidepressant effect.
Antidiabetics	Increased effect of primidone sedation.
Antihistamines	Increased effect of primidone sedation.
Aspirin	Decreased aspirin effect.
Contraceptives (oral)	Decreased contraceptive effect.
Cortisone drugs	Decreased cortisone effect.

Digitalis preparations	Decreased digitalis effect.
Griseofulvin	Decreased griseofulvin effect.
Isoniazid	Increased isoniazid effect.
MAO inhibitors	Increased effect of primidone sedation.
Mind-altering drugs	Increased effect of mind-altering drugs.
Narcotics	Increased narcotic effect.
Oxyphenbutazone	Decreased oxyphenbutazone effect.
Phenylbutazone	Decreased phenylbutazone effect.
Sedatives	Increased sedative effect.
Sleep inducers	Increased effect of sleep inducer.
Tranquilizers	Increased tranquilizer effect.

 POSSIBLE INTERACTION WITH OTHER SUBSTANCES

INTERACTS WITH	COMBINED EFFECT
Alcohol:	Dangerous sedative effect. Avoid.
Beverages:	None expected.
Cocaine:	Decreased primidone effect.
Foods:	Possible need for more vitamin D.
Marijuana:	Decreased anticonvulsant effect of primidone. Drowsiness, unsteadiness.
Tobacco:	None expected.

PROBENECID

BRAND NAMES

Benacen
Benemid
Benuryl
ColBENEMID

Col-Probenecid
Polycillin-PRB
Probalan
SK-Probenecid

BASIC INFORMATION

Habit forming? No
Prescription needed? Yes
Available as generic? Yes
Drug class: Antigout (uricosuric)

 USES

- Treatment for chronic gout.
- Increases blood levels of penicillins and cephalosporins.

 DOSAGE & USAGE INFORMATION

How to take:
Tablet or capsule—Swallow with liquid or food to lessen stomach irritation. If you can't swallow whole, crumble tablet or open capsule and take with liquid or food.

When to take:
At the same time each day.

If you forget a dose:
Take as soon as you remember up to 12 hours late. If more than 12 hours, wait for next scheduled dose (don't double this dose).

What drug does:
- Forces kidneys to excrete uric acid.
- Reduces amount of penicillin excreted in urine.

Time lapse before drug works:
May require several months of regular use to prevent acute gout.

Continued next column

 OVERDOSE

SYMPTOMS:
Breathing difficulty, severe nervous agitation, convulsions, delirium, coma.
WHAT TO DO:
- Dial 0 (operator) or 911 (emergency) for an ambulance or medical help. Then give first aid immediately.
- See emergency information on inside covers.

Don't take with:
- Non-prescription drugs containing aspirin or caffeine.
- See Interaction column and consult doctor.

 POSSIBLE ADVERSE REACTIONS OR SIDE EFFECTS

SYMPTOMS	WHAT TO DO
Life-threatening: None expected.	
Common: Headache, appetite loss, nausea, vomiting.	Continue. Call doctor when convenient.
Infrequent:	
• Blood in urine, low back pain.	Discontinue. Call doctor right away.
• Dizziness, flushed face, itchy skin.	Continue. Call doctor when convenient.
• Painful or frequent urination.	Continue. Tell doctor at next visit.
Rare: Sore throat; difficult breathing; unusual bleeding or bruising; red, painful joint; jaundice; fever.	Discontinue. Call doctor right away.

WARNINGS & PRECAUTIONS

Don't take if:
- You are allergic to any uricosuric.
- You have acute gout.
- Patient is younger than 2.

Before you start, consult your doctor:
- If you have had kidney stones or kidney disease.
- If you have a peptic ulcer.
- If you have bone-marrow or blood-cell disease.

Over age 60:
Adverse reactions and side effects may be more frequent and severe than in younger persons.

Pregnancy:
Studies inconclusive on harm to unborn child. Animal studies show fetal abnormalities. Decide with your doctor whether drug benefits justify risk to unborn child.

Breast-feeding:
No proven problems.

Infants & children:
Not recommended.

Prolonged use:
Possible kidney damage.

Skin & sunlight:
No problems expected.

Driving, piloting or hazardous work:
Avoid if you feel dizzy. Otherwise, no problems expected.

Discontinuing:
Don't discontinue without consulting doctor. Dose may require gradual reduction if you have taken drug for a long time. Doses of other drugs may also require adjustment.

Others:
If signs of gout attack develop while taking medicine, consult doctor.

POSSIBLE INTERACTION WITH OTHER DRUGS

GENERIC NAME OR DRUG CLASS	COMBINED EFFECT
Acetohexamide	Increased acetohexamide effect.
Anticoagulants (oral)	Increased anticoagulant effect.
Aspirin	Decreased probenecid effect.
Cephalosporins	Increased cephalosporin effect.
Dapsone	Increased dapsone effect. Increased toxicity.
Diuretics (thiazide)	Decreased probenecid effect.
Indapamide	Decreased probenecid effect.
Indomethacin	Increased adverse effects of indomethacin.
Methotrexate	Increased methotrexate toxicity.
Nitrofurantoin	Increased effect of nitrofurantoin.
Para-aminosalicylic acid (PAS)	Increased effect of para-aminosalicylic acid.
Penicillins	Enhanced penicillin effect.
Pyrazinamide	Decreased probenecid effect.
Salicylates	Decreased probenecid effect.
Sulfa drugs	Slows elimination. May cause harmful accumulation of sulfa.

POSSIBLE INTERACTION WITH OTHER SUBSTANCES

INTERACTS WITH	COMBINED EFFECT
Alcohol:	Decreased probenecid effect.
Beverages: Caffeine drinks.	Loss of probenecid effectiveness.
Cocaine:	None expected.
Foods:	None expected.
Marijuana:	Daily use—Decreased probenecid effect.
Tobacco:	None expected.

PROBENECID & COLCHICINE

BRAND NAMES

Colabid Proben-C
Col Benemid

BASIC INFORMATION

Habit forming? No
Prescription needed? Yes
Available as generic? Yes
Drug class: Antigout (uricosuric)

 ## USES

- Increases blood levels of penicillins and cephalosporins.
- Relieves joint pain, inflammation, swelling from gout.

 ## DOSAGE & USAGE INFORMATION

How to take:
Tablet or capsule—Swallow with liquid or food to lessen stomach irritation. If you can't swallow whole, crumble tablet or open capsule and take with liquid or food.

When to take:
At the same time each day.

If you forget a dose:
Take as soon as you remember up to 12 hours late. If more than 12 hours, wait for next scheduled dose (don't double this dose).

What drug does:
- Forces kidneys to excrete uric acid.
- Reduces amount of penicillin excreted in urine.
- Decreases acidity of joint tissues and prevents deposits of uric-acid crystals.

Continued next column

 ## OVERDOSE

SYMPTOMS:
Breathing difficulty, severe nervous agitation, convulsions, bloody urine, diarrhea, muscle weakness, fever, stupor, delirium, coma.
WHAT TO DO:
- Dial 0 (operator) or 911 (emergency) for an ambulance or medical help. Then give first aid immediately.
- See emergency information on inside covers.

Time lapse before drug works:
12 to 48 hours.

Don't take with:
- Non-prescription drugs containing aspirin or caffeine.
- See Interaction column and consult doctor.

 ## POSSIBLE ADVERSE REACTIONS OR SIDE EFFECTS

SYMPTOMS	WHAT TO DO
Life-threatening:	
Blood in urine; convulsions; severe muscle weakness; difficult breathing; burning feeling of stomach, throat or skin.	Discontinue. Seek emergency treatment.
Common:	
Diarrhea, headache, abdominal pain.	Discontinue. Call doctor right away.
Infrequent:	
• Back pain; painful, difficult urination.	Discontinue. Call doctor right away.
• Dizziness, red or flushed face, urgent urination, sore gums, hair loss.	Continue. Call doctor when convenient.
Rare:	
Sudden decrease in urine output; nausea; vomiting; mood change; fever; diarrhea; jaundice; numbness or tingling in hands or feet; rash; sore throat, fever, mouth sores; swollen feet and ankles; unexplained bleeding or bruising; weight gain or loss.	Discontinue. Call doctor right away.

WARNINGS & PRECAUTIONS

Don't take if:
You are allergic to any uricosuric or colchicine.

Before you start, consult your doctor:
- If you have had kidney stones, kidney disease, heart or liver disease, peptic ulcers or ulcerative colitis.
- If you have bone-marrow or blood-cell disease.
- If you will have surgery within 2 months, including dental surgery, requiring general or spinal anesthesia.

Over age 60:
Adverse reactions and side effects may be more frequent and severe than in younger persons. Colchicine has a narrow margin of safety for people in this age group.

Pregnancy:
Risk to unborn child outweighs drug benefits. Don't use.

Breast-feeding:
No problems expected, but consult doctor.

Infants & children:
Not recommended.

Prolonged use:
- Possible kidney damage.
- Permanent hair loss.
- Anemia. Request blood counts.
- Numbness or tingling in hands and feet.

Skin & sunlight:
No problems expected.

Driving, piloting or hazardous work:
Don't drive or pilot aircraft until you learn how medicine affects you. Don't work around dangerous machinery. Don't climb ladders or work in high places. Danger increases if you drink alcohol or take medicine affecting alertness and reflexes, such as antihistamines, tranquilizers, sedatives, pain medicine, narcotics and mind-altering drugs.

Discontinuing:
- May be unnecessary to finish medicine. Follow doctor's instructions.
- Stop taking if severe digestive upsets occur before symptoms are relieved.

Others:
- If signs of gout attack develop while taking medicine, consult doctor.
- Limit each course of treatment to 8 mg. Don't exceed 3 mg. per 24 hours.
- Possible sperm damage. May cause birth defects if child conceived while father taking colchicine.

POSSIBLE INTERACTION WITH OTHER DRUGS

GENERIC NAME OR DRUG CLASS	COMBINED EFFECT
Acetohexamide	Increased acetohexamide effect.
Amphetamines	Increased amphetamine effect.

Anticoagulants	Irregular effect on anticoagulation, sometimes increased, sometimes decreased. Follow prothrombin times.
Antidepressants	Oversedation.
Antihistamines	Oversedation.
Antihypertensives	Decreased antihypertensive effect.
Appetite suppressants	Increased suppressant effect.
Cephalosporins	Increased cephalosporin effect.
Dapsone	Increased dapsone effect. Increased toxicity.
Diuretics (thiazide)	Decreased probenecid effect.
Indapamide	Increased probenecid effect.
Indomethacin	Increased adverse effects of indomethacin.
Methotrexate	Increased methotrexate effect.
Mind-altering drugs	Oversedation.
Narcotics	Oversedation.
Nitrofurantoin	Increased nitrofurantoin effect.
Para-aminosalicylic acid (PAS)	Increased effect of para-aminosalicylic acid.
Penicillins	Enhanced penicillin effect.

Continued page 974

POSSIBLE INTERACTION WITH OTHER SUBSTANCES

INTERACTS WITH	COMBINED EFFECT
Alcohol:	Decreased probenecid effect.
Beverages: Caffeine drinks.	Loss of probenecid effectiveness.
Herbal teas.	Increased colchicine effect. Avoid.
Cocaine:	Overstimulation. Avoid.
Foods:	No proven problems.
Marijuana:	Decreased colchicine and probenecid effect.
Tobacco:	No proven problems.

PROBUCOL

BRAND NAMES

Lorelco

BASIC INFORMATION

Habit forming? No
Prescription needed? Yes
Available as generic? No
Drug class: Antihyperlipidemic

 ## USES

Lowers cholesterol level in blood in persons with type IIa hyperlipoproteinemia.

 ## DOSAGE & USAGE INFORMATION

How to take:
Tablet or capsule—Swallow with liquid. If you can't swallow whole, crumble tablet or open capsule and take with liquid or food.

When to take:
With morning and evening meals.

If you forget a dose:
Take as soon as you remember up to 2 hours late. If more than 2 hours, wait for next scheduled dose (don't double this dose).

What drug does:
Reduces serum cholesterol without reducing liver cholesterol.

Time lapse before drug works:
3 to 4 months.

Don't take with:
Other medicines or vitamins. Separate by 1 to 2 hours.

 ## OVERDOSE

SYMPTOMS:
None reported.
WHAT TO DO:
Overdose unlikely to threaten life. If person takes much larger amount than prescribed, call doctor, poison-control center or hospital emergency room for instructions.

 ## POSSIBLE ADVERSE REACTIONS OR SIDE EFFECTS

SYMPTOMS	WHAT TO DO
Life-threatening:	
None expected.	
Common:	
Bloating, diarrhea, nausea, vomiting, stomach pain.	Discontinue. Call doctor right away.
Infrequent:	
• Dizziness, headache.	Discontinue. Call doctor right away.
• Numbness or tingling in feet, toes, fingers, face.	Continue. Call doctor when convenient.
Rare:	
• Swelling of hands, face, feet, mouth.	Discontinue. Seek emergency treatment.
• Rash.	Discontinue. Call doctor right away.
• Insomnia, blurred vision, diminished taste.	Continue. Call doctor when convenient.

WARNINGS & PRECAUTIONS

Don't take if:
You are allergic to probucol.

Before you start, consult your doctor:
- If you have liver disease such as cirrhosis.
- If you have heartbeat irregularity.
- If you have congestive heart failure that is not under control.
- If you have gallstones.

Over age 60:
Adverse reactions and side effects may be more frequent and severe than in younger persons.

Pregnancy:
No proven problems. Avoid if possible. Continue using birth-control methods for 6 months after discontinuing medicine.

Breast-feeding:
Not recommended. Animal studies show drug passes into milk. Studies not available for human beings.

Infants & children:
Not recommended. Safety and dosage have not been established.

Prolonged use:
Request serum cholesterol and serum triglyceride laboratory studies every 2 to 4 months.

Skin & sunlight:
No problems expected.

Driving, piloting or hazardous work:
If medicine does not cause dizziness, no problems expected.

Discontinuing:
Don't discontinue without consulting doctor. Dose may require gradual reduction if you have taken drug for a long time. Doses of other drugs may also require adjustment.

Others:
Medicine works best in conjunction with low-fat, low-cholesterol diet and an active, regular exercise program.

POSSIBLE INTERACTION WITH OTHER DRUGS

GENERIC NAME OR DRUG CLASS	COMBINED EFFECT
Clofibrate	Combination no more effective than one drug only, so don't take both.

POSSIBLE INTERACTION WITH OTHER SUBSTANCES

INTERACTS WITH	COMBINED EFFECT
Alcohol:	May aggravate liver problems. Avoid.
Beverages:	None expected.
Cocaine:	None expected.
Foods:	None expected.
Marijuana:	None expected.
Tobacco:	None expected.

PROCAINAMIDE

BRAND NAMES

Procan	Pronestyl
Procan SR	Pronestyl SR
Procamide	Rhythmin
Procapan	Sub-Quin
Promine	

BASIC INFORMATION

Habit forming? No
Prescription needed? Yes
Available as generic? Yes
Drug class: Antiarrhythmic

USES

Stabilizes irregular heartbeat.

DOSAGE & USAGE INFORMATION

How to take:
- Tablet or capsule—Swallow with liquid.
- Extended-release tablets or capsules—Swallow each dose whole. If you take regular tablets, you may chew or crush them.

When to take:
Best taken on empty stomach, 1 hour before or 2 hours after meals. If necessary, may be taken with food or milk to lessen stomach upset.

If you forget a dose:
Take as soon as you remember up to 2 hours late. If more than 2 hours, wait for next scheduled dose (don't double this dose).

What drug does:
Slows activity of pacemaker (rhythm-control center of heart) and delays transmission of electrical impulses.

Time lapse before drug works:
30 to 60 minutes.

Don't take with:
See Interaction column and consult doctor.

OVERDOSE

SYMPTOMS:
Fast and irregular heartbeat, stupor, fainting, cardiac arrest.
WHAT TO DO:
- **Dial 0 (operator) or 911 (emergency) for an ambulance or medical help. Then give first aid immediately.**
- **See emergency information on inside covers.**

POSSIBLE ADVERSE REACTIONS OR SIDE EFFECTS

SYMPTOMS	WHAT TO DO
Life-threatening:	
None expected.	
Common:	
Diarrhea, appetite loss, nausea, vomiting.	Continue. Call doctor when convenient.
Infrequent:	
• Joint pain, painful breathing.	Discontinue. Call doctor right away.
• Dizziness.	Continue. Call doctor when convenient.
Rare:	
• Hallucinations, confusion, depression, itchy skin, rash, sore throat, fever.	Discontinue. Call doctor right away.
• Fatigue.	Continue. Call doctor when convenient.

WARNINGS & PRECAUTIONS

Don't take if:
- You are allergic to procainamide.
- You have myasthenia gravis.

Before you start, consult your doctor:
- If you are allergic to local anesthetics that end in "caine."
- If you have had liver or kidney disease or impaired kidney function.
- If you have had lupus.
- If you take digitalis preparations.
- If you will have surgery within 2 months, including dental surgery, requiring general or spinal anesthesia.

Over age 60:
Adverse reactions and side effects may be more frequent and severe than in younger persons.

Pregnancy:
No proven harm to unborn child. Avoid if possible.

Breast-feeding:
No proven problems. Consult doctor.

Infants & children:
Not recommended.

Prolonged use:
May cause lupus-like illness.

Skin & sunlight:
No problems expected.

Driving, piloting or hazardous work:
Use caution if you feel dizzy or weak. Otherwise, no problems expected.

Discontinuing:
Don't discontinue without doctor's advice until you complete prescribed dose, even though symptoms diminish or disappear.

Others:
No problems expected.

 ## POSSIBLE INTERACTION WITH OTHER DRUGS

GENERIC NAME OR DRUG CLASS	COMBINED EFFECT
Acetazolamide	Increased procainamide effect.
Ambenonium	Decreased ambenonium effect.
Antihypertensives	Increased antihypertensive effect.
Antimyasthenics	Decreased antimyasthenic effect.
Anticholinergics	Increased anticholinergic effect.
Flecainide	Possible irregular heartbeat.
Kanamycin	Severe muscle weakness, impaired breathing.
Neomycin	Severe muscle weakness, impaired breathing.
Tocainide	Increased likelihood of adverse reactions with either drug.

 ## POSSIBLE INTERACTION WITH OTHER SUBSTANCES

INTERACTS WITH	COMBINED EFFECT
Alcohol:	None expected.
Beverages: Caffeine drinks, iced drinks.	Irregular heartbeat.
Cocaine:	Decreased procainamide effect.
Foods:	None expected.
Marijuana:	None expected.
Tobacco:	Decreased procainamide effect.

PROCARBAZINE

BRAND NAMES

Matulane   Natulan

BASIC INFORMATION

Habit forming? No
Prescription needed? Yes
Available as generic? No
Drug class: Antineoplastic

 USES

Treatment for some kinds of cancer.

 DOSAGE & USAGE INFORMATION

How to take:
Tablet or capsule—Swallow with liquid after light meal. Don't drink fluids with meals. Drink extra fluids between meals. Avoid sweet or fatty foods.

When to take:
At the same time each day.

If you forget a dose:
Take as soon as you remember. Don't double dose ever.

What drug does:
Inhibits abnormal cell reproduction. Procarbazine is an alkylating agent and a MAO inhibitor.

Time lapse before drug works:
Up to 6 weeks for full effect.

Don't take with:
See Interaction column and consult doctor.

 OVERDOSE

SYMPTOMS:
Restlessness, agitation, fever, convulsions, bleeding.
WHAT TO DO:
- Dial 0 (operator) or 911 (emergency) for an ambulance or medical help. Then give first aid immediately.
- If patient is unconscious and not breathing, give mouth-to-mouth breathing. If there is no heartbeat, use cardiac massage and mouth-to-mouth breathing (CPR). Don't try to make patient vomit. If you can't get help quickly, take patient to nearest emergency facility.
- See emergency information on inside covers.

 POSSIBLE ADVERSE REACTIONS OR SIDE EFFECTS

SYMPTOMS	WHAT TO DO
Life-threatening:	
None expected.	
Common:	
• Fatigue, weakness.	Continue. Call doctor when convenient.
• Dizziness when changing position, dry mouth, constipation, difficult urination.	Continue. Tell doctor at next visit.
Infrequent:	
• Fainting.	Discontinue. Seek emergency treatment.
• Severe headache, abnormal bleeding or bruising, chest pain.	Discontinue. Call doctor right away.
• Hallucinations, insomnia, nightmares, diarrhea, rapid or pounding heartbeat, swollen feet or legs.	Continue. Call doctor when convenient.
• Diminished sex drive.	Continue. Tell doctor at next visit.
Rare:	
Rash, nausea, vomiting, stiff neck, jaundice, fever.	Discontinue. Call doctor right away.

WARNINGS & PRECAUTIONS

Don't take if:
- You are allergic to any MAO inhibitor.
- You have heart disease, congestive heart failure, heart-rhythm irregularities or high blood pressure.
- You have liver or kidney disease.

Before you start, consult your doctor:
- If you are alcoholic.
- If you have asthma.
- If you have had a stroke.
- If you have diabetes or epilepsy.
- If you have overactive thyroid.
- If you have schizophrenia.
- If you have Parkinson's disease.
- If you have adrenal-gland tumor.
- If you will have surgery within 2 months, including dental surgery, requiring general or spinal anesthesia.

Over age 60:
Not recommended.

Pregnancy:
Avoid if possible.

Breast-feeding:
Safety not established. Consult doctor.

Infants & children:
Not recommended.

Prolonged use:
May be toxic to liver.

Skin & sunlight:
May cause rash or intensify sunburn in areas exposed to sun or sunlamp.

Driving, piloting or hazardous work:
Don't drive or pilot aircraft until you learn how medicine affects you. Don't work around dangerous machinery. Don't climb ladders or work in high places. Danger increases if you drink alcohol or take medicine affecting alertness and reflexes.

Discontinuing:
- Don't discontinue without doctor's advice until you complete prescribed dose, even though symptoms diminish or disappear.
- Follow precautions regarding foods, drinks and other medicines for 2 weeks after discontinuing.

Others:
- May affect blood-sugar levels in patients with diabetes.
- Fever may indicate that MAO inhibitor dose requires adjustment.

POSSIBLE INTERACTION WITH OTHER DRUGS

GENERIC NAME OR DRUG CLASS	COMBINED EFFECT
Amphetamines	Blood-pressure rise to life-threatening level.
Anticonvulsants	Changed seizure pattern.
Antidepressants (tricyclic)	Blood-pressure rise to life-threatening level.
Antidiabetics (oral and insulin)	Excessively low blood sugar.
Caffeine	Irregular heartbeat or high blood pressure.
Carbamazepine	Fever, seizures. Avoid.
Cyclobenzaprine	Fever, seizures. Avoid.
Diuretics	Excessively low blood pressure.
Guanethidine	Blood-pressure rise to life-threatening level.
Levodopa	Sudden, severe blood-pressure rise.
MAO inhibitors (other)	High fever, convulsions, death.

POSSIBLE INTERACTION WITH OTHER SUBSTANCES

INTERACTS WITH	COMBINED EFFECT
Alcohol:	Increased sedation to dangerous level.
Beverages: Caffeine drinks.	Irregular heartbeat or high blood pressure.
Drinks containing tyramine (see Glossary).	Blood-pressure rise to life-threatening level.
Cocaine:	Overstimulation. Possibly fatal.
Foods: Foods containing tyramine (see Glossary).	Blood-pressure rise to life-threatening level.
Marijuana:	Overstimulation. Avoid.
Tobacco:	No proven problems.

PROCHLORPERAZINE

BRAND NAMES

Chlorazine
Combid
Compazine
Eskatrol

Prochlor-Iso
Pro-Iso
Stemetil

BASIC INFORMATION

Habit forming? No
Prescription needed? Yes
Available as generic? Yes
Drug class: Tranquilizer, antiemetic (phenothiazine)

USES

• Stops nausea, vomiting.
• Reduces anxiety, agitation.

DOSAGE & USAGE INFORMATION

How to take:
• Tablet or capsule—Swallow with liquid or food to lessen stomach irritation.
• Suppositories—Remove wrapper and moisten suppository with water. Gently insert into rectum, large end first.
• Drops or liquid—Dilute dose in beverage.

When to take:
• Nervous and mental disorders—Take at the same times each day.
• Nausea and vomiting—Take as needed, no more often than every 4 hours.

If you forget a dose:
• Nervous and mental disorders—Take up to 2 hours late. If more than 2 hours, wait for next scheduled dose (don't double this dose).
• Nausea and vomiting—Take as soon as you remember. Wait 4 hours for next dose.

Continued next column

OVERDOSE

SYMPTOMS:
Stupor, convulsions, coma.
WHAT TO DO:
• Dial 0 (operator) or 911 (emergency) for an ambulance or medical help. Then give first aid immediately.
• See emergency information on inside covers.

What drug does:
• Suppresses brain's vomiting center.
• Suppresses brain centers that control abnormal emotions and behavior.

Time lapse before drug works:
• Nausea and vomiting—1 hour or less.
• Nervous and mental disorders—4-6 weeks.

Don't take with:
• Antacid or medicine for diarrhea.
• Non-prescription drug for cough, cold or allergy.
• See Interaction column and consult doctor.

POSSIBLE ADVERSE REACTIONS OR SIDE EFFECTS

SYMPTOMS	WHAT TO DO
Life-threatening: None expected.	
Common:	
• Muscle spasms of face and neck, unsteady gait.	Discontinue. Seek emergency treatment.
• Restlessness, tremor, drowsiness.	Discontinue. Call doctor right away.
• Decreased sweating, dry mouth, runny nose, constipation.	Continue. Call doctor when convenient.
Infrequent:	
• Fainting.	Discontinue. Seek emergency treatment.
• Rash.	Discontinue. Call doctor right away.
• Difficult urination, diminished sex drive, swollen breasts, menstrual irregularities.	Continue. Call doctor when convenient.
Rare:	
Change in vision, sore throat, fever, jaundice.	Discontinue. Call doctor right away.

WARNINGS & PRECAUTIONS

Don't take if:
- You are allergic to any phenothiazine.
- You have a blood or bone-marrow disease.

Before you start, consult your doctor:
- If you will have surgery within 2 months, including dental surgery, requiring general or spinal anesthesia.
- If you have asthma, emphysema or other lung disorder.
- If you take non-prescription ulcer medicine, asthma medicine or amphetamines.

Over age 60:
Adverse reactions and side effects may be more frequent and severe than in younger persons. More likely to develop involuntary movement of jaws, lips, tongue, chewing. Report this to your doctor immediately. Early treatment can help.

Pregnancy:
Risk to unborn child outweighs drug benefits. Don't use.

Breast-feeding:
Drug passes into milk. Avoid drug or discontinue nursing until you finish medicine. Consult doctor for advice on maintaining milk supply.

Infants & children:
Don't give to children younger than 2.

Prolonged use:
May lead to tardive dyskinesia (involuntary movement of jaws, lips, tongue, chewing).

Skin & sunlight:
May cause rash or intensify sunburn in areas exposed to sun or sunlamp. Skin may remain sensitive for 3 months after discontinuing.

Driving, piloting or hazardous work:
Don't drive or pilot aircraft until you learn how medicine affects you. Don't work around dangerous machinery. Don't climb ladders or work in high places. Danger increases if you drink alcohol or take medicine affecting alertness and reflexes.

Discontinuing:
- Nervous and mental disorders—Don't discontinue without doctor's advice until you complete prescribed dose, even though symptoms diminish or disappear.
- Nausea and vomiting—May be unnecessary to finish medicine. Follow doctor's instructions.

POSSIBLE INTERACTION WITH OTHER DRUGS

GENERIC NAME OR DRUG CLASS	COMBINED EFFECT
Anticholinergics	Increased anticholinergic effect.
Antidepressants (tricyclic)	Increased prochlorperazine effect.
Antihistamines	Increased antihistamine effect.
Appetite suppressants	Decreased suppressant effect.
Dronabinol	Increased effects of both drugs. Avoid.
Levodopa	Decreased levodopa effect.
Mind-altering drugs	Increased effect of mind-altering drugs.
Molindone	Increased tranquilizer effect.
Narcotics	Increased narcotic effect.
Phenytoin	Increased phenytoin effect.
Quinidine	Impaired heart function. Dangerous mixture.
Sedatives	Increased sedative effect.
Tranquilizers (other)	Increased tranquilizer effect.

POSSIBLE INTERACTION WITH OTHER SUBSTANCES

INTERACTS WITH	COMBINED EFFECT
Alcohol:	Dangerous oversedation.
Beverages:	None expected.
Cocaine:	Decreased prochlorperazine effect. Avoid.
Foods:	None expected.
Marijuana:	Drowsiness. May increase antinausea effect.
Tobacco:	None expected.

PROCHLORPERAZINE & ISOPROPAMIDE

BRAND NAMES

Combid Spansules

BASIC INFORMATION

Habit forming? No
Prescription needed? Yes
Available as generic? No
Drug class: Antispasmodic, antiemetic,
                tranquilizer (phenothiazine)

 USES

- Stops nausea, vomiting.
- Reduces anxiety, agitation.
- Reduces spasms of digestive system.

 DOSAGE & USAGE INFORMATION

How to take:

- Tablet or capsule—Swallow with liquid or food to lessen stomach irritation.
- Extended-release tablets or capsules—Swallow each dose whole. If you take regular tablets, you may chew or crush them.

When to take:
30 minutes before meals (unless directed otherwise by doctor).

If you forget a dose:
Take as soon as you remember up to 2 hours late. If more than 2 hours, wait for next scheduled dose (don't double this dose).

Continued next column

 OVERDOSE

SYMPTOMS:
Dilated pupils, rapid pulse and breathing, dizziness, fever, hallucinations, confusion, slurred speech, agitation, flushed face, convulsions, stupor, coma.
WHAT TO DO:

- **Dial 0 (operator) or 911 (emergency) for an ambulance or medical help. Then give first aid immediately.**
- **See emergency information on inside covers.**

What drug does:

- Suppresses brain's vomiting center.
- Suppresses brain centers that control abnormal emotions and behavior.
- Blocks nerve impulses at parasympathetic nerve endings, preventing muscle contractions and gland secretions of organs involved.

Time lapse before drug works:
15 to 30 minutes.

Don't take with:

- Antacid or medicine for diarrhea.
- Non-prescription drugs for cough, cold or allergy.
- See Interaction column and consult doctor.

 POSSIBLE ADVERSE REACTIONS OR SIDE EFFECTS

SYMPTOMS	WHAT TO DO
Life-threatening:	
Fainting, dilated pupils, rapid pulse, hallucinations, muscle spasms, unsteady gait.	Discontinue. Seek emergency treatment.
Common:	
• Restlessness, tremor, confusion, drowsiness, rash.	Discontinue. Call doctor right away.
• Decreased sweating, dry mouth, runny nose, constipation, nausea.	Continue. Call doctor when convenient.
Infrequent:	
• Painful, difficult urination; vomiting.	Discontinue. Call doctor right away.
• Headache, diminished sex drive, swollen breasts, menstrual irregularities.	Continue. Call doctor when convenient.
Rare:	
Hives; change in vision; eye pain; sore throat, fever, mouth sores.	Discontinue. Call doctor right away.

 WARNINGS & PRECAUTIONS

Don't take if:

- You are allergic to any anticholinergic or phenothiazine.
- You have trouble with stomach bloating, difficulty emptying your bladder completely, narrow-angle glaucoma, severe ulcerative colitis, a blood or bone-marrow disease.

PROCHLORPERAZINE & ISOPROPAMIDE

Before you start, consult your doctor:
- If you have open-angle glaucoma, angina, chronic bronchitis or asthma, hiatal hernia, liver disease, enlarged prostate, myasthenia gravis, peptic ulcer, emphysema or other lung disorder.
- If you take non-prescription ulcer medicine, asthma medicine or amphetamines.
- If you will have surgery within 2 months, including dental surgery, requiring general or spinal anesthesia.

Over age 60:
Adverse reactions and side effects may be more frequent and severe than in younger persons. More likely to develop involuntary movement of jaws, lips, tongue, chewing. Report this to your doctor immediately. Early treatment can help.

Pregnancy:
Risk to unborn child outweighs drug benefits. Don't use.

Breast-feeding:
Drug passes into milk. Avoid drug or discontinue nursing until you finish medicine. Consult doctor for advice on maintaining milk supply.

Infants & children:
Use only under medical supervision.

Prolonged use:
- Chronic constipation, possible fecal impaction.
- May lead to tardive dyskinesia (involuntary movement of jaws, lips, tongue, chewing).

Skin & sunlight:
May cause rash or intensify sunburn in areas exposed to sun or sunlamp. Skin may remain sensitive for 3 months after discontinuing.

Driving, piloting or hazardous work:
Don't drive or pilot aircraft until you learn how medicine affects you. Don't work around dangerous machinery. Don't climb ladders or work in high places. Danger increases if you drink alcohol or take medicine affecting alertness and reflexes, such as antihistamines, tranquilizers, sedatives, pain medicine, narcotics and mind-altering drugs.

Discontinuing:
- May be unnecessary to finish medicine. Follow doctor's instructions.
- If you develop withdrawal symptoms of hallucinations, agitation or sleeplessness after discontinuing, call doctor right away.

Others:
No problems expected.

 ## POSSIBLE INTERACTION WITH OTHER DRUGS

GENERIC NAME OR DRUG CLASS	COMBINED EFFECT
Amantadine	Increased isopropamide effect.
Anticholinergics	Increased anticholingeric effect.
Antidepressants (tricyclic)	Increased atropine effect. Increased sedation.
Antihistamines	Increased isopropamide effect.
Appetite suppressants	Decreased suppressant effect.
Cortisone drugs	Increased internal-eye pressure.
Dronabinol	Increased effect of both drugs. Avoid.
Haloperidol	Increased internal-eye pressure.
Levodopa	Decreased levodopa effect.
MAO inhibitors	Increased isopropamide effect.
Meperidine	Increased isopropamide effect.
Methylphenidate	Increased isopropamide effect.
Mind-altering drugs	Increased effect of mind-altering drugs.
Narcotics	Increased narcotic effect.

Continued page 974

 ## POSSIBLE INTERACTION WITH OTHER SUBSTANCES

INTERACTS WITH	COMBINED EFFECT
Alcohol:	Dangerous oversedation.
Beverages:	None expected.
Cocaine:	Excessively rapid heartbeat. Avoid.
Foods:	None expected.
Marijuana:	Drowsiness and dry mouth. May increase antinausea effect.
Tobacco:	None expected.

PROCYCLIDINE

BRAND NAMES

Kemadrin   Procyclid
PMS Procyclidine

BASIC INFORMATION

Habit forming? No
Prescription needed? Yes
Available as generic? No
Drug class: Antidyskinetic, antiparkinsonism

 ## USES

- Treatment of Parkinson's disease.
- Treatment of adverse effects of phenothiazines.

 ## DOSAGE & USAGE INFORMATION

How to take:
Tablets or capsules—Take with food to lessen stomach irritation.

When to take:
At the same times each day.

If you forget a dose:
Take as soon as you remember up to 2 hours late. If more than 2 hours, wait for next scheduled dose (don't double this dose).

What drug does:
- Balances chemical reactions necessary to send nerve impulses within base of brain.
- Improves muscle control and reduces stiffness.

Continued next column

 ## OVERDOSE

SYMPTOMS:
Agitation, dilated pupils, hallucinations, dry mouth, rapid heartbeat, sleepiness.
WHAT TO DO:
- **Dial 0 (operator) or 911 (emergency) for an ambulance or medical help. Then give first aid immediately.**
- **If patient is unconscious and not breathing, give mouth-to-mouth breathing. If there is no heartbeat, use cardiac massage and mouth-to-mouth breathing (CPR). Don't try to make patient vomit. If you can't get help quickly, take patient to nearest emergency facility.**
- **See emergency information on inside covers.**

Time lapse before drug works:
1 to 2 hours.

Don't take with:
- Non-prescription drugs for colds, cough or allergy.
- See Interaction column and consult doctor.

 ## POSSIBLE ADVERSE REACTIONS OR SIDE EFFECTS

SYMPTOMS	WHAT TO DO
Life-threatening: None expected.	
Common:	
• Blurred vision, light sensitivity, constipation, nausea, vomiting.	Continue. Call doctor when convenient.
• Frequent, painful or difficult urination.	Continue. Tell doctor at next visit.
Infrequent: None expected.	
Rare:	
• Rash, eye pain.	Discontinue. Call doctor right away.
• Confusion, dizziness, sore mouth or tongue, muscle cramps, numbness or weakness in hands or feet.	Continue. Call doctor when convenient.

WARNINGS & PRECAUTIONS

Don't take if:
You are allergic to any antidyskinetic.

Before you start, consult your doctor:
- If you have had glaucoma.
- If you have had high blood pressure or heart disease.
- If you have had impaired liver function.
- If you have had kidney disease or urination difficulty.

Over age 60:
More sensitive to drug. Aggravates symptoms of enlarged prostate. Causes impaired thinking, hallucinations, nightmares. Consult doctor about any of these.

Pregnancy:
Studies inconclusive on harm to unborn child. Animal studies show fetal abnormalities. Decide with your doctor whether drug benefits justify risk to unborn child.

Breast-feeding:
No problems expected.

Infants & children:
Not recommended for children 3 and younger. Use for older children only under doctor's supervision.

Prolonged use:
Possible glaucoma.

Skin & sunlight:
No problems expected.

Driving, piloting or hazardous work:
Don't drive or pilot aircraft until you learn how medicine affects you. Don't work around dangerous machinery. Don't climb ladders or work in high places. Danger increases if you drink alcohol or take medicine affecting alertness and reflexes, such as antihistamines, tranquilizers, sedatives, pain medicine, narcotics and mind-altering drugs.

Discontinuing:
Don't discontinue without consulting doctor. Dose may require gradual reduction if you have taken drug for a long time. Doses of other drugs may also require adjustment.

Others:
- Internal eye pressure should be measured regularly.
- Avoid becoming overheated.

POSSIBLE INTERACTION WITH OTHER DRUGS

GENERIC NAME OR DRUG CLASS	COMBINED EFFECT
Amantadine	Increased amantadine effect.
Antidepressants (tricyclic)	Increased procyclidine effect. May cause glaucoma.
Antihistamines	Increased procyclidine effect.
Levodopa	Increased levodopa effect. Improved results in treating Parkinson's disease.
Meperidine	Increased procyclidine effect.
MAO inhibitors	Increased procyclidine effect.
Orphenadrine	Increased procyclidine effect.
Phenothiazines	Behavior changes.
Primidone	Excessive sedation.
Procainamide	Increased procainamide effect.
Quinidine	Increased procyclidine effect.
Tranquilizers	Excessive sedation.

POSSIBLE INTERACTION WITH OTHER SUBSTANCES

INTERACTS WITH	COMBINED EFFECT
Alcohol:	None expected.
Beverages:	None expected.
Cocaine:	Decreased procyclidine effect. Avoid.
Foods:	None expected.
Marijuana:	None expected.
Tobacco:	None expected.

PROMAZINE

BRAND NAMES

Norzine
Promanyl

Prozine
Sparine

BASIC INFORMATION

Habit forming? No
Prescription needed? Yes
Available as generic? Yes
Drug class: Tranquilizer, antiemetic
(phenothiazine)

 ## USES

- Stops nausea, vomiting.
- Reduces anxiety, agitation.

 ## DOSAGE & USAGE INFORMATION

How to take:

- Tablet or capsule—Swallow with liquid or food to lessen stomach irritation.
- Suppositories—Remove wrapper and moisten suppository with water. Gently insert into rectum, large end first.
- Drops or liquid—Dilute dose in beverage.

When to take:

- Nervous and mental disorders—Take at the same times each day.
- Nausea and vomiting—Take as needed, no more often than every 4 hours.

If you forget a dose:

- Nervous and mental disorders—Take up to 2 hours late. If more than 2 hours, wait for next scheduled dose (don't double this dose).
- Nausea and vomiting—Take as soon as you remember. Wait 4 hours for next dose.

What drug does:

- Suppresses brain's vomiting center.
- Suppresses brain centers that control abnormal emotions and behavior.

Continued next column

 ## OVERDOSE

SYMPTOMS:
Stupor, convulsions, coma.
WHAT TO DO:

- **Dial 0 (operator) or 911 (emergency) for an ambulance or medical help. Then give first aid immediately.**
- **See emergency information on inside covers.**

Time lapse before drug works:

- Nausea and vomiting—1 hour or less.
- Nervous and mental disorders—4-6 weeks.

Don't take with:

- Antacid or medicine for diarrhea.
- Non-prescription drug for cough, cold or allergy.
- See Interaction column and consult doctor.

 ## POSSIBLE ADVERSE REACTIONS OR SIDE EFFECTS

SYMPTOMS	WHAT TO DO
Life-threatening:	
None expected.	
Common:	
• Muscle spasms of face and neck, unsteady gait.	Discontinue. Seek emergency treatment.
• Restlessness, tremor, drowsiness.	Discontinue. Call doctor right away.
• Decreased sweating, dry mouth, runny nose, constipation.	Continue. Call doctor when convenient.
Infrequent:	
• Fainting.	Discontinue. Seek emergency treatment.
• Rash.	Discontinue. Call doctor right away.
• Difficult urination, diminished sex drive, swollen breasts, menstrual irregularities.	Continue. Call doctor when convenient.
Rare:	
Change in vision, sore throat, fever, jaundice.	Discontinue. Call doctor right away.

WARNINGS & PRECAUTIONS

Don't take if:
- You are allergic to any phenothiazine.
- You have a blood or bone-marrow disease.

Before you start, consult your doctor:
- If you will have surgery within 2 months, including dental surgery, requiring general or spinal anesthesia.
- If you have asthma, emphysema or other lung disorder.
- If you take non-prescription ulcer medicine, asthma medicine or amphetamines.

Over age 60:
Adverse reactions and side effects may be more frequent and severe than in younger persons. More likely to develop involuntary movement of jaws, lips, tongue, chewing. Report this to your doctor immediately. Early treatment can help.

Pregnancy:
Risk to unborn child outweighs drug benefits. Don't use.

Breast-feeding:
Drug passes into milk. Avoid drug or discontinue nursing until you finish medicine. Consult doctor for advice on maintaining milk supply.

Infants & children:
Don't give to children younger than 2.

Prolonged use:
May lead to tardive dyskinesia (involuntary movement of jaws, lips, tongue, chewing).

Skin & sunlight:
May cause rash or intensify sunburn in areas exposed to sun or sunlamp. Skin may remain sensitive for 3 months after discontinuing.

Driving, piloting or hazardous work:
Don't drive or pilot aircraft until you learn how medicine affects you. Don't work around dangerous machinery. Don't climb ladders or work in high places. Danger increases if you drink alcohol or take medicine affecting alertness and reflexes.

Discontinuing:
- Nervous and mental disorders—Don't discontinue without doctor's advice until you complete prescribed dose, even though symptoms diminish or disappear.
- Nausea and vomiting—May be unnecessary to finish medicine. Follow doctor's instructions.

POSSIBLE INTERACTION WITH OTHER DRUGS

GENERIC NAME OR DRUG CLASS	COMBINED EFFECT
Anticholinergics	Increased anticholinergic effect.
Antidepressants (tricyclic)	Increased promazine effect.
Antihistamines	Increased antihistamine effect.
Appetite suppressants	Decreased suppressant effect.
Dronabinol	Increased effects of both drugs. Avoid.
Levodopa	Decreased levodopa effect.
Mind-altering drugs	Increased effect of mind-altering drugs.
Molindone	Increased tranquilizer effect.
Narcotics	Increased narcotic effect.
Phenytoin	Increased phenytoin effect.
Quinidine	Impaired heart function. Dangerous mixture.
Sedatives	Increased sedative effect.
Tranquilizers (other)	Increased tranquilizer effect.

POSSIBLE INTERACTION WITH OTHER SUBSTANCES

INTERACTS WITH	COMBINED EFFECT
Alcohol:	Dangerous oversedation.
Beverages:	None expected.
Cocaine:	Decreased promazine effect. Avoid.
Foods:	None expected.
Marijuana:	Drowsiness. May increase antinausea effect.
Tobacco:	None expected.

PROMETHAZINE

BRAND NAMES

See complete list of brand names in the *Brand Name Directory*, page 955.

BASIC INFORMATION

Habit forming? No
Prescription needed? Yes
Available as generic? Yes
Drug class: Antihistamine, tranquilizer (phenothiazine)

 USES

- Stops nausea, vomiting and dizziness of motion sickness.
- Produces mild sedation and light sleep.
- Reduces allergic symptoms of hay fever and hives.

 DOSAGE & USAGE INFORMATION

How to take:
- Tablets or liquid—Swallow with water.
- Suppositories—Remove wrapper and moisten suppository with water. Gently insert larger end into rectum. Push well into rectum with finger.

When to take:
Take as needed, no more often than every 12 hours.

If you forget a dose:
Take as soon as you remember. Wait 12 hours for next dose.

What drug does:
- Blocks stimulation of brain's vomiting center.
- Suppresses brain centers that control abnormal emotions and behavior.
- Blocks histamine action in sensitized cells.

Time lapse before drug works:
1 to 2 hours.

Continued next column

 OVERDOSE

SYMPTOMS:
Stupor, convulsions, coma.
WHAT TO DO:
- Dial 0 (operator) or 911 (emergency) for an ambulance or medical help. Then give first aid immediately.
- See emergency information on inside covers.

Don't take with:
- Antacid or medicine for diarrhea.
- Non-prescription drug for cough, cold or allergy.
- See Interaction column and consult doctor.

 POSSIBLE ADVERSE REACTIONS OR SIDE EFFECTS

SYMPTOMS	WHAT TO DO
Life-threatening: None expected.	
Common:	
• Restlessness, tremor, drowsiness.	Discontinue. Call doctor right away.
• Decreased sweating, dry mouth, runny nose, constipation.	Continue. Call doctor when convenient.
Infrequent:	
• Fainting.	Discontinue. Seek emergency treatment.
• Rash, muscle spasms of face and neck, unsteady gait.	Discontinue. Call doctor right away.
• Difficult urination, diminished sex drive, swollen breasts, menstrual irregularities.	Continue. Call doctor when convenient.
Rare: Change in vision, sore throat, fever, jaundice.	Discontinue. Call doctor right away.

 WARNINGS & PRECAUTIONS

Don't take if:
- You are allergic to any phenothiazine.
- You have a blood or bone-marrow disease.

Before you start, consult your doctor:
- If you will have surgery within 2 months, including dental surgery, requiring general or spinal anesthesia.
- If you have asthma, emphysema or other lung disorder.
- If you take non-prescription ulcer medicine, asthma medicine or amphetamines.

Over age 60:
Adverse reactions and side effects may be more frequent and severe than in younger persons. More likely to develop tardive dyskinesia (involuntary movement of jaws, lips, tongue, chewing). Report this to your doctor immediately. Early treatment can help.

Pregnancy:
Risk to unborn child outweighs drug benefits. Don't use.

Breast-feeding:
Drug passes into milk. Avoid drug or discontinue nursing until you finish medicine. Consult doctor for advice on maintaining milk supply.

Infants & children:
Don't give to children younger than 2.

Prolonged use:
May lead to tardive dyskinesia (involuntary movement of jaws, lips, tongue, chewing).

Skin & sunlight:
May cause rash or intensify sunburn in areas exposed to sun or sunlamp. Skin may remain sensitive for 3 months after discontinuing.

Driving, piloting or hazardous work:
Don't drive or pilot aircraft until you learn how medicine affects you. Don't work around dangerous machinery. Don't climb ladders or work in high places. Danger increases if you drink alcohol or take medicine affecting alertness and reflexes.

Discontinuing:
- Nervous and mental disorders—Don't discontinue without doctor's advice until you complete prescribed dose, even though symptoms diminish or disappear.
- Nausea, vomiting or allergy—May be unnecessary to finish medicine. Follow doctor's instructions.

Others:
No problems expected.

POSSIBLE INTERACTION WITH OTHER DRUGS

GENERIC NAME OR DRUG CLASS	COMBINED EFFECT
Antacids	Decreased promethazine effect.
Anticholinergics	Increased anticholinergic effect.
Anticonvulsants (hydantoin)	Increased anticonvulsant effect.
Antidepressants (tricyclic)	Increased promethazine effect.
Antihistamines (other)	Increased antihistamine effect.
Appetite suppressants	Decreased suppressant effect.
Barbiturates	Oversedation.
Dronabinol	Increased effects of both drugs. Avoid.
Glycopyrrolate	Possible increased glycopyrrolate effect.
Guanethidine	Decreased guanethidine effect.
Levodopa	Decreased levodopa effect.
MAO inhibitors	Increased promethazine effect.
Mind-altering drugs	Increased effect of mind-altering drugs.
Molindone	Increased sedative and antihistamine effect.
Narcotics	Increased narcotic effect.
Sedatives	Increased sedative effect.
Terfenadine	Possible oversedation.
Tranquilizers (other)	Increased tranquilizer effect.

POSSIBLE INTERACTION WITH OTHER SUBSTANCES

INTERACTS WITH	COMBINED EFFECT
Alcohol:	Dangerous sedation.
Beverages:	None expected.
Cocaine:	Decreased effect of promethazine. Avoid.
Foods:	None expected.
Marijuana:	Drowsiness. May increase antinausea effect.
Tobacco:	None expected.

PROPANTHELINE

BRAND NAMES

Banlin
Norpanth
Novopropanthil
Pro-Banthine
Pro-Banthine with
  Phenobarbital
Propanthel
Ropanth
SK-Propantheline

BASIC INFORMATION

Habit forming? No
Prescription needed?
  High strength: Yes
  Low strength: No
Available as generic? Yes
Drug class: Antispasmodic, anticholinergic

 ## USES

Reduces spasms of digestive system, bladder and urethra.

 ## DOSAGE & USAGE INFORMATION

How to take:
Tablet—Swallow with liquid or food to lessen stomach irritation.

When to take:
30 minutes before meals (unless directed otherwise by doctor).

If you forget a dose:
Take as soon as you remember up to 2 hours late. If more than 2 hours, wait for next scheduled dose (don't double this dose).

What drug does:
Blocks nerve impulses at parasympathetic nerve endings, preventing muscle contractions and gland secretions of organs involved.

Time lapse before drug works:
15 to 30 minutes.

Don't take with:
See Interaction column and consult doctor.

 ## OVERDOSE

SYMPTOMS:
Dilated pupils, rapid pulse and breathing, dizziness, fever, hallucinations, confusion, slurred speech, agitation, flushed face, convulsions, coma.
WHAT TO DO:
- Dial 0 (operator) or 911 (emergency) for an ambulance or medical help. Then give first aid immediately.
- See emergency information on inside covers.

 ## POSSIBLE ADVERSE REACTIONS OR SIDE EFFECTS

SYMPTOMS	WHAT TO DO
Life-threatening: None expected.	
Common:	
• Confusion, delirium, rapid heartbeat.	Discontinue. Call doctor right away.
• Nausea, vomiting, decreased sweating.	Continue. Call doctor when convenient.
• Constipation.	Continue. Tell doctor at next visit.
• Dry ears, nose, throat.	No action necessary.
Infrequent: Headache, difficult urination.	Continue. Call doctor when convenient.
Rare: Rash or hives, pain, blurred vision.	Discontinue. Call doctor right away.

 ## WARNINGS & PRECAUTIONS

Don't take if:
- You are allergic to any anticholinergic.
- You have trouble with stomach bloating.
- You have difficulty emptying your bladder completely.
- You have narrow-angle glaucoma.
- You have severe ulcerative colitis.

Before you start, consult your doctor:
- If you have open-angle glaucoma.
- If you have angina.
- If you have chronic bronchitis or asthma.
- If you have hiatal hernia.
- If you have liver disease.
- If you have enlarged prostate.
- If you have myasthenia gravis.
- If you have peptic ulcer.
- If you will have surgery within 2 months, including dental surgery, requiring general or spinal anesthesia.

Over age 60:
Adverse reactions and side effects may be more frequent and severe than in younger persons.

Pregnancy:
Studies inconclusive on harm to unborn child. Animal studies show fetal abnormalities. Decide with your doctor whether drug benefits justify risk to unborn child.

Breast-feeding:
Drug passes into milk and decreases milk flow. Avoid drug or discontinue nursing until you finish medicine. Consult doctor for advice on maintaining milk supply.

Infants & children:
Use only under medical supervision.

Prolonged use:
Chronic constipation, possible fecal impaction. Consult doctor immediately.

Skin & sunlight:
No problems expected.

Driving, piloting or hazardous work:
Use disqualifies you for piloting aircraft. Otherwise, no problems expected.

Discontinuing:
May be unnecessary to finish medicine. Follow doctor's instructions.

Others:
No problems expected.

POSSIBLE INTERACTION WITH OTHER DRUGS

GENERIC NAME OR DRUG CLASS	COMBINED EFFECT
Amantadine	Increased propantheline effect.
Anticholinergics (other)	Increased propantheline effect.
Antidepressants (tricyclic)	Increased propantheline effect. Increased sedation.
Antihistamines	Increased propantheline effect.
Cortisone drugs	Increased internal eye pressure.
Haloperidol	Increased internal eye pressure.
MAO inhibitors	Increased propantheline effect.
Meperidine	Increased propantheline effect.
Methylphenidate	Increased propantheline effect.
Molindone	Increased anticholinergic effect.
Nitrates	Increased internal-eye pressure.
Orphenadrine	Increased propantheline effect.
Phenothiazines	Increased propantheline effect.
Pilocarpine	Loss of pilocarpine effect in glaucoma treatment.
Potassium supplements	Increased possibility of intestinal ulcers with oral potassium tablets.
Terfenadine	Possible increased propantheline effect.
Vitamin C	Decreased propantheline effect. Avoid large doses of vitamin C.

POSSIBLE INTERACTION WITH OTHER SUBSTANCES

INTERACTS WITH	COMBINED EFFECT
Alcohol:	None expected.
Beverages:	None expected.
Cocaine:	Excessively rapid heartbeat. Avoid.
Foods:	None expected.
Marijuana:	Drowsiness and dry mouth.
Tobacco:	None expected.

PROPRANOLOL

BRAND NAMES

Apo-Propranolol	Inderide
Detensol	Novopranol
Inderal	Panolol
Inderal LA	pms-Propranolol

BASIC INFORMATION

Habit forming? No
Prescription needed? Yes
Available as generic? Yes
Drug class: Beta-adrenergic blocker

USES

- Reduces angina attacks.
- Stabilizes irregular heartbeat.
- Lowers blood pressure.
- Reduces frequency of migraine headaches. (Does not relieve headache pain.)
- Other uses prescribed by your doctor.

DOSAGE & USAGE INFORMATION

How to take:
Tablet or capsule—Swallow with liquid. If you can't swallow whole, crumble tablet or open capsule and take with liquid or food.

When to take:
With meals or immediately after.

If you forget a dose:
Take as soon as you remember. Return to regular schedule, but allow 3 hours between doses.

What drug does:
- Blocks certain actions of sympathetic nervous system.
- Lowers heart's oxygen requirements.
- Slows nerve impulses through heart.
- Reduces blood vessel contraction in heart, scalp and other body parts.

Continued next column

OVERDOSE

SYMPTOMS:
Weakness, slow or weak pulse, blood-pressure drop, fainting, convulsions, cold and sweaty skin.
WHAT TO DO:
- **Dial 0 (operator) or 911 (emergency) for an ambulance or medical help. Then give first aid immediately.**
- **See emergency information on inside covers.**

Time lapse before drug works:
1 to 4 hours.

Don't take with:
Non-prescription drugs or drugs in Interaction column without consulting doctor.

POSSIBLE ADVERSE REACTIONS OR SIDE EFFECTS

SYMPTOMS	WHAT TO DO
Life-threatening:	
None expected.	
Common:	
● Pulse slower than 50 beats per minute.	Discontinue. Call doctor right away.
● Drowsiness, numbness or tingling of fingers or toes, dizziness, diarrhea, nausea, fatigue, weakness.	Continue. Call doctor when convenient.
● Cold hands or feet; dry mouth, eyes and skin.	Continue. Tell doctor at next visit.
Infrequent:	
● Hallucinations, nightmares, insomnia, headache, difficult breathing, joint pain.	Discontinue. Call doctor right away.
● Confusion, depression, reduced alertness, impotence.	Continue. Call doctor when convenient.
● Constipation.	Continue. Tell doctor at next visit.
Rare:	
● Rash, sore throat, fever.	Discontinue. Call doctor right away.
● Unusual bleeding and bruising.	Continue. Call doctor when convenient.

WARNINGS & PRECAUTIONS

Don't take if:
- You are allergic to any beta-adrenergic blocker.
- You have asthma.
- You have hay fever symptoms.
- You have taken MAO inhibitors in past 2 weeks.

Before you start, consult your doctor:
- If you have heart disease or poor circulation to the extremities.
- If you have hay fever, asthma, chronic bronchitis, emphysema.
- If you have overactive thyroid function.
- If you have impaired liver or kidney function.
- If you will have surgery within 2 months, including dental surgery, requiring general or spinal anesthesia.
- If you have diabetes or hypoglycemia.

Over age 60:
Adverse reactions and side effects may be more frequent and severe than in younger persons.

Pregnancy:
Risk to unborn child outweighs drug benefits. Don't use.

Breast-feeding:
Drug passes into milk. Avoid drug or discontinue nursing until you finish medicine. Consult doctor for advice on maintaining milk supply.

Infants & children:
Not recommended.

Prolonged use:
Weakens heart muscle contractions.

Skin & sunlight:
No problems expected.

Driving, piloting or hazardous work:
Don't drive or pilot aircraft until you learn how medicine affects you. Don't work around dangerous machinery. Don't climb ladders or work in high places. Danger increases if you drink alcohol or take medicine affecting alertness and reflexes.

Discontinuing:
Don't discontinue without consulting doctor. Dose may require gradual reduction if you have taken drug for a long time. Doses of other drugs may also require adjustment.

Others:
May mask hypoglycemia.

POSSIBLE INTERACTION WITH OTHER DRUGS

GENERIC NAME OR DRUG CLASS	COMBINED EFFECT
Acebutolol	Increased antihypertensive effects of both drugs. Dosages may require adjustment.
Albuterol	Decreased Albuterol effect and Beta-adrenergic blocking effect

Antidiabetics	Increased antidiabetic effect.
Antihistamines	Decreased antihistamine effect.
Antihypertensives	Increased antihypertensive effect.
Anti-inflammatory drugs	Decreased anti-inflammatory effect.
Barbiturates	Increased barbiturate effect. Dangerous sedation.
Digitalis preparations	Can either increase or decrease heart rate. Improves irregular heartbeat.
Molindone	Increased tranquilizer effect.
Narcotics	Increased narcotic effect. Dangerous sedation.
Nitrates	Possible excessive blood-pressure drop.
Pentoxifylline	Increased antihypertensive effect.
Phenytoin	Increased propranolol effect.
Quinidine	Slows heart excessively.
Reserpine	Increased reserpine effect. Excessive sedation and depression.
Tocainide	May worsen congestive heart failure.

POSSIBLE INTERACTION WITH OTHER SUBSTANCES

INTERACTS WITH	COMBINED EFFECT
Alcohol:	Excessive blood-pressure drop. Avoid.
Beverages:	None expected.
Cocaine:	Irregular heartbeat. Avoid.
Foods:	None expected.
Marijuana:	Daily use—Impaired circulation to hands and feet.
Tobacco:	Possible irregular heartbeat.

PSEUDOEPHEDRINE

BRAND NAMES

See complete list of brand names in the *Brand Name Directory,* page 955.

BASIC INFORMATION

Habit forming? No
Prescription needed?
  U.S.: High strength—Yes
       Low strength—No
  Canada: No
Available as generic? Yes
Drug class: Sympathomimetic

 USES

Reduces congestion of nose, sinuses and throat from allergies and infections.

 DOSAGE & USAGE INFORMATION

How to take:
- Tablet or capsule—Swallow with liquid. You may chew or crush tablet.
- Extended-release tablets or capsules—Swallow each dose whole.
- Syrup—Take as directed on label.

When to take:
- At the same times each day.
- To prevent insomnia, take last dose of day a few hours before bedtime.

If you forget a dose:
Take up to 2 hours late. If more than 2 hours, wait for next dose (don't double this dose).

What drug does:
Decreases blood volume in nasal tissues, shrinking tissues and enlarging airways.

Continued next column

 OVERDOSE

SYMPTOMS:
Nervousness, restlessness, headache, rapid or irregular heartbeat, sweating, nausea, vomiting, anxiety, confusion, delirium, muscle tremors.
WHAT TO DO:
- **Dial 0 (operator) or 911 (emergency) for an ambulance or medical help. Then give first aid immediately.**
- **See emergency information on inside covers.**

Time lapse before drug works:
15 to 20 minutes.

Don't take with:
- See Interaction column and consult doctor.
- Non-prescription drugs with caffeine without consulting doctor.

 POSSIBLE ADVERSE REACTIONS OR SIDE EFFECTS

SYMPTOMS	WHAT TO DO
Life-threatening:	
None expected.	
Common:	
Agitation, insomnia.	Continue. Tell doctor at next visit.
Infrequent:	
• Nausea or vomiting, irregular or slow heartbeat, difficult breathing, unusually fast or pounding heartbeat, painful or difficult urination, increased sweating.	Discontinue. Call doctor right away.
• Dizziness, headache, shakiness, weakness.	Continue. Call doctor when convenient.
• Paleness.	Continue. Tell doctor at next visit.
Rare:	
Hallucinations, seizures.	Discontinue. Seek emergency treatment.

WARNINGS & PRECAUTIONS

Don't take if:
You are allergic to any sympathomimetic drug.

Before you start, consult your doctor:
- If you have overactive thyroid or diabetes.
- If you have taken any MAO inhibitors in past 2 weeks.
- If you take digitalis preparations or have high blood pressure or heart disease.
- If you will have surgery within 2 months, including dental surgery, requiring general or spinal anesthesia.
- If you have urination difficulty.

Over age 60:
Adverse reactions and side effects may be more frequent and severe than in younger persons.

Pregnancy:
No proven harm to unborn child. Avoid if possible.

Breast-feeding:
Drug passes into milk. Avoid drug or discontinue nursing until you finish medicine. Consult doctor for advice on maintaining milk supply.

Infants & children:
Keep dose low or avoid.

Prolonged use:
No proven problems.

Skin & sunlight:
No problems expected.

Driving, piloting or hazardous work:
Avoid if you feel dizzy. Otherwise, no problems expected..

Discontinuing:
May be unnecessary to finish medicine. Follow doctor's instructions.

Others:
No problems expected.

POSSIBLE INTERACTION WITH OTHER DRUGS

GENERIC NAME OR DRUG CLASS	COMBINED EFFECT
Antidepressants (tricyclic)	Increased pseudoephedrine effect.
Antihypertensives	Decreased antihypertensive effect.
Beta-adrenergic blockers	Decreased effects of both drugs.
Calcium supplements	Increased pseudoephedrine effect.
Digitalis preparations	Irregular heartbeat.
Epinephrine	Increased epinephrine effect. Excessive heart stimulation and blood-pressure increase.
Ergot preparations	Serious blood-pressure rise.
Guanethidine	Decreased effect of both drugs.
MAO inhibitors	Increased pseudoephedrine effect.
Nitrates	Possible decreased effects of both drugs.

POSSIBLE INTERACTION WITH OTHER SUBSTANCES

INTERACTS WITH	COMBINED EFFECT
Alcohol:	None expected.
Beverages: Caffeine drinks.	Nervousness or insomnia.
Cocaine:	Dangerous stimulation. Avoid.
Foods:	None expected.
Marijuana:	Rapid heartbeat.
Tobacco:	None expected.

PSORALENS

BRAND AND GENERIC NAMES

METHOXSALEN
Methoxsalen Lotion
  (Topical)
Oxsoralen

Oxsoralen (Topical)
TRIOXSALEN
Trisoralen

BASIC INFORMATION

Habit forming? No
Prescription needed? Yes
Available as generic? No
Drug class: Repigmenting agent (psoralen)

 ## USES

- Repigmenting skin affected with vitiligo (absence of skin pigment).
- Treatment for psoriasis, when other treatments haven't helped.
- Treatment for mycosis fungoides.

 ## DOSAGE & USAGE INFORMATION

How to take or apply:
- Tablet or capsule—Swallow with liquid or food to lessen stomach irritation.
- Topical—As directed by doctor.

When to take or apply:
2 to 4 hours before exposure to sunlight or sunlamp.

If you forget a dose:
Take as soon as you remember. Delay sun exposure for at least 2 hours after taking.

What drug does:
Helps pigment cells when used in conjunction with ultraviolet light.

Time lapse before drug works:
- For vitiligo, up to 6 months.
- For psoriasis, 10 weeks or longer.
- For tanning, 3 to 4 days.

Don't take with:
Any other medicine which causes skin sensitivity to sun. Ask pharmacist.

 ## OVERDOSE

SYMPTOMS:
Blistering skin, swelling feet and legs.
WHAT TO DO:
Overdose unlikely to threaten life. If person takes much larger amount than prescribed, call doctor, poison-control center or hospital emergency room for instructions.

 ## POSSIBLE ADVERSE REACTIONS OR SIDE EFFECTS

SYMPTOMS	WHAT TO DO
Life-threatening: None expected.	
Always:	
• Increased skin sensitivity to sun.	Always protect from overexposure.
• Increased eye sensitivity to sunlight.	Always protect with wrap-around sunglasses.
Infrequent: None expected.	
Rare: Hepatitis with jaundice, blistering and peeling.	Discontinue. Call doctor right away.

 ## WARNINGS & PRECAUTIONS

Don't take if:
- You are allergic to any other psoralen.
- You are unwilling or unable to remain under close medical supervision.

Before you start, consult your doctor:
- If you have heart or liver disease.
- If you have allergy to sunlight.
- If you have cataracts.
- If you have albinism.
- If you have lupus erythematosis, porphyria, chronic infection, skin cancer or peptic ulcer.
- If you will have surgery within 2 months, including dental surgery, requiring general or spinal anesthesia.

Over age 60:
Adverse reactions and side effects may be more frequent and severe than in younger persons.

Pregnancy:
Risk to unborn child outweighs drug benefits. Don't use.

Breast-feeding:
Drug passes into milk. Avoid drug or discontinue nursing until you finish medicine. Consult doctor for advice on maintaining milk supply.

Infants & children:
Not recommended.

Prolonged use:
Increased chance of toxic effects.

Skin & sunlight:
Too much can burn skin. Cover skin for 24 hours before and 8 hours following treatments.

Driving, piloting or hazardous work:
No problems expected. Protect eyes and skin from bright light.

Discontinuing:
Skin may remain sensitive for some time after treatment stops. Use extra protection from sun.

Others:
- Use sunblock on lips.
- Don't use just to make skin tan.

POSSIBLE INTERACTION WITH OTHER DRUGS

GENERIC NAME OR DRUG CLASS	COMBINED EFFECT
Any medicine causing sensitization to sunlight, such as: acetohexamide, amitriptyline, anthralin, barbiturates, bendroflumethiazide, carbamazepine, chlordiazepoxide, chloroquine, chlorothiazide, chloropromazine, chloropropamide, chlortetracycline, chlorthalidone, clindamycin, coal tar derivatives, cyproheptadine, demeclocycline, desipramine, diethylstilbrestrol, diphenhydramine, doxepin, doxycycline, estrogen, fluphenazine, gold preparations, glyburide, griseofulvin, hydrochlorothiazide, hydroflumethiazide, imipramine, lincomycin, mesoridazine, methacycline, nalidixic acid, nortriptyline, oral contraceptives, oxyphenbutazone, oxytetracycline,	Greatly increased likelihood of extreme sensitivity to sunlight.

perphenazine, phenobarbital, phenylbutazone, phenytoin, prochlorperazine, promazine, promethazine, protriptyline, pyrazinamide, sulfonamides, tetracycline, thioridazine, thiazide diuretics, tolazamide, tolbutamide, tranylcypromine, triamterene, trifluoperazine, trimeprazine, trimipramine, triprolidine.

POSSIBLE INTERACTION WITH OTHER SUBSTANCES

INTERACTS WITH	COMBINED EFFECT
Alcohol:	May increase chance of liver toxicity.
Beverages: Lime drinks.	Avoid—toxic.
Cocaine:	Increased chance of toxicity. Avoid.
Foods: Those containing furocoumarin (limes, parsley, figs, parsnips, carrots, celery, mustard).	May cause toxic effects to psoralens.
Marijuana:	Increased chance of toxicity. Avoid.
Tobacco:	May cause uneven absorption of medicine. Avoid.

PSYLLIUM

BRAND NAMES

See complete list of brand names in the *Brand Name Directory*, page 956.

BASIC INFORMATION

Habit forming? No
Prescription needed? No
Available as generic? Yes
Drug class: Laxative (bulk-forming)

 ## USES

Relieves constipation and prevents straining for bowel movement.

 ## DOSAGE & USAGE INFORMATION

How to take:
Powder, flakes or granules—Dilute dose in 8 oz. cold water or fruit juice.

When to take:
At the same time each day, preferably morning.

If you forget a dose:
Take as soon as you remember. Resume regular schedule.

What drug does:
Absorbs water, stimulating the bowel to form a soft, bulky stool.

Time lapse before drug works:
May require 2 or 3 days to begin, then works in 12 to 24 hours.

Don't take with:
- See Interaction column and consult doctor.
- Don't take within 2 hours of taking another medicine.

 ## OVERDOSE

SYMPTOMS:
None expected.
WHAT TO DO:
Overdose unlikely to threaten life. If person takes much larger amount than prescribed, call doctor, poison-control center or hospital emergency room for instructions.

 ## POSSIBLE ADVERSE REACTIONS OR SIDE EFFECTS

SYMPTOMS	WHAT TO DO
Life-threatening None expected.	
Common: None expected.	
Infrequent: Swallowing difficulty, "lump in throat" sensation.	Continue. Call doctor when convenient.
Rare: Rash, itchy skin, intestinal blockage, asthma.	Discontinue. Call doctor right away.

WARNINGS & PRECAUTIONS

Don't take if:
- You are allergic to any bulk-forming laxative.
- You have symptoms of appendicitis, inflamed bowel or intestinal blockage.
- You have missed a bowel movement for only 1 or 2 days.

Before you start, consult your doctor:
- If you have diabetes.
- If you have kidney disease.
- If you have a laxative habit.
- If you have rectal bleeding.
- If you have difficulty swallowing.
- If you take other laxatives.

Over age 60:
Adverse reactions and side effects may be more frequent and severe than in younger persons.

Pregnancy:
Most bulk-forming laxatives contain sodium or sugars which may cause fluid retention. Avoid if possible.

Breast-feeding:
No problems expected.

Infants & children:
Use only under medical supervision.

Prolonged use:
Don't take for more than 1 week unless under a doctor's supervision. May cause laxative dependence.

Skin & sunlight:
No problems expected.

Driving, piloting or hazardous work:
No problems expected.

Discontinuing:
May be unnecessary to finish medicine. Follow doctor's instructions.

Others:
Don't take to "flush out" your system, or as a "tonic."

 ## POSSIBLE INTERACTION WITH OTHER DRUGS

GENERIC NAME OR DRUG CLASS	COMBINED EFFECT
Antibiotics	Decreased antibiotic effect.
Anticoagulants	Decreased anticoagulant effect.
Digitalis preparations	Decreased digitalis effect.
Salicylates (including aspirin)	Decreased salicylate effect.

 ## POSSIBLE INTERACTION WITH OTHER SUBSTANCES

INTERACTS WITH	COMBINED EFFECT
Alcohol:	None expected.
Beverages:	None expected.
Cocaine:	None expected.
Foods:	None expected.
Marijuana:	None expected.
Tobacco:	None expected.

PYRIDOSTIGMINE

BRAND NAMES

Mestinon   Regonol
Mestinon Timespans

BASIC INFORMATION

Habit forming? No
Prescription needed? Yes
Available as generic? Yes
Drug class: Cholinergic (anticholinesterase)

USES

- Treatment of myasthenia gravis.
- Treatment of urinary retention and abdominal distention.
- Antidote to adverse effects of muscle relaxants used in surgery.

DOSAGE & USAGE INFORMATION

How to take:
- Tablet or syrup—Swallow with liquid or food to lessen stomach irritation.
- Extended-release tablets or capsules—Swallow each dose whole. If you take regular tablets, you may chew or crush them.

When to take:
As directed, usually 3 or 4 times a day.

If you forget a dose:
Take as soon as you remember up to 2 hours late. If more than 2 hours, wait for next scheduled dose (don't double this dose).

Continued next column

OVERDOSE

SYMPTOMS:
Muscle weakness, cramps, twitching or clumsiness; severe diarrhea, nausea, vomiting, stomach cramps or pain; breathing difficulty; confusion, irritability, nervousness, restlessness, fear; unusually slow heartbeat; seizures.
WHAT TO DO:
- **Dial 0 (operator) or 911 (emergency) for an ambulance or medical help. Then give first aid immediately.**
- **See emergency information on inside covers.**

What drug does:
Inhibits the chemical activity of an enzyme (cholinesterase) so nerve impulses can cross the junction of nerves and muscles.

Time lapse before drug works:
3 hours.

Don't take with:
See Interaction column and consult doctor.

POSSIBLE ADVERSE REACTIONS OR SIDE EFFECTS

SYMPTOMS	WHAT TO DO
Life-threatening:	
None expected.	
Common:	
• Mild diarrhea, nausea, vomiting, stomach cramps or pain.	Discontinue. Call doctor right away.
• Excess saliva, unusual sweating.	Continue. Call doctor when convenient.
Infrequent:	
• Confusion, irritability.	Discontinue. Seek emergency treatment.
• Constricted pupils, watery eyes, lung congestion, frequent urge to urinate.	Continue. Call doctor when convenient.
Rare:	
None expected.	

WARNINGS & PRECAUTIONS

Don't take if:
- You are allergic to any cholinergic or bromide.
- You take mecamylamine.

Before you start, consult your doctor:
- If you plan to become pregnant within medication period.
- If you have bronchial asthma.
- If you have heartbeat irregularities.
- If you have urinary obstruction or urinary-tract infection.

Over age 60:
Adverse reactions and side effects may be more frequent and severe than in younger persons.

Pregnancy:
No proven harm to unborn child. Avoid if possible. May increase uterus contractions close to delivery.

Breast-feeding:
No problems expected, but consult doctor.

Infants & children:
Not recommended.

Prolonged use:
Medication may lose effectiveness. Discontinuing for a few days may restore effect.

Skin & sunlight:
No problems expected.

Driving, piloting or hazardous work:
Don't drive or pilot aircraft until you learn how medicine affects you. Don't work around dangerous machinery. Don't climb ladders or work in high places. Danger increases if you drink alcohol or take medicine affecting alertness and reflexes, such as antihistamines, tranquilizers, sedatives, pain medicine, narcotics and mind-altering drugs.

Discontinuing:
Don't discontinue without doctor's advice until you complete prescribed dose, even though symptoms diminish or disappear.

Others:
No problems expected.

POSSIBLE INTERACTION WITH OTHER DRUGS

GENERIC NAME OR DRUG CLASS	COMBINED EFFECT
Anesthetics (local or general)	Decreased pyridostigmine effect.
Antiarrhythmics	Decreased pyridostigmine effect.
Antibiotics	Decreased pyridostigmine effect.
Anticholinergics	Decreased pyridostigmine effect. May mask severe side effects.
Cholinergics (other)	Reduced intestinal-tract function. Possible brain and nervous-system toxicity.
Mecamylamine	Decreased pyridostigmine effect.
Nitrates	Decreased pyridostigmine effect.
Quinidine	Decreased pyridostigmine effect.

POSSIBLE INTERACTION WITH OTHER SUBSTANCES

INTERACTS WITH	COMBINED EFFECT
Alcohol:	No proven problems with small doses.
Beverages:	None expected.
Cocaine:	Decreased pyridostigmine effect. Avoid.
Foods:	None expected.
Marijuana:	No proven problems.
Tobacco:	No proven problems.

PYRIDOXINE (VITAMIN B-6)

BRAND NAMES

Alba-Lybe	Hexa-Betalin
Al-Vite	Hexacrest
Beelith	Hexavibex
Beesix	Mega-B
Bendectin	Nu-Iron-V
Eldertonic	Pyroxine
Glutofac	Rodex
Hemo-vite	Tex Six T.R.
Herpecin-L	Vicon

BASIC INFORMATION

Habit forming? No
Prescription needed?
  High strength: Yes
  Low strength: No
Available as generic? Yes
Drug class: Vitamin supplement

 USES

- Prevention and treatment of pyridoxine deficiency.
- Treatment of some forms of anemia.

 DOSAGE & USAGE INFORMATION

How to take:
- Tablets—Swallow with liquid.
- Extended-release tablets—Swallow each dose whole with liquid.

When to take:
At the same times each day.

If you forget a dose:
Take as soon as you remember, then resume regular schedule.

What drug does:
Acts as co-enzyme in carbohydrate, protein and fat metabolism.

Time lapse before drug works:
15 to 20 minutes.

Don't take with:
- Levodopa—Small amounts of pyridoxine will nullify levodopa effect. Carbidopa-levodopa combination not affected by this interaction.
- See Interaction column and consult doctor.

 OVERDOSE

SYMPTOMS:
None expected.
WHAT TO DO:
Overdose unlikely to threaten life.

 POSSIBLE ADVERSE REACTIONS OR SIDE EFFECTS

SYMPTOMS	WHAT TO DO
Life-threatening: None expected.	
Common: None expected.	
Infrequent: None expected.	
Rare: None expected.	

WARNINGS & PRECAUTIONS

Don't take if:
You are allergic to pyridoxine.

Before you start, consult your doctor:
If you are pregnant or breast-feeding.

Over age 60:
No problems expected.

Pregnancy:
Don't exceed recommended dose.

Breast-feeding:
Don't exceed recommended dose.

Infants & children:
Don't exceed recommended dose.

Prolonged use:
Large doses for more than 1 month may cause toxicity.

Skin & sunlight:
No problems expected.

Driving, piloting or hazardous work:
No problems expected.

Discontinuing:
No problems expected.

Others:
Regular pyridoxine supplements recommended if you take chloramphenicol, cycloserine, ethionamide, hydralazine, immunosuppressants, isoniazid or penicillamine. These decrease pyridoxine absorption and can cause anemia or tingling and numbness in hands and feet.

POSSIBLE INTERACTION WITH OTHER DRUGS

GENERIC NAME OR DRUG CLASS	COMBINED EFFECT
Chloramphenicol	Decreased pyridoxine effect.
Contraceptives (oral)	Decreased pyridoxine effect.
Cycloserine	Decreased pyridoxine effect.
Ethionamide	Decreased pyridoxine effect.
Hydralazine	Decreased pyridoxine effect.
Hypnotics (barbiturates)	Decreased hypnotic effect.
Immunosuppressants	Decreased pyridoxine effect.
Isoniazid	Decreased pyridoxine effect.
Levodopa	Decreased levodopa effect.
Penicillamine	Decreased pyridoxine effect.
Phenytoin	Decreased phenytoin effect.

POSSIBLE INTERACTION WITH OTHER SUBSTANCES

INTERACTS WITH	COMBINED EFFECT
Alcohol:	None expected.
Beverages:	None expected.
Cocaine:	None expected.
Foods:	None expected.
Marijuana:	None expected.
Tobacco:	May decrease pyridoxine absorption. Decreased pyridoxine effect.

PYRILAMINE

BRAND NAMES

See complete list of brand names in the
Brand Name Directory, page 956.

BASIC INFORMATION

Habit forming? No
Prescription needed? No
Available as generic? Yes
Drug class: Antihistamine

 ## USES

- Reduces allergic symptoms such as hay fever, hives, rash or itching.
- Prevents motion sickness, nausea, vomiting.
- Induces sleep.

 ## DOSAGE & USAGE INFORMATION

How to take:
Tablet or capsule—Swallow with liquid or food to lessen stomach irritation.

When to take:
Varies with form. Follow label directions.

If you forget a dose:
Take as soon as you remember up to 2 hours late. If more than 2 hours, wait for next scheduled dose (don't double this dose).

What drug does:
Blocks action of histamine after an allergic response triggers histamine release in sensitive cells.

Continued next column

 ## OVERDOSE

SYMPTOMS:
Convulsions, red face, hallucinations, coma.
WHAT TO DO:
- Dial 0 (operator) or 911 (emergency) for an ambulance or medical help. Then give first aid immediately.
- If patient is unconscious and not breathing, give mouth-to-mouth breathing. If there is no heartbeat, use cardiac massage and mouth-to-mouth breathing (CPR). Don't try to make patient vomit. If you can't get help quickly, take patient to nearest emergency facility.
- See emergency information on inside covers.

Time lapse before drug works:
30 minutes.

Don't take with:
See Interaction column and consult doctor.

 ## POSSIBLE ADVERSE REACTIONS OR SIDE EFFECTS

SYMPTOMS	WHAT TO DO
Life-threatening: None expected.	
Common: Drowsiness; dizziness; dry mouth, nose and throat; nausea.	Continue. Tell doctor at next visit.
Infrequent:	
• Change in vision.	Discontinue. Call doctor right away.
• Less tolerance for contact lenses, urination difficulty.	Continue. Call doctor when convenient.
• Appetite loss.	Continue. Tell doctor at next visit.
Rare: Nightmares, agitation, irritability, sore throat, fever, rapid heartbeat, unusual bleeding or bruising, fatigue, weakness.	Discontinue. Call doctor right away.

WARNINGS & PRECAUTIONS

Don't take if:
You are allergic to any antihistamine.

Before you start, consult your doctor:
- If you have glaucoma.
- If you have enlarged prostate.
- If you have asthma.
- If you have kidney disease.
- If you have peptic ulcer.
- If you will have surgery within 2 months, including dental surgery, requiring general or spinal anesthesia.

Over age 60:
Don't exceed recommended dose. Adverse reactions and side effects may be more frequent and severe than in younger persons, especially urination difficulty, diminished alertness and other brain and nervous-system symptoms.

Pregnancy:
No proven harm to unborn child. Avoid if possible.

Breast-feeding:
Drug passes into milk. Avoid drug or discontinue nursing until you finish medicine. Consult doctor for advice on maintaining milk supply.

Infants & children:
Not recommended for premature or newborn infants. Otherwise, no problems expected.

Prolonged use:
Avoid. May damage bone marrow and nerve cells.

Skin & sunlight:
May cause rash or intensify sunburn in areas exposed to sun or sunlamp.

Driving, piloting or hazardous work:
Don't drive or pilot aircraft until you learn how medicine affects you. Don't work around dangerous machinery. Don't climb ladders or work in high places. Danger increases if you drink alcohol or take medicine affecting alertness and reflexes, such as antihistamines, tranquilizers, sedatives, pain medicine, narcotics and mind-altering drugs.

Discontinuing:
No problems expected.

Others:
May mask symptoms of hearing damage from aspirin, other salicylates, cisplatin, paromomycin, vancomycin or anticonvulsants. Consult doctor if you use these.

POSSIBLE INTERACTION WITH OTHER DRUGS

GENERIC NAME OR DRUG CLASS	COMBINED EFFECT
Anticholinergics	Increased anticholinergic effect.
Antidepressants (tricyclic)	Increased pyrilamine effect. Excess sedation.
Antihistamines (other)	Excess sedation. Avoid.
Dronabinol	Increased effects of both drugs. Avoid.
Hypnotics	Excess sedation. Avoid.
MAO inhibitors	Increased pyrilamine effect.
Mind-altering drugs	Excess sedation. Avoid.
Molindone	Increased sedative and antihistamine effect.
Narcotics	Excess sedation. Avoid.
Sedatives	Excess sedation. Avoid.
Sleep inducers	Excess sedation. Avoid.
Tranquilizers	Excess sedation. Avoid.

POSSIBLE INTERACTION WITH OTHER SUBSTANCES

INTERACTS WITH	COMBINED EFFECT
Alcohol:	Excess sedation. Avoid.
Beverages: Caffeine drinks.	Less pyrilamine sedation.
Cocaine:	Decreased pyrilamine effect. Avoid.
Foods:	None expected.
Marijuana:	Excess sedation. Avoid.
Tobacco:	None expected.

PYRILAMINE & PENTOBARBITAL

BRAND NAMES

Wans

BASIC INFORMATION

Habit forming? Yes
Prescription needed? Yes
Available as generic? No
Drug class: Antihistamine, sedative
(barbiturate)

 USES

- Prevents and relieves motion sickness, nausea, vomiting.
- Induces sleep.

 DOSAGE & USAGE INFORMATION

How to take:
Suppositories—Remove wrapper and moisten suppository with water. Gently insert larger end into rectum. Push well into rectum with finger.

When to take:
As directed when needed.

If you forget a dose:
Take as soon as you remember up to 2 hours late. If more than 2 hours, wait for next scheduled dose (don't double this dose).

Continued next column

 OVERDOSE

SYMPTOMS:
Deep sleep, weak pulse, convulsions, red face, hallucinations, coma.
WHAT TO DO:
- **Dial 0 (operator) or 911 (emergency) for an ambulance or medical help. Then give first aid immediately.**
- **If patient is unconscious and not breathing, give mouth-to-mouth breathing. If there is no heartbeat, use cardiac massage and mouth-to-mouth breathing (CPR). Don't try to make patient vomit. If you can't get help quickly, take patient to nearest emergency facility.**
- **See emergency information on inside covers.**

What drug does:
- May partially block nerve impulses at nerve-cell connections in nausea center of brain.
- Blocks action of histamine after an allergic response triggers histamine release in sensitive cells.

Time lapse before drug works:
30 minutes.

Don't take with:
- Non-prescription drugs without consulting doctor.
- See Interaction column and consult doctor.

 POSSIBLE ADVERSE REACTIONS OR SIDE EFFECTS

SYMPTOMS	WHAT TO DO
Life-threatening:	
Slow or fast heartbeat, difficult breathing.	Discontinue. Seek emergency treatment.
Common:	
• Drowsiness, agitation.	Discontinue. Call doctor right away.
• Dizziness, "hangover" effect, dry mouth.	Continue. Call doctor when convenient.
Infrequent:	
• Rash; swelling of face, lip or eyelid; change in vision; nausea; vomiting; diarrhea; appetite loss.	Discontinue. Call doctor right away.
• Less tolerance for contact lens, joint or muscle pain, frequent urination.	Continue. Call doctor when convenient.
Rare:	
Sore throat, fever, mouth sores; urgent urination; jaundice.	Discontinue. Call doctor right away.

 WARNINGS & PRECAUTIONS

Don't take if:
- You are allergic to any antihistamine or barbiturate.
- You have porphyria.

Before you start, consult your doctor:
- If you have glaucoma, enlarged prostate, peptic ulcer, epilepsy, kidney or liver damage, asthma, anemia, chronic pain.
- If you will have surgery within 2 months, including dental surgery, requiring general or spinal anesthesia.

Over age 60:
Don't exceed recommended dose. Adverse reactions and side effects may be more frequent and severe than in younger persons, especially urination difficulty, diminished alertness and other brain and nervous-system symptoms.

Pregnancy:
Risk to unborn child outweighs drug benefits. Don't use.

Breast-feeding:
Drug passes into milk. Avoid drug or discontinue nursing until you finish medicine. Consult doctor for advice on maintaining milk supply.

Infants & children:
Not recommended for premature or newborn infants. Use only under doctor's supervision.

Prolonged use:
- May damage bone marrow and nerve cells. Avoid.
- May cause addiction, anemia, chronic intoxication.
- May lower body temperature, making exposure to cold temperatures hazardous.

Skin & sunlight:
May cause rash or intensify sunburn in areas exposed to sun or sunlamp.

Driving, piloting or hazardous work:
Don't drive or pilot aircraft until you learn how medicine affects you. Don't work around dangerous machinery. Don't climb ladders or work in high places. Danger increases if you drink alcohol or take medicine affecting alertness and reflexes, such as antihistamines, tranquilizers, sedatives, pain medicine, narcotics and mind-altering drugs.

Discontinuing:
- May be unnecessary to finish medicine. Follow doctor's instructions.
- If you develop withdrawal symptoms of hallucinations, agitation or sleeplessness after discontinuing, call doctor right away.

Others:
- May mask symptoms of hearing damage from aspirin, other salicylates, cisplatin, paromomycin, vancomycin or anticonvulsants. Consult your doctor if you use these.
- Great potential for abuse.

POSSIBLE INTERACTION WITH OTHER DRUGS

GENERIC NAME OR DRUG CLASS	COMBINED EFFECT
Anticholinergics	Increased anticholinergics effect.
Anticoagulants	Decreased anticoagulant effect.
Anticonvulsants	Changed seizure patterns.
Antidepressants (tricyclics)	Possible dangerous oversedation. Increased pyrilamine effect.
Antidiabetics	Increased pentobarbital effect.
Antihistamines	Dangerous sedation. Avoid.
Anti-inflammatory drugs (non-steroidal)	Decreased anti-inflammatory effect.
Aspirin	Decreased aspirin effect.
Beta-adrenergic blockers	Decreased effect of beta-adrenergic blocker.
Contraceptives (oral)	Decreased contraceptive effect.
Cortisone drugs	Decreased cortisone effect.
Digitoxin	Decreased digitoxin effect.
Doxycycline	Decreased doxycycline effect.
Dronabinol	Increased effect of both drugs.

Continued page 974

POSSIBLE INTERACTION WITH OTHER SUBSTANCES

INTERACTS WITH	COMBINED EFFECT
Alcohol:	Possible fatal oversedation. Avoid.
Beverages: Caffeine drinks.	Less pyrilamine sedation.
Cocaine:	Decreased Wans effect. Avoid.
Foods:	None expected.
Marijuana:	Excessive sedation. Avoid.
Tobacco:	None expected.

PYRVINIUM

BRAND NAMES

Pamovin   Vanquin
Povan   Viprynium
Pyr-pam

BASIC INFORMATION

Habit forming? No
Prescription needed? Yes
Available as generic? No
Drug class: Antihelminthic (antiworm medication)

 USES

Treatment for pinworm infestation.

 DOSAGE & USAGE INFORMATION

How to take:
- Tablet—Swallow whole with food or liquid. Don't crush or chew tablet.
- Liquid—Take with food or liquid.

When to take:
According to label instructions. Usually a single dose, which may be repeated in 2 or 3 weeks.

If you forget a dose:
Take when remembered.

What drug does:
Interferes with a metabolic process in the infecting parasite and kills it.

Time lapse before drug works:
12 hours.

Don't take with:
Non-prescription drugs for pinworms.

 OVERDOSE

SYMPTOMS:
Increased severity of adverse reactions and side effects.
WHAT TO DO:
Overdose unlikely to threaten life. If person takes much larger amount than prescribed, call doctor, poison-control center or hospital emergency room for instructions.

 POSSIBLE ADVERSE REACTIONS OR SIDE EFFECTS

SYMPTOMS	WHAT TO DO
Life-threatening: None expected.	
Common: None expected.	
Infrequent: None expected.	
Rare:	
• Rash.	Discontinue. Call doctor right away.
• Dizziness, stomach cramps, nausea, vomiting.	Continue. Call doctor when convenient.

WARNINGS & PRECAUTIONS

Don't take if:
You are allergic to any antihelminthic drug.

Before you start, consult your doctor:
- If you have kidney or liver disease.
- If you have a bowel disease or inflammation.

Over age 60:
Adverse reactions and side effects may be more frequent and severe than in younger persons.

Pregnancy:
No proven harm to unborn child. Avoid if possible.

Breast-feeding:
No problems expected, but consult doctor.

Infants & children:
No problems expected.

Prolonged use:
Not recommended.

Skin & sunlight:
May cause rash or intensify sunburn in areas exposed to sun or sunlamp.

Driving, piloting or hazardous work:
Avoid if you feel dizzy. Otherwise, no problems expected.

Discontinuing:
Don't discontinue without doctor's advice until you complete prescribed dose, even though symptoms diminish or disappear.

Others:
- This medicine is a dye that permanently stains most materials. Teeth will be stained a few days. Stool and vomit may be red.
- Pinworm infestations are highly contagious. All family members should be treated at the same time.

POSSIBLE INTERACTION WITH OTHER DRUGS

GENERIC NAME OR DRUG CLASS	COMBINED EFFECT
None	

POSSIBLE INTERACTION WITH OTHER SUBSTANCES

INTERACTS WITH	COMBINED EFFECT
Alcohol:	None expected.
Beverages:	None expected.
Cocaine:	None expected.
Foods:	None expected.
Marijuana:	None expected.
Tobacco:	None expected.

BRAND NAMES

Estrovis

BASIC INFORMATION

Habit forming? No
Prescription needed? Yes
Available as generic? Yes
Drug class: Female sex hormone (estrogen)

 ## USES

- Treatment for symptoms of menopause and menstrual-cycle irregularity.
- Replacement for female hormone deficiency.

 ## DOSAGE & USAGE INFORMATION

How to take:
Tablet—Swallow with liquid. If you can't swallow whole, crumble tablet and take with liquid or food.

When to take:
At the same time each day.

If you forget a dose:
Take as soon as you remember up to 12 hours late. If more than 12 hours, wait for next scheduled dose (don't double this dose).

What drug does:
Restores normal estrogen level in tissues.

Time lapse before drug works:
10 to 20 days.

Don't take with:
See Interaction column and consult doctor.

 ## OVERDOSE

SYMPTOMS:
Nausea, vomiting, fluid retention, breast enlargement and discomfort, abnormal vaginal bleeding.
WHAT TO DO:
Overdose unlikely to threaten life. If person takes much larger amount than prescribed, call doctor, poison-control center or hospital emergency room for instructions.

 ## POSSIBLE ADVERSE REACTIONS OR SIDE EFFECTS

SYMPTOMS	WHAT TO DO
Life-threatening:	
None expected.	
Common:	
• Stomach cramps.	Discontinue. Call doctor right away.
• Appetite loss.	Continue. Call doctor when convenient.
• Nausea; diarrhea; swollen ankles, feet; swollen, tender breasts.	Continue. Tell doctor at next visit.
Infrequent:	
• Rash, stomach or side pain.	Discontinue. Call doctor right away.
• Depression, dizziness, irritability, vomiting, breast lumps.	Continue. Call doctor when convenient.
• Brown blotches, hair loss, vaginal discharge or bleeding, changes in sex drive.	Continue. Tell doctor at next visit.
Rare:	
Jaundice.	Discontinue. Call doctor right away.

WARNINGS & PRECAUTIONS

Don't take if:
- You are allergic to any estrogen-containing drugs.
- You have impaired liver function.
- You have had blood clots, stroke or heart attack.
- You have unexplained vaginal bleeding.

Before you start, consult your doctor:
- If you have had cancer of breast or reproductive organs, fibrocystic breast disease, fibroid tumors of the uterus or endometriosis.
- If you have had migraine headaches, epilepsy or porphyria.
- If you have diabetes, high blood pressure, asthma, congestive heart failure, kidney disease or gallstones.
- If you plan to become pregnant within 3 months.

Over age 60:
Controversial. You and your doctor must decide if drug risks outweigh benefits.

Pregnancy:
Risk to unborn child outweighs drug benefits. Don't use.

Breast-feeding:
Drug filters into milk. May harm child. Avoid.

Infants & children:
Not recommended.

Prolonged use:
Increased growth of fibroid tumors of uterus. Possible association with cancer of uterus.

Skin & sunlight:
May cause rash or intensify sunburn in areas exposed to sun or sunlamp.

Driving, piloting or hazardous work:
No problems expected.

Discontinuing:
You may need to discontinue quinestrol periodically. Consult your doctor.

Others:
In rare instances, may cause blood clot in lung, brain or leg. Symptoms are *sudden* severe headache, coordination loss, vision change, chest pain, breathing difficulty, slurred speech, pain in legs or groin. Seek emergency treatment immediately.

 ## POSSIBLE INTERACTION WITH OTHER DRUGS

GENERIC NAME OR DRUG CLASS	COMBINED EFFECT
Anticoagulants (oral)	Decreased anticoagulant effect.
Anticonvulsants (hydantoin)	Increased seizures.
Antidiabetics (oral)	Unpredictable increase or decrease in blood sugar.
Carbamazepine	Increased seizures.
Clofibrate	Decreased clofibrate effect.
Meprobamate	Increased quinestrol effect.
Phenobarbital	Decreased quinestrol effect.
Primidone	Decreased quinestrol effect.
Rifampin	Decreased quinestrol effect.
Thyroid hormones	Decreased thyroid effect.

 ## POSSIBLE INTERACTION WITH OTHER SUBSTANCES

INTERACTS WITH	COMBINED EFFECT
Alcohol:	None expected.
Beverages:	None expected.
Cocaine:	No proven problems.
Foods:	None expected.
Marijuana:	Possible menstrual irregularities and bleeding between periods.
Tobacco:	Increased risk of blood clots leading to stroke or heart attack.

QUINETHAZONE

BRAND NAMES

Aquamox | Hydromox

BASIC INFORMATION

Habit forming? No
Prescription needed? Yes
Available as generic? Yes
Drug class: Antihypertensive, diuretic (thiazide)

 USES

- Controls, but doesn't cure, high blood pressure.
- Reduces fluid retention (edema) caused by conditions such as heart disorders and liver disease.

 DOSAGE & USAGE INFORMATION

How to take:
Tablet or capsule—Swallow with liquid. If you can't swallow whole, crumble tablet or open capsule and take with liquid or food. Don't exceed dose.

When to take:
At the same time each day.

If you forget a dose:
Take as soon as you remember up to 2 hours late. If more than 2 hours, wait for next scheduled dose (don't double this dose).

What drug does:
- Forces sodium and water excretion, reducing body fluid.
- Relaxes muscle cells of small arteries.
- Reduced body fluid and relaxed arteries lower blood pressure.

Continued next column

 OVERDOSE

SYMPTOMS:
Cramps, weakness, drowsiness, weak pulse, coma.
WHAT TO DO:
- Dial 0 (operator) or 911 (emergency) for an ambulance or medical help. Then give first aid immediately.
- See emergency information on inside covers.

Time lapse before drug works:
4 to 6 hours. May require several weeks to lower blood pressure.

Don't take with:
- See Interaction column and consult doctor.
- Non-prescription drugs without consulting doctor.

 POSSIBLE ADVERSE REACTIONS OR SIDE EFFECTS

SYMPTOMS	WHAT TO DO
Life-threatening: None expected.	
Common: None expected.	
Infrequent:	
• Blurred vision, severe abdominal pain, nausea, vomiting, irregular heartbeat, weak pulse.	Discontinue. Call doctor right away.
• Dizziness, mood change, headache, weakness, tiredness, weight changes.	Continue. Call doctor when convenient.
• Dry mouth, thirst.	Continue. Tell doctor at next visit.
Rare:	
• Rash or hives.	Discontinue. Seek emergency treatment.
• Sore throat, fever, jaundice.	Discontinue. Call doctor right away.

 WARNINGS & PRECAUTIONS

Don't take if:
You are allergic to any thiazide diuretic drug.

Before you start, consult your doctor:
- If you are allergic to any sulfa drug.
- If you have gout.
- If you have liver, pancreas or liver disorder.

Over age 60:
Adverse reactions and side effects may be more frequent and severe than in younger persons, especially dizziness and excessive potassium loss.

Pregnancy:
Risk to unborn child outweighs drug benefits. Don't use.

Breast-feeding:
Drug passes into milk. Avoid drug or discontinue nursing.

Infants & children:
No problems expected.

Prolonged use:
You may need medicine to treat high blood pressure for the rest of your life.

Skin & sunlight:
May cause rash or intensify sunburn in areas exposed to sun or sunlamp.

Driving, piloting or hazardous work:
Don't drive or pilot aircraft until you learn how medicine affects you. Don't work around dangerous machinery. Don't climb ladders or work in high places. Danger increases if you drink alcohol or take medicine affecting alertness and reflexes, such as antihistamines, tranquilizers, sedatives, pain medicine, narcotics and mind-altering drugs.

Discontinuing:
Don't discontinue without medical advice.

Others:
- Hot weather and fever may cause dehydration and drop in blood pressure. Dose may require temporary adjustment. Weigh daily and report any unexpected weight decreases to your doctor.
- May cause rise in uric acid, leading to gout.
- May cause blood-sugar rise in diabetics.

POSSIBLE INTERACTION WITH OTHER DRUGS

GENERIC NAME OR DRUG CLASS	COMBINED EFFECT
Acebutolol	Increased antihypertensive effect. Dosages of both drugs may require adjustments.
Allopurinol	Decreased allopurinol effect.
Amiodarone	Increased risk of heartbeat irregularity due to low potassium.
Antidepressants (tricyclic)	Dangerous drop in blood pressure. Avoid combination unless under medical supervision.
Barbiturates	Increased quinethazone effect.
Calcium supplements	Increased calcium in blood.
Cholestyramine	Decreased quinethazone effect.
Cortisone drugs	Excessive potassium loss that causes dangerous heart rhythms.
Digitalis preparations	Excessive potassium loss that causes dangerous heart rhythms.
Diuretics (thiazide)	Increased effect of other thiazide diuretics.
Enalapril	Possible excessive potassium in blood.
Indapamide	Increased diuretic effect.
Labetolol	Increased antihypertensive effects.
Lithium	Increased effect of lithium.
MAO inhibitors	Increased quinethazone effect.
Nitrates	Excessive blood-pressure drop.
Oxprenolol	Increased antihypertensive effect. Dosages of both drugs may require adjustments.
Potassium supplements	Decreased potassium effect.
Probenecid	Decreased probenecid effect.

POSSIBLE INTERACTION WITH OTHER SUBSTANCES

INTERACTS WITH	COMBINED EFFECT
Alcohol:	Dangerous blood-pressure drop.
Beverages:	None expected.
Cocaine:	None expected.
Foods: Licorice.	Excessive potassium loss that causes dangerous heart rhythms.
Marijuana:	May increase blood pressure.
Tobacco:	None expected.

QUINIDINE

BRAND NAMES

Apo-Quinidine	Quinalan
Biquin Durules	Quinate
Cardioquin	Quinidex Extentabs
Cin-Quin	Quinobarb
Duraquin	Quinora
Novoquinidin	SK-Quinidine Sulfate
Quinaglute Dura-Tabs	

BASIC INFORMATION

Habit forming? No
Prescription needed?
  U.S.: Yes
  Canada: No
Available as generic? Yes
Drug class: Antiarrhythmic

 USES

Corrects heart-rhythm disorders.

 DOSAGE & USAGE INFORMATION

How to take:
- Tablet or capsule—Swallow with liquid or food to lessen stomach irritation.
- Extended-release tablets or capsules—Swallow each dose whole. If you take regular tablets, you may chew or crush them.

When to take:
At the same times each day.

If you forget a dose:
Take as soon as you remember up to 2 hours late. If more than 2 hours, wait for next scheduled dose (don't double this dose).

Continued next column

 OVERDOSE

SYMPTOMS:
Confusion, severe blood-pressure drop, breathing difficulty, fainting.
WHAT TO DO:
- Dial 0 (operator) or 911 (emergency) for an ambulance or medical help. Then give first aid immediately.
- If patient is unconscious and not breathing, give mouth-to-mouth breathing. If there is no heartbeat, use cardiac massage and mouth-to-mouth breathing (CPR). Don't try to make patient vomit. If you can't get help quickly, take patient to nearest emergency facility.
- See emergency information on inside covers.

What drug does:
Delays nerve impulses to the heart to regulate heartbeat.

Time lapse before drug works:
2 to 4 hours.

Don't take with:
See Interaction column and consult doctor.

 POSSIBLE ADVERSE REACTIONS OR SIDE EFFECTS

SYMPTOMS	WHAT TO DO
Life-threatening: None expected.	
Common: Bitter taste, diarrhea, nausea, vomiting.	Discontinue. Call doctor right away.
Infrequent:	
• Dizziness, lightheadedness, fainting, headache, confusion, rash, change in vision, difficult breathing, rapid heartbeat.	Discontinue. Call doctor right away.
• Ringing in ears.	Continue. Call doctor when convenient.
Rare:	
• Unusual bleeding or bruising.	Discontinue. Call doctor right away.
• Weakness.	Continue. Call doctor when convenient.

WARNINGS & PRECAUTIONS

Don't take if:
- You are allergic to quinidine.
- You have an active infection.

Before you start, consult your doctor:
About any drug you take, including non-prescription drugs.

Over age 60:
Adverse reactions and side effects may be more frequent and severe than in younger persons.

Pregnancy:
Risk to unborn child outweighs drug benefits. Don't use.

Breast-feeding:
Drug filters into milk. May harm child. Avoid.

Infants & children:
No problems expected.

Prolonged use:
No problems expected.

Skin & sunlight:
No problems expected.

Driving, piloting or hazardous work:
Don't drive or pilot aircraft until you learn how medicine affects you. Don't work around dangerous machinery. Don't climb ladders or work in high places. Danger increases if you drink alcohol or take medicine affecting alertness and reflexes, such as antihistamines, tranquilizers, sedatives, pain medicine, narcotics and mind-altering drugs.

Discontinuing:
Don't discontinue without doctor's advice until you complete prescribed dose, even though symptoms diminish or disappear.

Others:
No problems expected.

POSSIBLE INTERACTION WITH OTHER DRUGS

GENERIC NAME OR DRUG CLASS	COMBINED EFFECT
Anticholinergics	Increased anticholinergic effect.
Anticoagulants	Increased anticoagulant effect.
Antidepressants (tricyclic)	Irregular heartbeat.
Antihypertensives	Increased antihypertensive effect.
Calcium supplements	Increased quinidine effect.
Cholinergics	Decreased cholinergic effect.
Citrates	Prolongs citrate effect.
Digitalis preparations	Slows heartbeat excessively.
Flecainide	Possible irregular heartbeat.
Molindone	Impaired heart function. Dangerous mixture.
Phenytoin	Increased quinidine effect.
Propranolol	Slows heartbeat excessively.
Pyrimethamine	Increased quinidine effect.
Rauwolfia alkaloids	Seriously disturbs heart rhythms.
Tocainide	Increased possibility of adverse reactions from either drug.

POSSIBLE INTERACTION WITH OTHER SUBSTANCES

INTERACTS WITH	COMBINED EFFECT
Alcohol:	None expected.
Beverages: Caffeine drinks.	Causes rapid heartbeat. Use sparingly.
Cocaine:	Irregular heartbeat. Avoid.
Foods:	None expected.
Marijuana:	Can cause fainting.
Tobacco:	Irregular heartbeat. Avoid.

QUININE

BRAND NAMES

Coco-Quinine	Quindan
Kinine	Quine
NovoQuinie	Quinite
Quinamm	Strema

BASIC INFORMATION

Habit forming? No
Prescription needed?
  High strength: Yes
  Low strength: No
Available as generic? Yes
Drug class: Antiprotozoal

 ## USES

- Treatment or prevention of malaria.
- Relief of muscle cramps.

 ## DOSAGE & USAGE INFORMATION

How to take:
Liquid, tablet or capsule—Swallow with liquid or food to lessen stomach irritation.

When to take:
- Prevention—At the same time each day, usually at bedtime.
- Treatment—At the same times each day in evenly spaced doses.

If you forget a dose:
- Prevention—Take as soon as you remember up to 12 hours late. If more than 12 hours, wait for next scheduled dose (don't double this dose).
- Treatment—Take as soon as you remember up to 2 hours late. If more than 2 hours, wait for next scheduled dose (don't double this dose).

Continued next column

 ## OVERDOSE

SYMPTOMS:
Severe impairment of vision and hearing; severe nausea, vomiting, diarrhea; shallow breathing, fast heartbeat; apprehension, confusion, delirium.
WHAT TO DO:
Dial 0 (operator) or 911 (emergency) for an ambulance or medical help. Then give first aid immediately.

What drug does:
- Reduces contractions of skeletal muscles.
- Increases blood flow.
- Interferes with genes in malaria micro-organisms.

Time lapse before drug works:
May require several days or weeks for maximum effect.

Don't take with:
See Interaction column and consult doctor.

 ## POSSIBLE ADVERSE REACTIONS OR SIDE EFFECTS

SYMPTOMS	WHAT TO DO
Life-threatening:	
None expected.	
Common:	
Blurred vision or change in vision.	Discontinue. Call doctor right away.
Dizziness, headache, stomach discomfort, mild nausea, vomiting, diarrhea.	Continue. Call doctor when convenient.
Ringing or buzzing in ears, impaired hearing.	Continue. Tell doctor at next visit.
Infrequent:	
Rash, hives, itchy skin, difficult breathing.	Discontinue. Call doctor right away.
Rare:	
Sore throat, fever, unusual bleeding or bruising, unusual tiredness or weakness.	Discontinue. Call doctor right away.

WARNINGS & PRECAUTIONS

Don't take if:
You are allergic to quinine or quinidine.

Before you start, consult your doctor:
- If you plan to become pregnant within medication period.
- If you have asthma.
- If you have eye disease, hearing problems or ringing in the ears.
- If you have heart disease.
- If you have myasthenia gravis.

Over age 60:
Adverse reactions and side effects may be more frequent and severe than in younger persons.

Pregnancy:
Risk to unborn child outweighs drug benefits. Don't use.

Breast-feeding:
Drug filters into milk. May harm child. Avoid.

Infants & children:
Use only under medical supervision.

Prolonged use:
May develop headache, blurred vision, nausea, temporary hearing loss, but seldom need to discontinue because of these symptoms.

Skin & sunlight:
No problems expected.

Driving, piloting or hazardous work:
Avoid if you feel dizzy or have blurred vision. Otherwise, no problems expected.

Discontinuing:
Don't discontinue without doctor's advice until you complete prescribed dose, even though symptoms diminish or disappear.

Others:
Don't confuse with quinidine, a medicine for heart-rhythm problems.

POSSIBLE INTERACTION WITH OTHER DRUGS

GENERIC NAME OR DRUG CLASS	COMBINED EFFECT
Antacids (with aluminum hydroxide)	Decreased quinine effect.
Anticoagulants	Increased anticoagulant effect.
Quinidine	Possible toxic effects of quinine.
Sodium bicarbonate	Possible toxic effects of quinine.

POSSIBLE INTERACTION WITH OTHER SUBSTANCES

INTERACTS WITH	COMBINED EFFECT
Alcohol:	No proven problems.
Beverages:	None expected.
Cocaine:	No proven problems.
Foods:	None expected.
Marijuana:	No proven problems.
Tobacco:	None expected.

RADIO-PHARMACEUTICALS

BRAND NAMES

See complete list of brand names in the *Brand Name Directory*, page 956.

BASIC INFORMATION

Habit forming? No
Prescription needed? Yes
Available as generic? Yes
Drug class: Radio-pharmaceuticals

 USES

To help establish an accurate diagnosis for many medical problems, such as pernicious anemia, malabsorption, iron metabolism, cancer, abscess, infection, cerebrospinal fluid flow, blood volume, kidney diseases, lung diseases, pancreas diseases, red blood cell disorders, spleen diseases, thyroid diseases, thyroid cancer, brain diseases or tumor, bladder diseases, eye tumors, liver diseases, heart diseases, bone diseases, bone marrow diseases.

 DOSAGE & USAGE INFORMATION

How to take:
- As directed by nuclear medicine specialist. Most are given intravenously by the doctor, some are taken by mouth.
- Drink lots of liquids and urinate often after test to decrease possible radiation effect on the urinary bladder.

When to take:
According to individual instructions.

If you forget a dose:
Take as soon as you remember.

What drug does:
Very small quantities of radioactive substances concentrate in various organs of the body and become measurable. Pictures or readings of the organ or system under study become possible.

Time lapse before drug works:
Varies between products.

Don't take with:
Any other medicine without consulting doctor.

 OVERDOSE

SYMPTOMS:
None expected.
WHAT TO DO:
None expected.

 POSSIBLE ADVERSE REACTIONS OR SIDE EFFECTS

SYMPTOMS	WHAT TO DO
Life-threatening: None expected.	
Common: None expected.	
Infrequent: Drowsiness; fast heartbeat; swollen feet, ankles, hands or throat; abdominal pain; rash; hives; nausea; vomiting, headache; red or flushed face; fever; fainting.	Discontinue. Call doctor right away.
Rare: None expected.	

WARNINGS & PRECAUTIONS

Don't take if:
You are allergic to the prescribed drug.

Before you start, consult your doctor:
- If you have had allergic reactions to human serum albumin.
- If you are allergic to anything.

Over age 60:
Adverse reactions and side effects may be more frequent and severe than in younger persons. Ask doctor about smaller doses.

Pregnancy:
Avoid during pregnancy if possible.

Breast-feeding:
Drug passes into milk. Avoid drug or discontinue nursing until you finish medicine. Consult doctor for advice on maintaining milk supply.

Infants & children:
No problems expected.

Prolonged use:
Not intended for prolonged use.

Skin & sunlight:
No problems expected.

Driving, piloting or hazardous work:
No problems expected.

Discontinuing:
No problems expected.

Others:
Some of these agents may accumulate in the urinary bladder. To decrease chance of excessive radiation, drink 8 oz. of fluid every 1 hour for 10-12 hours following the test, unless otherwise specified by your doctor.

POSSIBLE INTERACTION WITH OTHER DRUGS

GENERIC NAME OR DRUG CLASS	COMBINED EFFECT
None expected.	

POSSIBLE INTERACTION WITH OTHER SUBSTANCES

INTERACTS WITH	COMBINED EFFECT
Alcohol:	None expected.
Beverages:	None expected.
Cocaine:	None expected.
Foods:	None expected.
Marijuana:	None expected.
Tobacco:	None expected.

RANITIDINE

BRAND NAMES

Zantac

BASIC INFORMATION

Habit forming? No
Prescription needed? Yes
Available as generic? No
Drug class: Histamine H2 antagonist

 USES

- Treatment for duodenal ulcer.
- Decreases acid in stomach.

 DOSAGE & USAGE INFORMATION

How to take:
Tablets—Swallow with liquid.

When to take:
At same times each day.

If you forget a dose:
Take as soon as you remember up to 2 hours late. If more than 2 hours, wait for next scheduled dose (don't double this dose).

What drug does:
Decreases stomach-acid production.

Time lapse before drug works:
2 to 3 hours.

Don't take with:
- Alcohol.
- See Interaction column and consult doctor.

 OVERDOSE

SYMPTOMS:
Muscular tremors, vomiting, rapid breathing, coma.
WHAT TO DO:
- Dial 0 (operator) or 911 (emergency) for an ambulance or medical help. Then give first aid immediately.
- If patient is unconscious and not breathing, give mouth-to-mouth breathing. If there is no heartbeat, use cardiac massage and mouth-to-mouth breathing (CPR). Don't try to make patient vomit. If you can't get help quickly, take patient to nearest emergency facility.
- See emergency information on inside covers.

 POSSIBLE ADVERSE REACTIONS OR SIDE EFFECTS

SYMPTOMS	WHAT TO DO
Life-threatening: None expected.	
Common: None expected.	
Infrequent:	
• Rash.	Discontinue. Call doctor right away.
• Headache, dizziness, constipation, abdominal pain, nausea.	Continue. Call doctor when convenient.
Rare: Jaundice.	Discontinue. Call doctor right away.

WARNINGS & PRECAUTIONS

Don't take if:
You are allergic to any histamine H2 antagonist.

Before you start, consult your doctor:
If you have kidney disease.

Over age 60:
Adverse reactions and side effects may be more frequent and severe than in younger persons.

Pregnancy:
No proven harm to unborn child. Avoid if possible.

Breast-feeding:
Drug passes into milk. Avoid drug or discontinue nursing until you finish medicine. Consult doctor for advice on maintaining milk supply.

Infants & children:
Not recommended.

Prolonged use:
Not recommended. Use for short term only.

Skin & sunlight:
No problems expected.

Driving, piloting or hazardous work:
Avoid if you feel dizzy. Otherwise, no problems expected.

Discontinuing:
Don't discontinue without consulting doctor until you finish prescribed dose, even though symptoms diminish or disappear.

Others:
No problems expected.

 ## POSSIBLE INTERACTION WITH OTHER DRUGS

GENERIC NAME OR DRUG CLASS	COMBINED EFFECT
Antacids	Decreased absorption of ranitidine if taken simultaneously.
Ketoconazole	Decreased absorption of ranitidine.

 ## POSSIBLE INTERACTION WITH OTHER SUBSTANCES

INTERACTS WITH	COMBINED EFFECT
Alcohol:	Decreased ranitidine effect.
Beverages:	None expected.
Cocaine:	No proven problems.
Foods:	None expected.
Marijuana:	No proven problems.
Tobacco:	Decreased ranitidine effect.

RAUWOLFIA ALKALOIDS

BRAND AND GENERIC NAMES

See complete list of brand and generic names in the *Brand Name Directory,* page 956.

BASIC INFORMATION

Habit forming? No
Prescription needed? Yes
Available as generic? Yes
Drug class: Antihypertensive, tranquilizer (rauwolfia alkaloid)

USES

- Treatment for high blood pressure.
- Tranquilizer for mental and emotional disturbances.

DOSAGE & USAGE INFORMATION

How to take:
Tablet—Swallow with liquid or food to lessen stomach irritation. If you can't swallow whole, crumble tablet and take with liquid or food.

When to take:
At the same times each day.

If you forget a dose:
Take as soon as you remember up to 2 hours late. If more than 2 hours, wait for next scheduled dose (don't double this dose).

What drug does:
- Interferes with nerve impulses and relaxes blood-vessel muscles, reducing blood pressure.
- Suppresses brain centers that control emotions.

Time lapse before drug works:
3 weeks continual use required to determine effectiveness.

Don't take with:
See Interaction column and consult doctor.

OVERDOSE

SYMPTOMS:
Drowsiness; slow, weak pulse; slow, shallow breathing; diarrhea; coma; flush; low body temperature.
WHAT TO DO:
- **Dial 0 (operator) or 911 (emergency) for an ambulance or medical help. Then give first aid immediately.**
- **See emergency information on inside covers.**

POSSIBLE ADVERSE REACTIONS OR SIDE EFFECTS

SYMPTOMS	WHAT TO DO
Life-threatening:	
None expected.	
Common:	
• Depression.	Continue. Call doctor when convenient.
• Headache, drowsiness or faintness, lethargy, eye redness, stuffy nose, impotence, diminished sex drive.	Continue. Tell doctor at next visit.
Infrequent:	
• Black stool; bloody vomit; chest pain; shortness of breath; irregular or slow heartbeat; stiffness in muscles, bones, joints.	Discontinue. Call doctor right away.
• Trembling hands.	Continue. Call doctor when convenient.
Rare:	
• Rash or itchy skin, sore throat, fever, stomach pain, nausea, vomiting, unusual bleeding or bruising, jaundice.	Discontinue. Call doctor right away.
• Painful urination.	Continue. Call doctor when convenient.

WARNINGS & PRECAUTIONS

Don't take if:
- You are allergic to any rauwolfia alkaloid.
- You are depressed.
- You have active peptic ulcer.
- You have ulcerative colitis.

Before you start, consult your doctor:
- If you have been depressed.
- If you have had peptic ulcer, ulcerative colitis or gallstones.
- If you have epilepsy.
- If you will have surgery within 2 months, including dental surgery, requiring general or spinal anesthesia.

Over age 60:
Adverse reactions and side effects may be more frequent and severe than in younger persons.

Pregnancy:
Studies inconclusive on harm to unborn child.
Animal studies show fetal abnormalities. Decide
with your doctor whether drug benefits justify
risk to unborn child.

Breast-feeding:
Drug passes into milk. Avoid drug or
discontinue nursing until you finish medicine.
Consult doctor for advice on maintaining milk
supply.

Infants & children:
Not recommended.

Prolonged use:
Causes cancer in laboratory animals. Consult
your doctor if you have family or personal
history of cancer.

Skin & sunlight:
No problems expected.

Driving, piloting or hazardous work:
Avoid if you feel drowsy, dizzy or faint.
Otherwise, no problems expected.

Discontinuing:
Don't discontinue without consulting doctor.
Dose may require gradual reduction if you have
taken drug for a long time. Doses of other drugs
may also require adjustment.

Others:
Consult your doctor if you do isometric
exercises. These raise blood pressure. Drug
may intensify blood-pressure rise.

POSSIBLE INTERACTION WITH OTHER DRUGS

GENERIC NAME OR DRUG CLASS	COMBINED EFFECT
Acebutolol	Possible increased effects of both drugs, causing excessively low blood pressure and slow heartbeat.
Anticoagulants (oral)	Unpredictable increased or decreased effect of anticoagulant.
Anticonvulsants	Serious change in seizure pattern.
Antidepressants	Increased antidepressant effect.
Antihistamines	Increased antihistamine effect.
Aspirin	Decreased aspirin effect.

Beta-adrenergic blockers	Increased effect of rauwolfia alkaloids. Excessive sedation.
Digitalis preparations	Irregular heartbeat.
Dronabinol	Increased effects of both drugs. Avoid.
Levodopa	Decreased levodopa effect.
MAO inhibitors	Severe depression.
Mind-altering drugs	Excessive sedation.
Pentoxifylline	Increased antihypertensive effect.

POSSIBLE INTERACTION WITH OTHER SUBSTANCES

INTERACTS WITH	COMBINED EFFECT
Alcohol:	Increased intoxication. Use with extreme caution.
Beverages: Carbonated drinks.	Decreased rauwolfia alkaloids effect.
Cocaine:	Decreased rauwolfia alkaloids effect.
Foods: Spicy foods.	Possible digestive upset.
Marijuana:	Occasional use—Mild drowsiness. Daily use—Moderate drowsiness, low blood pressure, depression.
Tobacco:	No problems expected.

RAUWOLFIA & THIAZIDE DIURETICS

BRAND NAMES

See complete list of brand names in the *Brand Name Directory,* page 957.

BASIC INFORMATION

Habit forming? No
Prescription needed? Yes
Available as generic? Yes
Drug class: Antihypertensive, diuretic, tranquilizer

 ## USES

- Controls, but doesn't cure, high blood pressure.
- Reduces fluid retention (edema).

 ## DOSAGE & USAGE INFORMATION

How to take:
Tablet or capsule—Swallow with liquid. If you can't swallow whole, crumble tablet or open capsule and take with liquid or food.

When to take:
At the same time each day.

If you forget a dose:
Take as soon as you remember up to 2 hours late. If more than 2 hours, wait for next scheduled dose (don't double this dose).

What drug does:
- Forces sodium and water excretion, reducing body fluid.
- Reduced body fluid and relaxed arteries lower blood pressure.
- Interferes with nerve impulses and relaxes blood-vessel muscles, reducing blood pressure.
- Suppresses brain centers that control emotion.

Continued next column

 ## OVERDOSE

SYMPTOMS:
Cramps; weakness; drowsiness; slow, weak pulse; slow, shallow breathing; diarrhea; flush; low body temperature; coma.
WHAT TO DO:
- **Dial 0 (operator) or 911 (emergency) for an ambulance or medical help. Then give first aid immediately.**
- **See emergency information on inside covers.**

Time lapse before drug works:
3 weeks continual use required to determine effectiveness.

Don't take with:
- Non-prescription drugs without consulting doctor.
- See Interaction column and consult doctor.

 ## POSSIBLE ADVERSE REACTIONS OR SIDE EFFECTS

SYMPTOMS	WHAT TO DO
Life-threatening:	
Irregular heartbeat, weak pulse, hives, black stool, bloody vomit.	Discontinue. Seek emergency treatment.
Common:	
Lethargy, drowsiness, tremor, depression, red eyes, runny nose.	Continue. Call doctor when convenient.
Infrequent:	
• Blurred vision, abdominal pain, nausea, vomiting, irregular heartbeat, joint pain.	Discontinue. Call doctor right away.
• Dizziness, mood change, headache, dry mouth, weakness, tiredness, weight gain or loss.	Continue. Call doctor when convenient.
Rare:	
• Sore throat, fever, mouth sores; jaundice; unexplained bleeding or bruising.	Discontinue. Call doctor right away.
• Rash, painful or difficult urination, tremor, impotence.	Continue. Call doctor when convenient.

 ## WARNINGS & PRECAUTIONS

Don't take if:
- You are allergic to any thiazide diuretic drug or any rauwolfia alkaloid.
- You are depressed.
- You have active peptic ulcer or ulcerative colitis.

782

RAUWOLFIA & THIAZIDE DIURETICS

Before you start, consult your doctor:
- If you are allergic to any sulfa drug.
- If you have gout, liver, pancreas or kidney disorder, epilepsy.
- If you have had peptic ulcer, ulcerative colitis or gallstones.
- If you have been depressed.
- If you will have surgery within 2 months, including dental surgery, requiring general or spinal anesthesia.

Over age 60:
Adverse reactions and side effects may be more frequent and severe than in younger persons, especially dizziness and excessive potassium loss.

Pregnancy:
Risk to unborn child outweighs drug benefits. Don't use.

Breast-feeding:
Drug passes into milk. Avoid drug or discontinue nursing until you finish medicine. Consult doctor for advice on maintaining milk supply.

Infants & children:
Not recommended.

Prolonged use:
- You may need medicine to treat high blood pressure for the rest of your life.
- Causes cancer in laboratory animals. Consult your doctor if you have family or personal history of cancer.

Skin & sunlight:
May cause rash or intensify sunburn in areas exposed to sun or sunlamp.

Driving, piloting or hazardous work:
Don't drive or pilot aircraft until you learn how medicine affects you. Don't work around dangerous machinery. Don't climb ladders or work in high places. Danger increases if you drink alcohol or take medicine affecting alertness and reflexes, such as antihistamines, tranquilizers, sedatives, pain medicine, narcotics and mind-altering drugs.

Discontinuing:
Don't discontinue without consulting doctor. Dose may require gradual reduction if you have taken drug for a long time. Doses of other drugs may also require adjustment.

Others:
- Hot weather and fever may cause dehydration and drop in blood pressure. Dose may require temporary adjustment. Weigh daily and report any unexpected weight decreases to your doctor.
- May cause rise in uric acid, leading to gout.
- May cause blood-sugar rise in diabetics.
- Consult your doctor if you do isometric exercises. These raise blood pressure. Drug may intensify blood-pressure rise.

POSSIBLE INTERACTION WITH OTHER DRUGS

GENERIC NAME OR DRUG CLASS	COMBINED EFFECT
Acebutolol	Possible increased effect of both drugs, causing excessively low blood pressure and slow heartbeat.
Anticoagulants (oral)	Unpredictable increased or decreased effect of anticoagulant.
Anticonvulsants	Serious change in seizure pattern.
Antidepressants (tricyclic)	Dangerous drop in blood pressure. Avoid combination unless under medical supervision.
Antihistamines	Increased antihistamine effect.
Aspirin	Decreased aspirin effect.
Barbiturates	Increased hydrochlorothiazide effect.

Continued page 974

POSSIBLE INTERACTION WITH OTHER SUBSTANCES

INTERACTS WITH	COMBINED EFFECT
Alcohol:	Increased intoxication. Dangerous blood-pressure drop. Avoid.
Beverages: Carbonated drinks.	Decreased rauwolfia effect.
Cocaine:	Decreased rauwolfia effect.
Foods: Spicy foods.	Possible digestive upset.
Licorice.	Excessive potassium loss that causes dangerous heart rhythms.
Marijuana:	Occasional use—Mild drowsiness. Daily use—Moderate drowsiness, low blood pressure, depression.
Tobacco:	No proven problems.

RESERPINE & HYDRALAZINE

BRAND NAMES

Serpasil-Apresoline

BASIC INFORMATION

Habit forming? No
Prescription needed? Yes
Available as generic? No
Drug class: Antihypertensive, tranquilizer
(rauwolfia alkaloid)

 USES

Treatment for high blood pressure and congestive heart failure.

 DOSAGE & USAGE INFORMATION

How to take:
Tablet—Swallow with liquid or food to lessen stomach irritation. If you can't swallow whole, crumble tablet and take with liquid or food.

When to take:
At the same times each day.

If you forget a dose:
Take as soon as you remember up to 2 hours late. If more than 2 hours, wait for next scheduled dose (don't double this dose).

Continued next column

 OVERDOSE

SYMPTOMS:
Drowsiness, slow, shallow breathing; diarrhea; flush; low body temperature; rapid, weak heartbeat; fainting; extreme weakness; cold, sweaty skin; coma.
WHAT TO DO:
- **Dial 0 (operator) or 911 (emergency) for an ambulance or medical help. Then give first aid immediately.**
- **If patient is unconscious and not breathing, give mouth-to-mouth breathing. If there is no heartbeat, use cardiac massage and mouth-to-mouth breathing (CPR). Don't try to make patient vomit. If you can't get help quickly, take patient to nearest emergency facility.**
- **See emergency information on inside covers.**

What drug does:
- Interferes with nerve impulses and relaxes blood-vessel muscles, reducing blood pressure.
- Suppresses brain centers that control emotions.

Time lapse before drug works:
Regular use for several weeks may be necessary to determine drug's effectiveness.

Don't take with:
- Non-prescription drugs containing alcohol without consulting doctor.
- See Interaction column and consult doctor.

 POSSIBLE ADVERSE REACTIONS OR SIDE EFFECTS

SYMPTOMS	WHAT TO DO
Life-threatening:	
Fainting, black stool, black vomit, chest pain, rapid or irregular heartbeat.	Discontinue. Seek emergency treatment.
Common:	
• Nausea, vomiting.	Discontinue. Call doctor right away.
• Headache, drowsiness, runny nose, diarrhea, appetite loss.	Continue. Call doctor when convenient.
Infrequent:	
• Rash, hives, joint pain.	Discontinue. Call doctor right away.
• Confusion; dizziness; red or flushed face; irritated, red, watery eyes; constipation; joint stiffness; weakness.	Continue. Call doctor when convenient.
Rare:	
Unexplained bleeding or bruising, sore throat, abdominal pain, jaundice, swollen lymph glands.	Discontinue. Call doctor right away.

WARNINGS & PRECAUTIONS

Don't take if:
- If you are allergic to any rauwolfia alkaloid or hydralazine.
- You are depressed.
- You have active peptic ulcer, ulcerative colitis, or history of coronary-artery disease or rheumatic heart disease.

Before you start, consult your doctor:
- If you have been depressed.
- If you have had peptic ulcer, ulcerative colitis, gallstones, lupus, a stroke, kidney disease or impaired kidney function.
- If you have epilepsy.
- If you will have surgery within 2 months, including dental surgery, requiring general or spinal anesthesia.

Over age 60:
Adverse reactions and side effects may be more frequent and severe than in younger persons.

Pregnancy:
Risk to unborn child outweighs drug benefits. Don't use.

Breast-feeding:
Drug passes into milk. Avoid drug or discontinue nursing until you finish medicine. Consult doctor for advice on maintaining milk supply.

Infants & children:
Not recommended.

Prolonged use:
- Causes cancer in laboratory animals. Consult your doctor if you have family or personal history of cancer.
- May cause lupus (a connective tissue illness with arthritis, anemia and kidney malfunction).
- Possible psychosis.
- May cause numbness, tingling in hands or feet.

Skin & sunlight:
No problems expected.

Driving, piloting or hazardous work:
Don't drive or pilot aircraft until you learn how medicine affects you. Don't work around dangerous machinery. Don't climb ladders or work in high places. Danger increases if you drink alcohol or take medicine affecting alertness and reflexes, such as antihistamines, tranquilizers, sedatives, pain medicine, narcotics and mind-altering drugs.

Discontinuing:
Don't discontinue without consulting doctor. Dose may require gradual reduction if you have taken drug for a long time. Doses of other drugs may also require adjustment.

Others:
- Consult your doctor if you do isometric exercises. These raise blood pressure. Drug may intensify blood-pressure rise.
- Vitamin B-6 diet supplement may be advisable. Consult doctor.

POSSIBLE INTERACTION WITH OTHER DRUGS

GENERIC NAME OR DRUG CLASS	COMBINED EFFECT
Acebutolol	Possible increased effect of both drugs, causing excessively low blood pressure and slow heartbeat.
Amphetamines	Decreased hydralazine effect.
Anticoagulants (oral)	Unpredictable increased or decreased effect of anticoagulant.
Anticonvulsants	Serious change in seizure pattern.
Antidepressants	Increased antidepressant effect.
Antihistamines	Increased antihistamine effect.
Antihypertensives (other)	Increased antihypertensive effect.

Continued page 975

POSSIBLE INTERACTION WITH OTHER SUBSTANCES

INTERACTS WITH	COMBINED EFFECT
Alcohol:	Increased intoxication. Avoid.
Beverages: Carbonated drinks.	Decreased rauwolfia alkaloids effect.
Cocaine:	Dangerous blood-pressure rise. Avoid.
Foods: Spicy foods.	Possible digestive upset.
Marijuana:	Occasional use—Mild drowsiness. Daily use—Moderate drowsiness, low blood pressure, depression.
Tobacco:	Possible angina attacks.

RESERPINE, HYDRALAZINE & HYDROCHLOROTHIAZIDE

BRAND NAMES

Hydrap-Es
Hyserp
R-HCTZ-H

Ser-Ap-Es
Tri-Hydroserpine
Unipres

BASIC INFORMATION

Habit forming? No
Prescription needed? Yes
Available as generic? No
Drug class: Antihypertensive

USES

- Treatment for high blood pressure and congestive heart failure.
- Reduces fluid retention (edema).

DOSAGE & USAGE INFORMATION

How to take:
Tablet or capsule—Swallow with liquid. If you can't swallow whole, crumble tablet or open capsule and take with liquid or food.

When to take:
At the same times each day.

If you forget a dose:
Take as soon as you remember up to 2 hours late. If more than 2 hours, wait for next scheduled dose (don't double this dose).

Continued next column

OVERDOSE

SYMPTOMS:
Drowsiness; slow, shallow breathing; diarrhea; flush; low body temperature; rapid, weak heartbeat; fainting; extreme weakness; cold, sweaty skin; cramps, coma.
WHAT TO DO:
- **Dial 0 (operator) or 911 (emergency) for an ambulance or medical help. Then give first aid immediately.**
- **If patient is unconscious and not breathing, give mouth-to-mouth breathing. If there is no heartbeat, use cardiac massage and mouth-to-mouth breathing (CPR). Don't try to make patient vomit. If you can't get help quickly, take patient to nearest emergency facility.**
- **See emergency information on inside covers.**

What drug does:
- Interferes with nerve impulses and relaxes blood-vessel muscles, reducing blood pressure.
- Suppresses brain centers that control emotions.
- Forces sodium and water excretion, reducing body fluid.
- Reduced body fluid and relaxed arteries lower blood pressure.

Time lapse before drug works:
Regular use for several weeks may be necessary to determine drug's effectiveness.

Don't take with:
- Non-prescription drugs containing alcohol without consulting doctor.
- See Interaction column and consult doctor.

POSSIBLE ADVERSE REACTIONS OR SIDE EFFECTS

SYMPTOMS	WHAT TO DO
Life-threatening:	
Rapid or irregular heartbeat, weak pulse, fainting, black stool, black or bloody vomit, chest pain.	Discontinue. Seek emergency treatment.
Common:	
• Nausea, vomiting.	Discontinue. Call doctor right away.
• Headache, drowsiness, runny nose, diarrhea, appetite loss.	Continue. Call doctor when convenient.
Infrequent:	
• Blurred vision, abdominal pain, rash, hives, joint pain.	Discontinue. Call doctor right away.
• Dizziness; mood change; headache; dry mouth; weakness; tiredness; weight gain or loss; eyes red, watery, irritated; confusion; constipation; red or flushed face; joint stiffness.	Continue. Call doctor when convenient.
Rare:	
Sore throat; jaundice; unexplained bleeding or bruising; sore throat, fever, mouth sores.	Discontinue. Call doctor right away.

WARNINGS & PRECAUTIONS

Don't take if:
- You are allergic to any rauwolfia alkaloid, hydralazine, or any thiazide diuretic drug.
- You are depressed.
- You have active peptic ulcer, ulcerative colitis, history of coronary-artery disease or rheumatic heart disease.

Before you start, consult your doctor:
- If you have been depressed.
- If you have had peptic ulcer, ulcerative colitis, gallstones, kidney disease or impaired kidney function, lupus or a stroke.
- If you have epilepsy, gout, liver, pancreas or kidney disorder.
- If you feel pain in chest, neck or arms on physical exertion.
- If you are allergic to any sulfa drug.
- If you will have surgery within 2 months, including dental surgery, requiring general or spinal anesthesia.

Over age 60:
Adverse reactions and side effects may be more frequent and severe than in younger persons, especially dizziness and excessive potassium loss.

Pregnancy:
Risk to unborn child outweighs drug benefits. Don't use.

Breast-feeding:
Drug passes into milk. Avoid drug or discontinue nursing until you finish medicine.

Infants & children:
Not recommended.

Prolonged use:
- Causes cancer in laboratory animals. Consult your doctor if you have family or personal history of cancer.
- May cause lupus.
- Possible psychosis.
- May cause numbness, tingling in hands or feet.

Skin & sunlight:
May cause rash or intensify sunburn in areas exposed to sun or sunlamp.

Driving, piloting or hazardous work:
Don't drive or pilot aircraft until you learn how medicine affects you. Don't work around dangerous machinery. Don't climb ladders or work in high places. Danger increases if you drink alcohol or take medicine affecting alertness and reflexes.

Discontinuing:
Don't discontinue without consulting doctor. Dose may require gradual reduction if you have taken drug for a long time. Doses of other drugs may also require adjustment.

Others:
- Consult your doctor if you do isometric exercises. These raise blood pressure. Drug may intensify blood-pressure rise.
- Vitamin B-6 supplement may be advisable. Consult doctor.
- Hot weather and fever may cause dehydration and drop in blood pressure. Dose may require temporary adjustment. Weigh daily and report any unexpected weight decreases to your doctor.
- May cause rise in uric acid, leading to gout.
- May cause blood-sugar rise in diabetics.

POSSIBLE INTERACTION WITH OTHER DRUGS

GENERIC NAME OR DRUG CLASS	COMBINED EFFECT
Acebutolol	Possible increased effects of drugs.

Continued page 975

POSSIBLE INTERACTION WITH OTHER SUBSTANCES

INTERACTS WITH	COMBINED EFFECT
Alcohol:	Increased intoxication. Avoid.
Beverages: Carbonated drinks.	Decreased rauwolfia alkaloids effect.
Cocaine:	Dangerous blood-pressure rise. Avoid.
Foods: Spicy foods.	Possible digestive upset.
Licorice.	Excessive potassium loss that causes dangerous heart rhythms.
Marijuana:	Weakness on standing. May increase blood pressure. Occasional use—Mild drowsiness. Daily use—Moderate drowsiness, low blood pressure, depression.
Tobacco:	Possible angina attacks.

RIBAVIRIN

BRAND NAMES

Tribavirin   Viramid
Vilona   Virazole

BASIC INFORMATION

Habit forming? No
Prescription needed? Yes
Available as generic? No
Drug class: Antiviral

 USES

- Treats severe viral pneumonia.
- Treats influenza A and B.
- It does *not* treat other viruses such as the common cold.

 DOSAGE & USAGE INFORMATION

How to take:
By inhalation of a fine mist through mouth. Requires a special sprayer attached to oxygen mask, face mask for infants or hood.

When to take:
As ordered by your doctor.

If you forget a dose:
Use as soon as you remember.

What drug does:
Kills virus or prevents its growth.

Time lapse before drug works:
Begins working in 1 hour. May require treatment for 12 to 18 hours per day for 3 to 7 days.

Don't take with:
See Interaction column and consult doctor.

 OVERDOSE

SYMPTOMS:
None expected.
WHAT TO DO:
Overdose unlikely to threaten life. If person takes much larger amount than prescribed, call doctor, poison-control center or hospital emergency room for instructions.

 POSSIBLE ADVERSE REACTIONS OR SIDE EFFECTS

SYMPTOMS	WHAT TO DO
Life-threatening:	
None expected.	
Common:	
None expected.	
Infrequent:	
Blurred vision; dizziness; fainting; eye irritation; eyes more sensitive to light; red, swollen or itchy eyes.	Discontinue. Call doctor right away.
Rare:	
None expected.	

WARNINGS & PRECAUTIONS

Don't take if:
You are allergic to ribavirin.

Before you start, consult your doctor:
If you are now on low-salt, low-sugar or any special diet.

Over age 60:
Adverse reactions and side effects may be more frequent and severe than in younger persons. Ask doctor about smaller doses.

Pregnancy:
Risk to unborn child outweighs drug benefits. Don't use.

Breast-feeding:
Drug passes into milk. Avoid drug or discontinue nursing until you finish medicine. Consult doctor for advice on maintaining milk supply.

Infants & children:
Use only under close medical supervision.

Prolonged use:
No problems expected.

Skin & sunlight:
No problems expected.

Driving, piloting or hazardous work:
Don't drive or pilot aircraft until you learn how medicine affects you. Don't work around dangerous machinery. Don't climb ladders or work in high places. Danger increases if you drink alcohol or take medicine affecting alertness and reflexes, such as antihistamines, tranquilizers, sedatives, pain medicine, narcotics and mind-altering drugs.

Discontinuing:
Don't discontinue without consulting doctor. Dose may require gradual reduction if you have taken drug for a long time. Doses of other drugs may also require adjustment.

Others:
No problems expected.

POSSIBLE INTERACTION WITH OTHER DRUGS

GENERIC NAME OR DRUG CLASS	COMBINED EFFECT
None expected.	

POSSIBLE INTERACTION WITH OTHER SUBSTANCES

INTERACTS WITH	COMBINED EFFECT
Alcohol:	None expected.
Beverages:	None expected.
Cocaine:	None expected.
Foods:	None expected.
Marijuana:	None expected.
Tobacco:	None expected.

RIBOFLAVIN (VITAMIN B-2)

BRAND NAMES

Riobin-50   Many multivitamin
                 preparations.

BASIC INFORMATION

Habit forming? No
Prescription needed? No
Available as generic? Yes
Drug class: Vitamin supplement

 ## USES

- Dietary supplement to ensure normal growth and health.
- Dietary supplement to treat symptoms caused by deficiency of B-2: sores in mouth, eyes sensitive to light, itching and peeling skin.
- Infections, stomach problems, burns, alcoholism, liver disease.
- Overactive thyroid may cause need for extra Vitamin B-2.

 ## DOSAGE & USAGE INFORMATION

How to take:
Tablet or capsule—Swallow with liquid or food to lessen stomach irritation. If you can't swallow whole, crumble tablet or open capsule and take with liquid or food.

When to take:
At the same times each day.

If you forget a dose:
Take as soon as you remember. Resume regular schedule. Don't double dose.

What drug does:
Promotes normal growth and health.

Time lapse before drug works:
Requires continual intake.

Don't take with:
See Interaction column and consult doctor.

 ## OVERDOSE

SYMPTOMS:
Dark urine, nausea, vomiting.
WHAT TO DO:
Overdose unlikely to threaten life. If person takes much larger amount than prescribed, call doctor, poison-control center or hospital emergency room for instructions.

 ## POSSIBLE ADVERSE REACTIONS OR SIDE EFFECTS

SYMPTOMS	WHAT TO DO
Life-threatening:	
None expected.	
Common:	
Urine yellow in color.	No action necessary.
Infrequent:	
None expected.	
Rare:	
None expected.	

**WARNINGS &
PRECAUTIONS**

Don't take if:
- You are allergic to any B vitamin.
- You have chronic kidney failure.

Before you start, consult your doctor:
If you are pregnant or plan pregnancy.

Over age 60:
No problems expected.

Pregnancy:
Recommended. Consult doctor.

Breast-feeding:
Recommended. Consult doctor.

Infants & children:
Consult doctor.

Prolonged use:
No problems expected.

Skin & sunlight:
No problems expected.

Driving, piloting or hazardous work:
No problems expected.

Discontinuing:
No problems expected.

Others:
A balanced diet should provide all the vitamin B-2 a healthy person needs and make supplements unnecessary during periods of good health. Best sources are milk, meats and green leafy vegetables.

 **POSSIBLE INTERACTION
WITH OTHER DRUGS**

GENERIC NAME OR DRUG CLASS	COMBINED EFFECT
Antidepressants (tricyclic)	Decreased riboflavin effect.
Phenothiazines	Decreased riboflavin effect.
Probenecid	Decreased riboflavin effect.

 **POSSIBLE INTERACTION
WITH OTHER SUBSTANCES**

INTERACTS WITH	COMBINED EFFECT
Alcohol:	Prevents uptake and absorption of vitamin B-2.
Beverages:	No problems expected.
Cocaine:	No problems expected.
Foods:	No problems expected.
Marijuana:	No problems expected.
Tobacco:	Prevents absorption of vitamin B-2 and other vitamins and nutrients.

RIFAMPIN

BRAND NAMES

Rifadin
Rifamate
Rifampicin

Rifomycin
Rimactane
Rofact

BASIC INFORMATION

Habit forming? No
Prescription needed? Yes
Available as generic? No
Drug class: Antibiotic (rifamycin)

USES

Treatment for tuberculosis and other infections.
Requires daily use for 1 to 2 years.

DOSAGE & USAGE INFORMATION

How to take:
Capsule—Swallow with liquid. If you can't
swallow whole, open capsule and take with
liquid or small amount of food. For child, mix
with small amount of applesauce or jelly.

When to take:
1 hour before or 2 hours after a meal.

If you forget a dose:
Take as soon as you remember up to 2 hours
late. If more than 2 hours, wait for next
scheduled dose (don't double this dose).

What drug does:
Prevents multiplication of tuberculosis germs.

Continued next column

OVERDOSE

SYMPTOMS:
Slow, shallow breathing; weak, rapid pulse;
cold, sweaty skin; coma.
WHAT TO DO:
- Dial 0 (operator) or 911 (emergency) for an
  ambulance or medical help. Then give first
  aid immediately.
- If patient is unconscious and not
  breathing, give mouth-to-mouth breathing.
  If there is no heartbeat, use cardiac
  massage and mouth-to-mouth breathing
  (CPR). Don't try to make patient vomit. If
  you can't get help quickly, take patient to
  nearest emergency facility.
- See emergency information on inside
  covers.

Time lapse before drug works:
Usually 2 weeks. May require 1 to 2 years
without missed doses for maximum benefit.

Don't take with:
See Interaction column and consult doctor.

POSSIBLE ADVERSE REACTIONS OR SIDE EFFECTS

SYMPTOMS	WHAT TO DO
Life-threatening: None expected.	
Common: Diarrhea; reddish urine, stool, saliva, sweat and tears.	Continue. Call doctor when convenient.
Infrequent: • Rash, itchy skin, blurred vision, difficult breathing.	Discontinue. Call doctor right away.
• Dizziness, unsteady gait, confusion, muscle or bone pain.	Continue. Call doctor when convenient.
• Headache.	Continue. Tell doctor at next visit.
Rare: • Sore throat, mouth or tongue; jaundice.	Discontinue. Call doctor right away.
• Appetite loss, vomiting, less urination.	Continue. Call doctor when convenient.

WARNINGS & PRECAUTIONS

Don't take if:
- You are allergic to rifampin.
- You wear soft contact lenses.

Before you start, consult your doctor:
If you are alcoholic or have liver disease.

Over age 60:
Adverse reactions and side effects may be more frequent and severe than in younger persons.

Pregnancy:
Studies inconclusive on harm to unborn child. Animal studies show fetal abnormalities. Decide with your doctor whether drug benefits justify risk to unborn child.

Breast-feeding:
No proven problems. Consult doctor.

Infants & children:
Use only under medical supervision.

Prolonged use:
You may become more susceptible to infections caused by germs not responsive to rifampin.

Skin & sunlight:
No problems expected.

Driving, piloting or hazardous work:
Don't drive or pilot aircraft until you learn how medicine affects you. Don't work around dangerous machinery. Don't climb ladders or work in high places. Danger increases if you drink alcohol or take medicine affecting alertness and reflexes, such as antihistamines, tranquilizers, sedatives, pain medicine, narcotics and mind-altering drugs.

Discontinuing:
Don't discontinue without doctor's advice until you complete prescribed dose, even though symptoms diminish or disappear.

Others:
No problems expected.

POSSIBLE INTERACTION WITH OTHER DRUGS

GENERIC NAME OR DRUG CLASS	COMBINED EFFECT
Anticoagulants (oral)	Decreased anticoagulant effect.
Barbiturates	Decreased barbiturate effect.
Contraceptives (oral)	Decreased contraceptive effect.
Cortisone drugs	Decreased effect of cortisone drugs.
Dapsone	Decreased dapsone effect.
Digitoxin	Decreased digitoxin effect.
Flecainide	Possible decreased blood-cell production in bone marrow.
Isoniazid	Possible toxicity to liver.
Methadone	Decreased methadone effect.
Para-aminosalicylic acid (PAS)	Decreased rifampin effect.
Probenecid	Possible toxicity to liver.
Tocainide	Possible decreased blood-cell production in bone marrow.
Tolbutamide	Decreased tolbutamide effect.
Trimethoprim	Decreased trimethoprim effect.

POSSIBLE INTERACTION WITH OTHER SUBSTANCES

INTERACTS WITH	COMBINED EFFECT
Alcohol:	Possible toxicity to liver.
Beverages:	None expected.
Cocaine:	No proven problems.
Foods:	None expected.
Marijuana:	No proven problems.
Tobacco:	None expected.

RITODRINE

BRAND NAMES

Yutopar

BASIC INFORMATION

Habit forming? No
Prescription needed? Yes
Available as generic? No
Drug class: Labor inhibitor; Beta-adrenergic stimulator

USES

Halts premature labor in pregnancies of 20 or more weeks.

DOSAGE & USAGE INFORMATION

How to take:
Tablet or capsule—Swallow with liquid or food to lessen stomach irritation. If you can't swallow whole, crumble tablet or open capsule and take with liquid or food.

When to take:
Every 4 to 6 hours until term.

If you forget a dose:
Take as soon as you remember up to 2 hours late. If more than 2 hours, wait for next scheduled dose (don't double this dose).

What drug does:
Inhibits contractions of uterus (womb).

Continued next column

OVERDOSE

SYMPTOMS:
Rapid, irregular heartbeat to 120 or more; shortness of breath.
WHAT TO DO:
- Dial 0 (operator) or 911 (emergency) for an ambulance or medical help. Then give first aid immediately.
- If patient is unconscious and not breathing, give mouth-to-mouth breathing. If there is no heartbeat, use cardiac massage and mouth-to-mouth breathing (CPR). Don't try to make patient vomit. If you can't get help quickly, take patient to nearest emergency facility.
- See emergency information on inside covers.

Time lapse before drug works:
30 to 60 minutes (oral form). Faster intravenously.

Don't take with:
See Interaction column and consult doctor.

POSSIBLE ADVERSE REACTIONS OR SIDE EFFECTS

SYMPTOMS	WHAT TO DO
Life-threatening:	
None expected.	
Always:	
Increased heart rate.	Continue. Call doctor when convenient.
Common:	
• Irregular heartbeat.	Discontinue. Call doctor right away.
• Increased systolic blood pressure.	Continue. Tell doctor at next visit.
Infrequent:	
• Shortness of breath.	Discontinue. Call doctor right away.
• Nervousness, trembling, headache, nausea, vomiting.	Continue. Call doctor when convenient.
Rare:	
Rash.	Discontinue. Call doctor right away.

WARNINGS & PRECAUTIONS

Don't take if:
- You have heart disease.
- You have eclampsia.
- You have lung congestion.
- You have infection in the uterus.
- You have an overactive thyroid.
- You have a bleeding disorder.

Before you start, consult your doctor:
- If you have asthma.
- If you have diabetes.
- If you have high blood pressure.
- If you have pre-eclampsia.

Over age 60:
Not used.

Pregnancy:
Ritodrine crosses placenta, but animal studies show that it causes no effects on fetuses. Benefits versus risks must be assessed by you and your doctor.

Breast-feeding:
Not applicable.

Infants & children:
Not used.

Prolonged use:
Request blood sugar and electrolytes measurements.

Skin & sunlight:
No problems expected.

Driving, piloting or hazardous work:
Don't drive or pilot aircraft until you learn how medicine affects you. Don't work around dangerous machinery. Don't climb ladders or work in high places. Danger increases if you drink alcohol or take medicine affecting alertness and reflexes, such as antihistamines, tranquilizers, sedatives, pain medicine, narcotics and mind-altering drugs.

Discontinuing:
Don't discontinue without consulting doctor. Dose may require gradual reduction if you have taken drug for a long time. Doses of other drugs may also require adjustment.

Others:
No problems expected.

POSSIBLE INTERACTION WITH OTHER DRUGS

GENERIC NAME OR DRUG CLASS	COMBINED EFFECT
Adrenal corticosteroids	Increased chance of fluid in lungs of mother. Avoid.
Beta-adrenergic blockers	Decreased effect of ritodrine.
Sympathomimetics	Increased side effects of both.

POSSIBLE INTERACTION WITH OTHER SUBSTANCES

INTERACTS WITH	COMBINED EFFECT
Alcohol:	Increased adverse effects. Avoid.
Beverages:	No problems expected.
Cocaine:	Injury to fetus. Avoid.
Foods:	No problems expected.
Marijuana:	Injury to fetus. Avoid.
Tobacco:	Injury to fetus. Avoid.

SALICYLATES

BRAND AND GENERIC NAMES

See complete list of brand and generic names in the *Brand Name Directory,* page 957.

BASIC INFORMATION

Habit forming? No
Prescription needed? No
Available as generic? Yes
Drug class: Analgesic, anti-inflammatory
(salicylate)

USES

- Reduces pain, fever, inflammation.
- Relieves swelling, stiffness, joint pain of arthritis or rheumatism.

DOSAGE & USAGE INFORMATION

How to take:
- Tablet or capsule—Swallow with liquid.
- Extended-release tablets or capsules—Swallow each dose whole.
- Suppositories—Remove wrapper and moisten suppository with water. Gently insert into rectum, large end first.

When to take:
Pain, fever, inflammation—As needed, no more often than every 4 hours.

If you forget a dose:
- Pain, fever—Take as soon as you remember. Wait 4 hours for next dose.
- Arthritis—Take as soon as you remember up to 2 hours late. Return to regular schedule.

Continued next column

OVERDOSE

SYMPTOMS:
Ringing in ears; nausea; vomiting; dizziness; fever; deep, rapid breathing; hallucinations; convulsions; coma.
WHAT TO DO:
- **Dial 0 (operator) or 911 (emergency) for an ambulance or medical help. Then give first aid immediately.**
- **See emergency information on inside covers.**

What drug does:
- Affects hypothalamus, the part of the brain that regulates temperature by dilating small blood vessels in skin.
- Prevents clumping of platelets (small blood cells) so blood vessels remain open.
- Decreases prostaglandin effect.
- Suppresses body's pain messages.

Time lapse before drug works:
30 minutes for pain, fever, arthritis.

Don't take with:
- Tetracyclines. Space doses 1 hour apart.
- See Interaction column and consult doctor.

POSSIBLE ADVERSE REACTIONS OR SIDE EFFECTS

SYMPTOMS	WHAT TO DO
Life-threatening:	
Hives, rash, intense itching, faintness soon after a dose (anaphylaxis); black or bloody vomit; blood in urine.	Seek emergency treatment immediately.
Common:	
• Nausea, vomiting, abdominal pain.	Discontinue. Seek emergency treatment.
• Heartburn, indigestion.	Continue. Call doctor when convenient.
• Ringing in ears.	Continue. Tell doctor at next visit.
Infrequent:	
None expected.	
Rare:	
• Black stools, unexplained fever.	Discontinue. Seek emergency treatment.
• Rash, hives, itchy skin, diminished vision, shortness of breath, wheezing, jaundice.	Discontinue. Call doctor right away.
• Drowsiness.	Continue. Call doctor when convenient.

WARNINGS & PRECAUTIONS

Don't take if:
- You need to restrict sodium in your diet. Buffered effervescent tablets and sodium salicylate are high in sodium.
- Salicylates have a strong vinegar-like odor, which means it has decomposed.
- You have a peptic ulcer of stomach or duodenum.
- You have a bleeding disorder.

Before you start, consult your doctor:
- If you have had stomach or duodenal ulcers.
- If you have had gout.
- If you have asthma or nasal polyps.

Over age 60:
More likely to cause hidden bleeding in stomach or intestines. Watch for dark stools.

Pregnancy:
Risk to unborn child outweighs drug benefits. Don't use.

Breast-feeding:
Drug passes into milk. Avoid drug or discontinue nursing until you finish medicine. Consult doctor for advice on maintaining milk supply.

Infants & children:
Overdose frequent and severe. Keep bottles out of children's reach.

Prolonged use:
Kidney damage. Periodic kidney-function test recommended.

Skin & sunlight:
Aspirin combined with sunscreen may decrease sunburn.

Driving, piloting or hazardous work:
No restrictions unless you feel drowsy.

Discontinuing:
For chronic illness—Don't discontinue without doctor's advice until you complete prescribed dose, even though symptoms diminish or disappear.

Others:
- Salicylates can complicate surgery, pregnancy, labor and delivery, and illness.
- For arthritis—Don't change dose without consulting doctor.
- Urine tests for blood sugar may be inaccurate.

POSSIBLE INTERACTION WITH OTHER DRUGS

GENERIC NAME OR DRUG CLASS	COMBINED EFFECT
Acebutolol	Decreased antihypertensive effect of acebutolol.
Allopurinol	Decreased allopurinol effect.
Antacids	Decreased salicylate effect.
Anticoagulants	Increased anticoagulant effect. Abnormal bleeding.
Antidiabetics (oral)	Low blood sugar.

Anti-inflammatory drugs (non-steroid)	Risk of stomach bleeding and ulcers.
Aspirin (other)	Likely salicylate toxicity.
Calcium supplements	Increased salicylate effect.
Cortisone drugs	Increased cortisone effect. Risk of ulcers and stomach bleeding.
Furosemide	Possible salicylate toxicity.
Gold compounds	Increased likelihood of kidney damage.
Indomethacin	Risk of stomach bleeding and ulcers.
Ketoprofen	Increased possibility of internal bleeding.
Methotrexate	Increased methotrexate effect.
Minoxidil	Decreased minoxidil effect.
Oxprenolol	Decreased antihypertensive effect of oxprenolol.
Para-aminosalicylic acid (PAS)	Possible salicylate toxicity.
Penicillins	Increased effect of both drugs.
Phenobarbital	Decreased salicylate effect.
Phenytoin	Increased phenytoin effect.
Probenecid	Decreased probenecid effect.

Continued page 976

POSSIBLE INTERACTION WITH OTHER SUBSTANCES

INTERACTS WITH	COMBINED EFFECT
Alcohol:	Possible stomach irritation and bleeding. Avoid.
Beverages:	None expected.
Cocaine:	None expected.
Foods:	None expected.
Marijuana:	Possible increased pain relief, but marijuana may slow body's recovery. Avoid.
Tobacco:	None expected.

SCOPOLAMINE (HYOSCINE)

BRAND NAMES

See complete list of brand names in the *Brand Name Directory,* page 957.

BASIC INFORMATION

Habit forming? No
Prescription needed?
  High strength: Yes
  Low strength: No
Available as generic? Yes
Drug class: Antispasmodic, anticholinergic

USES

- Reduces spasms of digestive system, bladder and urethra.
- Relieves painful menstruation.
- Prevents motion sickness.

DOSAGE & USAGE INFORMATION

How to take:
- Tablet or capsule—Swallow with liquid or food to lessen stomach irritation.
- Extended-release tablets or capsules—Swallow each dose whole.
- Drops—Dilute dose in beverage.
- Skin discs—Clean application site. Change application sites with each dose.

When to take:
- Motion sickness—Apply disc 30 minutes before departure.
- Other uses—Take 30 minutes before meals (unless directed otherwise by doctor).

If you forget a dose:
Take up to 2 hours late. If more than 2 hours, wait for next dose (don't double this dose).

Continued next column

OVERDOSE

SYMPTOMS:
Dilated pupils, rapid pulse and breathing, dizziness, fever, hallucinations, confusion, slurred speech, agitation, flushed face, convulsions, coma.
WHAT TO DO:
- **Dial 0 (operator) or 911 (emergency) for an ambulance or medical help. Then give first aid immediately.**
- **See emergency information on inside covers.**

What drug does:
Blocks nerve impulses at parasympathetic nerve endings, preventing muscle contractions and gland secretions of organs involved.

Time lapse before drug works:
15 to 30 minutes.

Don't take with:
See Interaction column and consult doctor.

POSSIBLE ADVERSE REACTIONS OR SIDE EFFECTS

SYMPTOMS	WHAT TO DO
Life-threatening:	
None expected.	
Common:	
• Confusion, delirium, rapid heartbeat.	Discontinue. Call doctor right away.
• Nausea, vomiting, decreased sweating.	Continue. Call doctor when convenient.
• Constipation.	Continue. Tell doctor at next visit.
• Dryness in ears, nose, throat.	No action necessary.
Infrequent:	
Headache, difficult urination.	Continue. Call doctor when convenient.
Rare:	
Rash or hives, pain, blurred vision.	Discontinue. Call doctor right away.

WARNINGS & PRECAUTIONS

Don't take if:
- You are allergic to any anticholinergic.
- You have trouble with stomach bloating.
- You have difficulty emptying your bladder completely.
- You have narrow-angle glaucoma.
- You have severe ulcerative colitis.

Before you start, consult your doctor:
- If you have open-angle glaucoma.
- If you have angina.
- If you have chronic bronchitis or asthma.
- If you have hiatal hernia.
- If you have liver disease.
- If you have enlarged prostate.
- If you have myasthenia gravis.
- If you have peptic ulcer.
- If you will have surgery within 2 months, including dental surgery, requiring general or spinal anesthesia.

Over age 60:
Adverse reactions and side effects may be more frequent and severe than in younger persons.

Pregnancy:
Studies inconclusive on harm to unborn child. Animal studies show fetal abnormalities. Decide with your doctor whether drug benefits justify risk to unborn child.

Breast-feeding:
Drug passes into milk and decreases milk flow. Avoid drug or discontinue nursing until you finish medicine. Consult doctor for advice on maintaining milk supply.

Infants & children:
Use only under medical supervision.

Prolonged use:
Chronic constipation, possible fecal impaction. Consult doctor immediately.

Skin & sunlight:
No problems expected.

Driving, piloting or hazardous work:
Use disqualifies you for piloting aircraft. Otherwise, no problems expected.

Discontinuing:
May be unnecessary to finish medicine. Follow doctor's instructions.

Others:
No problems expected.

POSSIBLE INTERACTION WITH OTHER DRUGS

GENERIC NAME OR DRUG CLASS	COMBINED EFFECT
Amantadine	Increased scopolamine effect.
Anticholinergics (other)	Increased scopolamine effect.
Antidepressants (tricyclic)	Increased scopolamine effect. Increased sedation.

Antihistamines	Increased scopolamine effect.
Cortisone drugs	Increased internal-eye pressure.
Haloperidol	Increased internal-eye pressure.
MAO inhibitors	Increased scopolamine effect.
Meperidine	Increased scopolamine effect.
Methylphenidate	Increased scopolamine effect.
Molindone	Increased anticholinergic effect.
Nitrates	Increased internal-eye pressure.
Orphenadrine	Increased scopolamine effect.
Phenothiazines	Increased scopolamine effect.
Pilocarpine	Loss of pilocarpine effect in glaucoma treatment.
Potassium supplements	Possible intestinal ulcers with oral potassium tablets.
Vitamin C	Decreased scopolamine effect. Avoid large doses of vitamin C.

POSSIBLE INTERACTION WITH OTHER SUBSTANCES

INTERACTS WITH	COMBINED EFFECT
Alcohol:	None expected.
Beverages:	None expected.
Cocaine:	Excessively rapid heartbeat. Avoid.
Foods:	None expected.
Marijuana:	Drowsiness, dry mouth.
Tobacco:	None expected.

SECOBARBITAL

BRAND NAMES

Novo Secobarb   Seral
Secogen   Tuinal
Seconal

BASIC INFORMATION

Habit forming? Yes
Prescription needed? Yes
Available as generic? Yes
Drug class: Sedative, hypnotic (barbiturate)

USES

- Reduces anxiety or nervous tension (low dose).
- Relieves insomnia (higher bedtime dose).

DOSAGE & USAGE INFORMATION

How to take:
- Tablet, capsule or liquid—Swallow with food or liquid to lessen stomach irritation. If you can't swallow whole, crumble tablet or open capsule and take with liquid or food.
- Suppositories—Remove wrapper and moisten suppository with water. Gently insert larger end into rectum. Push well into rectum with finger.

When to take:
At the same times each day.

If you forget a dose:
Take as soon as you remember up to 2 hours late. If more than 2 hours, wait for next scheduled dose (don't double this dose).

What drug does:
May partially block nerve impulses at nerve-cell connections.

Time lapse before drug works:
60 minutes.

Don't take with:
- Non-prescription drugs without consulting doctor.
- See Interaction column and consult doctor.

OVERDOSE

SYMPTOMS:
Deep sleep, weak pulse, coma.
WHAT TO DO:
- Dial 0 (operator) or 911 (emergency) for an ambulance or medical help. Then give first aid immediately.
- See emergency information on inside covers.

POSSIBLE ADVERSE REACTIONS OR SIDE EFFECTS

SYMPTOMS	WHAT TO DO
Life-threatening:	
None expected.	
Common:	
Dizziness, drowsiness, "hangover" effect.	Continue. Call doctor when convenient.
Infrequent:	
• Rash or hives; swollen face, lip or eyelids; sore throat, fever.	Discontinue. Call doctor right away.
• Depression, confusion, slurred speech, diarrhea, nausea, vomiting, joint or muscle pain.	Continue. Call doctor when convenient.
Rare:	
• Agitation, slow heartbeat, difficult breathing, jaundice.	Discontinue. Call doctor right away.
• Unexplained bleeding or bruising.	Continue. Call doctor when convenient.

WARNINGS & PRECAUTIONS

Don't take if:
- You are allergic to any barbiturate.
- You have porphyria.

Before you start, consult your doctor:
- If you have epilepsy.
- If you have kidney or liver damage.
- If you have asthma.
- If you have anemia.
- If you have chronic pain.
- If you will have surgery within 2 months, including dental surgery, requiring general or spinal anesthesia.

Over age 60:
Adverse reactions and side effects may be more frequent and severe than in younger persons. Use small doses.

Pregnancy:
Risk to unborn child outweighs drug benefits. Don't use.

Breast-feeding:
Drug passes into milk. Avoid drug or discontinue nursing until you finish medicine. Consult doctor for advice on maintaining milk supply.

Infants & children:
Use only under doctor's supervision.

Prolonged use:
- May cause addiction, anemia, chronic intoxication.
- May lower body temperature, making exposure to cold temperatures hazardous.

Skin & sunlight:
May cause rash or intensify sunburn in areas exposed to sun or sunlamp.

Driving, piloting or hazardous work:
Don't drive or pilot aircraft until you learn how medicine affects you. Don't work around dangerous machinery. Don't climb ladders or work in high places. Danger increases if you drink alcohol or take medicine affecting alertness and reflexes.

Discontinuing:
May be unnecessary to finish medicine. Follow doctor's instructions. If you develop withdrawal symptoms of hallucinations, agitation or sleeplessness after discontinuing, call doctor right away.

Others:
Great potential for abuse.

 ## POSSIBLE INTERACTION WITH OTHER DRUGS

GENERIC NAME OR DRUG CLASS	COMBINED EFFECT
Anticoagulants (oral)	Decreased anticoagulant effect.
Anticonvulsants	Changed seizure patterns.
Antidepressants (tricyclics)	Decreased antidepressant effect. Increased sedation.
Antidiabetics (oral)	Increased secobarbital effect.
Antihistamines	Dangerous sedation. Avoid.
Anti-inflammatory drugs (non-steroidal)	Decreased anti-inflammatory effect.
Aspirin	Decreased aspirin effect.
Beta-adrenergic blockers	Decreased effect of beta-adrenergic blocker.
Contraceptives (oral)	Decreased contraceptive effect.
Cortisone drugs	Decreased cortisone effect.
Digitoxin	Decreased digitoxin effect.
Doxycycline	Decreased doxycycline effect.
Dronabinol	Increased effects of both drugs. Avoid.
Griseofulvin	Decreased griseofulvin effect.
Indapamide	Increased indapamide effect.
MAO inhibitors	Increased secobarbital effect.
Mind-altering drugs	Dangerous sedation. Avoid.
Molindone	Increased sedative effect.
Narcotics	Dangerous sedation. Avoid.
Pain relievers	Dangerous sedation. Avoid.
Sedatives	Dangerous sedation. Avoid.
Sleep inducers	Dangerous sedation. Avoid.
Tranquilizers	Dangerous sedation. Avoid.
Valproic acid	Increased secobarbital effect.

 ## POSSIBLE INTERACTION WITH OTHER SUBSTANCES

INTERACTS WITH	COMBINED EFFECT
Alcohol:	Possible fatal oversedation. Avoid.
Beverages:	None expected.
Cocaine:	Decreased secobarbital effect.
Foods:	None expected.
Marijuana:	Excessive sedation. Avoid.
Tobacco:	None expected.

SENNA

BRAND NAMES

Black Draught	Fletcher's Castoria
Black-Draught Lax	Senexon
Senna	Senokot
Casa-Fru	Senolax
Dr. Caldwell's Senna	Swiss Kriss
Laxative	X-Prep

BASIC INFORMATION

Habit forming? No
Prescription needed? No
Available as generic? Yes
Drug class: Laxative (stimulant)

 USES

Constipation relief.

 DOSAGE & USAGE INFORMATION

How to take:
- Tablet—Swallow with liquid. If you can't swallow whole, chew or crumble tablet and take with liquid or food.
- Liquid, granules—Drink 6 to 8 glasses of water each day, in addition to one taken with each dose.

When to take:
Usually at bedtime with a snack, unless directed otherwise.

If you forget a dose:
Take as soon as you remember.

What drug does:
Acts on smooth muscles of intestine wall to cause vigorous bowel movement.

Time lapse before drug works:
6 to 10 hours.

Don't take with:
- See Interaction column and consult doctor.
- Don't take within 2 hours of taking another medicine. Laxative interferes with medicine absorption.

 OVERDOSE

SYMPTOMS:
Vomiting, electrolyte depletion.
WHAT TO DO:
Overdose unlikely to threaten life. If person takes much larger amount than prescribed, call doctor, poison-control center or hospital emergency room for instructions.

 POSSIBLE ADVERSE REACTIONS OR SIDE EFFECTS

SYMPTOMS	WHAT TO DO
Life-threatening:	
None expected.	
Common:	
• Rectal irritation.	Continue. Call doctor when convenient.
• Yellow-brown or red-violet urine.	No action necessary.
Infrequent:	
• Dangerous potassium loss.	Discontinue. Call doctor right away.
• Belching, cramps, nausea.	Continue. Call doctor when convenient.
Rare:	
• Irritability, confusion, headache, rash, difficult breathing, irregular heartbeat, muscle cramps, unusual tiredness or weakness.	Discontinue. Call doctor right away.
• Burning on urination.	Continue. Call doctor when convenient.

WARNINGS & PRECAUTIONS

Don't take if:
- You have symptoms of appendicitis, inflamed bowel or intestinal blockage.
- You are allergic to a stimulant laxative.
- You have missed a bowel movement for only 1 or 2 days.

Before you start, consult your doctor:
- If you have a colostomy or ileostomy.
- If you have congestive heart disease.
- If you have diabetes.
- If you have high blood pressure.
- If you have a laxative habit.
- If you have rectal bleeding.
- If you take other laxatives.

Over age 60:
Adverse reactions and side effects may be more frequent and severe than in younger persons.

Pregnancy:
Risk to mother and unborn child outweighs drug benefits. Don't use.

Breast-feeding:
Drug passes into milk. Avoid drug or discontinue nursing until you finish medicine. Consult doctor for advice on maintaining milk supply.

Infants & children:
Use only under medical supervision.

Prolonged use:
Don't take for more than 1 week unless under a doctor's supervision. May cause laxative dependence.

Skin & sunlight:
No problems expected.

Driving, piloting or hazardous work:
No problems expected.

Discontinuing:
May be unnecessary to finish medicine. Follow doctor's instructions.

Others:
Don't take to "flush out" your system or as a "tonic."

POSSIBLE INTERACTION WITH OTHER DRUGS

GENERIC NAME OR DRUG CLASS	COMBINED EFFECT
Antihypertensives	May cause dangerous low potassium level.
Diuretics	May cause dangerous low potassium level.

POSSIBLE INTERACTION WITH OTHER SUBSTANCES

INTERACTS WITH	COMBINED EFFECT
Alcohol:	None expected.
Beverages:	None expected.
Cocaine:	None expected.
Foods:	None expected.
Marijuana:	None expected.
Tobacco:	None expected.

SENNOSIDES A & B

BRAND NAMES

Glysennid   Senokot
Nytilax   X-Prep

BASIC INFORMATION

Habit forming? No
Prescription needed? No
Available as generic? Yes
Drug class: Laxative (stimulant)

USES

Constipation relief.

DOSAGE & USAGE INFORMATION

How to take:
- Tablet—Swallow with liquid. If you can't swallow whole, chew or crumble tablet and take with liquid or food.
- Liquid, granules—Drink 6 to 8 glasses of water each day, in addition to one taken with each dose.

When to take:
Usually at bedtime with a snack, unless directed otherwise.

If you forget a dose:
Take as soon as you remember.

What drug does:
Acts on smooth muscles of intestine wall to cause vigorous bowel movement.

Time lapse before drug works:
6 to 10 hours.

Don't take with:
- See Interaction column and consult doctor.
- Don't take within 2 hours of taking another medicine. Laxative interferes with medicine absorption.

OVERDOSE

SYMPTOMS:
Vomiting, electrolyte depletion.
WHAT TO DO:
Overdose unlikely to threaten life. If person takes much larger amount than prescribed, call doctor, poison-control center or hospital emergency room for instructions.

POSSIBLE ADVERSE REACTIONS OR SIDE EFFECTS

SYMPTOMS	WHAT TO DO
Life-threatening:	
None expected.	
Common:	
• Rectal irritation.	Continue. Call doctor when convenient.
• Yellow-brown or red-violet urine.	No action necessary.
Infrequent:	
• Dangerous potassium loss.	Discontinue. Call doctor right away.
• Belching, cramps, nausea.	Continue. Call doctor when convenient.
Rare:	
• Irritability, confusion, headache, rash, difficult breathing, irregular heartbeat, muscle cramps, unusual tiredness or weakness.	Discontinue. Call doctor right away.
• Burning on urination.	Continue. Call doctor when convenient.

WARNINGS & PRECAUTIONS

Don't take if:
- You have symptoms of appendicitis, inflamed bowel or intestinal blockage.
- You are allergic to a stimulant laxative.
- You have missed a bowel movement for only 1 or 2 days.

Before you start, consult your doctor:
- If you have a colostomy or ileostomy.
- If you have congestive heart disease.
- If you have diabetes.
- If you have high blood pressure.
- If you have a laxative habit.
- If you have rectal bleeding.
- If you take other laxatives.

Over age 60:
Adverse reactions and side effects may be more frequent and severe than in younger persons.

Pregnancy:
Risk to mother and unborn child outweighs drug benefits. Don't use.

Breast-feeding:
Drug passes into milk. Avoid drug or discontinue nursing until you finish medicine. Consult doctor for advice on maintaining milk supply.

Infants & children:
Use only under medical supervision.

Prolonged use:
Don't take for more than 1 week unless under a doctor's supervision. May cause laxative dependence.

Skin & sunlight:
No problems expected.

Driving, piloting or hazardous work:
No problems expected.

Discontinuing:
May be unnecessary to finish medicine. Follow doctor's instructions.

Others:
Don't take to "flush out" your system or as a "tonic."

POSSIBLE INTERACTION WITH OTHER DRUGS

GENERIC NAME OR DRUG CLASS	COMBINED EFFECT
Antihypertensives	May cause dangerous low potassium level.
Diuretics	May cause dangerous low potassium level.

POSSIBLE INTERACTION WITH OTHER SUBSTANCES

INTERACTS WITH	COMBINED EFFECT
Alcohol:	None expected.
Beverages:	None expected.
Cocaine:	None expected.
Foods:	None expected.
Marijuana:	None expected.
Tobacco:	None expected.

SIMETHICONE

BRAND NAMES

Barriere
Celluzyme
Di-Gel
Gas-X
Gelusil
Mygel
Mylanta
Mylicon

Ovol
Phazyme
Phazyme 125
Riopan Plus
Simeco
Silain
Tri-Cone

BASIC INFORMATION

Habit forming? No
Prescription needed? No
Available as generic? Yes
Drug class: Antiflatulent

 ## USES

- Treatment for retention of abdominal gas.
- Used prior to x-ray of abdomen to reduce gas shadows.

 ## DOSAGE & USAGE INFORMATION

How to take:
- Tablet—Swallow with liquid.
- Liquid—Dissolve in water. Drink complete dose.
- Chewable tablets—Chew completely. Don't swallow whole.

When to take:
After meals and at bedtime.

If you forget a dose:
Take when remembered if needed.

What drug does:
Reduces surface tension of gas bubbles in stomach.

Time lapse before drug works:
10 minutes.

Don't take with:
No restrictions.

 ## OVERDOSE

SYMPTOMS:
None expected.
WHAT TO DO:
Overdose unlikely to threaten life.

 ## POSSIBLE ADVERSE REACTIONS OR SIDE EFFECTS

SYMPTOMS	WHAT TO DO
Life-threatening: None expected.	
Common: None expected.	
Infrequent: None expected.	
Rare: None expected.	

WARNINGS & PRECAUTIONS

Don't take if:
You are allergic to simethicone.

Before you start, consult your doctor:
No problems expected.

Over age 60:
No problems expected.

Pregnancy:
No proven harm to unborn child. Avoid if possible.

Breast-feeding:
No problems expected.

Infants & children:
Not recommended.

Prolonged use:
No problems expected.

Skin & sunlight:
No problems expected.

Driving, piloting or hazardous work:
No problems expected.

Discontinuing:
May be unnecessary to finish medicine. Discontinue when symptoms disappear.

Others:
No problems expected.

POSSIBLE INTERACTION WITH OTHER DRUGS

GENERIC NAME OR DRUG CLASS	COMBINED EFFECT
None	

POSSIBLE INTERACTION WITH OTHER SUBSTANCES

INTERACTS WITH	COMBINED EFFECT
Alcohol:	None expected.
Beverages:	None expected.
Cocaine:	None expected.
Foods:	None expected.
Marijuana:	None expected.
Tobacco:	None expected.

SODIUM BICARBONATE

BRAND NAMES

Alka-Citrate Compound	Ceo-Two
	Chembicarb
Alka-Seltzer Antacid	Citrocarbonate
Arm and Hammer Baking Soda	Eno
	Fizrin
Bell/ans	Infalyte
Bisodol	Neut
Bisodol Powder	Seidlitz Powder
Brioschi	Soda Mint
Bromo Seltzer	

BASIC INFORMATION

Habit forming? No
Prescription needed? No
Available as generic? Yes
Drug class: Antacid

USES

Treatment for hyperacidity in upper gastrointestinal tract, including stomach and esophagus. Symptoms may be heartburn or acid indigestion. Diseases include peptic ulcer, gastritis, esophagitis, hiatal hernia.

DOSAGE & USAGE INFORMATION

How to take:
- Tablet—Swallow with liquid.
- Chewable tablets or wafers—Chew well before swallowing.
- Powder—Dilute dose in beverage before swallowing.

When to take:
1 to 3 hours after meals unless directed otherwise by your doctor.

If you forget a dose:
Take as soon as you remember.

What drug does:
- Neutralizes some of the hydrochloric acid in the stomach.
- Reduces action of pepsin, a digestive enzyme.

Continued next column

OVERDOSE

SYMPTOMS:
Weakness, fatigue, dizziness.
WHAT TO DO:
Overdose unlikely to threaten life. If person takes much larger amount than prescribed, call doctor, poison-control center or hospital emergency room for instructions.

Time lapse before drug works:
15 minutes.

Don't take with:
Other medicines at the same time. Decreases absorption of other drugs.

POSSIBLE ADVERSE REACTIONS OR SIDE EFFECTS

SYMPTOMS	WHAT TO DO
Life-threatening:	
None expected.	
Common:	
• Constipation, appetite loss, weight gain.	Continue. Call doctor when convenient.
• Belching.	Continue. Tell doctor at next visit.
Infrequent:	
• Lower abdominal pain and swelling, bone pain, muscle weakness, swollen wrists or ankles.	Discontinue. Call doctor right away.
• Mood change, nausea, vomiting, weight loss.	Continue. Call doctor when convenient.
Rare:	
None expected.	

SODIUM BICARBONATE

 ## WARNINGS & PRECAUTIONS

Don't take if:
You are allergic to any antacid.

Before you start, consult your doctor:
- If you have kidney disease, liver disease, high blood pressure or congestive heart failure.
- If you have chronic constipation or diarrhea.
- If you have symptoms of appendicitis.
- If you have stomach or intestinal bleeding.

Over age 60:
Adverse reactions and side effects may be more frequent and severe than in younger persons. Diarrhea or constipation particularly likely.

Pregnancy:
Risk to unborn child outweighs drug benefits. Don't use.

Breast-feeding:
Drug passes into milk. Avoid drug or discontinue nursing until you finish medicine. Consult doctor for advice on maintaining milk supply.

Infants & children:
Use only under medical supervision.

Prolonged use:
Prolonged use with calcium supplements or milk leads to too much calcium in blood.

Skin & sunlight:
No problems expected.

Driving, piloting or hazardous work:
No problems expected.

Discontinuing:
May be unnecessary to finish medicine. Follow doctor's instructions.

Others:
Don't take longer than 2 weeks unless under medical supervision.

 ## POSSIBLE INTERACTION WITH OTHER DRUGS

GENERIC NAME OR DRUG CLASS	COMBINED EFFECT
Amphetamine	Increased amphetamine effect.
Anticoagulants	Decreased anticoagulant effect.
Iron supplements	Decreased iron effect.
Meperidine	Increased meperidine effect.
Mexiletine	May slow elimination of mexiletine and cause need to adjust dosage.
Nalidixic acid	Decreased effect of nalidixic acid.
Oxyphenbutazone	Decreased oxyphenbutazone effect.
Para-aminosalicylic acid (PAS)	Decreased PAS effect.
Penicillins	Decreased penicillin effect.
Pentobarbital	Decreased pentobarbital effect.
Phenylbutazone	Decreased phenylbutazone effect.
Pseudoephedrine	Increased pseudoephedrine effect.
Quinidine	Increased quinidine effect.
Salicylates	Decreased salicylate effect.
Sulfa drugs	Decreased sulfa effect.
Tetracyclines	Decreased tetracycline effect.

 ## POSSIBLE INTERACTION WITH OTHER SUBSTANCES

INTERACTS WITH	COMBINED EFFECT
Alcohol:	Decreased antacid effect.
Beverages:	No proven problems.
Cocaine:	No proven problems.
Foods:	Decreased antacid effect. Wait 1 hour after eating.
Marijuana:	No proven problems.
Tobacco:	Decreased antacid effect.

SODIUM CARBONATE

BRAND NAMES

Rolaids

BASIC INFORMATION

Habit forming? No
Prescription needed? No
Available as generic? Yes
Drug class: Antacid

 USES

Treatment for hyperacidity in upper gastrointestinal tract, including stomach and esophagus. Symptoms may be heartburn or acid indigestion. Diseases include peptic ulcer, gastritis, esophagitis, hiatal hernia.

 DOSAGE & USAGE INFORMATION

How to take:
Chewable tablets or wafers—Chew well before swallowing.

When to take:
1 to 3 hours after meals unless directed otherwise by your doctor.

If you forget a dose:
Take as soon as you remember.

What drug does:
- Neutralizes some of the hydrochloric acid in the stomach.
- Reduces action of pepsin, a digestive enzyme.

Time lapse before drug works:
15 minutes.

Don't take with:
Other medicines at the same time. Decreases absorption of other drugs.

 OVERDOSE

SYMPTOMS:
Weakness, fatigue, dizziness.
WHAT TO DO:
Overdose unlikely to threaten life. If person takes much larger amount than prescribed, call doctor, poison-control center or hospital emergency room for instructions.

 POSSIBLE ADVERSE REACTIONS OR SIDE EFFECTS

SYMPTOMS	WHAT TO DO
Life-threatening: None expected.	
Common: Constipation, appetite loss.	Continue. Call doctor when convenient.
Infrequent:	
• Lower abdominal pain and swelling, bone pain, muscle weakness, swollen wrists or ankles.	Discontinue. Call doctor right away.
• Mood change, nausea, vomiting, weight loss.	Continue. Call doctor when convenient.
Rare: None expected.	

WARNINGS & PRECAUTIONS

Don't take if:
You are allergic to any antacid.

Before you start, consult your doctor:
- If you have kidney disease, liver disease, high blood pressure or congestive heart failure.
- If you have chronic constipation or diarrhea.
- If you have symptoms of appendicitis.
- If you have stomach or intestinal bleeding.

Over age 60:
Adverse reactions and side effects may be more frequent and severe than in younger persons. Diarrhea or constipation particularly likely.

Pregnancy:
Risk to unborn child outweighs drug benefits. Don't use.

Breast-feeding:
Drug passes into milk. Avoid drug or discontinue nursing until you finish medicine. Consult doctor for advice on maintaining milk supply.

Infants & children:
Use only under medical supervision.

Prolonged use:
Fluid retention.

Skin & sunlight:
No problems expected.

Driving, piloting or hazardous work:
No problems expected.

Discontinuing:
May be unnecessary to finish medicine. Follow doctor's instructions.

Others:
Don't take longer than 2 weeks unless under medical supervision.

 ## POSSIBLE INTERACTION WITH OTHER DRUGS

GENERIC NAME OR DRUG CLASS	COMBINED EFFECT
Anticoagulants	Decreased anticoagulant effect.
Chlorpromazine	Decreased chlorpromazine effect.
Digitalis preparations	Decreased digitalis effect.
Iron supplements	Decreased iron effect.
Meperidine	Increased meperidine effect.
Nalidixic acid	Decreased effect of nalidixic acid.
Oxyphenbutazone	Decreased oxyphenbutazone effect.
Para-aminosalicylic acid (PAS)	Decreased PAS effect.
Penicillins	Decreased penicillin effect.
Pentobarbital	Decreased pentobarbital effect.
Phenylbutazone	Decreased phenylbutazone effect.
Pseudoephedrine	Increased pseudoephedrine effect.
Sulfa drugs	Decreased sulfa effect.
Tetracyclines	Decreased tetracycline effect.
Vitamins A and C	Decreased vitamin effect.

 ## POSSIBLE INTERACTION WITH OTHER SUBSTANCES

INTERACTS WITH	COMBINED EFFECT
Alcohol:	Decreased antacid effect.
Beverages:	No proven problems.
Cocaine:	No proven problems.
Foods:	Decreased antacid effect. Wait 1 hour after eating.
Marijuana:	No proven problems.
Tobacco:	Decreased antacid effect.

SODIUM FLUORIDE

BRAND NAMES

Denta-Fl	Luride-SF
Flo-Tab	Nafeen
Fluor-A-Day	Pediaflor
Fluorident	Pedi-Dent
Fluoritab	Solu-Flur
Fluorodex	Stay-Flo
Flura	Studaflor
Karidium	Thera-Flur
Luride	

Numerous other multiple vitamin-mineral supplements.

BASIC INFORMATION

Habit forming? No
Prescription needed? Yes
Available as generic? Yes
Drug class: Mineral supplement (fluoride)

USES

Reduces tooth cavities.

DOSAGE & USAGE INFORMATION

How to take:
- Tablet—Swallow with liquid or crumble tablet and take with liquid (*not* milk) or food.
- Liquid—Measure with dropper and take directly or with liquid.
- Chewable tablets—Chew slowly and thoroughly before swallowing.

When to take:
Usually at bedtime after teeth are thoroughly brushed.

If you forget a dose:
Take as soon as you remember. Don't double a forgotten dose. Return to schedule.

Continued next column

OVERDOSE

SYMPTOMS:
Stomach cramps or pain, nausea, faintness, vomiting (possibly bloody), diarrhea, black stools, shallow breathing.
WHAT TO DO:
- **Dial 0 (operator) or 911 (emergency) for an ambulance or medical help. Then give first aid immediately.**
- **See emergency information on inside covers.**

What drug does:
Provides supplemental fluoride to combat tooth decay.

Time lapse before drug works:
8 weeks to provide maximum effect.

Don't take with:
- Other medicine simultaneously.
- See Interaction column.

POSSIBLE ADVERSE REACTIONS OR SIDE EFFECTS

SYMPTOMS	WHAT TO DO
Life-threatening: None expected.	
Common: None expected.	
Infrequent: Rash.	Discontinue. Call doctor right away.
Rare: • Severe upsets (digestive) only with overdose.	Discontinue. Seek emergency treatment.
• Sores in mouth and lips.	Discontinue. Call doctor right away.

SODIUM FLUORIDE

 WARNINGS & PRECAUTIONS

Don't take if:
- Your water supply contains 0.7 parts fluoride per million. Too much fluoride stains teeth permanently.
- You are allergic to any fluoride-containing product.
- You have underactive thyroid.

Before you start, consult your doctor:
Not necessary.

Over age 60:
No problems expected.

Pregnancy:
No problems expected.

Breast-feeding:
No problems expected.

Infants & children:
No problems expected except accidental overdose. Keep vitamin-mineral supplements out of children's reach.

Prolonged use:
Excess may cause discolored teeth and decreased calcium in blood.

Skin & sunlight:
No problems expected.

Driving, piloting or hazardous work:
No problems expected.

Discontinuing:
No problems expected.

Others:
Store in original plastic container. Fluoride decomposes glass.

 POSSIBLE INTERACTION WITH OTHER DRUGS

GENERIC NAME OR DRUG CLASS	COMBINED EFFECT
None	

POSSIBLE INTERACTION WITH OTHER SUBSTANCES

INTERACTS WITH	COMBINED EFFECT
Alcohol:	None expected.
Beverages: Milk.	Prevents absorption of fluoride. Space dose 2 hours before or after milk.
Cocaine:	None expected.
Foods:	None expected.
Marijuana:	None expected.
Tobacco:	None expected.

SODIUM PHOSPHATE

BRAND NAMES

Fleet Phospho-Soda   Sal Hepatica
Phospho-Soda

BASIC INFORMATION

Habit forming? No
Prescription needed? No
Available as generic? Yes
Drug class: Laxative (hyperosmotic)

 USES

Constipation relief.

 DOSAGE & USAGE INFORMATION

How to take:
Liquid, effervescent tablet or powder—Dilute dose in beverage before swallowing.

When to take:
Usually once a day, preferably in the morning.

If you forget a dose:
Take as soon as you remember up to 8 hours before bedtime. If later, wait for next scheduled dose (don't double this dose). Don't take at bedtime.

What drug does:
Draws water into bowel from other body tissues. Causes distention through fluid accumulation, which promotes soft stool and accelerates bowel motion.

Time lapse before drug works:
30 minutes to 3 hours.

Don't take with:
See Interaction column and consult doctor.

 OVERDOSE

SYMPTOMS:
Fluid depletion, weakness, vomiting, fainting.
WHAT TO DO:
Overdose unlikely to threaten life. If person takes much larger amount than prescribed, call doctor, poison-control center or hospital emergency room for instructions.

 POSSIBLE ADVERSE REACTIONS OR SIDE EFFECTS

SYMPTOMS	WHAT TO DO
Life-threatening:	
None expected.	
Common:	
None expected.	
Infrequent:	
• Irregular heartbeat.	Discontinue. Call doctor right away.
• Increased thirst, cramps, nausea, diarrhea, gaseousness.	Continue. Tell doctor at next visit.
Rare:	
Dizziness, confusion, tiredness or weakness.	Continue. Call doctor when convenient.

WARNINGS & PRECAUTIONS

Don't take if:
- You are allergic to any hyperosmotic laxative.
- You have symptoms of appendicitis, inflamed bowel or intestinal blockage.
- You have missed a bowel movement for only 1 or 2 days.

Before you start, consult your doctor:
- If you have congestive heart disease.
- If you have diabetes.
- If you have high blood pressure.
- If you have a colostomy or ileostomy.
- If you have kidney disease.
- If you have a laxative habit.
- If you have rectal bleeding.
- If you take another laxative.

Over age 60:
Adverse reactions and side effects may be more frequent and severe than in younger persons.

Pregnancy:
Salt content may cause fluid retention and swelling. Avoid if possible.

Breast-feeding:
No problems expected.

Infants & children:
Use only under medical supervision.

Prolonged use:
Don't take for more than 1 week unless under a doctor's supervision. May cause laxative dependence.

Skin & sunlight:
No problems expected.

Driving, piloting or hazardous work:
No problems expected.

Discontinuing:
May be unnecessary to finish medicine. Follow doctor's instructions.

Others:
- Don't take to "flush out" your system or as a "tonic."
- Don't take within 2 hours of taking another medicine.

POSSIBLE INTERACTION WITH OTHER DRUGS

GENERIC NAME OR DRUG CLASS	COMBINED EFFECT
Chlordiazepoxide	Decreased chlordiazepoxide effect.
Chlorpromazine	Decreased chlorpromazine effect.
Dicumarol	Decreased dicumarol effect.
Digoxin	Decreased digoxin effect.
Isoniazid	Decreased isoniazid effect.
Mexiletine	May decrease effectiveness of mexiletine.
Tetracyclines	Possible intestinal blockage.

POSSIBLE INTERACTION WITH OTHER SUBSTANCES

INTERACTS WITH	COMBINED EFFECT
Alcohol:	None expected.
Beverages:	None expected.
Cocaine:	None expected.
Foods:	None expected.
Marijuana:	None expected.
Tobacco:	None expected.

SPIRONOLACTONE

BRAND NAMES

Aldactazide	Sincomen
Aldactone	Spironazide
Novospiroton	

BASIC INFORMATION

Habit forming? No
Prescription needed? Yes
Available as generic? Yes
Drug class: Antihypertensive, diuretic

USES

- Reduces high blood pressure.
- Prevents fluid retention.

DOSAGE & USAGE INFORMATION

How to take:
Tablet—Swallow with liquid or food to lessen stomach irritation. If you can't swallow whole, crumble tablet and take with liquid or food.

When to take:
- 1 dose a day—Take after breakfast.
- More than 1 dose a day—Take last dose no later than 6 p.m.

If you forget a dose:
- 1 dose a day—Take as soon as you remember up to 12 hours late. If more than 12 hours, wait for next scheduled dose (don't double this dose).
- More than 1 dose a day—Take as soon as you remember. Wait 6 hours for next dose.

What drug does:
- Increases sodium and water excretion through increased urine production, decreasing body fluid and blood pressure.
- Retains potassium.

Continued next column

OVERDOSE

SYMPTOMS:
Thirst, drowsiness, confusion, fatigue, weakness, nausea, vomiting, irregular heartbeat, excessive blood-pressure drop.
WHAT TO DO:
- **Dial 0 (operator) or 911 (emergency) for an ambulance or medical help. Then give first aid immediately.**
- **See emergency information on inside covers.**

Time lapse before drug works:
3 to 5 days.

Don't take with:
See Interaction column and consult doctor.

POSSIBLE ADVERSE REACTIONS OR SIDE EFFECTS

SYMPTOMS	WHAT TO DO
Life-threatening: None expected.	
Common: Drowsiness or headache, thirst, nausea, vomiting, diarrhea.	Continue. Call doctor when convenient.
Infrequent:	
• Confusion, irregular heartbeat, shortness of breath, unusual sweating.	Discontinue. Call doctor right away.
• Numbness, tingling in hands and feet; menstrual irregularities; tender breasts; change in sex drive.	Continue. Call doctor when convenient.
Rare:	
• Rash or itchy skin.	Discontinue. Call doctor right away.
• Deep voice in women.	Continue. Tell doctor at next visit.

WARNINGS & PRECAUTIONS

Don't take if:
- You are allergic to spironolactone.
- You have impaired kidney function.
- Your serum potassium level is high.

Before you start, consult your doctor:
- If you have had kidney or liver disease.
- If you will have surgery within 2 months, including dental surgery, requiring general or spinal anesthesia.

Over age 60:
- Limit use to 2 to 3 weeks if possible.
- Adverse reactions and side effects may be more frequent and severe than in younger persons.
- Heat or fever can reduce blood pressure. May require dose adjustment.
- Overdose and extended use may cause blood clots.

Pregnancy:
No proven harm to unborn child. Avoid if possible.

Breast-feeding:
No proven problems. Consult doctor.

Infants & children:
Use only under medical supervision.

Prolonged use:
Potassium retention with irregular heartbeat, unusual weakness and confusion.

Skin & sunlight:
No problems expected.

Driving, piloting or hazardous work:
Avoid if you feel drowsy. Otherwise, no problems expected.

Discontinuing:
Consult doctor about adjusting doses of other drugs.

Others:
No problems expected.

POSSIBLE INTERACTION WITH OTHER DRUGS

GENERIC NAME OR DRUG CLASS	COMBINED EFFECT
Acebutolol	Increased antihypertensive effect. Dosages of both drugs may require adjustment.
Amiodarone	Increased risk of heartbeat irregularity due to low potassium.
Anticoagulants (oral)	Decreased anticoagulant effect.
Antihypertensives (other)	Increased antihypertensive effect.
Aspirin	Decreased spironolactone effect.
Calcium supplements	Increased calcium in blood.
Digitalis preparations	Decreased digitalis effect.
Diuretics (other)	Increased effect of both drugs. Beneficial if needed and dose is correct.

Enalapril	Possible excessive potassium in blood.
Labetolol	Increased antihypertensive effects.
Laxatives	Reduced potassium levels.
Lithium	Likely lithium toxicity.
Nitrates	Excessive blood-pressure drop.
Oxprenolol	Increased antihypertensive effect. Dosages of both drugs may require adjustment.
Pentoxifylline	Increased antihypertensive effect.
Potassium supplements	Dangerous potassium retention, causing possible heartbeat irregularity.
Sodium bicarbonate	Reduces high potassium levels.
Triamterene	Dangerous potassium retention.

POSSIBLE INTERACTION WITH OTHER SUBSTANCES

INTERACTS WITH	COMBINED EFFECT
Alcohol:	None expected.
Beverages: Low-salt milk.	Possible potassium toxicity.
Cocaine:	Decreased spironolactone effect.
Foods: Salt.	Don't restrict unless directed by doctor.
Salt substitutes.	Possible potassium toxicity.
Marijuana:	Increased thirst, fainting.
Tobacco:	None expected.

SPIRONOLACTONE & HYDROCHLOROTHIAZIDE

BRAND NAMES

Aldactazide

BASIC INFORMATION

Habit forming? Yes
Prescription needed? Yes
Available as generic? No
Drug class: Antihypertensive, diuretic
    (thiazide)

USES

- Controls, but doesn't cure, high blood pressure.
- Reduces fluid retention (edema).

DOSAGE & USAGE INFORMATION

How to take:
Tablet or capsule—Swallow with liquid. If you can't swallow whole, crumble tablet or open capsule and take with liquid or food.

When to take:
- 1 dose a day—Take after breakfast.
- More than 1 dose a day—Take last dose no later than 6 p.m.

If you forget a dose:
- 1 dose a day—Take as soon as you remember up to 12 hours late. If more than 12 hours, wait for next scheduled dose (don't double this dose).
- More than 1 dose a day—Take as soon as you remember. Wait 6 hours for next dose.

Continued next column

OVERDOSE

SYMPTOMS:
Thirst, drowsiness, confusion, fatigue, weakness, nausea, vomiting, cramps, irregular heartbeat, weak pulse, excessive blood-pressure drop, coma.
WHAT TO DO:
- **Dial 0 (operator) or 911 (emergency) for an ambulance or medical help. Then give first aid immediately.**
- **See emergency information on inside covers.**

What drug does:
- Increases sodium and water excretion through increased urine production.
- Retains potassium.
- Relaxes muscle cells of small arteries.
- Reduced body fluid and relaxed arteries lower blood pressure.

Time lapse before drug works:
4 to 6 hours. May require several weeks to lower blood pressure.

Don't take with:
- See Interaction column and consult doctor.
- Non-prescription drugs without consulting doctor.

POSSIBLE ADVERSE REACTIONS OR SIDE EFFECTS

SYMPTOMS	WHAT TO DO
Life-threatening:	
Irregular heartbeat, weak pulse, shortness of breath.	Discontinue. Seek emergency treatment.
Common:	
Drowsiness, headache, thirst.	Continue. Call doctor when convenient.
Infrequent:	
• Blurred vision, abdominal pain, nausea, vomiting.	Discontinue. Call doctor right away.
• Dizziness, mood change, headache, dry mouth, menstrual irregularities, tender breasts, diminished sex drive, increased sweating, weakness, tiredness, weight gain or loss, confusion, numbness or tingling in hands or feet, diarrhea.	Continue. Call doctor when convenient.
Rare:	
• Sore throat, jaundice, rash.	Discontinue. Call doctor right away.
• Deepening of voice in women.	Continue. Call doctor when convenient.

WARNINGS & PRECAUTIONS

Don't take if:
You are allergic to any thiazide diuretic drug.

Before you start, consult your doctor:
- If you are allergic to any sulfa drug.
- If you have gout, liver, pancreas or kidney disorder.
- If you have had kidney or liver disease.
- If you will have surgery within 2 months, including dental surgery, requiring general or spinal anesthesia.

Over age 60:
- Adverse reactions and side effects may be more frequent and severe than in younger persons, especially dizziness and excessive potassium loss.
- Limit use to 2 to 3 weeks if possible.
- Heat or fever can reduce blood pressure. May require dose adjustment.
- Overdose and extended use may cause blood clots.

Pregnancy:
Risk to unborn child outweighs drug benefits. Don't use.

Breast-feeding:
Drug passes into milk. Avoid drug or discontinue nursing until you finish medicine.

Infants & children:
Use only under medical supervision.

Prolonged use:
- You may need medicine to treat high blood pressure for the rest of your life.
- Potassium retention with irregular heartbeat, unusual weakness and confusion.

Skin & sunlight:
May cause rash or intensify sunburn in areas exposed to sun or sunlamp.

Driving, piloting or hazardous work:
Don't drive or pilot aircraft until you learn how medicine affects you. Don't work around dangerous machinery. Don't climb ladders or work in high places. Danger increases if you drink alcohol or take medicine affecting alertness and reflexes.

Discontinuing:
- Don't discontinue without medical advice.
- Consult doctor about adjusting doses of other drugs.

Others:
- Hot weather and fever may cause dehydration and drop in blood pressure. Dose may require temporary adjustment. Weigh daily and report any unexpected weight decreases to your doctor.
- May cause rise in uric acid, leading to gout.
- May cause blood-sugar rise in diabetics.

POSSIBLE INTERACTION WITH OTHER DRUGS

GENERIC NAME OR DRUG CLASS	COMBINED EFFECT
Acebutolol	Increased antihypertensive effect. Dosages of both drugs may require adjustment.
Allopurinol	Decreased allopurinol effect.
Anticoagulants (oral)	Decreased anticoagulant effect.
Antidepressants (tricyclic)	Dangerous drop in blood pressure. Avoid combination unless under medical supervision.

Continued page 976

POSSIBLE INTERACTION WITH OTHER SUBSTANCES

INTERACTS WITH	COMBINED EFFECT
Alcohol:	Dangerous blood-pressure drop.
Beverages: Low-salt milk.	Possible potassium toxicity.
Cocaine:	Decreased spironolactone effect.
Foods: Salt.	Don't restrict unless directed by doctor.
Salt substitutes.	Possible potassium toxicity.
Marijuana:	May increase blood pressure. Increased thirst, fainting.
Tobacco:	None expected.

SUCRALFATE

BRAND NAMES

Carafate   Sulcrate

BASIC INFORMATION

Habit forming? No
Prescription needed? Yes
Available as generic? No
Drug class: Anti-ulcer

 ## USES

Treatment of duodenal ulcer.

 ## DOSAGE & USAGE INFORMATION

How to take:
Tablet or capsule—Swallow with liquid or food to lessen stomach irritation. If you can't swallow whole, crumble tablet or open capsule and take with liquid or food.

When to take:
1 hour before meals and at bedtime. Allow 2 hours to elapse before taking other prescription medicines.

If you forget a dose:
Take as soon as you remember up to 2 hours late. If more than 2 hours, wait for next scheduled dose (don't double this dose).

What drug does:
Covers ulcer site and protects from acid, enzymes and bile salts.

Time lapse before drug works:
Begins in 30 minutes. May require several days to relieve pain.

Don't take with:
See Interaction column and consult doctor.

 ## OVERDOSE

SYMPTOMS:
No data available yet for this new drug.
WHAT TO DO:
Overdose unlikely to threaten life. If person takes much larger amount than prescribed, call doctor, poison-control center or hospital emergency room for instructions.

 ## POSSIBLE ADVERSE REACTIONS OR SIDE EFFECTS

SYMPTOMS	WHAT TO DO
Life-threatening: None expected.	
Common: Constipation.	Continue. Call doctor when convenient.
Infrequent: Dizziness, sleepiness, rash, itchy skin, abdominal pain, nausea, vomiting, indigestion, back pain.	Continue. Call doctor when convenient.
Rare: None expected.	

SUCRALFATE

WARNINGS & PRECAUTIONS

Don't take if:
You are allergic to sucralfate.

Before you start, consult your doctor:
If you will have surgery within 2 months, including dental surgery, requiring general or spinal anesthesia.

Over age 60:
Adverse reactions and side effects may be more frequent and severe than in younger persons.

Pregnancy:
No proven harm to unborn child. Avoid if possible.

Breast-feeding:
Unknown effects.

Infants & children:
Safety not established.

Prolonged use:
Request blood counts if medicine needed longer than 8 weeks.

Skin & sunlight:
No problems expected.

Driving, piloting or hazardous work:
Don't drive or pilot aircraft until you learn how medicine affects you. Don't work around dangerous machinery. Don't climb ladders or work in high places. Danger increases if you drink alcohol or take medicine affecting alertness and reflexes, such as antihistamines, tranquilizers, sedatives, pain medicine, narcotics and mind-altering drugs.

Discontinuing:
Don't discontinue without consulting doctor. Dose may require gradual reduction if you have taken drug for a long time. Doses of other drugs may also require adjustment.

Others:
No problems expected.

POSSIBLE INTERACTION WITH OTHER DRUGS

GENERIC NAME OR DRUG CLASS	COMBINED EFFECT
Cimetidine	Decreased absorption of cimetidine if taken simultaneously.
Phenytoin	Decreased absorption of phenytoin if taken simultaneously.
Tetracyclines	Decreased absorption of tetracycline if taken simultaneously.

POSSIBLE INTERACTION WITH OTHER SUBSTANCES

INTERACTS WITH	COMBINED EFFECT
Alcohol:	Irritates ulcer. Avoid.
Beverages: Caffeine.	Irritates ulcer. Avoid.
Cocaine:	May make ulcer worse. Avoid.
Foods:	No problems expected.
Marijuana:	May make ulcer worse. Avoid.
Tobacco:	May make ulcer worse. Avoid.

SULFACYTINE

BRAND NAMES

Renoquid

BASIC INFORMATION

Habit forming? No
Prescription needed? Yes
Available as generic? Yes
Drug class: Sulfa (sulfonamide)

 USES

Treatment for infections responsive to this drug.

 DOSAGE & USAGE INFORMATION

How to take:
Tablet—Swallow with liquid. Instructions to take on empty stomach mean 1 hour before or 2 hours after eating.

When to take:
At the same times each day, evenly spaced.

If you forget a dose:
Take as soon as you remember up to 2 hours late. If more than 2 hours, wait for next scheduled dose (don't double this dose).

What drug does:
Interferes with a nutrient (folic acid) necessary for growth and reproduction of bacteria. Will not attack viruses.

Time lapse before drug works:
2 to 5 days to affect infection.

Don't take with:
See Interaction column and consult doctor.

 OVERDOSE

SYMPTOMS:
Less urine, bloody urine, coma.
WHAT TO DO:
- **Dial 0 (operator) or 911 (emergency) for an ambulance or medical help. Then give first aid immediately.**
- **See emergency information on inside covers.**

 POSSIBLE ADVERSE REACTIONS OR SIDE EFFECTS

SYMPTOMS	WHAT TO DO
Life-threatening: None expected.	
Common:	
• Itchy skin, rash.	Discontinue. Call doctor right away.
• Headache, dizziness, appetite loss, nausea, vomiting, diarrhea.	Continue. Call doctor when convenient.
Infrequent: Red, peeling or blistering skin; sore throat; fever; swallowing difficulty; unusual bruising; aching joints or muscles; jaundice.	Discontinue. Call doctor right away.
Rare: Painful urination, low back pain.	Discontinue. Call doctor right away.

WARNINGS & PRECAUTIONS

Don't take if:
You are allergic to any sulfa drug.

Before you start, consult your doctor:
- If you are allergic to carbonic anhydrase inhibitors, oral antidiabetics or thiazide diuretics.
- If you are allergic by nature.
- If you have liver or kidney disease.
- If you have porphyria.
- If you have developed anemia from use of any drug.

Over age 60:
Adverse reactions and side effects may be more frequent and severe than in younger persons.

Pregnancy:
Risk to unborn child outweighs drug benefits. Don't use.

Breast-feeding:
Drug passes into milk. Avoid drug or discontinue nursing until you finish medicine. Consult doctor for advice on maintaining milk supply.

Infants & children:
Don't give to infants younger than 1 month.

Prolonged use:
- May enlarge thyroid gland.
- You may become more susceptible to infections caused by germs not responsive to this drug.
- Request frequent blood counts, liver- and kidney-function studies.

Skin & sunlight:
May cause rash or intensify sunburn in areas exposed to sun or sunlamp.

Driving, piloting or hazardous work:
Avoid if you feel dizzy. Otherwise, no problems expected.

Discontinuing:
Don't discontinue without doctor's advice until you complete prescribed dose, even though symptoms diminish or disappear.

Others:
- Drink 2 quarts of liquid each day to prevent adverse reactions.
- If you require surgery, tell anesthetist you take sulfa. Pentothal anesthesia should not be used.

POSSIBLE INTERACTION WITH OTHER DRUGS

GENERIC NAME OR DRUG CLASS	COMBINED EFFECT
Aminobenzoate potassium	Possible decreased sulfa effect.
Anticoagulants (oral)	Increased anticoagulant effect.
Anticonvulsants (hydantoin)	Toxic effect on brain.
Aspirin	Increased sulfa effect.
Calcium supplements	Decreased sulfa effect.
Isoniazid	Possible anemia.
Methenamine	Possible kidney blockage.
Methotrexate	Increased methotrexate effect.
Oxyphenbutazone	Increased sulfa effect.
Para-aminosalicylic acid (PAS)	Decreased sulfa effect.
Penicillins	Decreased penicillin effect.
Phenylbutazone	Increased sulfa effect.
Probenecid	Increased sulfa effect.
Sulfinpyrazone	Increased sulfa effect.
Trimethoprim	Increased sulfa effect.

POSSIBLE INTERACTION WITH OTHER SUBSTANCES

INTERACTS WITH	COMBINED EFFECT
Alcohol:	Increased alcohol effect.
Beverages: Less than 2 quarts of fluid daily.	Kidney damage.
Cocaine:	None expected.
Foods:	None expected.
Marijuana:	None expected.
Tobacco:	None expected.

SULFAMETHOXAZOLE

BRAND NAMES

Apo-Sulfamethoxazole
Apo-Sulfatrim
Azo Gantanol
Bactrim
Cetamide
Cotrim
Cotrim D.S.
Co-trimoxazole
Gantanol
Gantrisin
Methoxanol
Novotrimel
Protrin
Roubac
Septra
SMZ-TMP
Sulfamethoprim

BASIC INFORMATION

Habit forming? No
Prescription needed? Yes
Available as generic? Yes
Drug class: Sulfa (sulfonamide)

USES

Treatment for infections responsive to this drug.

DOSAGE & USAGE INFORMATION

How to take:
- Tablet—Swallow with liquid. Instructions to take on empty stomach mean 1 hour before or 2 hours after eating.
- Liquid—Shake carefully before measuring.

When to take:
At the same times each day, evenly spaced.

If you forget a dose:
Take as soon as you remember up to 2 hours late. If more than 2 hours, wait for next scheduled dose (don't double this dose).

What drug does:
Interferes with a nutrient (folic acid) necessary for growth and reproduction of bacteria. Will not attack viruses.

Continued next column

OVERDOSE

SYMPTOMS:
Less urine, bloody urine, coma.
WHAT TO DO:
- Dial 0 (operator) or 911 (emergency) for an ambulance or medical help. Then give first aid immediately.
- See emergency information on inside covers.

Time lapse before drug works:
2 to 5 days to affect infection.

Don't take with:
See Interaction column and consult doctor.

POSSIBLE ADVERSE REACTIONS OR SIDE EFFECTS

SYMPTOMS	WHAT TO DO
Life-threatening:	
None expected.	
Common:	
● Itchy skin, rash.	Discontinue. Call doctor right away.
● Headache, dizziness, appetite loss, nausea, vomiting, diarrhea.	Continue. Call doctor when convenient.
Infrequent:	
Red, peeling or blistering skin; sore throat; fever; swallowing difficulty; unusual bruising; aching joints or muscles; jaundice.	Discontinue. Call doctor right away.
Rare:	
Painful urination, low back pain.	Discontinue. Call doctor right away.

WARNINGS & PRECAUTIONS

Don't take if:
You are allergic to any sulfa drug.

Before you start, consult your doctor:
- If you are allergic to carbonic anhydrase inhibitors, oral antidiabetics or thiazide diuretics.
- If you are allergic by nature.
- If you have liver or kidney disease.
- If you have porphyria.
- If you have developed anemia from use of any drug.

Over age 60:
Adverse reactions and side effects may be more frequent and severe than in younger persons.

Pregnancy:
Risk to unborn child outweighs drug benefits. Don't use.

Breast-feeding:
Drug passes into milk. Avoid drug or discontinue nursing until you finish medicine. Consult doctor for advice on maintaining milk supply.

Infants & children:
Don't give to infants younger than 1 month.

Prolonged use:
- May enlarge thyroid gland.
- You may become more susceptible to infections caused by germs not responsive to this drug.
- Request frequent blood counts, liver- and kidney-function studies.

Skin & sunlight:
May cause rash or intensify sunburn in areas exposed to sun or sunlamp.

Driving, piloting or hazardous work:
Avoid if you feel dizzy. Otherwise, no problems expected.

Discontinuing:
Don't discontinue without doctor's advice until you complete prescribed dose, even though symptoms diminish or disappear.

Others:
- Drink 2 quarts of liquid each day to prevent adverse reactions.
- If you require surgery, tell anesthetist you take sulfa. Pentothal anesthesia should not be used.

POSSIBLE INTERACTION WITH OTHER DRUGS

GENERIC NAME OR DRUG CLASS	COMBINED EFFECT
Aminobenzoate potassium	Possible decreased sulfa effect.
Anticoagulants (oral)	Increased anticoagulant effect.
Anticonvulsants (hydantoin)	Toxic effect on brain.
Aspirin	Increased sulfa effect.
Calcium supplements	Decreased sulfa effect.
Isoniazid	Possible anemia.
Methenamine	Possible kidney blockage.
Methotrexate	Increased methotrexate effect.
Oxyphenbutazone	Increased sulfa effect.
Para-aminosalicylic acid (PAS)	Decreased sulfa effect.
Penicillins	Decreased penicillin effect.
Phenylbutazone	Increased sulfa effect.
Probenecid	Increased sulfa effect.
Sulfinpyrazone	Increased sulfa effect.
Trimethoprim	Increased sulfa effect.

POSSIBLE INTERACTION WITH OTHER SUBSTANCES

INTERACTS WITH	COMBINED EFFECT
Alcohol:	Increased alcohol effect.
Beverages: Less than 2 quarts of fluid daily.	Kidney damage.
Cocaine:	None expected.
Foods:	None expected.
Marijuana:	None expected.
Tobacco:	None expected.

SULFASALAZINE

BRAND NAMES

Azulfidine   Salazopyrin
Azulfidine En-Tabs   SAS-500

BASIC INFORMATION

Habit forming? No
Prescription needed? Yes
Available as generic? Yes
Drug class: Sulfa (sulfonamide)

 USES

Treatment for ulceration and bleeding during active phase of ulcerative colitis.

 DOSAGE & USAGE INFORMATION

How to take:
- Tablet—Swallow with liquid. Instructions to take on empty stomach mean 1 hour before or 2 hours after eating.
- Liquid—Shake carefully before measuring.

When to take:
At the same times each day, evenly spaced.

If you forget a dose:
Take as soon as you remember up to 2 hours late. If more than 2 hours, wait for next scheduled dose (don't double this dose).

What drug does:
Anti-inflammatory action reduces tissue destruction in colon.

Time lapse before drug works:
2 to 5 days.

Don't take with:
See Interaction column and consult doctor.

 OVERDOSE

SYMPTOMS:
Less urine, bloody urine, coma.
WHAT TO DO:
- Dial 0 (operator) or 911 (emergency) for an ambulance or medical help. Then give first aid immediately.
- See emergency information on inside covers.

 POSSIBLE ADVERSE REACTIONS OR SIDE EFFECTS

SYMPTOMS	WHAT TO DO
Life-threatening:	
None expected.	
Common:	
• Itchy skin, rash.	Discontinue. Call doctor right away.
• Headache, dizziness, appetite loss, nausea, vomiting, diarrhea.	Continue. Call doctor when convenient.
• Orange urine.	Continue. Tell doctor at next visit.
Infrequent:	
Red, peeling or blistering skin; sore throat; fever; swallowing difficulty; unusual bruising; aching joints or muscles; jaundice.	Discontinue. Call doctor right away.
Rare:	
Painful urination, low back pain.	Discontinue. Call doctor right away.

WARNINGS & PRECAUTIONS

Don't take if:
You are allergic to any sulfa drug.

Before you start, consult your doctor:
- If you are allergic to carbonic anhydrase inhibitors, oral antidiabetics or thiazide diuretics.
- If you are allergic by nature.
- If you have liver or kidney disease.
- If you have porphyria.
- If you have developed anemia from use of any drug.

Over age 60:
Adverse reactions and side effects may be more frequent and severe than in younger persons.

Pregnancy:
Risk to unborn child outweighs drug benefits. Don't use.

Breast-feeding:
Drug passes into milk. Avoid drug or discontinue nursing until you finish medicine. Consult doctor for advice on maintaining milk supply.

Infants & children:
Don't give to infants younger than 1 month.

Prolonged use:
- May enlarge thyroid gland.
- You may become more susceptible to infections caused by germs not responsive to this drug.
- Request frequent blood counts, liver- and kidney-function studies.

Skin & sunlight:
May cause rash or intensify sunburn in areas exposed to sun or sunlamp.

Driving, piloting or hazardous work:
Avoid if you feel dizzy. Otherwise, no problems expected.

Discontinuing:
Don't discontinue without doctor's advice until you complete prescribed dose, even though symptoms diminish or disappear.

Others:
- Drink 2 quarts of liquid each day to prevent adverse reactions.
- If you require surgery, tell anesthetist you take sulfa. Pentothal anesthesia should not be used.

POSSIBLE INTERACTION WITH OTHER DRUGS

GENERIC NAME OR DRUG CLASS	COMBINED EFFECT
Aminobenzoate potassium	Possible decreased sulfa effect.
Antibiotics	Decreased sulfa effect.
Anticoagulants (oral)	Increased anticoagulant effect.
Anticonvulsants (hydantoin)	Toxic effect on brain.
Aspirin	Increased sulfa effect.
Calcium supplements	Decreased sulfa efffect.
Digoxin	Decreased digoxin effect.
Iron supplements	Decreased sulfa effect.
Isoniazid	Possible anemia.
Methenamine	Possible kidney blockage.
Methotrexate	Increased methotrexate effect.
Oxyphenbutazone	Increased sulfa effect.
Para-aminosalicylic acid (PAS)	Decreased sulfa effect.
Penicillins	Decreased penicillin effect.
Phenylbutazone	Increased sulfa effect.
Probenecid	Increased sulfa effect.
Sulfinpyrazone	Increased sulfa effect.
Trimethoprim	Increased sulfa effect.
Vitamin C	Possible kidney damage. Avoid large doses of vitamin C.

POSSIBLE INTERACTION WITH OTHER SUBSTANCES

INTERACTS WITH	COMBINED EFFECT
Alcohol:	Increased alcohol effect.
Beverages: Less than 2 quarts of fluid daily.	Kidney damage.
Cocaine:	None expected.
Foods:	None expected.
Marijuana:	None expected.
Tobacco:	None expected.

SULFINPYRAZONE

BRAND NAMES

Antazone
Anturan
Anturane
Apo-Sulfinpyrazone

Aprazone
Novopyrazone
Zynol

BASIC INFORMATION

Habit forming? No
Prescription needed? Yes
Available as generic? Yes
Drug class: Antigout (uricosuric)

 ## USES

- Treatment for chronic gout.
- Reduces severity of recurrent heart attack. (This use is experimental and not yet approved by F.D.A.)

 ## DOSAGE & USAGE INFORMATION

How to take:
Tablet or capsule—Swallow with liquid or food to lessen stomach irritation. If you can't swallow whole, crumble tablet or open capsule and take with liquid or food.

When to take:
At the same times each day.

If you forget a dose:
Take as soon as you remember up to 2 hours late. If more than 2 hours, wait for next scheduled dose (don't double this dose).

Continued next column

 ## OVERDOSE

SYMPTOMS:
Breathing difficulty, imbalance, convulsions, coma.
WHAT TO DO:
- Dial 0 (operator) or 911 (emergency) for an ambulance or medical help. Then give first aid immediately.
- If patient is unconscious and not breathing, give mouth-to-mouth breathing. If there is no heartbeat, use cardiac massage and mouth-to-mouth breathing (CPR). Don't try to make patient vomit. If you can't get help quickly, take patient to nearest emergency facility.
- See emergency information on inside covers.

What drug does:
Reduces uric-acid level in blood and tissues by increasing amount of uric acid secreted in urine by kidneys.

Time lapse before drug works:
May require 6 months to prevent gout attacks.

Don't take with:
See Interaction column and consult doctor.

 ## POSSIBLE ADVERSE REACTIONS OR SIDE EFFECTS

SYMPTOMS	WHAT TO DO
Life-threatening: None expected.	
Common: None expected.	
Infrequent:	
• Painful or difficult urination.	Discontinue. Call doctor right away.
• Rash, nausea, vomiting, stomach pain, low back pain.	Continue. Call doctor when convenient.
Rare:	
• Black, bloody or tarry stools.	Discontinue. Seek emergency treatment.
• Sore throat; fever; unusual bleeding or bruising; red, painful joints; blood in urine; fatigue or weakness.	Discontinue. Call doctor right away.

WARNINGS & PRECAUTIONS

Don't take if:
- You are allergic to any uricosuric.
- You have acute gout.
- You have active ulcers (stomach or duodenal), enteritis or ulcerative colitis.
- You have blood-cell disorders.
- You are allergic to oxyphenbutazone or phenylbutazone.

Before you start, consult your doctor:
If you have kidney or blood disease.

Over age 60:
Adverse reactions and side effects may be more frequent and severe than in younger persons. You require lower dose because of decreased kidney function.

Pregnancy:
Studies inconclusive on harm to unborn child. Animal studies show fetal abnormalities. Decide with your doctor whether drug benefits justify risk to unborn child.

Breast-feeding:
No proven problems. Consult doctor.

Infants & children:
Not recommended.

Prolonged use:
Possible kidney damage.

Skin & sunlight:
No problems expected.

Driving, piloting or hazardous work:
No problems expected.

Discontinuing:
Don't discontinue without consulting doctor. Dose may require gradual reduction if you have taken drug for a long time. Doses of other drugs may also require adjustment.

Others:
- Drink 10 to 12 glasses of water each day you take this medicine.
- Periodic blood and urine laboratory tests recommended.

POSSIBLE INTERACTION WITH OTHER DRUGS

GENERIC NAME OR DRUG CLASS	COMBINED EFFECT
Anticoagulants (oral)	Increased anticoagulant effect.
Antidiabetics (oral)	Increased antidiabetic effect.
Aspirin	Bleeding tendency. Decreased sulfinpyrazone effect.
Cephalexin	Increased effect of cephalexin.
Cephradine	Increased effect of cephradine.
Contraceptives (oral)	Increased bleeding between menstrual periods.
Diuretics	Decreased sulfinpyrazone effect.
Flecainide	Possible decreased blood-cell production in bone marrow.
Insulin	Increased insulin effect.
Penicillins	Increased penicillin effect.
Probenecid	Possible increased sulfinpyrazone effect.
Salicylates	Bleeding tendency. Decreased sulfinpyrazone effect.
Sulfa drugs	Increased effect of sulfa drugs.
Tocainide	Possible decreased blood-cell production in bone marrow.

POSSIBLE INTERACTION WITH OTHER SUBSTANCES

INTERACTS WITH	COMBINED EFFECT
Alcohol:	Decreased sulfinpyrazone effect.
Beverages: Caffeine drinks.	Decreased sulfinpyrazone effect.
Cocaine:	None expected.
Foods:	None expected.
Marijuana:	Occasional use—None expected. Daily use—May increase blood level of uric acid.
Tobacco:	None expected.

SULFISOXAZOLE

BRAND NAMES

See complete list of brand names in the *Brand Name Directory,* page 957.

BASIC INFORMATION

Habit forming? No
Prescription needed? Yes
Available as generic? Yes
Drug class: Sulfa (sulfonamide)

 USES

Treatment for infections responsive to this drug.

 DOSAGE & USAGE INFORMATION

How to take:
- Tablet—Swallow with liquid. Instructions to take on empty stomach mean 1 hour before or 2 hours after eating.
- Liquid—Shake carefully before measuring.

When to take:
At the same times each day, evenly spaced.

If you forget a dose:
Take as soon as you remember up to 2 hours late. If more than 2 hours, wait for next scheduled dose (don't double this dose).

What drug does:
Interferes with a nutrient (folic acid) necessary for growth and reproduction of bacteria. Will not attack viruses.

Time lapse before drug works:
2 to 5 days to affect infection.

Don't take with:
See Interaction column and consult doctor.

 OVERDOSE

SYMPTOMS:
Less urine, bloody urine, coma.
WHAT TO DO:
- **Dial 0 (operator) or 911 (emergency) for an ambulance or medical help. Then give first aid immediately.**
- **See emergency information on inside covers.**

 POSSIBLE ADVERSE REACTIONS OR SIDE EFFECTS

SYMPTOMS	WHAT TO DO
Life-threatening: None expected.	
Common:	
• Itchy skin, rash.	Discontinue. Call doctor right away.
• Headache, dizziness, appetite loss, nausea, vomiting, diarrhea.	Continue. Call doctor when convenient.
Infrequent: Red, peeling or blistering skin; sore throat; fever; swallowing difficulty; unusual bruising; aching joints or muscles; jaundice.	Discontinue. Call doctor right away.
Rare: Painful urination, low back pain.	Discontinue. Call doctor right away.

WARNINGS & PRECAUTIONS

Don't take if:
You are allergic to any sulfa drug.

Before you start, consult your doctor:
- If you are allergic to carbonic anhydrase inhibitors, oral antidiabetics or thiazide diuretics.
- If you are allergic by nature.
- If you have liver or kidney disease.
- If you have porphyria.
- If you have developed anemia from use of any drug.

Over age 60:
Adverse reactions and side effects may be more frequent and severe than in younger persons.

Pregnancy:
Risk to unborn child outweighs drug benefits. Don't use.

Breast-feeding:
Drug passes into milk. Avoid drug or discontinue nursing until you finish medicine. Consult doctor for advice on maintaining milk supply.

Infants & children:
Don't give to infants younger than 1 month.

Prolonged use:
- May enlarge thyroid gland.
- You may become more susceptible to infections caused by germs not responsive to this drug.
- Request frequent blood counts, liver- and kidney-function studies.

Skin & sunlight:
May cause rash or intensify sunburn in areas exposed to sun or sunlamp.

Driving, piloting or hazardous work:
Avoid if you feel dizzy. Otherwise, no problems expected.

Discontinuing:
Don't discontinue without doctor's advice until you complete prescribed dose, even though symptoms diminish or disappear.

Others:
- Drink 2 quarts of liquid each day to prevent adverse reactions.
- If you require surgery, tell anesthetist you take sulfa.

POSSIBLE INTERACTION WITH OTHER DRUGS

GENERIC NAME OR DRUG CLASS	COMBINED EFFECT
Aminobenzoate potassium	Possible decreased sulfisoxazole effect.
Anticoagulants (oral)	Increased anticoagulant effect.
Anticonvulsants (hydantoin)	Toxic effect on brain.
Aspirin	Increased sulfa effect.
Calcium supplements	Decreased sulfa effect.
Flecainide	Possible decreased blood-cell production in bone marrow.
Isoniazid	Possible anemia.
Methenamine	Possible kidney blockage.
Methotrexate	Increased possibility of toxic side effects from methotrexate.
Oxyphenbutazone	Increased sulfa effect.
Para-aminosalicylic acid (PAS)	Decreased sulfa effect.
Penicillins	Decreased penicillin effect.
Phenylbutazone	Increased sulfa effect.
Probenecid	Increased sulfa effect.
Sulfinpyrazone	Increased sulfa effect.
Tocainide	Possible decreased blood-cell production in bone marrow.
Trimethoprim	Increased sulfa effect.

POSSIBLE INTERACTION WITH OTHER SUBSTANCES

INTERACTS WITH	COMBINED EFFECT
Alcohol:	Increased alcohol effect.
Beverages: Less than 2 quarts of fluid daily.	Kidney damage.
Cocaine:	None expected.
Foods:	None expected.
Marijuana:	None expected.
Tobacco:	None expected.

SULFONAMIDES & PHENAZOPYRIDINE

BRAND AND GENERIC NAMES

Azo Gantanol
Azo Gantrisin
Azo-Soxazole
Azo-Sulfamethoxazole
Azo-Sulfisoxazole
Suldiazo

Sulfafurazole &
  Phenazopyridine
SULFAMETHOXAZOLE
  & PHENAZOPYRIDINE
SULFISOXAZOLE &
  PHENAZOPYRIDINE

BASIC INFORMATION

Habit forming? No
Prescription needed? Yes
Available as generic? Yes
Drug class: Analgesic (urinary) sulfonamide

 USES

- Treatment for infections responsive to this drug.
- Relieves pain of lower urinary-tract irritation, as in cystitis, urethritis or prostatitis.

 DOSAGE & USAGE INFORMATION

How to take:
Tablet—Swallow with liquid. Instructions to take on empty stomach mean 1 hour before or 2 hours after eating.

When to take:
At the same times each day, evenly spaced.

If you forget a dose:
Take as soon as you remember up to 2 hours late. If more than 2 hours, wait for next scheduled dose (don't double this dose).

Continued next column

 OVERDOSE

SYMPTOMS:
Less urine, bloody urine, shortness of breath, weakness, coma.
WHAT TO DO:
- Dial 0 (operator) or 911 (emergency) for an ambulance or medical help. Then give first aid immediately.
- See emergency information on inside covers.

What drug does:
- Interferes with a nutrient (folic acid) necessary for growth and reproduction of bacteria. Will not attack viruses.
- Anesthetizes lower urinary tract. Relieves pain, burning, pressure and urgency to urinate.

Time lapse before drug works:
2 to 5 days to affect infection.

Don't take with:
See Interaction column and consult doctor.

 POSSIBLE ADVERSE REACTIONS OR SIDE EFFECTS

SYMPTOMS	WHAT TO DO
Life-threatening:	
None expected.	
Common:	
• Rash, itchy skin.	Discontinue. Call doctor right away.
• Dizziness, diarrhea, headache, appetite loss, nausea, vomiting.	Continue. Call doctor when convenient.
Infrequent:	
• Joint pain; swallowing difficulty; pale skin; blistering; peeling of skin; sore throat, fever, mouth sores; unexplained bleeding or bruising; weakness; jaundice; increased sun sensitivity.	Discontinue. Call doctor right away.
• Abdominal pain, indigestion.	Continue. Call doctor when convenient.
Rare:	
Back pain, neck swelling.	Discontinue. Call doctor right away.

WARNINGS & PRECAUTIONS

Don't take if:
- You are allergic to any sulfa drug or urinary analgesic.
- You have hepatitis.

Before you start, consult your doctor:
- If you are allergic to carbonic anhydrase inhibitors, oral antidiabetics or thiazide diuretics.
- If you are allergic by nature.
- If you have liver or kidney disease, porphyria.
- If you have developed anemia from use of any drug.

Over age 60:
Adverse reactions and side effects may be more frequent and severe than in younger persons.

Pregnancy:
Risk to unborn child outweighs drug benefits. Don't use.

Breast-feeding:
Drug passes into milk. Avoid drug or discontinue nursing until you finish medicine. Consult doctor for advice on maintaining milk supply.

Infants & children:
Don't give to infants younger than 1 month.

Prolonged use:
- May enlarge thyroid gland.
- You may become more susceptible to infections caused by germs not responsive to this drug.
- Request frequent blood counts, liver- and kidney-function studies.
- Orange or yellow skin.
- Anemia. Occasional blood studies recommended.

Skin & sunlight:
May cause rash or intensify sunburn in areas exposed to sun or sunlamp.

Driving, piloting or hazardous work:
Avoid if you feel dizzy. Otherwise, no problems expected.

Discontinuing:
Don't discontinue without doctor's advice until you complete prescribed dose, even though symptoms diminish or disappear.

Others:
- Drink 2 quarts of liquid each day to prevent adverse reactions.
- If you require surgery, tell anesthetist you take sulfa.
- Will probably cause urine to be reddish orange. Requires no action.

POSSIBLE INTERACTION WITH OTHER DRUGS

GENERIC NAME OR DRUG CLASS	COMBINED EFFECT
Aminobenzoate potassium	Possible decreased sulfa effect.
Anticoagulants (oral)	Increased anticoagulant effect.
Anticonvulsants (hydantoin)	Toxic effect on brain.
Aspirin	Increased sulfa effect.
Isoniazid	Possible anemia.
Methenamine	Possible kidney blockage.
Methotrexate	Increased methotrexate effect.
Oxyphenbutazone	Increased sulfa effect.
Para-aminosalicylic acid (PAS)	Decreased sulfa effect.
Penicillins	Decreased penicillin effect.
Phenylbutazone	Increased sulfa effect.
Probenecid	Increased sulfa effect.
Sulfinpyrazone	Increased sulfa effect.
Trimethoprim	Increased sulfa effect.

POSSIBLE INTERACTION WITH OTHER SUBSTANCES

INTERACTS WITH	COMBINED EFFECT
Alcohol:	Increased alcohol effect.
Beverages: Less than 2 quarts of fluid daily.	Kidney damage.
Cocaine:	None expected.
Foods:	None expected.
Marijuana:	None expected.
Tobacco:	None expected.

SULINDAC

BRAND NAMES

Clinoril

BASIC INFORMATION

Habit forming? No
Available as generic? Yes
Prescription needed? Yes
Drug class: Anti-inflammatory (non-steroid)

 USES

- Treatment for joint pain, stiffness, inflammation and swelling of arthritis and gout.
- Pain reliever.

 DOSAGE & USAGE INFORMATION

How to take:
Tablet—Swallow with liquid or food to lessen stomach irritation. If you can't swallow whole, crumble tablet and take with liquid or food.

When to take:
At the same times each day.

If you forget a dose:
Take as soon as you remember up to 2 hours late. If more than 2 hours, wait for next scheduled dose (don't double this dose).

What drug does:
Reduces tissue concentration of prostaglandins (hormones which produce inflammation and pain).

Time lapse before drug works:
Begins in 4 to 24 hours. May require 3 weeks regular use for maximum benefit.

Don't take with:
See Interaction column and consult doctor.

 OVERDOSE

SYMPTOMS:
Confusion, agitation, incoherence, convulsions, possible hemorrhage from stomach or intestine, coma.
WHAT TO DO:
- Dial 0 (operator) or 911 (emergency) for an ambulance or medical help. Then give first aid immediately.
- See emergency information on inside covers.

 POSSIBLE ADVERSE REACTIONS OR SIDE EFFECTS

SYMPTOMS	WHAT TO DO
Life-threatening: None expected.	
Common:	
• Dizziness, nausea, pain.	Continue. Call doctor when convenient.
• Headache.	Continue. Tell doctor at next visit.
Infrequent: Depression, drowsiness, ringing in ears, constipation or diarrhea, vomiting, swollen feet or legs.	Continue. Call doctor when convenient.
Rare:	
• Convulsions; confusion; rash, hives or itchy skin; blurred vision; black, bloody or tarry stool; difficult breathing; tightness in chest; rapid heartbeat; unusual bleeding or bruising; blood in urine; jaundice.	Discontinue. Call doctor right away.
• Frequent, painful or difficult urination; fatigue; weakness.	Continue. Call doctor when convenient.

WARNINGS & PRECAUTIONS

Don't take if:
- You are allergic to aspirin or any non-steroid, anti-inflammatory drug.
- You have gastritis, peptic ulcer, enteritis, ileitis, ulcerative colitis, asthma, heart failure, high blood pressure or bleeding problems.
- You have had recent rectal bleeding and suppository form has been prescribed.
- Patient is younger than 15.

Before you start, consult your doctor:
- If you have epilepsy.
- If you have Parkinson's disease.
- If you have been mentally ill.
- If you have had kidney disease or impaired kidney function.

Over age 60:
Adverse reactions and side effects may be more frequent and severe than in younger persons.

Pregnancy:
Studies inconclusive on harm to unborn child. Decide with your doctor whether drug benefits justify risk to unborn child.

Breast-feeding:
May harm child. Avoid.

Infants & children:
Not recommended for those younger than 15. Use only under medical supervision.

Prolonged use:
- Eye damage.
- Reduced hearing.
- Sore throat, fever.
- Weight gain.

Skin & sunlight:
No problems expected.

Driving, piloting or hazardous work:
Don't drive or pilot aircraft until you learn how medicine affects you. Don't work around dangerous machinery. Don't climb ladders or work in high places. Danger increases if you drink alcohol or take medicine affecting alertness and reflexes, such as antihistamines, tranquilizers, sedatives, pain medicine, narcotics and mind-altering drugs.

Discontinuing:
Don't discontinue without consulting doctor. Dose may require gradual reduction if you have taken drug for a long time. Doses of other drugs may also require adjustment.

Others:
No problems expected.

POSSIBLE INTERACTION WITH OTHER DRUGS

GENERIC NAME OR DRUG CLASS	COMBINED EFFECT
Acebutolol	Decreased antihypertensive effect of acebutolol.
Anticoagulants (oral)	Increased risk of bleeding.
Aspirin	Increased risk of stomach ulcer.
Cortisone drugs	Increased risk of stomach ulcer.
Furosemide	Decreased diuretic effect of furosemide.
Gold compounds	Possible increased likelihood of kidney damage.
Ketoprofen	Increased possibility of internal bleeding.
Minoxidil	Decreased minoxidil effect.
Oxprenolol	Decreased antihypertensive effect of oxprenolol.
Oxyphenbutazone	Possible stomach ulcer.
Phenylbutazone	Possible stomach ulcer.
Probenecid	Increased sulindac effect.
Thyroid hormones	Rapid heartbeat, blood-pressure rise.

POSSIBLE INTERACTION WITH OTHER SUBSTANCES

INTERACTS WITH	COMBINED EFFECT
Alcohol:	Possible stomach ulcer or bleeding.
Beverages:	None expected.
Cocaine:	None expected.
Foods:	None expected.
Marijuana:	Increased pain relief from sulindac.
Tobacco:	None expected.

SUPROFEN

BRAND NAMES

Suprol

BASIC INFORMATION

Habit forming? No
Prescription needed? Yes
Available as generic? No
Drug class: Analgesic, antidysmenorreal
(non-steroidal anti-inflammatory
analgesic [NSAIA])

 USES

- Treatment of pain.
- Treatment of soft-tissue athletic injuries.
- Treats dysmenorrhea.

 DOSAGE & USAGE INFORMATION

How to take:
Capsules—Take with full glass of water while
sitting or standing upright. Take on an empty
stomach, either 1/2 hour before or 2 hours after
meals. If stomach irritation occurs, may take
with food or aluminum hydroxide or magnesium
hydroxide antacids.

When to take:
At the same times each day.

If you forget a dose:
Take as soon as you remember up to 2 hours
late. If more than 2 hours, wait for next
scheduled dose (don't double this dose).

What drug does:
Reduces tissue concentration of prostaglandins
(hormones which produce inflammation and
pain).

Time lapse before drug works:
Begins in 4 to 24 hours. May require 3 weeks
regular use for maximum benefit.

Continued next column

 OVERDOSE

SYMPTOMS:
**Confusion, agitation, incoherence,
convulsions, possible hemorrhage from
stomach or intestine, coma.**
WHAT TO DO
- **Dial 0 (operator) or 911 (emergency) for an
  ambulance or medical help. Then give first
  aid immediately.**
- **See emergency information on inside
  covers.**

Don't take with:
- Large doses of acetaminophen. Combination
  increases possibility of kidney damage.
- See Interaction column and consult doctor.

 POSSIBLE ADVERSE REACTIONS OR SIDE EFFECTS

SYMPTOMS	WHAT TO DO
Life-threatening:	
Hives, rash, intense itching, faintness soon after a dose (anaphylaxis); breathing difficulty; tightness in chest; rapid heartbeat.	Discontinue. Seek emergency treatment.
Common:	
Dizziness, headache, nausea, pain, depression, drowsiness, ringing in ears.	Continue. Call doctor when convenient.
Infrequent:	
• Flank pain.	Discontinue. Call doctor right away.
• Constipation or diarrhea, vomiting.	Continue. Call doctor when convenient.
Rare:	
• Bloody or black, tarry stools; convulsions; confusion; rash, hives or itch; blurred vision; unusual bleeding or bruising; jaundice; blood in urine; difficult, painful or frequent urination.	Discontinue. Call doctor right away.
• Fatigue, weakness.	Continue. Call doctor when convenient.

 WARNINGS & PRECAUTIONS

Don't take if:
- You are allergic to suprofen, aspirin or any
  non-steroid, anti-inflammatory drug.
- You have gastritis, peptic ulcer, enteritis,
  ileitis, ulcerative colitis, asthma, heart failure,
  high blood pressure or bleeding problems.
- Patient is younger than 15.

Before you start, consult your doctor:
- If you have epilepsy or Parkinson's disease.
- If you have been mentally ill.
- If you have had kidney disease or impaired
  kidney function.

Over age 60:
Adverse reactions and side effects may be more frequent and severe than in younger persons.

Pregnancy:
Studies inconclusive on harm to unborn child. Decide with your doctor whether drug benefits justify risk to unborn child.

Breast-feeding:
May harm child. Avoid.

Infants & children:
Not recommended for anyone younger than 15. Use only under medical supervision.

Prolonged use:
- Eye damage.
- Reduced hearing.
- Sore throat, fever.
- Weight gain.

Skin & sunlight:
No problems expected.

Driving, piloting or hazardous work:
Don't drive or pilot aircraft until you learn how medicine affects you. Don't work around dangerous machinery. Don't climb ladders or work in high places. Danger increases if you drink alcohol or take medicine affecting alertness and reflexes, such as antihistamines, tranquilizers, sedatives, pain medicine, narcotics and mind-altering drugs.

Discontinuing:
Don't discontinue without consulting doctor. Dose may require gradual reduction if you have taken drug for a long time. Doses of other drugs may also require adjustment.

Others:
No problems expected.

POSSIBLE INTERACTION WITH OTHER DRUGS

GENERIC NAME OR DRUG CLASS	COMBINED EFFECT
Acebutolol	Decreased antihypertensive effect of acebutolol.
Anticoagulants (oral)	Increased risk of bleeding.
Any other non-steroidal anti-inflammatory analgesic, such as oxyphenbutazone, phenylbutazone, fenoprofen, ibuprofen, indomethacin, meclofenamate, naproxen, salicylates, sulindac, tolmetin	Increased possibility of internal bleeding.
Aspirin	Increased risk of stomach ulcer.
Cortisone drugs	Increased risk of stomach ulcer and bleeding.
Furosemide	Decreased diuretic effect of furosemide.
Gold compounds	Possible increased likelihood of kidney damage.
Lithium	May increase lithium in blood.
Minoxidil	Decreased minoxidil effect.
Nifedipine	Increases chance of nifedipine toxicity
Oxprenolol	Increased antihypertensive effect of oxprenolol.
Oxyphenbutazone	Possible stomach ulcer.
Phenylbutazone	Possible stomach ulcer.
Probenecid	Increased suprofen effect.
Thyroid hormones	Rapid heartbeat, blood-pressure rise.
Verapamil	Increases chance of verapamil toxicity.

POSSIBLE INTERACTION WITH OTHER SUBSTANCES

INTERACTS WITH	COMBINED EFFECT
Alcohol:	Possible stomach ulcer or bleeding. Avoid.
Beverages:	None expected.
Cocaine:	None expected.
Foods:	None expected.
Marijuana:	Increased pain relief from suprofen.
Tobacco:	None expected.

TALBUTAL (BUTALBITAL)

BRAND NAMES

Axotal
Buff-A-Comp
Butal Compound
Fiorinal
Isollyl
Lanorinal

Lotusate
Marnal
Plexonal
Protensin
Sandoptal
Tenstan

BASIC INFORMATION

Habit forming? Yes
Prescription needed? Yes
Available as generic? Yes
Drug class: Sedative, hypnotic (barbiturate)

 ## USES

- Reduces anxiety or nervous tension (low dose).
- Relieves insomnia (higher bedtime dose).

 ## DOSAGE & USAGE INFORMATION

How to take:
Tablet or capsule—Swallow with liquid or food to lessen stomach irritation. If you can't swallow whole, crumble tablet or open capsule and take with liquid or food.

When to take:
At the same times each day.

If you forget a dose:
Take as soon as you remember up to 2 hours late. If more than 2 hours, wait for next scheduled dose (don't double this dose).

What drug does:
May partially block nerve impulses at nerve-cell connections.

Time lapse before drug works:
60 minutes.

Don't take with:
- Non-prescription drugs without consulting doctor.
- See Interaction column and consult doctor.

 ## OVERDOSE

SYMPTOMS:
Deep sleep, weak pulse, coma.
WHAT TO DO:
- **Dial 0 (operator) or 911 (emergency) for an ambulance or medical help. Then give first aid immediately.**
- **See emergency information on inside covers.**

 ## POSSIBLE ADVERSE REACTIONS OR SIDE EFFECTS

SYMPTOMS	WHAT TO DO
Life-threatening: None expected.	
Common: Dizziness, drowsiness, "hangover" effect.	Continue. Call doctor when convenient.
Infrequent: • Rash or hives; swollen face, lip, eyelids; sore throat; fever.	Discontinue. Call doctor right away.
• Depression, confusion, slurred speech, diarrhea, nausea, vomiting, joint or muscle pain.	Continue. Call doctor when convenient.
Rare: • Agitation, slow heartbeat, difficult breathing, jaundice.	Discontinue. Call doctor right away.
• Unexplained bleeding or bruising.	Continue. Call doctor when convenient.

 ## WARNINGS & PRECAUTIONS

Don't take if:
- You are allergic to any barbiturate.
- You have porphyria.

Before you start, consult your doctor:
- If you have epilepsy, kidney or liver damage, asthma, anemia, or chronic pain.
- If you will have surgery within 2 months, including dental surgery, requiring general or spinal anesthesia.

Over age 60:
Adverse reactions and side effects may be more frequent and severe than in younger persons. Use small doses.

Pregnancy:
Risk to unborn child outweighs drug benefits. Don't use.

Breast-feeding:
Drug passes into milk. Avoid drug or discontinue nursing until you finish medicine. Consult doctor for advice on maintaining milk supply.

Infants & children:
Use only under doctor's supervision.

Prolonged use:
- May cause addiction, anemia, chronic intoxication.
- May lower body temperature, making exposure to cold temperatures hazardous.

Skin & sunlight:
May cause rash or intensify sunburn in areas exposed to sun or sunlamp.

Driving, piloting or hazardous work:
Don't drive or pilot aircraft until you learn how medicine affects you. Don't work around dangerous machinery. Don't climb ladders or work in high places. Danger increases if you drink alcohol or take medicine affecting alertness and reflexes.

Discontinuing:
May be unnecessary to finish medicine. Follow doctor's instructions. If you develop withdrawal symptoms of hallucinations, agitation or sleeplessness after discontinuing, call doctor right away.

Others:
No problems expected.

 POSSIBLE INTERACTION WITH OTHER DRUGS

GENERIC NAME OR DRUG CLASS	COMBINED EFFECT
Anticoagulants (oral)	Decreased anticoagulant effect.
Anticonvulsants	Changed seizure patterns.
Antidepressants (tricyclics)	Decreased antidepressant effect. Possible dangerous oversedation.
Antidiabetics (oral)	Increased talbutal (butalbital) effect.
Antihistamines	Dangerous sedation. Avoid.
Anti-inflammatory drugs (non-steroidal)	Decreased anti-inflammatory effect.
Aspirin	Decreased aspirin effect.
Beta-adrenergic blockers	Decreased effect of beta-adrenergic blocker.
Contraceptives (oral)	Decreased contraceptive effect.
Cortisone drugs	Decreased cortisone effect.
Digitoxin	Decreased digitoxin effect.
Doxycycline	Decreased doxycycline effect.
Dronabinol	Increased effects of both drugs. Avoid.
Griseofulvin	Decreased griseofulvin effect.
Indapamide	Increased indapamide effect.
MAO inhibitors	Increased talbutal (butalbital) effect.
Mind-altering drugs	Dangerous sedation. Avoid.
Molindone	Increased sedative effect.
Narcotics	Dangerous sedation. Avoid.
Pain relievers	Dangerous sedation. Avoid.
Sedatives	Dangerous sedation. Avoid.
Sleep inducers	Dangerous sedation. Avoid.
Tranquilizers	Dangerous sedation. Avoid.
Valproic acid	Increased talbutal (butalbital) effect.

 POSSIBLE INTERACTION WITH OTHER SUBSTANCES

INTERACTS WITH	COMBINED EFFECT
Alcohol:	Possible fatal oversedation. Avoid.
Beverages:	None expected.
Cocaine:	Decreased talbutal (butalbital) effect.
Foods:	None expected.
Marijuana:	Excessive sedation. Avoid.
Tobacco:	None expected.

TEMAZEPAM

BRAND NAMES

Restoril

BASIC INFORMATION

Habit forming? Yes
Prescription needed? Yes
Available as generic? Yes
Drug class: Tranquilizer (benzodiazepine)

 USES

Treatment for insomnia.

 DOSAGE & USAGE INFORMATION

How to take:
Tablet or capsule—Swallow with liquid. If you can't swallow whole, crumble tablet or open capsule and take with liquid or food.

When to take:
At the same time each day, according to instructions on prescription label.

If you forget a dose:
Take as soon as you remember up to 2 hours late. If more than 2 hours, wait for next scheduled dose (don't double this dose).

What drug does:
Affects limbic system of brain—part that controls emotions. Induces near-normal sleep pattern.

Time lapse before drug works:
30 minutes.

Don't take with:
See Interaction column and consult doctor.

 OVERDOSE

SYMPTOMS:
Drowsiness, weakness, tremor, stupor, coma.
WHAT TO DO:
- **Dial 0 (operator) or 911 (emergency) for an ambulance or medical help. Then give first aid immediately.**
- **If patient is unconscious and not breathing, give mouth-to-mouth breathing. If there is no heartbeat, use cardiac massage and mouth-to-mouth breathing (CPR). Don't try to make patient vomit. If you can't get help quickly, take patient to nearest emergency facility.**
- **See emergency information on inside covers.**

 POSSIBLE ADVERSE REACTIONS OR SIDE EFFECTS

SYMPTOMS	WHAT TO DO
Life-threatening:	
None expected.	
Common:	
Clumsiness, drowsiness, dizziness.	Continue. Call doctor when convenient.
Infrequent:	
● Hallucinations, confusion, depression, irritability, rash, itchy skin, change in vision.	Discontinue. Call doctor right away.
● Constipation or diarrhea, nausea, vomiting, difficult urination.	Continue. Call doctor when convenient.
Rare:	
● Slow heartbeat, difficult breathing.	Discontinue. Seek emergency treatment.
● Mouth or throat ulcers, jaundice.	Discontinue. Call doctor right away.

WARNINGS & PRECAUTIONS

Don't take if:
- You are allergic to any benzodiazepine.
- You have myasthenia gravis.
- You are active or recovering alcoholic.
- Patient is younger than 6 months.

Before you start, consult your doctor:
- If you have liver, kidney or lung disease.
- If you have diabetes, epilepsy or porphyria.

Over age 60:
Adverse reactions and side effects may be more frequent and severe than in younger persons. May develop agitation, rage or "hangover" effect.

Pregnancy:
Risk to unborn child outweighs drug benefits. Don't use.

Breast-feeding:
Drug passes into milk. Avoid drug or discontinue nursing until you finish medicine. Consult doctor for advice on maintaining milk supply.

Infants & children:
Use only under medical supervision for children older than 6 months.

Prolonged use:
May impair liver function.

Skin & sunlight:
No problems expected.

Driving, piloting or hazardous work:
Don't drive or pilot aircraft until you learn how medicine affects you. Don't work around dangerous machinery. Don't climb ladders or work in high places. Danger increases if you drink alcohol or take medicine affecting alertness and reflexes.

Discontinuing:
Don't discontinue without doctor's advice until you complete prescribed dose, even though symptoms diminish or disappear.

Others:
- Hot weather, heavy exercise and profuse sweat may reduce excretion and cause overdose.
- Blood sugar may rise in diabetics, requiring insulin adjustment.

POSSIBLE INTERACTION WITH OTHER DRUGS

GENERIC NAME OR DRUG CLASS	COMBINED EFFECT
Anticonvulsants	Change in seizure frequency or severity.
Antidepressants	Increased sedative effect of both drugs.
Antihistamines	Increased sedative effect of both drugs.
Antihypertensives	Excessively low blood pressure.
Cimetidine	Excess sedation.
Disulfiram	Increased temazepam effect.
Dronabinol	Increased effects of both drugs. Avoid.
MAO inhibitors	Convulsions, deep sedation, rage.
Molindone	Increased sedative effect.
Narcotics	Increased sedative effect of both drugs.
Sedatives	Increased sedative effect of both drugs.
Tranquilizers	Increased sedative effect of both drugs.

POSSIBLE INTERACTION WITH OTHER SUBSTANCES

INTERACTS WITH	COMBINED EFFECT
Alcohol:	Heavy sedation. Avoid.
Beverages:	None expected.
Cocaine:	Decreased temazepam effect.
Foods:	None expected.
Marijuana:	Heavy sedation. Avoid.
Tobacco:	Decreased temazepam effect.

TERBUTALINE

BRAND NAMES

Brethaire   Bricanyl
Brethine

BASIC INFORMATION

Habit forming? No
Prescription needed? Yes
Available as generic? No
Drug class: Sympathomimetic

 USES

Treatment of bronchial asthma, bronchitis and emphysema.

 DOSAGE & USAGE INFORMATION

How to take:
Tablet or capsule—Swallow with liquid or food to lessen stomach irritation.

When to take:
At the same times each day.

If you forget a dose:
Take as soon as you remember up to 2 hours late. If more than 2 hours, wait for next scheduled dose (don't double this dose).

What drug does:
Dilates constricted bronchial tubes.

Time lapse before drug works:
30 minutes.

Don't take with:
See Interaction column and consult doctor.

 OVERDOSE

SYMPTOMS:
Rapid heartbeat, chest pain, tremors.
WHAT TO DO:
- Dial 0 (operator) or 911 (emergency) for an ambulance or medical help. Then give first aid immediately.
- If patient is unconscious and not breathing, give mouth-to-mouth breathing. If there is no heartbeat, use cardiac massage and mouth-to-mouth breathing (CPR). Don't try to make patient vomit. If you can't get help quickly, take patient to nearest emergency facility.
- See emergency information on inside covers.

 POSSIBLE ADVERSE REACTIONS OR SIDE EFFECTS

SYMPTOMS	WHAT TO DO
Life-threatening: None expected.	
Common: Headache, nervousness, restlessness, trembling.	Continue. Call doctor when convenient.
Infrequent:	
• Drowsiness, nausea, vomiting, fast or pounding heartbeat, cramps, weakness.	Discontinue. Call doctor right away.
• Unusual sweating.	Continue. Call doctor when convenient.
Rare: None expected.	

WARNINGS & PRECAUTIONS

Don't take if:
You are allergic to any sympathomimetic.

Before you start, consult your doctor:
- If you have diabetes.
- If you have heart disease or high blood pressure.
- If you have overactive thyroid.
- If you have had seizures.
- If you take non-prescription amphetamines or other asthma medicines.

Over age 60:
Adverse reactions and side effects may be more frequent and severe than in younger persons.

Pregnancy:
No proven harm to unborn child. Avoid if possible. May prolong labor and delivery.

Breast-feeding:
No proven problems. Avoid if possible.

Infants & children:
Use only under medical supervision.

Prolonged use:
No problems expected.

Skin & sunlight:
No problems expected.

Driving, piloting or hazardous work:
Avoid if you feel drowsy. Otherwise, no problems expected.

Discontinuing:
May be unnecessary to finish medicine. Follow doctor's instructions.

Others:
If troubled breathing does not improve or worsens after using medicine, don't increase dose. Consult doctor.

POSSIBLE INTERACTION WITH OTHER DRUGS

GENERIC NAME OR DRUG CLASS	COMBINED EFFECT
Albuterol	Increased effect of both drugs, especially harmful side effects.
Antidepressants (tricyclics)	Increased terbutaline effect.
Beta-adrenergic blockers	Decreased effects of both drugs.
Ephedrine	Increased terbutaline effect. Excess heart stimulation.
Epinephrine	Increased terbutaline effect. Excess heart stimulation.
MAO inhibitors	Increased terbutaline effect. Dangerous. Avoid.
Minoxidil	Decreased minoxidil effect.
Nitrates	Possible decreased effects of both drugs.
Sympathomimetics	Increased terbutaline effect.

POSSIBLE INTERACTION WITH OTHER SUBSTANCES

INTERACTS WITH	COMBINED EFFECT
Alcohol:	None expected.
Beverages:	None expected.
Cocaine:	Overstimulation.
Foods:	None expected.
Marijuana:	Possible increased therapeutic effect of terbutaline. May cause lung disorders to worsen.
Tobacco:	No interactions expected, but smoking may slow body's recovery. Avoid.

TERFENADINE

BRAND NAMES

Seldane   Vantac

BASIC INFORMATION

Habit forming? No
Prescription needed? No
Available as generic? No
Drug class: Antihistamine

 USES

Reduces allergic symptoms such as hay fever, hives, rash or itching. Less likely to cause drowsiness than most other antihistamines.

 DOSAGE & USAGE INFORMATION

How to take:
Tablet—Swallow with water or food to lessen stomach irritation.

When to take:
Follow prescription instructions.

If you forget a dose:
Take as soon as you remember up to 2 hours late. If more than 2 hours, wait for next scheduled dose (don't double this dose).

What drug does:
Blocks effects of histamine, a chemical produced by the body as a result of contact with an allergen.

Time lapse before drug works:
1 to 2 hours; maximum effect at 3 to 4 hours.

Don't take with:
See Interaction column and consult doctor.

 OVERDOSE

SYMPTOMS:
Flushed face, hallucinations.
WHAT TO DO:
- **Dial 0 (operator) or 911 (emergency) for an ambulance or medical help. Then give first aid immediately.**
- **See emergency information on inside covers.**

 POSSIBLE ADVERSE REACTIONS OR SIDE EFFECTS

SYMPTOMS	WHAT TO DO
Life-threatening: None expected.	
Common: None expected.	
Infrequent: None expected.	
Rare:	
• Swollen lips.	Discontinue. Seek emergency treatment.
• Rapid heart rate.	Discontinue. Call doctor right away.
• Nightmares, mild visual disturbances, nausea, vomiting, change in bowel habits, hair loss.	Continue. Call doctor when convenient.
• Depression, difficulty in falling asleep, sore throat, irregular heartbeat, frequent urination, mildly painful menstruation.	Continue. Tell doctor at next visit.

WARNINGS & PRECAUTIONS

Don't take if:
- You are allergic to terfenadine.
- You have urinary-tract blockage.

Before you start, consult your doctor:
- If you are allergic to other antihistamines.
- If you are under age 12.
- If you are allergic to any substance or any medicine.
- If you are pregnant or expect to become pregnant.
- If you have asthma.
- If you will have surgery within 2 months, including dental surgery, requiring general or spinal anesthesia.
- If you plan to have skin tests for allergies.

Over age 60:
Don't exceed recommended dose. Adverse reactions and side effects may be more frequent and severe than in younger persons, especially urination difficulty, diminished alertness and other brain and nervous-system symptoms.

Pregnancy:
No proven harm to unborn child. Avoid if possible.

Breast-feeding:
Drug passes into milk. Avoid drug or discontinue nursing until you finish medicine. Consult doctor for advice on maintaining milk supply.

Infants & children:
Not recommended for premature or newborn infants. Otherwise, no problems expected.

Prolonged use:
Avoid. May damage bone marrow and nerve cells.

Skin & sunlight:
May cause rash or intensify sunburn in areas exposed to sun or sunlamp.

Driving, piloting or hazardous work:
Don't drive or pilot aircraft until you learn how medicine affects you. Sedation and dizziness are less likely to occur with terfenadine than with other antihistamines.

Discontinuing:
No problems expected.

Others:
May mask symptoms of hearing damage from aspirin, other salicylates, cisplatin, paramomycin, vancomycin or anticonvulsants. Consult doctor if you use these.

POSSIBLE INTERACTION WITH OTHER DRUGS

GENERIC NAME OR DRUG CLASS	COMBINED EFFECT
Aspirin in large doses regularly	Terfenadine may conceal overdose of aspirin, such as ringing in the ears.
Anticholinergics	Possible increased anticholinergic effect.
Antidepressants	Possible increased side effects of antidepressants.
Antihistamines (other)	Possible oversedation. Avoid.
Hypnotics	Possible oversedation.
MAO inhibitors	Increased side effects of MAO inhibitors.
Molindone	Increased antihistamine effect.
Narcotics	Possible oversedation.
Sedatives	Possible oversedation.
Sleep inducers	Possible oversedation.
Tranquilizers	Possible oversedation.

POSSIBLE INTERACTION WITH OTHER SUBSTANCES

INTERACTS WITH	COMBINED EFFECT
Alcohol:	Possible oversedation.
Beverages:	None expected.
Cocaine:	Decreased terfenadine effect.
Foods:	None expected.
Marijuana:	None expected.
Tobacco:	None expected.

TERPIN HYDRATE

BRAND NAMES

Cotussis
Prunicodeine
SK-Terpin Hydrate
  w/Codeine

Terpin Hydrate and
  Codeine Syrup
Terpin Hydrate Elixir

BASIC INFORMATION

Habit forming? Yes
Prescription needed? No
Available as generic? Yes
Drug class: Expectorant

USES

Decreases cough due to simple bronchial irritation.

DOSAGE & USAGE INFORMATION

How to take:
Follow each dose with 8 oz. water. Works better in combination with a cool-air vaporizer.

When to take:
3 to 4 times each day, spaced at least 4 hours apart.

If you forget a dose:
Take as soon as you remember. Wait 4 hours for next dose.

What drug does:
Loosens mucus in bronchial tubes to make mucus easier to cough up.

Time lapse before drug works:
10 to 15 minutes.

Don't take with:
See Interaction column and consult doctor.

OVERDOSE

SYMPTOMS:
Nausea, drowsiness.
WHAT TO DO:
Overdose unlikely to threaten life. If person takes much larger amount than prescribed, call doctor, poison-control center or hospital emergency room for instructions.

POSSIBLE ADVERSE REACTIONS OR SIDE EFFECTS

SYMPTOMS	WHAT TO DO
Life-threatening: None expected.	
Common: None expected.	
Infrequent: Nausea, vomiting, stomach pain.	Continue. Call doctor when convenient.
Rare: Symptoms of alcohol intoxication, especially in children.	Discontinue. Call doctor right away.

WARNINGS & PRECAUTIONS

Don't take if:
- You are allergic to terpin hydrate.
- You are a recovering or active alcoholic.

Before you start, consult your doctor:
If you plan to become pregnant within medication period.

Over age 60:
No problems expected.

Pregnancy:
Risk to unborn child outweighs drug benefits. Don't use.

Breast-feeding:
Drug filters into milk. May harm child. Avoid.

Infants & children:
Use only under medical supervision.

Prolonged use:
Habit forming.

Skin & sunlight:
No problems expected.

Driving, piloting or hazardous work:
Don't drive or pilot aircraft until you learn how medicine affects you. Don't work around dangerous machinery. Don't climb ladders or work in high places. Danger increases if you drink alcohol or take medicine affecting alertness and reflexes, such as antihistamines, tranquilizers, sedatives, pain medicine, narcotics and mind-altering drugs.

Discontinuing:
May be unnecessary to finish medicine. Follow doctor's instructions.

Others:
- Exceeding recommended doses may cause intoxication; drug is 42.5% alcohol.
- Frequently combined with codeine, which increases hazards.

POSSIBLE INTERACTION WITH OTHER DRUGS

GENERIC NAME OR DRUG CLASS	COMBINED EFFECT
Antidepressants	Increased effect of terpin hydrate.
Antihistamines	Increased effect of terpin hydrate.
Muscle relaxants	Increased effect of terpin hydrate.
Narcotics	Increased effect of terpin hydrate.
Sedatives	Increased effect of terpin hydrate.
Sleep inducers	Increased effect of terpin hydrate.
Tranquilizers	Increased effect of terpin hydrate.

POSSIBLE INTERACTION WITH OTHER SUBSTANCES

INTERACTS WITH	COMBINED EFFECT
Alcohol:	Increased sedative effect of both drugs. Avoid.
Beverages:	None expected.
Cocaine:	Unpredictable effect on nervous system. Avoid.
Foods:	None expected.
Marijuana:	Unpredictable effect on nervous system. Avoid.
Tobacco:	None expected.

BRAND NAMES

See complete list of brand names in the *Brand Name Directory,* page 957.

BASIC INFORMATION

Habit forming? No
Prescription needed? Yes
Available as generic? No
Drug class: Androgens-estrogens

 ## USES

- Prevents breast fullness in new mothers after childbirth.
- Relieves menopause symptoms such as unnecessary sweating, hot flashes, chills, faintness and dizziness.

 ## DOSAGE & USAGE INFORMATION

How to take:
Given by injection, deeply intramuscular.

When to take:
When directed.

If you forget a dose:
Check with your doctor.

What drug does:
- Restores normal estrogen level in tissues.
- Stimulates cells that produce male sex characteristics.
- Replaces hormone deficiencies.
- Stimulates red-blood-cell production.
- Suppresses production of estrogen.

Time lapse before drug works:
10 to 20 days.

Don't take with:
See Interaction column and consult doctor.

 ## OVERDOSE

SYMPTOMS:
Nausea, vomiting, fluid retention, breast enlargement and discomfort, abnormal vaginal bleeding.
WHAT TO DO:
Overdose unlikely to threaten life. If person takes much larger amount than prescribed, call doctor, poison-control center or hospital emergency room for instructions.

 ## POSSIBLE ADVERSE REACTIONS OR SIDE EFFECTS

SYMPTOMS	WHAT TO DO
Life-threatening:	
Hives, black stool, black or bloody vomit, intense itching, weakness, loss of consciousness.	Discontinue. Seek emergency treatment.
Common:	
• Red or flushed face; rash; swollen, tender breasts.	Discontinue. Call doctor right away.
• Depression, confusion, dizziness, irritability, acne or oily skin (females), enlarged clitoris, deepened voice, appetite loss, increased sex drive.	Continue. Call doctor when convenient.
Infrequent:	
• Nausea, vomiting, diarrhea, unusual vaginal bleeding or discharge.	Discontinue. Call doctor right away.
• Swollen feet and ankles, increased libido in some women.	Continue. Call doctor when convenient.
Rare:	
• Jaundice, abdominal pain.	Discontinue. Call doctor right away.
• Brown blotches on skin; hair loss; sore throat, fever, mouth sores.	Continue. Call doctor when convenient.

 ## WARNINGS & PRECAUTIONS

Don't take if:
- You are allergic to any male hormone or any estrogen-containing drugs.
- You have impaired liver function.
- You have had blood clots, stroke or heart attack.
- You have unexplained vaginal bleeding.

Before you start, consult your doctor:

- If you might be pregnant or plan to become pregnant within 3 months.
- If you have heart disease, arteriosclerosis, diabetes, liver disease, high blood pressure, asthma, congestive heart failure, kidney disease or gallstones.
- If you have high level of blood calcium.
- If you have had migraine headaches, epilepsy or porphyria.
- If you have had cancer of breast or reproductive organs, fibrocystic breast disease, fibroid tumors of the uterus or endometriosis.

Over age 60:

- May stimulate sexual activity.
- Can make high blood pressure or heart disease worse.
- Controversial. You and your doctor must decide if drug risks outweigh benefits.

Pregnancy:

Risk to unborn child outweighs drug benefits. Don't use.

Breast-feeding:

Drug passes into milk. Avoid drug or discontinue nursing until you finish medicine. Consult doctor for advice on maintaining milk supply.

Infants & children:

Not recommended.

Prolonged use:

- Increased growth of fibroid tumors of uterus.
- Possible kidney stones.
- Unnatural hair growth and deep voice in women.

Skin & sunlight:

May cause rash or intensify sunburn in areas exposed to sun or sunlamp.

Driving, piloting or hazardous work:

No problems expected.

Discontinuing:

You may need to discontinue estrogens periodically. Consult your doctor.

Others:

- In rare instances, may cause blood clot in lung, brain or leg. Symptoms are *sudden* severe headache, coordination loss, vision change, chest pain, breathing difficulty, slurred speech, pain in legs or groin. Seek emergency treatment immediately.
- Will not increase strength in athletes.
- Read carefully the paper delivered with your prescription called "Information for the Patient."

POSSIBLE INTERACTION WITH OTHER DRUGS

GENERIC NAME OR DRUG CLASS	COMBINED EFFECT
Anticonvulsants (hydantoin)	Increased seizures.
Antidiabetics (oral)	Unpredictable increase or decrease in blood sugar.
Carbamazepine	Increased seizures.
Chlorzoxazone	Decreased androgen effect.
Clofibrate	Decreased clofibrate effect.
Meprobamate	Increased estrogen effect.
Oxyphenbutazone	Decreased androgen effect.
Phenobarbital	Decreased androgen and estrogen effect.
Phenylbutazone	Decreased androgen effect.
Primidone	Decreased estrogen effect.
Rifampin	Decreased estrogen effect.
Thyroid hormones	Decreased thyroid effect.

POSSIBLE INTERACTION WITH OTHER SUBSTANCES

INTERACTS WITH	COMBINED EFFECT
Alcohol:	None expected.
Beverages:	None expected.
Cocaine:	No proven problems.
Foods: Salt.	Excessive fluid retention (edema). Decrease salt intake while taking male hormones.
Marijuana:	Decreased blood levels of androgens. Possible menstrual irregularities and bleeding between periods.
Tobacco:	Increased risk of blood clots leading to stroke or heart attack.

TETRACYCLINES

BRAND AND GENERIC NAMES

See complete list of brand and generic names in the *Brand Name Directory,* page 958.

BASIC INFORMATION

Habit forming? No
Prescription needed? Yes
Available as generic? Yes
Drug class: Antibiotic (tetracycline)

 USES

- Treatment for infections susceptible to any tetracycline. Will not cure virus infections such as colds or flu.
- Treatment for acne.

 DOSAGE & USAGE INFORMATION

How to take:
- Tablet or capsule—Take on empty stomach 1 hour before or 2 hours after eating. If you can't swallow whole, crumble tablet or open capsule and take with liquid or food.
- Liquid—Shake well. Take with measuring spoon.

When to take:
At the same times each day, evenly spaced.

If you forget a dose:
Take as soon as you remember up to 2 hours late. If more than 2 hours, wait for next scheduled dose (don't double this dose).

What drug does:
Prevents germ growth and reproduction.

Time lapse before drug works:
- Infections—May require 5 days to affect infection.
- Acne—May require 4 weeks to affect acne.

Don't take with:
- Non-prescription drugs without consulting doctor.
- See Interaction column and consult doctor.

 OVERDOSE

SYMPTOMS:
Severe nausea, vomiting, diarrhea.
WHAT TO DO:
Overdose unlikely to threaten life. If person takes much larger amount than prescribed, call doctor, poison-control center or hospital emergency room for instructions.

 POSSIBLE ADVERSE REACTIONS OR SIDE EFFECTS

SYMPTOMS	WHAT TO DO
Life-threatening: None expected.	
Common:	
• Sore mouth or tongue, nausea, vomiting, diarrhea, abdominal burning.	Discontinue. Seek emergency treatment.
• Itching around rectum and genitals.	Discontinue. Call doctor right away.
• Dark tongue.	Continue. Tell doctor at next visit.
Infrequent:	
• Headache, rash.	Discontinue. Call doctor right away.
• Excessive thirst, increased urination.	Continue. Call doctor when convenient.
Rare:	
Blurred vision, jaundice.	Discontinue. Call doctor right away.

WARNINGS & PRECAUTIONS

Don't take if:
You are allergic to any tetracycline antibiotic.

Before you start, consult your doctor:
- If you have kidney or liver disease.
- If you have lupus.
- If you have myasthenia gravis.

Over age 60:
Dosage usually less than in younger adults. More likely to cause itching around rectum. Ask your doctor how to prevent it.

Pregnancy:
Risk to unborn child outweighs drug benefits. Don't use.

Breast-feeding:
Drug passes into milk. Avoid drug or discontinue nursing until you finish medicine. Consult doctor for advice on maintaining milk supply.

Infants & children:
May cause permanent teeth malformation or discoloration in children less than 8 years old. Don't use.

Prolonged use:
- You may become more susceptible to infections caused by germs not responsive to tetracycline.
- May cause rare problems in liver, kidney or bone marrow. Periodic laboratory blood studies, liver- and kidney-function tests recommended if you use drug a long time.

Skin & sunlight:
May cause rash or intensify sunburn in areas exposed to sun or sunlamp.

Driving, piloting or hazardous work:
No problems expected.

Discontinuing:
Don't discontinue without doctor's advice until you complete prescribed dose, even though symptoms diminish or disappear.

Others:
No problems expected.

POSSIBLE INTERACTION WITH OTHER DRUGS

GENERIC NAME OR DRUG CLASS	COMBINED EFFECT
Antacids	Decreased tetracycline effect.
Anticoagulants (oral)	Increased anticoagulant effect.
Calcium supplements	Decreased tetracycline effect.
Contraceptives (oral)	Decreased contraceptive effect.
Digitalis preparations	Increased digitalis effect.
Lithium	Increased lithium effect.
Mineral supplements (iron, calcium, magnesium, zinc)	Decreased tetracycline absorption. Separate doses by 1 to 2 hours.
Penicillins	Decreased penicillin effect.
Sodium bicarbonate	Decreased tetracycline effect.

POSSIBLE INTERACTION WITH OTHER SUBSTANCES

INTERACTS WITH	COMBINED EFFECT
Alcohol:	Possible liver damage. Avoid.
Beverages: Milk.	Decreased tetracycline absorption. Take dose 2 hours after or 1 hour before drinking.
Cocaine:	No proven problems.
Foods: Dairy products.	Decreased tetracycline absorption. Take dose 2 hours after or 1 hour before eating.
Marijuana:	No interactions expected, but marijuana may slow body's recovery. Avoid.
Tobacco:	None expected.

THEOPHYLLINE, EPHEDRINE & BARBITURATES

BRAND NAMES

Azma Aid	T.E.P.
Ephenyllin	Thalfed
Lardet	Theocord
Primatene "P"	Theodrine
Formula	Theofedral
Tedral	Theophenyllin
Tedral SA	Theoral

BASIC INFORMATION

Habit forming? Yes
Prescription needed? Some yes, others no
Available as generic? Some yes, others no
Drug class: Bronchodilator,
**   sympathomimetic, barbiturate,**
**   sedative**

USES

- Treatment for bronchial asthma symptoms.
- Decreases congestion of breathing passages.
- Suppresses allergic reactions.
- Reduces anxiety or nervous tension (low dose).

DOSAGE & USAGE INFORMATION

How to take:
- Tablet or capsule—Swallow with liquid.
- Extended-release tablets or capsules—Swallow each dose whole. If you take regular tablets, you may chew or crush them

When to take:
Most effective taken on empty stomach 1 hour before or 2 hours after eating. However, may take with food to lessen stomach upset.

Continued next column

OVERDOSE

SYMPTOMS:
Restlessness, irritability, anxiety, confusion, delirium, muscle tremors, convulsions, rapid and irregular pulse, coma.
WHAT TO DO:
- **Dial 0 (operator) or 911 (emergency) for an ambulance or medical help. Then give first aid immediately.**
- **See emergency information on inside covers.**

If you forget a dose:
Take as soon as you remember up to 2 hours late. If more than 2 hours, wait for next scheduled dose (don't double this dose).

What drug does:
- Relaxes and expands bronchial tubes.
- Prevents cells from releasing allergy-causing chemicals (histamines).
- Decreases blood-vessel size and blood flow, thus causing decongestion.
- May partially block nerve impulses at nerve-cell connections.

Time lapse before drug works:
15 to 30 minutes.

Don't take with:
- See Interaction column and consult doctor.
- Non-prescription drugs with ephedrine, pseudoephedrine or epinephrine.
- Non-prescription drugs for cough, cold, allergy or asthma without consulting doctor.

POSSIBLE ADVERSE REACTIONS OR SIDE EFFECTS

SYMPTOMS	WHAT TO DO
Life-threatening:	
Difficult breathing, uncontrollable rapid heart rate, loss of consciousness.	Discontinue. Seek emergency treatment.
Common:	
• Headache, irritability, nervousness, restlessness, insomnia, nausea, vomiting, abdominal pain, "hangover" effect.	Discontinue. Call doctor right away.
• Dizziness, lightheadedness, paleness, irregular heartbeat.	Continue. Call doctor when convenient.
Infrequent:	
• Rash; hives; red or flushed face; appetite loss; diarrhea; cough; confusion; slurred speech; eyelid, face, lip swelling; joint pain.	Discontinue. Call doctor right away.
• Frequent urination.	Continue. Call doctor when convenient.
Rare:	
Agitation; sore throat, fever, mouth sores; jaundice.	Discontinue. Call doctor right away.

WARNINGS & PRECAUTIONS

Don't take if:
- You are allergic to any bronchodilator or barbiturate.
- You are allergic to ephedrine or any sympathomimetic drug.
- You have an active peptic ulcer or porphyria.

Before you start, consult your doctor:
- If you have gastritis, peptic ulcer, high blood pressure or heart disease, diabetes, overactive thyroid gland, difficulty urinating, epilepsy, kidney or liver damage, asthma, anemia, chronic pain, taken any MAO inhibitor in past 2 weeks, taken digitalis preparations in the last 7 days.
- If you have had impaired kidney or liver function.
- If you take medication for gout.
- If you will have surgery within 2 months, including dental surgery, requiring general or spinal anesthesia.

Over age 60:
- Adverse reactions and side effects may be more frequent and severe than in younger persons. Use small doses.
- More likely to develop high blood pressure, heart-rhythm disturbances, angina and to feel drug's stimulant effects.

Pregnancy:
Risk to unborn child outweighs drug benefits. Don't use.

Breast-feeding:
Drug passes into milk. Avoid drug or discontinue nursing until you finish medicine.

Infants & children:
Use only under medical supervision.

Prolonged use:
- Stomach irritation.
- Excessive doses—Rare toxic psychosis.
- Men with enlarged prostate gland may have more urination difficulty.
- May cause addiction, anemia, chronic intoxication.
- May lower body temperature, making exposure to cold temperatures hazardous.

Skin & sunlight:
May cause rash or intensify sunburn in areas exposed to sun or sunlamp.

Driving, piloting or hazardous work:
Don't drive or pilot aircraft until you learn how medicine affects you. Don't work around dangerous machinery. Don't climb ladders or work in high places. Danger increases if you drink alcohol or take medicine affecting alertness and reflexes.

Discontinuing:
- May be unnecessary to finish medicine. Follow doctor's instructions.
- If you develop withdrawal symptoms of hallucinations, agitation or sleeplessness after discontinuing, call doctor right away.

Others:
Potential for abuse.

POSSIBLE INTERACTION WITH OTHER DRUGS

GENERIC NAME OR DRUG CLASS	COMBINED EFFECT
Allopurinol	Decreased allopurinol effect.
Anticoagulants (oral)	Decreased anticoagulant effect.
Anticonvulsants	Changed seizure patterns.
Antidepressants (tricyclics)	Decreased antidepressant effect. Possible dangerous oversedation.
Antidiabetics (oral)	Increased phenobarbital effect.
Antihistamines	Dangerous sedation. Avoid.

Continued page 976

POSSIBLE INTERACTION WITH OTHER SUBSTANCES

INTERACTS WITH	COMBINED EFFECT
Alcohol:	Possible fatal oversedation. Avoid.
Beverages: Caffeine drinks.	Nervousness or insomnia.
Cocaine:	Rapid heartbeat. Avoid.
Foods:	None expected.
Marijuana:	Rapid heartbeat, possible heart-rhythm disturbance.
Tobacco:	Decreased bronchodilator effect.

THEOPHYLLINE, EPHEDRINE, GUAIFENESIN & BARBITURATES

BRAND NAMES

Bronkolixir
Bronkotabr
Guaiaphed

Lardet Expectorant
Mudrane GG
Quibron Plus

BASIC INFORMATION

Habit forming? Yes (barbiturates)
Prescription needed? Yes
Available as generic? No
Drug class: Bronchodilator (xanthine),
cough/cold preparation,
sympathomimetic, sedative

 ## USES

- Treatment for symptoms of bronchial asthma, emphysema, chronic bronchitis.
- Relieves wheezing, coughing and shortness of breath.

 ## DOSAGE & USAGE INFORMATION

How to take:
- Tablet or capsule—Swallow with liquid.
- Extended-release tablets or capsules—Swallow each dose whole. If you take regular tablets, you may chew or crush them.

When to take:
Most effective taken on empty stomach 1 hour before or 2 hours after eating. However, may take with food to lessen stomach upset.

Continued next column

 ## OVERDOSE

SYMPTOMS:
Restlessness, irritability, confusion, muscle tremors, severe anxiety, rapid and irregular pulse, mild weakness, nausea, vomiting, delirium, coma.
WHAT TO DO:
- **Overdose unlikely to threaten life. Depending on severity of symptoms and amount taken, call doctor, poison-control center or hospital emergency room for instructions.**
- **Dial 0 (operator) or 911 (emergency) for an ambulance or medical help. Then give first aid immediately.**
- **See emergency information on inside covers.**

If you forget a dose:
Take as soon as you remember up to 2 hours late. If more than 2 hours, wait for next scheduled dose (don't double this dose).

What drug does:
- Relaxes and expands bronchial tubes.
- Prevents cells from releasing allergy-causing chemicals (histamines).
- Relaxes muscles of bronchial tubes.
- Decreases blood-vessel size and blood flow, thus causing decongestion.
- Increases production of watery fluids to thin mucus so it can be coughed out or absorbed.
- May partially block nerve impulses at nerve-cell connections.

Time lapse before drug works:
30 to 60 minutes.

Don't take with:
- Non-prescription drugs with ephedrine, pseudoephedrine or epinephrine.
- Non-prescription drugs for cough, cold, allergy or asthma without consulting doctor.
- See Interaction column and consult doctor.

 ## POSSIBLE ADVERSE REACTIONS OR SIDE EFFECTS

SYMPTOMS	WHAT TO DO
Life-threatening:	
Difficult breathing, uncontrollable rapid heart rate, loss of consciousness.	Discontinue. Seek emergency treatment.
Common:	
• Headache, irritability, nervousness, restlessness, insomnia, nausea, vomiting, abdominal pain.	Discontinue. Call doctor right away.
• Dizziness, lightheadedness, paleness, irregular heartbeat.	Continue. Call doctor when convenient.
Infrequent:	
• Skin rash or hives, red or flushed face, appetite loss, diarrhea, abdominal pain.	Discontinue. Call doctor right away.
• Frequent urination.	Continue. Call doctor when convenient.
Rare:	
None expected.	

THEOPHYLLINE, EPHEDRINE, GUAIFENESIN & BARBITURATES

WARNINGS & PRECAUTIONS

Don't take if:
- You are allergic to any bronchodilator, ephedrine, any sympathomimetic drug, cough or cold preparation containing guaifenesin.
- You have an active peptic ulcer.

Before you start, consult your doctor:
- If you have had impaired kidney or liver function.
- If you have gastritis, peptic ulcer, high blood pressure, heart disease, diabetes, overactive thyroid gland, difficulty urinating, epilepsy, anemia, chronic pain, taken any MAO inhibitor in past 2 weeks, taken digitalis preparations in the last 7 days.
- If you take medication for gout.
- If you will have surgery within 2 months, including dental surgery, requiring general or spinal anesthesia.

Over age 60:
- Adverse reactions and side effects may be more frequent and severe than in younger persons. Use small doses. For drug to work, you must drink 8 to 10 glasses of fluid per day.
- More likely to develop high blood pressure, heart-rhythm disturbances, angina and to feel drug's stimulant effects.

Pregnancy:
Risk to unborn child outweighs drug benefits. Don't use.

Breast-feeding:
Drug passes into milk. Avoid drug or discontinue nursing until you finish medicine. Consult doctor for advice on maintaining milk supply.

Infants & children:
Use only under medical supervision.

Prolonged use:
- Stomach irritation.
- Excessive doses—Rare toxic psychosis.
- Men with enlarged prostate gland may have more urination difficulty.
- May cause addiction, anemia, chronic intoxication.
- May lower body temperature, making exposure to cold temperature hazardous.

Skin & sunlight:
May cause rash or intensify sunburn in areas exposed to sun or sunlamp.

Driving, piloting or hazardous work:
Don't drive or pilot aircraft until you learn how medicine affects you. Don't work around dangerous machinery. Don't climb ladders or work in high places. Danger increases if you drink alcohol or take medicine affecting alertness and reflexes, such as antihistamines, tranquilizers, sedatives, pain medicine, narcotics and mind-altering drugs.

Discontinuing:
- May be unnecessary to finish medicine. Follow doctor's instructions.
- If you develop withdrawal symptoms of hallucinations, agitation or sleeplessness after discontinuing, call doctor right away.

Others:
Great potential for abuse.

POSSIBLE INTERACTION WITH OTHER DRUGS

GENERIC NAME OR DRUG CLASS	COMBINED EFFECT
Allopurinol	Decreased allopurinol effect.
Anticonvulsants	Changed seizure patterns.

Continued page 977

POSSIBLE INTERACTION WITH OTHER SUBSTANCES

INTERACTS WITH	COMBINED EFFECT
Alcohol:	Possible fatal oversedation. Avoid.
Beverages:	You must drink 8 to 10 glasses of fluid per day for drug to work.
Caffeine drinks.	Nervousness and insomnia.
Cocaine:	Rapid heartbeat. Excess stimulation. Avoid.
Foods:	None expected.
Marijuana:	Excessive sedation, rapid heartbeat, possible heart-rhythm disturbance. Avoid.
Tobacco:	Decreased bronchodilator effect. Smoking is damaging to all problems this medicine treats. Avoid.

THEOPHYLLINE, EPHEDRINE & HYDROXYZINE

BRAND NAMES

Brophed	Marax D.F.
Hydromax	Moxy Compound
Hydrophed	T.E.H. Compound
Marax	Theozine

BASIC INFORMATION

Habit forming? No
Prescription needed? Yes
Available as generic? No
**Drug class: Bronchodilator (xanthine),
           sympathomimetic, antihistamine,
           tranquilizer**

 USES

- Treatment for symptoms of bronchial asthma, emphysema, chronic bronchitis.
- Relieves wheezing, coughing and shortness of breath.

 DOSAGE & USAGE INFORMATION

How to take:
- Tablet or capsule—Swallow with liquid.
- Extended-release tablets or capsules—Swallow each dose whole. If you take regular tablets, you may chew or crush them.

When to take:
Most effective taken on empty stomach 1 hour before or 2 hours after eating. However, may take with food to lessen stomach upset.

If you forget a dose:
Take as soon as you remember up to 2 hours late. If more than 2 hours, wait for next scheduled dose (don't double this dose).

Continued next column

 OVERDOSE

SYMPTOMS:
Restlessness, irritability, confusion, severe anxiety, muscle tremors, rapid and irregular pulse, agitation, purposeless movements, delirium, convulsions, coma.
WHAT TO DO:
- **Dial 0 (operator) or 911 (emergency) for an ambulance or medical help. Then give first aid immediately.**
- **See emergency information on inside covers.**

What drug does:
- Relaxes and expands bronchial tubes.
- Prevents cells from releasing allergy-causing chemicals (histamines).
- Relaxes muscles of bronchial tubes.
- Decreases blood-vessel size and blood flow, thus causing decongestion.
- May reduce activity in areas of the brain that influence emotional stability.

Time lapse before drug works:
15 to 60 minutes.

Don't take with:
- Non-prescription drugs with ephedrine, pseudoephedrine or epinephrine.
- Non-prescription drugs for cough, cold, allergy or asthma without consulting doctor.
- See Interaction column and consult doctor.

 POSSIBLE ADVERSE REACTIONS OR SIDE EFFECTS

SYMPTOMS	WHAT TO DO
Life-threatening:	
Difficult breathing, uncontrollable rapid heart rate, loss of consciousness.	Discontinue. Seek emergency treatment.
Common:	
• Headache, irritability, nervousness, restlessness, insomnia, nausea, vomiting, abdominal pain.	Discontinue. Call doctor right away.
• Dizziness, lightheadedness, paleness, irregular heartbeat.	Continue. Call doctor when convenient.
Infrequent:	
• Skin rash or hives, red or flushed face, appetite loss, diarrhea, abdominal pain.	Discontinue. Call doctor right away.
• Frequent urination.	Continue. Call doctor when convenient.
Rare:	
Tremor.	Discontinue. Call doctor right away.

WARNINGS & PRECAUTIONS

Don't take if:
- You are allergic to any bronchodilator, ephedrine, any sympathomimetic drug, or antihistamine.
- You have an active peptic ulcer.

Before you start, consult your doctor:
- If you have had impaired kidney or liver function.
- If you have gastritis, peptic ulcer, high blood pressure, heart disease, diabetes, overactive thyroid gland, difficulty urinating, epilepsy, taken any MAO inhibitor in past 2 weeks, taken digitalis preparations in the last 7 days.
- If you take medication for gout.
- If you will have surgery within 2 months, including dental surgery, requiring general or spinal anesthesia.

Over age 60:
- Adverse reactions and side effects may be more frequent and severe than in younger persons.
- More likely to develop increased urination difficulty, high blood pressure, heart-rhythm disturbances, angina and to feel drug's stimulant effects.

Pregnancy:
Risk to unborn child outweighs drug benefits. Don't use.

Breast-feeding:
Drug passes into milk. Avoid drug or discontinue nursing until you finish medicine. Consult doctor for advice on maintaining milk supply.

Infants & children:
Use only under medical supervision.

Prolonged use:
- Stomach irritation.
- Excessive doses—Rare toxic psychosis.
- Men with enlarged prostate gland may have more urination difficulty.
- Tolerance develops and reduces effectiveness.

Skin & sunlight:
No problems expected.

Driving, piloting or hazardous work:
Don't drive or pilot aircraft until you learn how medicine affects you. Don't work around dangerous machinery. Don't climb ladders or work in high places. Danger increases if you drink alcohol or take medicine affecting alertness and reflexes, such as antihistamines, tranquilizers, sedatives, pain medicine, narcotics and mind-altering drugs.

Discontinuing:
Don't discontinue without consulting doctor. Dose may require gradual reduction if you have taken drug for a long time. Doses of other drugs may also require adjustment.

Others:
No problems expected.

POSSIBLE INTERACTION WITH OTHER DRUGS

GENERIC NAME OR DRUG CLASS	COMBINED EFFECT
Allopurinol	Decreased allopurinol effect.
Anticoagulants (oral)	Increased anticoagulant effect.
Anticonvulsants (hydantoin)	Decreased anticonvulsant effect.
Antidepressants (tricyclics)	Increased effect of ephedrine. Excess stimulation of heart and blood pressure.
Antihistamines	Increased hydroxyzine effect.
Antihypertensives	Decreased antihypertensive effect.

Continued page 978

POSSIBLE INTERACTION WITH OTHER SUBSTANCES

INTERACTS WITH	COMBINED EFFECT
Alcohol:	Increased sedation and intoxication. Avoid.
Beverages: Caffeine drinks.	Nervousness and insomnia.
Cocaine:	Excess stimulation and rapid heartbeat. Avoid.
Foods:	None expected.
Marijuana:	Slightly increased antiasthmatic effect of bronchodilator. Rapid heartbeat, possible heart-rhythm disturbance.
Tobacco:	Decreased bronchodilator effect. Smoking is damaging to all problems this medicine treats. Avoid.

THEOPHYLLINE & GUAIFENESIN

BRAND NAMES

Asbcon G Inlay Tabs
Bronchial
Elixophyllin-GG
Glycery T
Lanophyllin-GG
Quibron

Slo-Phyllin GG
Syncophylate-GG
Theocolate
Theolair-Plus
Theolate

BASIC INFORMATION

Habit forming? No
Prescription needed? Yes
Available as generic? No
Drug class: Bronchodilator, expectorant

 USES

- Treatment for bronchial asthma symptoms.
- Loosens mucus in respiratory passages.
- Relieves coughing, wheezing, shortness of breath.

 DOSAGE & USAGE INFORMATION

How to take:
- Tablet or capsule—Swallow with liquid.
- Extended-release tablets or capsules—Swallow each dose whole. If you take regular tablets, you may chew or crush them.

When to take:
Most effective taken on empty stomach 1 hour before or 2 hours after eating. However, may take with food to lessen stomach upset.

If you forget a dose:
Take as soon as you remember up to 2 hours late. If more than 2 hours, wait for next scheduled dose (don't double this dose).

Continued next column

 OVERDOSE

SYMPTOMS:
Restlessness, irritability, confusion, drowsiness, mild weakness, nausea, vomiting, delirium, convulsions, rapid pulse, coma.
WHAT TO DO:
- Dial 0 (operator) or 911 (emergency) for an ambulance or medical help. Then give first aid immediately.
- See emergency information on inside covers.

What drug does:
- Relaxes and expands bronchial tubes.
- Increases production of watery fluids to thin mucus so it can be coughed out or absorbed.

Time lapse before drug works:
15 to 30 minutes.

Don't take with:
See Interaction column and consult doctor.

 POSSIBLE ADVERSE REACTIONS OR SIDE EFFECTS

SYMPTOMS	WHAT TO DO
Life-threatening:	
Difficult breathing, uncontrollable heart rate, loss of consciousness.	Discontinue. Seek emergency treatment.
Common:	
• Headache, irritability, nervousness, restlessness, insomnia, drowsiness, nausea, vomiting, abdominal pain.	Discontinue. Call doctor right away.
• Dizziness, lightheadedness, diarrhea, abdominal pain.	Continue. Call doctor when convenient.
Infrequent:	
Skin rash or hives, red or flushed face, appetite loss, diarrhea.	Discontinue. Call doctor right away.
Rare:	
None expected.	

WARNINGS & PRECAUTIONS

Don't take if:
- You are allergic to any bronchodilator or cough or cold preparation containing guaifenesin.
- You have an active peptic ulcer.

Before you start, consult your doctor:
- If you have had impaired kidney or liver function.
- If you have gastritis, peptic ulcer, high blood pressure or heart disease.
- If you take medication for gout.

Over age 60:
Adverse reactions and side effects may be more frequent and severe than in younger persons. For drug to work, you must drink 8 to 10 glasses of fluid per day.

Pregnancy:
Risk to unborn child outweighs drug benefits. Don't use.

Breast-feeding:
Drug passes into milk. Avoid drug or discontinue nursing until you finish medicine. Consult doctor for advice on maintaining milk supply.

Infants & children:
Use only under medical supervision.

Prolonged use:
Stomach irritation.

Skin & sunlight:
No problems expected.

Driving, piloting or hazardous work:
Avoid if lightheaded, drowsy or dizzy. Otherwise, no problems expected.

Discontinuing:
May be unnecessary to finish medicine. Follow doctor's instructions.

Others:
No problems expected.

POSSIBLE INTERACTION WITH OTHER DRUGS

GENERIC NAME OR DRUG CLASS	COMBINED EFFECT
Allopurinol	Decreased allopurinol effect.
Anticoagulants	Risk of bleeding.
Ephedrine	Increased effect of both drugs.
Epinephrine	Increased effect of both drugs.
Erythromycin	Increased bronchodilator effect.
Furosemide	Increased furosemide effect.
Lincomycins	Increased bronchodilator effect.
Lithium	Decreased lithium effect.
Probenecid	Decreased effect of both drugs.
Propranolol	Decreased bronchodilator effect.
Rauwolfia alkaloids	Rapid heartbeat.
Sulfinpyrazone	Decreased sulfinpyrazone effect.
Troleandomycin	Increased bronchodilator effect.

POSSIBLE INTERACTION WITH OTHER SUBSTANCES

INTERACTS WITH	COMBINED EFFECT
Alcohol:	No proven problems.
Beverages:	You must drink 8 to 10 glasses of fluid per day for drug to work.
Caffeine drinks.	Nervousness and insomnia.
Cocaine:	Excess stimulation. Avoid.
Foods:	None expected.
Marijuana:	Slightly increased antiasthmatic effect of bronchodilator.
Tobacco:	Decreased bronchodilator effect. Cigarette smoking makes worse all problems that this medicine treats. Avoid.

THIABENDAZOLE

BRAND NAMES

Foldan	Minzolum
Mintezol	Triasox
Mintezol (Topical)	

BASIC INFORMATION

Habit forming? No
Prescription needed? Yes
Available as generic? No
**Drug class: Antihelminthic (antiworm
    medication)**

USES

Treatment of parasite infestations.

DOSAGE & USAGE INFORMATION

How to take or apply:
- Tablet or capsule—Swallow with liquid or food to lessen stomach irritation.
- Topical suspension—Apply to end of each tunnel or burrow made by worm.

When to take or apply:
- Tablet or capsule—According to instructions on prescription, after meals.
- Topical—2 to 4 times daily up to 14 days.

If you forget a dose:
Take as soon as you remember up to 2 hours late. If more than 2 hours, wait for next scheduled dose (don't double this dose).

What drug does:
Kills larvae and adult worms.

Continued next column

OVERDOSE

SYMPTOMS:
Aching, fever, blistered skin, seizures.
WHAT TO DO:
- **Dial 0 (operator) or 911 (emergency) for an ambulance or medical help. Then give first aid immediately.**
- **If patient is unconscious and not breathing, give mouth-to-mouth breathing. If there is no heartbeat, use cardiac massage and mouth-to-mouth breathing (CPR). Don't try to make patient vomit. If you can't get help quickly, take patient to nearest emergency facility.**
- **See emergency information on inside covers.**

Time lapse before drug works:
Varies according to degree of infestation.

Don't take with:
See Interaction column and consult doctor.

POSSIBLE ADVERSE REACTIONS OR SIDE EFFECTS

SYMPTOMS	WHAT TO DO
Life-threatening:	
None expected.	
Common:	
• Nausea, vomiting, abdominal pain.	Discontinue. Call doctor right away.
• Dizziness, drowsiness, headache, nausea, appetite loss, bedwetting.	Continue. Call doctor when convenient.
• Asparagus-like odor of urine.	Continue. Tell doctor at next visit.
Infrequent:	
• Redness, blistering with fever, rash with itchy skin, aching joints and muscles.	Discontinue. Call doctor right away.
• Ringing or buzzing in ears, numbness or tingling in hands and feet.	Continue. Call doctor when convenient.
Rare:	
Blurred or yellow vision.	Discontinue. Call doctor right away.

WARNINGS & PRECAUTIONS

Don't take if:
You are allergic to thiabendazole.

Before you start, consult your doctor:
● If you have kidney disease.
● If you have liver disease.

Over age 60:
Adverse reactions and side effects may be more frequent and severe than in younger persons.

Pregnancy:
Risk to unborn child outweighs drug benefits. Don't use.

Breast-feeding:
Unknown effect. Consult doctor.

Infants & children:
Use only under medical supervision.

Prolonged use:
Request follow-up stool exams 2 to 3 weeks following treatment.

Skin & sunlight:
No problems expected.

Driving, piloting or hazardous work:
Don't drive or pilot aircraft until you learn how medicine affects you. Don't work around dangerous machinery. Don't climb ladders or work in high places. Danger increases if you drink alcohol or take medicine affecting alertness and reflexes, such as antihistamines, tranquilizers, sedatives, pain medicine, narcotics and mind-altering drugs.

Discontinuing:
May be unnecessary to finish medicine. Follow doctor's instructions.

Others:
To prevent reinfection: Deworm household pets regularly. Cover sand boxes. Cook all pork until well done.

POSSIBLE INTERACTION WITH OTHER DRUGS

GENERIC NAME OR DRUG CLASS	COMBINED EFFECT
None expected.	

POSSIBLE INTERACTION WITH OTHER SUBSTANCES

INTERACTS WITH	COMBINED EFFECT
Alcohol:	Decreased thiabendazole effect.
Beverages:	No problems expected.
Cocaine:	Decreased thiabendazole effect.
Foods:	Take with foods to decrease nausea.
Marijuana:	Decreased thiabendazole effect.
Tobacco:	May decrease absorption of medicine.

THIAMINE (VITAMIN B-1)

BRAND NAMES

Betalin S   Biamine
Betaxin   Pan-B-1
Bewon
Numerous other multiple vitamin-mineral supplements.

BASIC INFORMATION

Habit forming? No
Prescription needed? No
Available as generic? Yes
Drug class: Vitamin supplement

 ## USES

- Dietary supplement to promote normal growth, development and health.
- Treatment for beri-beri (a thiamine-deficiency disease).
- Dietary supplement for alcoholism, cirrhosis, overactive thyroid, infection, breast-feeding, absorption diseases, pregnancy, prolonged diarrhea, burns.

 ## DOSAGE & USAGE INFORMATION

How to take:
Tablet or liquid—Swallow with beverage or food to lessen stomach irritation.

When to take:
At the same time each day.

If you forget a dose:
Take when remembered. Return to regular schedule.

What drug does:
- Promotes normal growth and development.
- Combines with an enzyme to metabolize carbohydrates.

Time lapse before drug works:
15 minutes.

Don't take with:
See Interaction column and consult doctor.

 ## OVERDOSE

SYMPTOMS:
Increased severity of adverse reactions and side effects.
WHAT TO DO:
Overdose unlikely to threaten life. If person takes much larger amount than prescribed, call doctor, poison-control center or hospital emergency room for instructions.

 ## POSSIBLE ADVERSE REACTIONS OR SIDE EFFECTS

SYMPTOMS	WHAT TO DO
Life-threatening:	
Hives, rash, intense itching, faintness soon after a dose (anaphylaxis).	Seek emergency treatment immediately.
Common:	
None expected.	
Infrequent:	
None expected.	
Rare:	
• Wheezing.	Discontinue. Seek emergency treatment.
• Rash or itchy skin.	Discontinue. Call doctor right away.

WARNINGS & PRECAUTIONS

Don't take if:
You are allergic to any B vitamin.

Before you start, consult your doctor:
If you have liver or kidney disease.

Over age 60:
No problems expected.

Pregnancy:
No problems expected.

Breast-feeding:
No problems expected.

Infants & children:
No problems expected.

Prolonged use:
No problems expected.

Skin & sunlight:
No problems expected.

Driving, piloting or hazardous work:
No problems expected.

Discontinuing:
No problems expected.

Others:
A balanced diet should provide enough thiamine for healthy people to make supplement unnecessary. Best dietary sources of thiamine are whole-grain cereals and meats.

POSSIBLE INTERACTION WITH OTHER DRUGS

GENERIC NAME OR DRUG CLASS	COMBINED EFFECT
Barbiturates	Decreased thiamine effect.

POSSIBLE INTERACTION WITH OTHER SUBSTANCES

INTERACTS WITH	COMBINED EFFECT
Alcohol:	None expected.
Beverages: Carbonates, citrates (additives listed on many beverage labels).	Decreased thiamine effect.
Cocaine:	None expected.
Foods: Carbonates, citrates (additives listed on many food labels).	Decreased thiamine effect.
Marijuana:	None expected.
Tobacco:	None expected.

THIORIDAZINE

BRAND NAMES

Apo-Thioridazine
Mellaril
Mellaril S
Millazine
Novoridazine

PMS Thioridazine
SK-Thioridazine
  Hydrochloride
Thioril

BASIC INFORMATION

Habit forming? No
Prescription needed? Yes
Available as generic? Yes
Drug class: Tranquilizer, antiemetic
      (phenothiazine)

USES

- Stops nausea, vomiting.
- Reduces anxiety, agitation.

DOSAGE & USAGE INFORMATION

How to take:
- Tablet or capsule—Swallow with liquid or food to lessen stomach irritation.
- Suppositories—Remove wrapper and moisten suppository with water. Gently insert into rectum, large end first.
- Drops or liquid—Dilute dose in beverage.

When to take:
- Nervous and mental disorders—Take at the same times each day.
- Nausea and vomiting—Take as needed, no more often than every 4 hours.

If you forget a dose:
- Nervous and mental disorders—Take up to 2 hours late. If more than 2 hours, wait for next scheduled dose (don't double this dose).
- Nausea and vomiting—Take as soon as you remember. Wait 4 hours for next dose.

Continued next column

OVERDOSE

SYMPTOMS:
Stupor, convulsions, coma.
WHAT TO DO:
- Dial 0 (operator) or 911 (emergency) for an ambulance or medical help. Then give first aid immediately.
- See emergency information on inside covers.

What drug does:
- Suppresses brain's vomiting center.
- Suppresses brain centers that control abnormal emotions and behavior.

Time lapse before drug works:
- Nausea and vomiting—1 hour or less.
- Nervous and mental disorders—4-6 weeks.

Don't take with:
- Antacid or medicine for diarrhea.
- Non-prescription drug for cough, cold or allergy.
- See Interaction column and consult doctor.

POSSIBLE ADVERSE REACTIONS OR SIDE EFFECTS

SYMPTOMS	WHAT TO DO
Life-threatening: None expected.	
Common:	
• Muscle spasms of face and neck, unsteady gait.	Discontinue. Seek emergency treatment.
• Restlessness, tremor, drowsiness.	Discontinue. Call doctor right away.
• Decreased sweating, dry mouth, nasal congestion, constipation.	Continue. Call doctor when convenient.
Infrequent:	
• Fainting.	Discontinue. Seek emergency treatment.
• Rash.	Discontinue. Call doctor right away.
• Difficult urination, less interest in sex, swollen breasts, menstrual irregularities.	Continue. Call doctor when convenient.
Rare:	
Change in vision, jaundice, sore throat, fever.	Discontinue. Call doctor right away.

WARNINGS & PRECAUTIONS

Don't take if:
- You are allergic to any phenothiazine.
- You have a blood or bone-marrow disease.

Before you start, consult your doctor:
- If you will have surgery within 2 months, including dental surgery, requiring general or spinal anesthesia.
- If you have asthma, emphysema or other lung disorder.
- If you take non-prescription ulcer medicine, asthma medicine or amphetamines.

Over age 60:
Adverse reactions and side effects may be more frequent and severe than in younger persons. More likely to develop involuntary movement of jaws, lips, tongue, chewing. Report this to your doctor immediately. Early treatment can help.

Pregnancy:
Risk to unborn child outweighs drug benefits. Don't use.

Breast-feeding:
Drug passes into milk. Avoid drug or discontinue nursing until you finish medicine. Consult doctor for advice on maintaining milk supply.

Infants & children:
Don't give to children younger than 2.

Prolonged use:
May lead to tardive dyskinesia (involuntary movement of jaws, lips, tongue, chewing).

Skin & sunlight:
May cause rash or intensify sunburn in areas exposed to sun or sunlamp. Skin may remain sensitive for 3 months after discontinuing.

Driving, piloting or hazardous work:
Don't drive or pilot aircraft until you learn how medicine affects you. Don't work around dangerous machinery. Don't climb ladders or work in high places. Danger increases if you drink alcohol or take medicine affecting alertness and reflexes.

Discontinuing:
- Nervous and mental disorders—Don't discontinue without doctor's advice until you complete prescribed dose, even though symptoms diminish or disappear.
- Nausea and vomiting—May be unnecessary to finish medicine. Follow doctor's instructions.

Others:
No problems expected.

POSSIBLE INTERACTION WITH OTHER DRUGS

GENERIC NAME OR DRUG CLASS	COMBINED EFFECT
Anticholinergics	Increased anticholinergic effect.
Antidepressants (tricyclic)	Increased thioridazine effect.
Antihistamines	Increased antihistamine effect.
Appetite suppressants	Decreased suppressant effect.
Dronabinol	Increased effects of both drugs. Avoid.
Levodopa	Decreased levodopa effect.
Mind-altering drugs	Increased effect of mind-altering drugs.
Molindone	Increased tranquilizer effect.
Narcotics	Increased narcotic effect.
Phenytoin	Increased phenytoin effect.
Quinidine	Impaired heart function. Dangerous mixture.
Sedatives	Increased sedative effect.
Tranquilizers (other)	Increased tranquilizer effect.

POSSIBLE INTERACTION WITH OTHER SUBSTANCES

INTERACTS WITH	COMBINED EFFECT
Alcohol:	Dangerous oversedation.
Beverages:	None expected.
Cocaine:	Decreased thioridazine effect. Avoid.
Foods:	None expected.
Marijuana:	Drowsiness. May increase antinausea effect.
Tobacco:	None expected.

THIOTHIXENE

BRAND NAMES

Navane

BASIC INFORMATION

Habit forming? No
Prescription needed? Yes
Available as generic? No
Drug class: Tranquilizer (thioxanthine),
antiemetic

USES

- Reduces anxiety, agitation, psychosis.
- Stops vomiting.

DOSAGE & USAGE INFORMATION

How to take:
- Capsule—Swallow with liquid. If you can't swallow whole, open capsule and take with liquid or food.
- Syrup—Dilute dose in beverage before swallowing.

When to take:
At the same time each day.

If you forget a dose:
Take as soon as you remember up to 2 hours late. If more than 2 hours, wait for next scheduled dose (don't double this dose).

What drug does:
Corrects imbalance of nerve impulses.

Continued next column

OVERDOSE

SYMPTOMS:
Drowsiness, dizziness, weakness, muscle rigidity, twitching, tremors, confusion, dry mouth, blurred vision, rapid pulse, shallow breathing, low blood pressure, convulsions, coma.
WHAT TO DO:
- **Dial 0 (operator) or 911 (emergency) for an ambulance or medical help. Then give first aid immediately.**
- **If patient is unconscious and not breathing, give mouth-to-mouth breathing. If there is no heartbeat, use cardiac massage and mouth-to-mouth breathing (CPR). Don't try to make patient vomit. If you can't get help quickly, take patient to nearest emergency facility.**
- **See emergency information on inside covers.**

Time lapse before drug works:
3 weeks.

Don't take with:
See Interaction column and consult doctor.

POSSIBLE ADVERSE REACTIONS OR SIDE EFFECTS

SYMPTOMS	WHAT TO DO
Life-threatening: None expected.	
Common:	
• Fainting, restlessness, jerky and involuntary movements, blurred vision, rapid heartbeat.	Discontinue. Call doctor right away.
• Dizziness, drowsiness, constipation, muscle spasms, shuffling walk, decreased sweating.	Continue. Call doctor when convenient.
• Dry mouth, nasal congestion.	Continue. Tell doctor at next visit.
Infrequent:	
• Rash.	Discontinue. Call doctor right away.
• Less sexual ability, difficult urination.	Continue. Call doctor when convenient.
• Menstrual irregularities, swollen breasts.	Continue. Tell doctor at next visit.
Rare: Sore throat, fever, jaundice.	Discontinue. Call doctor right away.

WARNINGS & PRECAUTIONS

Don't take if:
- You are allergic to any thioxanthine or phenothiazine tranquilizer.
- You have serious blood disorder.
- You have Parkinson's disease.
- Patient is younger than 12.

Before you start, consult your doctor:
- If you have had liver or kidney disease.
- If you have epilepsy or glaucoma.
- If you have high blood pressure or heart disease (especially angina).
- If you use alcohol daily.
- If you will have surgery within 2 months, including dental surgery, requiring general or spinal anesthesia.

Over age 60:
Adverse reactions and side effects may be more frequent and severe than in younger persons.

Pregnancy:
No proven harm to unborn child. Avoid if possible.

Breast-feeding:
Studies inconclusive. Consult your doctor.

Infants & children:
Not recommended.

Prolonged use:
• Pigment deposits in lens and retina of eye.
• Involuntary movements of jaws, lips, tongue (tardive dyskinesia).

Skin & sunlight:
May cause rash or intensify sunburn in areas exposed to sun or sunlamp.

Driving, piloting or hazardous work:
Don't drive or pilot aircraft until you learn how medicine affects you. Don't work around dangerous machinery. Don't climb ladders or work in high places. Danger increases if you drink alcohol or take medicine affecting alertness and reflexes.

Discontinuing:
Don't discontinue without consulting doctor. Dose may require gradual reduction if you have taken drug for a long time. Doses of other drugs may also require adjustment.

Others:
Hot temperatures increase chance of heat stroke.

POSSIBLE INTERACTION WITH OTHER DRUGS

GENERIC NAME OR DRUG CLASS	COMBINED EFFECT
Anticholinergics	Increased anticholinergic effect.
Anticonvulsants	Change in seizure pattern.
Antidepressants (tricyclic)	Increased thiothixene effect. Excessive sedation.
Antihistamines	Increased thiothixene effect. Excessive sedation.
Antihypertensives	Excessively low blood pressure.
Barbiturates	Increased thiothixene effect. Excessive sedation.
Bethanechol	Decreased bethanechol effect.
Dronabinol	Increased effects of both drugs. Avoid.
Guanethidine	Decreased guanethidine effect.
Levodopa	Decreased levodopa effect.
MAO inhibitors	Excessive sedation.
Mind-altering drugs	Increased thiothixene effect. Excessive sedation.
Narcotics	Increased thiothixene effect. Excessive sedation.
Sedatives	Increased thiothixene effect. Excessive sedation.
Sleep inducers	Increased thiothixene effect. Excessive sedation.
Tranquilizers	Increased thiothixene effect. Excessive sedation.

POSSIBLE INTERACTION WITH OTHER SUBSTANCES

INTERACTS WITH	COMBINED EFFECT
Alcohol:	Excessive brain depression. Avoid.
Beverages:	None expected.
Cocaine:	Decreased thiothixene effect. Avoid.
Foods:	None expected.
Marijuana:	Daily use—Fainting likely, possible psychosis.
Tobacco:	None expected.

THYROGLOBULIN

BRAND NAMES

Proloid

BASIC INFORMATION

Habit forming? No
Prescription needed? Yes
Available as generic? Yes
Drug class: Thyroid hormone

 USES

Replacement for thyroid hormone deficiency.

 DOSAGE & USAGE INFORMATION

How to take:
- Tablet or capsule—Swallow with liquid.
- Extended-release tablets or capsules—Swallow each dose whole. If you take regular tablets, you may chew or crush them.

When to take:
At the same time each day before a meal or on awakening.

If you forget a dose:
Take as soon as you remember up to 12 hours late. If more than 12 hours, wait for next scheduled dose (don't double this dose).

What drug does:
Increases cell metabolism rate.

Time lapse before drug works:
48 hours.

Don't take with:
See Interaction column and consult doctor.

 OVERDOSE

SYMPTOMS:
"Hot" feeling, heart palpitations, nervousness, sweating, hand tremors, insomnia, rapid and irregular pulse, headache, irritability, diarrhea, weight loss, muscle cramps.
WHAT TO DO:
Overdose unlikely to threaten life. If person takes much larger amount than prescribed, call doctor, poison-control center or hospital emergency room for instructions.

 POSSIBLE ADVERSE REACTIONS OR SIDE EFFECTS

SYMPTOMS	WHAT TO DO
Life-threatening:	
None expected.	
Common:	
• Tremor, headache, irritability, insomnia.	Discontinue. Call doctor right away.
• Appetite change, diarrhea, leg cramps, menstrual irregularities, fever, heat sensitivity, unusual sweating, weight loss.	Continue. Call doctor when convenient.
Infrequent:	
Hives, rash, vomiting, chest pain, rapid and irregular heartbeat, shortness of breath.	Discontinue. Call doctor right away.
Rare:	
None expected.	

WARNINGS & PRECAUTIONS

Don't take if:
- You have had a heart attack within 6 weeks.
- You have no thyroid deficiency, but use this to lose weight.

Before you start, consult your doctor:
- If you have heart disease or high blood pressure.
- If you have diabetes.
- If you have Addison's disease, have had adrenal gland deficiency or use epinephrine, ephedrine or isoproterenol for asthma.

Over age 60:
More sensitive to thyroid hormone. May need smaller doses.

Pregnancy:
Considered safe if for thyroid deficiency only.

Breast-feeding:
Present in milk. Considered safe if dose is correct.

Infants & children:
Use only under medical supervision.

Prolonged use:
No problems expected, if dose is correct.

Skin & sunlight:
No problems expected.

Driving, piloting or hazardous work:
No problems expected.

Discontinuing:
Don't discontinue without consulting doctor. Dose may require gradual reduction if you have taken drug for a long time. Doses of other drugs may also require adjustment.

Others:
Digestive upsets, tremors, cramps, nervousness, insomnia or diarrhea may indicate need for dose adjustment.

POSSIBLE INTERACTION WITH OTHER DRUGS

GENERIC NAME OR DRUG CLASS	COMBINED EFFECT
Amphetamines	Increased amphetamine effect.
Anticoagulants (oral)	Increased anticoagulant effect.
Antidepressants (tricyclic)	Increased antidepressant effect. Irregular heartbeat.
Antidiabetics	Antidiabetic may require adjustment.
Aspirin (large doses, continuous use)	Increased thyroglobulin effect.
Barbiturates	Decreased barbiturate effect.
Cholestyramine	Decreased thyroglobulin effect.
Contraceptives (oral)	Decreased thyroglobulin effect.
Cortisone drugs	Requires dose adjustment to prevent cortisone deficiency.
Digitalis preparations	Increased digitalis effect.
Ephedrine	Increased ephedrine effect.
Epinephrine	Increased epinephrine effect.
Methylphenidate	Increased methylphenidate effect.
Phenytoin	Increased thyroglobulin effect.

POSSIBLE INTERACTION WITH OTHER SUBSTANCES

INTERACTS WITH	COMBINED EFFECT
Alcohol:	None expected.
Beverages:	None expected.
Cocaine:	Excess stimulation. Avoid.
Foods: Soybeans.	Heavy consumption interferes with thyroid function.
Marijuana:	None expected.
Tobacco:	None expected.

THYROID

BRAND NAMES

Armour
Cytomel
Euthroid
Levothroid
Proloid

S-P-T
Synthroid
Thyrar
Thyrocrine

BASIC INFORMATION

Habit forming? No
Prescription needed? Yes
Available as generic? Yes
Drug class: Thyroid hormone

 ## USES

Replacement for thyroid hormone deficiency.

 ## DOSAGE & USAGE INFORMATION

How to take:
- Tablet or capsule—Swallow with liquid.
- Extended-release tablets or capsules—Swallow each dose whole. If you take regular tablets, you may chew or crush them.

When to take:
At the same time each day before a meal or on awakening.

If you forget a dose:
Take as soon as you remember up to 12 hours late. If more than 12 hours, wait for next scheduled dose (don't double this dose).

What drug does:
Increases cell metabolism rate.

Time lapse before drug works:
48 hours.

Don't take with:
See Interaction column and consult doctor.

 ## OVERDOSE

SYMPTOMS:
"Hot" feeling, heart palpitations, nervousness, sweating, hand tremors, insomnia, rapid and irregular pulse, headache, irritability, diarrhea, weight loss, muscle cramps.
WHAT TO DO:
Overdose unlikely to threaten life. If person takes much larger amount than prescribed, call doctor, poison-control center or hospital emergency room for instructions.

 ## POSSIBLE ADVERSE REACTIONS OR SIDE EFFECTS

SYMPTOMS	WHAT TO DO
Life-threatening: None expected.	
Common:	
• Tremor, headache, irritability, insomnia.	Discontinue. Call doctor right away.
• Appetite change, diarrhea, leg cramps, menstrual irregularities, fever, heat sensitivity, unusual sweating, weight loss.	Continue. Call doctor when convenient.
Infrequent: Hives, rash, vomiting, chest pain, rapid and irregular heartbeat, shortness of breath.	Discontinue. Call doctor right away.
Rare: None expected.	

WARNINGS & PRECAUTIONS

Don't take if:
- You have had a heart attack within 6 weeks.
- You have no thyroid deficiency, but use this to lose weight.

Before you start, consult your doctor:
- If you have heart disease or high blood pressure.
- If you have diabetes.
- If you have Addison's disease, have had adrenal gland deficiency or use epinephrine, ephedrine or isoproterenol for asthma.

Over age 60:
More sensitive to thyroid hormone. May need smaller doses.

Pregnancy:
Considered safe if for thyroid deficiency only.

Breast-feeding:
Present in milk. Considered safe if dose is correct.

Infants & children:
Use only under medical supervision.

Prolonged use:
No problems expected, if dose is correct.

Skin & sunlight:
No problems expected.

Driving, piloting or hazardous work:
No problems expected.

Discontinuing:
Don't discontinue without consulting doctor. Dose may require gradual reduction if you have taken drug for a long time. Doses of other drugs may also require adjustment.

Others:
Digestive upsets, tremors, cramps, nervousness, insomnia or diarrhea may indicate need for dose adjustment.

POSSIBLE INTERACTION WITH OTHER DRUGS

GENERIC NAME OR DRUG CLASS	COMBINED EFFECT
Amphetamines	Increased amphetamine effect.
Anticoagulants (oral)	Increased anticoagulant effect.
Antidepressants (tricyclic)	Increased antidepressant effect. Irregular heartbeat.
Antidiabetics	Antidiabetic may require adjustment.
Aspirin (large doses, continuous use)	Increased thyroid effect.
Barbiturates	Decreased barbiturate effect.
Cholestyramine	Decreased thyroid effect.
Contraceptives (oral)	Decreased thyroid effect.
Cortisone drugs	Requires dose adjustment to prevent cortisone deficiency.
Digitalis preparations	Increased digitalis effect.
Ephedrine	Increased ephedrine effect.
Epinephrine	Increased epinephrine effect.
Methylphenidate	Increased methylphenidate effect.
Phenytoin	Increased thyroid effect.

POSSIBLE INTERACTION WITH OTHER SUBSTANCES

INTERACTS WITH	COMBINED EFFECT
Alcohol:	None expected.
Beverages:	None expected.
Cocaine:	Excess stimulation. Avoid.
Foods: Soybeans.	Heavy consumption interferes with thyroid function.
Marijuana:	None expected.
Tobacco:	None expected.

THYROXINE (T-4, LEVOTHYROXINE)

BRAND NAMES

Choloxin
Cytolen
Elthroxin
Euthroid
Letter
Levoid
Levothroid

L-Thyroxine
L-T-S
Noroxine
Ro-Thyroxine
Synthroid
Thyrolar

BASIC INFORMATION

Habit forming? No
Prescription needed? Yes
Available as generic? Yes
Drug class: Thyroid hormone

 USES

Replacement for thyroid hormone deficiency.

 DOSAGE & USAGE INFORMATION

How to take:
- Tablet or capsule—Swallow with liquid.
- Extended-release tablets or capsules—Swallow each dose whole. If you take regular tablets, you may chew or crush them.

When to take:
At the same time each day before a meal or on awakening.

If you forget a dose:
Take as soon as you remember up to 12 hours late. If more than 12 hours, wait for next scheduled dose (don't double this dose).

What drug does:
Increases cell metabolism rate.

Time lapse before drug works:
48 hours.

Don't take with:
See Interaction column and consult doctor.

 OVERDOSE

SYMPTOMS:
"Hot" feeling, heart palpitations, nervousness, sweating, hand tremors, insomnia, rapid and irregular pulse, headache, irritability, diarrhea, weight loss, muscle cramps.
WHAT TO DO:
Overdose unlikely to threaten life. If person takes much larger amount than prescribed, call doctor, poison-control center or hospital emergency room for instructions.

 POSSIBLE ADVERSE REACTIONS OR SIDE EFFECTS

SYMPTOMS	WHAT TO DO
Life-threatening: None expected.	
Common:	
• Tremor, headache, irritability, insomnia.	Discontinue. Call doctor right away.
• Appetite change, diarrhea, leg cramps, menstrual irregularities, fever, heat sensitivity, unusual sweating, weight loss.	Continue. Call doctor when convenient.
Infrequent: Hives, rash, vomiting, chest pain, rapid and irregular heartbeat, shortness of breath.	Discontinue. Call doctor right away.
Rare: None expected.	

WARNINGS & PRECAUTIONS

Don't take if:
- You have had a heart attack within 6 weeks.
- You have no thyroid deficiency, but use this to lose weight.

Before you start, consult your doctor:
- If you have heart disease or high blood pressure.
- If you have diabetes.
- If you have Addison's disease, have had adrenal gland deficiency or use epinephrine, ephedrine or isoproterenol for asthma.

Over age 60:
More sensitive to thyroid hormone. May need smaller doses.

Pregnancy:
Considered safe if for thyroid deficiency only.

Breast-feeding:
Present in milk. Considered safe if dose is correct.

Infants & children:
Use only under medical supervision.

Prolonged use:
No problems expected, if dose is correct.

Skin & sunlight:
No problems expected.

Driving, piloting or hazardous work:
No problems expected.

Discontinuing:
Don't discontinue without consulting doctor. Dose may require gradual reduction if you have taken drug for a long time. Doses of other drugs may also require adjustment.

Others:
Digestive upsets, tremors, cramps, nervousness, insomnia or diarrhea may indicate need for dose adjustment.

POSSIBLE INTERACTION WITH OTHER DRUGS

GENERIC NAME OR DRUG CLASS	COMBINED EFFECT
Amphetamines	Increased amphetamine effect.
Anticoagulants (oral)	Increased anticoagulant effect.
Antidepressants (tricyclic)	Increased antidepressant effect. Irregular heartbeat.
Antidiabetics	Antidiabetic may require adjustment.
Aspirin (large doses, continuous use)	Increased thyroxine effect.
Barbiturates	Decreased barbiturate effect.
Cholestyramine	Decreased thyroxine effect.
Contraceptives (oral)	Decreased thyroxine effect.
Cortisone drugs	Requires dose adjustment to prevent cortisone deficiency.
Digitalis preparations	Increased digitalis effect.
Ephedrine	Increased ephedrine effect.
Epinephrine	Increased epinephrine effect.
Methylphenidate	Increased methylphenidate effect.
Phenytoin	Increased thyroxine effect.

POSSIBLE INTERACTION WITH OTHER SUBSTANCES

INTERACTS WITH	COMBINED EFFECT
Alcohol:	None expected.
Beverages:	None expected.
Cocaine:	Excess stimulation. Avoid.
Foods: Soybeans.	Heavy consumption interferes with thyroid function.
Marijuana:	None expected.
Tobacco:	None expected.

TICARCILLIN

BRAND NAMES

Ticar

BASIC INFORMATION

Habit forming? No
Prescription needed? Yes
Available as generic? Yes
Drug class: Antibiotic (penicillin)

 USES

Treatment of bacterial infections that are susceptible to ticarcillin.

 DOSAGE & USAGE INFORMATION

How to take:
By injection only.

When to take:
Follow doctor's instructions.

If you forget a dose:
Consult doctor.

What drug does:
Destroys susceptible bacteria. Does not kill viruses.

Time lapse before drug works:
May be several days before medicine affects infection.

Don't take with:
See Interaction column and consult doctor.

 OVERDOSE

SYMPTOMS:
Severe diarrhea, nausea, edema or vomiting.
WHAT TO DO:
Overdose unlikely to threaten life. If person takes much larger amount than prescribed, call doctor, poison-control center or hospital emergency room for instructions.

 POSSIBLE ADVERSE REACTIONS OR SIDE EFFECTS

SYMPTOMS	WHAT TO DO
Life-threatening: Hives, rash, intense itching, faintness soon after a dose (anaphylaxis).	Seek emergency treatment immediately.
Common: Dark or discolored tongue.	Continue. Tell doctor at next visit.
Infrequent: Mild nausea, vomiting, diarrhea.	Continue. Call doctor when convenient.
Rare: Unexplained bleeding.	Discontinue. Call doctor right away.

WARNINGS & PRECAUTIONS

Don't take if:
You are allergic to ticarcillin, cephalosporin antibiotics, other penicillins or penicillamine. Life-threatening reaction may occur.

Before you start, consult your doctor:
If you are allergic to any substance or drug.

Over age 60:
You may have skin reactions, particularly around genitals and anus.

Pregnancy:
Studies inconclusive on harm to unborn child. Animal studies show fetal abnormalities. Decide with your doctor whether drug benefits justify risk to unborn child.

Breast-feeding:
Drug passes into milk. Child may become sensitive to penicillins and have allergic reactions to penicillin drugs. Avoid ticarcillin or discontinue nursing until you finish medicine. Consult doctor for advice on maintaining milk supply.

Infants & children:
No problems expected.

Prolonged use:
You may become more susceptible to infections caused by germs not responsive to ticarcillin.

Skin & sunlight:
No problems expected.

Driving, piloting or hazardous work:
Usually not dangerous. Most hazardous reactions likely to occur a few minutes after taking ticarcillin.

Discontinuing:
Don't discontinue without doctor's advice until you complete prescribed dose, even though symptoms diminish or disappear.

Others:
No problems expected.

POSSIBLE INTERACTION WITH OTHER DRUGS

GENERIC NAME OR DRUG CLASS	COMBINED EFFECT
Beta-adrenergic blockers	Increased chance of anaphylaxis (see emergency information on inside front cover).
Chloramphenicol	Decreased effect of both drugs.
Erythromycins	Decreased effect of both drugs.
Loperamide	Decreased ticarcillin effect.
Paromomycin	Decreased effect of both drugs.
Tetracyclines	Decreased effect of both drugs.
Troleandomycin	Decreased effect of both drugs.

POSSIBLE INTERACTION WITH OTHER SUBSTANCES

INTERACTS WITH	COMBINED EFFECT
Alcohol:	Occasional stomach irritation.
Beverages:	None expected.
Cocaine:	No proven problems.
Foods:	None expected.
Marijuana:	No proven problems.
Tobacco:	None expected.

TIMOLOL

BRAND NAMES

Blocadren   Timoptic
Timolide

BASIC INFORMATION

Habit forming? No
Prescription needed? Yes
Available as generic? No
Drug class: Beta-adrenergic blocker,
          antiglaucoma agent

 USES

- Reduces angina attacks.
- Stabilizes irregular heartbeat.
- Lowers blood pressure.
- Reduces frequency of migraine headaches. (Does not relieve headache pain.)
- Decreases internal-eye pressure of glaucoma (ophthalmic drops).

 DOSAGE & USAGE INFORMATION

How to take:
- Eye drops—Wash hands. Apply slight pressure with finger to inside corner of eye. Pull lower eyelid down. Put drop just above lowered eyelid. Close eye gently for 2 minutes. Don't blink.
- Tablet or capsule—Swallow with liquid or crumble and take with food.

When to take:
- Tablet or capsule—With meals or immediately after.
- Eye drops—Follow prescription directions.

If you forget a dose:
Take as soon as you remember. Return to regular schedule, but allow 3 hours between doses.

Continued next column

 OVERDOSE

SYMPTOMS:
Weakness; slow or weak pulse; blood-pressure drop; fainting; convulsions; cold, sweaty skin.
WHAT TO DO:
- Dial 0 (operator) or 911 (emergency) for an ambulance or medical help. Then give first aid immediately.
- See emergency information on inside covers.

What drug does:
- Blocks certain actions of sympathetic nervous system.
- Lowers heart's oxygen requirements.
- Slows nerve impulses through heart.
- Reduces blood vessel contraction in heart, scalp and other body parts.
- Eye drops lower pressure inside eye.

Time lapse before drug works:
1 to 4 hours.

Don't take with:
Non-prescription drugs or drugs in Interaction column without consulting doctor.

 POSSIBLE ADVERSE REACTIONS OR SIDE EFFECTS

SYMPTOMS	WHAT TO DO
Life-threatening:	
None expected.	
Common:	
• Pulse slower than 50 beats per minute.	Discontinue. Call doctor right away.
• Drowsiness, numbness or tingling of fingers or toes, dizziness, diarrhea, nausea, fatigue, weakness.	Continue. Call doctor when convenient.
• Cold hands or feet; dry mouth, eyes and skin.	Continue. Tell doctor at next visit.
Infrequent:	
• Hallucinations, nightmares, insomnia, headache, difficult breathing.	Discontinue. Call doctor right away.
• Confusion, depression, reduced alertness, impotence.	Continue. Call doctor when convenient.
• Constipation.	Continue. Tell doctor at next visit.
Rare:	
• Rash, sore throat, fever.	Discontinue. Call doctor right away.
• Unusual bleeding or bruising.	Continue. Call doctor when convenient.

 WARNINGS & PRECAUTIONS

Don't take if:
- You are allergic to any beta-adrenergic blocker.
- You have asthma.
- You have hay fever symptoms.
- You have taken MAO inhibitors in past 2 weeks.

Before you start, consult your doctor:
- If you have heart disease or poor circulation to the extremities.
- If you have hay fever, asthma, chronic bronchitis, emphysema.
- If you have overactive thyroid function.
- If you have impaired liver or kidney function.
- If you will have surgery within 2 months, including dental surgery, requiring general or spinal anesthesia.
- If you have diabetes or hypoglycemia.

Over age 60:
Adverse reactions and side effects may be more frequent and severe than in younger persons.

Pregnancy:
Risk to unborn child outweighs drug benefits. Don't use.

Breast-feeding:
Drug passes into milk. Avoid drug or discontinue nursing until you finish medicine. Consult doctor about maintaining milk supply.

Infants & children:
Not recommended.

Prolonged use:
Weakens heart muscle contractions.

Skin & sunlight:
No problems expected.

Driving, piloting or hazardous work:
Don't drive or pilot aircraft until you learn how medicine affects you. Don't work around dangerous machinery. Don't climb ladders or work in high places. Danger increases if you drink alcohol or take medicine affecting alertness and reflexes.

Discontinuing:
Don't discontinue without consulting doctor. Dose may require gradual reduction if you have taken drug for a long time. Doses of other drugs may also require adjustment.

Others:
- May mask hypoglycemia.
- Side effects, such as burning or stinging of the eye, may also occur with timolol used as eye drops.

POSSIBLE INTERACTION WITH OTHER DRUGS

GENERIC NAME OR DRUG CLASS	COMBINED EFFECT
Acebutolol	Increased antihypertensive effects of both drugs. Dosages may require adjustment.
Albuterol	Decreased albuterol effect and beta-adrenergic blocking effect.
Antidiabetics	Increased antidiabetic effect.
Antihistamines	Decreased antihistamine effect.
Antihypertensives	Increased antihypertensive effect.
Anti-inflammatory drugs	Decreased effect of anti-inflammatory.
Barbiturates	Increased barbiturate effect. Dangerous sedation.
Digitalis preparations	Increased or decreased heart rate. Improves irregular heartbeat.
Narcotics	Increased narcotic effect. Dangerous sedation.
Nitrates	Possible excessive blood-pressure drop.
Pentoxifylline	Increased antihypertensive effect.
Phenytoin	Increased timolol effect.
Quinidine	Slows heart excessively.
Reserpine	Increased reserpine effect. Excessive sedation, depression.
Tocainide	May worsen congestive heart failure.

POSSIBLE INTERACTION WITH OTHER SUBSTANCES

INTERACTS WITH	COMBINED EFFECT
Alcohol:	Excessive blood-pressure drop. Avoid.
Beverages:	None expected.
Cocaine:	Irregular heartbeat. Avoid.
Foods:	None expected.
Marijuana:	Daily use—Impaired circulation to hands and feet.
Tobacco:	Possible irregular heartbeat.

TOCAINIDE

BRAND NAMES

Tonocard

BASIC INFORMATION

Habit forming? No
Prescription needed? Yes
Available as generic? No
Drug class: Antiarrhythmic

 USES

Stabilizes irregular heartbeat, particularly irregular contractions of the ventricles of the heart or a too rapid heart rate.

 DOSAGE & USAGE INFORMATION

How to take:
Tablet—Swallow with food, water or milk. Dosage may need to be changed according to individual response.

When to take:
Take at regular times each day. For example, instructions to take 3 times a day means every 8 hours.

If you forget a dose:
Take as soon as you remember up to 4 hours late. If more than 4 hours, wait for next scheduled dose (don't double this dose).

What drug does:
Decreases excitability of cells of heart muscle.

Time lapse before drug works:
30 minutes to 2 hours.

Don't take with:
- See Interaction column and consult doctor.
- Wear identification information that states that you take this medicine so during an emergency a physician will know to avoid additional medicines that might be harmful or dangerous.

 OVERDOSE

SYMPTOMS:
Convulsions, depressed breathing, cardiac arrest.
WHAT TO DO:
- **Dial 0 (operator) or 911 (emergency) for an ambulance or medical help. Then give first aid immediately.**
- **See emergency information on inside covers.**

 POSSIBLE ADVERSE REACTIONS OR SIDE EFFECTS

SYMPTOMS	WHAT TO DO
Life-threatening: None expected.	
Common: Nausea, vomiting.	Discontinue. Call doctor right away.
Infrequent:	
• Trembling.	Discontinue. Call doctor right away.
• Lightheadedness.	Continue. Call doctor when convenient.
Rare:	
• Sore throat, red tongue, mouth ulcers, unexplained bleeding or bruising, fever, chills.	Discontinue. Seek emergency treatment.
• Blurred vision, may accelerate heart rate or worsen irregular heartbeat, cough, difficult breathing, wheezing, may decrease white blood-cell count.	Discontinue. Call doctor right away.
• Numbness or tingling in hands or feet, rash, joint pain, swollen feet and ankles, unusual sweating.	Continue. Call doctor when convenient.

WARNINGS & PRECAUTIONS

Don't take if:
- You are allergic to tocainide or anesthetics whose names end in "caine."
- You have myasthenia gravis.

Before you start, consult your doctor:
- If you have congestive heart failure.
- If you are pregnant or plan to become pregnant.
- If you take anticancer drugs, trimethoprim, pyrimethamine, primaquine, phenylbutazone, penicillamine or oxyphenbutazone. These may affect blood-cell production in bone marrow.
- If you take any other heart medicine such as digitalis, flucystosine, colchicine, chloramphenicol, beta-adrenergic blockers or azathioprine. These can worsen heartbeat irregularity.
- If you will have surgery within 2 months, including dental surgery, requiring general, local or spinal anesthesia.
- If you have liver or kidney disease.

Over age 60:
Adverse reactions and side effects may be more frequent and severe than in younger persons.

Pregnancy:
No proven harm to unborn child. Nevertheless, avoid if possible.

Breast-feeding:
Avoid if possible.

Infants & children:
Not recommended. Safety and dosage have not been established.

Prolonged use:
Request periodic lab studies on blood, liver function, potassium levels.

Skin & sunlight:
No problems expected.

Driving, piloting or hazardous work:
Use caution if medicine causes you to feel dizzy or weak. Otherwise, no problems expected.

Discontinuing:
Don't discontinue without consulting doctor, even though symptoms diminish or disappear.

Others:
No problems expected.

POSSIBLE INTERACTION WITH OTHER DRUGS

GENERIC NAME OR DRUG CLASS	COMBINED EFFECT
Antiarrhythmics (others)	Increased possibility of adverse reactions from either drug.
Beta-adrenergic blockers	Possible irregular heartbeat. May worsen congestive heart failure.
Bone-marrow depressants, such as anticancer drugs, azathyoprine, chloramphenicol, colchicine, flucytosine, oxyphenbutazone, penicillamine, phenylbutazone, primaquine, pyrimethamine, trimethoprim.	Possible decreased production of blood cells in bone marrow.

POSSIBLE INTERACTION WITH OTHER SUBSTANCES

INTERACTS WITH	COMBINED EFFECT
Alcohol:	Possible irregular heartbeat. Avoid.
Beverages: Caffeine drinks, iced drinks.	Possible irregular heartbeat.
Cocaine:	Possible lightheadedness, dizziness, quivering, convulsions.
Foods:	None expected.
Marijuana:	None expected.
Tobacco:	Possible irregular heartbeat.

TOLAZAMIDE

BRAND NAMES

Ronase   Tolinase

BASIC INFORMATION

Habit forming? No
Prescription needed? Yes
Available as generic? Yes
Drug class: Antidiabetic (oral), sulfonurea

USES

Treatment for diabetes in adults who can't control blood sugar by diet, weight loss and exercise.

DOSAGE & USAGE INFORMATION

How to take:
Tablet—Swallow with liquid or food to lessen stomach irritation. If you can't swallow whole, crumble tablet and take with liquid or food.

When to take:
At the same times each day.

If you forget a dose:
Take as soon as you remember up to 2 hours late. If more than 2 hours, wait for next scheduled dose (don't double this dose).

What drug does:
Stimulates pancreas to produce more insulin. Insulin in blood forces cells to use sugar in blood.

Time lapse before drug works:
3 to 4 hours. May require 2 weeks for maximum benefit.

Don't take with:
See Interaction column and consult doctor.

OVERDOSE

SYMPTOMS:
Excessive hunger, nausea, anxiety, cool skin, cold sweats, drowsiness, rapid heartbeat, weakness, unconsciousness, coma.
WHAT TO DO:
- **Dial 0 (operator) or 911 (emergency) for an ambulance or medical help. Then give first aid immediately.**
- **See emergency information on inside covers.**

POSSIBLE ADVERSE REACTIONS OR SIDE EFFECTS

SYMPTOMS	WHAT TO DO
Life-threatening: None expected.	
Common:	
• Dizziness.	Discontinue. Call doctor right away.
• Diarrhea, appetite loss, nausea, stomach pain, heartburn.	Continue. Call doctor when convenient.
Infrequent: Low blood sugar (hunger, anxiety, cold sweats, rapid pulse).	Discontinue. Seek emergency treatment.
Rare: Fatigue, itchy skin or rash, sore throat, fever, ringing in ears, unusual bleeding or bruising, jaundice.	Discontinue. Call doctor right away.

WARNINGS & PRECAUTIONS

Don't take if:
- You are allergic to any sulfonurea.
- You have impaired kidney or liver function.

Before you start, consult your doctor:
- If you have a severe infection.
- If you have thyroid disease.
- If you take insulin.
- If you have heart disease.

Over age 60:
Dose usually smaller than for younger adults. Avoid "low-blood-sugar" episodes because repeated ones can damage brain permanently.

Pregnancy:
No proven harm to unborn child. Avoid if possible.

Breast-feeding:
Drug filters into milk. May lower baby's blood sugar. Avoid.

Infants & children:
Don't give to infants or children.

Prolonged use:
None expected.

Skin & sunlight:
May cause rash or intensify sunburn in areas exposed to sun or sunlamp.

Driving, piloting or hazardous work:
No problems expected unless you develop hypoglycemia (low blood sugar). If so, avoid driving or hazardous activity.

Discontinuing:
Don't discontinue without consulting doctor. Dose may require gradual reduction if you have taken drug for a long time. Doses of other drugs may also require adjustment.

Others:
Don't exceed recommended dose.
Hypoglycemia (low blood sugar) may occur, even with proper dose schedule. You must balance medicine, diet and exercise.

POSSIBLE INTERACTION WITH OTHER DRUGS

GENERIC NAME OR DRUG CLASS	COMBINED EFFECT
Androgens	Increased tolazamide effect.
Anticoagulants (oral)	Unpredictable prothrombin times.
Anticonvulsants (hydantoin)	Decreased tolazamide effect.
Anti-inflammatory drugs (non-steroidal)	Increased tolazamide effect.
Aspirin	Increased tolazamide effect.
Beta-adrenergic blockers	Increased tolazamide effect. Possible increased difficulty in regulating blood-sugar levels.
Chloramphenicol	Increased tolazamide effect.
Clofibrate	Increased tolazamide effect.
Contraceptives (oral)	Decreased tolazamide effect.
Cortisone drugs	Decreased tolazamide effect.
Diuretics (thiazide)	Decreased tolazamide effect.
Epinephrine	Decreased tolazamide effect.
Estrogens	Increased tolazamide effect.
Guanethidine	Unpredictable tolazamide effect.
Isoniazid	Decreased tolazamide effect.
Labetolol	Increased antidiabetic effect, may mask hypoglycemia.
MAO inhibitors	Increased tolazamide effect.
Oxyphenbutazone	Increased tolazamide effect.
Phenylbutazone	Increased tolazamide effect.
Phenyramidol	Increased tolazamide effect.
Probenecid	Increased tolazamide effect.
Pyrazinamide	Decreased tolazamide effect.
Sulfaphenazole	Increased tolazamide effect.
Sulfa drugs	Increased tolazamide effect.
Thyroid hormones	Decreased tolazamide effect.

POSSIBLE INTERACTION WITH OTHER SUBSTANCES

INTERACTS WITH	COMBINED EFFECT
Alcohol:	Disulfiram reaction (see Glossary). Avoid.
Beverages:	None expected.
Cocaine:	No proven problems.
Foods:	None expected.
Marijuana:	Decreased tolazamide effect. Avoid.
Tobacco:	None expected.

TOLBUTAMIDE

BRAND NAMES

Apo-Tolbutamide	Oramide
Mobenol	Orinase
Neo-Dibetic	SK-Tolbutamide
Novobutamide	Tolbutone

BASIC INFORMATION

Habit forming? No
Prescription needed? Yes
Available as generic? Yes
Drug class: Antidiabetic (oral), sulfonurea

 ## USES

Treatment for diabetes in adults who can't control blood sugar by diet, weight loss and exercise.

 ## DOSAGE & USAGE INFORMATION

How to take:
Tablet—Swallow with liquid or food to lessen stomach irritation. If you can't swallow whole, crumble tablet and take with liquid or food.

When to take:
At the same times each day.

If you forget a dose:
Take as soon as you remember up to 2 hours late. If more than 2 hours, wait for next scheduled dose (don't double this dose).

What drug does:
Stimulates pancreas to produce more insulin. Insulin in blood forces cells to use sugar in blood.

Time lapse before drug works:
3 to 4 hours. May require 2 weeks for maximum benefit.

Don't take with:
See Interaction column and consult doctor.

 ## OVERDOSE

SYMPTOMS:
Excessive hunger, nausea, anxiety, cool skin, cold sweats, drowsiness, rapid heartbeat, weakness, unconsciousness, coma.
WHAT TO DO:
- **Dial 0 (operator) or 911 (emergency) for an ambulance or medical help. Then give first aid immediately.**
- **See emergency information on inside covers.**

 ## POSSIBLE ADVERSE REACTIONS OR SIDE EFFECTS

SYMPTOMS	WHAT TO DO
Life-threatening: None expected.	
Common:	
• Dizziness.	Discontinue. Call doctor right away.
• Diarrhea, appetite loss, nausea, stomach pain, heartburn.	Continue. Call doctor when convenient.
Infrequent: Low blood sugar (hunger, anxiety, cold sweats, rapid pulse).	Discontinue. Seek emergency treatment.
Rare: Fatigue, itchy skin or rash, sore throat, fever, ringing in ears, unusual bleeding or bruising, jaundice.	Discontinue. Call doctor right away.

 ## WARNINGS & PRECAUTIONS

Don't take if:
- You are allergic to any sulfonurea.
- You have impaired kidney or liver function.

Before you start, consult your doctor:
- If you have a severe infection.
- If you have thyroid disease.
- If you take insulin.
- If you have heart disease.

Over age 60:
Dose usually smaller than for younger adults. Avoid "low-blood-sugar" episodes because repeated ones can damage brain permanently.

Pregnancy:
No proven harm to unborn child. Avoid if possible.

Breast-feeding:
Drug filters into milk. May lower baby's blood sugar. Avoid.

Infants & children:
Don't give to infants or children.

Prolonged use:
None expected.

Skin & sunlight:
May cause rash or intensify sunburn in areas exposed to sun or sunlamp.

Driving, piloting or hazardous work:
No problems expected unless you develop hypoglycemia (low blood sugar). If so, avoid driving or hazardous activity.

Discontinuing:
Don't discontinue without consulting doctor. Dose may require gradual reduction if you have taken drug for a long time. Doses of other drugs may also require adjustment.

Others:
Don't exceed recommended dose. Hypoglycemia (low blood sugar) may occur, even with proper dose schedule. You must balance medicine, diet and exercise.

POSSIBLE INTERACTION WITH OTHER DRUGS

GENERIC NAME OR DRUG CLASS	COMBINED EFFECT
Androgens	Increased tolbutamide effect.
Anticoagulants (oral)	Unpredictable prothrombin times.
Anticonvulsants (hydantoin)	Decreased tolbutamide effect.
Anti-inflammatory drugs (non-steroidal)	Increased tolbutamide effect.
Aspirin	Increased tolbutamide effect.
Beta-adrenergic blockers	Increased tolbutamide effect. Possible increased difficulty in regulating blood-sugar levels.
Chloramphenicol	Increased tolbutamide effect.
Clofibrate	Increased tolbutamide effect.
Contraceptives (oral)	Decreased tolbutamide effect.
Cortisone drugs	Decreased tolbutamide effect.
Diuretics (thiazide)	Decreased tolbutamide effect.
Epinephrine	Decreased tolbutamide effect.
Estrogens	Increased tolbutamide effect.
Guanethidine	Unpredictable tolbutamide effect.
Isoniazid	Decreased tolbutamide effect.
Labetolol	Increased antidiabetic effect, may mask hypoglycemia.
MAO inhibitors	Increased tolbutamide effect.
Oxyphenbutazone	Increased tolbutamide effect.
Phenylbutazone	Increased tolbutamide effect.
Phenyramidol	Increased tolbutamide effect.
Probenecid	Increased tolbutamide effect.
Pyrazinamide	Decreased tolbutamide effect.
Sulfa drugs	Increased tolbutamide effect.
Sulfaphenazole	Increased tolbutamide effect.
Thyroid hormones	Decreased tolbutamide effect.

POSSIBLE INTERACTION WITH OTHER SUBSTANCES

INTERACTS WITH	COMBINED EFFECT
Alcohol:	Disulfiram reaction (see Glossary). Avoid.
Beverages:	None expected.
Cocaine:	No proven problems.
Foods:	None expected.
Marijuana:	Decreased tolbutamide effect. Avoid.
Tobacco:	None expected.

TOLMETIN

BRAND NAMES

Tolectin   Tolectin DS

BASIC INFORMATION

Habit forming? No
Prescription needed? Yes
Available as generic? No
Drug class: Anti-inflammatory (non-steroid)

 USES

- Treatment for joint pain, stiffness, inflammation and swelling of arthritis and gout.
- Pain reliever.

 DOSAGE & USAGE INFORMATION

How to take:
Tablet or capsule—Swallow with liquid or food to lessen stomach irritation. If you can't swallow whole, crumble tablet or open capsule and take with liquid or food.

When to take:
At the same times each day.

If you forget a dose:
Take as soon as you remember up to 2 hours late. If more than 2 hours, wait for next scheduled dose (don't double this dose).

What drug does:
Reduces tissue concentration of prostaglandins (hormones which produce inflammation and pain).

Time lapse before drug works:
Begins in 4 to 24 hours. May require 3 weeks regular use for maximum benefit.

Don't take with:
See Interaction column and consult doctor.

 OVERDOSE

SYMPTOMS:
Confusion, agitation, incoherence, convulsions, possible hemorrhage from stomach or intestine, coma.
WHAT TO DO:
- Dial 0 (operator) or 911 (emergency) for an ambulance or medical help. Then give first aid immediately.
- See emergency information on inside covers.

 POSSIBLE ADVERSE REACTIONS OR SIDE EFFECTS

SYMPTOMS	WHAT TO DO
Life-threatening: None expected.	
Common:	
● Dizziness, nausea, pain.	Continue. Call doctor when convenient.
● Headache.	Continue. Tell doctor at next visit.
Infrequent: Depression, drowsiness, ringing in ears, swollen feet or legs, constipation or diarrhea, vomiting.	Continue. Call doctor when convenient.
Rare:	
● Convulsions; confusion; rash, hives or itchy skin; blurred vision; black, bloody or tarry stools; difficult breathing; tightness in chest; rapid heartbeat; unusual bleeding or bruising; blood in urine; jaundice.	Discontinue. Call doctor right away.
● Painful or difficult urination, fatigue, weakness.	Continue. Call doctor when convenient.

WARNINGS & PRECAUTIONS

Don't take if:
- You are allergic to aspirin or any non-steroid, anti-inflammatory drug.
- You have gastritis, peptic ulcer, enteritis, ileitis, ulcerative colitis, asthma, heart failure, high blood pressure or bleeding problems.
- Patient is younger than 15.

Before you start, consult your doctor:
- If you have epilepsy.
- If you have Parkinson's disease.
- If you have been mentally ill.
- If you have had kidney disease or impaired kidney function.

Over age 60:
Adverse reactions and side effects may be more frequent and severe than in younger persons.

Pregnancy:
Studies inconclusive on harm to unborn child. Decide with your doctor whether drug benefits justify risk to unborn child.

Breast-feeding:
May harm child. Avoid.

Infants & children:
Not recommended for anyone younger than 15. Use only under medical supervision.

Prolonged use:
- Eye damage.
- Reduced hearing.
- Sore throat, fever.
- Weight gain.

Skin & sunlight:
No problems expected.

Driving, piloting or hazardous work:
Don't drive or pilot aircraft until you learn how medicine affects you. Don't work around dangerous machinery. Don't climb ladders or work in high places. Danger increases if you drink alcohol or take medicine affecting alertness and reflexes, such as antihistamines, tranquilizers, sedatives, pain medicine, narcotics and mind-altering drugs.

Discontinuing:
Don't discontinue without consulting doctor. Dose may require gradual reduction if you have taken drug for a long time. Doses of other drugs may also require adjustment.

Others:
No problems expected.

POSSIBLE INTERACTION WITH OTHER DRUGS

GENERIC NAME OR DRUG CLASS	COMBINED EFFECT
Acebutolol	Decreased antihypertensive effect of acebutolol.
Anticoagulants (oral)	Increased risk of bleeding.
Aspirin	Increased risk of stomach ulcer.
Cortisone drugs	Increased risk of stomach ulcer.
Furosemide	Decreased diuretic effect of furosemide.
Gold compounds	Possible increased likelihood of kidney damage.
Ketoprofen	Increased possibility of internal bleeding.
Minoxidil	Decreased minoxidil effect.
Oxprenolol	Decreased antihypertensive effect of oxprenolol.
Oxyphenbutazone	Possible stomach ulcer.
Phenylbutazone	Possible stomach ulcer.
Probenecid	Increased tolmetin effect.
Thyroid hormones	Rapid heartbeat, blood-pressure rise.

POSSIBLE INTERACTION WITH OTHER SUBSTANCES

INTERACTS WITH	COMBINED EFFECT
Alcohol:	Possible stomach ulcer or bleeding.
Beverages:	None expected.
Cocaine:	None expected.
Foods:	None expected.
Marijuana:	Increased pain relief from tolmetin.
Tobacco:	None expected.

TRAZODONE

BRAND NAMES

Desyrel   Desyrel Dividose

BASIC INFORMATION

Habit forming? No
Prescription needed? Yes
Available as generic? No
Drug class: Antidepressant (non-tricyclic)

 ## USES

- Treats mental depression.
- Treats anxiety.

 ## DOSAGE & USAGE INFORMATION

How to take:
Tablet or capsule—Swallow with liquid or food to lessen stomach irritation. If you can't swallow whole, crumble tablet or open capsule and take with liquid or food.

When to take:
According to prescription directions. Bedtime dose usually higher than other doses.

If you forget a dose:
Take as soon as you remember up to 2 hours late. If more than 2 hours, wait for next scheduled dose (don't double this dose).

What drug does:
Inhibits serotonin uptake in brain cells.

Time lapse before drug works:
2 to 4 weeks for full effect.

Don't take with:
See Interaction column and consult doctor.

 ## OVERDOSE

SYMPTOMS:
Fainting, irregular heartbeat, chest pain, seizures, coma.
WHAT TO DO:
- Dial 0 (operator) or 911 (emergency) for an ambulance or medical help. Then give first aid immediately.
- If patient is unconscious and not breathing, give mouth-to-mouth breathing. If there is no heartbeat, use cardiac massage and mouth-to-mouth breathing (CPR). Don't try to make patient vomit. If you can't get help quickly, take patient to nearest emergency facility.
- See emergency information on inside covers.

 ## POSSIBLE ADVERSE REACTIONS OR SIDE EFFECTS

SYMPTOMS	WHAT TO DO
Life-threatening: None expected.	
Common: None expected.	
Infrequent:	
• Tremor, incoordination, blood pressue rise or drop, rapid heartbeat, shortness of breath, fainting.	Discontinue. Call doctor right away.
• Dizziness on standing, confusion, disorientation, drowsiness, excitement, fatigue, headache, nervousness, rash, itchy skin, blurred vision, ringing in ears, dry mouth, bad taste, diarrhea, nausea, vomiting, constipation, aching, prolonged penile erections, menstrual changes, diminished sex drive.	Continue. Call doctor when convenient.
Rare: None expected.	

WARNINGS & PRECAUTIONS

Don't take if:
- You are allergic to trazodone.
- You are thinking about suicide.

Before you start, consult your doctor:
- If you have heart rhythm problem.
- If you have any heart disease.
- If you will have surgery within 2 months, including dental surgery, requiring general or spinal anesthesia.

Over age 60:
Adverse reactions and side effects may be more frequent and severe than in younger persons.

Pregnancy:
Risk to unborn child outweighs drug benefits. Don't use.

Breast-feeding:
Drug passes into milk. Avoid drug or discontinue nursing until you finish medicine. Consult doctor for advice on maintaining milk supply.

Infants & children:
Not recommended.

Prolonged use:
Occasional blood counts, especially if you have fever and sore throat.

Skin & sunlight:
No problems expected.

Driving, piloting or hazardous work:
Don't drive or pilot aircraft until you learn how medicine affects you. Don't work around dangerous machinery. Don't climb ladders or work in high places. Danger increases if you drink alcohol or take medicine affecting alertness and reflexes, such as antihistamines, tranquilizers, sedatives, pain medicine, narcotics and mind-altering drugs.

Discontinuing:
Don't discontinue without consulting doctor. Dose may require gradual reduction if you have taken drug for a long time. Doses of other drugs may also require adjustment.

Others:
Electroshock therapy should be avoided.

POSSIBLE INTERACTION WITH OTHER DRUGS

GENERIC NAME OR DRUG CLASS	COMBINED EFFECT
Antidepressants (other)	Excess drowsiness.
Antihistamines	Excess drowsiness.
Antihypertensives	Too low blood pressure. Avoid.
Barbiturates	Too low blood pressure. Avoid.
Digitalis preparations	Increased digitalis level in blood.
MAO inhibitors	May add to toxic effect of each.
Narcotics	Excess drowsiness.
Phenytoin	Increased phenytoin level in blood.
Sedatives	Excess drowsiness.
Tranquilizers	Excess drowsiness.

POSSIBLE INTERACTION WITH OTHER SUBSTANCES

INTERACTS WITH	COMBINED EFFECT
Alcohol:	Excess sedation. Avoid.
Beverages: Caffeine.	May add to heartbeat irregularity. Avoid.
Cocaine:	May add to heartbeat irregularity. Avoid.
Foods:	No problems expected.
Marijuana:	May add to heartbeat irregularity. Avoid.
Tobacco:	May add to heartbeat irregularity. Avoid.

TRETINOIN

BRAND NAMES

Retin-A   StieVAA
Retinoic Acid   Vitamin A Acid

BASIC INFORMATION

Habit forming? No
Prescription needed? Yes
Available as generic? Yes
Drug class: Antiacne (topical)

 ## USES

Treatment for acne, psoriasis, ichthyosis, keratosis, folliculitis, flat warts.

 ## DOSAGE & USAGE INFORMATION

How to use:
Wash skin with non-medicated soap, pat dry, wait 20 minutes before applying.
- Cream or gel—Apply to affected areas with fingertips and rub in gently.
- Solution—Apply to affected areas with gauze pad or cotton swab. Avoid getting too wet so medicine doesn't drip into eyes, mouth, lips or inside nose.
- Follow manufacturer's directions on container.

When to use:
At the same time each day.

If you forget an application:
Use as soon as you remember.

What drug does:
Increases skin-cell turnover so skin layer peels off more easily.

Time lapse before drug works:
2 to 3 weeks. May require 6 weeks for maximum improvement.

Don't use with:
- Benzoyl peroxide. Apply 12 hours apart.
- See Interaction column and consult doctor.

 ## OVERDOSE

SYMPTOMS:
None expected.
WHAT TO DO:
If person swallows drug, call doctor, poison-control center or hospital emergency room for instructions.

 ## POSSIBLE ADVERSE REACTIONS OR SIDE EFFECTS

SYMPTOMS	WHAT TO DO
Life-threatening: None expected.	
Common:	
• Pigment change in treated area, warmth or stinging, peeling.	Continue. Tell doctor at next visit.
• Senstivity to wind or cold.	No action necessary.
Infrequent: Blistering, crusting, severe burning, swelling.	Discontinue. Call doctor right away.
Rare: None expected.	

WARNINGS & PRECAUTIONS

Don't take if:
- You are allergic to tretinoin.
- You are sunburned, windburned or have an open skin wound.

Before you start, consult your doctor:
If you have eczema.

Over age 60:
Not recommended.

Pregnancy:
No proven harm to unborn child. Avoid if possible.

Breast-feeding:
No problems expected.

Infants & children:
Not recommended.

Prolonged use:
No problems expected.

Skin & sunlight:
- May cause rash or intensify sunburn in areas exposed to sun or sunlamp.
- In some animal studies, tretinoin caused skin tumors to develop faster when treated area was exposed to ultraviolet light (sunlight or sunlamp). No proven similar effects in humans.

Driving, piloting or hazardous work:
No problems expected.

Discontinuing:
Don't discontinue without doctor's advice until you complete prescribed dose, even though symptoms diminish or disappear.

Others:
Acne may get worse before improvement starts in 2 or 3 weeks. Don't wash face more than 2 or 3 times daily.

POSSIBLE INTERACTION WITH OTHER DRUGS

GENERIC NAME OR DRUG CLASS	COMBINED EFFECT
Antiacne topical preparations (other)	Severe skin irritation.
Cosmetics (medicated)	Severe skin irritation.
Skin preparations with alcohol	Severe skin irritation.
Soaps or cleansers (abrasive)	Severe skin irritation.

POSSIBLE INTERACTION WITH OTHER SUBSTANCES

INTERACTS WITH	COMBINED EFFECT
Alcohol:	None expected.
Beverages:	None expected.
Cocaine:	None expected.
Foods:	None expected.
Marijuana:	None expected.
Tobacco:	None expected.

BRAND NAMES

See complete list of brand names in the
Brand Name Directory, page 958.

BASIC INFORMATION

Habit forming? No
Prescription needed? Yes
Available as generic? Yes
**Drug class: Cortisone drug (adrenal
corticosteroid)**

 USES

- Reduces inflammation caused by many
  different medical problems.
- Treatment for some allergic diseases, blood
  disorders, kidney diseases, asthma and
  emphysema.
- Replaces corticosteroid deficiencies.

 DOSAGE & USAGE
INFORMATION

How to take:
Tablet or syrup—Swallow with liquid or food to
lessen stomach irritation. If you can't swallow
whole, crumble tablet.

When to take:
At the same times each day. Take once-a-day
or once-every-other-day doses in mornings.

If you forget a dose:
- Several-doses-per-day prescription—Take as
  soon as you remember up to 2 hours late. If
  more than 2 hours, wait for next scheduled
  dose (don't double this dose).
- Once-a-day dose or less—Wait for next dose.
  Double this dose.

What drug does:
Decreases inflammatory responses.

Time lapse before drug works:
2 to 4 days.

Don't take with:
See Interaction column and consult doctor.

 OVERDOSE

SYMPTOMS:
Headache, convulsions, heart failure.
WHAT TO DO:
- **Dial 0 (operator) or 911 (emergency) for an
  ambulance or medical help. Then give first
  aid immediately.**
- **See emergency information on inside
  covers.**

 POSSIBLE
ADVERSE REACTIONS
OR SIDE EFFECTS

SYMPTOMS	WHAT TO DO
Life-threatening:	
None expected.	
Common:	
Acne, thirst, indigestion, nausea, vomiting, poor wound healing.	Continue. Call doctor when convenient.
Infrequent:	
● Black, bloody or tarry stool.	Discontinue. Seek emergency treatment.
● Blurred vision, halos around lights, muscle cramps, swollen legs and feet, sore throat, fever.	Discontinue. Call doctor right away.
● Mood change, insomnia, restlessness, frequent urination, weight gain, round face, fatigue, weakness, TB recurrence, menstrual irregularities.	Continue. Call doctor when convenient.
Rare:	
● Irregular heartbeat.	Discontinue. Seek emergency treatment.
● Rash.	Discontinue. Call doctor right away.

 WARNINGS &
PRECAUTIONS

Don't take if:
- You are allergic to any cortisone drug.
- You have tuberculosis or fungus infection.
- You have herpes infection of eyes, lips or
  genitals.

Before you start, consult your doctor:
- If you have had tuberculosis.
- If you have congestive heart failure.
- If you have diabetes.
- If you have peptic ulcer.
- If you have glaucoma.
- If you have underactive thyroid.
- If you have high blood pressure.
- If you have myasthenia gravis.
- If you have blood clots in legs or lungs.

Over age 60:
Adverse reactions and side effects may be
more frequent and severe than in younger
persons. Likely to aggravate edema, diabetes or
ulcers. Likely to cause cataracts and
osteoporosis (softening of the bones).

Pregnancy:
Risk to unborn child outweighs drug benefits.
Don't use.

Breast-feeding:
Drug passes into milk. Avoid drug or
discontinue nursing until you finish medicine.
Consult doctor for advice on maintaining milk
supply.

Infants & children:
Use only under medical supervision.

Prolonged use:
• Retards growth in children.
• Possible glaucoma, cataracts, diabetes,
  fragile bones and thin skin.
• Functional dependence.

Skin & sunlight:
No problems expected.

Driving, piloting or hazardous work:
No problems expected.

Discontinuing:
• Don't discontinue without doctor's advice until
  you complete prescribed dose, even though
  symptoms diminish or disappear.
• Drug affects your response to surgery, illness,
  injury or stress for 2 years after discontinuing.
  Tell anyone who takes medical care of you
  within 2 years about drug.

Others:
Avoid immunizations if possible.

POSSIBLE INTERACTION WITH OTHER DRUGS

GENERIC NAME OR DRUG CLASS	COMBINED EFFECT
Amphoterecin B	Potassium depletion.
Anticholinergics	Possible glaucoma.
Anticoagulants (oral)	Decreased anticoagulant effect.
Anticonvulsants (hydantoin)	Decreased triamcinolone effect.
Antidiabetics (oral)	Decreased antidiabetic effect.
Antihistamines	Decreased triamcinolone effect.
Aspirin	Increased triamcinolone effect.
Barbiturates	Decreased triamcinolone effect. Oversedation.
Beta-adrenergic blockers	Decreased triamcinolone effect.
Chloral hydrate	Decreased triamcinolone effect.
Chlorthalidone	Potassium depletion.

Cholinergics	Decreased cholinergic effect.
Contraceptives (oral)	Increased triamcinolone effect.
Digitalis preparations	Dangerous potassium depletion. Possible digitalis toxicity.
Diuretics (thiazide)	Potassium depletion.
Ephedrine	Decreased triamcinolone effect.
Estrogens	Increased triamcinolone effect.
Ethacrynic acid	Potassium depletion.
Furosemide	Potassium depletion.
Glutethimide	Decreased triamcinolone effect.
Indapamide	Possible excessive potassium loss, causing dangerous heartbeat irregularity.
Indomethacin	Increased triamcinolone effect.
Insulin	Decreased insulin effect.
Isoniazid	Decreased isoniazid effect.
Oxyphenbutazone	Possible ulcers.
Phenylbutazone	Possible ulcers.
Potassium supplements	Decreased potassium effect.
Rifampin	Decreased triamcinolone effect.
Sympathomimetics	Possible glaucoma.

POSSIBLE INTERACTION WITH OTHER SUBSTANCES

INTERACTS WITH	COMBINED EFFECT
Alcohol:	Risk of stomach ulcers.
Beverages:	No proven problems.
Cocaine:	Overstimulation. Avoid.
Foods:	No proven problems.
Marijuana:	Decreased immunity.
Tobacco:	Increased triamcinolone effect. Possible toxicity.

TRIAMTERENE

BRAND NAMES

Dyazide   Maxzide
Dyrenium

BASIC INFORMATION

Habit forming? No
Prescription needed? Yes
Available as generic? No
Drug class: Antihypertensive, diuretic

 USES

- Reduces fluid retention (edema).
- Reduces potassium loss.

 DOSAGE & USAGE INFORMATION

How to take:
Tablet or capsule—Swallow with liquid or food to lessen stomach irritation. If you can't swallow whole, crumble tablet or open capsule and take with liquid or food.

When to take:
- 1 dose per day—Take after breakfast.
- More than 1 dose per day—Take last dose no later than 6 p.m.

If you forget a dose:
Take as soon as you remember up to 6 hours late. If more than 6 hours, wait for next scheduled dose (don't double this dose).

What drug does:
Increases urine production to eliminate sodium and water from body while conserving potassium.

Continued next column

 OVERDOSE

SYMPTOMS:
Lethargy, irregular heartbeat, coma.
WHAT TO DO:
- **Dial 0 (operator) or 911 (emergency) for an ambulance or medical help. Then give first aid immediately.**
- **If patient is unconscious and not breathing, give mouth-to-mouth breathing. If there is no heartbeat, use cardiac massage and mouth-to-mouth breathing (CPR). Don't try to make patient vomit. If you can't get help quickly, take patient to nearest emergency facility.**
- **See emergency information on inside covers.**

Time lapse before drug works:
2 hours. May require 2 to 3 days for maximum benefit.

Don't take with:
See Interaction column and consult doctor.

 POSSIBLE ADVERSE REACTIONS OR SIDE EFFECTS

SYMPTOMS	WHAT TO DO
Life-threatening: None expected.	
Common: None expected.	
Infrequent:	
• Drowsiness, confusion, dry mouth, thirst, irregular heartbeat, shortness of breath, unusual tiredness, weakness.	Discontinue. Call doctor right away.
• Diarrhea.	Continue. Call doctor when convenient.
• Anxiety.	Continue. Tell doctor at next visit.
Rare:	
• Rash, sore throat, fever, red or inflamed tongue, unusual bleeding or bruising.	Discontinue. Call doctor right away.
• Headache.	Continue. Tell doctor at next visit.

WARNINGS & PRECAUTIONS

Don't take if:
- You are allergic to triamterene.
- You have had severe liver or kidney disease.

Before you start, consult your doctor:
- If you have gout.
- If you have diabetes.
- If you will have surgery within 2 months, including dental surgery, requiring general or spinal anesthesia.

Over age 60:
- Warm weather or fever can decrease blood pressure. Dose may require adjustment.
- Extended use can increase blood clots.

Pregnancy:
No proven harm to unborn child. Avoid if possible.

Breast-feeding:
Present in milk. Avoid.

Infants & children:
Used infrequently. Use only under medical supervision.

Prolonged use:
Potassium retention which may lead to heart-rhythm problems.

Skin & sunlight:
May cause rash or intensify sunburn in areas exposed to sun or sunlamp.

Driving, piloting or hazardous work:
Avoid if you feel drowsy or confused. Otherwise, no problems expected.

Discontinuing:
Don't discontinue without consulting doctor. Dose may require gradual reduction if you have taken drug for a long time. Doses of other drugs may also require adjustment.

Others:
No problems expected.

 POSSIBLE INTERACTION WITH OTHER DRUGS

GENERIC NAME OR DRUG CLASS	COMBINED EFFECT
Acebutolol	Increased antihypertensive effect. Dosages may require adjustment.
Amiodarone	Increased risk of heartbeat irregularity due to low potassium.
Antidiabetics (oral)	Decreased antidiabetic effect.
Antihypertensives (other)	Increased effect of other antihypertensives.
Calcium supplements	Increased calcium in blood.
Digitalis preparations	Decreased digitalis effect.
Enalapril	Possible excessive potassium in blood.
Labetolol	Increased antihypertensive effects.
Lithium	Increased lithium effect.
Nitrates	Excessive blood-pressure drop.
Oxprenolol	Increased antihypertensive effect. Dosages may require adjustment.
Potassium supplements	Possible excessive potassium retention.
Spironolactone	Dangerous retention of potassium.

 POSSIBLE INTERACTION WITH OTHER SUBSTANCES

INTERACTS WITH	COMBINED EFFECT
Alcohol:	None expected.
Beverages:	None expected.
Cocaine:	Decreased triamterene effect.
Foods: Salt.	Don't restrict unless directed by doctor.
Marijuana:	Daily use—Fainting likely.
Tobacco:	None expected.

TRIAMTERENE & HYDROCHLOROTHIAZIDE

BRAND NAMES

Dyazide   Maxzide

BASIC INFORMATION

Habit forming? No
Prescription needed? Yes
Available as generic? No
Drug class: Diuretic

 USES

- Reduces fluid retention (edema).
- Reduces potassium loss.
- Controls, but doesn't cure, high blood pressure.

 DOSAGE & USAGE INFORMATION

How to take:
Tablet or capsule—Swallow with liquid. If you can't swallow whole, crumble tablet or open capsule and take with liquid or food.

When to take:
- 1 dose per day—Take after breakfast.
- More than 1 dose per day—Take last dose no later than 6 p.m.

If you forget a dose:
Take as soon as you remember up to 6 hours late. If more than 6 hours, wait for next scheduled dose (don't double this dose).

What drug does:
- Increases urine production to eliminate sodium and water from body while conserving potassium.

Continued next column

 OVERDOSE

SYMPTOMS:
Lethargy, irregular heartbeat, cramps, weakness, drowsiness, weak pulse, coma.
WHAT TO DO:
- **Dial 0 (operator) or 911 (emergency) for an ambulance or medical help. Then give first aid immediately.**
- **If patient is unconscious and not breathing, give mouth-to-mouth breathing. If there is no heartbeat, use cardiac massage and mouth-to-mouth breathing (CPR). Don't try to make patient vomit. If you can't get help quickly, take patient to nearest emergency facility.**
- **See emergency information on inside covers.**

- Forces sodium and water excretion, reducing body fluid.
- Relaxes muscle cells of small arteries.
- Reduced body fluid and relaxed arteries lower blood pressure.

Time lapse before drug works:
4 to 6 hours. May require several weeks to lower blood pressure.

Don't take with:
- Non-prescription drugs without consulting doctor.
- See Interaction column and consult doctor.

 POSSIBLE ADVERSE REACTIONS OR SIDE EFFECTS

SYMPTOMS	WHAT TO DO
Life-threatening:	
Irregular heartbeat, weak pulse, shortness of breath.	Discontinue. Seek emergency treatment.
Common:	
• Mood change, muscle cramps.	Discontinue. Call doctor right away.
• Numbness or tingling in hands or feet.	Continue. Call doctor when convenient.
Infrequent:	
• Blurred vision, abdominal pain, nausea, vomiting.	Discontinue. Call doctor right away.
• Dizziness, mood change, headache, dry mouth, weakness, tiredness, weight gain or loss.	Continue. Call doctor when convenient.
Rare:	
• Sore throat, fever, mouth sores; jaundice; rash; joint or muscle pain; hives; unexplained bleeding or bruising.	Discontinue. Call doctor right away.
• Corners of mouth cracked, weakness.	Continue. Call doctor when convenient.

 WARNINGS & PRECAUTIONS

Don't take if:
- If you are allergic to triamterene or any thiazide diuretic drug.
- If you have had severe liver or kidney disease.

Before you start, consult your doctor:
- If you have gout, diabetes, liver, pancreas or kidney disorder.
- You are allergic to any sulfa drug.
- If you will have surgery within 2 months, including dental surgery, requiring general or spinal anesthesia.

Over age 60:
- Adverse reactions and side effects may be more frequent and severe than in younger persons, especially dizziness and excessive potassium loss.
- Warm weather or fever can decrease blood pressure. Dose may require adjustment.
- Extended use can increase blood clots.

Pregnancy:
Risk to unborn child outweighs drug benefits. Don't use.

Breast-feeding:
Drug passes into milk. Avoid drug or discontinue nursing until you finish medicine. Consult doctor for advice on maintaining milk supply.

Infants & children:
Used infrequently. Use only under medical supervision.

Prolonged use:
Potassium retention which may lead to heart-rhythm problems.

Skin & sunlight:
May cause rash or intensify sunburn in areas exposed to sun or sunlamp.

Driving, piloting or hazardous work:
Don't drive or pilot aircraft until you learn how medicine affects you. Don't work around dangerous machinery. Don't climb ladders or work in high places. Danger increases if you drink alcohol or take medicine affecting alertness and reflexes, such as antihistamines, tranquilizers, sedatives, pain medicine, narcotics and mind-altering drugs.

Discontinuing:
Don't discontinue without consulting doctor. Dose may require gradual reduction if you have taken drug for a long time. Doses of other drugs may also require adjustment.

Others:
- Hot weather and fever may cause dehydration and drop in blood pressure. Dose may require temporary adjustment. Weigh daily and report any unexpected weight decreases to your doctor.
- May cause rise in uric acid, leading to gout.
- May cause blood-sugar rise in diabetics.

 POSSIBLE INTERACTION WITH OTHER DRUGS

GENERIC NAME OR DRUG CLASS	COMBINED EFFECT
Acebutolol	Decreased antihypertensive effect of acebutolol.
Allopurinol	Decreased allopurinol effect.
Antidepressants	Dangerous drop in blood pressure. Avoid combination unless under medical supervision.
Antidiabetics (oral)	Decreased antidiabetic effect.
Barbiturates	Increased hydrochlorothiazide effect.
Cholestyramine	Decreased hydrochlorothiazide effect.
Cortisone drugs	Excessive potassium loss that causes dangerous heart rhythms.
Digitalis preparations	Excessive potassium loss that causes dangerous heart rhythms.
Diuretics (thiazide)	Increased effect of other thiazide diuretics.
Indapamide	Increased diuretic effect.
Lithium	Increased lithium effect.
MAO inhibitors	Increased hydrochlorothiazide effect.
Nitrates	Excessive blood-pressure drop.

Continued page 979

 POSSIBLE INTERACTION WITH OTHER SUBSTANCES

INTERACTS WITH	COMBINED EFFECT
Alcohol:	Dangerous blood-pressure drop.
Beverages:	None expected.
Cocaine:	Decreased triamterene effect.
Foods: Salt.	Don't restrict unless directed by doctor.
Marijuana:	Daily use—Fainting likely.
Tobacco:	Decreases drug's effectiveness.

TRIAZOLAM

BRAND NAMES

Halcion

BASIC INFORMATION

Habit forming? Yes
Prescription needed? Yes
Available as generic? No
Drug class: Tranquilizer (benzodiazepine)

 USES

Treatment of insomnia. Not recommended for
more than 2 weeks maximum.

 **DOSAGE & USAGE
INFORMATION**

How to take:
Tablet or capsule—Swallow with liquid. If you
can't swallow whole, crumble tablet or open
capsule and take with liquid or food.

When to take:
At the same time each day, according to
instructions on prescription label.

If you forget a dose:
Take as soon as you remember up to 2 hours
late. If more than 2 hours, wait for next
scheduled dose (don't double this dose).

What drug does:
Affects limbic system, the part of the brain that
controls emotions.

Time lapse before drug works:
2 hours. May take 6 weeks for full benefit.

Don't take with:
See Interaction column and consult doctor.

 OVERDOSE

SYMPTOMS:
**Drowsiness, weakness, tremor, stupor,
coma.**
WHAT TO DO:
- **Dial 0 (operator) or 911 (emergency) for an
  ambulance or medical help. Then give first
  aid immediately.**
- **If patient is unconscious and not
  breathing, give mouth-to-mouth breathing.
  If there is no heartbeat, use cardiac
  massage and mouth-to-mouth breathing
  (CPR). Don't try to make patient vomit. If
  you can't get help quickly, take patient to
  nearest emergency facility.**
- **See emergency information on inside
  covers.**

 **POSSIBLE
ADVERSE REACTIONS
OR SIDE EFFECTS**

SYMPTOMS	WHAT TO DO
Life-threatening:	
None expected.	
Common:	
Clumsiness,	Continue. Call doctor
drowsiness, dizziness.	when convenient.
Infrequent:	
• Hallucinations, confusion, depression, irritability, rash, itchy skin, change in vision.	Discontinue. Call doctor right away.
• Constipation or diarrhea, nausea, vomiting, difficult urination.	Continue. Call doctor when convenient.
Rare:	
• Slow heartbeat, difficult breathing.	Discontinue. Seek emergency treatment.
• Mouth or throat ulcers, jaundice.	Discontinue. Call doctor right away.

WARNINGS & PRECAUTIONS

Don't take if:
- You are allergic to any benzodiazepine.
- You have myasthenia gravis.
- You are active or recovering alcoholic.
- Patient is younger than 6 months.

Before you start, consult your doctor:
- If you have liver, kidney or lung disease.
- If you have diabetes, epilepsy or porphyria.
- If you will have surgery within 2 months, including dental surgery, requiring general or spinal anesthesia.

Over age 60:
Adverse reactions and side effects may be more frequent and severe than in younger persons. You need smaller doses for shorter periods of time. May develop agitation, rage or "hangover" effect.

Pregnancy:
Risk to unborn child outweighs drug benefits. Don't use.

Breast-feeding:
Drug passes into milk. Avoid drug or discontinue nursing until you finish medicine. Consult doctor for advice on maintaining milk supply.

Infants & children:
Use only under medical supervision for children older than 6 months.

Prolonged use:
May impair liver function.

Skin & sunlight:
No problems expected.

Driving, piloting or hazardous work:
Don't drive or pilot aircraft until you learn how medicine affects you. Don't work around dangerous machinery. Don't climb ladders or work in high places. Danger increases if you drink alcohol or take medicine affecting alertness and reflexes.

Discontinuing:
Don't discontinue without consulting doctor. Dose may require gradual reduction if you have taken drug for a long time. Doses of other drugs may also require adjustment.

Others:
- Hot weather, heavy exercise and profuse sweat may reduce excretion and cause overdose.
- Blood sugar may rise in diabetics, requiring insulin adjustment.

POSSIBLE INTERACTION WITH OTHER DRUGS

GENERIC NAME OR DRUG CLASS	COMBINED EFFECT
Anticonvulsants	Change in seizure frequency or severity.
Antidepressants	Increased sedative effect of both drugs.
Antihistamines	Increased sedative effect of both drugs.
Antihypertensives	Excessively low blood pressure.
Cimetidine	Excess sedation.
Disulfiram	Increased triazolam effect.
Dronabinol	Increased effects of both drugs. Avoid.
MAO inhibitors	Convulsions, deep sedation, rage.
Molindone	Increased sedative effect.
Narcotics	Increased sedative effect of both drugs.
Sedatives	Increased sedative effect of both drugs.
Sleep inducers	Increased sedative effect of both drugs.
Tranquilizers	Increased sedative effect of both drugs.

POSSIBLE INTERACTION WITH OTHER SUBSTANCES

INTERACTS WITH	COMBINED EFFECT
Alcohol:	Heavy sedation. Avoid.
Beverages:	None expected.
Cocaine:	Decreased triazolam effect.
Foods:	None expected.
Marijuana:	Heavy sedation. Avoid.
Tobacco:	Decreased triazolam effect.

TRICHLORMETHIAZIDE

BRAND NAMES

Metahydrin	Naqua
Metatensin	Naquival

BASIC INFORMATION

Habit forming? No
Prescription needed? Yes
Available as generic? Yes
Drug class: Antihypertensive, diuretic
(thiazide)

USES

- Controls, but doesn't cure, high blood pressure.
- Reduces fluid retention (edema) caused by conditions such as heart disorders and liver disease.

DOSAGE & USAGE INFORMATION

How to take:
Tablet or capsule—Swallow with liquid. If you can't swallow whole, crumble tablet or open capsule and take with liquid or food. Don't exceed dose.

When to take:
At the same time each day.

If you forget a dose:
Take as soon as you remember up to 2 hours late. If more than 2 hours, wait for next scheduled dose (don't double this dose).

What drug does:
- Forces sodium and water excretion, reducing body fluid.
- Relaxes muscle cells of small arteries.
- Reduced body fluid and relaxed arteries lower blood pressure.

Time lapse before drug works:
4 to 6 hours. May require several weeks to lower blood pressure.

Continued next column

OVERDOSE

SYMPTOMS:
Cramps, weakness, drowsiness, weak pulse, coma.
WHAT TO DO:
- Dial 0 (operator) or 911 (emergency) for an ambulance or medical help. Then give first aid immediately.
- See emergency information on inside covers.

Don't take with:
- See Interaction column and consult doctor.
- Non-prescription drugs without consulting doctor.

POSSIBLE ADVERSE REACTIONS OR SIDE EFFECTS

SYMPTOMS	WHAT TO DO
Life-threatening: None expected.	
Common: None expected.	
Infrequent:	
• Blurred vision, severe abdominal pain, nausea, vomiting, irregular heartbeat, weak pulse, sore throat, fever.	Discontinue. Call doctor right away.
• Dizziness, mood change, headache, weakness, tiredness, weight changes.	Continue. Call doctor when convenient.
• Dry mouth, thirst.	Continue. Tell doctor at next visit.
Rare:	
• Rash or hives.	Discontinue. Seek emergency treatment.
• Jaundice.	Discontinue. Call doctor right away.

WARNINGS & PRECAUTIONS

Don't take if:
You are allergic to any thiazide diuretic drug.

Before you start, consult your doctor:
- If you are allergic to any sulfa drug.
- If you have gout.
- If you have liver, pancreas or kidney disorder.

Over age 60:
Adverse reactions and side effects may be more frequent and severe than in younger persons, especially dizziness and excessive potassium loss.

Pregnancy:
Risk to unborn child outweighs drug benefits. Don't use.

Breast-feeding:
Drug passes into milk. Avoid drug or discontinue nursing.

Infants & children:
No problems expected.

Prolonged use:
You may need medicine to treat high blood pressure for the rest of your life.

Skin & sunlight:
May cause rash or intensify sunburn in areas exposed to sun or sunlamp.

Driving, piloting or hazardous work:
Don't drive or pilot aircraft until you learn how medicine affects you. Don't work around dangerous machinery. Don't climb ladders or work in high places. Danger increases if you drink alcohol or take medicine affecting alertness and reflexes, such as antihistamines, tranquilizers, sedatives, pain medicine, narcotics and mind-altering drugs.

Discontinuing:
Don't discontinue without medical advice.

Others:
- Hot weather and fever may cause dehydration and drop in blood pressure. Dose may require temporary adjustment. Weigh daily and report any unexpected weight decreases to your doctor.
- May cause rise in uric acid, leading to gout.
- May cause blood-sugar rise in diabetics.

POSSIBLE INTERACTION WITH OTHER DRUGS

GENERIC NAME OR DRUG CLASS	COMBINED EFFECT
Acebutolol	Increased antihypertensive effect. Dosages of both drugs may require adjustments.
Allopurinol	Decreased allopurinol effect.
Amiodarone	Increased risk of heartbeat irregularity due to low potassium.
Antidepressants (tricyclic)	Dangerous drop in blood pressure. Avoid combination unless under medical supervision.
Barbiturates	Increased trichlormethiazide effect.
Calcium supplements	Increased calcium in blood.
Cholestyramine	Decreased trichlormethiazide effect.
Cortisone drugs	Excessive potassium loss that causes dangerous heart rhythms.

Digitalis preparations	Excessive potassium loss that causes dangerous heart rhythms.
Diuretics (thiazide)	Increased effect of other thiazide diuretics.
Indapamide	Increased diuretic effect.
Labetolol	Increased antihypertensive effects.
Lithium	Increased effect of lithium.
MAO inhibitors	Increased trichlormethiazide effect.
Nitrates	Excessive blood-pressure drop.
Oxprenolol	Increased antihypertensive effect. Dosages of both drugs may require adjustments.
Potassium supplements	Decreased potassium effect.
Probenecid	Decreased probenecid effect.

POSSIBLE INTERACTION WITH OTHER SUBSTANCES

INTERACTS WITH	COMBINED EFFECT
Alcohol:	Dangerous blood-pressure drop.
Beverages:	None expected.
Cocaine:	None expected.
Foods: Licorice.	Excessive potassium loss that causes dangerous heart rhythms.
Marijuana:	May increase blood pressure.
Tobacco:	None expected.

TRICYCLIC ANTIDEPRESSANTS

BRAND NAMES

See complete list of brand names in the *Brand Name Directory,* page 958.

BASIC INFORMATION

Habit forming? No
Prescription needed? Yes
Available as generic? Yes
Drug class: Antidepressant (tricyclic)

 ## USES

- Gradually relieves, but doesn't cure, symptoms of depression.
- Imipramine is also used to decrease bedwetting.

 ## DOSAGE & USAGE INFORMATION

How to take:
Tablet or capsule—Swallow with liquid.

When to take:
At the same time each day, usually at bedtime.

If you forget a dose:
Bedtime dose—If you forget your once-a-day bedtime dose, don't take it more than 3 hours late. If more than 3 hours, wait for next scheduled dose. Don't double this dose.

What drug does:
Probably affects part of brain that controls messages between nerve cells.

Time lapse before drug works:
Begins in 1 to 2 weeks. May require 4 to 6 weeks for maximum benefit.

Continued next column

 ## OVERDOSE

SYMPTOMS:
Hallucinations, convulsions, coma.
WHAT TO DO:
- **Dial 0 (operator) or 911 (emergency) for an ambulance or medical help. Then give first aid immediately.**
- **If patient is unconscious and not breathing, give mouth-to-mouth breathing. If there is no heartbeat, use cardiac massage and mouth-to-mouth breathing (CPR). Don't try to make patient vomit. If you can't get help quickly, take patient to nearest emergency facility.**
- **See emergency information on inside covers.**

Don't take with:
- Non-prescription drugs without consulting doctor.
- See Interaction column and consult doctor.

 ## POSSIBLE ADVERSE REACTIONS OR SIDE EFFECTS

SYMPTOMS	WHAT TO DO
Life-threatening:	
Seizures.	Seek emergency treatment immediately.
Common:	
• Headache, dry mouth or unpleasant taste, constipation or diarrhea, nausea, indigestion, fatigue, weakness.	Continue. Call doctor when convenient.
• Insomnia, "sweet tooth."	Continue. Tell doctor at next visit.
Infrequent:	
• Hallucinations, shakiness, dizziness, fainting, blurred vision, eye pain, vomiting, irregular heartbeat or slow pulse.	Discontinue. Call doctor right away.
• Difficult urination.	Continue. Call doctor when convenient.
Rare:	
Rash, itchy skin, sore throat, jaundice, fever.	Discontinue. Call doctor right away.

 ## WARNINGS & PRECAUTIONS

Don't take if:
- You are allergic to any tricyclic antidepressant.
- You drink alcohol.
- You have had a heart attack within 6 weeks.
- You have glaucoma.
- You have taken MAO inhibitors within 2 weeks.
- Patient is younger than 12.

Before you start, consult your doctor:

- If you will have surgery within 2 months, including dental surgery, requiring general or spinal anesthesia.
- If you have an enlarged prostate.
- If you have heart disease or high blood pressure.
- If you have stomach or intestinal problems.
- If you have an overactive thyroid.
- If you have asthma.
- If you have liver disease.

Over age 60:

More likely to develop urination difficulty and side effects such as seizures, hallucinations, shaking, dizziness, fainting, headache, insomnia.

Pregnancy:

Studies inconclusive on harm to unborn child. Animal studies show fetal abnormalities. Decide with your doctor whether drug benefits justify risk to unborn child.

Breast-feeding:

Drug passes into milk. Avoid drug or discontinue nursing until you finish medicine. Consult doctor about maintaining milk supply.

Infants & children:

Don't give to children younger than 12.

Prolonged use:

No problems expected.

Skin & sunlight:

May cause rash or intensify sunburn in areas exposed to sun or sunlamp.

Driving, piloting or hazardous work:

Don't drive or pilot aircraft until you learn how medicine affects you. Don't work around dangerous machinery. Don't climb ladders or work in high places. Danger increases if you drink alcohol or take medicine affecting alertness and reflexes.

Discontinuing:

Don't discontinue without consulting doctor. Dose may require gradual reduction if you have taken drug for a long time. Doses of other drugs may also require adjustment.

Others:

No problems expected.

POSSIBLE INTERACTION WITH OTHER DRUGS

GENERIC NAME OR DRUG CLASS	COMBINED EFFECT
Anticoagulants (oral)	Increased anticoagulant effect.
Anticholinergics	Increased sedation.
Antihistamines	Increased antihistamine effect.
Barbiturates	Decreased antidepressant effect.
Clonidine	Decreased clonidine effect.
Diuretics (thiazide)	Increased antidepressant effect.
Ethchlorvynol	Delirium.
Guanethidine	Decreased guanethidine effect.
MAO inhibitors	Fever, delirium, convulsions.
Methyldopa	Decreased methyldopa effect.
Molindone	Increased molindone effect.
Narcotics	Dangerous oversedation.
Phenytoin	Decreased phenytoin effect.
Quinidine	Irregular heartbeat.
Sedatives	Dangerous oversedation.
Sympathomimetics	Increased sympathomimetic effect.
Thyroid hormones	Irregular heartbeat.

POSSIBLE INTERACTION WITH OTHER SUBSTANCES

INTERACTS WITH	COMBINED EFFECT
Alcohol: Beverages or medicines with alcohol.	Excessive intoxication. Avoid.
Beverages:	None expected.
Cocaine:	Excessive intoxication. Avoid.
Foods:	None expected.
Marijuana:	Excessive drowsiness. Avoid.
Tobacco:	None expected.

TRIDIHEXETHYL

BRAND NAMES

Milpath   Pathilon
Pathibamate

BASIC INFORMATION

Habit forming? No
Prescription needed?
  Low strength: No
  High strength: Yes
Available as generic? Yes
Drug class: Antispasmodic, anticholinergic

 USES

Reduces spasms of digestive system, bladder
and urethra.

DOSAGE & USAGE INFORMATION

How to take:
Tablet—Swallow with liquid or food to lessen
stomach irritation.

When to take:
30 minutes before meals (unless directed
otherwise by doctor).

If you forget a dose:
Take as soon as you remember up to 2 hours
late. If more than 2 hours, wait for next
scheduled dose (don't double this dose).

What drug does:
Blocks nerve impulses at parasympathetic nerve
endings, preventing muscle contractions and
gland secretions of organs involved.

Time lapse before drug works:
15 to 30 minutes.

Don't take with:
See Interaction column and consult doctor.

 OVERDOSE

SYMPTOMS:
**Dilated pupils, rapid pulse and breathing,
dizziness, fever, hallucinations, confusion,
slurred speech, agitation, flushed face,
convulsions, coma.**
WHAT TO DO:
- **Dial 0 (operator) or 911 (emergency) for an
  ambulance or medical help. Then give first
  aid immediately.**
- **See emergency information on inside
  covers.**

POSSIBLE ADVERSE REACTIONS OR SIDE EFFECTS

SYMPTOMS	WHAT TO DO
Life-threatening:	
None expected.	
Common:	
• Confusion, delirium, rapid heartbeat.	Discontinue. Call doctor right away.
• Nausea, vomiting, decreased sweating.	Continue. Call doctor when convenient.
• Constipation.	Continue. Tell doctor at next visit.
• Dryness in ears, nose, throat.	No action necessary.
Infrequent:	
Difficult urination, headache.	Continue. Call doctor when convenient.
Rare:	
Rash or hives, pain, blurred vision.	Discontinue. Call doctor right away.

WARNINGS & PRECAUTIONS

Don't take if:
- You are allergic to any anticholinergic.
- You have trouble with stomach bloating.
- You have difficulty emptying your bladder
  completely.
- You have narrow-angle glaucoma.
- You have severe ulcerative colitis.

Before you start, consult your doctor:
- If you have open-angle glaucoma.
- If you have angina.
- If you have chronic bronchitis or asthma.
- If you have hiatal hernia.
- If you have liver disease.
- If you have enlarged prostate.
- If you have myasthenia gravis.
- If you have peptic ulcer.
- If you will have surgery within 2 months,
  including dental surgery, requiring general or
  spinal anesthesia.

Over age 60:
Adverse reactions and side effects may be
more frequent and severe than in younger
persons.

Pregnancy:
Studies inconclusive on harm to unborn child.
Animal studies show fetal abnormalities. Decide
with your doctor whether drug benefits justify
risk to unborn child.

Breast-feeding:
Drug passes into milk and decreases milk flow. Avoid drug or discontinue nursing until you finish medicine. Consult doctor for advice on maintaining milk supply.

Infants & children:
Use only under medical supervision.

Prolonged use:
Chronic constipation, possible fecal impaction. Consult doctor immediately.

Skin & sunlight:
No problems expected.

Driving, piloting or hazardous work:
Use disqualifies you for piloting aircraft. Otherwise, no problems expected.

Discontinuing:
May be unnecessary to finish medicine. Follow doctor's instructions.

Others:
No problems expected.

POSSIBLE INTERACTION WITH OTHER DRUGS

GENERIC NAME OR DRUG CLASS	COMBINED EFFECT
Amantadine	Increased tridihexethyl effect.
Anticholinergics (other)	Increased tridihexethyl effect.
Antidepressants (tricyclic)	Increased tridihexethyl effect. Increased sedation.
Antihistamines	Increased tridihexethyl effect.
Cortisone drugs	Increased internal-eye pressure.
Haloperidol	Increased internal-eye pressure.

MAO inhibitors	Increased tridihexethyl effect.
Meperidine	Increased tridihexethyl effect.
Methylphenidate	Increased tridihexethyl effect.
Nitrates	Increased internal-eye pressure.
Orphenadrine	Increased tridihexethyl effect.
Phenothiazines	Increased tridihexethyl effect.
Pilocarpine	Loss of pilocarpine effect in glaucoma treatment.
Potassium supplements	Possible intestinal ulcers with oral potassium tablets.
Vitamin C	Decreased tridihexethyl effect. Avoid large doses of vitamin C.

POSSIBLE INTERACTION WITH OTHER SUBSTANCES

INTERACTS WITH	COMBINED EFFECT
Alcohol:	None expected.
Beverages:	None expected.
Cocaine:	Excessively rapid heartbeat. Avoid.
Foods:	None expected.
Marijuana:	Drowsiness and dry mouth.
Tobacco:	None expected.

TRIFLUOPERAZINE

BRAND NAMES

Apo-Trifluoperazine	Stelazine
Clinazine	Suprazine
Novoflurazine	Terfluzine
Pentazine	Triflurin
Solazine	Tripazine

BASIC INFORMATION

Habit forming? No
Prescription needed? Yes
Available as generic? Yes
Drug class: Tranquilizer, antiemetic
(phenothiazine)

USES

- Stops nausea, vomiting.
- Reduces anxiety, agitation.

DOSAGE & USAGE INFORMATION

How to take:
- Tablet or capsule—Swallow with liquid or food to lessen stomach irritation.
- Suppositories—Remove wrapper and moisten suppository with water. Gently insert into rectum, large end first.
- Drops or liquid—Dilute dose in beverage.

When to take:
- Nervous and mental disorders—Take at the same times each day.
- Nausea and vomiting—Take as needed, no more often than every 4 hours.

If you forget a dose:
- Nervous and mental disorders—Take up to 2 hours late. If more than 2 hours, wait for next scheduled dose (don't double this dose).
- Nausea and vomiting—Take as soon as you remember. Wait 4 hours for next dose.

What drug does:
- Suppresses brain's vomiting center.
- Suppresses brain centers that control abnormal emotions and behavior.

Continued next column

OVERDOSE

SYMPTOMS:
Stupor, convulsions, coma.
WHAT TO DO:
- **Dial 0 (operator) or 911 (emergency) for an ambulance or medical help. Then give first aid immediately.**
- **See emergency information on inside covers.**

Time lapse before drug works:
- Nausea and vomiting—1 hour or less.
- Nervous and mental disorders—4-6 weeks.

Don't take with:
- Antacid or medicine for diarrhea.
- Non-prescription drug for cough, cold or allergy.
- See Interaction column and consult doctor.

POSSIBLE ADVERSE REACTIONS OR SIDE EFFECTS

SYMPTOMS	WHAT TO DO
Life-threatening: None expected.	
Common:	
• Muscle spasms of face and neck, unsteady gait.	Discontinue. Seek emergency treatment.
• Restlessness, tremor, drowsiness.	Discontinue. Call doctor right away.
• Decreased sweating, dry mouth, nasal congestion, constipation.	Continue. Call doctor when convenient.
Infrequent:	
• Fainting.	Discontinue. Seek emergency treatment.
• Rash.	Discontinue. Call doctor right away.
• Difficult urination, less interest in sex, swollen breasts, menstrual irregularities.	Continue. Call doctor when convenient.
Rare:	
Change in vision, sore throat, fever, jaundice.	Discontinue. Call doctor right away.

WARNINGS & PRECAUTIONS

Don't take if:
- You are allergic to any phenothiazine.
- You have a blood or bone-marrow disease.

Before you start, consult your doctor:
- If you will have surgery within 2 months, including dental surgery, requiring general or spinal anesthesia.
- If you have asthma, emphysema or other lung disorder.
- If you take non-prescription ulcer medicine, asthma medicine or amphetamines.

Over age 60:
Adverse reactions and side effects may be more frequent and severe than in younger persons. More likely to develop involuntary movement of jaws, lips, tongue, chewing. Report this to your doctor immediately. Early treatment can help.

Pregnancy:
Risk to unborn child outweighs drug benefits. Don't use.

Breast-feeding:
Drug passes into milk. Avoid drug or discontinue nursing until you finish medicine. Consult doctor for advice on maintaining milk supply.

Infants & children:
Don't give to children younger than 2.

Prolonged use:
May lead to tardive dyskinesia (involuntary movement of jaws, lips, tongue, chewing).

Skin & sunlight:
May cause rash or intensify sunburn in areas exposed to sun or sunlamp. Skin may remain sensitive for 3 months after discontinuing.

Driving, piloting or hazardous work:
Don't drive or pilot aircraft until you learn how medicine affects you. Don't work around dangerous machinery. Don't climb ladders or work in high places. Danger increases if you drink alcohol or take medicine affecting alertness and reflexes.

Discontinuing:
- Nervous and mental disorders—Don't discontinue without doctor's advice until you complete prescribed dose, even though symptoms diminish or disappear.
- Nausea and vomiting—May be unnecessary to finish medicine. Follow doctor's instructions.

Others:
No problems expected.

POSSIBLE INTERACTION WITH OTHER DRUGS

GENERIC NAME OR DRUG CLASS	COMBINED EFFECT
Anticholinergics	Increased anticholinergic effect.
Antidepressants (tricyclic)	Increased trifluoperazine effect.
Antihistamines	Increased antihistamine effect.
Appetite suppressants	Decreased suppressant effect.
Dronabinol	Increased effects of both drugs. Avoid.
Levodopa	Decreased levodopa effect.
Mind-altering drugs	Increased effect of mind-altering drugs.
Molindone	Increased tranquilizer effect.
Narcotics	Increased narcotic effect.
Phenytoin	Increased phenytoin effect.
Quinidine	Impaired heart function. Dangerous mixture.
Sedatives	Increased sedative effect.
Tranquilizers (other)	Increased tranquilizer effect.

POSSIBLE INTERACTION WITH OTHER SUBSTANCES

INTERACTS WITH	COMBINED EFFECT
Alcohol:	Dangerous oversedation.
Beverages:	None expected.
Cocaine:	Decreased trifluoperazine effect. Avoid.
Foods:	None expected.
Marijuana:	Drowsiness. May increase antinausea effect.
Tobacco:	None expected.

TRIFLUPROMAZINE

BRAND NAMES

Psyquil   **Vesprin**

BASIC INFORMATION

Habit forming? No
Prescription needed? Yes
Available as generic? Yes
Drug class: Tranquilizer, antiemetic
          (phenothiazine)

 USES

- Stops nausea, vomiting.
- Reduces anxiety, agitation.

 DOSAGE & USAGE INFORMATION

How to take:
- Tablet or capsule—Swallow with liquid or food to lessen stomach irritation.
- Suppositories—Remove wrapper and moisten suppository with water. Gently insert into rectum, large end first.
- Drops or liquid—Dilute dose in beverage.

When to take:
- Nervous and mental disorders—Take at the same times each day.
- Nausea and vomiting—Take as needed, no more often than every 4 hours.

If you forget a dose:
- Nervous and mental disorders—Take up to 2 hours late. If more than 2 hours, wait for next scheduled dose (don't double this dose).
- Nausea and vomiting—Take as soon as you remember. Wait 4 hours for next dose.

What drug does:
- Suppresses brain's vomiting center.
- Suppresses brain centers that control abnormal emotions and behavior.

Time lapse before drug works:
- Nausea and vomiting—1 hour or less.
- Nervous and mental disorders—4-6 weeks.

Continued next column

 OVERDOSE

SYMPTOMS:
Stupor, convulsions, coma.
WHAT TO DO:
- **Dial 0 (operator) or 911 (emergency) for an ambulance or medical help. Then give first aid immediately.**
- **See emergency information on inside covers.**

Don't take with:
- Antacid or medicine for diarrhea.
- Non-prescription drug for cough, cold or allergy.
- See Interaction column and consult doctor.

 POSSIBLE ADVERSE REACTIONS OR SIDE EFFECTS

SYMPTOMS	WHAT TO DO
Life-threatening:	
None expected.	
Common:	
• Muscle spasms of face and neck, unsteady gait.	Discontinue. Seek emergency treatment.
• Restlessness, tremor, drowsiness.	Discontinue. Call doctor right away.
• Decreased sweating, dry mouth, nasal congestion, constipation.	Continue. Call doctor when convenient.
Infrequent:	
• Fainting.	Discontinue. Seek emergency treatment.
• Rash.	Discontinue. Call doctor right away.
• Difficult urination, less interest in sex, swollen breasts, menstrual irregularities.	Continue. Call doctor when convenient.
Rare:	
Change in vision, sore throat, fever, jaundice.	Discontinue. Call doctor right away.

WARNINGS & PRECAUTIONS

Don't take if:
- You are allergic to any phenothiazine.
- You have a blood or bone-marrow disease.

Before you start, consult your doctor:
- If you will have surgery within 2 months, including dental surgery, requiring general or spinal anesthesia.
- If you have asthma, emphysema or other lung disorder.
- If you take non-prescription ulcer medicine, asthma medicine or amphetamines.

Over age 60:
Adverse reactions and side effects may be more frequent and severe than in younger persons. More likely to develop involuntary movement of jaws, lips, tongue, chewing. Report this to your doctor immediately. Early treatment can help.

Pregnancy:
Risk to unborn child outweighs drug benefits. Don't use.

Breast-feeding:
Drug passes into milk. Avoid drug or discontinue nursing until you finish medicine. Consult doctor for advice on maintaining milk supply.

Infants & children:
Don't give to children younger than 2.

Prolonged use:
May lead to tardive dyskinesia (involuntary movement of jaws, lips, tongue, chewing).

Skin & sunlight:
May cause rash or intensify sunburn in areas exposed to sun or sunlamp. Skin may remain sensitive for 3 months after discontinuing.

Driving, piloting or hazardous work:
Don't drive or pilot aircraft until you learn how medicine affects you. Don't work around dangerous machinery. Don't climb ladders or work in high places. Danger increases if you drink alcohol or take medicine affecting alertness and reflexes.

Discontinuing:
- Nervous and mental disorders—Don't discontinue without doctor's advice until you complete prescribed dose, even though symptoms diminish or disappear.
- Nausea and vomiting—May be unnecessary to finish medicine. Follow doctor's instructions.

Others:
No problems expected.

POSSIBLE INTERACTION WITH OTHER DRUGS

GENERIC NAME OR DRUG CLASS	COMBINED EFFECT
Anticholinergics	Increased anticholinergic effect.
Antidepressants (tricyclic)	Increased triflupromazine effect.
Antihistamines	Increased antihistamine effect.
Appetite suppressants	Decreased suppressant effect.
Dronabinol	Increased effects of both drugs. Avoid.
Levodopa	Decreased levodopa effect.
Mind-altering drugs	Increased effect of mind-altering drugs.
Molindone	Increased tranquilizer effect.
Narcotics	Increased narcotic effect.
Phenytoin	Increased phenytoin effect.
Quinidine	Impaired heart function. Dangerous mixture.
Sedatives	Increased sedative effect.
Tranquilizers (other)	Increased tranquilizer effect.

POSSIBLE INTERACTION WITH OTHER SUBSTANCES

INTERACTS WITH	COMBINED EFFECT
Alcohol:	Dangerous oversedation.
Beverages:	None expected.
Cocaine:	Decreased triflupromazine effect. Avoid.
Foods:	None expected.
Marijuana:	Drowsiness. May increase antinausea effect.
Tobacco:	None expected.

TRIHEXYPHENIDYL

BRAND NAMES

Aparkane	T.H.P.
Apo-Trihex	Tremin
Artane	Trihexane
Artane Sequels	Trihexidyl
Novohexidyl	Trihexy

BASIC INFORMATION

Habit forming? No
Prescription needed? Yes
Available as generic? Yes
Drug class: Antidyskinetic, antiparkinsonism

USES

- Treatment of Parkinson's disease.
- Treatment of adverse effects of phenothiazines.

DOSAGE & USAGE INFORMATION

How to take:
Tablets or capsules—Take with food to lessen stomach irritation.

When to take:
At the same times each day.

If you forget a dose:
Take as soon as you remember up to 2 hours late. If more than 2 hours, wait for next scheduled dose (don't double this dose).

What drug does:
- Balances chemical reactions necessary to send nerve impulses within base of brain.
- Improves muscle control and reduces stiffness.

Continued next column

OVERDOSE

SYMPTOMS:
Agitation, dilated pupils, hallucinations, dry mouth, rapid heartbeat, sleepiness.
WHAT TO DO:
- Dial 0 (operator) or 911 (emergency) for an ambulance or medical help. Then give first aid immediately.
- If patient is unconscious and not breathing, give mouth-to-mouth breathing. If there is no heartbeat, use cardiac massage and mouth-to-mouth breathing (CPR). Don't try to make patient vomit. If you can't get help quickly, take patient to nearest emergency facility.
- See emergency information on inside covers.

Time lapse before drug works:
1 to 2 hours.

Don't take with:
- Non-prescription drugs for colds, cough or allergy.
- See Interaction column and consult doctor.

POSSIBLE ADVERSE REACTIONS OR SIDE EFFECTS

SYMPTOMS	WHAT TO DO
Life-threatening: None expected.	
Common:	
• Blurred vision, light sensitivity, constipation, nausea, vomiting.	Continue. Call doctor when convenient.
• Painful or difficult urination.	Continue. Tell doctor at next visit.
Infrequent: None expected.	
Rare:	
• Rash, eye pain.	Discontinue. Call doctor right away.
• Confusion, dizziness, sore mouth or tongue, muscle cramps, numbness or tingling in hands or feet.	Continue. Call doctor when convenient.

WARNINGS & PRECAUTIONS

Don't take if:
You are allergic to any antidyskinetic.

Before you start, consult your doctor:
- If you have had glaucoma.
- If you have had high blood pressure or heart disease.
- If you have had impaired liver function.
- If you have had kidney disease or urination difficulty.

Over age 60:
More sensitive to drug. Aggravates symptoms of enlarged prostate. Causes impaired thinking, hallucinations, nightmares. Consult doctor about any of these.

Pregnancy:
Studies inconclusive on harm to unborn child. Animal studies show fetal abnormalities. Decide with your doctor whether drug benefits justify risk to unborn child.

Breast-feeding:
No problems expected.

Infants & children:
Not recommended for children 3 and younger. Use for older children only under doctor's supervision.

Prolonged use:
Possible glaucoma.

Skin & sunlight:
No problems expected.

Driving, piloting or hazardous work:
Don't drive or pilot aircraft until you learn how medicine affects you. Don't work around dangerous machinery. Don't climb ladders or work in high places. Danger increases if you drink alcohol or take medicine affecting alertness and reflexes, such as antihistamines, tranquilizers, sedatives, pain medicine, narcotics and mind-altering drugs.

Discontinuing:
Don't discontinue without consulting doctor. Dose may require gradual reduction if you have taken drug for a long time. Doses of other drugs may also require adjustment.

Others:
- Internal eye pressure should be measured regularly.
- Avoid becoming overheated.

POSSIBLE INTERACTION WITH OTHER DRUGS

GENERIC NAME OR DRUG CLASS	COMBINED EFFECT
Amantadine	Increased amantadine effect.
Antidepressants (tricyclic)	Increased trihexyphenidyl effect. May cause glaucoma.
Antihistamines	Increased trihexyphenidyl effect.
Levodopa	Increased levodopa effect. Improved results in treating Parkinson's disease.
MAO inhibitors	Increased trihexyphenidyl effect.
Meperidine	Increased trihexyphenidyl effect.
Orphenadrine	Increased trihexyphenidyl effect.
Phenothiazines	Behavior changes.
Primidone	Excessive sedation.
Procainamide	Increased procainamide effect.
Quinidine	Increased trihexyphenidyl effect.
Tranquilizers	Excessive sedation.

POSSIBLE INTERACTION WITH OTHER SUBSTANCES

INTERACTS WITH	COMBINED EFFECT
Alcohol:	None expected.
Beverages:	None expected.
Cocaine:	Decreased trihexyphenidyl effect. Avoid.
Foods:	None expected.
Marijuana:	None expected.
Tobacco:	None expected.

TRIMEPRAZINE

BRAND NAMES

Panectyl   Temaril

BASIC INFORMATION

Habit forming? No
Prescription needed? Yes
Available as generic? Yes
Drug class: Tranquilizer (phenothiazine),
**   antihistamine**

 USES

Relieves itching of hives, skin allergies, chickenpox.

 DOSAGE & USAGE INFORMATION

How to take:
- Tablet or syrup—Swallow with liquid or food to lessen stomach irritation.
- Extended-release capsules—Swallow each dose whole. If you take regular tablets, you may chew or crush them.

When to take:
At the same times each day.

If you forget a dose:
Take as soon as you remember up to 2 hours late. If more than 2 hours, wait for next scheduled dose (don't double this dose).

What drug does:
Blocks histamine action in skin.

Time lapse before drug works:
1 to 2 hours.

Don't take with:
- Antacid or medicine for diarrhea.
- Non-prescription drug for cough, cold or allergy.
- See Interaction column and consult doctor.

 OVERDOSE

SYMPTOMS:
Stupor, convulsions, coma.
WHAT TO DO:
- **Dial 0 (operator) or 911 (emergency) for an ambulance or medical help. Then give first aid immediately.**
- **See emergency information on inside covers.**

 POSSIBLE ADVERSE REACTIONS OR SIDE EFFECTS

SYMPTOMS	WHAT TO DO
Life-threatening: None expected.	
Common:	
• Restlessness, tremor, drowsiness.	Discontinue. Call doctor right away.
• Decreased sweating, dry mouth, nasal congestion, constipation.	Continue. Call doctor when convenient.
Infrequent:	
• Fainting.	Discontinue. Seek emergency treatment.
• Rash, muscle spasms of face and neck, unsteady gait.	Discontinue. Call doctor right away.
• Difficult urination, less interest in sex, swollen breasts, menstrual irregularities.	Continue. Call doctor when convenient.
Rare:	
Change in vision, sore throat, fever, jaundice.	Discontinue. Call doctor right away.

WARNINGS & PRECAUTIONS

Don't take if:
- You are allergic to any phenothiazine.
- You have a blood or bone-marrow disease.

Before you start, consult your doctor:
- If you will have surgery within 2 months, including dental surgery, requiring general or spinal anesthesia.
- If you have asthma, emphysema or other lung disorder.
- If you take non-prescription ulcer medicine, asthma medicine or amphetamines.

Over age 60:
Adverse reactions and side effects may be more frequent and severe than in younger persons. More likely to develop tardive dyskinesia (involuntary movement of jaws, lips, tongue, chewing). Report this to your doctor immediately. Early treatment can help.

Pregnancy:
Risk to unborn child outweighs drug benefits. Don't use.

Breast-feeding:
Drug passes into milk. Avoid drug or discontinue nursing until you finish medicine. Consult doctor for advice on maintaining milk supply.

Infants & children:
Don't give to children younger than 2.

Prolonged use:
May lead to tardive dyskinesia (involuntary movement of jaws, lips, tongue, chewing).

Skin & sunlight:
May cause rash or intensify sunburn in areas exposed to sun or sunlamp. Skin may remain sensitive for 3 months after discontinuing.

Driving, piloting or hazardous work:
Don't drive or pilot aircraft until you learn how medicine affects you. Don't work around dangerous machinery. Don't climb ladders or work in high places. Danger increases if you drink alcohol or take medicine affecting alertness and reflexes.

Discontinuing:
May be unnecessary to finish medicine. Follow doctor's instructions.

Others:
No problems expected.

POSSIBLE INTERACTION WITH OTHER DRUGS

GENERIC NAME OR DRUG CLASS	COMBINED EFFECT
Antacids	Decreased trimeprazine effect.
Anticholinergics	Increased anticholinergic effect.
Anticonvulsants (hydantoin)	Increased anticonvulsant effect.
Antidepressants (tricyclic)	Increased trimeprazine effect.
Antihistamines (other)	Increased antihistamine effect.
Appetite suppressants	Decreased suppressant effect.
Barbiturates	Oversedation.
Dronabinol	Increased effects of both drugs. Avoid.
Guanethidine	Decreased guanethidine effect.
Levodopa	Decreased levodopa effect.
MAO inhibitors	Increased trimeprazine effect.
Mind-altering drugs	Increased effect of mind-altering drugs.
Molindone	Increased sedative and antihistamine effect.
Narcotics	Increased narcotic effect.
Sedatives	Increased sedative effect.
Tranquilizers	Increased tranquilizer effect. Avoid.

POSSIBLE INTERACTION WITH OTHER SUBSTANCES

INTERACTS WITH	COMBINED EFFECT
Alcohol:	Dangerous oversedation.
Beverages:	None expected.
Cocaine:	Decreased effect of trimeprazine. Avoid.
Foods:	None expected.
Marijuana:	Drowsiness.
Tobacco:	None expected.

TRIMETHOBENZAMIDE

BRAND NAMES

Stemetic	Tigan
Tegamide	Tiject-20
Ticon	

BASIC INFORMATION

Habit forming? No
Prescription needed? Yes
Available as generic? Yes
Drug class: Antiemetic

 USES

Reduces nausea and vomiting.

 DOSAGE & USAGE INFORMATION

How to take:
- Capsule—Swallow with liquid. If you can't swallow whole, open capsule and take with liquid or food.
- Suppositories—Remove wrapper and moisten suppository with water. Gently insert larger end into rectum. Push well into rectum with finger.

When to take:
When needed, no more often than label directs.

If you forget a dose:
Take when you remember. Wait as long as label directs for next dose.

What drug does:
Possibly blocks nerve impulses to brain's vomiting centers.

Time lapse before drug works:
20 to 40 minutes.

Continued next column

 OVERDOSE

SYMPTOMS:
Confusion, convulsions, coma.
WHAT TO DO:
- Dial 0 (operator) or 911 (emergency) for an ambulance or medical help. Then give first aid immediately.
- If patient is unconscious and not breathing, give mouth-to-mouth breathing. If there is no heartbeat, use cardiac massage and mouth-to-mouth breathing (CPR). Don't try to make patient vomit. If you can't get help quickly, take patient to nearest emergency facility.
- See emergency information on inside covers.

Don't take with:
Non-prescription drugs or drugs in Interaction column without consulting doctor.

 POSSIBLE ADVERSE REACTIONS OR SIDE EFFECTS

SYMPTOMS	WHAT TO DO
Life-threatening:	
None expected.	
Common:	
None expected.	
Infrequent:	
• Rash, blurred vision, low blood pressure.	Discontinue. Call doctor right away.
• Dizziness, drowsiness, headache, diarrhea, muscle cramps, unusual tiredness.	Continue. Call doctor when convenient.
Rare:	
Seizures, tremor, depression, sore throat, fever, repeated vomiting, back pain, jaundice.	Discontinue. Call doctor right away.

WARNINGS & PRECAUTIONS

Don't take if:
- You are allergic to trimethobenzamide.
- You are allergic to local anesthetics and have suppository form.

Before you start, consult your doctor:
If you have reacted badly to antihistamines.

Over age 60:
More susceptible to low blood pressure and sedative effects of this drug.

Pregnancy:
No proven harm to unborn child. Avoid if possible.

Breast-feeding:
No proven problems. Avoid if possible.

Infants & children:
- Injectable form not recommended.
- Avoid during viral infections. Drug may contribute to Reyes' syndrome.

Prolonged use:
- Damages blood-cell production of bone marrow.
- Causes Parkinson-like symptoms of tremors, rigidity.

Skin & sunlight:
Possible sun sensitivity. Use caution.

Driving, piloting or hazardous work:
- Use disqualifies you for piloting aircraft.
- Don't drive until you learn how medicine affects you. Don't work around dangerous machinery. Don't climb ladders or work in high places. Danger increases if you drink alcohol or take medicine affecting alertness and reflexes, such as antihistamines, tranquilizers, sedatives, pain medicine, narcotics and mind-altering drugs.

Discontinuing:
May be unnecessary to finish medicine. Follow doctor's instructions.

Others:
No problems expected.

POSSIBLE INTERACTION WITH OTHER DRUGS

GENERIC NAME OR DRUG CLASS	COMBINED EFFECT
Antidepressants	Increased sedative effect.
Antihistamines	Increased sedative effect.
Barbiturates	Increased effect of both drugs.
Belladonna	Increased effect of both drugs.
Cholinergics	Increased effect of both drugs.
Mind-altering drugs	Increased effect of mind-altering drug.
Narcotics	Increased sedative effect.
Phenothiazines	Increased effect of both drugs.
Sedatives	Increased sedative effect.
Sleep inducers	Increased effect of sleep inducer.
Tranquilizers	Increased sedative effect.

POSSIBLE INTERACTION WITH OTHER SUBSTANCES

INTERACTS WITH	COMBINED EFFECT
Alcohol:	Oversedation. Avoid.
Beverages:	None expected.
Cocaine:	None expected.
Foods:	None expected.
Marijuana:	Increased antinausea effect.
Tobacco:	None expected.

TRIMETHOPRIM

BRAND NAMES

Apo-Sulfatrim	Rovbac
Bactrim	Septra
Cotrim	SMZ-TMP
Novotrimel	Syraprim
Proloprim	Trimpex
Protrin	

BASIC INFORMATION

Habit forming? No
Prescription needed? Yes
Available as generic? Yes
Drug class: Antimicrobial

 ## USES

- Treatment for urinary-tract infections susceptible to trimethoprim.
- Helps prevent recurrent urinary-tract infections if taken once a day.

 ## DOSAGE & USAGE INFORMATION

How to take:
- Tablet or capsule—Swallow with liquid or food to lessen stomach irritation.
- Drops—Dilute dose in beverage before swallowing.

When to take:
Space doses evenly in 24 hours to keep constant amount in urine.

If you forget a dose:
Take as soon as possible. Wait 5 to 6 hours before next dose. Then return to regular schedule.

What drug does:
Stops harmful bacterial germs from multiplying. Will not kill viruses.

Time lapse before drug works:
2 to 5 days.

Don't take with:
See Interaction column and consult doctor.

 ## OVERDOSE

SYMPTOMS:
Nausea, vomiting, diarrhea.
WHAT TO DO:
Overdose unlikely to threaten life. If person takes much larger amount than prescribed, call doctor, poison-control center or hospital emergency room for instructions.

 ## POSSIBLE ADVERSE REACTIONS OR SIDE EFFECTS

SYMPTOMS	WHAT TO DO
Life-threatening: None expected.	
Common: Rash, itchy skin.	Discontinue. Seek emergency treatment.
Infrequent: • Diarrhea, nausea, vomiting, abdominal pain.	Discontinue. Call doctor right away.
• Headache.	Continue. Call doctor when convenient.
Rare: • Blue fingernails, lips and skin; difficult breathing.	Discontinue. Seek emergency treatment.
• Sore throat, fever.	Discontinue. Call doctor right away.

WARNINGS & PRECAUTIONS

Don't take if:
You are allergic to trimethoprim or any sulfa drug.

Before you start, consult your doctor:
If you have had liver or kidney disease.

Over age 60:
- Reduced liver and kidney function may require reduced dose.
- More likely to have severe anal and genital itch.
- Increased susceptibility to anemia.

Pregnancy:
Studies inconclusive on harm to unborn child. Animal studies show fetal abnormalities. Decide with your doctor whether drug benefits justify risk to unborn child.

Breast-feeding:
No proven harm to unborn child. Avoid if possible.

Infants & children:
Use under medical supervision only.

Prolonged use:
Anemia.

Skin & sunlight:
May cause rash or intensify sunburn in areas exposed to sun or sunlamp.

Driving, piloting or hazardous work:
No problems expected.

Discontinuing:
Don't discontinue without doctor's advice until you complete prescribed dose, even though symptoms diminish or disappear.

Others:
No problems expected.

POSSIBLE INTERACTION WITH OTHER DRUGS

GENERIC NAME OR DRUG CLASS	COMBINED EFFECT
Diuretics (thiazide)	Unusual bleeding or bruising.
Flecainide	Possible decreased blood-cell production in bone marrow.
Sulfamethoxazole	Beneficial increase of sulfamethoxazole effect.
Tocainide	Possible decreased blood-cell production in bone marrow.

POSSIBLE INTERACTION WITH OTHER SUBSTANCES

INTERACTS WITH	COMBINED EFFECT
Alcohol:	Increased alcohol effect with Bactrim or Septra.
Beverages:	None expected.
Cocaine:	No proven problems.
Foods:	None expected.
Marijuana:	None expected.
Tobacco:	None expected.

TRIPELENNAMINE

BRAND NAMES

PBZ	Pyribenzamine
PBZ-SR	Ro-Hist

BASIC INFORMATION

Habit forming? No
Prescription needed?
  High strength: Yes
  Low strength: No
Available as generic? Yes
Drug class: Antihistamine

 ## USES

- Reduces allergic symptoms such as hay fever, hives, rash or itching.
- Induces sleep.

 ## DOSAGE & USAGE INFORMATION

How to take:
- Tablet or liquid—Swallow with liquid or food to lessen stomach irritation.
- Extended-release tablets—Swallow each dose whole.

When to take:
Varies with form. Follow label directions.

If you forget a dose:
Take as soon as you remember up to 2 hours late. If more than 2 hours, wait for next scheduled dose (don't double this dose).

What drug does:
Blocks action of histamine after an allergic response triggers histamine release in sensitive cells.

Continued next column

 ## OVERDOSE

SYMPTOMS:
Convulsions, red face, hallucinations, coma.
WHAT TO DO:
- Dial 0 (operator) or 911 (emergency) for an ambulance or medical help. Then give first aid immediately.
- If patient is unconscious and not breathing, give mouth-to-mouth breathing. If there is no heartbeat, use cardiac massage and mouth-to-mouth breathing (CPR). Don't try to make patient vomit. If you can't get help quickly, take patient to nearest emergency facility.
- See emergency information on inside covers.

Time lapse before drug works:
30 minutes.

Don't take with:
See Interaction column and consult doctor.

 ## POSSIBLE ADVERSE REACTIONS OR SIDE EFFECTS

SYMPTOMS	WHAT TO DO
Life-threatening: None expected.	
Common: Drowsiness; dizziness; dry mouth, nose and throat; nausea.	Continue. Tell doctor at next visit.
Infrequent:	
• Change in vision.	Discontinue. Call doctor right away.
• Less tolerance for contact lenses, difficult urination.	Continue. Call doctor when convenient.
• Appetite loss.	Continue. Tell doctor at next visit.
Rare: Nightmares, agitation, irritability, sore throat, fever, rapid heartbeat, unusual bleeding or bruising, fatigue, weakness.	Discontinue. Call doctor right away.

WARNINGS & PRECAUTIONS

Don't take if:
You are allergic to any antihistamine.

Before you start, consult your doctor:
- If you have glaucoma.
- If you have enlarged prostate.
- If you have asthma.
- If you have kidney disease.
- If you have peptic ulcer.
- If you will have surgery within 2 months, including dental surgery, requiring general or spinal anesthesia.

Over age 60:
Don't exceed recommended dose. Adverse reactions and side effects may be more frequent and severe than in younger persons, especially urination difficulty, diminished alertness and other brain and nervous-system symptoms.

Pregnancy:
No proven harm to unborn child. Avoid if possible.

Breast-feeding:
Drug passes into milk. Avoid drug or discontinue nursing until you finish medicine. Consult doctor for advice on maintaining milk supply.

Infants & children:
Not recommended for premature or newborn infants. Otherwise, no problems expected.

Prolonged use:
Avoid. May damage bone marrow and nerve cells.

Skin & sunlight:
May cause rash or intensify sunburn in areas exposed to sun or sunlamp.

Driving, piloting or hazardous work:
Don't drive or pilot aircraft until you learn how medicine affects you. Don't work around dangerous machinery. Don't climb ladders or work in high places. Danger increases if you drink alcohol or take medicine affecting alertness and reflexes, such as antihistamines, tranquilizers, sedatives, pain medicine, narcotics and mind-altering drugs.

Discontinuing:
No problems expected.

Others:
May mask symptoms of hearing damage from aspirin, other salicylates, cisplatin, paromomycin, vancomycin or anticonvulsants. Consult doctor if you use these.

POSSIBLE INTERACTION WITH OTHER DRUGS

GENERIC NAME OR DRUG CLASS	COMBINED EFFECT
Anticholinergics	Increased anticholinergic effect.
Antidepressants (tricyclic)	Increased tripelennamine effect. Excess sedation.
Antihistamines (other)	Excess sedation. Avoid.
Dronabinol	Increased effects of both drugs. Avoid.
Hypnotics	Excess sedation. Avoid.
MAO inhibitors	Increased tripelennamine effect.
Mind-altering drugs	Excess sedation. Avoid.
Molindone	Increased antihistamine effect.
Narcotics	Excess sedation. Avoid.
Sedatives	Excess sedation. Avoid.
Sleep inducers	Excess sedation. Avoid.
Tranquilizers	Excess sedation. Avoid.

POSSIBLE INTERACTION WITH OTHER SUBSTANCES

INTERACTS WITH	COMBINED EFFECT
Alcohol:	Excess sedation. Avoid.
Beverages: Caffeine drinks.	Less tripelennamine sedation.
Cocaine:	Decreased tripelennamine effect. Avoid.
Foods:	None expected.
Marijuana:	Excess sedation. Avoid.
Tobacco:	None expected.

TRIPROLIDINE

BRAND NAMES

Actidil	Triafed-C
Actifed	Trifed
Bayidyl	Tripodrine
Eldafed	

BASIC INFORMATION

Habit forming? No
Prescription needed?
  High Strength: Yes
  Low strength: No
Available as generic? Yes
Drug class: Antihistamine

USES

- Reduces allergic symptoms such as hay fever, hives, rash or itching.
- Induces sleep.

DOSAGE & USAGE INFORMATION

How to take:
Tablet or syrup—Swallow with liquid or food to lessen stomach irritation.

When to take:
Varies with form. Follow label directions.

If you forget a dose:
Take as soon as you remember up to 2 hours late. If more than 2 hours, wait for next scheduled dose (don't double this dose).

What drug does:
Blocks action of histamine after an allergic response triggers histamine release in sensitive cells.

Continued next column

OVERDOSE

SYMPTOMS:
Convulsions, red face, hallucinations, coma.
WHAT TO DO:
- Dial 0 (operator) or 911 (emergency) for an ambulance or medical help. Then give first aid immediately.
- If patient is unconscious and not breathing, give mouth-to-mouth breathing. If there is no heartbeat, use cardiac massage and mouth-to-mouth breathing (CPR). Don't try to make patient vomit. If you can't get help quickly, take patient to nearest emergency facility.
- See emergency information on inside covers.

Time lapse before drug works:
30 minutes.

Don't take with:
See Interaction column and consult doctor.

POSSIBLE ADVERSE REACTIONS OR SIDE EFFECTS

SYMPTOMS	WHAT TO DO
Life-threatening: None expected.	
Common: Drowsiness; dizziness; dry mouth, nose and throat; nausea.	Continue. Tell doctor at next visit.
Infrequent: • Change in vision.	Discontinue. Call doctor right away.
• Less tolerance for contact lenses, difficult urination.	Continue. Call doctor when convenient.
• Appetite loss.	Continue. Tell doctor at next visit.
Rare: Nightmares, agitation, irritability, sore throat, fever, rapid heartbeat, unusual bleeding or bruising, fatigue, weakness.	Discontinue. Call doctor right away.

WARNINGS & PRECAUTIONS

Don't take if:
You are allergic to any antihistamine.

Before you start, consult your doctor:
- If you have glaucoma.
- If you have enlarged prostate.
- If you have asthma.
- If you have kidney disease.
- If you have peptic ulcer.
- If you will have surgery within 2 months, including dental surgery, requiring general or spinal anesthesia.

Over age 60:
Don't exceed recommended dose. Adverse reactions and side effects may be more frequent and severe than in younger persons, especially urination difficulty, diminished alertness and other brain and nervous-system symptoms.

Pregnancy:
No proven harm to unborn child. Avoid if possible.

Breast-feeding:
Drug passes into milk. Avoid drug or discontinue nursing until you finish medicine. Consult doctor for advice on maintaining milk supply.

Infants & children:
Not recommended for premature or newborn infants. Otherwise, no problems expected.

Prolonged use:
Avoid. May damage bone marrow and nerve cells.

Skin & sunlight:
May cause rash or intensify sunburn in areas exposed to sun or sunlamp.

Driving, piloting or hazardous work:
Don't drive or pilot aircraft until you learn how medicine affects you. Don't work around dangerous machinery. Don't climb ladders or work in high places. Danger increases if you drink alcohol or take medicine affecting alertness and reflexes, such as antihistamines, tranquilizers, sedatives, pain medicine, narcotics and mind-altering drugs.

Discontinuing:
No problems expected.

Others:
May mask symptoms of hearing damage from aspirin, other salicylates, cisplatin, paromomycin, vancomycin or anticonvulsants. Consult doctor if you use these.

POSSIBLE INTERACTION WITH OTHER DRUGS

GENERIC NAME OR DRUG CLASS	COMBINED EFFECT
Anticholinergics	Increased anticholinergic effect.
Antidepressants (tricyclic)	Increased triprolidine effect. Excess sedation.
Antihistamines (other)	Excess sedation. Avoid.
Dronabinol	Increased effects of both drugs. Avoid.
Hypnotics	Excess sedation. Avoid.
MAO inhibitors	Increased triprolidine effect.
Mind-altering drugs	Excess sedation. Avoid.
Molindone	Increased antihistamine effect.
Narcotics	Excess sedation. Avoid.
Sedatives	Excess sedation. Avoid.
Sleep inducers	Excess sedation. Avoid.
Tranquilizers	Excess sedation. Avoid.

POSSIBLE INTERACTION WITH OTHER SUBSTANCES

INTERACTS WITH	COMBINED EFFECT
Alcohol:	Excess sedation. Avoid.
Beverages: Caffeine drinks.	Less triprolidine sedation.
Cocaine:	Decreased triprolidine effect. Avoid.
Foods:	None expected.
Marijuana:	Excess sedation. Avoid.
Tobacco:	None expected.

VALPROIC ACID (DIPROPYLACETIC ACID)

BRAND NAMES

Depakene   Epival
Depakote

BASIC INFORMATION

Habit forming? No
Prescription needed? Yes
Available as generic? Yes
Drug class: Anticonvulsant

USES

Controls petit mal (absence) seizures in treatment of epilepsy.

DOSAGE & USAGE INFORMATION

How to take:
Tablet or capsule—Swallow with liquid or food to lessen stomach irritation.

When to take:
Once a day.

If you forget a dose:
Take as soon as you remember. Don't ever double dose.

What drug does:
Increases concentration of gamma aminobutyric acid, which inhibits nerve transmission in parts of brain.

Time lapse before drug works:
1 to 4 hours.

Don't take with:
See Interaction column and consult doctor.

OVERDOSE

SYMPTOMS:
Coma
WHAT TO DO:
- Dial 0 (operator) or 911 (emergency) for an ambulance or medical help. Then give first aid immediately.
- If patient is unconscious and not breathing, give mouth-to-mouth breathing. If there is no heartbeat, use cardiac massage and mouth-to-mouth breathing (CPR). Don't try to make patient vomit. If you can't get help quickly, take patient to nearest emergency facility.
- See emergency information on inside covers.

POSSIBLE ADVERSE REACTIONS OR SIDE EFFECTS

SYMPTOMS	WHAT TO DO
Life-threatening:	
None expected.	
Common:	
Menstrual irregularities.	Continue. Call doctor when convenient.
Infrequent:	
• Rash, blood spots under skin, hair loss, bleeding (heart and lungs), easy bruising.	Discontinue. Call doctor right away.
• Sleepiness, weakness, easily upset emotionally, depression, psychic changes, headache, incoordination, nausea, vomiting, abdominal cramps, appetite change.	Continue. Call doctor when convenient.
Rare:	
• Double vision, unusual movements of eyes (nystagmus).	Discontinue. Call doctor right away.
• Anemia.	Continue. Call doctor when convenient.

VALPROIC ACID (DIPROPYLACETIC ACID)

 ## WARNINGS & PRECAUTIONS

Don't take if:
You are allergic to valproic acid.

Before you start, consult your doctor:
- If you have blood, kidney or liver disease.
- If you will have surgery within 2 months, including dental surgery, requiring general or spinal anesthesia.

Over age 60:
Adverse reactions and side effects may be more frequent and severe than in younger persons.

Pregnancy:
No proven harm to unborn child. Avoid if possible.

Breast-feeding:
Unknown effect.

Infants & children:
Under close medical supervision only.

Prolonged use:
Request periodic blood tests, liver and kidney function tests.

Skin & sunlight:
No problems expected.

Driving, piloting or hazardous work:
Don't drive or pilot aircraft until you learn how medicine affects you. Don't work around dangerous machinery. Don't climb ladders or work in high places. Danger increases if you drink alcohol or take medicine affecting alertness and reflexes, such as antihistamines, tranquilizers, sedatives, pain medicine, narcotics and mind-altering drugs.

Discontinuing:
Don't discontinue without consulting doctor. Dose may require gradual reduction if you have taken drug for a long time. Doses of other drugs may also require adjustment.

Others:
No problems expected.

 ## POSSIBLE INTERACTION WITH OTHER DRUGS

GENERIC NAME OR DRUG CLASS	COMBINED EFFECT
Anticoagulants	Increased chance of bleeding.
Aspirin	Increased chance of bleeding.
Central nervous system depressants: Antidepressants, antihistamines, narcotics, sedatives, sleeping pills, tranquilizers, muscle relaxants	Increased sedative effect.
Clonazepam	May prolong seizure.
Dypiradamole	Increased chance of bleeding.
Flecainide	Possible decreased blood-cell production in bone marrow.
MAO inhibitors	Increased sedative effect.
Phenytoin	Unpredictable. Dose may require adjustment.
Primidone	Increased chance of toxicity.
Sulfinpyrazone	Increased chance of bleeding.
Tocainide	Possible decreased blood-cell production in bone marrow.

 ## POSSIBLE INTERACTION WITH OTHER SUBSTANCES

INTERACTS WITH	COMBINED EFFECT
Alcohol:	Deep sedation. Avoid.
Beverages:	No problems expected.
Cocaine:	Increased brain sensitivity. Avoid.
Foods:	No problems expected.
Marijuana:	Increased brain sensitivity. Avoid.
Tobacco:	Decreased valproic acid effect.

VERAPAMIL

BRAND NAMES

Calan   Isoptin

BASIC INFORMATION

Habit forming? No
Prescription needed? Yes
Available as generic? No
Drug class: Calcium-channel blocker,
        antiarrhythmic, antianginal

 ## USES

- Prevents angina attacks.
- Stabilizes irregular heartbeat.

 ## DOSAGE & USAGE INFORMATION

How to take:
Tablet—Swallow with liquid.

When to take:
At the same times each day 1 hour before or 2
hours after eating.

If you forget a dose:
Take as soon as you remember up to 2 hours
late. If more than 2 hours, wait for next
scheduled dose (don't double this dose).

What drug does:
- Reduces work that heart must perform.
- Reduces normal artery pressure.
- Increases oxygen to heart muscle.

Time lapse before drug works:
1 to 2 hours.

Don't take with:
See Interaction column and consult doctor.

 ## OVERDOSE

SYMPTOMS:
Unusually fast or unusually slow heartbeat,
loss of consciousness, cardiac arrest.
WHAT TO DO:
- Dial 0 (operator) or 911 (emergency) for an
  ambulance or medical help. Then give first
  aid immediately.
- If patient is unconscious and not
  breathing, give mouth-to-mouth breathing.
  If there is no heartbeat, use cardiac
  massage and mouth-to-mouth breathing
  (CPR). Don't try to make patient vomit. If
  you can't get help quickly, take patient to
  nearest emergency facility.
- See emergency information on inside
  covers.

 ## POSSIBLE ADVERSE REACTIONS OR SIDE EFFECTS

SYMPTOMS	WHAT TO DO
Life-threatening: None expected.	
Common: Tiredness.	Continue. Tell doctor at next visit.
Infrequent: • Unusually fast or unusually slow heartbeat, wheezing, cough, shortness of breath.	Discontinue. Call doctor right away.
• Dizziness; numbness or tingling in hands and feet; swollen feet, ankles or legs; difficult urination.	Continue. Call doctor when convenient.
• Nausea, constipation.	Continue. Tell doctor at next visit.
Rare: • Fainting.	Discontinue. Call doctor right away.
• Headache.	Continue. Tell doctor at next visit.

 ## WARNINGS & PRECAUTIONS

Don't take if:
- You are allergic to verapamil.
- You have very low blood pressure.

Before you start, consult your doctor:
- If you have kidney or liver disease.
- If you have high blood pressure.
- If you have heart disease other than
  coronary-artery disease.

Over age 60:
Adverse reactions and side effects may be
more frequent and severe than in younger
persons.

Pregnancy:
No proven harm to unborn child. Avoid if
possible.

Breast-feeding:
Safety not established. Avoid if possible.

Infants & children:
Not recommended.

Prolonged use:
No problems expected.

Skin & sunlight:
No problems expected.

Driving, piloting or hazardous work:
Avoid if you feel dizzy. Otherwise, no problems expected.

Discontinuing:
Don't discontinue without doctor's advice until you complete prescribed dose, even though symptoms diminish or disappear.

Others:
Learn to check your own pulse rate. If it drops to 50 beats per minute or lower, don't take verapamil until your consult your doctor.

POSSIBLE INTERACTION WITH OTHER DRUGS

GENERIC NAME OR DRUG CLASS	COMBINED EFFECT
Amiodarone	Increased likelihood of slow heartbeat.
Anticoagulants (oral)	Increased anticoagulant effect.
Anticonvulsants (hydantoin)	Increased anticonvulsant effect.
Antihypertensives	Dangerous blood-pressure drop.
Beta-adrenergic blockers	Possible irregular heartbeat.
Calcium (large doses)	Decreased verapamil effect.
Digitalis preparations	Increased digitalis effect. May need to reduce dose.
Disopyramide	May cause dangerously slow, fast or irregular heartbeat.
Diuretics	Dangerous blood-pressure drop.
Enalapril	Possible excessive potassium in blood.
Flecainide	Possible irregular heartbeat.
Ketoprofen	Increased chance of toxicity of verapamil.
Nitrates	Reduced angina attacks.
Oxprenolol	Possible greater difficulty in treating patients with congestive heart failure.
Pentoxifylline	Increased antihypertensive effect.
Quinidine	Increased quinidine effect.

Suprofen	Increased chance of toxicity of verapamil.
Tocainide	Possible irregular heartbeat.
Vitamin D (large doses)	Decreased verapamil effect.

POSSIBLE INTERACTION WITH OTHER SUBSTANCES

INTERACTS WITH	COMBINED EFFECT
Alcohol:	Dangerously low blood pressure. Avoid.
Beverages:	None expected.
Cocaine:	Possible irregular heartbeat. Avoid.
Foods:	None expected.
Marijuana:	Possible irregular heartbeat. Avoid.
Tobacco:	Possible rapid heartbeat. Avoid.

VITAMIN A

BRAND NAMES

Acon
Afaxin
Alphalin
Aquasol A
Dispatabs
Sust-A
Numerous multiple vitamin-mineral supplements.

BASIC INFORMATION

Habit forming? No
Prescription needed? No
Available as generic? Yes
Drug class: Vitamin supplement

USES

Dietary supplement to ensure normal growth and health, especially eyes and skin.

DOSAGE & USAGE INFORMATION

How to take:
Tablet or capsule—Swallow with liquid. If you can't swallow whole, crumble tablet or open capsule and take with liquid or food.

When to take:
At the same time each day.

If you forget a dose:
Take as soon as you remember. Resume regular schedule.

What drug does:
• Prevents night blindness.
• Promotes normal growth and health.

Time lapse before drug works:
Requires continual intake.

Don't take with:
See Interaction column and consult doctor.

OVERDOSE

SYMPTOMS:
Increased adverse reactions and side effects. Jaundice (rare, but may occur with large doses).
WHAT TO DO:
Overdose unlikely to threaten life. If person takes much larger amount than prescribed, call doctor, poison-control center or hospital emergency room for instructions.

POSSIBLE ADVERSE REACTIONS OR SIDE EFFECTS

SYMPTOMS	WHAT TO DO
Life-threatening: None expected.	
Common: None expected.	
Infrequent: Confusion, dizziness, drowsiness, headache, irritability, dry lips, peeling skin, hair loss.	Continue. Call doctor when convenient.
Rare: • Bulging soft spot on baby's head, double vision.	Discontinue. Call doctor right away.
• Diarrhea, appetite loss, nausea, vomiting.	Continue. Call doctor when convenient.

WARNINGS & PRECAUTIONS

Don't take if:
You have chronic kidney failure.

Before you start, consult your doctor:
If you have any kidney disorder.

Over age 60:
No problems expected.

Pregnancy:
Don't take more than 6,000 units daily.

Breast-feeding:
No problems expected.

Infants & children:
• Avoid large doses.
• Keep vitamin-mineral supplements out of children's reach.

Prolonged use:
No problems expected.

Skin & sunlight:
No problems expected.

Driving, piloting or hazardous work:
No problems expected.

Discontinuing:
Don't discontinue without doctor's advice until you complete prescribed dose, even though symptoms diminish or disappear.

Others:
• Don't exceed dose. Too much over a long time may be harmful.
• A balanced diet should provide all the vitamin A a healthy person needs and prevent need for supplements. Best sources are liver, yellow-orange fruits and vegetables, dark-green, leafy vegetables, milk, butter and margarine.

POSSIBLE INTERACTION WITH OTHER DRUGS

GENERIC NAME OR DRUG CLASS	COMBINED EFFECT
Anticoagulants	Increased anticoagulant effect with large doses (over 10,000 I.U.) of vitamin A.
Calcium supplements	Decreased vitamin effect.
Cholestyramine	Decreased vitamin A absorption.
Colestipol	Decreased vitamin absorption.
Mineral oil (long term)	Decreased vitamin A absorption.
Neomycin	Decreased vitamin absorption.
Vitamin E (excess dose)	Vitamin A depletion.

POSSIBLE INTERACTION WITH OTHER SUBSTANCES

INTERACTS WITH	COMBINED EFFECT
Alcohol:	None expected.
Beverages:	None expected.
Cocaine:	None expected.
Foods:	None expected.
Marijuana:	None expected.
Tobacco:	None expected.

VITAMIN B-12 (CYANOCOBALAMIN)

BRAND NAMES

See complete list of brand names in the *Brand Name Directory,* page 958.

BASIC INFORMATION

Habit forming? No
Prescription needed? No
Available as generic? Yes
Drug class: Vitamin supplement

USES

- Dietary supplement for normal growth, development and health.
- Treatment for nerve damage.
- Treatment for pernicious anemia.
- Treatment and prevention of vitamin B-12 deficiencies in people who have had stomach or intestines surgically removed.
- Prevention of vitamin B-12 deficiency in strict vegetarians and persons with absorption diseases.

DOSAGE & USAGE INFORMATION

How to take:
- Tablets—Swallow with liquid.
- Injection—Follow doctor's directions.

When to take:
- Oral—At the same time each day.
- Injection—Follow doctor's directions.

If you forget a dose:
Take when remembered. Don't double next dose. Resume regular schedule.

What drug does:
Acts as enzyme to promote normal fat and carbohydrate metabolism and protein synthesis.

Time lapse before drug works:
15 minutes.

Don't take with:
See Interaction column and consult doctor.

OVERDOSE

SYMPTOMS:
Increased adverse reactions and side effects.
WHAT TO DO:
Overdose unlikely to threaten life. If person takes much larger amount than prescribed, call doctor, poison-control center or hospital emergency room for instructions.

POSSIBLE ADVERSE REACTIONS OR SIDE EFFECTS

SYMPTOMS	WHAT TO DO
Life-threatening:	
Hives, rash, intense itching, faintness soon after a dose (anaphylaxis).	Seek emergency treatment immediately.
Common:	
None expected.	
Infrequent:	
None expected.	
Rare:	
• Itchy skin, wheezing.	Discontinue. Call doctor right away.
• Diarrhea.	Continue. Call doctor when convenient.

WARNINGS & PRECAUTIONS

Don't take if:
You have Leber's disease (optic nerve atrophy).

Before you start, consult your doctor:
- If you have gout.
- If you have heart disease.

Over age 60:
Don't take more than 100mg per day unless prescribed by your doctor.

Pregnancy:
No problems expected.

Breast-feeding:
No problems expected.

Infants & children:
No problems expected.

Prolonged use:
No problems expected.

Skin & sunlight:
No problems expected.

Driving, piloting or hazardous work:
No problems expected.

Discontinuing:
Don't discontinue without doctor's advice until you complete prescribed dose, even though symptoms diminish or disappear.

Others:
- A balanced diet should provide all the vitamin B-12 a healthy person needs and make supplements unnecessary. Best sources are meat, fish, egg yolk and cheese.
- Tablets should be used only for diet supplements. All other uses of vitamin B-12 require injections.
- Don't take large doses of vitamin C (1,000mg or more per day) unless prescribed by your doctor.

POSSIBLE INTERACTION WITH OTHER DRUGS

GENERIC NAME OR DRUG CLASS	COMBINED EFFECT
Anticonvulsants	Decreased absorption of vitamin B-12.
Aspirin	Decreased absorption of vitamin B-12.
Chloramphenicol	Decreased vitamin B-12 effect.
Colchicine	Decreased absorption of vitamin B-12.
Neomycin	Decreased absorption of vitamin B-12.
Potassium (extended-release forms)	Decreased absorption of vitamin B-12.
Vitamin C (ascorbic acid)	Destroys vitamin B-12 if taken at same time. Take 2 hours apart.

POSSIBLE INTERACTION WITH OTHER SUBSTANCES

INTERACTS WITH	COMBINED EFFECT
Alcohol:	Decreased absorption of vitamin B-12.
Beverages:	None expected.
Cocaine:	None expected.
Foods:	None expected.
Marijuana:	None expected.
Tobacco:	None expected.

BRAND NAMES

See complete list of brand names in the *Brand Name Directory,* page 958.

BASIC INFORMATION

Habit forming? No
Prescription needed? No
Available as generic? Yes
Drug class: Vitamin supplement

 ## USES

- Prevention and treatment of scurvy and other vitamin-C deficiencies.
- Treatment of anemia.
- Maintenance of acid urine.

 ## DOSAGE & USAGE INFORMATION

How to take:
- Tablets, capsules, liquid—Swallow with 8 oz. water.
- Extended-release tablets—Swallow whole.
- Drops—Squirt directly into mouth or mix with liquid or food.

When to take:
1, 2 or 3 times per day, as prescribed on label.

If you forget a dose:
Take as soon as you remember. Return to regular schedule.

What drug does:
- May help form collagen.
- Increases iron absorption from intestine.
- Contributes to hemoglobin and red-blood-cell production in bone marrow.

Time lapse before drug works:
1 week.

Don't take with:
See Interaction column and consult doctor.

 ## OVERDOSE

SYMPTOMS:
Diarrhea, vomiting, dizziness.
WHAT TO DO:
Overdose unlikely to threaten life. If person takes much larger amount than prescribed, call doctor, poison-control center or hospital emergency room for instructions.

 ## POSSIBLE ADVERSE REACTIONS OR SIDE EFFECTS

SYMPTOMS	WHAT TO DO
Life-threatening:	
None expected.	
Common:	
None expected.	
Infrequent:	
• Mild diarrhea, nausea, vomiting.	Discontinue. Call doctor right away.
• Flushed face.	Continue. Call doctor when convenient.
Rare:	
• Kidney stones with high doses, anemia.	Discontinue. Call doctor right away.
• Headache.	Continue. Tell doctor at next visit.

WARNINGS & PRECAUTIONS

Don't take if:
You are allergic to vitamin C.

Before you start, consult your doctor:
- If you have sickle-cell or other anemia.
- If you have had kidney stones.
- If you have gout.

Over age 60:
Don't take more than 100mg per day unless prescribed by your doctor.

Pregnancy:
No proven harm to unborn child. Avoid large doses.

Breast-feeding:
Avoid large doses.

Infants & children:
- Avoid large doses.
- Keep vitamin-mineral supplements out of children's reach.

Prolonged use:
Large doses for longer than 2 months may cause kidney stones.

Skin & sunlight:
No problems expected.

Driving, piloting or hazardous work:
No problems expected.

Discontinuing:
No problems expected.

Others:
- Store in cool, dry place.
- May cause inaccurate tests for sugar in urine or blood in stool.
- May cause crisis in patients with sickle-cell anemia.
- A balanced diet should provide all the vitamin C a healthy person needs and make supplements unnecessary. Best sources are citrus, strawberries, cantaloupe and raw peppers.
- Don't take large doses of vitamin C (1,000mg or more per day) unless prescribed by your doctor.

POSSIBLE INTERACTION WITH OTHER DRUGS

GENERIC NAME OR DRUG CLASS	COMBINED EFFECT
Anticholinergics	Decreased anticholinergic effect.
Anticoagulants (oral)	Decreased anticoagulant effect.
Aspirin	Decreased vitamin C effect.
Barbiturates	Decreased vitamin C effect. Increased barbiturate effect.
Contraceptives (oral)	Decreased vitamin C effect.
Estrogens	Increased likelihood of adverse effects from estrogen with 1gm or more of vitamin C per day.
Iron supplements	Increased iron effect.
Mexiletine	May decrease effectiveness of mexiletine.
Mineral oil	Decreased vitamin C effect.
Quinidine	Decreased quinidine effect.
Salicylates	Decreased vitamin C effect.
Tetracyclines	Decreased vitamin C effect.
Tranquilizers (phenothiazine)	Decreased phenothiazine effect if no vitamin C deficiency exists.

POSSIBLE INTERACTION WITH OTHER SUBSTANCES

INTERACTS WITH	COMBINED EFFECT
Alcohol:	None expected.
Beverages:	None expected.
Cocaine:	None expected.
Foods:	None expected.
Marijuana:	None expected.
Tobacco:	Increased requirement for vitamin C.

VITAMIN D

BRAND NAMES

Calciferol
Calcifidiol
Calcitriol
Calderol
Deltalin
DHT
Dihydrotachysterol

Drisdol
Ergocalciferol
Hytakerol
Ostoforte
Radiostol
Radiostol Forte
Rocaltrol

Numerous other multiple vitamin-mineral
supplements.

BASIC INFORMATION

Habit forming? No
Prescription needed?
  Low strength: No
  High strength: Yes
Available as generic? Yes
Drug class: Vitamin supplement

 USES

- Dietary supplement.
- Prevention of rickets (bone disease).
- Treatment for hypocalcemia (low blood calcium) in kidney disease.
- Treatment for postoperative muscle contractions.

 DOSAGE & USAGE INFORMATION

How to take:
- Tablet or capsule—Swallow with liquid.
- Drops—Dilute dose in beverage.

When to take:
As directed, usually once a day at the same time each day.

If you forget a dose:
Take up to 12 hours late. If more than 12 hours, wait for next dose (don't double this dose).

Continued next column

 OVERDOSE

SYMPTOMS:
Severe stomach pain, nausea, vomiting, weight loss; bone and muscle pain; increased urination, cloudy urine; mood or mental changes (possible psychosis); high blood pressure, irregular heartbeat; eye irritation or light sensitivity; itchy skin.
WHAT TO DO:
Overdose unlikely to threaten life. If person takes much larger amount than prescribed, call doctor, poison-control center or hospital emergency room for instructions.

What drug does:
Maintains growth and health. Prevents rickets. Essential so body can use calcium and phosphate.

Time lapse before drug works:
2 hours. May require 2 to 3 weeks of continual use for maximum effect.

Don't take with:
Non-prescription drugs or drugs in Interaction column without consulting doctor.

 POSSIBLE ADVERSE REACTIONS OR SIDE EFFECTS

SYMPTOMS	WHAT TO DO
Life-threatening: None expected.	
Common: None expected.	
Infrequent: Headache, metallic taste in mouth, thirst, dry mouth, constipation, appetite loss, nausea, vomiting.	Continue. Call doctor when convenient.
Rare: None expected.	

WARNINGS & PRECAUTIONS

Don't take if:
You are allergic to medicine containing vitamin D.

Before you start, consult your doctor:
- If you plan to become pregnant while taking vitamin D.
- If you have epilepsy.
- If you have heart or blood-vessel disease.
- If you have kidney disease.

Over age 60:
Adverse reactions and side effects may be more frequent and severe than in younger persons.

Pregnancy:
Risk to unborn child outweighs drug benefits. Don't use.

Breast-feeding:
No problems expected, but consult doctor.

Infants & children:
- Avoid large doses.
- Keep vitamins out of children's reach.

Prolonged use:
No problems expected.

Skin & sunlight:
No problems expected.

Driving, piloting or hazardous work:
No problems expected.

Discontinuing:
Don't discontinue without doctor's advice until you complete prescribed dose, even though symptoms diminish or disappear.

Others:
- Don't exceed dose. Too much over a long time may be harmful.
- A balanced diet should provide all the vitamin D a healthy person needs and make supplements unnecessary. Best sources are fish and vitamin-D fortified milk and bread.

POSSIBLE INTERACTION WITH OTHER DRUGS

GENERIC NAME OR DRUG CLASS	COMBINED EFFECT
Antacids (magnesium-containing)	Possible excess magnesium.
Anticonvulsants (hydantoin)	Decreased vitamin D effect.
Calcium (high doses)	Excess calcium in blood.
Calcium-channel blockers	Decreased effect of calcium-channel blockers.
Calcium supplements	Excessive absorption of vitamin D.
Cholestyramine	Decreased vitamin D effect.
Colestipol	Decreased vitamin D absorption.
Digitalis preparations	Heartbeat irregularities.
Mineral oil	Decreased vitamin D effect.
Neomycin	Decreased vitamin D absorption.
Phenobarbital	Decreased vitamin D effect.
Phosphorous preparations	Accumulation of excess phosphorous.
Vitamin D (other)	Possible toxicity.

POSSIBLE INTERACTION WITH OTHER SUBSTANCES

INTERACTS WITH	COMBINED EFFECT
Alcohol:	None expected.
Beverages:	None expected.
Cocaine:	None expected.
Foods:	None expected.
Marijuana:	None expected.
Tobacco:	None expected.

VITAMIN E

BRAND NAMES

Aquasol E
Chew-E
Daltose
Eferol

Eprolin
Epsilan-M
Pheryl-E
Viterra E

Numerous other multiple vitamin-mineral supplements.

BASIC INFORMATION

Habit forming? No
Prescription needed? No
Available as generic? Yes
Drug class: Vitamin supplement

 ## USES

- Dietary supplement to promote normal growth, development and health.
- Treatment and prevention of vitamin-E deficiency, especially in premature or low birth-weight infants.
- Treatment for fibrocystic disease of the breast.
- Treatment for circulatory problems to the lower extremities.
- Treatment for sickle-cell anemia.
- Treatment for lung toxicity from air pollution.

 ## DOSAGE & USAGE INFORMATION

How to take:
- Tablet, capsule or chewable tablets—Swallow with liquid or food to lessen stomach irritation.
- Drops—Dilute dose in beverage before swallowing or squirt directly into mouth.

When to take:
At the same times each day.

If you forget a dose:
Take when you remember. Don't double next dose.

What drug does:
- Promotes normal growth and development.
- Prevents oxidation in body.

Continued next column

 ## OVERDOSE

SYMPTOMS:
Nausea, vomiting.
WHAT TO DO:
Overdose unlikely to threaten life. If person takes much larger amount than prescribed, call doctor, poison-control center or hospital emergency room for instructions.

Time lapse before drug works:
Not determined.

Don't take with:
See Interaction column and consult doctor.

 ## POSSIBLE ADVERSE REACTIONS OR SIDE EFFECTS

SYMPTOMS	WHAT TO DO
Life-threatening: None expected.	
Common: None expected.	
Infrequent: Nausea, stomach pain, muscle aches, pain in lower legs, fever, tiredness, weakness.	Continue. Call doctor when convenient.
Rare: None expected.	

WARNINGS & PRECAUTIONS

Don't take if:
You are allergic to vitamin E.

Before you start, consult your doctor:
- If you have had blood clots in leg veins (thrombophlebitis).
- If you have liver disease.

Over age 60:
No problems expected. Avoid excessive doses.

Pregnancy:
No problems expected with normal daily requirements. Don't exceed prescribed dose.

Breast-feeding:
No problems expected.

Infants & children:
Use only under medical supervision.

Prolonged use:
Toxic accumulation of vitamin E. Don't exceed recommended dose.

Skin & sunlight:
No problems expected.

Driving, piloting or hazardous work:
No problems expected.

Discontinuing:
No problems expected.

Others:
A balanced diet should provide all the vitamin E a healthy person needs and make supplements unnecessary. Best sources are vegetable oils, whole-grain cereals, liver.

POSSIBLE INTERACTION WITH OTHER DRUGS

GENERIC NAME OR DRUG CLASS	COMBINED EFFECT
Anticoagulants (oral)	Increased anticoagulant effect.
Cholestyramine	Decreased vitamin E absorption.
Colestipol	Decreased vitamin E absorption.
Iron supplements	Decreased effect of iron supplement in patients with iron-deficiency anemia. Decreased vitamin E effect in healthy persons.
Neomycin	Decreased vitamin E absorption.
Vitamin A	Recommended dose of vitamin E— Increased benefit and decreased toxicity of vitamin A. Excess dose of vitamin E—Vitamin A depletion.

POSSIBLE INTERACTION WITH OTHER SUBSTANCES

INTERACTS WITH	COMBINED EFFECT
Alcohol:	None expected.
Beverages:	None expected.
Cocaine:	None expected.
Foods:	None expected.
Marijuana:	None expected.
Tobacco:	None expected.

VITAMIN K

BRAND NAMES

Konakion
Menadione
Menadiol

Mephyton
Phytonadione
Synkayvite

BASIC INFORMATION

Habit forming? No
Prescription needed? No
Available as generic? Yes
Drug class: Vitamin supplement

USES

- Dietary supplement.
- Treatment for bleeding disorders and malabsorption diseases due to vitamin K deficiency.
- Treatment for hemorrhagic disease of the newborn.
- Treatment for bleeding due to overdose of oral anticoagulants.

DOSAGE & USAGE INFORMATION

How to take:
Tablet—Swallow with liquid. If you can't swallow whole, crumble tablet or open capsule and take with liquid or food.

When to take:
At the same time each day.

If you forget a dose:
Take as soon as you remember up to 12 hours late. If more than 12 hours, wait for next scheduled dose (don't double this dose).

What drug does:
- Promotes growth, development and good health.
- Supplies a necessary ingredient for blood clotting.

Time lapse before drug works:
15 to 30 minutes to support blood clotting.

Don't take with:
See Interaction column and consult doctor.

OVERDOSE

SYMPTOMS:
Nausea, vomiting.
WHAT TO DO:
Overdose unlikely to threaten life. If person takes much larger amount than prescribed, call doctor, poison-control center or hospital emergency room for instructions.

POSSIBLE ADVERSE REACTIONS OR SIDE EFFECTS

SYMPTOMS	WHAT TO DO
Life-threatening: None expected.	
Common: None expected.	
Infrequent: Unusual taste.	Continue. Call doctor when convenient.
Rare: None expected.	

WARNINGS & PRECAUTIONS

Don't take if:
- You are allergic to vitamin K.
- You have G6PD deficiency.
- You have liver disease.

Before you start, consult your doctor:
If you are pregnant.

Over age 60:
No problems expected.

Pregnancy:
Don't exceed dose.

Breast-feeding:
No problems expected.

Infants & children:
Phytonadione is the preferred form for hemorrhagic disease of the newborn.

Prolonged use:
No problems expected.

Skin & sunlight:
No problems expected.

Driving, piloting or hazardous work:
No problems expected.

Discontinuing:
No problems expected.

Others:
- Tell all doctors and dentists you consult that you take this medicine.
- Don't exceed dose. Too much over a long time may be harmful.
- A balanced diet should provide all the vitamin K a healthy person needs and make supplements unnecessary. Best sources are green, leafy vegetables, meat or dairy products.

POSSIBLE INTERACTION WITH OTHER DRUGS

GENERIC NAME OR DRUG CLASS	COMBINED EFFECT
Anticoagulants (oral)	Decreased anticoagulant effect.
Cholestyramine	Decreased vitamin K effect.
Colestipol	Decreased vitamin K absorption.
Mineral oil (long term)	Vitamin K deficiency.
Neomycin	Decreased vitamin K absorption.
Sulfa drugs	Vitamin K deficiency.

POSSIBLE INTERACTION WITH OTHER SUBSTANCES

INTERACTS WITH	COMBINED EFFECT
Alcohol:	None expected.
Beverages:	None expected.
Cocaine:	None expected.
Foods:	None expected.
Marijuana:	None expected.
Tobacco:	None expected.

VITAMINS & FLUORIDE

BRAND AND GENERIC NAMES

Adeflor
Cari-Tab
Mulvidren-F
Poly-Vi-Flor
MULTIPLE VITAMINS & FLUORIDE
VITAMINS A, D & C & FLUORIDE

Tri-Vi-Flor
Vi-Daylin/F
Vi-Penta F

BASIC INFORMATION

Habit forming? No
Prescription needed? Yes
Available as generic? No
Drug class: Vitamins, minerals

 USES

- Reduces incidence of tooth cavities (fluoride). Children who need supplements should take until age 16.
- Prevents deficiencies of vitamin included in formula (some contain multiple vitamins whose content varies among products, others contain only vitamins A, D and C).

 DOSAGE & USAGE INFORMATION

How to take:
- Chewable tablets—Chew or crush before swallowing.
- Oral liquid—Take by mouth measured with specially marked dropper. May mix with food, fruit juice, cereal.

When to take:
- Bedtime or with or just after meals.
- If at bedtime, brush teeth first.

If you forget a dose:
Take as soon as you remember up to 2 hours late. If more than 2 hours, wait for next scheduled dose (don't double this dose).

Continued next column

 OVERDOSE

SYMPTOMS:
Minor overdose—Black, brown or white spots on teeth.
Massive overdose—Shallow breathing, black or tarry stools, bloody vomit.
WHAT TO DO:
- Dial 0 (operator) or 911 (emergency) for an ambulance or medical help. Then give first aid immediately.
- See emergency information on inside covers.

What drug does:
Provides supplemental fluoride to combat tooth decay.

Time lapse before drug works:
8 weeks to provide maximum benefit.

Don't take with:
- Other medicine simultaneously.
- See Interaction column and consult doctor.

 POSSIBLE ADVERSE REACTIONS OR SIDE EFFECTS

SYMPTOMS	WHAT TO DO
Life-threatening:	
Fainting, bloody vomit, bloody or black stool.	Discontinue. Seek emergency treatment.
Common:	
White, black or brown spots on teeth; nausea; vomiting.	Discontinue. Call doctor right away.
Infrequent:	
• Drowsiness; abdominal pain; increased salivation; watery eyes; weight loss; sore throat, fever, mouth sores; constipation; bone pain; rash; muscle stiffness; weakness; tremor; agitation.	Discontinue. Call doctor right away.
• Diarrhea.	Continue. Call doctor when convenient.
Rare:	
None expected.	

WARNINGS & PRECAUTIONS

Don't take if:
- Your water supply contains 0.7 parts fluoride per million. Too much fluoride stains teeth permanently.
- You are allergic to any fluoride-containing product.
- You have underactive thyroid.

Before you start, consult your doctor or dentist:
For proper dosage.

Over age 60:
No problems expected.

Pregnancy:
No problems expected.

Breast-feeding:
No problems expected.

Infants & children:
No problems expected in children over 3 years of age except accidental overdose. Keep vitamin-mineral supplements out of children's reach.

Prolonged use:
Excess may cause discolored teeth and decreased calcium in blood.

Skin & sunlight:
No problems expected.

Driving, piloting or hazardous work:
No problems expected.

Discontinuing:
No problems expected.

Others:
- Store in original plastic container. Fluoride decomposes glass.
- Check with dentist once or twice a year to keep cavities at a minimum. Topical applications of fluoride may also be helpful.
- Fluoride probably not necessary if water contains about 1 part per million of fluoride or more. Check with health department.
- Don't freeze.
- Don't keep outdated medicine.

POSSIBLE INTERACTION WITH OTHER DRUGS

GENERIC NAME OR DRUG CLASS	COMBINED EFFECT
Anticoagulants	Decreased anticoagulant effect.
Iron supplements	Decreased effect of any vitamin E if present in multivitamin product.
Vitamin D	May lead to vitamin D toxicity if vitamin D is in combination.

POSSIBLE INTERACTION WITH OTHER SUBSTANCES

INTERACTS WITH	COMBINED EFFECT
Alcohol:	None expected.
Beverages: Milk.	Prevents absorption of fluoride. Space dose 2 hours before or after milk.
Cocaine:	None expected.
Foods:	None expected.
Marijuana:	None expected.
Tobacco:	None expected.

XANTHINE BRONCHODILATORS

BRAND NAMES

See complete list of brand names in the *Brand Name Directory*, page 959.

BASIC INFORMATION

Habit forming? No
Prescription needed?
  Canada—No
  U.S.: High strength—Yes
      Low strength—No
Available as generic? Yes
Drug class: Bronchodilator (xanthine)

 ## USES

Treatment for bronchial asthma symptoms.

 ## DOSAGE & USAGE INFORMATION

How to take:
- Tablet or capsule—Swallow with liquid.
- Extended-release tablets or capsules—Swallow each dose whole. If you take regular tablets, you may chew or crush them.
- Suppositories—Remove wrapper and moisten suppository with water. Gently insert larger end into rectum. Push well into rectum with finger.
- Syrup—Take as directed on bottle.
- Enema—Use as directed on label.

When to take:
Most effective taken on empty stomach 1 hour before or 2 hours after eating. However, may take with food to lessen stomach upset.

If you forget a dose:
Take as soon as you remember up to 2 hours late. If more than 2 hours, wait for next scheduled dose (don't double this dose).

What drug does:
Relaxes and expands bronchial tubes.

Continued next column

 ## OVERDOSE

SYMPTOMS:
Restlessness, irritability, confusion, delirium, convulsions, rapid pulse, coma.
WHAT TO DO:
- **Dial 0 (operator) or 911 (emergency) for an ambulance or medical help. Then give first aid immediately.**
- **See emergency information on inside covers.**

Time lapse before drug works:
15 to 30 minutes.

Don't take with:
See Interaction column and consult doctor.

 ## POSSIBLE ADVERSE REACTIONS OR SIDE EFFECTS

SYMPTOMS	WHAT TO DO
Life-threatening: None expected.	
Common: Headache, irritability, nervousness, restlessness, insomnia, nausea, vomiting, stomach pain.	Continue. Call doctor when convenient.
Infrequent:	
• Rash or hives, flushed face, diarrhea, appetite loss, rapid breathing, irregular heartbeat.	Discontinue. Call doctor right away.
• Dizziness or lightheadedness.	Continue. Call doctor when convenient.
Rare: None expected.	

WARNINGS & PRECAUTIONS

Don't take if:
- You are allergic to any bronchodilator.
- You have an active peptic ulcer.

Before you start, consult your doctor:
- If you have had impaired kidney or liver function.
- If you have gastritis.
- If you have a peptic ulcer.
- If you have high blood pressure or heart disease.
- If you take medication for gout.

Over age 60:
Adverse reactions and side effects may be more frequent and severe than in younger persons.

Pregnancy:
Risk to unborn child outweighs drug benefits. Don't use.

Breast-feeding:
Drug passes into milk. Avoid drug or discontinue nursing until you finish medicine. Consult doctor for advice on maintaining milk supply.

Infants & children:
Use only under medical supervision.

Prolonged use:
Stomach irritation.

Skin & sunlight:
No problems expected.

Driving, piloting or hazardous work:
Avoid if lightheaded or dizzy. Otherwise, no problems expected.

Discontinuing:
May be unnecessary to finish medicine. Follow doctor's instructions.

Others:
No problems expected.

POSSIBLE INTERACTION WITH OTHER DRUGS

GENERIC NAME OR DRUG CLASS	COMBINED EFFECT
Allopurinol	Decreased allopurinol effect.
Ephedrine	Increased effect of both drugs.
Epinephrine	Increased effect of both drugs.
Erythromycin	Increased bronchodilator effect.
Furosemide	Increased furosemide effect.
Lincomycins	Increased bronchodilator effect.
Lithiuim	Decreased lithiuim effect.
Probenecid	Decreased effect of both drugs.
Propranolol	Decreased bronchodilator effect.
Rauwolfia alkaloids	Rapid heartbeat.
Sulfinpyrazone	Decreased sulfinpyrazone effect.
Troleandomycin	Increased bronchodilator effect.

POSSIBLE INTERACTION WITH OTHER SUBSTANCES

INTERACTS WITH	COMBINED EFFECT
Alcohol:	None expected.
Beverages: Caffeine drinks.	Nervousness and insomnia.
Cocaine:	Excess stimulation. Avoid.
Foods:	None expected.
Marijuana:	Slightly increased antiasthmatic effect of bronchodilator.
Tobacco:	Decreased bronchodilator effect.

Brand Name Directory

The following drugs are alphabetized by generic name or drug class, shown in large capital letters. The brand and gneeric names that follow each title in this list are the complete list referred to on the drug charts. Generic names are in all capital letters on the lists.

ACETAMINOPHEN

A'Cenol
Acephen
Aceta
Ace-Tabs
Aceta w/Codeine
Acetaco
Acetaminophen w/Codeine
Actamin
Algisin
Amacodone
Amaphen
Amphenol
Anacin-3
Anapap
Anaphen
Anoquan
Anuphen
Apamide Tablets
APAP
Apo-Acetaminophen
Arthralgen
Aspirin-Free Excedrin
Atasol
Axotal
Bancap w/Codeine
Banesin
Banesin Forte
Bayapap
Bromo-Seltzer
C2A
Campain
Capital
Capital w/Codeine
Chlorzone Forte
Co-Gesic
Co-Tylenol
Coastaldyne
Coastalgesic
Codalan
Codap
Colrex
Compal
Comtrex
Conacetol
Congespirin
Covangesic
D-Sinus
Dapa
Dapase
Darvocet-N
Datril
Dia-Gesic
Dialog
Dolacet
Dolanex
Dolene AP-65
Dolor
Dolprin
Dorcol
Dorcol Children's Fever and Pain
   Reducer
Dristan
Duadacin

Dularin
Duradyne DHC
Dynosal
Empracet w/Codeine
Endecon
Esgic
Excedrin
Exdol
Febrigesic
Febrinol
Febrogesic
Fendol
G-1
G-2
G-3
Gaysal
Genapap
Genebs
Genetabs
Guaiamine
Halenol
Hasacode
Hi-Temp
Hyco-Pap
Hycomine Compound
Korigesic
Liquiprin
Liquix-C
Lorcet
Lyteca
Meda Cap
Meda Tab
Mejoral without aspirin
Mejoralito
Metrogesic
Midol PMS
Midrin
Migralam
Minotal
Naldegesic
NAPAP
Nebs
Neopap
Oraphen-PD
Ornex
Ossonate-Plus
Pacaps
Pain Relief without aspirin
Panadol
Panasorb
Panex
Paracetamol
Parafon Forte
Paraphen
Pavadon
Pedric
Peedee Dose Aspirin
Percocet-5
Percogesic
Phenaphen
Phenaphen w/Codeine
Phendex
Phrenilin
Presalin

Prodolor
Protid
Proval
Repan
Rhinocaps
Robigesic
Ronuvex
Rounox
S-A-C
SK-65 APAP
SK-APAP
SK-Oxycodone w/Acetaminophen
Salatin
Saleto
Salimeph Forte
Salphenyl
Sedapap
Sinarest
Sine-Aid
Sine-Off
Singlet
Sinubid
Sinulin
Sinutab
St. Joseph Aspirin Free
Stopayne
Strascogesic
Sudoprin
Summit
Supac
Suppap
Sylapar
T.P.I.
Talacen
Tapanol
Tapar
Temlo
Tempra
Tenlap
Tenol
Triaminicin
Trigesic
Trind Sryup
Two-Dyne
Ty-tabs
Tylenol
Tylenol w/Codeine
Tylox
Valadol
Valorin
Vanquish
Vicodin
Wygesic

ACETAMINOPHEN & SALICYLATES

445 Anti-Pain Compound
Accurate Forte
ACETAMINOPHEN & ASPIRIN
ACETAMINOPHEN, ASPIRIN &
   SALICYLAMIDE
ACETAMINOPHEN &
   SALICYLAMIDE

ACETAMINOPHEN & SODIUM SALICYLATE

APAP Fortified
Arthralgen
Banesin
Buffets II
Dinol
Double-A
Duoprin
Duoprin-S
Duradyne
Dynosal
Excedrin
Gaysal-S
Gemnisyn
Goody's Extra Strength Tablets
Goody's Headache Powders
Presalin
Rid-A-Pain Compound
S-A-C
Salatin
Saleto
Salimeph Forte
Salocol
Supac
Tisma
Trigesic
Vanquish

ADRENOCORTICOIDS (TOPICAL)

Acticort
Adcortyl
Aeroseb-Dex
Aeroseb-HC
Alphatrex
Aristocort
Aristocort A
Aristocort C
Aristocort D
Aristocort R
Bactine Hydrocortisone
Barriere-HC
Beben
Benisone
Beta-Val
Betacort
Betacort Scalp Lotion
Betaderm
Betaderm Scalp Lotion
Betatrex
Betnovate
CaldeCORT
Caldecort Anti-Itch
Carmol-HC
Celestoderm-V
Celestone
Cetacort
Clinicort
Cloderm
Cordran
Cordran SP
Cort-Dome
Cortaid
Cortate
Cortef
Corticosporin
Corticreme
Cortifoam
Cortiment
Cortisol

Cortizone
Cortril
Cremocort
Cyclocort
Decaderm
Decadron
Decaspray
Delacort
Dermacort
DermiCort
Dermolate
Dermophyl
Dermovate
Dermovate Scalp Application
Dermtex HC
DesOwen
Dioderm
Diprolene
Diprosone
Drenison
EF cortelan
Ectosone
Ectosone Scalp Lotion
Eldecort
Emo-Cort
Epifoam
Florone
Fluocet
Fluoderm
Fluolar
Fluolean
Fluonid
Fluonide
Flurosyn
Flutex
Flutone
Gynecort
H2 Cort
HC-Jel
Halciderm
Halog
Halog E
Hexadrol
Hi-Cor
Hi-Cort
Hyderm
Hydro-Corilean
Hydro-Tex
Hydrocortone
Hytone
Kenalog
Kenalog-E
Kenalog-H
Lacticare-HC
Lanacort
Lidemol
Lidex
Lidex-E
Locoid
Locacorten
Lyderm
Maxiflor
Medrol
Metaderm
Meti-Derm
Metosyn
Metosyn FAPG
Neo-Cortef
Neo-Decadron
Novobetamet
Novohydrocort
Nutracort

Oxylone
Penecort
Pharma-Cort
Proctocort
Psorcon
Psorcon-E
Racet-SE
Rhulicort
Spencort
Stie-Cort
Synacort
Synalar
Synamol
Synandone
Synemol
Temovate
Texacort
Topicort
Topsyn
Triacet
Triaderm
Trianide
Tridesilon
Trymex
Unicort
Uticort
Valisone
Valisone Scalp Lotion
Vioform
Westcort
Some of these brands are available as oral medicine. Look under specific generic name for each brand.

ALUMINUM HYDROXIDE

Alagel
Algenic Alka
Alka-mag
ALternaGEL
Alu-Cap
Alu-Tab
Aludrox
Alumid
Aluscop
Amphojel
Basaljel
Bisodol
Camalox
Chemgel
Creamalin
De Witts
Delcid
Di-Gel
Dialume
Dioval Ex
Ducon
Estomul-m
Gaviscon
Gelusil
Kolantyl
Kolantyl Wafers
Kudrox
Lowsium
Maalox
Magmalin
Magnagel
Magnatril
Maox
Marblen
Max-Ox 40

Maxamag
M.O.M.
Mucotin
Mygel
Mylanta
Neosorb Plus
Nephrox
Neutracomp
Neutralca-S
Par-mag
Pepsogel
Phillips Milk of Magnesia
Ratic
Riopan
Robalate
Rolaids
Rulox
Spastoced
Sterazolidin
Tralmag
Univol
Uro-Mag
Vanquish
Win Gel

ALUMINUM & MAGNESIUM ANTACIDS

Algenic Alka
Alka-Med
Alma-Mag
Aludrox
Alumid
ALUMINA & MAGNESIA
ALUMINA & MAGENSIUM
  CARBONATE
ALUMINA, MAGNESIUM
  CARBONATE & MAGNESIUM
  OXIDE
ALUMINA & MAGNESIUM
  TRISILICATE
Aluscop
Creamalin
Delcid
DIHYDROXYALUMINUM
  AMINOACETATE & MAGNESIA
DIHYDROXYALUMINUM
  AMINOACETATE, MAGNESIA &
  ALUMINA
Diovol Ex
Estomul-M
Gaviscon
Kolantyl
Kudrox
Lowsium
Maalox
Maalox TC
Magmalin
Magnagel
Magnatril
MAGNESIUM TRISILICATE,
  ALUMINA & MAGNESIA
Neosorb Plus
Neutracomp
Neutralca-S
Riopan
Rolox
Rulox
Tralmag
Univol
WinGel

ALUMINUM, MAGNESIUM, MAGALDRATE & SIME-THICONE ANTACIDS

Alma-Mag 4 Improved
Almacone
Alumid Plus
ALUMINA, MAGNESIA &
  SIMETHICONE
Amphojel Plus
Di-Gel
Diovol
Gelusil
Maalox Plus
MAGALDRATE & SIMETHICONE
Mygel
Mylanta
Mylanta-2
Mylanta-2 Extra Strength
Riopan Plus
Silain-Gel
Simaal Gel
Simeco
SIMETHICONE, ALUMINA,
  MAGNESIUM CARBONATE
  & MAGNESIA

|

ANDROGENS

Anabolin
Anabolin LA 100
Anadrol-50
Anapolon 50
Anavar
Andro
Andro-Cyp
Andro-LA
Android
Android-F
Android-T
Androlone
Andron
Andronaq
Andronaq-LA
Andronate
Androyd
Andryl
Bay-Testone
Danabol
Deca-Durabolin
Delatestryl
Dep Andro
Depo-Testosterone
Depotest
Dianabol
Durabolin
Duratest
Durathate
ETHYLESTRENOL
Everone
FLUOXYMESTERONE
Halotestin
Histerone
Malogen
Malogex
Maxibolin
Metandren
Metandren Linguets
METHANDROSTENOLONE
METHYLTESTOSTERONE
NANDROLONE
Ora-Testryl

Oratestin
Oreton Methyl
OXANDROLONE
OXYMETHOLONE
STANOZOLOL
T-Cypionate
Tesionate
Testa-C
Testaqua
Testex
Testoject
Testoject-LA
Testolin
Testone L.A.
TESTOSTERONE
Testostroval P.A.
Testred
Testrin P.A.
T-Iontae
Virilon
Winstrol

ANESTHETICS (TOPICAL

Aero Caine
Aero Caine Aerosol
Aerotherm
Americaine
Americaine Aerosol
Americaine Ointment
Anbesol
Anestacon
Bactine
Benzocaine
Benzocaine Topical
Benzocal
BiCozene
Burntame
BUTACAINE
BUTAMBEN
Butesin Picrate
Butyl aminobenzoate
Butyn Sulfate
Caine Spray
Cal-Vi-Nol
Cetacaine
Cetacine
Chiggerex
Chiggertox
Clinicaine
Cyclaine
Cyclaine Solution
CYCLOMETHYCAINE
Derma-Medicone
Dermacoat
Dermo-Gen
Dermoplast
Dibucaine
Diothane
DIPERODON
Dyclone
DYCLONINE
Ethyl Aminobenzoate
Foille
Hexathricin Aerospra
HEXYLCAINE
Hurricaine
Isotraine
Ivy-Dry Cream
Lanacane
Lida-Mantle
Lidocaine

Lidocaine Ointment
Lignocaine
Medicone
Medicone Dressing
Mercurochrome II
Morusan
Nupercainal
Nupercainal Cream
Nupercainal Ointment
Nupercainal Spray
Panthocal A & D
Perifoam
Pontocaine
Pontocaine Cream
Pontocaine Ointment
PRAMOXINE
Prax
Proctodon
Proctofoam
Proxine
Quotane
Rectal Medicone
Soft-N-Soothe
Solarcaine
Surfacaine
Tega-Caine
Tega-Dyne
TETRACAINE
Tronolane
Tronothane
Unguentine
Unguentine Plus
Unguentine Spray
Urolocaine
Velvacaine
Xylocaine
Xylocaine Ointment

APPETITE SUPPRESSANTS

Adipex-D
Adipex-P
Adipost
Adphen
Anorex
Bacarate
BENZPHETAMINE
B.O.F.
Bontril PDM
Bontril Slow Release
Chlor-Tripolon
Chlorophen
CHLORPHENTERMINE
CLORTERMINE
Dapex
Dapex-37.5
Delcozine
D.E.P.—75
Depletite
Dexatrim
Di-Ap-Trol
Didrex
Dietec
DIETHYLPROPION
Dyrexan-OD
Elephemet
Ex-Obese
Fastin
FENFLURAMINE
Hyrex

Hyrex-105
Inifast Unicelles
Ionamin
Limit
Limitite
MASINDOL
Mazanor
Melfiat
Menrium
Metra
Minus
Nobesine
Nobesine-75
Nu-Dispoz
Obalan
Obe-Nil TR
Obe-Nix
Obephen
Obermine
Obestin
Obestin-30
Obestrol
Obeval
Obezine
Oby-Trim
Parmine
Penderal Pacaps
Phendiet
PHENDIMETRAZINE
PHENMETRAZINE
Phentamine
PHENTERMINE
Phentrol
Phenzine
Plegine
Ponderal
Pondimin
Pre-Sate
Prelu-2
Preludin
Propion
P.S.P.R.X. 1,2 &3
Reducto
Regibon
Ro-Diet
Sanorex
Slim-Tabs
Slynn-LL
Span-RD
Sprx-1
Sprx-105
Sprx-3
Statobex
Statobex-G
Symetra
Tenuate
Tenuate Dospan
Tepanil
Tepanil Ten-Tab
Teramine
Tora
Trimcaps
Trimstat
Trimtabs
Unicelles
Unifast
Voranil
Wehless
Weightrol
Wilpowr
X-Trozine
X-Trozine LA

ASPIRIN

4-Way Cold Tablets
8-Hour Bayer Timed Release
Acetophen
Acetylsalicylic Acid
Alka Seltzer
Alka-Seltzer
Alka-Seltzer Effervescent Pain
    Reliever & Antacid
Aluminum ASA
Amytal and Aspirin
Anacin
Anaphen
Ancasal
Anexsia w/Codeine
A.P.C.
A.P.C w/Codeine
Apo-Asen
Arthritis Bayer Timed-Release
Arthritis Pain Formula
A.S.A.
A.S.A. & Codeine Compound
A.S.A. Compound
A.S.A. Enseals
Ascodeen-30
Ascriptin
Ascriptin A/D
Ascriptin w/Codeine
Asperbuf
Aspergum
Aspir-10
Aspirin Compound w/Codeine
Aspirjen Jr.
Astrin
Axotal
Bancap w/Codeine
Bayer
Bayer Timed-Release Arthritic Pain
    Formula
Bexophene
Buff-A
Buff-A-Comp
Buffaprin
Buffered ASA
Bufferin
Buffex
Buffinol
Buf-Tabs
Calciphen
Cama Arthritis Pain Reliever
Cama Inlay
Causalin
Cefinal
Cirin
Codalan
Codasa
Congespirin
Coralsone
Coricidin D
Coryphen
Cosprin
Darvon Compound
Dasicon
Decagesic
Dia-Gesic
Dihydrocodein Compound
Dolene Compound-65
Dolor
Dolprn #3
Dynosal
Easprin

943

Ecotrin
Elder 65 Compound
Emagrin
Empirin
Empirin Compound
Empirin Compound w/Codeine
Emprazil
Encaprin
Entrophen
Equagesic
Excedrin
Fiorinal
Fiorinal w/Codeine
Hiprin
Histadyl and ASA Compound
Hyco-Pap
ICN 65 Compound
Kengesin
Lanorinal
Lemidyne w/Codeine
Magnaprin
Maprin
Maprin I-B
Measurin
Mepro Compound
Metrogesic
Mobidin
Norgesic
Norwich Aspirin
Nova-Phase
Novasen
Pabirin Buffered
P-A-C Compound
P-A-C Compound w/Codeine
Pargesic Compound 65
Percodan
Persistin
Phenodyne w/Codeine
Poxy Compound-65
Presalin
Progesic Compound-65
Propoxychel Compound
Propoxyphene HCl Compound
Repro Compound 65
Rhinocaps
Riphen-10
Safety Coated APF Arthritis Pain
  Formula
St. Joseph
St. Joseph Aspirin for Children
Sal-Adult
Salatin
Salatin w/Codeine
Saleto
Salimeph Forte
Sal-Infant
Salocol
Salsprin
SK-65 Compound
Soma Compound
Soma Compound w/Codeine
Stero-Darvon
Supac
Supasa
Synalgos
Talwin Compound
Triaminic
Triaphen-10
Trigesic
Vanquish
Verin
Wesprin Buffered

Zorprin

ATROPINE

Almezyme
Amocine
Antrocol
Arco-Lase
Atrobarbital
Atromal
Atropine Bufopto
Atropisol
Atrosed
Barbella
Barbeloid
Barbidonna
Barbidonna-CR
Bar-Cy-Amine
Bar-Cy-A-Tab
Bar-Don
Bar-Tropin
Belbutal
Belkaloids
Belladenal
Bellergal-S
Bioxatphen
Briabell
Briaspaz
Brobella
Buren
Butibel
Cerebel
Chardonna
Comhist
Contac
Copin
Dallergy
Ditropan
Donnacin
Donnagel
Donnamine
Donnatal
Donnazyme
Drinus
Eldonal
G.B.S.
HASP
Haponal
Harvitrate
Hyatal
Hybephen
Hycodan
Hyonal
Hyonatol
Hytrona
Isopto Atropine
Kalmedic
Kinesed
Koryza
Levamine
Lyopine Vari-Dose
Magnased
Magnox
Maso-Donna
Neogel w/Sulfa
Nilspasm
Oxybutynin
P & A
Palbar No. 2
PAMA
Peece
Prydon
Renalgin

Ro Trim
Ru-Tuss
Sedamine
Sedapar
Sedatabs
Sedralex
Seds
SK-Diphenoxylate
SMP Atropine
Spabelin
Spasaid
Spasdel
Spasidon
Spasloids
Spasmate
Spasmolin
Spasquid
Spastolate
Spastosed
Stannitol
Thitrate
Trac
Unitral
Urised
Uriseptin
Urogesic
Zemarine

BELLADONNA

Amobel
Atrocap
Atrosed
Barbidonna
Bebetab
Belap
Belatol
Belbarb
Bellachar
Belladenal
Bellafedrol
Bellergal
Bellkatal
Bello-phen
Belphen
B & O Supprettes
B-Sed
Butabar
Butabar Elixir
Butibel
Butibel Elixir
Butibel-Zyme
Chardonna
Comhist
Coryztime
Decobel
Donabarb
Donnafed Jr.
Donnatal
Donnazyme
Fitacol
Gastrolic
Gelcomul
Hycoff Cold Caps
Hynaldyne
Kamabel
Kinesed
Lanothal
Mallenzyme
Medi-Spas
Nilspasm
Phebe
Phen-o-bel

Rectacort
Sedapar
Sedatromine
Spabelin
Spasnil
Trac 2X
Ultabs
Urilief
Urised
U-Tract
Wigraine
Woltac
Wyanoids

BELLADONNA ALKALOIDS & BARBITURATES

Amobell
Anaspaz PB
Antrocol
ATROPINE, HYOSCYAMINE, SCOPOLAMINE & BUTABARBITAL
ATROPINE, HYOSCYAMINE, SCOPOLAMINE & PHENOBARBITAL
ATROPINE & PHENOBARBITAL
Barbidonna
Barophen
Bay-Ase
Belap
BELLADONNA & AMOBARBITAL
BELLADONNA & BUTABARBITAL
Bellalphen
Bellastal
Bellkatal
Chardonna-2
Donna-Sed
Donnapine
Donnatal
Donnatal Extentabs
Donphen
Hybephen
HYOSCYAMINE & PHENOBARBITAL
Hyosophen
Kinesed
Levsin-PB
Levsin with Phenobarbital
Levsinex with Phenobarbital Timecaps
Malatal
Palbar
Palbar No. 2
Pheno-Bella
Relaxadon
Seds
Spaslin
Spasmolin
Spasmophen
Spasquid
Susano
Vanatal
Vanodonnal

BENZOYL PEROXIDE

Acetoxyl
Acne-Aid
Allercreme Clear-Up
Alquam-X
Ben-Aqua

Benoxyl
Benzac
Benzac W
Benzagel
Buf-Oxal
Clear By Design
Clearasil
Clearasil BP(M)
Cuticura Acne
Dermodex
Dermoxyl
Desquam-X
Dry and Clean
Dry and Clear
Eloxyl
Epi-Clear
Fostex
Fostex BPO
H_2Oxyl
Intraderm-19
Loroxide
Neutrogena Acne Mask
Oxyderm
Oxy-5
Oxy-10
PanOxyl
PanOxyl AQ
Persadox
Persadox HP
Persa-Gel
Persa-Gel W
PHisoAc BP
Porox 7
Propa P.H.
Propa P.H. Porox
Teen
Topex
Vanoxide
Vanoxide-HC
Xerac BP
Zeroxin

BETAMETHASONE

17-Valerate Celestone
17-Valerate Diprosone
Alphatrex
Beben
Benzoate
Beta-Val
Betacort
Betnelan
Betnesol
Betratrex
B-S-P
Celestoderm
Celestoject
Celestone
Cel-U-Sec
Dipropinate Metaderm
Diprosone
Disodium Phosphate Betnovate
Lotrisone
Uticort
Valerate Betaderm
Valerate Novobetamet
Valisone
Vancerace

BROMPHENIRAMINE

Brocon
Bromamine

Brombay
Bromepath
Bromfed
Bromphen
Dehist
Dimetane
Dimetane Extentabs
Dimetane-Ten
Dimetapp
Disophrol Chronotabs
Drixoral
Dura Tap-PD
Eldatapp
E.N.T. Syrup
Histaject modified
Histatapp
Nasahist B
ND-Stat Revised
Oraminic II
Poly-Histine
Ralabromophen
Rynatapp
S-T Decongestant
Symptom 3
Taltapp
Tamine S.R.
Tapp
Tolabromophen
Veltane
Veltap

BUTABARBITAL

Broncholate
Brondilate
Butabell HMB
Butalan
Butaserpazide
Butatran
Butibel
Buticaps
Butisol
Butizide
Cyclo-Bell
Cytospaz-SR
Day-Barb
Levamine
Neo-Barb
Numa-Dura-Tablets
Pyridium Plus
Quibron Plus
Sarisol No. 2
Scolate
Sidonna
Sinate-M
Tedral

CAFFEINE

Amaphen
Amaphen w/Codeine #3
Anacin
Anaphen
Anexsia w/Codeine
Anoquan
A.P.C.
A.S.A. Compound
Asphac-G
Aspirin Compound w/Codeine
Ban-Drow 2
Bexophene
Buff-A-Comp
Buffadyne

Butigetic
Cafacetin
Cafecon
Cafergot
Cafermine
Cafetrate
Cefinal
Cenagesic
Citrated Caffeine
Coastalgesic
Codalan #3
Colrex
Compal
Coryban D
Coryzaid
Darvon Compound
Dasicon
Dexatrim
Dexitac
Dia-Gesic
Dihydrocodeine Compound
Dolor
Duadacin
Dularin
Dynosal
Elder 65 Compound
Emagrin
Empirin Compound
Emprazil
Esgic
Excedrin Extra Strength
Fendol
Fiorinal
G-1 Capsules
Hista-Derfule
Histadyl Compound
ICN 65 Compound
Kengesin
Kirkaffeine
Korigesic
Lanorinal
Lemidyne w/Codeine
Midol
Migralam
Nodaca
Nodoz
Pacaps
P-A-C Compound w/Codeine
Pargesic Compound 65
Percodan
Phenodyne
Phenodyne w/Codeine
Phensal
Phrenilin
Poxy Compound-65
Prodolor
Progesic Compound-65
Propoxychel Compound-65
Propoxyphene Compound
Pyrroxate
Quick Pep
Repro Compound 65
S-A-C
Salatin
Salatin w/Codeine
Saleto
Salocol
Sinarest
SK-65 Compound
Supac
Synalgos
Synalgos-DC

Tirend
Triaminic
Triaminicin
Trigesic
Two-Dyne
Vanquish
Vivarin
Wigraine

CALCIUM CARBONATE

Alka-mints
Alka-2
Alkets
Amitone
Bio Cal
Calcet
Calcilac
Calcitrate 600
Calglycine
Cal-Sup
Caltrate
Camalox
Chooz
Dicarbosil
Ducon
El-Da-Mint
Equilet
Fosfree
Gustalac
Iromin-G
Mallamint
Mission
Natacomp-FA
Natalins
Nu-Iron-V
Os-Cal
Os-Cal 500
Pama No. 1
Pramet FA
Pramilet FA
Prenate 90
Ratio
Suplical
Theracal
Titracid
Titralac
Trialka
Tums
Tums E-X
Zenate

CALCIUM SUPPLEMENTS

BioCal
CALCIUM CARBONATE (also used
    as an antacid)
CALCIUM CITRATE
CALCIUM GLUBIONATE
CALCIUM GLUCONATE
CALCIUM GLYCEROPHOSPHATE
    & CALCIUM LACTATE
CALCIUM LACTATE
Calphosan
Cal-Sup
Caltrate
Citracal
DIBASIC CALCIUM PHOSPHATE
Neo-Calglucon
Os-Cal 500
Posture
Suplical
Theracal

TRIBASIC CALCIUM PHOSPHATE
Tums
Tums E-X

CHLORDIAZEPOXIDE & CLIDINIUM

Apo-Chlorax
Clindex
Clinoxide
Clipoxide
Corium
Librax
Lidox

CHLORPHENIRAMINE

4-Way Cold Tablets
Acutuss
Acutuss Expectorant w/Codeine
Alermine
Alka-Seltzer Plus
Aller-chlor
Allerbid Tymcaps
Allerest
Allerform
Allergesic
Allerid - O.D.
AL-R
Alumadrine
Anafed
Anamine
Anatuss
Antagonate
Brexin
Bronkotuss
Cerose Compound
Children's Allerest
Chlo-Amine
Chlorafed
Chloramate Unicelles
Chlor-Histine
Chlor-MAL
Chlormine
Chlor-Niramine
Chlor-100
Chlorphen
Chlor-PRO
Chlor-Span
Chlortab
Chlor-Trimeton
Chlor-Trimeton w/Codeine
Chlor-Trimeton Repetabs
Chlor-Tripolon
Ciramine
Ciriforte
Citra Forte
Codimal
Coldene
Colrex
Comhist
Comtrex
Conex w/Codeine
Conex-DA
Cophene-X
Co-Pyronil 2
Coricidin
Coricidin "D"
Corilin
Coryban-D
Coryzaid

Cosea
Co-Tylenol
Covanamine
Covangesic
Dallergy
Deconamine
Dehist
Demazin
Dextromal
Dextro-Tussin
DM Plus
Donatussin
Dorcol
Drinus
Dristan
Drize M
Duadacin
Duphrene
Dura-Vent/A
E.N.T.
Expectrosed
Extendryl
Fedahist
Fernhist
Ginsopan
Guaiahist TT
Guaiamine
Guistrey Fortis
Hal-Chlor
Histalet
Histalon
Histamic
Histaspan
Hista-Vadrin
Histex
Histor-D Timecelles
Historal
Histrey
Hycoff
Hycomine Compound
Iophen-C
Isoclor
Korigesic
Koryza
Kronofed-A
Kronohist Kronocaps
Lanatuss
Marhist
Naldecon
Naldetuss
Napril Plateau
Narine Gyrocaps
Narspan
Nasahist
Neo-Codenyl-M
Neotep Granucaps
Nilcol
Nolamine
Novafed A
Novahistine
Novopheniram
Omni-Tuss
Ornade Spansule
P.R. Syrup
P-V-Tussin
Palohist
Partuss T.D.
Pediacof
Phenacol-DM
Phenate
Phenetron
Phenetron Lanacaps

Polaramine
Probahist
Protid Improved Formula
Pseudo-Hist
Pyma
Pyrroxate
Pyrroxate w/Codeine
Quadrahist
Quelidrine
Queltuss
Resaid T.D.
Rhinex
Rhinolar
Rhinolar-EX
Ru-Tuss
Rynatan
Rynatuss
Salphenyl
Scot-Tussin
Sinarest
Singlet
Sinovan
Sinulin
T.D. Alermine
Tedral Anti-H
Teldrin
Teldrin Spansules
T.P.I.
Triaminicin
Trymegen
Tusquelin
Tuss-Ornade
Tussar
Tussi-Organidin
U.R.I.
Wesmatic Forte

CONTRACEPTIVES (ORAL)

Anoryol
Brevicon
Demulen
Enovid
Loestrin
Lo-Ovral
Micronor
Min-Ovral
Modacon
Modicon
Nordette
Norlestrin
Norinyl
Nor-Q.D.
Ortho-Novum
Ovcon
Ovral
Ovrette
Ovulen
Tri-Norinyl
Triphasil

DEXAMETHASONE

Aeroseb-Dex
Ak-Dex
Congespirin
Cremacoat 1
Dalalone
Dalalon L.A.
Decaderm
Decadrol
Decadron
Decadron L.A.

Decadron Respihaler
Decadron Turbinaire
Decadron with Xylocaine
Decajet
Decameth
Decaspray
Delsym
Demo-Cineol
Deronil
Dexacen
Dexasone
Dexon
Dexone
DM Cough
Extend-12
Hexadrol
Hexandrol
Hold
Maxidex
Mediquell
Oradexon
Pedia Care 1
Pertussin 8 Hour Cough Formula
SK-Dexamethasone
Solurex
Sucrets

DEXTROMETHORPHAN

2/C-DM
216 DM
Anti-Tuss DM
Balminil DM
Benylin DM
Broncho-Grippol-DM
Cheracol
Congespirin
Contratuss
Cosanyl DM
Cremacoat 1
Delsym
Delsym Polistirex
Demo-Cineol
Dextro-Tussin GG
DM Cough
DM Syrup
Dormethan
Dristan
Dristan Cough Formula
Duad Koff Balls
Endotussin-NN
Extend-12
Formula 44-D
Glycotuss-dM
Guiatuss D-M
Hold
Hold Cough Suppressant
Koffex
Lixaminol AT
Mediquell
Neo-DM
Novahistine DMX
Nyquil
Ornacol
Pedia Care 1
Pertussin 8 Hour Cough Formula
Queltuss
Robidex
Robitussin
Robitussin-DM
Romilar
Romilar CF

Romilar Children's Cough
Sedatuss
Silence is Golden
Silexin
Sorbase
Sorbutuss
St. Joseph
St. Joseph Cough Syrup
St. Joseph for Children
Sucrets
Trind DM
Trocal
Tussagesic
Tussaminic
Unproco
Vicks
Vicks Cough Syrup

DICYCLOMINE

Antispas
A-Spas
Baycyclomine
Bentyl
Bentylol
Byclomine
Cyclobec
Cyclocen
Dibent
Dicen
Dilomine
Di-Spaz
Dyspas
Formulex
Lomine
Menospasm
Neoquess
Nospaz
Or-Tyl
Protylol
Spasmoban
Spasmoject
Triactin
Viscerol

DIMENHYDRINATE

Apo-Dimenhydrinate
Calm X
Dimentabs
Dinate
Dommanate
Dramaban
Dramamine
Dramilin
Dramocen
Dramoject
Dymenate
Eldodram
Gravol
Hydrate
Marine
Marmine
Motion-Aid
Nauseatol
Novodimenate
PMS-Dimenhydrinate
Reidamine
Travamine
Trav-Arex
Vertiban
Wehamine

DIPHENHYDRAMINE

Allerdryl
Ambenyl Expectorant
Bena-D
Benadryl
Benadryl Children's Allergy
Benadryl Complete Allergy
Benahist
Bendylate
Benoject-10
Benylin Cough Syrup
Caladryl
Compoz
Diahist
Dihydrex
Diphen
Diphenacen
Diphenadril
Eldadryl
Fenylhist
Fynex
Hydramine
Hydril
Hyrexin-50
Insomnal
Nervine Nighttime Sleep-Aid
Noradryl
Nordryl
Nytol
Nytol with DPH
Phen-Amin
Robalyn
SK-Diphenhydramine
Sleep-Eze
Sleep-Eze 3
Sominex
Sominex Formula 2
SominiFere
Tusstat
Twilite
Valdrene
Wehydryl

DOCUSATE SODIUM

Afko-Lube
Bilax
Bu-Lax
Colace
Colax
Coloctyl
Dialose
Dilax
Diocto
Dioctyl Sodium Sulfosuccinate
Dioeze
DioMedicone
Diosuccin
Dio-Sul
Disonate
Di-Sosul
Doctate
Doss
Doxidan
Doxinate
D-S-S
Duosol
Ferro-sequels
Geriplex-FS
Laxagel
Laxinate
Liqui-Doss

Modane Plus
Modane Soft
Molatoc
Neolax
Peri-Colase
Peritinic
Prenate 90
Pro-Sof 100
Regulex
Regutol
Senokot-S
Stulex
Trilax

EPHEDRINE

Acet-Am
Aladrine
Amesec
Amodrine
Asminyl
Benadryl w/Ephedrine
Broncholate
Brondilate
Bronkaid
Bronkolixir
Bronkotabs
Bronkotuss
Calcidrine
Coryza Brengle
Co-Xan Elixir
Dainite
Derma Medicone-HC
Duovent
Ectasule III
Ectasule Minus
Ephed-Organidin
Ephedrine and Amytal
Ephedrine and Nembutal-25
Ephedrine and Seconal
Ephedrol
Ephedrol w/Codeine
Epragen
Iso-Asminyl
Isuprel
Luasmin
Lufyllin-EPG
Marax
Mudrane
Numa-Dura-Tablets
Nyquil
Phyldrox
Primatene
Pyribenazmine w/Ephedrine
Quadrinal
Quelidrine
Quibron Plus
Slo-Fedrin A-60
Tedfern
Tedral
T.E.H.
T-E-P
Thalfed
Theofedral
Theotabs
Theozine
Wesmatic
Wyanoids

EPINEPHRINE

Adrenalin
Asmolin
Asthma Haler

Asthma Nefrin
Ayerst Epitrate
Bronitin
Bronkaid
Bronkaid Mist
Dysne-Inhal
Epifrin
EpiPen-Epinephrine Auto-Injector
Epi-Pen Jr.
Epitrate
Eppy
Glaucon
Marcaine Hydrochloride
   w/Epinephrine
Medihaler-Epi
microNEFRIN
Murocoll
Mytrate
Primatene
Primatene Mist
Simplene
Sus-phrine
Vaponefrin

ERYTHROMYCINS

Apo-Erythro-S
A/T/S
Bristamycin
Dowmycin
E-Biotic
E.E.S.
E-Mycin
E-Mycin E
Eryc
Ery-derm
EryPed
Erymax
Erypar
Ery-Tab
Erythrocin
Erythrocin Ethyl Succinate
Erythromid
ERYTHROMYCIN
ERYTHROMYCIN ESTOLATE
ERYTHROMYCIN
   ETHYLSUCCINATE
ERYTHROMYCIN GLUCEPTATE
ERYTHROMYCIN LACTOBIONATE
ERYTHROMYCIN STEARATE
Ethril
Ilosone
Ilosone Estolate
Ilotycin
Ilotycin Gluceptate
Kesso-mycin
Novorythro
Pediazole
Pediamycin
Pendiamycin
Pfizer-E
Robimycin
RP-Mycin
SK-Erythromycin
Staticin
T-Star
Wyamycin
Wyamycin E
Wyamycin S

ESTROGEN

Amnestrogen
Clinestrone

Delestrogen
DES
DIENESTROL (vaginal)
DV (vaginal)
Estinyl
Estomed
Estrace
Estrace (vaginal)
ESTRADIOL (vaginal)
Estraguard (vaginal)
Estratab
Estrocon
ESTROGENS, CONJUGATED
   (vaginal)
ESTRONE (vaginal)
ESTROPIPATE (vaginal)
Estrovis
Evex
Feminone
Femogen
Formatrix
Hormonin
Menest
Menotrol
Menrium
Milprem
Oagen
Oestrilin
Oestrilin (vaginal)
Ogen
Ogen (vaginal)
Ortho Dienestrol (vaginal)
Piperazine Estrone Sulfate (vaginal)
PMB-200
PMB-400
Premarin
Premarin (vaginal)
Progens
Stilphostrol
Theogen

FERROUS FUMARATE

Cevi-Fer
Chromagen
Feco-T
Femiron
Feostat
Ferancee
Ferrofume
Ferro-sequels
Fersamal
Fetrin
Fumasorb
Fumerin
Hemocyte
Hemo-Vite
Ircon
Ircon-FA
Laud-Iron
Maniron
Natalins
Neo-Fer
Neo-Fer-50
Novofumar
Palafer
Palmiron
Poly-Vi-Flor
Pramilet FA
Prenate 90
Stuartinic
Toleron
Tolfrinic

Tolifer
Trinsicon
Vitron C
Zenate

FERROUS SULFATE

Apo-Ferrous Sulfate
Feosol
Fer-In-Sol
Fer-Iron
Fero-folic-500
Fero-Grad
Fero-Grad-500
Fero-Gradumet
Ferospace
Ferralyn
Fesofor
Geritol Tablets
Hematinic
Iberet
Iberet-500
Iberet-Folic-500
Iromal
Mol-Iron
Novoferrosulfa
PMS Ferrous Sulfate
Slow-Fe

GUAIFENESIN

2/G
2/G-DM
Actol
Ambenyl
Anti-Tuss
Asbron
Asma
Balminil
Baytussin
Breonesin
Brexin
Bromphen
Broncholate
Brondecon
Bronkolizir
Bronkotabs
Bronkotuss
Caldrex Expectorant
Cetro Cirose
Cheracol
Cheracol Cough
Chlor-Trimeton
Codimal
Coditrate
Colrex Expectorant
Conar
Conex
Conex w/Codeine
Congess Jr. & Sr.
Corutol
Coryban-D
Co-Xan
Cremacoat
Cremacoat 2
Deproist w/Codeine
Detussin
Dilaudid
Dilor-G
Dimetane
Donatussin
Dorcol
Dristan
Dristan Cough

Duovent
Dura-Vent
Elixophyllin-GG
Emfaseen
Entex
Entuss-D
Expectorant
Fedahist
Formula
Formula 44-D
Gee-Gee
GG-CEN
Glyceryl Guaiacolate
Glycotuss
Glytuss
Guaiahist
Guaifed
Guiamid
Guiatuss
Gylate
Halotussin
Histalet X
Hycotuss
Hytuss
Hytuss-2X
Luftodil
Lufyllin
Malotuss
Mudrane GG
Naldecon
Neo-Spec
Neospect
Neothyllin-G
Nortussin
Novahistine
Nucofed
Pee Dee Dose Expectorant
Poly-Histine
P-V-Tussin
Queltuss
Quibron
Respaire-SR
Resyl
Robafen
Robitussin
Scot-Tussin Sugar-Free
Silexin
Sinufed Timecelles
Slo-Phyllin GG
Sorbase
Sorbutuss
S-T Expectorant
S-T Forte
Synophylate-GG
Syrup
Tedral
Theo-Guaia
Theolair-Plus
Triafed-C
Triaminic
Triaminic w/Codeine
Trind
Tussar
Tussend
Uproco
Vicks
Vicks Cough
Zephrex

HYDROCHLOROTHIAZIDE

Aldactazide
Aldoril

Apo-Hydro
Butaserpazide
Butizide
Diuchlor H
Diupres
Dyazide
Esidrix
Esimil
H-H-R
Hydrid
Hydro-Aquil
HydroDIURIL
Hydropres
Hydroserp
Hydroserpine
Hydrotensin
Hydrozide-Z-50
Hyperetic
Inderide
Mallopress
Maxzide
Moduretic
Naquival
Natrimax
Nefrol
Neo-Codema
Novohydrazide
Oretic
Oreticyl
Reserpazide
Ser-Ap-Es
Serpasil-Esidrix
Singoserp-Esidrix
SK-Hydrochlorothiazide
Spironazide
Thiuretic
Timolide
Timolol and Hydrochlorothiazide
Tri-Hydroserpine
Unipres
Urozide
Zide

HYDROCORTISONE (CORTISOL)

Aeroseb-HC
A-hydroCort
Barseb
Biosone
Cortaid
Cortamed
Cortate
Cort-Dome
Cortef
Cortef Fluid
Cortenema
Corticreme
Cortifoam
Cortiment
Cortisol
Cortoderm
Cortril
Dermacort
Emo-Cort
Fernisone
Hyderm
Hydro-Cortilean
Hydrocortone
Hytone
Microcort
Novohydrocort

Orabase HCA
Proctocort
Rectoid
Restocort
Solu-Cortef
Texacort
Unicort
Westcort

HYDROXYZINE

Anxanil
Atarax
Ataraxoid
Atozine
Cartrax
Durrax
Enarax
E-Vista
Hydroxacen
Hy-Pam
Hyzine
Marax
Multipax
Neucalm 50
Orgatrax
Quiess
T.E.H. Tablets
Theozine
Vamate
Vistacon
Vistaject
Vistaquel
Vistaril
Vistazine
Vistrax

HYOSCYAMINE

Almezyme
Anaspa 3
Anaspaz
Anaspaz PB
Arco-Lase Plus
Barbella
Barbeloid
Barbidonna-CR
Bar-Cy-Amine
Bar-Cy-A-Tab
Bar-Don
Belbutal
Belkaloids
Bellafoline
Bellaspaz
Brobella-PB
Buren
Cytospa
De Tal
Donnacin
Donnagel
Donnamine
Donnatal
Donnazyme
Eldonal
Elixiril
Ergobel
Floramine
Gylanphen
Haponal
Hyatal
Hybephen
Hyonal
Hyonatol

Hytrona
Kinesed
Koryza
Kutrase
Levamine
Levsin
Levsinex
Levsinex Timecaps
Maso-Donna
Neoquess
Nevrotase
Nilspasm
Omnibel
Peece
Pyridium Plus
Renalgin
Restophen
Ru-Tuss
Sedajen
Sedamine
Sedapar
Sedatromine
Sedralex
Seds
Spabelin
Spasaid
Spasdel
Spasloids
Spasmolin
Spasquid
Spastolate
Trac 2X
Ultabs
Urised
Uriseptin
Urogesic
Zemarine

INSULIN

Actrapid
Globin Insulin
Humulin
Humulin BR
Humulin L
Humulin N
Humulin R
Insulatard
Insultard NPH
Lentard
Lente
Lente Iletin I
Lente Iletin II
Lente Insulin
Mixtard
Monotard
NPH
NPH Iletin I
NPH Iletin II
Novolin
Novolin L
Novolin N
Novolin R
Novolin 70/30
PZI
Protamine Zinc & Iletin
Protamine Zinc & Iletin I
Protamine Zinc & Iletin II
Protophane NPH
Regular
Regular (Concentrated) Iletin
Regular (Concentrated) Iletin II,
   U-500

Regular Iletin I
Regular Iletin II
Regular Insulin
Semilente
Semilente Iletin
Semilente Iletin I
Semitard
Ultralente
Ultratard
Utralente Iletin I
Velosulin
Velosulin Human

MAGNESIUM HYDROXIDE

Aludrox
Arthritis Pain Formula
Camalox
Creamalin
Delcid
Di-Gel
Dolprn   3
Ducon
Gelusil
Kolantyl
Maalox
Magnatril
Maxamag
Milk of Magnesia
M.O.M.
Mucotin
Mygel
Mylanta
Phillips' Milk of Magnesia
Silain-Gel
Simeco
Univol
Vanquish
Win-Gel

MEPROBAMATE

Apo-Meprobamate
Arcoban
Bamate
Bamo 400
Coprobate
Deprol
Equagesic
Equanil
Equanil Wyseals
Evenol
Kalmn
Lan-Dol
Medi-Tran
Mep-E
Mepriam
Mepro Compound
Meprocon
Meprospan
Meprotabs
Meribam
Miltown
Neo-Tran
Neuramate
Neurate
Novo-Mepro
Novomepro
Pathibamate
Pax 400
PMB
Protran
Quietal

Robam
Robamate
Sedabamate
SK-Bamate
Tranmep

METHYLPREDNISOLONE

A-methaPred
dep Medalone
Depoject
Depo-Medrol
Depo-medrone
Depopred
Depo-Pred-40
Depo-Pred-80
Duralone
Duralone-40
Duralone-80
Durameth
Medralone
Medralone-40
Medralone-80
Medrol
Medrol Enpak
Medrone
Medrone-80
Mepred-40
Methylone
m-Prednisol
Pre-Dep
Pro-Dep-40
Pro-Dep-80
Rep-Pred
Solu-Medrol
Solu-medrone

NARCOTIC &
ACETAMINOPHEN

ACETAMINOPHEN & CODEINE
Aceta with Codeine
Amacodone
Atasol with Codeine
Bancap-HC
Bayapap with Codeine
Capital with Codeine
Codap
Co-gesic
Cotabs
Darvocet-N
Demerol-APAP
Dolacet
Dolene-AP
Dolo-Pap
Duradyne DHC
Empracet with Codeine
Exdol with Codeine
Hycodaphen
HYDROCODONE &
   ACETAMINOPHEN
Hydrogesic
Lortab 5
Lortab 7
MEPERIDINE & ACETAMINOPHEN
Norcet
Oxycocet
OXYCODONE & ACETAMINOPHEN
PENTAZOCINE &
   ACETAMINOPHEN
Percocet
Percocet-Demi
Phenaphen with Codeine

PROPOXYPHENE &
  ACETAMINOPHEN
Proval
SK-APAP with Codeine
SK-Oxycodone and Acetaminophen
SK-65 APAP
Talacen
T-Gesic Forte
Tylenol with Codeine
Tylox
Ty-Tabs
Vicodin
Wygesic

NARCOTIC ANALGESICS

642
Aceta w/Codeine
Acetaco
Acetaminophen w/Codeine
Actifed-C
Actifed-C Expectorant
Adatuss
Algodex
Ambenyl
Anaphen
A.P.C. w/Codeine Phosphate
  Tablets
A.P.C. w/Codeine Phosphate
Arthralgen
Ascriptin w/Codeine
Aspirin Compound w/Codeine
Axotal
Bancap w/Codeine
Banesin Forte
BUTORPHANOL
Calcidrine
Calcidrine Syrup
Capital w/Codeine
Cetro Cirose
Cheracol
Coastaldyne
Coastalgesic
Codalan
Codalex
Codap
CODEINE
Codeine Sulfate
Codimal PH
Coditrate
Codone
Colrex Compound
Copavin
Corutol DH
Cotussis
Co-Xan
Dapase
Darvocet-N 100
Darvon
Demer-Idine
Demerol
Depronal-SA
Dialog
Dicodid
Dihydromorphinone
Dilaudid
Dilaudid-HP
Dimetane-DC
Dimetane Expectorant-DC
Dolene
Dolophine
Dolor

Doxaphene
Dromoran
Dularin
Duramorph PF
Dynosal
Empirin w/Codeine
Empracet w/Codeine
Emprazil-C
Ephedrol w/Codeine
Epimorph
Esgic
FL-Tussex
Fiorinal w/Codeine
Fortral
Gaysal
G-2
G-3
Hasacode
Hycodan
Hycotuss
HYDROCODONE
HYDROMORPHONE
Isoclor
Levo-Dromoran
Levorphan
LEVORPHANOL
Liquix-C
Lo-Tussin
Maxigesic
Mepergan Fortis
MEPERIDINE
METHADONE
Methadose
Metrogesic
Minotal
MORPHINE
Morphitec
M.O.S. Syrup
MS Contin
MSIR
MST Continus
NALBUPHINE
Novahistine DH
Novahistine Expectorant
Novopropoxyn
Nubain
Numorphan
OPIUM
Ossonate-Plus
OXYCODONE
OXYMORPHONE
Pantapon
PAREGORIC
Pargesic
Pavadon
Paveral
Pediacof
PENTAZOCINE
Percodan
Pethadol
Pethidine
Phenaphen w/Codeine
Phenergan
Phrenilin
Physeptone
Poly-Histine w/Codeine
Presalin
Prodolor
Profene
Promethazine HCl w/Codeine
PROPOXYPHENE
Pro-65

Proxagesic
Proxene
Prunicodeine
RMS Uniserts
Robidone
Robitussin A-C
Roxanol
Roxanol SR
S-A-C
Salatin
Saleto
Salimeph Forte
Sedapap
SK-65
SK-APAP w/Codeine
Soma Compound w/Codeine
Sorbase II
Stadol
Statex
Strascogesic
Supac
Supeudol
Sylapar
Synalgos-DC
Talwin
Talwin-NX
Terpin Hydrate w/Codeine
Triaminic w/Codeine
Trigesic
Tussar
Tussend
Tussi-Organidin
Tylenol w/Codeine
Tylox
Vicodin
Wygesic

NARCOTIC & ASPIRIN

222
282
292
A&C with Codeine
A.C.&C.
Ancasal
Anexsia with Codeine
Anexsia-D
A.S.A. and Codeine Compound
Ascriptin with Codeine
ASPIRIN & CODEINE
ASPIRIN, CODEINE & CAFFEINE
Bexophene
BUFFERED ASPIRIN & CODEINE
Codoxy
Coryphen with Codeine
C2 with Codeine
Damason-P
Darvon Compound
Darvon with A.S.A.
Darvon-N with A.S.A.
Dolene Compound
Doxaphene Compound
DROCODE, ASPIRIN & CAFFEINE
Emcodeine
Empirin with Codeine
HYDROCODONE, ASPIRIN &
  CAFFEINE
Instantine Plus
Novo AC&C
Oxycodan
OXYCODONE & ASPIRIN
PENTAZOCINE & ASPIRIN
Percodan

Percodan-Demi
PROPOXYPHENE & ASPIRIN
PROPOXYPHENE ASPIRIN &
CAFFEINE
SK-65 Compound
SK-Oxycodone with Aspirin
Synalgos-DC
Talwin Compound

NIACIN (NICOTINIC ACID)

Diacin
N-Caps
Niac
Niacin
Nicalex
Nico-400
Nico-Span
Nicobid
Nicocap
Nicolar
Nicotinex
Nicotinyl alcohol
Nicotym
Novoniacin
SK-Niacin
Span-Niacin
Tega-Span
Vasotherm
Numerous other multiple
vitamin-mineral supplements.

NITRATES

Ang-O-Span
Cardilate
Coronex
Dilatrate-SR
Duotrate
ERYTHRITYL TETRANITRATE
Glyceryl Trinitrate
Iso-Bid
Isochron
Isogard
Isonate
Isonate TR
Isordil
ISOSORBIDE DINITRATE
Isotrate
Kaytrate
Klavikordal
Naptrate
N-G-C
Niong
Nitro-Bid
Nitrobon
Nitrocap
Nitrocap T.D.
Nitrocardin
Nitrodisc
Nitro-Dur
Nitrogard-SR
NITROGLYCERIN (GLYCERYL
TRINITRATE)
Nitroglyn
Nitrol
Nitrolin
Nitro-Long
Nitronet
Nitrong
Nitrospan
Nitrostablin
Nitrostat

Nitro-Time
Novosorbide
Onset
PENTAERYTHRITOL
TETRANITRATE
Pentestan
Pentol
Pentol S.A.
Pentraspan
Pentraspan SR
Pentritol
Pentylan
Peritrate
Peritrate SA
P.E.T.N.
Sorate
Sorbide
Sorbide T.D.
Sorbitrate
Sorbitrate SA
Susadrin
Tranderm-Nitro
Trates
Tridil
Vaso-80
Vasoglyn

OXYMETAZOLINE

4-Way Long-Acting Nasal
Afrin
Bayfrin
Dristan Long Lasting
Duramist Plus
Duration
Nafrine
Neo-Synephrine 12 Hour
Nostrilla
NTZ Long Lasting Nasal
Ocuclear
Otrivin
Oxymeta-12 Nasal Spray
Sinex Long-Lasting
St. Joseph Decongestant for
Children

PAPAVERINE

Cerebid
Cerespan
Copavin
Dipav
Durapav
Dylate
Hyobid
Kavrin
Lapav
Myobid
Octapav
Orapav
P-200
P-A-V
Pavabid
Pavabid HP
Pavacap
Pavadon
Pavadur
Pavagen
Pavakey
Pavased
Pavasule
Pavatest
Pavatran

Pavatym
Paverolan
Payadur
Ro-Papan
Sustaverine
Therapav
Vasal
Vasospan

PHENOBARBITAL

Aminophylline-Phenobarbital
Anaspaz-PB
Antrocol
Asminyl
Banthine w/Phenobarbital
Barbidonna
Barbita
Bardase Filmseal
Bar-Tropin
Belap
Belbarb
Belladenal
Bellergal
Bellkatal
Bentyl Phenobarbital
Bronkolixir
Bronkotabs
Cantil w/Phenobarbital
Chardonna
Cyclo-Bell
Dactil Phenobarbital
Dainite-KI
Daricon PB
Donna-Lix
Donnatal
Duovent
Eskabarb
Gardenal
Gastrolic
HASP
Hybephen
Hytrona
Iso-Asminyl
Isuprel Compound
Kinesed
Levsin PB
Levsin w/Phenobarbital
Luasmin
Luftodil
Lufyllin-EPG
Luminal
Matropinal
Mesopin PB
Mudrane
Neospect
Nova-Pheno
Oxoids
Pamine PB
Pathilon w/Phenobarbital
PBR/12
Phyldrox
Primatene, P Formula
Pro-Banthine w/Phenobarbital
Probital
Pyrdonnal Spansules
Quadrinal
Robinul-PH
Sedadrops
SK-Phenobarbital
Solfoton
Spasdel
Spasticol

Tedral
T-E-P
Thalfed
Theofedral
Theotabs
Tral w/Phenobarbital
Valpin-PB

PHENYLEPHRINE

4-Way Nasal Spray
4-Way Tablets
Albatussin
Alconefrin
Alka-Seltzer Plus
Anamine T.D.
Bromepaph
Bromphen Compound
Callergy
Cenagesic
Children's Allerest
Chlor-Histine
Chlor-Trimeton
Citra
Clistin D
Codalex
Codimal
Colrex
Comhist
Conar
Congespirin
Contac
Coricidin
Coricidin Mist
Coryban-D
Coryban-D Cough Syrup
Coryzaid
Cosea-D
Co-Tylenol
Covanamine
Covangesic
Dallergy
Dehist
Demazin
Dimetapp
doKtors Nose Drops
Donatussin DC
Dri-Hist No. Meta-Caps
Drinus Graduals
Dristan Advanced Formula
Dristan Nasal Spray
Drize M
Duadacin
Duo-Medihaler
Duphrene
Dura Tap-PD
Duration Mild
Dura-Vent/DA
Emagrin Forte
E.N.T.
Entex
Extendryl
Fendol
Fernhist
Ginospan
Guaiahist
Hista-Vadrin
Histabid Duracaps
Histalet
Histaspan
Histatapp
Histor-D Timecelles
Historal No. 2

Hycomine Compound
Isophrin
Korigesic
Koryza
Marhist
Mydrin
Naldecon
Napril Plateau
Narine Cyrocaps
Narspan
Nasahist
Neo-Mist
Neo-Synephrine
NeoSynephrin Compound
Neotep Granucaps
Nostril
Novahistine
Palohist
Pediacof
Phenate
Phenergan VC
Phenergan VC w/Codeine
Prefrin
Protid Improved Formula
P-V-Tussin
Pyma Timed
Pyracort-D
Quelidrine
Rhinall
Rhinex
Rolabromophen
Rolahist
Ru-Tuss
Rynatan
Rynatapp
Salphenyl
Sinarest Nasal
Sinex
Singlet
Sinophen Intransal
Sinoran
S-T Forte
Super Anahist
Synasal
Taltapp
Tamine S.R.
Tapp
T.P.I.
Tussar DM
Tussirex
Tympagesic
U.R.I.
Vacon
Veltar

PHENYLPROPANOLAMINE

4-Way Cold Tablets
4-Way Nasal Spray
Acutrim Maximum Strength
Alka-Seltzer Plus
Allerest
Alumadrine
Asbron
Axon
Bayer Cold Tablets
Bayer Cough Syrup
Blu-Hist
Bromphen Compound
Caldecon
Children's Allerest
Cinsospan
Citra

Codimal
Coffee-Break
Colrex
Comtrex
Conex-DA
Congespirin
Conhist
Contac
Control
Coricidin "D" Decongestant
Cornex Plus
Coryban-D
Coryztime
CoTylenol Children's Liquid Cold
  Formula
Covanamine
Cremacoat
Dal-Sinus
Decongestant-P
Dehist
Dex-A-Diet
Dexatrim
Diadox
Dietac
Dieutrim
Dimetane
Dimetapp
Dri-Hist Meta-Kaps
Drinus Syrup
D-Sinus
Dura Tap-PD
Dura-Vent, /A

Efed II
Eldatapp
Endecon
E.N.T
Entex
Fiogesic
Formula 44-D
Help
Histalet Forte
Histapp
Histatapp
Hycomine
Korigesic
Koryza
Kronohist Kronocaps
MSC Triaminic
Naldecon
Napril Plateau
Nasahist
Nolamine
Novahistine
Obestat
Ornacol
Ornade
Ornex
Partuss T.D.
Phenate
Phenylin
Poly-Histine-D
PPA
Prolamine
Prolamine, Maximum Strength
Propadrine
Propagest
Quadrahist
Resaid T.D.
Rescaps-D T.D.
Resolution I Maximum Strength
Resolution II Half-Stregth
Rhindecon

Rhinex Ty-Med
Rhinidrin
Rhinocaps
Rhinolar
Robitussin-CF
Rolabromophen
Ru-Tuss
Rynatapp
Saleto-D
Sinarest
Sine-Off
Sinubid
Sinulin
Sinutab
S-T Decongestant
S-T Forte
Symtrol
Taltapp
Tapp
Tavist-D
T.P.I.
Triaminic
Triaminicin
Triaminicol
Tuss-Ade
Tussagesic
Tussaminic
Tuss-Ornade
Unitrol
U.R.I.
Ursinus
Veltap
Vernata Granucaps
Westrim
Westrim LA

PHENYLTOLOXAMINE

Amaril D
Amaril D Spantab
Comhist
Condecal
Decongestabs
Kutrase
Magsal
Naldecol
Naldecon
Naldelate
Percogesic
Poly-Histine-D
Quadra Hist
Sinocon
Sinubid
Sinutab
Trihista-Phen-25
Tri-Phen-Chlor
Tudecon
Tussionex

POTASSIUM SUPPLEMENTS

Apo-K
Bayon
Bi-K
Cena-K
CHLORIDE
EM-K-10%
Infacyte
K-10
Kalium Durules
Kaochlor
Kaochlor S-F

Kaochlor-Eff
Kaon
Kaon-Cl
Kaon-Cl 10
Kaon-Cl 20
Kao-Nor
Kato
Kay Ciel
Kaylixir
KCL
K-Dur
KEFF
K-G Elixir
K-Long
K-Lor
Klor-10%
Klor-Con
Klor-Con/EF
Klor Con/25
Klorvess
Klotrix
K-Lyte
K-Lyte DS
K-Lyte/Cl
K-Lyte/Cl 50
Kolyum
K-Tab
Micro-K
Micro-K 10
Neo-K
Novo-Lente-K
Pfiklor
Potachlor
Potage
Potasalan
Potassine
POTASSIUM ACETATE
POTASSIUM BICARBONATE
POTASSIUM BICARBONATE &
  POTASSIUM CHLORIDE
POTASSIUM BICARBONATE &
  POTASSIUM CITRATE
POTASSIUM CHLORIDE
POTASSIUM CHLORIDE,
  POTASSIUM BICARBONATE &
  POTASSIUM CITRATE
POTASSIUM GLUCONATE
POTASSIUM GLUCONATE &
  POTASSIUM CHLORIDE
POTASSIUM GLUCONATE &
  POTASSIUM CITRATE
POTASSIUM GLUCONATE,
  POTASSIUM CITRATE &
  AMMONIUM
Potassium Triplex
Potassium-Rougier
Potassium-Sandoz
Roychlor
Royonate
Rum-K
SK-Potassium Chloride
Slo-Pot
Slow-K
Tri-K
TRIKATES
Twin-K
Twin-K-Cl

PREDNISOLONE

Ak-Pred
Ak-Tate
Articulose

Codesol
Cortalone
Delta-Cortef
Deltastab
Econopred
Fernisolone-P
Hydeltrasol
Hydeltra-TBA
Inflamase
Key-Pred
Metalone-TBA
Meticortelone
Meti-Derm
Metimyd
Metreton
Nor-Pred-TBA
Nova-Pred
Novaprednisolone
Predaject
Predate
Predcor
Pred Cor-TBA
Pred Forte
Pred Mild
Prednisol TBA
Predulose
Prelone
PSP-IV
Savacort 50 & 100
Sterane

PROMETHAZINE

Anergan
Baymethazine
Dihydrocodeine Compound
Fellozine
Ganphen
Histantil
Historest
K-Phen
Mallergan
Mepergan Fortis
Phenazine
Phencen-50
Phenoject-50
Pentazine
Phenameth
Phenergan
Phenerhist
PMS Promethazine
Promet 50
Prometh
Prorex
Prosedin
Prothazine
Provigan
Remsed
V-Gan
ZiPan

PSEUDOEPHEDRINE

Actifed
Afrinol
Afrinol Repetabs
Ambenyl-D
Anafed
Anamine
Brexin
Bromfed
Bronchobid
Cardec DM

955

Cenafed
Children's Sudafed Liquid
Chlorafed
Chlor-Trimeton
Codimal
Co-Pyronil 2
Cosanyl
Co-Tylenol
Cotrol-D
Decofed
Deconamine
D-Feda
Deproist w/Codeine
Detussin
Dimacol
Disobrom
Disophrol
Dorcol
Dorcol Pediatric Formula
Drixoral
Eltor
Emprazil
Entuss-D
Fedahist
Fedrazil
Guaifed
Halofed
Hista-Clopane
Histalet DM
Histamic
Historal
Isoclor
Kronofed-A Kronocaps
Naldegesic
Neo-Synephrinol Day Relief
Neobid
Neofed
Novafed A
Novahistine DMX
Nucofed
PediaCare
Peedee Dose Decongestant
Phenergan
Phenergan-D
Poly-Histine-DX
Probahist
Pseudo-Hist
Pseudofrin
Redahist Gyrocaps
Respaire-SR
Ro-Fedrin
Robidrine
Robitussin-DAC
Rondec
Sherafed
Sine-Aid Sinus Headache Tablets
Sinufed
Sinufed Timecelles
Sudafed
Sudafed S.A.
Sudagest
Sudahist
Suda-Prol
Sudolin
Sudrin
Triafed
Trifed
Trinalin Repetabs
Triphed
Tripodrine
Tussend

Tylenol Maximum Strength Sinus
  Medicine
Zephrex

PSYLLIUM

Cillium
Effersyllium
Fiberall
Hydrocil
Konsyl
Konsyl-D
L.A. Formula
Metamucil
Modane Bulk
Mucillium
Mucilose
Naturacil
Perdiem Plain
Plova
Pro-Lax
Prompt
Regacilium
Reguloid
Saraka
Senokot with Psyllium
Serutan
Siblin
Sof-Cil
Syllact
V-Lax

PYRILAMINE

4-Way Nasal Spray
Albatussin
Allerstat
Allertoc
Citra Forte
Codimal DH, DM, PH
Covanamine
Dormarex
Duphrene
Excedrin P.M.
Fiogesic
Histalet Forte
Kronohist Kronocaps
Midol PMS
Napril Plateau
Nervine Nighttime Sleep-Aid
Panadyl
Poly-Histine D
Primatene, M Formula
P-V-Tussin
Relemine
Ru-Tuss
Rynatan
Sominex
Somnicaps
Triaminic
Trihista-Phen-25
Tussanil

RADIO-
PHARMACEUTICALS

Cyanocobalamin Co 57
Cyanocobalamin Co 60
Ferrous Citrate Fe 59
Gallium Citrate Ga 67
Indium In 111 Pentetate
Iodinated I 131 Albumin
Iodohippurate Sodium I 123
Iodohippurate Sodium I 131

Iothalamate Sodium I 125
Krypton Kr 81m
Selenomethionine Se 75
Sodium Chromate Cr 51
Sodium Iodide I 123
Sodium Iodide I 131
Sodium Pertechnetate Tc 99m
Sodium Phosphate P 32
Technetium Tc 99m Albumin
  Aggregated
Technetium Tc 99m Disofenin
Technetium Tc 99m Gluceptate
Technetium Tc 99m Human Serum
  Albumin
Technetium Tc 99m Medronate
Technetium Tc 99m Oxidronate
Technetium Tc 99m Pentetate
Technetium Tc 99m Pyrophosphate
Technetium Tc 99m Succimer
Technetium Tc 99m Sulfur Colloid
Thallous Chloride Tl 201
Xenon Xe 127
Xenon Xe 133

RAUWOLFIA ALKALOIDS

Alkarau
ALSEROXYLON
Bonapene
Broserpine
Butiserpazide-50 Prestabs
Buytizide-25 Prestabs
Chloroserpine
Demi-Regroton
DESERPIDINE
Diupres
Diutensin-R
Dralserp
Enduronyl
Harmonyl
Harmonyl-D
H-H-R
Hydro-Fluserpine
Hydromox R
Hydropres
Hydroserp
Hydroserpine
Hydrotensin-50
Mallopress
Metatensin
Naquival
Novoreserpine
Oreticyl
Raudixin
Raulfia
Raunormine
Raupoid
Rauraine
Rau-Sed
Rauserpa
Rautrax
Rauverid
Rauwiloid
Rauzide
RAUWOLFIA SERPENTINA
Regroton
Releserp-5
Renese-R
Reserfia
Reserpazide
RESERPINE
Reserpoid

Salutensin
Sandril
Ser-Ap-Es
Serpalan
Serpanray
Serpasil
Serpasil-Apresoline
Serpasil-Esidrix
SK-Reserpine
Serpate
Singoserp-Eisdrix
T-Serp
Unipres
Wolfina

RAUWOLFIA & THIAZIDE DIURETICS

Demi-Regroton
DESERPIDINE &
    HYDROCHLOROTHIAZIDE
DESERPIDINE &
    METHYCLOTHIAZIDE
Diupres
Diutensen-R
Enduronyl
Hydromox-R
Hydropres
Metatensin
Naquival
Oreticyl
Oreticyl Forte
RAUWOLFIA SERPENTINA &
    BENDROFLUMETHIAZIDE
Rauzide
Regroton
Renese-R
RESERPINE & CHLOROTHIAZIDE
RESERPINE & CHLORTHALIDONE
RESERPINE &
    HYDROCHLOROTHIAZIDE
RESERPINE &
    HYDROFLUMETHIAZIDE
RESERPINE &
    METHYCLOTHIAZIDE
RESERPINE & POLYTHIAZIDE
RESERPINE & QUINETHAZONE
RESERPINE &
    TRICHLORMETHIAZIDE
Salutensin
Salutensin-Demi
Serpasil-Esidrix

SALICYLATES

Arcylate
Artha-G
Arthropan
CHOLINE MAGNESIUM
    SALICYLATES
Choline Magnesium Trisalicylate
CHOLINE SALICYLATE
DIFLUNISAL
Disalcid
Doan's Pills
Durasil
Magan
MAGNESIUM SALICYLATE
Mobidin
SALICYLAMIDE
SALSALATE
SODIUM SALICYLATE
S-60

Uracel
Uromide

SCOPOLAMINE (HYOSCINE)

Allerspan
Almezyme
Aluscop
Bar-Cy-Amine
Bar-Cy-A-Tab
Barbella
Barbeloid
Barbidonna
Barbidonna-CR
Bar-Don
Belbutal
Belkaloids
Bobid
Brobella-PB
Buren
Cenahist
Chlorpel
Conalsyn
Dallergy
Donnacin
Donnagel
Donnamine
Donnatal
Donnazyme
Drinus
Drize
Eldonal
Eulcin
Extendryl
Haponal
Histaspan-D
Historal
Hyatal
Hybephen
Hydrochol-Plus
Hyonal
Hyonatol
Hytrona
Kinesed
Kleer
Kleer-Tuss
Koryza
Levamine
Maso-Donna
Methnite
MSC Triaminic
Narine
Narspan
Nilspasm
Omnibel
Pamine
Pamine PB
Paraspan
Renalgin
Ru-Tuss
Sanhist
Scoline
Scoline-Amobarbital
Scopolamine Trans-Derm
Scotnord
Sedamine
Sedapar
Sedralex
Seds
Sinaprel
Sinodec

Sinoran
Sinunil
Spabelin
Spasdel
Spasloids
Spasmid
Spasmolin
Spasquid
Spastolate
Symptrol
Transderm
Transderm-Scop
Transderm-V
Triptone
Trisohist
Uriseptin
Urogesic
Vanodonnal
Zemarine

SULFISOXAZOLE

Apo-Sulfisoxazole
Azo-Gantrisin
Azo-Soxazole
Barazole
Chemovag
Gantrisin
G-Sox
Lipo Gantrisin
Koro-Sulf
Novosoxazole
Pediazole
Rosoxol
SK-Soxazole
Sosol
Soxa
Sulfafurazole
Sulfagen
Sulfizin
Sulfizole
Urisoxin

TESTOSTERONE & ESTRADIOL

Andrest
Andro-Estro
Andro/Fem
Androgyn L.A.
De-Comberol
Deladumone
Deladumone OB
depAndrogyn
Depo-Testadiol
Depotestogen
Ditate
Ditate DS
Duo-Cyp
Duo-Gen L.A.
Duoval PA
Duratestrin
Estra-Testrin
Menoject-L.A.
Span-Est-Test
Teev
T.E.-Ionate P.A.
Testadiate-Depo
Test-Estra-C
Test-Estro Cypionates
TESTOSTERONE CYPIONATE &
    ESTRADIOL CYPIONATE

TESTOSTERONE ENANTHATE & ESTRADIOL VALERATE

Testradiol
Valertest

TETRACYCLINES

Achromycin
Achromycin V
Achrostatin V
Apo-Tetra
Bicycline
Bio-Tetra
Bristacycline
Cefracycline
Centet
Comycin
Cyclopar
Declomycin
DEMECLOCYCLINE
Desamycin
Doxy
Doxy-Caps
Doxychel
DOXYCYCLINE
Doxy-Lemmon
Doxy-Tabs
Fed-Mycin
G-Mycin
Kesso-Tetra
Lemtrex
Maytrex-BID
Medicycline
METHACYCLINE
Minocin
MINOCYCLINE
Muracine
Mysteclin F
Neo-Tetrine
Nor-Tet
Novotetra
Oxlopar
Oxy-Kesso-Tetra
OXYTETRACYCLINE
Paltet
Panmycin
Piracaps
PMS Tetracycline
Q'Dtet
Retet
Retet-S
Robitet
Ro-Cycline
Rondomycin
Sarocyclin
Scotrex
SK-Tetracycline
Sumycin
T-Caps
TETRACYCLINE
Terramycin
Tet-Cy
Tetet
Tetrachel
Tetra-Co
Tetracrine
Tetracyn
Tetracyrine
Tetralean
Tetram
Tetramax
Tetramine
Tetrastatin (M)

Tetrex
Tetrex-S
Topicycline
Trexin
Ultramycin
Urobiotic
Vibramycin
Vibratabs

TRIAMCINOLONE

Acetospan
Amcort
Aristocort
Aristospan
Articulose-L.A.
Azmacort
Cenocort
Cenocort Forte
Cinalone 40
Cino-40
Cinonide 40
Cremocort
Kenacort
Kenaject
Kenalog
Kenalog in Orabase
Kenalog-E
Kenalone
Ledercort
Lederspan
Mycolog
Myco-Triacet
Mytrex
Nust-Olone
Spencort
Tramacort
Triacet
Triacort
Triaderm
Trialean Acetonide
Triam
Triamcinair
Triamonide
Tri-Kort
Trilog
Trilone
Trimalone
Tristoject
Trymex

Some of these brands are available as topical medicines (ointments, creams or lotions).
See ADRENOCORTICOIDS (TOPICAL), page 16.

TRICYCLIC ANTIDEPRESSANTS

Adapin
Amitid
Amitril
AMITRYPTILINE
AMOXAPINE
Anafranil
Anemtyl
Apo-Amitriptyline
Apo-Imipramine
Ascendin
Aventyl
CLOMIPRAMINE
DESIPRAMINE
Elavil
Emitrip

Endep
Enovil
Etrafon
IMIPRAMINE
Impril
Janimine
Levate
Meravil
Norpramin
NORTRIPTYLINE
Novopramine
Novotriptyn
Pamelor
Pertofrane
Presamine
PROTRIPTYLINE
Sinequan
SK-Amitriptyline
SK-Pramine
Surmontil
Tipramine
Tofranil
Tofranil-PM
Triadapin
Triavil
TRIMIPRAMINE
Triptil
Vivactil

VITAMIN B-12 (CYANOCOBALAMIN)

Alphamin
Alpha Redisol
Anocobin
Bedoz
Berubigen
Betalin 12
Betalin 12 Crystalline
Cyanabin
Kaybovite
Kaybovite-1000
Neo-Betalin
Neo-Rubex
Redisol
Rubion
Rubramin
Rubramin-PC
Sytobex
Numerous other multiple vitamin-mineral supplements.

VITAMIN C (ASCORBIC ACID)

Adenex
Apo-C
Arco-Cee
Ascorbajen
Ascorbicap
Ascoril
Calscorbate
Cecon
Cemill
Cenolate
Ceri-Bid
Cetane
Cevalin
Cevi-Bid
Ce-Vi-Sol
Cevita
C-Ject
Flavorcee

Liqui-Cee
Megascorb
Redoxon
Numerous other multiple
vitamin-mineral supplements.

XANTHINE
BRONCHODILATORS

Accurbron
Aerolate
Aerophylline
Airet
Amesec
Aminodur
Aminodur Dura-tabs
Aminophyl
Aminophyllin
AMINOPHYLLINE
Aminophylline and Amytal
Aminophylline-Phenobarbital
Amodrine
Amoline
Amophylline
Apo-Oxtriphylline
Aquaphyllin
Asbron
Asma
Asmalix
Asminyl
Asthmophylline
Bronchobid Duracaps
Broncholate
Brondecon
Brondilate
Bronkodyl
Bronkodyl S-R
Bronkolixir
Bronkotabs
Brosema
Choledyl
Choledyl SA
Chophylline
Constant-T
Corophyllin
Corophylline
Co-Xan
Dilin
Dilor
Dilor-G
Droxine
Droxine L.A.
Droxine S.F.
Duovent
Duraphyl
Dyflex
Dylline
DYPHILLINE
Dy-Phyl-Lin
Elixicon
Elixomin
Elixophyllin
Elixophyllin SR
Emfaseem
G-Bron
Iso-Asminyl
Isuprel Compound
Klophyllin
LABID
Lanophyllin
Liquophylline
Lixaminol
Lixaminol AT

Lixolin
Lodrane
Luasmin
Luftodil
Lufyllin
Marax
Marax DF
Mersalyl-Theophylline
Mini-Lix
Mudrane
Neospect
Neothylline
Neothylline-G
Novotriphyl
Numa-Dura-Tabs
Orthoxine & Aminophylline
OXTRIPHYLLINE
Oxystat
Palaron
Phenylin
Phyldrox
Phyllocontin
Physpan
PMS Theophylline
Primatene, M Formula
Primatene, P Formula
Protophylline
Pulmophylline
Quadrinal
Quibron
Quibron Plus
Quibron-T
Quibron-T/SR Dividose
Respbid
Slo-Phyllin GG
Slo-bid Gyrocaps
Slophyllin
Somophyllin
Somophyllin-12
Somophyllin-CRT
Somophyllin-DF
Somophyllin-T
Sudolin
Sustaire
Synophylate-GG
Tedfern
Tedral
T.E.H.
Thalfed
Theobid
Theobid Duracaps
Theobid Jr. Duracaps
Theochron
Theoclear
Theoclear L.A. Cenules
Theo-Dur
Theo-Dur Sprinkle
Theofedral
Theo-Guaia
Theolair
Theolair-Plus
Theolair-SR
Theolixir
Theon
Theo-Nar 100
Theo-Organidin
Theophyl
Theophyl-SR
THEOPHYLLINE
Theophylline Choline
Theospan
Theospan SR

Theostat
Theostate 80
Theotabs
Theo-Time
Theo-24
Theovent Long-acting
Theozine
Truphylline
Uniphyl

Additional Drug Interactions

The following lists of drugs and their interactions with other drugs are continuations of lists found in the alphabetized drug charts beginning on page 2. These lists are alphabetized by generic name or drug class name, shown in large capital letters. Only those lists too long for the drug charts are included in this section. For complete information about any generic drug, see the alphabetized charts.

GENERIC NAME OR DRUG CLASS	COMBINED EFFECT	GENERIC NAME OR DRUG CLASS	COMBINED EFFECT

ACETAMINOPHEN & SALICYLATES

Phenytoin	Increased phenytoin effect.	Sulfinpyrazone	Decreased sulfinpyrazone effect.
Probenecid	Decreased probenecid effect.	Tetracyclines (effervescent granules or tablets)	May slow tetracycline absorption. Space doses 2 hours apart.
Propranolol	Decreased aspirin effect.	Vancomycin	Hearing loss.
Rauwolfia alkaloids	Decreased aspirin effect.	Verapamil	Increased risk of toxicity.
Spironolactone	Decreased spironolactone effect.	Vitamin C (large doses)	Possible aspirin toxicity.

ASPIRIN

Spironolactone	Decreased spironolactone effect.	Terfenadine	May conceal symptoms of aspirin overdose, such as ringing in ears.
Sulfinpyrazone	Decreased sulfinpyrazone effect.	Vitamin C (large doses)	Possible aspirin toxicity.
Suprofen	Increased risk of stomach ulcer.		

ATROPINE, HYOSCYAMINE, METHENAMINE, METHYLENE BLUE, PHENYLSALICYLATE & BENZOIC ACID

Meperidine	Increased atropine and hyoscyamine effect.	Phenothiazines	Increased atropine and hyoscyamine effect.
Methylphenidate	Increased atropine and hyoscyamine effect.	Phenytoin	Increased phenytoin effect.
Minoxidil	Decreased minoxidil effect.	Pilocarpine	Loss of pilocarpine effect in glaucoma treatment.
Orphenadrine	Increased atropine and hyoscyamine effect.	Potassium supplements	Possible intestinal ulcers with oral potassium tablets.
Oxprenolol	Decreased antihypertensive effect of oxprenolol.	Probenecid	Decreased probenecid effect.
Para-aminosalicylic acid (PAS)	Possible salicylate toxicity.	Propranolol	Decreased salicylate effect.
Penicillins	Increased effect of both drugs.	Rauwolfia alkaloids	Decreased salicylate effect.
Phenobarbital	Decreased salicylate effect.	Salicylates (other)	Likely salicylate toxicity.

GENERIC NAME OR DRUG CLASS	COMBINED EFFECT	GENERIC NAME OR DRUG CLASS	COMBINED EFFECT

ATROPINE, HYOSCYAMINE, METHENAMINE, METHYLENE BLUE, PHENYLSALICYLATE & BENZOIC ACID continued

Sodium bicarbonate	Decreased methenamine effect.	Terfenadine	May conceal symptoms of salicylate overdose, such as ringing in ears.
Spironolactone	Decreased spironolactone effect.	Vitamin C (1 to 4 grams per day)	Increased effect of methenamine, contributing to urine acidity; decreased atropine effect; possible salicylate toxicity.
Sulfa drugs	Possible kidney damage.		
Sulfinpyrazone	Decreased sulfinpyrazone effect.		

BELLADONNA ALKALOIDS & BARBITURATES

Meperidine	Increased belladonna effect.	Pilocarpine	Loss of pilocarpine effect in glaucoma treatment.
Methylphenidate	Increased belladonna effect.	Potassium supplements	Possible intestinal ulcers with oral potassium tablets.
Mind-altering drugs	Dangerous sedation. Avoid.	Sedatives	Dangerous sedation. Avoid.
Narcotics	Dangerous sedation. Avoid.	Sleep inducers	Dangerous sedation. Avoid.
Nitrates	Increased internal-eye pressure.	Tranquilizers	Dangerous sedation. Avoid.
Orphenadrine	Increased belladonna effect.	Valproic acid	Increased barbiturate effect.
Pain relievers	Dangerous sedation. Avoid.	Vitamin C	Decreased belladonna effect. Avoid large doses of vitamin C.
Phenothiazines	Increased belladonna effect. Danger of oversedation.		

BETA-ADRENERGIC BLOCKING AGENTS & THIAZIDE DIURETICS

Antidiabetics	Increased antidiabetic effect.	Digitalis preparations	Excessive potassium loss that causes dangerous heart rhythms. Can either increase or decrease heart rate. Improves irregular heartbeat.
Antihistamines	Decreased antihistamine effect.		
Antihypertensives	Increased antihypertensive effect.		
Anti-inflammatory drugs	Decreased anti-inflammatory effect.	Diuretics (thiazide)	Increased effect of other thiazide diuretics.
Barbiturates	Increased barbiturate effect. Dangerous sedation.	Indapamide	Increased diuretic effect.
Cholestyramine	Decreased hydrochlorothiazide effect.	MAO inhibitors	Increased hydrochlorothiazide effect.
Cortisone drugs	Excessive potassium loss that causes dangerous heart rhythms.	Narcotics	Increased narcotic effect. Dangerous sedation.

GENERIC NAME OR DRUG CLASS	COMBINED EFFECT	GENERIC NAME OR DRUG CLASS	COMBINED EFFECT

BETA-ADRENERGIC BLOCKING AGENTS & THIAZIDE DIURETICS continued

GENERIC NAME OR DRUG CLASS	COMBINED EFFECT	GENERIC NAME OR DRUG CLASS	COMBINED EFFECT
Nitrates	Excessive blood-pressure drop.	Probenecid	Decreased probenecid effect.
Oxprenolol	Increased antihypertensive effect. Dosages of both drugs may require adjustment.	Quinidine	Slows heart excessively.
		Reserpine	Increased reserpine effect. Excessive sedation and depression.
Phenytoin	Increased beta-adrenergic effect.		
Potassium supplements	Decreased potassium effect.	Tocainide	May worsen congestive heart failure.

BUTALBITAL & ASPIRIN (Also contains caffeine)

GENERIC NAME OR DRUG CLASS	COMBINED EFFECT	GENERIC NAME OR DRUG CLASS	COMBINED EFFECT
Anti-inflammatory drugs (non-steroid)	Risk of stomach bleeding and ulcers.	Mind-altering drugs	Dangerous sedation. Avoid.
Aspirin (other)	Likely aspirin toxicity.	Minoxidil	Decreased minoxidil effect.
Beta-adrenergic blockers	Decreased effect of beta-adrenergic blocker.	Narcotics	Dangerous sedation. Avoid.
Contraceptives (oral)	Decreased contraceptive effect.	Pain relievers	Dangerous sedation. Avoid.
Cortisone drugs	Increased cortisone effect. Risk of ulcer and stomach bleeding.	Salicylates (others)	Likely aspirin toxicity.
		Sedatives	Dangerous sedation. Avoid.
Digitoxin	Decreased digitoxin effect.	Sleep inducers	Dangerous sedation. Avoid.
Doxycycline	Decreased doxycycline effect.	Spironolactone	Decreased spironolactone effect.
Dronabinol	Increased effect of both drugs.	Sulfinpyrazone	Decreased sulfinpyrazone effect.
Furosemide	Possible aspirin toxicity.	Terfenadine	May conceal symptoms of aspirin overdose, such as ringing in ears.
Gold compounds	Increased likelihood of kidney damage.		
Griseofulvin	Decreased griseofulvin effect.	Tranquilizers	Dangerous sedation. Avoid.
Indapamide	Increased indapamide effect.	Valproic acid	Increased butalbital effect.
Indomethacin	Risk of stomach bleeding and ulcers.	Vitamin C (large doses)	Possible aspirin toxicity.
MAO inhibitors	Increased butalbital effect.		
Methotrexate	Increased methotrexate effect.		

BUTALBITAL, ASPIRIN & CODEINE (Also contains caffeine)

GENERIC NAME OR DRUG CLASS	COMBINED EFFECT	GENERIC NAME OR DRUG CLASS	COMBINED EFFECT
Antidepressants	Decreased antidepressant effect. Possible dangerous oversedation.	Antidiabetics (oral)	Increased butalbital effect. Low blood sugar.
		Antihistamines	Dangerous sedation. Avoid.

BUTALBITAL & ASPIRIN (Also contains caffeine) continued

GENERIC NAME OR DRUG CLASS	COMBINED EFFECT	GENERIC NAME OR DRUG CLASS	COMBINED EFFECT
Anti-inflammatory drugs (non-steroid)	Risk of stomach bleeding and ulcers.	Pain relievers	Dangerous sedation. Avoid.
Aspirin (other)	Likely aspirin toxicity.	Para-aminosalicylic acid (PAS)	Possible aspirin toxicity.
Beta-adrenergic blockers	Decreased effect of beta-adrenergic blocker.	Penicillins	Increased effect of drugs.
Contraceptives (oral)	Decreased contraceptive effect.	Phenobarbital	Decreased aspirin effect.
Cortisone drugs	Increased cortisone effect. Risk of ulcer and stomach bleeding.	Phenothiazines	Increased phenothiazine effect.
Digitoxin	Decreased digitoxin effect.	Phenytoin	Increased phenytoin effect.
Doxycycline	Decreased doxycycline effect.	Probenecid	Decreased probenecid effect.
Dronabinol	Increased effect of drugs.	Propranolol	Decreased aspirin effect.
Furosemide	Possible aspirin toxicity.	Rauwolfia alkaloids	Decreased aspirin effect.
Gold compounds	Increased likelihood of kidney damage.	Salicylates (others)	Likely aspirin toxicity.
Griseofulvin	Decreased griseofulvin effect.	Sedatives	Dangerous sedation. Avoid.
Indapamide	Increased indapamide effect.	Sleep inducers	Dangerous sedation. Avoid.
Indomethacin	Risk of stomach bleeding and ulcers.	Spironolactone	Decreased spironolactone effect.
MAO inhibitors	Increased butalbital effect.	Sulfinpyrazone	Decreased sulfinpyrazone effect.
Methotrexate	Increased methotrexate effect.	Terfenadine	May conceal symptoms of aspirin overdose, such as ringing in ears.
Mind-altering drugs	Dangerous sedation. Avoid.	Tranquilizers	Dangerous sedation. Avoid.
Minoxidil	Decreased minoxidil effect.	Valproic acid	Increased phenobarbital effect.
Narcotics	Dangerous sedation. Avoid.	Vitamin C (large doses)	Possible aspirin toxicity.
Nitrates	Excessive blood-pressure drop.		

CAPTOPRIL & HYDROCHLOROTHIAZIDE

GENERIC NAME OR DRUG CLASS	COMBINED EFFECT	GENERIC NAME OR DRUG CLASS	COMBINED EFFECT
Nitrates	Excessive blood-pressure drop.	Potassium supplements	Excessive potassium in blood.
Oxprenolol	Increased antihypertensive effect. Dosages of both drugs may require adjustments.	Probenecid	Decreased probenecid effect.
		Spironolactone	Possible excessive potassium in blood.
		Triamterene	Possible excessive potassium in blood.

CHLORDIAZEPOXIDE & AMITRIPTYLINE

Thyroid hormones	Irregular heartbeat.	Tranquilizers	Increased sedative effect of both drugs.

CHLORDIAZEPOXIDE & CLIDINIUM

Pilocarpine	Loss of pilocarpine effect in glaucoma treatment.	Sleep inducers	Increased sedative effect of both drugs.
Potassium supplements	Possible intestinal ulcers with oral potassium tablets.	Tranquilizers	Increased sedative effect of both drugs.
		Vitamin C	Decreased clidinium effect. Avoid large doses of vitamin C.
Sedatives	Increased sedative effect of both drugs.		

CLONIDINE & CHLORTHALIDONE

Digitalis preparations	Excessive potassium loss that causes dangerous heart rhythms.	MAO inhibitors	Increased chlorthalidone effect.
		Nitrates	Possible excessive blood-pressure drop.
Diuretics	Excessive blood-pressure drop.	Oxprenolol	Increased antihypertensive effect. Dosages of both drugs may require adjustments.
Fenfluramine	Possible increased clonidine effect.		
Indapamide	Increased diuretic effect.		
		Potassium supplements	Decreased potassium effect.
Lithium	Increased effect of lithium.	Probenecid	Decreased probenecid effect.

CORTISONE

Suprofen	Increased risk of stomach ulcer and bleeding.	Sympathomimetics	Possible glaucoma.

DEXAMETHASONE

Rifampin	Decreased dexamethasone effect.	Sympathomimetics	Possible glaucoma.

ENALAPRIL & HYDROCHLOROTHIAZIDE

Potassium supplements	Excessive potassium in blood.	Spironolactone	Possible excessive potassium in blood.
Probenecid	Decreased probenecid effect.	Triamterene	Possible excessive potassium in blood.

ERGOTAMINE, BELLADONNA & PHENOBARBITAL

Contraceptives (oral)	Decreased contraceptive effect.	Cortisone drugs	Decreased cortisone effect. Increased internal-eye pressure.

ADDITIONAL DRUG INTERACTIONS

ERGOTAMINE, BELLADONNA & PHENOBARBITAL continued

GENERIC NAME OR DRUG CLASS	COMBINED EFFECT	GENERIC NAME OR DRUG CLASS	COMBINED EFFECT
Digitoxin	Decreased digitoxin effect.	Nitrates	Increased internal-eye pressure.
Doxycycline	Decreased doxycycline effect.	Orphenadrine	Increased belladonna effect.
Dronabinol	Increased effect of drugs.	Pain relievers	Dangerous sedation. Avoid.
Ephedrine	Dangerous blood-pressure rise.	Phenothiazines	Increased belladonna effect.
Epinephrine	Dangerous blood-pressure rise.	Pilocarpine	Loss of pilocarpine effect in glaucoma treatment.
Griseofulvin	Decreased griseofulvin effect.	Potassium supplements	Possible intestinal ulcers with oral potassium tablets.
Haloperidol	Increased internal-eye pressure.		
Indapamide	Increased indapamide effect.	Sedatives	Dangerous sedation. Avoid.
MAO inhibitors	Increased belladonna and phenobarbital effect.	Sleep inducers	Dangerous sedation. Avoid.
Meperidine	Increased belladonna effect.	Tranquilizers	Dangerous sedation. Avoid.
Methylphenidate	Increased belladonna effect.	Troleandomycin	Increased adverse reactions of ergotamine.
Mind-altering drugs	Dangerous sedation. Avoid.	Valproic acid	Increased phenobarbital effect.
Narcotics	Dangerous sedation. Avoid.	Vitamin C	Decreased belladonna effect. Avoid large doses of vitamin C.

ERGOTAMINE, CAFFEINE, BELLADONNA & PENTOBARBITAL

GENERIC NAME OR DRUG CLASS	COMBINED EFFECT	GENERIC NAME OR DRUG CLASS	COMBINED EFFECT
Anticoagulants (oral)	Decreased anticoagulant effect.	Beta-adrenergic blockers	Decreased effect of beta-adrenergic blocker.
Anticonvulsants	Changed seizure patterns.	Contraceptives (oral)	Decreased contraceptive effect.
Antidepressants (tricyclics)	Decreased antidepressant effect. Possible dangerous oversedation.	Cortisone drugs	Decreased cortisone effect. Increased internal-eye pressure.
Antidiabetics (oral)	Increased pentobarbital effect.	Digitoxin	Decreased digitoxin effect.
Antihistamines	Dangerous sedation. Avoid.	Doxycycline	Decreased doxycycline effect.
Anti-inflammatory drugs (non-steroidal)	Decreased anti-inflammatory effect.	Dronabinol	Increased effect of drugs.
Aspirin	Decreased aspirin effect.	Ephedrine	Dangerous blood-pressure rise.
		Epinephrine	Dangerous blood-pressure rise.

GENERIC NAME OR DRUG CLASS	COMBINED EFFECT	GENERIC NAME OR DRUG CLASS	COMBINED EFFECT

ERGOTAMINE, CAFFEINE, BELLADONNA & PENTOBARBITAL continued

GENERIC NAME OR DRUG CLASS	COMBINED EFFECT	GENERIC NAME OR DRUG CLASS	COMBINED EFFECT
Griseofulvin	Decreased griseofulvin effect.	Phenothiazines	Increased belladonna effect.
Haloperidol	Increased internal-eye pressure.	Pilocarpine	Loss of pilocarpine effect in glaucoma treatment.
Indapamide	Increased indapamide effect.	Potassium supplements	Possible intestinal ulcers with oral potassium tablets.
Isoniazid	Increased caffeine effect.		
MAO inhibitors	Increased belladonna effect, dangerous blood-pressure rise.	Sedatives	Dangerous sedation. Avoid.
Meperidine	Increased belladonna effect.	Sleep inducers	Dangerous sedation. Avoid.
Methylphenidate	Increased belladonna effect.	Sympathomimetics	Overstimulation, blood-pressure rise.
Mind-altering drugs	Dangerous sedation. Avoid.	Thyroid hormones	Increased thyroid effect.
		Tranquilizers	Dangerous sedation. Avoid.
Narcotics	Dangerous sedation. Avoid.	Troleandomycin	Increased adverse reactions of ergotamine.
Nitrates	Increased internal-eye pressure.	Valproic acid	Increased pentobarbital effect.
Orphenadrine	Increased belladonna effect.	Vitamin C	Decreased belladonna effect. Avoid large doses of vitamin C.
Pain relievers	Dangerous sedation. Avoid.		

GUANETHIDINE & HYDROCHLOROTHIAZIDE

GENERIC NAME OR DRUG CLASS	COMBINED EFFECT	GENERIC NAME OR DRUG CLASS	COMBINED EFFECT
Indapamide	Possible increased effects of both drugs. When monitored carefully, combination may be beneficial in controlling hypertension.	Nitrates	Excessive blood-pressure drop.
		Oxprenolol	Increased antihypertensive effect. Dosages of both drugs may require adjustments.
Lithium	Increased lithium effect.		
MAO inhibitors	Increased hydrochlorothiazide effect.	Potassium supplements	Decreased potassium effect.
		Probenecid	Decreased probenecid effect.
Minoxidil	Dosage adjustments may be necessary to keep blood pressure at proper level.		

HYDRALAZINE & HYDROCHLOROTHIAZIDE

GENERIC NAME OR DRUG CLASS	COMBINED EFFECT	GENERIC NAME OR DRUG CLASS	COMBINED EFFECT
Lithium	Increased effect of lithium.	Oxprenolol	Increased antihypertensive effect. Dosages of both drugs may require adjustments.
MAO inhibitors	Increased effect of drugs.		
Nitrates	Excessive blood-pressure drop.		

GENERIC NAME OR DRUG CLASS	COMBINED EFFECT	GENERIC NAME OR DRUG CLASS	COMBINED EFFECT

HYDRALAZINE & HYDROCHLOROTHIAZIDE continued

Potassium supplements	Decreased potassium effect.	Probenecid	Decreased probenecid effect.

KAOLIN, PECTIN, BELLADONNA & OPIUM

Mind-altering drugs	Increased sedative effect.	Potassium supplements	Possible intestinal ulcers with oral potassium tablets.
Narcotics (other)	Increased narcotic effect.	Sedatives	Excessive sedation.
Nitrates	Increased internal-eye pressure.	Sleep inducers	Increased effect of sleep inducers.
Orphenadrine	Increased belladonna effect.	Tranquilizers	Increased tranquilizer effect.
Phenothiazines	Increased sedative effect of paregoric.	Vitamin C	Decreased belladonna effect. Avoid large doses of vitamin C.
Pilocarpine	Loss of pilocarpine effect in glaucoma treatment.	All other oral medicines	Decreases absorption of other medicines. Separate doses by at least 2 hours.

MEPROBAMATE & ASPIRIN

Para-aminosalicylic acid (PAS)	Possible aspirin toxicity.	Sleep inducers	Increased effect of sleep inducer.
Penicillins	Increased effect of both drugs.	Spironolactone	Decreased spironolactone effect.
Phenobarbital	Decreased aspirin effect.	Sulfinpyrazone	Decreased sulfinpyrazone effect.
Phenytoin	Increased phenytoin effect.	Terfenadine	Possible excessive sedation. May conceal symptoms of aspirin overdose, such as ringing in ears.
Probenecid	Decreased probenecid effect.		
Propranolol	Decreased aspirin effect.	Tranquilizers	Increased tranquilizer effect.
Rauwolfia alkaloids	Decreased aspirin effect.	Vitamin C (large doses)	Possible aspirin toxicity.
Salicylates (other)	Likely aspirin toxicity.		
Sedatives	Increased sedative effect.		

METHYLDOPA & THIAZIDE DIURETICS

MAO inhibitors	Dangerous blood-pressure changes.	Oxprenolol	Increased antihypertensive effect. Dosages of both drugs may require adjustments.
Nitrates	Excessive blood-pressure drop.		
		Potassium supplements	Decreased potassium effect.

METHYLPREDNISOLONE

Generic Name or Drug Class	Combined Effect
Potassium supplements	Decreased potassium effect.
Rifampin	Decreased methylprednisolone effect.
Sympathomimetics	Possible glaucoma.

NARCOTIC & ASPIRIN

Generic Name or Drug Class	Combined Effect
Phenobarbital	Decreased aspirin effect.
Phenytoin	Increased phenytoin effect.
Probenecid	Decreased probenecid effect.
Propranolol	Decreased aspirin effect.
Rauwolfia alkaloids	Decreased aspirin effect.
Salicylates (other)	Likely aspirin toxicity.
Sedatives	Increased sedative effect.
Sleep inducers	Increased sedative effect. sleep inducer.
Spironolactone	Decreased spironolactone effect.
Sulfinpyrazone	Decreased sulfinpyrazone effect.
Terfenadine	Possible excessive sedation. May conceal symptoms of aspirin overdose, such as ringing in ears.
Tranquilizers	Increased sedative effect.
Vitamin C (large doses)	Possible aspirin toxicity.

ORPHENADRINE, ASPIRIN & CAFFEINE

Generic Name or Drug Class	Combined Effect
Antidepressants (tricyclic)	Increased sedation.
Antidiabetics (oral)	Low blood sugar.
Anti-inflammatory drugs (non-steroid)	Risk of stomach bleeding and ulcers.
Aspirin (other)	Likely aspirin toxicity.
Chlorpromazine	Hypoglycemia (low blood sugar).
Contraceptives (oral)	Increased caffeine effect.
Cortisone drugs	Increased cortisone effect. Risk of ulcers and stomach bleeding.
Furosemide	Possible aspirin toxicity.
Gold compounds	Increased likelihood of kidney damage.
Griseofulvin	Decreased griseofulvin effect.
Indomethacin	Risk of stomach bleeding and ulcers.
Isoniazid	Increased caffeine effect.
Levodopa	Increased effect of levodopa. (Improves effectiveness in treating Parkinson's disease.)
MAO inhibitors	Dangerous blood-pressure rise.
Methotrexate	Increased methotrexate effect.
Minoxidil	Decreased minoxidil effect.
Nitrates	Increased internal-eye pressure.
Oxprenolol	Decreased antihypertensive effect of oxprenolol.
Para-aminosalicylic acid (PAS)	Possible aspirin toxicity.
Penicillins	Increased effect of drugs.
Phenobarbital	Decreased aspirin effect.
Potassium supplements	Increased possibility of intestinal ulcers with oral potassium tablets.

GENERIC NAME OR DRUG CLASS	COMBINED EFFECT	GENERIC NAME OR DRUG CLASS	COMBINED EFFECT

ORPHENADRINE, ASPIRIN & CAFFEINE continued

GENERIC NAME OR DRUG CLASS	COMBINED EFFECT	GENERIC NAME OR DRUG CLASS	COMBINED EFFECT
Probenecid	Decreased probenecid effect.	Sulfinpyrazone	Decreased sulfinpyrazone effect.
Propoxyphene	Possible confusion, nervousness, tremors.	Sympathomimetics	Overstimulation.
Propranolol	Decreased aspirin effect.	Terfenadine	May conceal symptoms of aspirin overdose, such as ringing in ears. Possible increased orphenadrine effect.
Rauwolfia alkaloids	Decreased aspirin effect.		
Salicylates (other)	Likely aspirin toxicity.	Thyroid hormones	Increased thyroid effect.
Sedatives	Decreased sedative effect.	Tranquilizers	Decreased tranquilizer effect.
Sleep inducers	Decreased sedative effect.	Vitamin C (large doses)	Possible aspirin toxicity.
Spironolactone	Decreased spironolactone effect.		

PANCREATIN, PEPSIN, BILE SALTS, HYOSCYAMINE, ATROPINE, SCOPOLAMINE & PHENOBARBITAL

GENERIC NAME OR DRUG CLASS	COMBINED EFFECT	GENERIC NAME OR DRUG CLASS	COMBINED EFFECT
Indapamide	Increased indapamide effect.	Pilocarpine	Loss of pilocarpine effect in glaucoma treatment.
MAO inhibitors	Increased atropine effect.	Potassium supplements	Possible intestinal ulcers with oral potassium tablets.
Meperidine	Increased atropine effect.		
Methylphenidate	Increased atropine effect.	Sedatives	Dangerous sedation. Avoid.
Mind-altering drugs	Dangerous sedation. Avoid.	Sleep inducers	Dangerous sedation. Avoid.
Narcotics	Dangerous sedation. Avoid.	Tranquilizers	Dangerous sedation. Avoid.
Nitrates	Increased internal-eye pressure.	Valproic acid	Increased phenobarbital effect.
Orphenadrine	Increased atropine effect.	Vitamin C	Decreased atropine effect. Avoid large doses of vitamin C.
Phenothiazines	Increased atropine effect.		

PARGYLINE & METHYCLOTHIAZIDE

GENERIC NAME OR DRUG CLASS	COMBINED EFFECT	GENERIC NAME OR DRUG CLASS	COMBINED EFFECT
Antihypertensives	Excessively low blood pressure.	Cortisone drugs	Excessive potassium loss that causes dangerous heart rhythms.
Barbiturates	Increased methyclothiazide effect.		
Caffeine	Irregular heartbeat or high blood pressure.	Cyclobenzaprine	Fever, seizures. Avoid.
Carbamazepine	Fever, seizures. Avoid.	Digitalis preparations	Excessive potassium loss that causes dangerous heart rhythms.
Cholestyramine	Decreased methyclothiazide effect.		

GENERIC NAME OR DRUG CLASS	COMBINED EFFECT	GENERIC NAME OR DRUG CLASS	COMBINED EFFECT

PARGYLINE & METHYCLOTHIAZIDE continued

GENERIC NAME OR DRUG CLASS	COMBINED EFFECT	GENERIC NAME OR DRUG CLASS	COMBINED EFFECT
Diuretics (other)	Excessively low blood pressure.	Nitrates	Excessive blood-pressure drop.
Guanethidine	Blood-pressure rise to life-threatening level.	Oxprenolol	Possible blood-pressure rise if MAO inhibitor is discontinued after simultaneous use with oxprenolol.
Indapamide	Increased indapamide and diuretic effect.		
Levodopa	Sudden, severe blood-pressure rise.	Potassium supplements	Decreased potassium effect.
Lithium	Increased effect of lithium.	Probenecid	Decreased probenecid effect.
MAO inhibitors (other, when taken together)	High fever, convulsions, death. Increased methyclothiazide effect.	Terfenadine	Increased side effects of MAO inhibitors.

PERPHENAZINE & AMITRIPTYLINE

GENERIC NAME OR DRUG CLASS	COMBINED EFFECT	GENERIC NAME OR DRUG CLASS	COMBINED EFFECT
Guanethidine	Decreased guanethidine effect.	Quinidine	Impaired heart function. Dangerous mixture.
Levodopa	Decreased levodopa effect.	Sedatives	Dangerous oversedation.
MAO inhibitors	Fever, delirium, convulsions.	Sympathomimetics	Increased sympathomimetics effect.
Methyldopa	Decreased methyldopa effect.	Thyroid hormones	Irregular heartbeat.
Mind-altering drugs	Increased effect of mind-altering drugs.	Tranquilizers (other)	Increased tranquilizer effect.
Narcotics	Increased narcotic effect and dangerous sedation.		

PHENPROCOUMON

GENERIC NAME OR DRUG CLASS	COMBINED EFFECT	GENERIC NAME OR DRUG CLASS	COMBINED EFFECT
Chloramphenicol	Increased phenprocoumon effect.	Digitalis preparations	Decreased phenprocoumon effect.
Chlorpromazine	Decreased phenprocoumon effect.	Disulfiram	Increased phenprocoumon effect.
Cholestyramine	Unpredictable increased or decreased phenprocoumon effect.	Estrogens	Decreased phenprocoumon effect.
Cimetidine	Increased phenprocoumon effect.	Ethacrynic acid	Increased phenprocoumon effect.
Clofibrate	Unpredictable increased or decreased phenprocoumon effect.	Ethchlorvynol	Decreased phenprocoumon effect.
Contraceptives (oral)	Unpredictable increased or decreased phenprocoumon effect.	Furosemide	Decreased phenprocoumon effect.
Cortisone drugs	Unpredictable increased or decreased phenprocoumon effect.	Glucagon	Increased phenprocoumon effect.
		Glutethimide	Decreased phenprocoumon effect.
		Griseofulvin	Decreased phenprocoumon effect.

GENERIC NAME OR DRUG CLASS	COMBINED EFFECT	GENERIC NAME OR DRUG CLASS	COMBINED EFFECT

PHENPROCOUMON continued

Guanethidine	Increased phenprocoumon effect.	Phenylbutazone	Unpredictable increased or decreased phenprocoumon effect.
Haloperidol	Decreased phenprocoumon effect.	Phenylpropanolamine	Decreased anticoagulant effect.
Hydroxyzine	Increased phenprocoumon effect.	Phenyramidol	Increased phenprocoumon effect.
Indomethacin	Increased phenprocoumon effect.	Probenecid	Increased phenprocoumon effect.
Insulin	Increased insulin effect.	Propoxyphene	Increased phenprocoumon effect.
Isocarboxazid	Increased phenprocoumon effect.	Propylthiouracil	Increased phenprocoumon effect.
Isoniazid	Increased phenprocoumon effect.	Quinidine	Increased phenprocoumon effect.
Mefenamic acid	Increased phenprocoumon effect.	Rauwolfia alkaloids	Unpredictable increased or decreased phenprocoumon effect.
Meprobamate	Decreased phenprocoumon effect.	Salicylates (including aspirin)	Increased phenprocoumon effect.
Mercaptopurine	Increased phenprocoumon effect.	Sulfa drugs	Increased phenprocoumon effect.
Methyldopa	Increased phenprocoumon effect.	Sulfinpyrazone	Increased phenprocoumon effect.
Methylphenidate	Increased phenprocoumon effect.	Tetracyclines	Increased phenprocoumon effect.
Metronidazole	Increased phenprocoumon effect.	Thyroid hormones	Increased phenprocoumon effect.
Nalidixic acid	Increased phenprocoumon effect.	Trimethoprim	Increased phenprocoumon effect.
Nortriptyline	Increased phenprocoumon effect.	Vitamin C (large doses)	Decreased phenprocoumon effect.
Oxyphenbutazone	Increased phenprocoumon effect.	Vitamin E (large doses)	Increased phenprocoumon effect.
Para-aminosalicylic acid (PAS)	Increased phenprocoumon effect.		
Phenelzine	Increased phenprocoumon effect.		

PHENYTOIN

Gold compounds	Increased phenytoin blood levels. Phenytoin dose may require adjustment.	Methotrexate	Increased methotrexate effect.
Griseofulvin	Increased griseofulvin effect.	Methylphenidate	Increased phenytoin effect.
Isoniazid	Increased phenytoin effect.	Molindone	Increased phenytoin effect.
MAO inhibitors	Increased polythiazide effect.	Nitrates	Excessive blood-pressure drop.
Methadone	Decreased methadone effect.	Oxyphenbutazone	Increased phenytoin effect.

GENERIC NAME OR DRUG CLASS	COMBINED EFFECT	GENERIC NAME OR DRUG CLASS	COMBINED EFFECT

PHENYTOIN continued

Oxprenolol	Increased antihypertensive effect. Dosages of both drugs may require adjustments.	Probenecid	Decreased probenecid effect.
Para-aminosalicylic acid (PAS)	Increased phenytoin effect.	Propranolol	Increased propranolol effect.
Phenothiazines	Increased phenytoin effect.	Quinidine	Increased quinidine effect.
Phenylbutazone	Increased phenytoin effect.	Sedatives	Increased sedative effect.
Potassium supplements	Decreased potassium effect.	Sulfa drugs	Increased phenytoin effect.
		Theophylline	Reduced anticonvulsant effect.

PRAZOSIN & POLYTHIAZIDE

Cholestyramine	Decreased polythiazide effect.	Lithium	Increased effect of lithium.
Chlorpromazine	Acute agitation.	MAO inhibitors	Blood-pressure drop. Increased polythiazide effect.
Cortisone drugs	Excessive potassium loss that causes dangerous heart rhythms.	Nitrates	Possible excessive blood-pressure drop.
Digitalis preparations	Excessive potassium loss that causes dangerous heart rhythms.	Oxprenolol	Increased antihypertensive effect. Dosages may require adjustments.
Diuretics (other)	Increased effect of other thiazide diuretics.	Potassium	Decreased potassium effect.
Indapamide	Increased diuretic effect.	Probenecid	Decreased probenecid effect.

PREDNISONE

Ethacrynic acid	Potassium depletion.	Isoniazid	Decreased isoniazid effect.
Furosemide	Potassium depletion.		
Glutethimide	Decreased prednisone effect.	Oxyphenbutazone	Possible ulcers.
		Phenylbutazone	Possible ulcers.
Indapamide	Possible excessive potassium loss, causing dangerous heartbeat irregularity.	Potassium supplements	Decreased potassium effect.
		Rifampin	Decreased prednisone effect.
Indomethacin	Increased prednisone effect.	Sympathomimetics	Possible glaucoma.
Insulin	Decreased insulin effect.		

PROBENECID & COLCHICINE

Generic Name or Drug Class	Combined Effect	Generic Name or Drug Class	Combined Effect
Pyrazinamide	Decreased probenecid effect.	Sleep inducers	Oversedation.
Salicylates	Decreased probenecid effect.	Sulfa drugs	Slows elimination. May cause harmful accumulation of sulfa.
Sedatives	Oversedation.	Tranquilizers	Oversedation.

PROCHLORPERAZINE & ISOPROPAMIDE

Generic Name or Drug Class	Combined Effect	Generic Name or Drug Class	Combined Effect
Nitrates	Increased internal-eye pressure.	supplements	ulcers with oral potassium tablets.
Orphenadrine	Increased isopropamide effect.	Quinidine	Impaired heart function. Dangerous mixture.
Phenothiazines	Increased isopropamide effect.	Sedatives	Increased sedative effect.
Phenytoin	Increased phenytoin effect.	Tranquilizers (other)	Increased tranquilizer effect.
Pilocarpine	Loss of pilocarpine effect in glaucoma treatment.	Vitamin C	Decreased isopropamide effect. Avoid large doses of vitamin C.

PYRILAMINE & PENTOBARBITAL

Generic Name or Drug Class	Combined Effect	Generic Name or Drug Class	Combined Effect
Griseofulvin	Decreased griseofulvin effect.	Pain relievers	Dangerous sedation. Avoid.
Hypnotics	Excess sedation. Avoid.	Sedatives	Dangerous sedation. Avoid.
Indapamide	Increased indapamide effect.	Sleep inducers	Dangerous sedation. Avoid.
MAO inhibitors	Increased pentobarbital effect. Avoid mixture. May be toxic.	Tranquilizers	Dangerous sedation. Avoid.
Mind-altering drugs	Dangerous sedation. Avoid.	Valproic acid	Dangerous sedation. Avoid.
Narcotics	Dangerous sedation. Avoid.		

RAUWOLFIA & THIAZIDE DIURETICS

Generic Name or Drug Class	Combined Effect	Generic Name or Drug Class	Combined Effect
Beta-adrenergic blockers	Increased effect of rauwolfia alkaloids. Excessive sedation.	Digitalis preparations	Excessive potassium loss that causes dangerous heart rhythms.
Cholestyramine	Decreased hydrocholorthiazide effect.	Diuretics (thiazide)	Increased effect of other thiazide diuretics.
Cortisone drugs	Excessive potassium loss that causes dangerous heart rhythms.	Dronabinol	Increased effect of both drugs. Avoid.
		Indapamide	Increased diuretic effect.
		Levodopa	Decreased levodopa effect.

GENERIC NAME OR DRUG CLASS	COMBINED EFFECT	GENERIC NAME OR DRUG CLASS	COMBINED EFFECT

RAUWOLFIA & THIAZIDE DIURETICS continued

GENERIC NAME OR DRUG CLASS	COMBINED EFFECT	GENERIC NAME OR DRUG CLASS	COMBINED EFFECT
Lithium	Increased effect of lithium.	Oxprenolol	Increased antihypertensive effect. Dosages of both drugs may require adjustments.
MAO inhibitors	Increased hydrochlorothiazide effect. Severe depression.		
Mind-altering drugs	Excessive sedation.	Potassium supplements	Decreased potassium effect.
Nitrates	Excessive blood-pressure drop.	Probenecid	Decreased probenecid effect.

RESERPINE & HYDRALAZINE

GENERIC NAME OR DRUG CLASS	COMBINED EFFECT	GENERIC NAME OR DRUG CLASS	COMBINED EFFECT
Aspirin	Decreased aspirin effect.	Dronabinol	Increased effect of both drugs. Avoid.
Beta-adrenergic blockers	Increased effect of rauwolfia alkaloids. Excessive sedation.	Levodopa	Decreased levodopa effect.
Digitalis preparations	Irregular heartbeat.	MAO inhibitors	Severe depression.
		Mind-altering drugs	Excessive sedation.
Diuretics (oral)	Increased effect of both drugs. When monitored carefully, combination may be beneficial in controlling hypertension.		

RESERPINE, HYDRALAZINE & HYDROCHLOROTHIAZIDE

GENERIC NAME OR DRUG CLASS	COMBINED EFFECT	GENERIC NAME OR DRUG CLASS	COMBINED EFFECT
Allopurinol	Decreased allopurinol effect.	Beta-adrenergic blockers	Increased effect of rauwolfia alkaloids. Excessive sedation.
Amphetamines	Decreased hydralazine effect.	Cholestyramine	Decreased hydrochlorothiazide effect.
Anticoagulants (oral)	Unpredictable increased or decreased effect of anticoagulant.	Cortisone drugs	Excessive potassium loss that causes dangerous heart rhythms.
Anticonvulsants	Serious change in seizure pattern.		
Antidepressants (tricyclic)	Dangerous drop in blood pressure. Avoid combination unless under medical supervision.	Digitalis preparations	Excessive potassium loss that causes dangerous heart rhythms.
Antihistamines	Increased antihistamine effect.	Diuretics (oral)	Increased effects of drugs. When monitored carefully, combination may be beneficial in controlling hypertension.
Antihypertensives (other)	Increased antihypertensive effect.		
Aspirin	Decreased aspirin effect.	Dronabinol	Increased effects of drugs.
Barbiturates	Increased hydrochlorothiazide effect.	Indapamide	Increased diuretic effect.

GENERIC NAME OR DRUG CLASS	COMBINED EFFECT	GENERIC NAME OR DRUG CLASS	COMBINED EFFECT

RESERPINE, HYDRALAZINE & HYDROCHLOROTHIAZIDE continued

GENERIC NAME OR DRUG CLASS	COMBINED EFFECT	GENERIC NAME OR DRUG CLASS	COMBINED EFFECT
Levodopa	Decreased levodopa effect.	Oxprenolol	Increased antihypertensive effect. Dosages of drug may require adjustments.
Lithium	Increased lithium effect.		
MAO inhibitors	Increased effects of drugs. Severe depression.	Potassium supplements	Decreased potassium effect.
Mind-altering drugs	Excessive sedation.	Probenecid	Decreased probenecid effect.
Nitrates	Excessive blood-pressure drop.		

SALICYLATES

GENERIC NAME OR DRUG CLASS	COMBINED EFFECT	GENERIC NAME OR DRUG CLASS	COMBINED EFFECT
Propranolol	Decreased salicylate effect.	Spironolactone	Decreased spironolactone effect.
Rauwolfia alkaloids	Decreased salicylate effect.	Sulfinpyrazone	Decreased sulfinpyrazone effect.
Salicylates (other)	Likely salicylate toxicity.	Vitamin C (large doses)	Possible salicylate toxicity.

SPIRONOLACTONE & HYDROCHLOROTHIAZIDE

GENERIC NAME OR DRUG CLASS	COMBINED EFFECT	GENERIC NAME OR DRUG CLASS	COMBINED EFFECT
Antihypertensives (other)	Increased antihypertensive effect.	Lithium	Increased effect of lithium. Likely lithium toxicity.
Aspirin	Decreased spironolactone effect.	MAO inhibitors	Increased hydrochlorothiazide effect.
Barbiturates	Increased hydrochlorothiazide effect.		
Cholestyramine	Decreased hydrochlorothiazide effect.	Nitrates	Excessive blood-pressure drop.
		Oxprenolol	Increased antihypertensive effect. Dosages of both drugs may require adjustment.
Cortisone drugs	Excessive potassium loss that causes dangerous heart rhythms.		
Diuretics (other)	Increased effect of both drugs. Beneficial if needed and dose is correct.	Potassium supplements	Decreased potassium effect. Dangerous potassium retention, causing possible heartbeat irregularity.
Indapamide	Increased diuretic effect.	Probenecid	Decreased probenecid effect.
Laxatives	Reduced potassium levels.	Sodium bicarbonate	Reduces high potassium levels.
		Triamterene	Dangerous potassium retention.

THEOPHYLLINE, EPHEDRINE, & BARBITURATES

GENERIC NAME OR DRUG CLASS	COMBINED EFFECT	GENERIC NAME OR DRUG CLASS	COMBINED EFFECT
Antihypertensives	Decreased antihypertensive effect.	Anti-inflammatory drugs (non-steroidal)	Decreased anti-inflammatory effect.

THEOPHYLLINE, EPHEDRINE, & BARBITURATES continued

GENERIC NAME OR DRUG CLASS	COMBINED EFFECT	GENERIC NAME OR DRUG CLASS	COMBINED EFFECT
Aspirin	Decreased aspirin effect.	Indapamide	Increased indapamide effect.
Beta-adrenergic blockers	Decreased effect of drugs.	Lincomycins	Increased bronchodilator effect.
Contraceptives (oral)	Decreased contraceptive effect.	Lithium	Decreased lithium effect.
Cortisone drugs	Decreased cortisone effect.	MAO inhibitors	Increased ephedrine effect. Dangerous blood-pressure rise.
Digitalis preparations	Serious heart-rhythm disturbances.	Mind-altering drugs	Dangerous sedation. Avoid.
Doxycycline	Decreased doxycycline effect.	Narcotics	Dangerous sedation. Avoid.
Dronabinol	Increased effect of drugs. Avoid.	Nitrates	Possible decreased effect of drugs.
Ephedrine	Increased effect of drugs.	Probenecid	Decreased effect of drugs.
Epinephrine	Increased effect of drugs.	Propranolol	Decreased bronchodilator effect.
Ergot preparations	Serious blood-pressure rise.	Pseudoephedrine	Increased pseudoephedrine effect.
Erythromycin	Increased bronchodilator effect.	Rauwolfia alkaloids	Rapid heartbeat.
Furosemide	Increased furosemide effect.	Sulfinpyrazone	Decreased sulfinpyrazone effect.
Griseofulvin	Decreased griseofulvin effect.	Troleandomycin	Increased bronchodilator effect.
Guanethidine	Decreased effect of drugs.	Valproic acid	Increased barbiturate effect.

THEOPHYLLINE, EPHEDRINE, GUAIFENESIN & BARBITURATES

GENERIC NAME OR DRUG CLASS	COMBINED EFFECT	GENERIC NAME OR DRUG CLASS	COMBINED EFFECT
Antidepressants (tricyclics)	Decreased antidepressant effect.	Digitalis preparations	Serious heart-rhythm disturbances.
Antidiabetics (oral)	Increased phenobarbital effect.	Digitoxin	Decreased digitoxin effect.
Antihistamines	Dangerous sedation. Avoid.	Doxycycline	Decreased doxycycline effect.
Anti-inflammatory drugs (non-steroid)	Decreased anti-inflammatory effect.	Dronabinol	Increased effect of drugs.
Aspirin (other)	Decreased aspirin effect.	Ephedrine	Increased effect of drugs.
Beta-adrenergic blockers	Decreased effect of drugs.	Ergot preparations	Serious blood-pressure rise.
Contraceptives (oral)	Decreased contraceptive effect.	Erythromycin	Increased bronchodilator effect.
Cortisone drugs	Increased cortisone effect.	Furosemide	Increased furosemide effect.

GENERIC NAME OR DRUG CLASS	COMBINED EFFECT	GENERIC NAME OR DRUG CLASS	COMBINED EFFECT

THEOPHYLLINE, EPHEDRINE, GUAIFENESIN & BARBITURATES continued

GENERIC NAME OR DRUG CLASS	COMBINED EFFECT	GENERIC NAME OR DRUG CLASS	COMBINED EFFECT
Griseofulvin	Decreased griseofulvin effect.	Probenecid	Decreased effect of drugs.
Guanethidine	Decreased effect of drugs.	Propranolol	Decreased bronchodilator effect.
Indapamide	Increased indapamide effect.	Pseudoephedrine	Increased pseudoephedrine effect.
Lincomycins	Increased bronchodilator effect.	Rauwolfia alkaloids	Rapid heartbeat.
Lithium	Decreased lithium effect.	Sedatives	Dangerous sedation. Avoid.
MAO inhibitors	Increased phenobarbital effect.	Sleep inducers	Dangerous sedation. Avoid.
Mind-altering drugs	Dangerous sedation. Avoid.	Sulfinpyrazone	Decreased sulfinpyrazone effect.
Narcotics	Dangerous sedation. Avoid.	Tranquilizers	Dangerous sedation. Avoid.
Nitrates	Possible decreased effect of drugs.	Troleandomycin	Increased bronchodilator effect.
Pain relievers	Dangerous sedation. Avoid.	Valproic acid	Increased phenobarbital effect.

THEOPHYLLINE, EPHEDRINE & HYDROXYZINE

GENERIC NAME OR DRUG CLASS	COMBINED EFFECT	GENERIC NAME OR DRUG CLASS	COMBINED EFFECT
Beta-adrenergic blockers	Decreased effect of drugs.	MAO inhibitors	Increased ephedrine effect. Dangerous blood-pressure rise.
Digitalis preparations	Serious heart-rhythm disturbances.	Nitrates	Possible decreased effect of drugs.
Dronabinol	Increased effect of drugs.	Pain relievers	Increased effect of drugs.
Ephedrine	Increased effect of drugs.	Probenecid	Decreased effect of drugs.
Epinephrine	Increased effect of drugs.	Propranolol	Decreased bronchodilator effect.
Ergot preparations	Serious blood-pressure rise.	Pseudoephedrine	Increased pseudoephedrine effect.
Erythromycin	Increased bronchodilator effect.	Rauwolfia alkaloids	Rapid heartbeat.
Furosemide	Increased furosemide effect.	Sulfinpyrazone	Decreased sulfinpyrazone effect.
Guanethidine	Decreased effect of drugs.	Tranquilizers	Increased effect of drugs.
Lincomycins	Increased bronchodilator effect.	Troleandomycin	Increased bronchodilator effect.
Lithium	Decreased lithium effect.		

TRIAMETERINE & HYDROCHOLOROTHIAZIDE

GENERIC NAME OR DRUG CLASS	COMBINED EFFECT	GENERIC NAME OR DRUG CLASS	COMBINED EFFECT
Oxprenolol	Increased antihypertensive effect. Dosages may require adjustments.	**Probenecid**	Decreased probenecid effect.
Potassium supplements	Possible excessive potassium retention. Decreased potassium effect.	**Spironolactone**	Dangerous retention of potassium.

ADDITIONAL DRUG INTERACTIONS

Glossary
The following medical terms are found in the drug charts.

A

A.C.E. inhibitor—Angiotensin-converting enzyme (A.C.E.) inhibitor reduces aldosterone secretion and reduces blood pressure. The inhibitors decrease the rate of conversion of Angiotensin I into Angiotensin II, which is the normal process for the angiotensin-converting enzyme.

Acute—Having a short and relatively severe course.

Addiction—Psychological or physiological dependence upon a drug.

Addison's Disease—Changes in the body caused by a deficiency of hormones manufactured by the adrenal gland. Usually fatal .if untreated.

Adrenal Cortex—Center of the adrenal gland.

Adrenal Gland—Gland next to the kidney that produces cortisone and epinephrine (adrenalin).

Alkylating Agent—Chemical used to treat malignant diseases.

Allergy—Excessive sensitivity to a substance.

Amebiasis—Infection with amoeba, one-celled organisms. Causes diarrhea, fever and abdominal cramps.

Amphetamine—Drug that stimulates the brain and central nervous system, increases blood pressure, reduces nasal congestion and is habit-forming.

Analgesic—Agent that reduces pain without reducing consciousness.

Anaphylaxis—Severe allergic response to a substance. Symptoms are wheezing, itching, hives, nasal congestion, intense burning of hands and feet, collapse, loss of consciousness and cardiac arrest. Symptoms appear within a few seconds or minutes after exposure. Anaphylaxis is a severe medical emergency. Without appropriate treatment, it can cause death. Instructions for home treatment for anaphylaxis are on the front inside cover.

Anemia—Not enough healthy red-blood cells in the bloodstream or too little hemoglobin in the red-blood cells. Anemia is caused by imbalance of blood loss and blood production.

Anemia, Hemolytic—Anemia caused by a shortened life span of red-blood cells. The body can't manufacture new cells fast enough to replace old cells.

Anemia, Iron-Deficiency—Anemia caused when iron necessary to manufacture red-blood cells is not available.

Anemia, Pernicious—Anemia caused by a vitamin B-12 deficiency. Symptoms include weakness, fatigue, numbness and tingling of the hands or feet, and degeneration of the central nervous system.

Anemia, Sickle-Cell—Anemia caused by defective hemoglobin that deprives red-blood cells of oxygen, making them sickle-shaped.

Anesthetic—Drug that eliminates the sensation of pain.

Angina (Angina Pectoris)—Chest pain with a sensation of suffocation and impending death. Caused by a temporary reduction in the amount of oxygen to the heart muscle through diseased coronary arteries.

Antacid—Chemical that neutralizes acid, usually in the stomach.

Antibiotic—Chemical that inhibits the growth of or kills germs.

Anticholinergic—Drug that chemically inhibits nerve impulses through the parasympathetic nervous system.

Anticoagulant—Drug that inhibits blood clotting.

Antiemetic—Drug that prevents or stops nausea and vomiting.

Antihypertensive—Medication to reduce blood pressure.

Appendicitis—Inflammation or infection of the appendix. Symptoms include loss of appetite, nausea, low-grade fever and tenderness in the lower right of the abdomen.

Artery—Blood vessel carrying blood away from the heart.

Asthma—Recurrent attacks of breathing difficulty due to spasms and contractions of the bronchial tubes.

B

Bacteria—Microscopic organism. Some bacteria contribute to health; others (germs) cause disease.

Basal Area of Brain—Part of the brain that regulates muscle control and tone.

Blood Count—Laboratory studies to count white-blood cells, red-blood cells, platelets and other elements of the blood.

Blood Pressure, Diastolic—Pressure (usually recorded in millimeters of mercury) in the large arteries of the body when the heart muscle is relaxed and filling for the next contraction.

Blood Pressure, Systolic—Pressure (usually recorded in millimeters of mercury) in the large arteries of the body at the instant the heart muscle contracts.

Blood Sugar (Blood Glucose)—Necessary element in the blood to sustain life.

C

Cataract—Loss of transparency in the lens of the eye.

Cell—Unit of protoplasm, the essential living matter of all plants and animals.

Cephalosporin—Antibiotic that kills many bacterial germs that penicillin and sulfa drugs can't destroy.

Cholinergic (also Parasympathomimetic)—Chemical that facilitates passage of nerve impulses through the parasympathetic nervous system.

Cirrhosis—Disease that scars and destroys liver tissue.

Cold Urticaria—Hives that appear in areas of the body exposed to the cold.

Colitis, Ulcerative—Chronic, recurring ulcers of the colon for unknown reasons.

Collagen—Support tissue of skin, tendon, bone, cartilage and connective tissue.

Colostomy—Surgical opening from the colon, the large intestine, to the outside of the body.

Congestive—Excess accumulation of blood. In congestive heart failure, congestion occurs in the lungs, liver, kidney and other parts to cause shortness of breath, swelling of the ankles and feet, rapid heartbeat and other symptoms.

Constriction—Tightness or pressure.

Contraceptive—Something that prevents pregnancy.

Convulsions—Violent, uncontrollable contractions of the voluntary muscles.

Corticosteroid (Adrenocorticosteroid)—Steroid hormones produced by the body's adrenal cortex or their synthetic equivalents.

Cystitis—Inflammation of the urinary bladder.

D

Delirium—Temporary mental disturbance characterized by hallucinations, agitation and incoherence.

Diabetes—Metabolic disorder in which the body can't use carbohydrates efficiently. This leads to a dangerously high level of glucose (a carbohydrate) in the blood.

Dialysis—Procedure to filter waste products from the bloodstream of patients with kidney failure.

Dilation—Enlargement.

Disulfiram Reaction—Disulfiram (Antabuse) is a drug to treat alcoholism. When alcohol in the bloodstream interacts with disulfiram, it causes a flushed face, severe headache, chest pains, shortness of breath, nausea, vomiting, sweating and weakness. Severe reactions may cause death.

A disulfiram reaction is the interaction of any drug with alcohol or another drug to produce these symptoms.

Duodenum—The first 12 inches of the small intestine.

E

Eczema—Disorder of the skin with redness, itching, blisters, weeping and abnormal pigmentation.

Electrolyte—Substance that can transmit electrical impulses when dissolved in body fluids.

Embolism—Sudden blockage of an artery by a clot or foreign material in the blood.

Emphysema—Disease in which the lung's air sacs lose elasticity, and air accumulates in the lungs.

Endometriosis—Condition in which uterus tissue is found outside the uterus. Can cause pain, abnormal menstruation and infertility.

Enzyme—Protein chemical that can accelerate a chemical reaction in the body.

Epilepsy—Episodes of brain disturbance that cause convulsions and loss of consciousness.

Esophagitis—Inflammation of the lower part of the esophagus, the tube connecting the throat and the stomach.

Estrogens—Female sex hormones that stimulate female characteristics and prepare the uterus for fertilization.

Eustachian Tube—Small passage from the middle ear to the sinuses and nasal passages.

Extremity—Arm, leg, hand or foot.

F

Fecal Impaction—Condition in which feces become firmly wedged in the rectum.

Fibrocystic Breast Disease—Overgrowth of fibrous tissue in the breast, producing non-malignant cysts.

Fibroid Tumors—Non-malignant tumors of the muscular layer of the uterus.

Flu (Influenza)—A virus infection of the respiratory tract that lasts three to ten days. Symptoms include headache, fever, runny nose, cough, tiredness and muscle aches.

Folliculitis—Inflammation of a follicle.

G

G6PD—Deficiency of glucose 6-phosphate, necessary for glucose metabolism.

Gastritis—Inflammation of the stomach.

Gastrointestinal—Stomach and intestinal tract.

Gland—Cells that manufacture and excrete materials not required for their own metabolic needs.

Glaucoma—Eye disease in which increased pressure inside the eye damages the optic nerve, causes pain and changes vision.

Glucagon—Injectable drug that immediately elevates blood sugar by mobilizing glycogen from the liver.

H

Hangover Effect—The same feelings as a "hangover" after too much alcohol consumption. Symptoms include headache, irritability and nausea.

Hemochromatosis—Disorder of iron metabolism in which excessive iron is deposited in and damages body tissues, particularly liver and pancreas.

Hemoglobin—Pigment that carries oxygen in red-blood cells.

Hemorrhage—Heavy bleeding.

Hemosiderosis—Increase of iron deposits in body tissues without tissue damage.

Hepatitis—Inflammation of liver cells, usually accompanied by jaundice.

Hiatal Hernia—Section of stomach that protrudes into the chest cavity.

Histamine—Chemical in body tissues that dilates the smallest blood vessels, constricts the smooth muscle surrounding the bronchial tubes and stimulates stomach secretions.

History—Past medical events in a patient's life.

Hives—Elevated patches on the skin that are redder or paler than surrounding skin and often itch severely.

Hormone—Chemical substance produced in the body to regulate other body functions.

Hypertension—High blood pressure.

Hypocalcemia—Abnormally low level of calcium in the blood.

Hypoglycemia—Low blood sugar (blood glucose). A critically low blood-sugar level will interfere with normal brain function and can damage the brain permanently.

I

Ichthyosis—Skin disorder with dryness, scaling and roughness.

Ileitis—Inflammation of the ileum, the last section of the small intestine.

Ileostomy—Surgical opening from the ileum, the end of the small intestine, to the outside of the body.

Impotence—Male's inability to achieve or sustain erection of the penis for sexual intercourse.

Insomnia—Sleeplessness.

Interaction—Change in the body's response to one drug when another is taken. Interaction may increase the effect of one or both drugs, decrease the effect of one or both drugs, or cause toxicity.

J

Jaundice—Symptoms of liver damage, bile obstruction or red-blood-cell destruction. Includes yellowed whites of the eyes, yellow skin, dark urine and light stool.

K

Keratosis—Growth that is an accumulation of cells from the outer skin layers.

Kidney Stones—Small, solid stones made from calcium, cholesterol, cysteine and other body chemicals.

L

Lupus—Serious disorder of connective tissue that primarily affects women. Varies in severity with skin eruptions, joint inflammation, low white-blood cell count and damage to internal organs, especially the kidney.

Lymph Glands—Glands in the lymph vessels throughout the body that trap foreign and infectious matter and protect the bloodstream from infection.

M

Manic-Depressive Illness—Psychosis with alternating cycles of excessive enthusiasm and depression.

Mast Cell—Connective-tissue cell.

Menopause—The end of menstruation in the female, often accompanied by irritability, hot flushes, changes in the skin and bones and vaginal dryness.

Metabolism—Process of using nutrients and energy to build and break down wastes.

Migraine—Periodic headaches caused by constriction of arteries to the skull. Symptoms include severe pain, vision disturbances, nausea, vomiting and light sensitivity.

Mind-Altering Drugs—Any drug that decreases alertness, perception, concentration, contact with reality or muscular coordination.

Myasthenia Gravis—Disease of the muscles characterized by fatigue and progressive paralysis. It is usually confined to muscles of the face, lips, tongue and neck.

N

Narcotic—Drug, usually addictive, that produces stupor.

O

Osteoporosis—Softening of bones caused by a loss of chemicals usually found in bone.

Ovary—Female sexual gland where eggs mature and ripen for fertilization.

P

Palpitations—Rapid heartbeat noticeable to the patient.

Pancreatitis—Serious inflammation or infection of the pancreas that causes upper abdominal pain.

Parkinson's Disease—Disease of the central nervous system. Characteristics are a fixed, emotionless expression of the face, tremor, slower muscle movements, weakness, changed gait and a peculiar posture.

Pellagra—Disease caused by a deficiency of the water-soluble vitamin, thiamine (vitamin B-1). Symptoms include brain disturbance, diarrhea and skin inflammation.

Penicillin—Chemical substance (antibiotic) originally discovered as a product of mold, which can kill some bacterial germs.

Phlegm—Thick mucus secreted by glands in the respiratory tract.

Pinworms—Common intestinal parasite that causes rectal itching and irritation.

Pituitary Gland—Gland at the base of the brain that secretes hormones to stimulate growth and other glands to produce hormones.

Platelet—Disc-shaped element of the blood, smaller than red- or white-blood cells, necessary for blood clotting.

Polyp—Growth on a mucous membrane.

Porphyria—Inherited metabolic disorder characterized by changes in the nervous system and kidney.

Post-partum—Following delivery of a baby.

Potassium—Important chemical found in body cells.

Potassium Foods—Foods high in potassium content, including dried apricots and peaches, lentils, raisins, citrus and whole-grain cereals.

Prostate—Gland in the male that surrounds the neck of the bladder and the urethra.

Prothrombin—Blood substance essential in clotting.

Prothrombin Time—Laboratory study used to follow prothrombin activity and keep coagulation safe.

Psoriasis—Chronic, inherited skin disease. Symptoms are lesions with silvery scales on the edges.

Psychosis—Mental disorder characterized by deranged personality, loss of contact with reality and possible delusions, hallucinations or illusions.

Purine Foods—Foods that are metabolized into uric acid. Foods high in purines include anchovies, liver, brains, sweetbreads, sardines, kidney, oysters, gravy and meat extracts.

R

RDA—Recommended daily allowance of a vitamin or mineral.

Rebound Effect—Return of a condition, often with increased severity, once the prescribed drug is withdrawn.

Renal—Pertaining to the kidney.

Retina—Innermost covering of the eyeball on which the image is formed.

Reye's Syndrome—Rare, sometimes fatal, disease of children that causes brain and liver damage.

Rickets—Bone disease caused by vitamin-D deficiency. Bones become bent and distorted during infancy or childhood.

S

Sedative—Drug that reduces excitement or anxiety.

Seizure—Brain disorder causing changes of consciousness or convulsions.

Sinusitis—Inflammation or infection of the sinus cavities in the skull.

Streptococcus—Bacteria that causes infections in the throat, respiratory system and skin. Improperly treated, can lead to disease in the heart, joints and kidneys.

Stroke—Sudden, severe attack. Usually sudden paralysis from injury to the brain or spinal cord caused by a blood clot or hemorrhage in the brain.

Stupor—Near unconsciousness.

Sublingual—Under the tongue. Some drugs are absorbed almost as quickly this way as by injection.

T

Tardive Dyskinesia—Involuntary movements of the jaw, lips and tongue caused by an unpredictable drug reaction.

Thrombophlebitis—Inflammation of a vein caused by a blood clot in the vein.

Thyroid—Gland in the neck that manufactures and secretes several hormones.

Tic-douloureaux—Painful condition caused by inflammation of a nerve in the face.

Toxicity—Poisonous reaction to a drug that impairs body functions or damages cells.

Tranquilizer—Drug that calms a person without clouding consciousness.

Tremor—Involuntary trembling.

Trichomoniasis—Infestation of the vagina by *trichomonas,* an infectious organism. The infection causes itching, vaginal discharge and irritation.

Triglyceride—Fatty chemical manufactured from carbohydrates for storage in fat cells.

Tyramine—Normal chemical component of the body that helps sustain blood pressure. Can rise to fatal levels in combination with some drugs.

Tyramine is found in many foods:

Beverages—Alcoholic beverages, especially Chianti or robust red wines, vermouth, ale, beer.

Breads—Homemade bread with a lot of yeast and breads or crackers containing cheese.

Fats—Sour cream.

Fruits—Bananas, red plums, avocados, figs, raisins.

Meats and meat substitutes—Aged game, liver, canned meats, salami, sausage, cheese, salted dried fish, pickled herring.

Vegetables—Italian broad beans, green-bean pods, eggplant.

Miscellaneous—Yeast concentrates or extracts, marmite, soup cubes, commercial gravy, soy sauce, any protein food that has been stored improperly or is spoiled.

U

Ulcer, Peptic—Open sore on the mucous membrane of the esophagus, stomach or duodenum caused by stomach acid.

Urethra—Hollow tube through which urine (and semen in men) is discharged.

Urethritis—Inflammation or infection of the urethra.

Uterus—Also called *womb*. A hollow muscular organ in the female in which the embryo develops into a fetus.

V
Vascular—Pertaining to blood vessels.
Virus—Infectious organism that reproduces in the cells of the infected host.

Y
Yeast—A single-cell organism that can cause infections of the mouth, vagina, skin and parts of the gastrointestinal system.

GUIDE TO INDEX

Alphabetical entries in the index include three categories—generic names, brand names and drug-class names.

1. Generic names appear in capital letter, followed by their chart page number:
   > ASPIRIN, 66

2. Brand names appear in *italic*, followed by their generic ingredient and chart page number.
   > *Bayer*—See ASPIRIN, 66

   Some brands contain two or more generic ingredients. These generic ingredients are listed in capital letters following the brand name:
   > *Cefinal*—See
   > ASPIRIN, 66
   > CAFFEINE, 128

   Some brands contain generic ingredients that are not included in this book because of space limitations. These generics are designated by (NL), which means "not listed."
   > *Fedrazil*—See
   > CHLORCYCLIZINE (NL)
   > PSEUDOEPHEDRINE, 752

3. Drug-class names appear in regular type, capital and lower-case letters. All generic drug names in this book that fall into a drug class are listed after the class name.
   > Analgesics
   > ACETAMINOPHEN, 4
   > ASPIRIN, 66
   > CARBAMAZEPINE, 140
   > PHENACETIN, 672
   > SALICYLATES, 796

PROPRANOLOL 750
Apo-Quinidine—See QUINIDINE 772
Apo-Sulfamethoxazole—See
  SULFAMETHOXAZOLE 824
Apo-Sulfatrim—See
  SULFAMETHOXAZOLE 824
  TRIMETHOPRIM 914
Apo-Sulfinpyrazone—See
  SULFINPYRAZONE 828
Apo-Sulfisoxazole—See
  SULFISOXAZOLE 830
Apo-Tetra—See TETRACYCLINES 850
Apo-Thioridazine—See
  THIORIDAZINE 864
Apo-Tolbutamide—See
  TOLBUTAMIDE 882
Apo-Trifluoperazine—See
  TRIFLUOPERAZINE 904
Apo-Trihex—See
  TRIHEXYPHENIDYL 908
A-poxide—See CHLORDIAZEPOXIDE 176
  CHLORDIAZEPOXIDE &
    CLIDINIUM 180
APPETITE SUPPRESSANTS 64
Aprazone—See SULFINPYRAZONE 828
Apresazide—See HYDRALAZINE &
    HYDROCHLOROTHIAZIDE 424
  HYDROCHLOROTHIAZIDE 426
Apresodez—See HYDRALAZINE &
    HYDROCHLOROTHIAZIDE 424
Apresoline—See HYDRALAZINE 422
Apresoline-Esidrix—See HYDRALAZINE &
    HYDROCHLOROTHIAZIDE 424
  HYDROCHLOROTHIAZIDE 426
Apsifen—See IBUPROFEN 438
Apsifen-F—See IBUPROFEN 438
Aquachloral—See
  CHLORAL HYDRATE 170
Aquachloral Suprettes—See
  CHLORAL HYDRATE 170
Aquamox—See QUINETHAZONE 770
Aquaphyllin—See XANTHINE
  BRONCHODILATORS 938
Aquasol A—See VITAMIN A 924
Aquasol E—See VITAMIN E 932
Aquastat—See BENZTHIAZIDE 92
Aquatag—See BENZTHIAZIDE 92
Aquatensen—See
  METHYCLOTHIAZIDE 550
Aralen—See CHLOROQUINE 182
Arcoban—See MEPROBAMATE 522
Arco-Cee—See ASCORBIC ACID
  (VITAMIN C) 928
Arco-Lase—See ATROPINE 70
Arco-Lase Plus—See
  HYOSCYAMINE 436
Arcylate—See SALICYLATES 796
Aristocort—See
  ADRENOCORTICOIDS (TOPICAL) 16
  TRIAMCINOLONE 890
Aristocort-A—See
  ADRENOCORTICOIDS (TOPICAL) 16
Aristocort C—See
  ADRENOCORTICOIDS (TOPICAL) 16
Aristocort D—See
  ADRENOCORTICOIDS (TOPICAL) 16
Aristocort R—See
  ADRENOCORTICOIDS (TOPICAL) 16
Aristospan—See TRIAMCINOLONE 890
Arlidin—See NYLIDRIN 620
Arlidin Forte—See NYLIDRIN 620
Arm-a-Char—See
  CHARCOAL, ACTIVATED 166
Arm-a-Med Isoetharine—See
  ISOETHARINE 450
Arm and Hammer Baking Soda—See
  SODIUM BICARBONATE 808
Armour—See THYROID 870
Aromatic Cascara Fluidextract—See
  CASCARA 154
Artane—See TRIHEXYPHENIDYL 908
Artane Sequels—See
  TRIHEXYPHENIDYL 908
Artha-G—See SALICYLATES 796
Arthralgen—See

ACETAMINOPHEN 4
ACETAMINOPHEN & SALICYLATES 6
NARCOTIC ANALGESICS 594
Arthritis Bayer Timed-Release—See
  ASPIRIN 66
Arthritis Pain Formula—See
  ASPIRIN 66
  MAGNESIUM HYDROXIDE 498
Arthropan—See SALICYLATES 796
Articulose—See PREDNISOLONE 722
Articulose-L.A.—See
  TRIAMCINOLONE 890
A.S.A. & Codeine Compound—See
  ASPIRIN 66
A.S.A. and Codeine Compound—See
  NARCOTIC & ASPIRIN 596
A.S.A. Compound—See
  ASPIRIN 66
  CAFFEINE 128
A.S.A. Enseals—See ASPIRIN 66
Asbcon G Inlay Tabs—See
  THEOPHYLLINE & GUAIFENESIN 858
Asbron—See
  UAIFENESIN 404
  PHENYLPROPANOLAMINE 690
  XANTHINE BRONCHODILATORS 938
Ascendin—See TRICYCLIC
  ANTIDEPRESSANTS 900
Ascodeen-30—See ASPIRIN 66
Ascorbajen—See ASCORBIC ACID
  (VITAMIN C) 928
ASCORBIC ACID (VITAMIN C) 928
Ascorbicap—See ASCORBIC ACID
  (VITAMIN C) 928
Ascoril—See
  ASCORBIC ACID (VITAMIN C) 928
Ascriptin—See ASPIRIN 66
Ascriptin A/D—See ASPIRIN 66
Ascriptin w/Codeine—See
  ASPIRIN 66
  NARCOTIC ANALGESICS 594
  NARCOTIC & ASPIRIN 596
Asma—See
  GUAIFENESIN 404
  XANTHINE BRONCHODILATORS 938
Asmalix—See XANTHINE
  BRONCHODILATORS 938
Asminly—See
  EPHEDRINE 326
  PHENOBARBITAL 678
  XANTHINE BRONCHODILATORS 938
Asmolin—See EPINEPHRINE 328
Aso-Sulfisoxazole—See SULFONAMIDES
  & PHENAZOPYRIDINE 832
A-Spas—See DICYCLOMINE 280
Asperbuf—See ASPIRIN 66
Aspergum—See ASPIRIN 66
Asphac-G—See CAFFEINE 128
Aspir-10—See ASPIRIN 66
ASPIRIN 66
ASPIRIN & BUTALBITAL (Also contains
  caffeine) 122
ASPIRIN, CAFFEINE &
  ORPHENADRINE 626
ASPIRIN & CODEINE—See NARCOTIC &
  ASPIRIN 596
ASPIRIN, CODEINE & BUTALBITAL (Also
  contains caffeine) 124
ASPIRIN, CODEINE & CAFFEINE—See
  NARCOTIC & ASPIRIN 596
Aspirin Compound w/Codeine—See
  ASPIRIN 66
  CAFFEINE 128
  NARCOTIC ANALGESICS 594
  PHENACETIN 672
Aspirin-Free Excedrin—See
  ACETAMINOPHEN 4
ASPIRIN & MEPROBAMATE 524
Aspirjen Jr.—See ASPIRIN 66
Asthma Haler—See EPINEPHRINE 328
Asthma Nefrin—See EPINEPHRINE 328
Asthmophylline—See XANTHINE
  BRONCHODILATORS 938
Astrin—See ASPIRIN 66
Atarax—See HYDROXYZINE 434

Ataraxoid—See HYDROXYZINE 434
Atasol—See ACETAMINOPHEN 4
Atasol with Codeine—See NARCOTIC &
  ACETAMINOPHEN 592
ATENOLOL & CHLORTHALIDONE—See
  BETA-ADRENERGIC BLOCKING
  AGENTS & THIAZIDE DIURETICS 96
Ativan—See LORAZEPAM 492
Atozine—See HYDROXYZINE 434
Atrobarbital—See ATROPINE 70
Atrocap—See BELLADONNA 84
Atromal—See ATROPINE 70
Atromid-S—See CLOFIBRATE 218
ATROPINE 70
Atropine Bufopto—See ATROPINE 70
ATROPINE & DIFENOXIN 284
ATROPINE & DIPHENOXYLATE 300
ATROPINE, HYOSCYAMINE,
  METHENAMINE, METHYLENE BLUE,
  PHENYLSALICYLATE & BENZOIC
  ACID 72
ATROPINE, HYOSCYAMINE,
  SCOPOLAMINE &
  BUTABARBITAL—See
  BELLADONNA
ATROPINE, HYOSCYAMINE,
  SCOPOLAMINE &
  PHENOBARBITAL—See BELLADONNA
  ALKALOIDS & BARBITURATES 86
ATROPINE & PHENOBARBITAL—See
  BELLADONNA ALKALOIDS &
  BARBITURATES 86
ATROPINE, SCOPOLAMINE,
  PHENOBARBITAL, PANCREATIN,
  PEPSIN, BILE SALTS &
  HYOSCYAMINE 640
Atropisol—See ATROPINE 70
Atrosed—See ATROPINE 70
  BELLADONNA 84
A/T/S—See ERYTHROMYCINS 342
Augmentin—See AMOXICILLIN 48
AURANOFIN (oral)—See
  GOLD COMPOUNDS 400
Aurothioglucose (injection)—See
  GOLD COMPOUNDS 400
Aventyl—See TRICYCLIC
  ANTIDEPRESSANTS 900
Avlosulfon—See DAPSONE 264
Axon—See
  PHENYLPROPANOLAMINE 690
Axotal—See ACETAMINOPHEN 4
  ASPIRIN 66
  NARCOTIC ANALGESICS 594
  TALBUTAL (BUTALBITAL) 838
Ayercillin—See PENICILLIN G 660
Ayerst Epitrate—See EPINEPHRINE 328
Aygestin—See
  NORETHINDRONE ACETATE 614
AZATADINE 74
AZIDOTHYMIDINE (AZT), Also Called
  ZIDOVUDINE 76
Azma Aid—See THEOPHYLLINE,
  EPHEDRINE & BARBITURATES 852
Azmacort—See TRIAMCINOLONE 890
Azo Gantanol—See
  SULFAMETHOXAZOLE 824
Azo Gantanol—See SULFONAMIDES &
  PHENAZOPYRIDINE 832
Azo Gantrisin—See SULFONAMIDES &
  PHENAZOPYRIDINE 832
Azo Sulfamethoxazole—See
  SULFONAMIDES &
  PHENAZOPYRIDINE 832
Azo-100—See PHENAZOPYRIDINE 674
Azodine—See PHENAZOPYRIDINE 674
Azo-Gantanol—See
  PHENAZOPYRIDINE 674
Azo-Gantrisin—See
  PHENAZOPYRIDINE 674
  SULFISOXAZOLE 830
Azolid—See PHENYLBUTAZONE 686
Azolinic Acid—See CINOXACIN 208
Azo-Mandelamine—See
  METHENAMINE 540

D

Dacodyl—See BISACODYL 104
Dactil Phenobarbital—See
   PHENOBARBITAL 678
Dainite—See EPHEDRINE 326
Dainite-KI—See PHENOBARBITAL 678
Dalacin C—See
   CLINDAMYCIN 216
   LINCOMYCIN 482
Dalalon L.A.—See
   DEXAMETHASONE 268
Dalalone—See DEXAMETHASONE 268
Dallergy—See
   ATROPINE 70
   CHLORPHENIRAMINE 190
   PHENYLEPHRINE 688
   SCOPOLAMINE (HYOSCINE) 798
Dalmane—See FLURAZEPAM 384
Dal-Sinus—See
   PHENYLPROPANOLAMINE 690
Daltose—See VITAMIN E 932

Damason-P—See NARCOTIC &
   ASPIRIN 596
Danabol—See ANDROGENS 54
DANAZOL 258
Danilone—See
   ANTICOAGULANTS (ORAL) 58
Danocrine—See DANAZOL 258
DANTHRON 260
Dantoin—See PHENYTOIN 694
Dantrium—See DANTROLENE 262
DANTROLENE 262
Dapa—See ACETAMINOPHEN 4
Dapase—See
   ACETAMINOPHEN 4
   NARCOTIC ANALGESICS 594
Dapex—See APPETITE
   SUPPRESSANTS 64
Dapex-37.5—See APPETITE
   SUPPRESSANTS 64
DAPSONE 264
Daranide—See CARBONATE
   ANHYDRASE INHIBITORS 148
Darbid—See ISOPROPAMIDE 456
Daricon PB—See PHENOBARBITAL 678
Darvocet-N—See
   ACETAMINOPHEN 4
   NARCOTIC & ACETAMINOPHEN 592
Darvocet-N 100—See NARCOTIC
   ANALGESICS 594
Darvon—See NARCOTIC
   ANALGESICS 594
Darvon Compound—See
   ASPIRIN 66
   CAFFEINE 128
   NARCOTIC & ASPIRIN 596
Darvon with A.S.A.—See NARCOTIC &
   ASPIRIN 596
Darvon-N with A.S.A.—See NARCOTIC &
   ASPIRIN 596
Dasicon—See
   ASPIRIN 66
   CAFFEINE 128
Datril—See ACETAMINOPHEN 4
Day-Barb—See BUTABARBITAL 120
Dazamide—See CARBONATE
   ANHYDRASE INHIBITORS 148
DDS—See DAPSONE 264
De Tal—See HYOSCYAMINE 436
De Witt's—See MAGNESIUM
   CARBONATE 494
De Witts—See ALUMINUM
   HYDROXIDE 26
Deapril-ST—See ERGOLOID
   MESYLATES 330
Decaderm—See
   ADRENOCORTICOIDS (TOPICAL) 16
Decaderm—See DEXAMETHASONE 268
Decadrol—See DEXAMETHASONE 268
Decadron—See
   ADRENOCORTICOIDS (TOPICAL) 16
   DEXAMETHASONE 268
Decadron L.A.—See
   DEXAMETHASONE 268

Decadron Respihaler—See
   DEXAMETHASONE 268
Decadron Turbinaire—See
   DEXAMETHASONE 268
Decadron with Xylocaine—See
   DEXAMETHASONE 268
Deca-Durabolin—See ANDROGENS 54
Decagesic—See ASPIRIN 66
Decajet—See DEXAMETHASONE 268
Decameth—See DEXAMETHASONE 268
Decapryn—See DOXYLAMINE 318
Decaspray—See
   ADRENOCORTICOIDS (TOPICAL) 16
   DEXAMETHASONE 268
Decholin—See
   DEHYDROCHOLIC ACID 266
Declobese—See
   AMPHETAMINE 50
   DEXTROAMPHETAMINE 272
Declomycin—See TETRACYCLINES 850
Declostatin—See NYSTATIN 622
Decobel—See BELLADONNA 84
Decofed—See PSEUDOEPHEDRINE 752
De-Comberol—See TESTOSTERONE &
   ESTRADIOL 848
Deconamine—See
   CHLORPHENIRAMINE 190
   PSEUDOEPHEDRINE 752
Decongestabs—See
   PHENYLTOLOXAMINE 692
Decongestant-P—See
   PHENYLPROPANOLAMINE 690

Dermacoat—See
   ANESTHETICS (TOPICAL) 56
   ADRENOCORTICOIDS (TOPICAL) 16
   HYDROCORTISONE (CORTISOL) 428
DermiCort—See
   ADRENOCORTICOIDS (TOPICAL) 16
Dermodex—See BENZOYL
   PEROXIDE 90
Dermo-Gen—See ANESTHETICS
   (TOPICAL) 56
Dermolate—See
   ADRENOCORTICOIDS (TOPICAL) 16
Derma-Medicone—See ANESTHETICS
   (TOPICAL) 56
Derma Medicone-HC—See
   EPHEDRINE 326
Dermophyl—See
   ADRENOCORTICOIDS (TOPICAL) 16
Dermoplast—See ANESTHETICS
   (TOPICAL) 56
Dermovate—See
   ADRENOCORTICOIDS (TOPICAL) 16
Dermovate Scalp Application—See
   ADRENOCORTICOIDS (TOPICAL) 16
Dermoxyl—See BENZOYL PEROXIDE 90
Dermtex HC—See
   ADRENOCORTICOIDS (TOPICAL) 16
Deronil—See DEXAMETHASONE 268
DES—See
   DIETHYLSTILBESTROL 282
   ESTROGEN 350
Desamycin—See TETRACYCLINES 850
DESERPIDINE—See
   RAUWOLFIA ALKALOIDS 780
DESERPIDINE &
   HYDROCHLOROTHIAZIDE—See
   RAUWOLFIA & THIAZIDE
   DIURETICS 782
DESERPIDINE &
   METHYCLOTHIAZIDE—See
   RAUWOLFIA & THIAZIDE
   DIURETICS 782
DESIPRAMINE—See TRICYCLIC
   ANTIDEPRESSANTS 900
DesOwen—See
   ADRENOCORTICOIDS (TOPICAL) 16
Desoxyn—See METHAMPHETAMINE 534
Desquam-X—See
   BENZOYL PEROXIDE 90
Desyrel—See TRAZODONE 886
Desyrel Dividose—See TRAZODONE 886

Detensol—See
   PROPRANOLOL 750
   GUAIFENESIN 404
Detussin—See PSEUDOEPHEDRINE 752
Deu-Gen L.A.—See
   TESTOSTERONE & ESTRADIOL 848
Dexacen—See DEXAMETHASONE 268
Dex-A-Diet—See
   PHENYLPROPANOLAMINE 690
DEXAMETHASONE 268
Dexampex—See
   DEXTROAMPHETAMINE 272
Dexamyl—See AMOBARBITAL 46
Dexasone—See DEXAMETHASONE 268
Dexatrim—See
   APPETITE SUPPRESSANTS 64
   CAFFEINE 128
   PHENYLPROPANOLAMINE 690
Dexchlor—See
   DEXCHLORPHENIRAMINE 270
DEXCHLORPHENIRAMINE 270
Dexedrine—See
   DEXTROAMPHETAMINE 272
Dexitac—See CAFFEINE 128
Dexol T.D.—See PANTOTHENIC ACID
   (VITAMIN B-5) 644
Dexon—See DEXAMETHASONE 268
Dexone—See DEXAMETHASONE 268
Dextromal—See
   CHLORPHENIRAMINE 190
   DEXTROAMPHETAMINE 272
   DEXTROMETHORPHAN 274
Dextro-Tussin—See
   CHLORPHENIRAMINE 190
Dextro-Tussin GG—See
   DEXTROMETHORPHAN 274
Dey-Dose Isoetharine—See
   ISOETHARINE 450
Dey-Lute Isoetharine—See
   ISOETHARINE 450
DHT—See VITAMIN D 930
D-Feda—See PSEUDOEPHEDRINE 752
Di-Phen—See PHENYTOIN 694
DiaBeta—See GLYBURIDE 396
Diabinese—See CHLORPROPAMIDE 194
Diacin—See NIACIN
   (NICOTINIC ACID) 602
Diadox—See
   PHENYLPROPANOLAMINE 690
Diafen—See DIPHENYLPYRALINE 302
Dia-Gesic—See ACETAMINOPHEN 4
   ASPIRIN 66
   CAFFEINE 128
Diagnostic aid—See GALLBLADDER
   X-RAY TEST DRUGS (   ) 390
Diahist—See DIPHENHYDRAMINE 296

Deficol—See BISACODYL 104
Dehist—See
   BROMPHENIRAMINE 110
   CHLORPHENIRAMINE 190
   PHENYLEPHRINE 688
   PHENYLPROPANOLAMINE 690
DEHYDROCHOLIC ACID 266
Delacort—See
   ADRENOCORTICOIDS (TOPICAL) 16
Deladumone—See
   TESTOSTERONE & ESTRADIOL 848
Deladumone OB—See
   TESTOSTERONE & ESTRADIOL 848
Delatestryl—See ANDROGENS 54
Delaxin—See METHOCARBAMOL 544
Delcid—See
   ALUMINUM & MAGNESIUM
   ANTACIDS 28
   ALUMINUM HYDROXIDE 26
   MAGNESIUM HYDROXIDE 498
Delcozine—See
   APPETITE SUPPRESSANTS 64
Delestrogen—See
   ESTRADIOL 348
   ESTROGEN 350
Delsym—See
   DEXAMETHASONE 268

INDEX

999

1001

INDEX

Neosar—See CYCLOPHOSPHAMIDE 250
Neosorb Plus—See
    ALUMINUM HYDROXIDE 26
    ALUMINUM & MAGNESIUM
        ANTACIDS 28
Neo-Spec—See GUAIFENESIN 404
Neospect—See
    GUAIFENESIN 404
    PHENOBARBITAL 678
    XANTHINE BRONCHODILATORS 938
NEOSTIGMINE 600
Neo-Synephrine—See PHENYLEPHRINE
    688
NeoSynephrine Compound—See
    PHENYLEPHRINE 688
Neo-Synephrine 12 Hour—See
    OXYMETAZOLINE 636
Neo-Synephrinol Day Relief—See
    PSEUDOEPHEDRINE 752
Neotep Granucaps—See
    CHLORPHENIRAMINE 190
    PHENYLEPHRINE 688
Neo-Tetrine—See TETRACYCLINES 850
Neothyllin-G—See GUAIFENESIN 404
Neothylline—See XANTHINE
    BRONCHODILATORS 938
Neothylline-G—See XANTHINE
    BRONCHODILATORS 938
Neo-Tran—See MEPROBAMATE 522
Neo-Tric—See METRONIDAZOLE 572
Neo-Zoline—See
    PHENYLBUTAZONE 686
Nephronex—See NITROFURANTOIN 610
Nephrox—See ALUMINUM
    HYDROXIDE 26
Neptazane—See CARBONATE
    ANHYDRASE INHIBITORS 148
Nervine Nighttime Sleep-Aid—See
    DIPHENHYDRAMINE 296
    PYRILAMINE 762
Neucalm 50—See HYDROXYZINE 434
Neuramate—See MEPROBAMATE 522
Neurate—See MEPROBAMATE 522
Neut—See SODIUM BICARBONATE 808
Neutracomp—See
    ALUMINUM HYDROXIDE 26
    ALUMINUM & MAGNESIUM
        ANTACIDS 28
Neutralca-S—See
    ALUMINUM HYDROXIDE 26
    ALUMINUM & MAGNESIUM
        ANTACIDS 28
Neutra-Phos—See POTASSIUM &
    SODIUM PHOSPHATES 712
Neutra-Phos K—See POTASSIUM
    PHOSPHATES 710
Neutrocomp—See MAGNESIUM
    TRISILICATE 502
Neutrogena Acne Mask—See BENZOYL
    PEROXIDE 90
Nevrotase—See HYOSCYAMINE 436
N-G-C—See NITRATES 608
Niac—See NIACIN (NICOTINIC
    ACID) 602
Niacin—See NIACIN (NICOTINIC
    ACID) 602
NIACIN (NICOTINIC ACID) 602
Nicalex—See NIACIN (NICOTINIC
    ACID) 602
Nico-400—See NIACIN (NICOTINIC
    ACID) 602
Nicobid—See NIACIN (NICOTINIC
    ACID) 602
Nicocap—See NIACIN (NICOTINIC
    ACID) 602
Nicolar—See NIACIN (NICOTINIC
    ACID) 602
Nicorette—See NICOTINE RESIN
    COMPLEX 604
Nico-Span—See NIACIN (NICOTINIC
    ACID) 602
NICOTINE RESIN COMPLEX 604
Nicotinex—See NIACIN (NICOTINIC
    ACID) 602
Nicotinyl alcohol—See NIACIN
    (NICOTINIC ACID) 602

Nicotym—See NIACIN (NICOTINIC
    ACID) 602
NIFEDIPINE 606
Niferex—See
    IRON-POLYSACCHARIDE 448
Nifuran—See NITROFURANTOIN 610
Nilcol—See CHLORPHENIRAMINE 190
Nilspasm—See
    ATROPINE 70
    BELLADONNA 84
    HYOSCYAMINE 436
    SCOPOLAMINE (HYOSCINE) 798
Nilstat—See NYSTATIN 622
Niong—See NITRATES 608
NITRATES 608
Nitrex—See NITROFURANTOIN 610
Nitro-Bid—See NITRATES 608
Nitrobon—See NITRATES 608
Nitrocap—See NITRATES 608
Nitrocap T.D.—See NITRATES 608
Nitrocardin—See NITRATES 608
Nitrodan—See NITROFURANTOIN 610
Nitrodisc—See NITRATES 608
Nitro-Dur—See NITRATES 608
NITROFURANTOIN 610
Nitrogard-SR—See NITRATES 608
NITROGLYCERIN (GLYCERYL
    TRINITRATE)—See NITRATES 608
Nitroglyn—See NITRATES 608
Nitrol—See NITRATES 608
Nitrolin—See NITRATES 608
Nitro-Long—See NITRATES 608
Nitronet—See NITRATES 608
Nitrong—See NITRATES 608
Nitrospan—See NITRATES 608
Nitrostablin—See NITRATES 608
Nitrostat—See NITRATES 608
Nitro-Time—See NITRATES 608
Nizoral—See KETOCONAZOLE 472
Nobesine—See APPETITE
    SUPPRESSANTS 64
Nobesine-75—See APPETITE
    SUPPRESSANTS 64
Noctec—See CHLORAL HYDRATE 170
Nodaca—See CAFFEINE 128
Nodoz—See CAFFEINE 128
Nolamine—See
    CHLORPHENIRAMINE 190
    PHENYLPROPANOLAMINE 690
Non-steroidal anti-inflammatory
    DIFLUNISAL 286
    FENOPROFEN 368
    IBUPROFEN 438
    INDOMETHACIN 443
    MECLOFENAMATE 510
    MEFANAMIC ACID 514
    NAPROXEN 590
    OXYPHENBUTAZONE 638
    PHENYLBUTAZONE 686
    PIROXICAM 702
    SULINDAC 834
    TOLMETIN 884
Non-steroidal anti-inflammatory
    (salicylates)—See ACETAMINOPHEN &
    SALICYLATES 6
Noradryl—See DIPHENHYDRAMINE 296
Norcet—See NARCOTIC &
    ACETAMINOPHEN 592
Nordette—See CONTRACEPTIVES
    (ORAL) 236
Nordryl—See DIPHENHYDRAMINE 296
NORETHINDRONE 612
NORETHINDRONE ACETATE 614
NORFLOXACIN 616
Norette—See ETHINYL ESTRADIOL 360
Norflex—See ORPHENADRINE 624
Norgesic—See
    ASPIRIN 66
    ORPHENADRINE, ASPIRIN &
        CAFFEINE 626
Norgesic Forte—See ORPHENADRINE,
    ASPIRIN & CAFFEINE 626
NORGESTREL 618
Norinyl—See ETHINYL ESTRADIOL 360
Norinyl 1 + 35 21-Day Tablets—See
    NORETHINDRONE 612

Norisodrine—See ISOPROTERENOL 458
Norisodrine Aerotrol—See
    ISOPROTERENOL 458
Norlestrin—See
    CONTRACEPTIVES (ORAL) 236
    ETHINYL ESTRADIOL 360
    NORETHINDRONE 612
Norlinyl—See CONTRACEPTIVES
    (ORAL) 236
Norlutate—See
    NORETHINDRONE 612
    NORETHINDRONE ACETATE 614
Norlutate Acetate—See
    NORETHINDRONE ACETATE 614
Norlutin—See
    NORETHINDRONE 612
    NORETHINDRONE ACETATE 614
Nor-Mil—See DIPHENOXYLATE &
    ATROPINE 300
Normodyne—See LABETOLOL 476
Nor-O.-D.—See NORETHINDRONE
    ACETATE 614
Noroxin—See NORFLOXACIN 616
Noroxine—See THYROXINE
    (T-4, LEVOTHYROXINE) 872
Norpace—See DISOPYRAMIDE 306
Norpace CR—See DISOPYRAMIDE 306
Norpanth—See PROPANTHELINE 748
Norpramin—See TRICYCLIC
    ANTIDEPRESSANTS 900
Nor-Pred-TBA—See
    PREDNISOLONE 722
Nor-Q.D.—See
    CONTRACEPTIVES (ORAL) 236
    NORETHINDRONE 612
Nor-Tet—See TETRACYCLINES 850
NORTRIPTYLINE—See TRICYCLIC
    ANTIDEPRESSANTS 900
Nortussin—See GUAIFENESIN 404
Norwich Aspirin—See ASPIRIN 66
Norzine—See PROMAZINE 744
Nospaz—See DICYCLOMINE 280
Nostril—See PHENYLEPHRINE 688
Nostrilla—See OXYMETAZOLINE 636
Nova-Carpine—See PILOCARPINE 696
Novafed A—See
    CHLORPHENIRAMINE 190
    PSEUDOEPHEDRINE 752
Novahistine DH—See NARCOTIC
    ANALGESICS 594
Novahistine DMX—See
    DEXTROMETHORPHAN 274
    PSEUDOEPHEDRINE 752
Novahistine Expectorant—See NARCOTIC
    ANALGESICS 594
Novahistine—See
    CHLORPHENIRAMINE 190
    GUAIFENESIN 404
    PHENYLEPHRINE 688
    PHENYLPROPANOLAMINE 690
Novamobarb—See AMOBARBITAL 46
Novamoxin—See AMOXICILLIN 48
Novapen V—See PENICILLIN V 662
Nova-Phase—See ASPIRIN 66
Nova-Phenicol—See
    CHLORAMPHENICOL 174
Nova-Pheno—See PHENOBARBITAL 678
Nova-Pred—See PREDNISOLONE 722
Novaprednisolone—See
    PREDNISOLONE 722
Nova-Rectal—See PENTOBARBITAL 664
Novasen—See ASPIRIN 66
Novo AC&C—See NARCOTIC &
    ASPIRIN 596
Novo-Ampicillin—See AMPICILLIN 52
Novobetamet—See
    ADRENOCORTICOIDS (TOPICAL) 16
Novobutamide—See TOLBUTAMIDE 882
Novobutazone—See
    PHENYLBUTAZONE 686
Novochlorhydrate—See CHLORAL
    HYDRATE 170
Novochlorocap—See
    CHLORAMPHENICOL 174
Novochlorpromazine—See
    CHLORPROMAZINE 192

INDEX

INDEX

Z

NOTES

NOTES

NOTES

NOTES

EMERGENCY GUIDE FOR OVERDOSE VICTIMS

This section lists *basic* steps in recognizing and treating immediate effects of drug overdose.

Study the information before you need it. If possible, take a course in first aid and learn external cardiac massage and mouth-to-mouth breathing techniques, called *cardiopulmonary resuscitation* (CPR).

For quick reference, list emergency telephone numbers in the spaces provided on the inside front cover for fire department paramedics, ambulance, poison-control center and your doctor. These numbers, except for doctor, are usually listed on the inside cover of your telephone directory.

IF VICTIM IS UNCONSCIOUS, NOT BREATHING:

1. Yell for help. Don't leave victim.

2. Begin mouth-to-mouth breathing immediately.

3. If there is no heartbeat, give external cardiac massage.

4. Have someone call 0 (operator) or 911 (emergency) for an ambulance or medical help.

5. Don't stop CPR until help arrives.

6. Don't try to make victim vomit.

7. If vomiting occurs, save vomit to take to emergency room for analysis.

8. Take medicine or empty bottles with you to emergency room.

IF VICTIM IS UNCONSCIOUS AND BREATHING:

1. Dial 0 (operator) or 911 (emergency) for an ambulance or medical help.

2. If you can't get help immediately, take victim to the nearest emergency room.

3. Don't try to make victim vomit.

4. If vomiting occurs, save vomit to take to emergency room for analysis.

5. Watch victim carefully on the way to the emergency room. If heart or breathing stops, use cardiac massage and mouth-to-mouth breathing (CPR).

6. Take medicine or empty bottles with you to emergency room.